# Fatty Acids in Health Promotion and Disease Causation

# Fatty Acids in Health Promotion and Disease Causation

Editor

**Ronald R. Watson**

AOCS PRESS
Urbana, Illinois

**AOCS Mission Statement**
To be a global forum to promote the exchange of ideas, information, and experience, to enhance personal excellence, and to provide high standards of quality among those with a professional interest in the science and technology of fats, oils, surfactants, and related materials.



AOCS Press, Urbana, IL 61802


ISBN 978-1-893997-65-3

**Library of Congress Cataloging-in-Publication Data**
Fatty acids in health : promotion and disease causation / editor, Ronald R. Watson.
p. cm.
Includes index.
ISBN 978-1-893997-65-3 (alk. paper)
1. Fatty acids in human nutrition. 2. Fatty acids--Health aspects. 3. Unsaturated fatty acids. 4. Essential fatty acids. I. Watson, Ronald R. (Ronald Ross)

QP752.F35F387 2008
612.3'97--dc22

2008046228

Printed in the United States of America.
13 12 11 10 6 5 4 3

The paper used in this book is acid-free and falls within the guidelines established to ensure permanence and durability.

# Contents

## Part 3 ● Fatty Acids and Health Promotion



## Part 4 ● Omega-3 Fatty Acids and Health

# Preface

With industrialization societies have and continue to change traditional dietary consumption of fats, frequently with adverse consequences to health and longevity. These include a more sedentary lifestyle with increased availability of high-energy foods. Dramatically increased use of corn oil with its n-6 polyunsaturated fatty acids, trans fatty acids, as well as animal products modified by diets high in these fatty acids occurred. Simultaneously use of n-3 fatty acids, commonly consumed in wild meats and foods, was reduced. The change has been about 10 fold, increased n-6 use compared to decreased n-3 consumption. In addition use of antioxidant containing foods was reduced, increased oxidative damage and lowering protection from industrial pollutants. The importance of fatty acids in gene regulation, homeostasis and overall all health is increasingly clear. The increased n-6/n-3 fatty acid intake has shown important correlation with early symptoms of degenerative diseases, common in the 20th century. However the prosperity and nutritional knowledge allow defined diets to promote health and prevent disease by regulating fatty acid intake, selectively. Thus the knowledge of fatty acids functions in health and methods to reverse this lifestyle are needed to promote health and survival. It is widely accepted that n-3 polyunsaturated fatty acids including conjugated linoleic isomers in fish oils protect against cardiovascular diseases. In addition they have effects on body composition, cancer development and immune regulation. However the primary dietary fatty acids for most Americans are n-6 which likely promotes such diseases. Interestingly cholesterol's role in disease promotion is being downgraded while its actions to promote health increasingly recognized. The role of dietary fatty acids as well as cholesterol in health becomes even more important in the aged who are at greater risk of premature death.

Previously immune and heart structural changes were attributed to the aging process with little if any recognition of the operating mechanism. Because of playing a key role in heart function cytokine polarization and its excessive inflammatory cytokines in seniors now become a target for regulation to prevent immune-mediated heart disease, using dietary fatty acids. Dietary supplements of n-3, n-6 and conjugated linoleic fatty acids as well as cholesterol are available in foods. Recently n-3 fatty acids have been added to eggs from hens and meat from cattle as a novel method to increase use. The book focuses on the role of omega-3 polyunsaturated fatty acids to promote health.

The book has four main focuses and sections. First there is a significant focus on heart disease and the role of fatty acids in its prevention as well as causation. Information on special populations, Native Americans, stroke and cardiac injury are examples of areas where fatty acids play a key role. As would be expected their actions in heart function in women, during diseases like diabetes and gene expression are described. The second main focus is on body composition, diabetic disease and health promotion, and actions after transformation by oxidation. Third there is a section on fatty acids in health promotion per se. This includes cancer, intestinal microbes, and membrane functions. Finally the actions of omega 3 fatty acids, the presumed health promoting ones are extensively investigate by experts from around the world. Clearly fatty acids fit the modern paradigm of being dangerous in the wrong amounts and types, while being health promoting otherwise, allowing people to make rational, science based choices in their diets to prevent and treat diseases which are prevalent in the 21st century due to our lifestyle changes from our ancestors.

*Ronald R. Watson*
*University of Arizona*

# PART 1

# Fatty Acids in Heart Disease

# 1

# *Trans* and Other Fatty Acids: Effects on Endothelial Functions

**Gholamreza Bahrami**

*Department of Pharmacology, School of Pharmacy, Kermanshah University of Medical Sciences, Kermanshah, Iran; Oil Research Center, Kermanshah University of Medical Sciences; Medical Biology Research Center, Kermanshah University of Medical Sciences; and Association of Cardiovascular Diseases Prevention (Iranian N.G.O. 2002)*

## Endothelial Functions

This chapter covers endothelial functions and the effect of fatty acids on them. A brief overview of endothelial functions is followed by descriptions of the effects of individual fatty acids, including: saturated fatty acids (SFAs), monounsaturated fatty acids (MUFAs), polyunsaturated fatty acids (PUFAs), and trans fatty acids (TFAs).

## Overview

Atherosclerosis remains the primary cause of death and disease-related disability in developed and many underdeveloped countries. It begins in childhood, progresses silently during the pre-clinical stage, and leads to adverse clinical outcomes such as stroke, myocardial infraction, and peripheral vascular diseases. However, several theories explain the pathogenesis of atherosclerosis; the current data indicate that it should be considered mainly as an inflammatory disease in which a change in the response of the vascular wall to various active chemical agents and different physiologic and pathologic conditions plays an important role (Lerman & Zeiher, 2005).

The vascular endothelium is not an inert, single-cell lining covering the internal surface of blood vessels, but it is the active and dynamic monolayer of cells that serves as a semi-permeable barrier between blood and tissue and plays a crucial role in the regulation of vascular tone and structure. The normal, healthy endothelium regulates several biological processes including vascular homeostasis, inflammation, and coagulation, and it exerts anticoagulant, finbrinolytic, antithrombotic, anti-inflammatory, antihypertrophic, and vasodilative properties.

The endothelium regulates vascular tone by synthesis and the release of several relaxing substances [e.g., nitric oxide (NO), heparan sulfonate, prostacyclin (PGI-2)] and contracting factors [e.g., thromboxane $A_2$ ($TXA_2$), endothelin, prostaglandin (PG) $H_2$, angiotensin II] (Davignon & Ganz, 2004; Landmesser et al., 2004; Shimokawa, 1999; Yang & Ming, 2006). The endothelium maintains the balance between vasodilatation and vasoconstriction, coagulation and fibrinolysis, homeostasis and thrombosis, as well as the inhibition and stimulation of smooth muscle cell (SMC) proliferation and migration. The upset of this balance leads to "endothelial dysfunction;" the term is now used for the endothelium-dependent changes of vascular tone.

In the vascular wall, a strong association exists between endothelial dysfunction and the development of atherosclerotic lesions and later clinical complications. Unlike the previous opinion, endothelial damage (in the form of focal desquamation or intimal denudation) is not necessarily required to begin the atherosclerotic process. Endothelial dysfunction can initiate the entire process. In fact, many risk factors for atherosclerosis (such as hyperlipidemia, hypertension, smoking, elevated plasma homocysteine levels, and diabetes) are associated with endothelial dysfunction. The term "endothelial activation" more specifically describes the functional changes that are produced in the vascular wall under the influence of various stimulations (Davignon & Ganz, 2004; De Caterina et al., 2000; Landmesser et al., 2004; Lerman & Zeiher, 2005; Shimokawa, 1999; Yang & Ming, 2006). This chapter reviews the effects of fatty acids on the endothelial functions.

## Healthy Endothelium

Endothelium plays a crucial role in regulating vascular tone and structure including antithrombotic, anti-inflammatory, anticoagulant, antihypertrophic, and vasodilatory actions. Many of these effects are mediated mainly by the action of nitrous oxide (NO)—originally called endothelial-derived relaxing factor (EDRF)—and PGI-2. Numerous other vasoactive substances, including endothelium-derived hyperpolarizing factor (EDHF) and endothelin, are released from endothelium under different physiologic and pathologic conditions (Behrendt & Ganz, 2002; Mitchell et al., 2007).

### *NO*

Joseph Pristly discovered NO in 1772, and reported its relaxant effect on strips of coronary artery in 1779. In 1980, Furchgott discovered that in vessels with intact endothelium, acetylcholine and a number of other agonists stimulate the release of an EDRF. In 1987, Moncada et al. and Ignarro et al. proved that "NO" and "EDRF" are two terms for a single substance (Yetik-Anacak & Catravas, 2006). By the action of a constitutive endothelial enzyme, namely a NO synthesizer (eNOS), which is activated by the $Ca^{2+}$/calmodulin complex in response to various stimuli, including fluid shear stress and exposure to several active agents such as acetylcholine, NO is formed in endothelial cells from its precursor L-arginine (Behrendt & Ganz, 2002; Yetik-Anacak & Catravas, 2006). It diffuses into the vascular SMCs and activates guanylate cyclase, which leads to the production of cGMP, thereby causing the relaxation of smooth muscles and arterial dilatation (Deanfield et al., 2007; Kawashima & Yokoyama, 2004).

### *PGI-2*

PGI-2 is the major product of vascular cyclooxygenase (COX), which is co-released with NO from the endothelial cells (Mitchell et al., 2007). The first step in the synthesis of a PGI-2 is the liberation of arachidonic acid (AA) from membrane-bound lipids by the action of a calcium-dependent enzyme phospholipase $A_2$. AA is then metabolized by the action of COX, which is present in two distinct isoforms, $COX_1$ and $COX_2$, to produce various eicosanoids. $COX_1$ is constitutively expressed and tends to be homeostatic in function, while $COX_2$ is induced during inflammation and tends to be facilitating the inflammatory response.

In healthy endothelial cells, $COX_1$ is the predominate isoform, which produces $PGG_2$ and then $H_2$ from AA in oxygenase and peroxidase steps, respectively. By the action of a range of downstream PG synthase enzymes, including PGI-2 synthetase, $PGH_2$ is further metabolized to PGI-2 in response to shear stress, hypoxia, and several mediators. PGI-2 is a potent inhibitor of platelet aggregation with an important vasodilator activity that acts by binding to smooth-muscle PGI-2 receptors and activating adenylate cyclase and/or intracellular peroxime proliferators–activated receptor (PPAR-β) (Mitchell et al., 2007). PGI-2 increases the synthesis of NO by endothelial cells, and, in turn, NO increases the activity of PGI-2 on smooth-muscle relaxation (O'Connell & Genest, 2001).

## Inflammation and Atherosclerosis

Accumulated data indicate that inflammation has a critical role in the initiation and progression of atherosclerosis (Call et al., 2004; Tousoulis et al., 2006). Epidemiologic studies suggest that infection and chronic inflammation may trigger endothelial dysfunction. Other potential causes of endothelial dysfunction are oxidative stress, mechanical stress, genetic background, hyperhomocysteinemia, and obesity and diabetes. Our knowledge indicates that atherosclerosis is not a simple disorder of lipid metabolism, but it is a complex process in which lipoproteins interact with inflammatory cells in the intima to produce foam cells rich in cholesteryl esters (Lemaitre et al., 2006). Four important stages occur in atherosclerosis in which inflammation and lipids accumulation have a critical role: (i) lesion initiation, (ii) monocyte infiltration and differentiation, (iii) lesion progression, and (iv) plaque rupture (Lemaitre et al., 2006).

Several protein families, each with distinct functions including—the selectin family of adhesion molecules, monocyte chemoattractant protein-1 (MCP-1), macrophage colony-stimulating factor (MCSF) (able to promote the activation and maturation of monocytes and macrophages), vascular cell adhesion molecule-1 (VCAM-1), intra-cellular adhesion molecule-1 (ICAM-1), as well as pro-inflammatory cytokines such as tumor necrosis factor-alpha (TNF-α), interleukin-1 (IL-1), IL-4, and IL-6—participate in the initiation and development of atherosclerosis (Frenette & Wagner, 1996).

A common pathologic mechanism is involved in the development of atherosclerosis by several risk factors, including hyperlipidemia, smoking, and hypertension. The activity of a select set of endothelial transcription factors [e.g., endothelial nuclear factor κB (NF-κB)] is modulated by a variety of pathologic stimuli with the common denominator apparently being reactive oxygen species (ROS). These stimuli cause phosphorylation and the proteolytic degradation of the inhibitory subunit of the factors, their translocation into the nucleus, and subsequent gene expression of many target genes in endothelial cells including the inflammatory cytokines and adhesion molecules. A second group of transcription factors involved in inflammation is the PPARs. The main members of this family are PPAR-α and PPAR-γ, which also are found in inflammatory cells, and are regulated by polyunsaturated fatty acids (PUFAs) and eicosanoid products. The activation of both forms inhibits the activation of inflammatory genes including TNF-α, IL-6, IL-8, and VCAM-1 (Calder, 2002; Deckelbaum et al., 2006b; Pegorier et al., 2004).

While blood leukocytes adhere poorly to the normal endothelium, one of the earliest events in the initiation of atherosclerotic lesions is leukocyte–endothelium interactions, which facilitate the impairment of the endothelial functions and have an important role in the process. Thus, among the earliest inflammatory steps of atherosclerosis are the slowing, tethering, rolling, and subsequent attachment of circulating leukocytes to the vascular endothelium. Several protein families, each with distinct mechanisms, provide traffic signals for leukocytes. A selection family of adhesion molecules, especially P-selectin, (which appear to interact with sialylated carbohydrates on leukocytes and endothelial cells) partly mediates this process (Ridker et al., 2001). However, adhesion is a multi-step process that starts with leukocyte rolling on the endothelial surface, potentiates with chemoattractants such as MCF-1 and IL-8, and subsequently firms by the interaction between immunoglobulin superfamily members (ICAM-1 and VCAM-1) on the endothelium and integrin ligands on the leukocyte surface.

Although leukocyte adhesion molecules, chemoattractants, and cytokines are three important products of endothelial activation for the initiation and progression of atherosclerotic lesions, one should consider other factors that regulate the expression of these signals. While normal endothelium cells express negligible amounts of these molecules, their gene expression is augmented several- fold in response to disturbed blood flow (e.g., branch points in arteries), bacterial endotoxins, and cytokines such as IL-1 and TNFs (Davis et al., 2007).

After the adhesion of the leukocytes to the endothelium and the penetration into the intima occur, the lymphocytes join macrophages during the progression of the lesion. A family of the T-cell chemoattractant may be involved in the recruitment of the lymphocytes into the intima.

MCSF and other mediators also promote the replication and differentiation of the macrophages within the lesion. The uptake and internalization of modified lipoproteins into the lesion by the action of scavenger receptors, with their expressions augmented by MCSF, lead to the formation of the foam cells. These cells are the main constituents of a fatty streak.

Low-density lipoprotein (LDL) concentration is a major determinant factor in plasma for the penetration of lipoproteins within the lesion and the development of atherosclerosis. Following penetration, LDL remains in the intima, in part, by binding to proteoglycans, and undergoes oxidative modification. Modified LDL promotes the release of lysophospholipids and oxidized phospholipids into the intimal space. These molecules further activate the endothelial cells, resulting in the expression of adhesion molecules, chemotactic agents, and cytokines, thereby converting a fatty streak into a complex plaque. The migration of SMCs, the formation of additional foam cells, and the production of extra- cellular matrix proteins then produce a fibrous cap over the plaque and further narrow the arterial lumen.

The modification of the apoprotein moieties of the lipoprotein particles renders them antigenic and further activates the immune response. The inflammatory process inhibits collagen synthesis and evokes the expression of collagenases by the foam cells within the intimal lesion. These changes thin the fibrous cap and make it susceptible to rupture. Exposing the thrombogenic contents of plaque to the bloodstream leads to the activation of coagulation systems, the formation of thrombus, and an acute myocardial infraction and stroke.

## Factors Affecting the Inflammatory Process of Atherosclerosis

### *LDL-oxidation*

Whereas LDL is considered an independent risk factor of cardiovascular artery disease (CAD), and despite the existence of a strong correlation between serum LDL-cholesterol concentrations and the risk of the disease, in vitro studies fail to demonstrate direct atherogenic effects for LDL particles (Keaney & Vita, 2002). Several lines of studies, however, indicate that LDL transfers cholesterol to the peripheral cells through the LDL receptor, which recognizes the ApoB-100 moiety of the lipid. As hypercholesterolemia down-regulates the LDL receptors, possibly, the native LDL and its receptors are not responsible for the formation of the foam cell.

The increased plasma level of LDL potentiates the rate of entry of LDL particles inside the arterial wall, and increases the intimal levels of the particles. While antioxidant compounds protect the particles from oxidation, LDL particles trapped within the intima are prone to oxidative damage (Osterud & Bjorklid, 2003). Before being completely oxidized, in the intima LDL particles have to undergo some modification and be minimally oxidized (MM-LDL). At first, native LDL particles contain intact apolipoprotein (Apo-B100), have no lipid peroxide, and are enriched in PUFAs and antioxidants. The oxidation of MM-LDL at this stage oxidizes the PUFAs and depletes antioxidant compounds, but the process is not so extensive that an Apo-B100 molecule is changed. Thus, the LDL receptor can still recognize MM-

LDL, although scavenger receptors of macrophage can not recognize it yet (Lapointe et al., 2006).

In the intimal location, the particles are brought into close proximity with endothelial cells that induce the expression of MCP-1 and MCSF, which promote the recruitment of monocytes into the artery wall and stimulate the differentiation of monocytes into macrophages. The presence of macrophages stimulates further the oxidation of the LDL in which Apo-B is modified into particles with more negative charges. These particles show a decreased affinity for LDL receptors and an increased affinity for scavenger receptors located on macrophages and other cell types (Stocker & Keaney, 2004).

The macrophages take up the now oxidized-LDL (Ox-LDL) in an up-regulated manner by the scavenger receptors, causing the accumulation of cholesterol and the production of the foam cell (Lapointe et al., 2006), followed by the activation of endothelial cells, the expression of the adhesion molecules, further recruitment of the monocytes within the artery wall, and thus the progression of atherosclerosis (Keaney & Vita, 2002; Lapointe et al., 2006; Stocker & Keaney, 2004).

Circulating Ox-LDL concentration was related to intima media thickness and the progression of atherosclerosis (Hulthe & Fagerberg, 2002; Metso et al., 2004; Wallenfeldt et al., 2004). While the oxidation of LDL has a critical role in the development of atherosclerosis, its effect on the initiation of foam-cell development was not established. Also, several different types of fatty acid oxidation products, such as the hydroxyl product of linoleic acid and arachidonic acid (AA), were present as cholesterol ester in human atherosclerotic lesions (e.g., cholesteryl linoleate and cholesteryl arachidonate) (Moreno & Mitjavila, 2003).

Lipid peroxidation appears to be a product of the inflammatory process, and plays an active role in the pathogenesis of atherosclerosis. An agent-limiting LDL oxidation also should limit the development of atherosclerosis. However, many large clinical antioxidant supplementation trials failed to demonstrate the important role of antioxidants in preventing or healing CAD (Keaney & Vita 2002).

### *Measuring Ox-LDL*

Several methods are available to assess LDL oxidation. In the most widely used of them, the susceptibility of isolated LDL particles to oxidation is measured by using lag time for the particles to resist copper-induced oxidation and by using spectrophotometric determination of conjugated dienes as a product of oxidation. "Lag time" is defined as the time between the addition of copper to the isolated LDL and the beginning of the oxidation; a longer lag time indicates a higher resistance to oxidation (Abuja & Albertini, 2001).

## High-density Lipoprotein (HDL)

HDLs are a heterogeneous group of small and dense lipoproteins. HDL or its major protein moiety Apo-A1 is anti-inflammatory in nature, and thus can prevent or reverse atherosclerosis and protect against CAD. Some of the cardioprotective mechanisms of HDL are: its ability to reverse the transport of cholesterol from the periphery back to the liver for disposal, inhibiting the formation of superoxide anions and the stimulation of the formation of NO and PGI-2 from the endothelial cells, which are potent platelet-aggregation inhibitors and vasodilators. Furthermore, HDL modifies the balance of PGI-2 to TX, and attenuates the expression of the adhesion molecules (VCAM-1, ICAM-1, and E-selectin) by TNF-$\alpha$. It counteracts OX-LDL-induced endothelial apoptosis and modulates the permeability of endothelium to LDL; it has long been known to be an important endothelial mitogen and vessel mender (O'Connell & Genest, 2001).

Recent studies indicate that endothelial lipase (EL), a new member of the lipase gene family that primarily shows phospholipase activity is a major determinant of HDL metabolism and concentration (Das, 2005). Overexpression of the gene for EL causes a decrease in HDL cholesterol, whereas suppressing its action increases the plasma concentration of HDL. Pro-inflammatory cytokines, such as TNF-$\alpha$ and interleukin-1 (IL-1), up-regulate EL in a dose-dependent manner. While, obesity, insulin resistance, hypertension, hyperlipidemia, and metabolic syndrome also increase the activation of EL, physical exercise and the consumption of fish oil decrease the activation of the enzyme and elevate plasma HDL levels (Das, 2005).

## *Hypertension*

Hypertension is a classic risk factor for atherosclerosis. Inflammation may involve and participate in hypertension, providing a pathophysiological link between hypertension and atherosclerosis (Libby et al., 2002). Increased plasma levels of primary (TNF-$\alpha$) and secondary (IL-6, ICAM-1, VCAM-1, and E-selectin) mediators of inflammation were frequently reported in hypertension (Madamanchi et al., 2005); thus, a high level of these markers (which have increased concentrations in atherosclerosis) is considered an independent risk factor of hypertension. Angiotensin is a potent vasoconstrictor agent, which also stimulates the proliferation of vascular cells, potentiates vascular inflammation by inducing oxidative stress, and contributes to the recruitment of the leukocyte within the inflammatory cells. Inhibition of its synthesis (by angiotensin-converting enzyme inhibitors) or its action (by angiotensin receptor blockers) reduces blood pressure and attenuates the progression of atherosclerosis (Savoia & Schiffrin, 2007).

## *Diabetes*

Like hypertension, inflammation links diabetes to atherosclerosis. Hyperglycemia may impair endothelial functions and increase oxidative stress. Endothelial dysfunction is an early finding of diabetic vascular abnormality. Atherosclerotic lesions in diabetic patients are more advanced than those in nondiabetic individuals, and the risk of CAD as well as the mortality rate in diabetic patients are generally more than in nondiabetic patients (Savoia & Schiffrin 2007).

## Hemostatic System

Hemostasis is a complex dynamic system of regulating the fluidity of the blood, repairing vascular injury, limiting blood loss, and at the same time inhibiting vascular occlusion (thrombosis). Three main biological systems involved in thrombus formation include platelet aggregation, coagulation, and fibrinolysis.

Platelets are responsible for initiating events leading to blood clotting by adhering to damaged blood vessels, following the activation by binding to any normally hidden subendothelial structural proteins at the site of an injury. The activation of platelets also releases several biologically active compounds to adhere to other platelets as well as to propagate a hemostatic response.

The coagulation system involves two independent pathways: (i) an intrinsic pathway including factors XII, XI, IX, and VIII and (ii) an extrinsic factor VII activated by the tissue factor (TF). With the exception of a small amount of circulating activated factor VII, other coagulation factors do not exist in active form in the blood. The initiating event is the exposure of the subendothelial TF which complexes with the activated factor VII to activate other coagulant factors in a cascading manner: conversion of prothrombin to thrombin leading to fibrin formation from fibrinogen, more platelet aggregation, and finally the production of a hemostatic plug.

The most important component of the fibrinolysis system is plasmin, an enzyme that circulates as inactive zymogen, plasminogen. The tissue plasminogen activator (tPA) is the major vascular activator of plasminogen, which is produced by endothelial cells. Also, endothelium can synthesize and store several inhibitors of fibrinolysis such as plasminogen-activator inhibitors (PAI-1) (Ajjan & Grant, 2006).

### *Regulatory Effects of Endothelium on Hemostatic System*

Intact healthy endothelium provides both anticoagulant properties as well as an anti- platelet deposition surface which are critical for the prevention of thrombosis in vascular lumen. In physiologic conditions, endothelium regulates platelet activity, the functions of coagulation factors, thrombosis, and fibrinolysis by the synthesis and expression of a large number of anticoagulant factors including NO, PGI-2, tPA, protein C, protein S, heparin, tissue factor pathway inhibitors (TFPIs), and thrombomodulin. Endothelium also plays a crucial role in the coagulation process by the production of numerous pro-thrombotic agents including the TF, von willebrand factor (vWF), PAI-1s, and factor V (Madamanchi et al., 2005).

NO inhibits platelet aggregation other than its anti-inflammatory and vasodilatory effects. Oxidative stress and inflammation reduce the production of NO, and impair vascular relaxation that leads to turbulence of blood flow, the activation of the platelet, and the coagulation cascade (Ajjan & Grant, 2006; Mensink, 2005). Also, reduced NO production potentiates the inflammatory process through an increase in leukocyte adhesion molecules and cytokines that produce a pro-coagulant surface in vascular lumen, and further activates a coagulation cascade (Landmesser et al.,

2004). Apart from its impact on vasodilation and inflammation, NO may relate to the inhibition of the PAI-1 expression and reduce platelet aggregation.

PGI-2 is a prostaglandin (PG) produced by endothelial cells that activates adenylate cyclase. It is a vasodilator that interacts synergically with NO, causing the inhibition of platelet adhesion and aggregation (O'Conell & Genest, 2001). PGI-2 increases the synthesis of NO by endothelial cells, and, in turn, NO enhances the vasodilator action of PGI-2 on smooth muscles. PGI-2 is formed in the intima, media, and adventitia in response to several parameters such as shear stress and hypoxia (Shimokawa, 1999).

$TXA_2$ is another eicosanoid produced by the endothelial cells which, unlike PGI-2 is a potent vasoconstrictor and a platelet aggregator. The ratio of PGI-2 to $TX A_2$ has an important role in cardiovascular health. Several factors, including fatty acids, can modify this balance (O'Connell & Genest, 2001).

The major natural anticoagulant pathways include: (i) protein C which is activated by thrombin bound to the endothelial cells and inhibits factors Va and VIIIa, (ii) TFPI which blocks the complex of TF VIIa, (iii) a heparin–antithrombin pathway which is the most effective at inhibiting thrombin and also inactivates factors IXa, Xa, and XIa, (iv) thrombomodulin and antithrombin that inhibit thrombin, and (v) factor X and the thrombin/thrombomodulin complex that activates protein C (Ajjan & Grant, 2006; Levi et al., 2002). All of these agents are products of endothelium which limit thrombin generation. Their decreased levels (e.g., because of the effects of inflammatory cytokines on their synthesis) are associated with increased thrombotic vascular diseases.

The TF is a transmembrane glycoprotein linked to factor VII and an important activator of the clotting cascade. It activates the coagulation system by forming a complex with factor VIIa. The TF is not detectable in normal endothelial cells but is found in atheromatous plaques, and its plasma levels are elevated in patients with CAD.

The TFPI is an inhibitory mechanism of thrombin generation which inhibits the TF–factor VIIa complex and exists in several pools, either endothelial-cell-associated or lipoprotein-bound in plasma (Ajjan & Grant, 2006; Levi et al., 2002; Vallet & Wiel, 2001; Warkentin et al., 2003).

The vWF is a coagulation factor, mainly produced by EC, and mediates platelet adhesion to damaged endothelium and stabilizes factor IIX. A positive relationship exists between vWF plasma levels and the progression of atherosclerosis (Ajjan & Grant, 2006).

## *Inflammation and Coagulation in Endothelium*

A combination of inflammatory and thrombotic processes contributes to the development of atherosclerosis. Endothelium has an important effect on the coagulation state through the production of different coagulant and anticoagulant agents; it also has a critical role in inflammation through the production of different cytokines. In fact, an important inter-relationship exists between the inflammation and the coagulation in endothelium because coagulation augments the inflammatory response, and inflammation produces a pro-coagulant surface on vascular intima that activates a coagulation cascade. In a healthy environment, a balance exists between these products. Endothelial dysfunction, however, upsets this balance to initiate events that lead to the progression of the atherosclerotic process (Ajjan & Grant, 2006).

## *Role of Oxidized LDL in Hemostasis*

Peroxidation of the lipids, such as LDL particles, augments the inflammatory process and plays an active role in the progression of atherosclerosis, not only by its pro-inflammatory effect but also through its significant effect on coagulation and platelet action. Ox-LDL increases the coagulability of the blood by enhancing the expression of the TF in vascular SMCs and the activation of several coagulation factors such as factors IIX and IX on the surface of macrophages and SMCs. Ox-LDL increases the aggregation and adhesion of platelets, enhances the formation of $TXA_2$ ($TXA_2$), and reduces the production of PGI-2. Ox-LDL also reduces the fibrinolytic activity in blood circulation by decreasing the formation of tPA and by increasing the generation of PAI-1 (Ajjan & Grant, 2006; Madamanchi et al., 2005).

## *Assessment of Endothelial Functions*

To improve our understanding of the vascular biology of endothelium, we must develop clinical tests to evaluate endothelial functions in normal and activated conditions. Ideally, such tests should be safe, noninvasive, reproducible, and cheap. No single test currently meets these requirements, and several tests (using both the measurement of endothelial-dependent vasomotion as well as circulating markers of endothelial functions) are therefore required to characterize endothelial functions. The gold-standard assessment involves the direct stimulation of the coronary endothelium with vasodilator agents such as acetylcholine and the measurement of endothelial reactivity with intra-coronary Doppler and angiography. Acetylcholine releases NO from vessels with an intact endothelium that leads to vasodilation, but causes vasoconstriction in subjects with endothelial dysfunction. Even though reliable results are obtained using this method, the test is invasive. The accepted noninvasive standard method is flow-mediated dilation (FMD) of the brachial artery. In this method, the brachial artery diameter is measured before and after an increase in shear stress which is induced by reactive hyperemia with high-resolution ultrasound imaging. FMD occurs predominantly as a result of a local endothelial release of NO. Data from several studies indicate that the FMD method correlates with the gold-standard measurement of the endothelium-mediated vasodilation of the coronary artery (Davis et al., 2007; Kasprzak et al., 2006; Lerman & Zeiher, 2005).

Endothelium regulates numerous vascular functions, including vascular tone, vascular SMC proliferation, and leukocyte migration. Thus, it is possible to assess endothelial functions using the measurement of the endothelial-origin molecule levels in circulating blood. These include the products of endothelial cells following their activation such as the measurement of NO biology, inflammatory cytokine adhesion molecules, and the regulators of thrombosis (Deanfield et al., 2007).

## Effect of Fatty Acids — Overview

Endothelial dysfunction is an important primary event in the progression of atherosclerosis. Inflammatory process, oxidative stress, and increased coagulability of the blood are known as key factors in endothelial dysfunction. High dietary-fat intake can significantly affect these parameters. However, various fat types have different health effects, and recent data indicate that types of fats have a more important role in determining the progression of atherosclerosis than the total amount of fat in the diet. Various fatty acids have different effects on the metabolism of lipoproteins, inflammatory processes, thrombosis, oxidative stress, and blood coagulation (Hennig et al., 2001a).

Whereas important limitations exist for the interpretation of conducted studies on the effect of different dietary fats on endothelial functions, we can evaluate these effects directly by using the measurement of inflammation indices either in tissue-culture studies or observational research and randomized trials. Furthermore, one can indirectly estimate these issues by using the effects of fatty acids on lipoprotein metabolism and peroxidation as well as on blood coagulability.

In these studies, however, one should control food intake and the total received calories with dietary fatty acids as the sole variable. Hence, one should replace individual fatty acid isoenergetically with another fatty acid or other nutrients (e.g., carbohydrates, proteins); it would otherwise be difficult to reliably identify the independent effects of fatty acids on endothelial functions. Thus, types of nutrients (e.g., carbohydrates, proteins, or other fatty acids) which are substituted have an important role in the obtained results, and the difficulty arises in separating the effect of the removal of the individual fatty acid from the diet, with the effects of substituted fats or other nutrients. Furthermore, one should rank other effects of fatty acids, for example, in the evaluation of the effects of fatty acids on lipoprotein metabolism; one should take into account an important effect of HDL cholesterol on endothelial functions other than total cholesterol (Calder, 2002; Mensink et al., 2003).

## Saturated Fatty Acids (SFAs)

The naturally occurring SFAs are functionally divided into short-, medium-, and long- chain fatty acids. The short- and medium-chain fatty acids (C4:0, C10:0) are known to exist in milk fat and dairy products. Lauric acid (C12:0) is the major component of some seed fats (palm, kernels, or coconut oil), and myristic acid (C14:0) is found in seed fats as well as in dairy products. Palmitic acid (C16:0) is the most prominent saturated fat occurring in animals and plants. Stearic acid (C18:0) is a minor component in vegetable fats, and mainly is found in the tallow of ruminants (Denke, 2006).

High intake (more than 15% of daily energy intake) of SFA is positively related to the rising of total cholesterol and LDL cholesterol, thereby risking CAD (Rioux & Legrand, 2007). Not enough data exist on the effect of individual fatty acids on plasma cholesterol levels in the range habitually consumed by humans, and a fatty acid balance of the diet seems to have a more important role than individual fatty acid intakes (Binkoski et al., 2005; Wilke & Clandinin, 2005). Individuals have supported the recommendation to decrease SFA for over 40 years. Although, this fact was questioned by a recent epidemiological study in a specific target population. An analysis of data from the Estrogen Replacement and Atherosclerosis (ERA) trial in postmenopausal women with relatively low-fat intake showed that a greater saturated-fat intake is associated with less progression of CAD compared to a greater carbohydrate intake (Mozaffarian et al., 2004b). Nonetheless, different diets may be recommended for different groups of postmenopausal women for the prevention of CAD (Griel & Kris-Etherton, 2006).

### *Direct Effects of SFA on Endothelial Functions*

Only a few data exist about the direct effects of SFA on endothelial functions (adhesion molecules, NO synthesis, coagulation state, and cellular oxidant/antioxidant equilibrium), and those that are available are controversial. Most of the published studies, however, evaluated the indirect effect of SFA on endothelial functions (e.g., the effect on LDL levels, HDL levels, and the sensitivity of LDL to oxidation).

Several studies report a pro-activating effect of SFA on endothelial functions (Brown & Hu, 2001; Christon, 2003; De Caterina et al., 1998; Hennig et al., 2000; Massaro et al., 1999). Long-term exposure of a human umbilical vein endothelial cell with palmitic acid resulted in a negative influence on endothelial functions as well as the activation of pro-apoptotic and inflammatory pathways (Ciapaite et al., 2007). The acetylcholine-induced, endothelium-dependent relaxation of rabbit aorta was inhibited by palmitic and stearic acids and to a lesser extent by myristic and lauric acids. In this study, however, unsaturated fatty acids with similar chain lengths produced a less inhibitory effect (Edirisinghe et al., 2006). In porcine endothelial cells, unlike oleic acid, stearic and linoleic acids (LAs), increased cellular oxidative stress and activated NF-$\kappa$ B as judged by the reduction of glutathione (GSH) levels and luciferase assay, respectively. However, in contrast to LA, pre-enrichment of endothelial cells with stearic, oleic, or linolenic acids followed by exposure to TNF-$\alpha$ was not associated with the enhancement of IL-6 (Hennig et al., 2000).

Feeding a diet rich in SFA reduces NO production, thereby causing the impairment of the endothelium-dependent relaxation of the vessels in the animals; thus, SFAs exert negative effects on endothelial NO production and resulted relaxation of vessels in pregnant rats, as well as in the offspring. In another study, however, the effects of the incorporation of different fatty acids, including myristic, palmitic, stearic, oleic, and LAs, into endothelial cells and NO synthesis were evaluated, and only LA reduced NO synthesis (Couloubaly et al., 2007).

One can assess the vascular functions of large vessels in relation to different diets by using the FMD method. Although, seemingly, no uniform standard exists in a used protocol and an ingested meal; however, several reports do exist which show that consuming a saturated fat-enriched diet is associated with a significant post-prandial impairment of vascular reactivity (Jackson et al., 2007; Nicholls et al., 2006).

A chronic intake of SFA increased factor VII, a key protein in thrombosis and a known thrombogenic risk factor for CAD. Also an acute intake of SFA was accompanied by the post-prandial activation of the coagulant factor (Marckmann et al., 1998). Nicholls et al. (2006) evaluated the effect of a single high-saturated-fat meal consumption on the anti-inflammatory properties of HDL cholesterol as judged by the expression of cell-surface adhesion molecules (ICAM-1 and VCAM-1) as well as the vascular functions of large vessels using FMD as a marker of vascular reactivity in healthy volunteers. Their study showed that HDLs collected after the saturated meal were less effective than HDLs isolated from fasting plasma, in terms of their ability to inhibit the expression of ICAM-1 and VCAM-1. They concluded that unlike PUFAs, a SFA diet reduced the anti-inflammatory properties of HDL and impaired endothelial functions and vascular reactivity (Nicholls et al., 2006).

## *Indirect Effects of SFA on Endothelial Functions*

Observational and epidemiological studies indicate that a high intake (more than 15% of daily energy intake) of SFAs—mainly palmitic (C16:0) and myristic (C14:0) acids, but not stearic (C18:0) acid (Kris-Etherton et al., 2005; Mensink, 2005; Tholstrup, 2005)—has a negative impact on plasma LDL cholesterol levels, the biomarkers of atherosclerosis and endothelial dysfunction (Rioux & Legrand, 2007; Wilke & Clandinin, 2005). SFAs raise plasma LDL by increasing the formation of LDL and decreasing its turnover and receptor activity (Fernandez & West, 2005; Rioux & Legrand, 2007). Even though the current dietary recommendation to decrease the risk of CAD is to keep SFA intake as low as possible, some considerations, however, should be taken into account:

1. In some studies, reducing SFA intake does not lower the incidence of nonfatal CAD or total mortality (Howard et al., 2006; Mozaffarian et al., 2004b), and the consumption of a low-fat diet (less than 20% energy) induces atherogenic dislipidemia. Thus, some studies recommend: "at this time, research on how specific saturated fatty acids contribute to CAD and on the role each specific saturated fatty acid plays in other health outcomes is not sufficient to make global recommendations for all persons to remove saturated fats from their diet." (German & Dillard, 2004; Volk, 2007).

2. Individual SFAs have different effects on plasma lipoproteins. Some evidence suggests that butyric acid (C4:0) reduces plasma cholesterol levels (Hara et al., 1999); caproic (C6:0), caprilic (C8:0), and capric (C10:0) acids are neutral with

respect to cholesterol-increasing properties (German & Dillard, 2004). Myristic acid (C14:0) is considered the most responsible for the increase of total plasma cholesterol levels or the equivalent of lauric (C12:0) and palmitic (C16:0) acids (German & Dillard, 2004), and stearic acid (C18:0) has minimal adverse effects on blood cholesterol (Kris-Etherton et al., 2005; Tholstrup, 2005).

3. Evidence indicates an increase in cholesterol from SFAs is related to an increase in both LDL and HDL cholesterol (German & Dillard, 2004; Rioux & Legrand, 2007). As convincing data indicate, increasing the concentration of HDL cholesterol through diet will lower the risk of CAD; the ratio of total to HDL cholesterol is now viewed as a more specific marker of CAD than LDL or total cholesterol alone. A meta-analysis of 60 selected trials on the effects of individual fatty acids on the ratio of total:HDL cholesterol reported that the ratio did not change if carbohydrates replaced SFAs. Based on this evaluation, lauric acid (C12:0) greatly increased total cholesterol, but much of its effect was on HDL cholesterol; it decreased the ratio of total:HDL cholesterol. Myristic (C14:0) and palmitic (C16:0) acids had little effect on the ratio, and stearic acid (C18:0) reduced the ratio slightly (Kris-Etherton et al., 2005; Mensink, 2005; Mensink et al., 2003). Samuelson et al. (2001) reported an inverse association between the estimated intake of SFAs mainly derived from milk fat and serum cholesterol in 15-year-old boys and girls.

4. Small dense (SD) LDL is an important predictor of CAD which correlates negatively with plasma HDL levels and positively with plasma triglycerides. The combination of SD-LDL, decreased HDL, and increased triglycerides is called an atherogenic lipoprotein phenotype. Some data showed a positive association between the intake of SFAs and the size of the LDL. An increase in the intake of SFAs, especially myristic acid, is associated with an increase in large LDL particles and a decrease in smaller LDL particles (Dreon et al., 1998).

5. While much data exist about the positive relationship between a high intake of SFAs (more than 15% of daily energy intake) and plasma cholesterol levels, at moderate levels and a usual intake range of SFAs, however, this association is difficult to prove (German & Dillard, 2004; Mozaffarian et al., 2004b; Rioux & Legrand, 2007; Wilke & Clandinin, 2005).

Also balance of the fatty acids in the diet is more important than the amounts of particular fatty acids (Wilke & Clandinin, 2005) [e.g., high levels of palmitic acid are not hypercholesterolemic when consumed linoleic acid is greater than 4.5% of energy (French et al., 2002)]. Furthermore, an imbalance in cellular oxidative stress/antioxidant status significantly affects atherogenicity and the inflammatory action of LDL (Hennig & Toborek, 2001b).

## *Monounsaturated Fatty Acids (MUFAs)*

More than 100 naturally occurring MUFAs were identified; however, most of them are very rare compounds. Oleic acid is one of the most widely distributed MUFAs, which is mainly found in olive oil, the major component of the Mediterranean diet. It also exists in a high amount in safflower oil, and canola, a form of rapeseed which is low in erucic acid (C22n-9), also contains considerable amounts of oleic acid.

Most natural sources of oleic acid are of the *cis* configuration; however, its *trans* forms are produced during the hydrogenation process to produce solid fats for margarine and shortening products. Although, the composition of olive oil is complex, the major compounds thought to contribute to its beneficial health effects include oleic acid, phenolic compounds, and squalene (Waterman & Lockwood, 2007).

Olive oil is unique with respect to its high oleic-acid content, high MUFA/PUFA ratio, less susceptibility to oxidation, and its antioxidant action.

Strong evidence indicates the existence of a negative association between a Mediterranean-style diet, in which olive oil is the main source of fat, and CAD. Although, minor compounds exist, including hydrocarbons, polyphenols, tocopherols, and sterols, in virgin olive oil, cumulative evidence shows that oleic acid may be the main component in this negative association (Hu, 2003). Oleic acid does not induce endothelial dysfunction; it modulates atherogenesis directly by affecting endothelial functions, hemostasis, coagulation, NO synthesis, and fibrinolysis, as well as indirectly by reducing LDLcholesterol and its susceptibility to oxidative modification (Willett, 2006a). Most studies (especially epidemiological studies and clinical trials), however, used an olive-oil-rich diet to evaluate the protective effect of dietary MUFA on atherosclerosis. As minor nonfatty acid constituents exist in the oil, separating the cardioprotective effects of oleic acid from the minor compounds of olive oil is difficult.

## *Direct Effects of MUFA on Endothelial Functions*

### *Endothelial Activation*

Oleic acid contributes to the prevention of atherosclerosis through a modulation of gene expression for endothelial leukocyte adhesion molecules (Basu et al.; 2006; Pérez-Jimenez et al., 2002; Ros, 2003). Oleic acid, when added to endothelial cells in a culture and under co-incubation with TNF-α, IL, and lipopolysaccharide (LPS), reduces the endothelial leukocyte adhesion molecules, including E-selectin, ICAM-1, and VCAM-1 in a concentration- and time-dependent manner (Carluccio et al., 1999). It also produced a quantitatively similar reduction in messenger ribonucleic acid (RNA) for this molecule and inhibited NF-κ B activation. Oleic acid inhibits the endothelial expression of adhesion molecules for monocytes, protects endothelial cells against cytokine-induced VCAM-1, ICAM-1 or E-selectin over-expression, exerts a direct vascular atheroprotective effect, and down-regulates the endothelial cell activation (Carluccio et al., 1999; Christon, 2003; Esposito et al., 2004, 2006; Hennig et al., 2000; Hennig & Toborek, 2001b; Massaro et al., 1999, 2002b; Perona et al., 2006; Toborek & Hennig, 1994 ). Some studies report similar anti-inflammatory effects for oleic acid and docosahexaenoic acid (DHA) (De Caterina et al., 2000).

A MUFA-rich diet significantly increased FMD which was accompanied by the decreasing of P-selection (Fuentes et al., 2001). Oleic acid exerts its anti-inflammatory activity by altering the $H_2O_2$ metabolism in vascular cells, reducing the enzymatic production of ROS, and/or by increasing their scavenging following production (Perona et al., 2006). When added to cytokine-stimulated endothelial cells, oleic acid prevented the depletion of GSH and increased the intracellular ROS in the cells without any change in the activity of GSH-related antioxidant enzymes, superoxide dismutase (SOD), and catalase (Massaro et a., 2002a). It also reduced the proliferation of SMCs and the oxidation of LDL (Hu, 2003).

***Effects of MUFA on Homeostasis, Coagulation, and Fibrinolysis***

Numerous studies evaluated the effects of n-3 fatty acids on these factors. Although, the effects of other fats, including MUFAs, on the formation of thrombi are less studied, convincing evidence in the literature indicates the anti-platelet and anticoagulant activities of MUFAs.

As it is true for n-3 long-chain fatty acids, oleic acid also decreases the in vitro production of $TXB_2$ in both rats and platelet samples obtained from humans with high-MUFA intake (Perez-Jimenez et al., 2002). Furthermore, an oleic acid-enriched diet reduced the urinary excretion of 11-dehydro-$TXB_2$, a metabolite of TX $B_2$ (Perez-Jimenez et al., 2002). Eicosatrienoic acid (C20:3n-3) which is produced from oleic acid, such as other long-chain omega-3 fatty acids, can shift the balance of eicosanoids toward a potentially less aggregator product (see below) (James et al., 2000).

The TF is a membrane-bound protein that is constitutively expressed on a number of cells throughout the body. In cells in contact with blood, TF expression is induced by the action of several compounds, including cytokines, C-reactive protein (CRP), and their advanced glycosylated end products. The TF expressed at the cell surface can interact with factor VII and activate it. The complex of factor VIIa-TF catalyzes the activation of factors IX and X. Factors IXa and Xa enhance the activation of factor X and prothrombin, respectively. Factor VII plays an important role in the initiation of a thrombus formation (Ajjan & Grant, 2006; Levi et al., 2002; Miller, 2005). Unlike SFA and n-6 PUFA, an oleic-acid-enriched diet reduced the activated form of factor VII in healthy volunteers (Kelly et al., 2001; Temme et al., 1999; Turpeinen & Mutanen, 1999). A comparison of a three-week intake with different diets enriched with olive oil, sunflower oil, or rapeseed oil in healthy volunteers followed by standardized high-fat meals shows that mean nonfasting peak concentrations of factor VIIa were lower after olive oil than either sunflower or rapeseed oils. However, no significant differences were noted between diets with respect to the nonfasting factor VII coagulant activities (Larsen et al., 1999). Similar to olive oil, rapeseed oil has a high content of oleic acid; however, unlike olive oil, this study failed to show any reduction by rapeseed oil in a thrombotic propensity associated with the consumption of fatty meals, possibly because of a higher content of PUFA in rapeseed and/or the minor nonfatty constituents of olive oil (Larsen et al., 1999). The isocaloric replacement of an SFA diet by a MUFA diet in healthy volunteers reduced the expression of the TF in monocytes (Perez-Jimenez et al., 2002).

Unlike a low-fat high-complex carbohydrate-enriched diet, the Mediterranean diet (containing 22% of calories as MUFA) significantly reduced the vWF plasma levels in healthy normolipemic subjects (Perez-Jimenez et al., 2002). Also in a study conducted in non-insulin-dependent diabetic subjects, a high-MUFA diet reduced the vWF plasma levels (Perez-Jimenez et al., 2002). Despite the addition of cholesterol to the diet, in the study conducted by Lopez-Segure et al., a MUFA-enriched diet reduced the PAI-1, the strong natural inhibitor of t-PA (Perez-Jimenez et al., 2002). However, the plasma levels of fibrinogen, thrombin–anti-thrombin complex, plasminogen, $\alpha$-$_2$ anti-plasmin, and t-PA did not alter in this study (Perez-Jimenez et al., 2002).

Other studies also reported the beneficial effects of the Mediterranean diet enriched in olive oil on the PAI-1 or factor VII in a healthy population (Avellone et al., 1998; Perez-Jimenez et al., 1999).

## Indirect Effects of MUFA on Endothelial Functions

### Effects of MUFA on Lipoprotein Metabolism

Olive oil and its major component, oleic acid, have beneficial effects in the prevention of CAD. The hypocholesterolemic and antioxidant effects of olive oil may contribute to these protective effects. Controversial reports exist about the effects of MUFAs on lipoprotein metabolism in the literature. Earlier studies report that oleic acid neither raises nor lowers plasma cholesterol levels (Hegsted et al., 1965; Mattson & Grundy, 1985). MUFAs were also considered to be neutral, regarding serum LDL concentrations. Numerous clinical trial and animal studies, however, show that oleic acid reduces total and LDL cholesterol levels in plasma (Fernandez & West, 2005; Kok & Kromhout, 2004; Mensink et al., 2003).

The ratio of total:HDL cholesterol is a more specific marker of CAD than the LDL or total cholesterol levels. Several meta-analyses evaluated the effects of dietary fatty acids on plasma lipid and lipoproteins (Davis et al., 2007; Howell et al., 1997; Mensink et al., 2003). Based on the meta-analysis of 224 studies published by Howell et al. (1997), changes in the intake of SFAs and PUFAs affect plasma LDL-cholesterol concentrations, whereas total fatty acids and SFAs are two major dietary determinants of changes in plasma HDL cholesterol, even though the degree of fatty acid unsaturation reduces this effect (Howell et al., 1997). The more recent meta-analysis, however, reported that by using the ratio of total:HDL cholesterol, the isoenergetic replacement of SFAs with carbohydrates does not improve the serum total:HDL cholesterol. An isoenergetic replacement of carbohydrates constituting 1% of dietary energy with an equal percentage of MUFAs reduces total:HDL cholesterol ($r$ = <0.001), total cholesterol ($r$ = 0.061), LDL cholesterol ($r$ = 0.004) and triglycerides

($r$ < 0.001), and increases HDL cholesterol ($r$ = <0.001) (Mensink et al., 2003). Based on this study, the replacement of 1% of energy in the form of a SFA, with an equal percentage in the form of a MUFA, is predicted to lower both LDL- and HDL-cholesterol concentrations.

In obese women, the comparison of two hypocaloric diets containing either high- complex carbohydrates (25% of energy from fat) or enriched MUFAs based (45% of energy from fat) on olive oil showed that the high-MUFA diet reduced the density of the LDL fraction (Zambon et al., 1999). This was supported by another study (Krauss, 2001), but in the other study with diabetic subjects, no difference was observed in the LDL size with diets varying in fat content up to 14% (Luscombe et al., 1999).

***Effects of MUFA on Lipid Peroxidation***

Protective effects of oleic acid in the oxidation of the LDL cholesterol received particular attention. The oleic-acid content of LDL particles in human subjects with a MUFA-rich diet is significantly higher than in individuals consuming other dietary protocols. An inverse correlation exists between the content of oleic acid in LDL particles and its sensitivity to oxidation (Tsimikas et al., 1999). In different studies, the resistance of LDL to different oxidant conditions was highest, whereas the induction of monocyte adhesion to endothelial cells was lowest with a MUFA-rich diet compared to a PUFA- or SFA-rich diet (Tsimikas et al., 1999), showing that LDL enriched with oleic acid may be less easily converted to inflammatory oxidized LDL. After the supplementation of human individuals with either oleic or LA, LDL particles isolated from the oleic-supplemented group when exposed to oxidative stress were more resistant to oxidation, and showed less monocyte adhesion (Tsimikas et al., 1999). Several studies report a higher resistance of MUFA-enriched LDL particles to oxidation as indicated by a long lag time (Ashton et al., 2001; Hargrove et al., 2001; Kratz et al., 2002; Lapointe et al., 2006; Mata et al., 1997; Nestel et al., 1997 ). Few studies, however, reported contrary results (Castro et al., 2000; Lapointe et al., 2006; Schwab et al., 1998).

As the oxidative modification of LDL cholesterol is critical for the initiation of atherosclerosis and also considering the protective effects of HDL cholesterol in endothelial activation (Nicholls et al., 2006), these findings suggest that MUFA also indirectly improves endothelial functions.

## Polyunsaturated Fatty Acids (PUFAs)

PUFAs contain two or more double bonds along the carbon chain, and are classified as n-3 or n-6 on the basis of the location of the last bond relative to the terminal methyl (omega) end of the molecule. LA (18:2n-6) is the most predominant PUFA in the diet. It is found in corn, soybean, sunflower, and safflower oils. LA is converted to AA (20:4n-6) which, along with other PUFAs, can serve as a precursor of eicosanoid products. α-linolenic acid (ALA, 18:3n-3) is another PUFA that is found in walnuts and in soybean, rapeseed, and flaxseed oils. Both LA and ALA cannot be synthesized de novo by human cells and are known as essential fatty acids. These essential fatty acids undergo a series of saturation, desaturation, and elongation steps from which other longer chain n-3 PUFAs are synthesized. Eicosapentaenoic acid (EPA, 20:5n-3) and DHA (22:6n-3) are two biologically important n-3 PUFAs which are synthesized from the essential fatty acids within the body and also are found in fish, marine oils, and fish products. They can be directly provided by the consumption of fish products, or synthesized from ALA. Large adipose-tissue reservoirs of LA slow down the conversion of ALA to EPA and DHA. In healthy volunteers, however, about 5–10% and 2–5% of dietary ALA are converted to EPA and DHA, respectively (Wijendran & Hayes, 2004).

CAD is rare in populations with a very high intake of fish, such as the South Pacific Islanders, the Japanese, and the indigenous Alaskans. The potatitive dietary component thought to reduce the CAD risk was the high level of dietary marine n-3 fatty acids. Numerous epidemiologic and experimental studies indicate that increased long-chain n-3 fatty acid consumption reduces the risk of CAD. However, insufficient clinical evidence is available regarding the effect of consuming ALA (Balk et al., 2006b). Although the intake of marine products or fish oil appears to have a modest beneficial effect on LDL cholesterol, HDL cholesterol, and triglyceride levels, the reduction in CAD is actually greater than what was expected on the basis of its effects on blood lipids (Balk et al., 2006b).

The exact cardioprotective mechanism of n-3 fatty acids is unclear; however, the exposure of endothelial cells to n-3 fatty acids as a result of fatty acid incorporation into the cellular phospholipids increases membrane fluidity, which can affect many aspects of the pathogenesis of CAD, including endothelial dysfunction. Long- chain n-3 PUFAs act both directly (e.g., by partial replacement for AA as an eicosanoid substrate in the cell membrane or the suppression of pro-inflammatory cytokine production) and indirectly (e.g., a change in lipoprotein metabolism) to reduce the incidence of CAD and other inflammatory diseases.

## Direct Effects of PUFA on Endothelial Functions

### *Effect of n-3 PUFA on Inflammatory Cytokines*

Although n-3 PUFAs exert many of their anti-inflammatory properties by an antagonistic effect on arachidonic acid metabolism (see below), they have numerous other anti-inflammatory characteristics that might occur independently from downstream of an altered eicosanoid metabolism. De Caterina et al. (2000) showed that incubation of the culture of human endothelial cells with DHA significantly reduced the cytokine-induced surface expression of ICAM-1, VCAM-1, and E-selectin (De Caterina et al., 2000). Based on their study, the effect was accompanied by a reduction in the adhesion of monocytes to cytokine-activated endothelium, and also seen for other cytokine-activated products (e.g., the soluble proteins IL-6 and IL-8) involved in the amplification of the inflammatory response and chemoattraction of the granulocytes (De Caterina et al., 2000). The effect of DHA is more potent than EPA (Mori & Woodman, 2006). However, each of them has a different metabolic role, with the DHA preferentially taken up by the cell membrane and the EPA utilized as a substrate for an eicosanoid (De Caterina et al., 2000).

By now, however, many studies in the literature, both in experimental animals and human subjects (Balk et al., 2006a, 2006b; Brazidec, 2007; Hjerkinn et al., 2005; Khan et al., 2003; Lopez-Garcia et al., 2004; Morgan et al., 2006; Sadeghi et al., 1999; Trebble et al., 2003; Wallace et al., 2003 ), show that n-3 fatty acids inhibit the expression of the adhesion molecules following different stimulations, decrease the circulating levels of soluble VCAM-1, inhibit the production of TNF-α and IL-1 by monocytes, and reduce the production of IL-6 and IL-8 by endothelial cells. They may affect the activation of other transcription factors (NF-κB and PPAR) (Calder, 2002; Jackson et al., 2007).

Several other studies, however, fail to show any significant inhibitory effects of n-3 PUFA on the production of inflammatory cytokines in humans, probably because low doses of the fatty acids are provided (Calder, 2006a; Kew et al., 2003; Thies et al., 2001; Wallace et al., 2003).

These modulatory effects on endothelial activation which have an important role in the clinical application of n-3 PUFA (e.g., rheumatoid arthritis, asthma, CAD, and inflammatory bowel diseases) may result from altered eicosanoid metabolism and/or other properties of the fatty acids. These effects were extensively reviewed (Calder, 2002, 2005, 2006a; Gebauer et al., 2006; Hartweg et al., 2007; Psota et al., 2006; Robinson & Stone, 2006 ).

A few studies evaluated the effects of ALA on inflammatory outcomes. While high amounts (13.7 g/day, 4 weeks) of ALA reduced the production of TNF-α and IL-1 in endotoxin-stimulated mononuclear cells, several studies using lower intakes of ALA (2–9.5 g/day) fail to show any significant effect on TNF-α, IL-6, IL-1, and ICAM-1 (Kew et al., 2003; Thies et al., 2001; Wallace et al., 2003). On a 1 g/day basis, it seems ALA is about nine times weaker than long-chain n-3 PUFAs with respect to the inflammatory markers in humans (Calder, 2006a). Thus, ALA does not appear to exert important anti-inflammatory effects with normal intake (Deckelbaum & Akabas, 2006a).

***Effect of n-6 PUFA on Inflammatory Cytokines***

The other class of PUFAs is the n-6 fatty acids comprised mainly of AA (20:4n-6) and its precursor LA (18:2n-6). Due to the lipid-lowering effect of LA, its consumption was promoted; however, numerous studies documented the harmful effects of LA, especially regarding endothelial functions (Hennig et al., 2001a; Hennig & Toborek, 2001b; Lima et al., 2007; Perez-Jimenez et al., 2002; Perona et al., 2006; Rodríguez-Lee et al., 2006).

The intake of LA causes endothelial dysfunction, and can potentiate TNF-mediated endothelial-cell injury. Moreover, it can cause an imbalance in cellular oxidative stress of the endothelium, thereby increasing the production of inflammatory cytokines and the expression of adhesion molecules. LA enhances platelet response to aggregation, suppresses the immune system, depletes cellular glutathione levels, activates NF-κ B, potentiates TNF-α-mediated apoptosis of cultured endothelial cells, and decreases NO synthesis (Toborek & Hennig, 1994).

In addition, an increased consumption of LA results in the accumulation of AA and the enhanced production of eicosanoids, which, in large quantities, can contribute to the formation of thrombi and atheroma. A positive correlation exists between the LA levels in the arterial wall of a human aorta artery and CAD (Bahrami et al., 2006). Furthermore, concentrations of LA in adipose tissue were positively correlated with the degree of the diseases (Bahrami et al., 2008; Hennig et al., 2001a).

***Effect of n-3 PUFA on Eicosanoid Products***

Among the key inflammatory mediators released by the endothelium, are the eicosanoids derived from the 20-atom carbon PUFA. Eicosanoids are oxygenated products of long-chain PUFAs which are liberated from cell-membrane phospholipids. They are biologically active in very small quantities, and their large amounts of production contribute to several pathologic conditions. The nature of the 20-carbon precursor that was esterified in specific membrane phospholipids is one of the most important determinants of the type of eicosanoids synthesized. Western-type diets typically contain high amounts of n-6 PUFAs, especially AA and its precursor LA, which is the dominant form of fatty acid in membrane phospholipids; thus, it is liberated and subsequently acts as a substrate for the enzymes that synthesize eicosanoids (Calder, 2006a). AA is the precursor for two different series of eicosanoids which have a wide range of effects on metabolic pathways relevant to endothelial functions. Several enzymatic systems include COX and the lypoxygenase oxygenate AA, following mobilization. Metabolism by the COX enzymes gives rise to the synthesis of the 2-series PGs and TX, while the 5-lipooxygenase pathway produces the 4-series LTs (Lotzer et al., 2005). Eicosanoids have a number of pro-inflammatory effects; among them is $TXA_2$, a platelet aggregator and vasoconstrictor. LTs, however, are linked to inflammation and atherogenesis, but the AA-derived PGI-2 is a potent vasodilator, and can inhibit platelet aggregation.

An increased intake of long-chain n-3 PUFAs, such as EPA and DHA which are found in marine products, leads to an increase in their proportion in inflammatory cell phospholipids, at the expense of AA in a dose-dependent manner. This dietary manipulation causes the alternative fatty acids to be metabolized and changes the final eicosanoid products of the process to the 3-series PGs and TXs as well as the 5-series LTs. The functional significance of this change is that the mediators formed from long-chain PUFAs are 10–100 times less potent than those formed from AA. For example $TXA_2$, which is synthesized from AA, is a powerful vasoconstrictor and platelet aggregator, while $TX_3$, which is produced from long-chain n-3 PUFAs, is relatively inactive. In addition, $LTB_5$ is 10- to 100-fold less potent as a neutrophil chemotactic agent than $LTB_4$. $PGE_2$ and $PGE_3$ have equivalent inhibitory effects on the production of TNF-α and IL-1 by human mononuclear cells stimulated with endotoxin; however, $PGE_3$ is a less- potent inducer of COX gene expression (Calder, 2006a). Also a new group of mediators termed "E-series resolvin" and "D-series resolvin" formed from EPA and DHA, respectively, with anti-inflammatory effects was identified. Thus, dietary EPA and DHA substitution for AA reduced endothelial dysfunction (Calder, 2006b; Psota et al., 2006; Robinson & Stone, 2006).

## *Indirect Effects of PUFA on Endothelial Functions*

### *Lipoprotein Metabolism*

The relationship between dietary fats and plasma-lipid concentrations was the subject of numerous studies during the last decades. Numerous researchers evaluated the effects of PUFAs, either n-3 or n-6, on lipids and lipoprotein metabolism. These studies were reviewed by several review articles and meta-analysis (Anil, 2007; Balk et al., 2006b; Denke, 2006; Harris et al., 2008; Howell et al., 1997; Mensink et al., 2003; Moreno & Mitjavila, 2003; Psota et al., 2006; Robinson & Stone, 2006; Ros & Mataix, 2006; Wang et al., 2006). However, some inconsistency remains in the literature regarding the effects of PUFAs on plasma-lipid concentrations.

The n-3 and n-6 PUFAs have different effects on plasma lipids. An intake of SFAs raises the serum concentrations of total, LDL, and HDL cholesterol as well as the total:HDL ratio. The isoenergetic substitution of PUFAs of the n-6 series has the opposite effect: it reduces total LDL and HDL cholesterol. The mechanisms of hypocholesterolemic effects of n-6 PUFAs are not fully understood. Although, the simple substituting of PUFAs for hypercholesterolemic fatty acids is involved, LA may reduce LDL cholesterol by up-regulating hepatic LDL receptors (Dietschy, 1998).

When dietary carbohydrate is replaced by n-6 PUFA, the LDL cholesterol does not change or is slightly reduced while HDL rises (Mensink et al., 2003). Indeed, all fatty acids elevate HDL cholesterol when substituted for carbohydrates, and the effect diminished with the increasing unsaturation of fatty acids (Mensink et al., 2003; Moreno & Mitjavila, 2003). Thus, effects of n-3 long-chain fatty acids (e.g., EPA or DHA) on HDL cholesterol are less than n-6 PUFAs. Compared with MUFA, n-6 PUFA leads to a slightly greater LDL-cholesterol reduction when substituted for SFA. Unlike n-6 PUFAs, fish oils have an insignificant effect on total cholesterol (Balk et al., 2006b), and their effects on the plasma levels of LDL cholesterol may be deleterious. Although they elevate LDL concentration (Anil, 2007; Balk et al., 2006b; Moreno & Mitjavila, 2003; Robinson & Stone, 2006), plasma-lipoprotein composition shifts to a less atherogenic pattern. Several studies reported that the supplementation with EPA or DHA decreases SD-LDL particles or increases the large buoyant LDL (Kris-Etherton et al., 2002; Mesa et al., 2004; Samuelson et al., 2001).

Although individual studies reported that no significant association exists between either a fish-oil dose or its duration of consumption and the effects on HDL, LDL, or total cholesterol levels; however, baseline total cholesterol as well as the dose and duration of the supplementation with the fatty acids are two important potential determinants of treatment effect: each 10 mg/dL increase in mean baseline total cholesterol is associated with an additional 0.8 mg/dL decrease after fish-oil consumption (Balk et al., 2006b). Hence, in the majority of studies the net effects of the parameters on total-, LDL-, and HDL-cholesterol levels were estimated as less than 5% (Balk et al., 2006b).

Several lines of evidence found at least a 15% net reduction in plasma triglyceride levels following supplementation with fish oil (Anil, 2007; Balk et al., 2006b; Kris-Etherton et al., 2004; Ros & Mataix, 2006). An independent association exists between the effect of fish-oil consumption on triglyceride levels and both the dose of fish oil used and the baseline triglyceride levels (Anil, 2007; Balk et al., 2006b). The n-3 fatty acids lower triglyceride by inhibiting the synthesis of very low density lipoproteins (VLDLs) in the liver (Anil, 2007; Harris et al, 2008; Ros & Mataix, 2006). Improved triglyceride metabolism, followed by the formation of less-dense LDL particles overall, leads to a less atherogenic lipid profile and off-setting of any adverse effect from an LDL-cholesterol elevation (Ros & Mataix, 2006; Satoh et al., 2007).

A few studies reported on the effect of ALA consumption on lipids. The studies were mostly of poor quality (Balk et al., 2006b); however, ALA does not share the hypotriglyceridemic effect of its marine counterparts, but its action on lipoproteins is similar to those of the n-6 PUFAs (Balk et al., 2006b; Ros & Mataix, 2006).

## Effects of PUFA on HDL Metabolism

Endothelial lipase (EL) plays a major role in atherosclerosis by using its ability to modulate the plasma concentrations of HDL cholesterol. Over-expression of the enzyme reduces plasma HDL concentrations, while its inactivation significantly elevates the HDL levels in plasma. Fish-oil supplementation reduces the activity of the enzyme that, in turn, augments HDL production. Although the exact mechanism of n-3 PUFA on EL is unclear, an adequate supply of n-3 PUFA in the endothelial cell increases the fluidity of the membrane, reduces the production of the cytokines and the formation of free radicals that, in turn, inhibits the activation of EL (Das 2005).

### *Lipid Peroxidation*

Many studies indicated that the type of fatty acid in the LDL particles significantly affects the susceptibility of LDL to oxidation. The presence of more double bonds increases the susceptibility to free-radical damage; thus, the susceptibility enhanced by increasing the unsaturation of fatty acids. Several studies compared the susceptibility of LDL to oxidation following supplementation with fish oil or n-6 PUFA, and reported that n-3 fatty acids from both marine and plant sources may increase the susceptibility of LDL to oxidation. Based on these studies, n-3 fatty acids reduced both lag time, an indicator of oxidizability, and the oxidation rate (Lapointe et al., 2006). The lipids present on the LDL surface are initially more readily oxidized in LDL particles obtained from individuals consuming fish oil, but the extent of oxidation is lower (Lapointe et al., 2006). Therefore, n-6 PUFA promotes LDL oxidation, while the effects of n-3 PUFA on LDL oxidation are not clearly identified (Anil, 2007; Lapointe et al., 2006; Robinson & Stone, 2006; Ros & Mataix, 2006).

Apparently, high-serum n-6 PUFAs, when insufficiently protected by antioxidants (e.g., vitamin E), may increase the risk of atherosclerosis (Hennig et al., 2000; Hennig & Toborek, 2001b). While n-6 PUFAs have desirable effects on lipid and lipoproteins, long-chain n-3 PUFAs exert their cardioprotective effects through changes in endothelial functions and AA metabolism. Thus, a balance between these two groups is important because it enables them to compete for the same enzyme systems involved in elongation and desaturation to synthesize more biologically active fatty acids. Furthermore, they also compete for COX and lypoxygenase involved in eicosanoid production that mediates a range of important endothelial and cardiovascular functions. An excessive intake of n-6 relative to n-3 fatty acids promotes the 2- and 4-series of eicosanoid products from AA which mediate pro-inflammatory and prothrombic effects.

## *Coagulation, Clotting Factors, and Plaque Stability*

Limited studies are available about the effects of PUFA supplementation on coagulation and clotting factors; however, these studies showed inconsistent findings about the effects of the fatty acids on coagulation and fibrinolysis pathways. The most consistent result is that long-chain PUFAs increase bleeding time especially when given in relatively large doses, probably due to the effect on platelet aggregation (Harris, 2007). Several clinical trials reported that supplementation with PUFA increases plasma concentration of factor V in healthy volunteers; however, this was not accompanied with a concomitant activation of factor X. The authors suggested that clotting was therefore not necessarily activated (Hartweg et al., 2007; Miller, 2005; Mutanen & Freese, 2001). Furthermore, factor VII activities are possibly related to habitual fat intake and plasma- triglyceride concentration which increases after the consumption of a high-fat meal, usually irrespective of the fat type (Mutanen & Freese, 2001).

The n-3 fatty acid supplementation, both long-chain fatty acids and ALA, leads to the harmful increasing of PAI-1, a potent inhibitor of fibrinolysis in plasma (Mutanen & Freese, 2001). Although insignificant changes in fibrinogen levels were reported by these fats (Hartweg et al., 2007), no effect on fibrinolysis and/or important change in coagulation markers are evident (Hartweg et al., 2007; Mutanen & Freese, 2001; Robinson & Stone, 2006).

The n-3 fatty acids increase systemic arterial compliance and tend to reduce pulse pressure and total vascular resistance (Nestel et al., 2002). They also reduce intima-media thickness, decrease the risk of stroke by increasing plaque stability, and change plaque morphology. These effects reduce the risk of acute plaque rupture by the ticking of the fibrous caps and reducing inflammation. The plaques from n-3 PUFA-supplemented individuals are less heavily infiltrated with macrophages and less likely to be thin, have an enflamed-cap, and be ruptured (Harris et al., 2008; Moreno & Mitjavila, 2003; Robinson & Stone, 2006).

In conclusion, these findings suggest that dietary supplementation with long-chain n-3 PUFAs has cardio-protective effects by improving endothelial functions, decreasing platelet aggregation, and lowering triglyceride levels. For supplementation with ALA, a decreasing effect on mortality has not been established (Wang et al., 2006); however, further studies are needed to elucidate its accurate cardiovascular effects. An intake of n-6 PUFAs is positively associated with a better lipid profile; however, their high consumption, especially with insufficient amounts of n-3 fatty acids adversely affects endothelial functions.

## ***Trans*** **Fatty Acids (TFAs)**

*Trans* fatty acids (TFAs)—which are formed during the hydrogenation of vegetable oils for use in margarines, food manufacturing, commercial cooking, and frying—are unsaturated fats with at least one carbon-carbon double bond in the *trans* configuration. They are also produced in small amounts by the action of gastric bacteria in cows, sheep, and other ruminants. During the process of the commercial hydrogenation of liquid vegetable oils or the bio-hydrogenation in ruminants, double bonds originally present at the *cis* position are modified in both conformation and position. The term "isometric fatty acids" refers to both of these types (positional and geometrical) as well as minor amounts of other fatty acids formed during hydrogenation. Positional isomers are formed when double bonds shift from their original position to other positions (for example, from position Δ-9 to Δ-12), and geometric isomers are produced when the naturally occurring *cis*-double bonds are isomerized to the more stable *trans* configuration.

In the *cis* form, the hydrogen atoms are on the same side of the double bond and have a "bent" structure. In the *trans* form, however, the hydrogen atoms are at opposite positions; the molecules are more linear and have a straight carbon chain resembling that of a SFA. Because the *trans* forms are more stable thermodynamically than the *cis* forms, they are more solid at room temperature with a higher melting point, are more stable during deep-frying, and have a longer shelf life. The predominant TFA isomer in industrially hydrogenated oils is *trans*-9 octadecanoic acid or elaidic acid, which accounts for up to 60% of all fatty acids and contributes to the hardness of partially hydrogenated oils.

A significant increase in TFA consumption occurred during World War II because of the widespread intake of partially hydrogenated oils, mainly due to economic dislocations. During the 1960s, margarines became viewed as the healthy alternative to butter to avoid saturated-fat consumption (Mozaffarian & Willett, 2007). This high intake of TFAs may be associated with a high rate of CAD during the second half of the twentieth century (Willett, 2006b).

Ruminant fatty acids, however, originate from milk, or the tissue fats of cows, sheep, and other ruminants, and only account for up to 5% of the total fatty acids

(Jakobsen et al., 2006; Pfeuffer & Schrezenmeir, 2006). Vaccinic acid (C18:1, 11*t*) is the most important ruminant *trans* fat which accounts for 1.0–6.0% of total milk and meat fatty acids (Mozaffarian & Willett, 2007). Smaller amounts of conjugated linoleic acid (CLA) are also formed. The term "CLA" refers to a mixture of positional and geometric isomers of LA with conjugated double bonds (e.g., C18:2, 10*t*–12*c*, C18:2, 10*t*–12*t*), but *cis* 9, *trans* 11 CLA is the main isomer accounting for over 90% of total CLA intake (Bhattacharya et al., 2006; Whigham et al., 2007).

Whereas consumption of TFAs increased enormously only during the past four or five decades, ruminant TFAs have been part of the human diet for thousands of years. Epidemiological studies show a strong positive association between the intake of industrially originated TFAs and the risk of CAD, but the ruminant TFAs may have different nutritional effects (Bhattacharya et al., 2006; Jakobsen et al., 2006; Pfeuffer & Schrezenmeir, 2006; Whigham et al., 2007). Thus, in contrast to ruminant fatty acids, a lot of data indicate that TFAs from partially hydrogenated oils have a wide range of detrimental effects on serum lipids, inflammation, and endothelial functions.

## *Effects of TFA from Partially Hydrogenated Oils on Endothelial Functions*

Prospective epidemiologic trials and case-control studies using the analysis of adipose tissue indicate that TFA has a major role in the risk of CAD. The magnitude of this association is considerably stronger than predicted by the effects of TFA on lipoprotein metabolism, and may be explained by the effect on inflammatory factors and endothelial functions. These effects were extensively reviewed (Ascherio, 2006; Hunter, 2006; Mozaffarian & Willett, 2007; Willett, 2006b). Both observational studies and randomized trials show that TFA has a unique cardio-metabolic imprint (Mozaffarian & Willett, 2007).

The intake of TFA is associated with higher circulating markers of systemic inflammation as well as endothelial dysfunction. A higher consumption of TFA was accompanied with higher levels of ICAM-1, VCAM-1, and E-selectin, the circulating markers of endothelial dysfunction (Lopez-Garcia et al., 2005). A randomized controlled trial in healthy volunteers (in whom oleic acid or carbohydrates were isoenergetically replaced with TFA) also showed similar harmful effects on endothelial functions (Baer et al., 2004).

Systemic inflammation is considered a strong nonlipid risk factor for CAD (Hunter, 2006). Different observational studies and randomized trials indicated that TFA promotes systemic inflammation. A high intake of TFA was associated with an increased activity of TNF-α and higher levels of IL-6 and CRP among overweight healthy women (Lopez-Garcia et al., 2005; Mozaffarian et al., 2004a). Among patients with established heart diseases, erythrocyte membrane TFA concentrations (a biomarker of dietary intake) were also positively associated with the activation of systemic inflammation responses, including higher levels of IL-6, TNF-α, and monocyte chemoattractant protein 1 (Mozaffarian et al., 2004a). In controlled feeding trials with 50 subjects, a high intake of TFA raised plasma CRP levels compared with isoenergetic oleic or carbohydrate diets (Baer et al., 2004). Among hypercholesterolemic subjects, TFA increased the production of IL-6 and TNF-α by cultured mono-nuclear cells compared with a soybean-oil diet (Han et al., 2002). In another randomized controlled trial, brachial-artery FMD was decreased by 20% with TFA consumption compared with the intake of saturated fats (De Roos et al., 2001).

The mechanisms of action of TFA on endothelial functions and systemic inflammation are not well-understood; however, TFAs are incorporated into endothelial cell membranes and directly affect the signaling pathway relating to inflammation (Mozaffarian, 2006).

## Effect of TFA on Serum Lipids

Several studies evaluated the effects of different amounts of TFA on the plasma concentrations of LDL and HDL. These studies were reviewed by Hunter (2006). TFAs have unique effects on serum lipids. Both SFAs and TFAs have LDL-cholesterol-raising effects when substituted for PUFAs or carbohydrates, but unlike SFAs, TFAs reduce HDL and increase the ratio of total:HDL cholesterol. Insufficient data exist about the effects of the consumption of low amounts of TFAs (<4% of energy in the diet). Their dietary levels necessary to decrease HDL cholesterol, however, appear to be around 5–6% of energy, and their amounts as low as 4% of energy significantly increase LDL cholesterol (Hunter, 2006).

In a meta-analysis of 60 controlled trials, TFA was considered the most harmful macro-nutrient in terms of the total:HDL cholesterol ratio (Mensink et al., 2003). A lot of controlled trials showed a dose-dependent relationship between TFA intake and the ratio. The magnitude of these effects is about twice greater for TFAs compared to SFAs, when they are used to replace other fats (e.g., MUFAs). Thus, the effects of the isocaloric replacement of 1% of energy from TFAs with a 1:1:1 mix of carbohydrates, MUFAs, and PUFAs on the rate of total:HDL cholesterol are equivalent to replacing SFAs constituting 1.8% of energy with such a mixture (Mensink et al., 2003). However, if TFAs are replaced exclusively with carbohydrates, the difference becomes even larger; hence, an isoenergetically replacement of 7.3% of energy from SFAs with carbohydrates is similar to substituting only 1% of energy from TFAs with carbohydrates (Mensink et al., 2003).

Little information is available about the effects of individual TFAs; however, in a randomized-trial, consumption of partially hydrogenated fish oil increased the ratio significantly more than isoenergetic amounts of partially hydrogenated soybean oil (Mozaffarian et al., 2004a). Also, the harmful effects of *trans* ALA (which is a product of oil deodorization and is found in refined liquid vegetable oils) are estimated to be six times greater than elaidic acid (Vermunt et al., 2001). Unlike *trans* 18:1, a positive relationship exists between the intake of *trans* 18:2 and sudden cardiac death (Lemaitre et al., 2006; Mozaffarian & Willett, 2007). In contrast to SFAs, the consumption of TFAs has a deleterious effect on LDL particle size, and increases SD-LDL cholesterol (Mauger et al., 2003). A higher intake of TFAs appears to predispose the body to accumulating fat, particularly abdominal fat (Mozaffarian & Willett, 2007), and inhibits the synthesis of essential PUFAs in the phospholipid of arterial cells (Kummerow et al., 2004).

A limited number of studies exists about the effects of TFAs on clotting factors and LDL oxidation, and the results of the available studies are inconsistent; however, it seems TFAs have no significant effect on lipid oxidation and clotting factors compared to dietary *cis* fatty acids.

TFAs exacerbate insulin resistance, and although further studies are needed to assess the accurate deleterious effects of TFAs on carbohydrate metabolism in both animal and human studies, the consumption of TFAs impairs carbohydrate metabolism (Lefevre et al., 2005; Mozaffarian & Willett, 2007). TFAs are transported across the placenta and enter human breast milk in proportion to their intake in the mother (Bahrami & Rahimi, 2005; Innis, 2006).

Generally, TFAs exert a wide range of adverse effects on human metabolism including the dysfunction of endothelium; lowering HDL cholesterol; raising LDL cholesterol, triglycerides, and VLDL; reducing the size of LDL particles; exacerbating insulin resistance; and increasing adiposity. Thus, they produce a unique cardio-metabolic imprint compared with other dietary nutrients (Mozaffarian & Willett, 2007).

In the literature, several studies exist about the healthy effects of ruminant TFAs (reviewed by Jakobsen et al., 2006 and Pfeuffer & Schrezenmeir, 2006).

Without a doubt, a need exists for controlled human studies comparing the effects of ruminant versus industrially produced TFA. The results from current epidemiological studies show that the intake of the ruminant *trans* fats does not have any adverse effects on CAD nor even significantly or insignificantly decreases the risk of the disease (Bhattacharya et al., 2006; Jakobsen et al., 2006; Pfeuffer & Schrezenmeir, 2006; Whigham et al., 2007).

## Conclusion

The endothelium plays an important role in the homeostasis of the circulation and vessels through the release of several mediators. Endothelial dysfunction is a key factor in the pathogenesis of atherosclerosis and CAD. Various risk factors such as hyperlipidemia, smoking, hypertension, and diabetes adversely affect endothelial functions. Regardless of the means of injury to the endothelium, the net results of endothelial dysfunction are vascular inflammation and atherosclerosis, which are characterized by reduced vasodilation, increased endothelium-dependent contraction, cell proliferation, platelet adhesion, and leukocyte–endothelial interaction.

Existing data emphasize the role of dietary factors, especially fatty acids, in modulating endothelial functions. In fact, various fatty acids affect all aspects of endothelial functions; however, individual fatty acids exert different effects. Whereas SFAs directly promote endothelial dysfunction, further studies are required to elucidate their indirect effects (e.g., total:HDL ratio, sensitivity of LDL to oxidation, size and density of LDL). MUFAs and long-chain n-3 PUFAs improve endothelial functions both directly and indirectly; however, in the case of n-6 PUFAs, in spite of their improving effects on lipid profiles, they directly exert harmful effects on endothelial functions especially when they are used with insufficient amounts of antioxidants or other biologically important fatty acids. *Trans* fats, however, have unique direct and indirect deleterious effects on endothelial functions and atherosclerosis.

## Acknowledgments

The author is indebted to Mrs. Bahareh Mohammadi from the Medical Biology Research Center, Kermanshah University of Medical Sciences, for constant assistance and valuable comments. The author also apologizes to those researchers whose important contributions to the field of endothelial functions could not be directly acknowledged due to the limited space available for this chapter.

### References

Abuja, P.M.; R. Albertini. Methods for monitoring oxidative stress, lipid per-oxidation and oxidation resistance of lipoproteins. *Clin. Chim. Acta* **2001,** *306,* 1–17.

Ajjan, R.; P.J. Grant. Coagulation and atherothrombotic disease. *Atherosclerosis* **2006,** *186,* 240–259.

Anil, E. The impact of EPA and DHA on blood lipids and lipoprotein metabolism: influence of apoE genotype. *Proc. Nutr. Soc.* **2007,** *66,* 60–68 .

Ascherio, A. *Trans* fatty acids and blood lipids. *Atherosclerosis* **2006,** *7,* 25–27.

Ashton, E.L.; J.D. Best; M.J. Ball. Effects of monounsaturated enriched sunflower oil on CHD risk factors including LDL size and copper-induced LDL oxidation. *J. Am. Coll. Nutr.* **2001,** *20,* 320–326.

Avellone, G.; V. Di Garbo; R. Cordova; L. Scalffidi; G.D. Bompiani. Effects of Mediterranean diet on lipid, coagulative and fibrinolytic parameters in two randomly selected population samples in Western Sicily. *Nutr. Metab. Cardiovasc. Dis.* **1998,** *8,* 287–296.

Baer, D.J.; J.T. Judd; B.A. Clevidence; R.P. Tracy. Dietary fatty acids affect plasma markers of inflammation in healthy men fed controlled diets: a randomized crossover study. *Am. J. Clin. Nutr.* **2004,** *79,* 969–973.

Bahrami, G.; E. Ghanbarian; M. Massoumi; Z. Rahimi; F. Rezwan madani. Comparison of fatty acid profiles of aorta and internal mammary arteries in patients with coronary artery disease. *Clin. Chim. Acta* **2006**, *370,* 143–146.

Bahrami, G.; M. Massoumi; Z. Rahimi. Co-existence of fatty acids changes in aorta artery and adipose tissue; comparison between CAD and non CAD patients. *J. Thromb. Thrombolysis* **2008.** (In press)

Bahrami, G.; Z. Rahimi. Fatty acid composition of human milk in Western Iran. *Eu. J. Clin. Nutr.* **2005**, *59,* 494-497.

Balk, E.M.; A.H. Lichtenstein; M. Chung; B. Kupelnick; P. Chew; J. Lau. Effects of omega-3 fatty acids on coronary restenosis, intima—media thickness, and exercise tolerance: A systematic review. *Atherosclerosis* **2006a,** *184,* 237–246.

Balk, E.M.; A.H. Lichtenstein; M. Chung; B. Kupelnick; P. Chew; J. Lau. Effects of omega-3 fatty acids on serum markers of cardiovascular disease risk: A systematic review. *Atherosclerosis* **2006b,** *189,* 19–30.

Basu, A.; S. Devaraj; I. Jialal. Dietary Factors That Promote or Retard Inflammation. *Arterioscler. Thromb. Vasc. Biol.* **2006,** *26,* 995–1001.

Behrendt, D.; P. Ganz. Endothelial Function: From Vascular Biology to Clinical Applications. *Am. J. Cardiol.* **2002,** *90,* 40L–48L.

Bhattacharya, A.; J. Banu; M. Rahman, J. Causey; G. Fernandes. Biological effects of conjugated linoleic acids in health and disease. *J. Nutr. Biochem.* **2006,** *17,* 789–810.

Binkoski, A.E.; P.M. Kris-Etherton; T.A. Wilson; M.L. Mountain; R.J. Nicolosi. Balance of Unsaturated Fatty Acids Is Important to a Cholesterol-Lowering Diet: Comparison of Mid-Oleic Sunflower Oil and Olive Oil on Cardiovascular Disease Risk Factors. *J. Am. Diet. Assoc.* **2005,** *105,* 1080–1086.

Brazidec, H.L. Lipoproteins and protection of the arterial wall against infection, The "response to the threat of infection" hypothesis. *Atherosclerosis* **2007,** *195,* e21–e31.

Brown, A.A.; F.B. Hu. Dietary modulation of endothelial function: implications for cardiovascular disease. *Am. J. Clin. Nutr.* **2001,** *73,* 673–686.

Calder, P.C. n-3 Polyunsaturated fatty acids, inflammation, and inflammatory diseases. *Am. J. Clin. Nutr.* **2006a,** *83,* 1505S–15019S.

Calder, P.C. Polyunsaturated fatty acids and inflammation. *Prostaglandins, LeukotrienesEssent. Fatty Acids* **2006b,** *75,* 197–202.

Calder, P.C. Dietary modification of inflammation with lipids. *Proc. Nutr. Soc.* **2002,** *61,* 345–358.

Calder, P.C. Polyunsaturated fatty acids and inflammation. *Biochem. Soc.Transactions* **2005,** *33,* 423–427.

Call, J.T.; E.N. Deliargyris; L.K. Newby. Focusing on Inflammation in the Treatment of Atherosclerosis. *Cardiology Rev.* **2004,** *12,* 194–200.

Carluccio, M.A.; M. Massaro; C. Bonfrate; L. Siculella; M. Maffia; G. Nicolardi; A. Distante; C. Storelli; R. De Caterina. Oleic Acid Inhibits Endothelial Activation, A Direct Vascular Anti-atherogenic Mechanism of a Nutritional, Component in the Mediterranean Diet. *Arterioscler. Thromb. Vasc. Biol.* **1999,** *19,* 220–228.

Castro, P.; J.L. Miranda; P. Gómez; D.M. Escalante; F.L. Segura; A. Martín; F. Fuentes; A. Blanco; J.M. Ordovás; F.P. Jiménez. Comparison of an oleic acid enriched-diet vs. NCEP-I diet on LDL susceptibility to oxidative modifications. *Eur. J. Clin. Nutr.* **2000,** *54,* 61–7.

Christon, R.A. Mechanisms of action of dietary fatty acids in regulating the activation of vascular endothelial cells during atherosclerosis. *Nutr. Rev.* **2003,** *61,* 272–279.

Ciapaite, J.; J.V. Bezu; G.V. Eikenhorst; S.J.L. Bakker; T. Teerlink; M. Diamant; R.J. Heine; K. Krab; H.V. Westerhoff; C.G. Schalkwijk. Palmitate and oleate have distinct effects on the inflammatory phenotype of human endothelial cells. *Biochim. Biophys. Acta* **2007,** *1771,* 147–154.

Couloubaly, S.; C. Deloménie ; D. Rousseau; J.L. Paul; A. Grynberg; M.L. Pourci. Fatty acid incorporation in endothelial cells and effects on endothelial nitric oxide synthase. *Eur. J. Clin. Invest* **2007,** *37,* 692–699.

Das, U.N. Long-chain polyunsaturated fatty acids, endothelial lipase and atherosclerosis. *Prostaglandins Leukotrienes Essent. Fatty Acids* **2005,** *72,* 173–179.

Davignon, J.; P. Ganz. Role of Endothelial Dysfunction in Atherosclerosis. *Circulation* **2004,** *109,* III27–III32.

Davis, N.; S. Katz; J.W. Rosett. The Effect of Diet on Endothelial Function. *Cardiology in Rev.* **2007,** *15,* 62–66.

Deanfield, J.E.; J.P. Halcox; T.J. Rabelink. Endothelial Function and Dysfunction, Testing and Clinical Relevance. *Circulation* **2007,** *115,* 1285–1295.

De Caterina, R.; W. Bernini; M.A. Carluccio; J.K. Liao; P. Libby. Structural requirements for inhibition of cytokine-induced endothelial activation by unsaturated fatty acids**.** *J. Lipid Res.* **1998,** *39,* 1062–1070.

De Caterina, R.; J.K. Liao; P. Libby. Fatty acid modulation of endothelial activation. *Am. J. Clin. Nutr.* **2000,** *71,* 213S–223S.

Deckelbaum, R.J.; S.R. Akabas. n-3 Fatty acids and cardiovascular disease: navigating toward recommendations. *Am. J. Clin. Nutr.* **2006a,** *84,* 1–2.

Deckelbaum, R.J.; T.S. Worgall; T. Seo. n-3 Fatty acids and gene expression. *Am. J. Clin. Nutr.* **2006b,** *83*(suppl), 1520S –5S.

Denke, M.A. Dietary Fats, Fatty Acids, and Their Effects on Lipoproteins. *Curr. Atheroscler. Reports* **2006,** *8,* 466–471.

De Roos, N.M.; M.L. Bots; M.B. Katan. Replacement of dietary saturated

fatty acids by *trans* fatty acids lowers serum HDL cholesterol and impairs endothelial function in healthy men and women. *Arterioscler. Thromb. Vasc. Biol.* **2001,** *21,* 1233–1237.

Dietschy, J.M. Dietary fatty acids and the regulation of plasma low density lipoprotein cholesterol concentration. *J. Nutr.* **1998,** *128,* 444s–448s.

Dreon, D.M.; H.A. Fernstrom; H. Campos; P. Blanche; P.T. Williams; R.M. Krauss. Change in dietary saturated fat intake is correlated with change in mass of large low-density-lipoprotein particles in men. *Am. J. Clin. Nutr.* **1998,** *67,* 828–836.

Edirisinghe, I.; K.M. Hallam; C. T. Kappagoda. Effect of fatty acids on endothelium-dependent relaxation in the rabbit aorta. *Clin. Sci.* **2006,** *111,* 145–151.

Esposito, K.; M.M. Ciotola; D. Giugliano. Mediterranean diet, endothelial function and vascular inflammatory markers. *Public Health Nutr.* **2006,** *9,* 1073–1076.

Esposito, K.; R. Marfella; M.M. Ciotola; C. Di Palo; F. Giugliano; G. Giugliano; M. D'Armiento; F. D'Andrea; D. Giugliano. Effect of a Mediterranean-Style Diet on Endothelial Dysfunction and Markers of Vascular Inflammation in the Metabolic Syndrome. *JAMA* **2004,** *292,* 1440–1446.

Fernandez, M.L.; K.L. West. Mechanisms by which Dietary Fatty Acids Modulate Plasma Lipids. *J. Nutr.* **2005,** *135,* 2075–2078.

French, M.A.; K.Sundram; M.T. Clandinin. Cholesterolaemic Effect of Palmitic Acid in Relation to Other Dietary Fatty Acids, *Asia Pac. J. Clin. Nutr.* **2002,** *11* (Suppl. 7), S401–S407.

Frenette, P.S.; D.D. Wagner. Molecular medicine, adhesion molecules. *New Engl. J. Med.* **1996,** *334,* 1526–1530.

Fuentes, F.; J. Lopez-Miranda; E. Sánchez; F. Sánchez; J. Paez; E. Paz-Rojas; et al. A Mediterranean and NCEP-I diet improve endothelial function in hypercholesterolemic males. *Ann. Intern. Med.* **2001,** *134,* 1115–1119.

Gebauer, S.K.; T.L. Psota; W.S. Harris; P.M. Kris-Etherton. n-3 Fatty acid dietary recommendations and food sources to achieve essentiality and cardiovascular benefits. *Am. J. Clin. Nutr.* **2006,** *83,* 1526S–1535S.

German, J.B.; C.J. Dillard. Saturated fats: what dietary intake? *Am. J. Clin. Nutr.* **2004,** *80,* 550–559.

Griel, A.E.; P.M. Kris-Etherton. Beyond Saturated Fat: The Importance of the Dietary Fatty Acid Profile on Cardiovascular Disease. *Nutr. Rev.* **2006,** *64,* 257–262.

Han, S.N.; L.S. Leka; A.H. Lichtenstein; et al. Effect of hydrogenated and saturated, relative to polyunsaturated, fat on immune and inflammatory responses of adults with moderate hypercholesterolemia. *J. Lipid Res.* **2002,** *43,* 445–452.

Hara, H.; S. Haga; Y. Aoyama; S. Kiriyama. Short Chain Fatty Acids Suppress Cholesterol Synthesis in Rat Liver and Intestine. *J. Nutr.* **1999,** *129,* 942–948.

Hargrove, R.L.; T.D. Etherton; T.A. Pearson; E.H. Harrison; P.M. Kris-Etherton. Low fat and high monounsaturated fat diets decrease human low density lipoprotein oxidative susceptibility in vitro. *J. Nutr.* **2001,** *131,* 1758–1763.

Harris, W.S. Expert Opinion: Omega-3 Fatty Acids and Bleeding Cause or Concern? *Am..J. Cardiol.* **2007,** *99,* 44C–46C.

Harris, W.S.; M. Miller; A.P. Tighe; M.H. Davidson; E.J. Schaefer. Omega-3 fatty acids and coronary heart disease risk: Clinical and mechanistic perspectives. *Atherosclerosis* **2008,** *197,* 12–24.

Hartweg, J.; A.J. Farmer; R.R. Holman; H.A.W. Neil. Meta-analysis of the effects of n-3 polyunsaturated fatty acids on haematological and thrombogenic factors in type 2 diabetes. *Diabetologia* **2007,** *50,* 250–258.

Hegsted, D.M.; R.B. McGandy; M.L. Myers, F.J. Stare. Quantitative effects of dietary fat on serum cholesterol in man. *Am. J. Clin. Nutr.* **1965,** *17,* 281–295.

Hennig, B.; P. Meerarani; P. Ramadass; B.A. Watkins; M. Toborek. Fatty Acid-Mediated Activation of Vascular Endothelial Cells. *Metabolism* **2000,** *49,* 1006–1013

Hennig, B.; M. Toborek. Nutrition and endothelial cell function: implications in atherosclerosis. *Nutr. Res.* **2001b,** *21,* 279–293.

Hennig, B.; M. Toborek; C.J. McClain. High-Energy Diets, Fatty Acids and Endothelial Cell Function: Implications for Atherosclerosis. *J. Am.College of Nutr.* **2001a,** *20,* 97–105.

Hjerkinn, E.M.; I. Seljeflot; I. Ellingsen; P. Berstad; I. Hjermann; L. Sandvik; H. Arnesen. Influence of long-term intervention with dietary counseling, long chain n-3 fatty acid supplements, or both on circulating markers of endothelial activation in men with long-standing hyperlipidemia. *Am. J. Clin. Nutr.* **2005,** *81,* 583–589.

Howard, B.V.; L. Van Horn; J. Hsia; J.E. Manson; M.L. Stefanick; S. Wassertheil-Smoller; L.H.

Kuller; A.Z. LaCroix; R.D. Longer; N.L. Lasser; et al. Low-Fat Dietary Pattern and Risk of Cardiovascular Disease The Women's Health Initiative Randomized Controlled Dietary Modification Trial. *JAMA* **2006,** *295,* 655–666.

Howell, W.H.; D.J. McNamara; M.A. Tosca; B.T. Smith; J.A. Gaines. Plasma lipid and lipoprotein responses to dietary fat and cholesterol: a meta-analysis. *Am. J. Clin. Nutr.* **1997,** *65,* 1747–1764.

Hu, F.B. The Mediterranean diet and mortality—olive oil and beyond. *N. Engl. J. Med.* **2003,** *348,* 2595–2596.

Hulthe, J.; B. Fagerberg. Circulating oxidized LDL is associated with subclinical atherosclerosis development and inflammatory cytokines. *Arterioscler. Thromb. Vasc. Biol.* **2002,** *22,* 1162–1167.

Hunter, J.E. Dietary *trans* Fatty Acids: Review of Recent Human Studies and Food Industry Response. *Lipids* **2006,** *41,* 967–992.

Innis, S.M. *Trans* fatty intakes during pregnancy, infancy and early childhood. *Atheroscler. Suppl.* **2006,** *7,* 17–20.

Jackson, K.G.; C.K. Armah; A.M. Minihane. Meal fatty acids and postprandial vascular reactivity. *Biochem. Soc.* **2007,** *35,* 451–454.

Jakobsen, M.U.; A. Bysted; N.L. Andersen; B.L. Heitmann; H.B. Hartkopp; T. Leth; K.Overvad; J. Dyerberg. Intake of ruminant *trans* fatty acids and risk of coronary heart disease. *Atherosclerosis* **2006,** *7,* 9–11.

James, M.J.; R.A. Gibson; L.G. Cleland. Dietary polyunsaturated fatty acids and inflammatory mediator production. *Am. J. Clin. Nutr.* **2000,** *71,* 343S–348S.

Kasprzak, J.D.; M. Ktosińska; J. Drozdz. Clinical aspects of assessment of endothelial function. *Pharmacol. Reports* **2006,** *58,* 33–40.

Kawashima, S.; M.Yokoyama. Dysfunction of Endothelial Nitric Oxide Synthase and Atherosclerosis. *Arterioscler. Thromb. Vasc. Biol.* **2004,** *24,* 998–1005.

Keaney, J.F.; J.A. Vita. Vascular Oxidative Stress and Antioxidant Protection in Atherosclerosis. *J. Cardiol. Rehab.* **2002,** *22,* 225–233.

Kelly, C.N.M.; R.D. Smith; C.M. Williams. Postgraduate Symposium Dietary monounsaturated fatty acids and haemostasis *Proceed. Nutr. Soc.* **2001,** *60,* 161–170.

Kew, S.; T. Banerjee; A.M. Minihane; Y.E. Finnegan; R. Muggli; R. Albers; C.M. Williams; P.C. Calder. Lack of effect of foods enriched with plant- or marine-derived n-3 fatty acids on human immune function. *Am. J. Clin. Nutr.* **2003,** *77,* 1287–1295.

Khan, F.; K. Elherik; C.B. Smith; R. Barr; A. Hill; I. Murrie; J.J.F. Belch. The effects of dietary fatty acid supplementation on endothelial function and vascular tone in healthy subjects. *Cardiovasc. Res.* **2003,** *59,* 955–962.

Kok, F.J.; D. Kromhout. Epidemiological studies on the health effects of a Mediterranean diet. *Eur. J. Nutr.* **2004,** *43,* I/2–I/5.

Kratz, M.; P. Cullen; F. Kannenberg; A. Kassner; M. Fobker; P.M. Abuja; G. Assmann; U. Wahrburg. Effects of dietary fatty acids on the composition and oxidizability of low-density lipoprotein. *Eur. J. Clin. Nutr.* **2002,** *56,* 72–81.

Krauss, R.M. Atherogenic lipoprotein phenotype and diet-gene interactions. *J. Nutr.* **2001,** *131,* 340S–343S.

Kris-Etherton, P.M.; A.E. Griel; T.L. Psota; S.K. Gebauer; J. Zhang; T.D. Etherton. Dietary Stearic Acid and Risk of Cardiovascular Disease: Intake, Sources, Digestion, and Absorption. *Lipids* **2005,** *40,* 1193–1200.

Kris-Etherton, P.M.; W.S. Harris; L.J. Appela. Fish consumption, fish oil, omega-3 fatty acids, and cardiovascular disease. *Circulation* **2002,** 106, 2747–2757.

Kris-Etherton, P.M.; K.D. Hecker; A.E. Binkoski. Polyunsaturated Fatty Acids and Cardiovascular Health. *Neutr. Rev.* **2004,** *62,* 414–426.

Kummerow, F.A.; Q. Zhou; M.M. Mahfouz; M.R. Smiricky; C.M. Grieshop; D.J. Schaeffer. *Trans* fatty acids in hydrogenated fat inhibited the synthesis of the polyunsaturated fatty acids in the phospholipid of arterial cells. *Life Sci.* **2004,** *74,* 2707–2723.

Landmesser, U.; B. Hornig; H. Drexler. Endothelial Function: A Critical Determinant in Atherosclerosis? *Circulation* **2004,** *109,* II-27–II-33.

Lapointe, A.; C. Couillard; S. Lemieux. Effects of dietary factors on oxidation of low-density lipoprotein particles. *J. Nutr. Biochem.* **2006,** *17,* 645–658.

Larsen, L.F.; J. Jespersen; P. Marckmann. Are olive oil diets antithrombotic? Diets enriched with olive, rapeseed, or sunflower oil affect postprandial factor VII differently. *Am. J. Clin. Nutr.* **1999,** *70,* 976–982.

Lefevre, M.; J.C. Lovejoy; S.R. Smith; J.P. Delany; C.Champagne; M.M. Most; Y. Denkins; L. de Jonge; J. Rood; G.A. Bray. Comparison of the acute response to meals enriched with cis or *trans* fatty acids on glucose and lipids in overweight individuals with differing FABP2 genotypes. *Metab. Clin. Exp.* **2005,** *54,* 1652–1658.

Lemaitre, R.N.; I.B. King; D. Mozaffarian; N. Sotoodehnia; T.D. Rea; L.H. Kuller; R.P. Tracy; D.S. Siscovick. Plasma Phospholipid *Trans* Fatty Acids, Fatal Ischemic Heart Disease, and Sudden Cardiac Death in Older Adults, The Cardiovascular Health Study. *Circulation* **2006,** *114,* 209–215.

Lerman, A.; A.M. Zeiher. Endothelial Function, Cardiac Events. *Circulation* **2005,** *111,* 363–368.

Levi, M.; H.T. Cate; T.V.D. Poll. Endothelium: Interface between coagulation and inflammation. *Crit. Care Med.* **2002,** *30,* S220–S224.

Libby, P.; P.M. Ridker; A. Maseri. Inflammation and Atherosclerosis. *Circulation* **2002,** *105,* 1135–1143.

Lima, T.M.D.; R. Gorjao; E. Hatanaka; M.F. Cury-Boaventura; E.P. Porttoli-silva; J. Procopio; R. Curi. Mechanisms by which fatty acids regulate leukocyte function. *Clin. Sci.* **2007,** *113,* 65–77.

Lopez-Garcia, E.; M.B. Schulze; J.E. Manson; J.B. Meigs; C.M. Albert; N. Rifai; W.C. Willett; F.B. Hu. Consumption of (n-3) Fatty Acids Is Related to Plasma Biomarkers of Inflammation and Endothelial Activation in Women. *J.Nutr.* **2004,** *134,* 1806–1811.

Lopez-Garcia, E.; M.B. Schulze; J.B. Meigs; J.E. Manson; N.Rifai; M.J. Stampfer; W.C. Willett; F.B. Hu. Consumption of *trans* fatty acids is related to plasma biomarkers of inflammation and endothelial dysfunction. *J. Nutr.* **2005,** *135,* 562–566.

Lotzer, K.; C.D. Funk; A.J.R. Habenicht. The 5-lipoxygenase pathway in arterial wall biology and atherosclerosis. *Biochim. Biophys. Acta* **2005,** *1736,* 30– 37.

Luscombe, N.D.; M. Noakes; P.M. Clifton. Diets high and low in glycemic index versus high monounsaturated fat diets: effects on glucose and lipid metabolism in NIDDM. *Eur. J. Clin. Nutr.* **1999**, *53,* 473–478.

Madamanchi, N.R.; A. Vendrov; M.S. Runge. Oxidative Stress and Vascular Disease. *Arterioscler. Thromb. Vasc. Biol.* **2005,** *25,* 29–38.

Marckmann, P.; E.M. Bladbjerg; J. Jespersen. Diet and blood coagulation factor VII/a key protein in arterial thrombosis. *Eur. J. Clin. Nutr.* **1998,** *52,* 75–84.

Massaro, M.; G. Basta; G. Lazzerini; M.A. Carluccio; F. Bosetti; G. Solaini; F. Visioli; A. Paolicchi; R. De Caterina. Quenching of intracellular ROS generation as a mechanism for oleate-induced reduction of endothelial activation and early atherogenesis. *Thromb. Haemost.* **2002a,** *88,* 335– 344.

Massaro, M.; M.A. Carluccio; A. Paolicchi; F. Bosetti; G. Solaini; R. De Caterina; G. Basta; R. De Caterina. Mechanisms for reduction of endothelial activation by oleate: inhibition of nuclear factor-kappaB through antioxidant effects. *Prostaglandins Leukotrienes Essent. Fatty Acids* **2002b,** *67,* 175–181.

Massaro, M.; M.A. Carluccio; C. Bonfrate; L. Siculella; G. Lazzerini; W. Bernini; G. Basta; R. De Caterina. The double bond in unsaturated fatty acids is the necessary and sufficient requirement for the inhibition of expression of endothelial leukocyte adhesion molecules through interference with nuclear factor-kappaB activation. *Lipids* **1999,** *34,* S213–S214.

Mata, P.; O. Varela; R. Alonso; C. Lahoz; M. de Oya; L. Badimon. Monounsaturated and polyunsaturated n-6 fatty acid-enriched diets modify LDL oxidation and decrease human coronary smooth muscle cell DNA synthesis. *Arterioscler. Thromb. Vasc. Biol.* **1997,** *17,* 2088–2095.

Mattson, F.H.; S.M. Grundy. Comparison of effects of dietary saturated, monounsaturated, and polyunsaturated fatty acids on plasma lipids and lipoproteins in man. *J. Lipid. Res.* **1985**, *26,* 194–202.

Mauger, J.F.; A.H. Lichtenstein; L.M. Ausman; S.M. Jalbert; M. Jauhiainen; C. Ehnholm; et al. Effect of different forms of dietary hydrogenated fats on LDL particle size. *Am. J. Clin. Nutr.* **2003,** *78,* 370–375.

Mensink, R.P. Effects of Stearic Acid on Plasma Lipid and Lipoproteins in Humans. *Lipids* **2005,** *40,* 1201–1205.

Mensink, R.P.; P.L. Zock; A.D.M. Kester; M.B. Katan. Effects of dietary fatty acids and carbohydrates on the ratio of serum total to HDL cholesterol and on serum lipids and apolipoproteins: a meta-analysis of 60 controlled trials. *Am. J. Clin. Nutr.* **2003,** *77,* 1146–1155.

Mesa, M.D.; R. Buckley; A.M. Minihane; P. Yaqoob. Effects of oils rich in eicosapentaenoic and docosahexaenoic acids on the oxidizability and thrombogenicity of low-density lipoprotein. *Atherosclerosis* **2004**, *175,* 333–343.

Metso, S.; A. Loimaala; M.F. Mercuri; A. Nenonen; I. Vuori; P. Oja; M.G. Bond; S. Laine; R. Rontu; T. Lehtimäki. Circulating oxidized low-density lipoprotein and common carotid artery intima-media thickness in a random sample of middle-aged men. *J. Biomed. Sci.* **2004,** *11,* 356–361.

Miller, G.J. Dietary fatty acids and the haemostatic system. *Atherosclerosis* **2005,** *179,* 213–227.

Mitchell, J.A.; F. Ali; L. Bailey; L. Moreno; L.S. Harrington. Role of nitric oxide and PGI-2 as vasoactive hormones released by the endothelium. *Exp. Physiol.* **2007,** *93,* 141–147.

Moreno, J.J.; M.T. Mitjavila. The degree of unsaturation of dietary fatty acids and the development of atherosclerosis. *J. Nutr. Biochem.* **2003,** *14,* 182–195.

Morgan, D.R.; L.J. Dixon; C.G. Hanratty; N. El-Sherbeeny; P.B. Hamilton; L.T. McGrath; W.J. Leahey; G.D. Johnston; G.E. McVeigh. Effects of Dietary Omega-3 Fatty Acid Supplementation on Endothelium-Dependent Vasodilation in Patients with Chronic Heart Failure. *Am. J. Cardiol.* **2006,** *97,* 547–551.

Mori, T.A.; R.J. Woodman. The independent effects of eicosapentaenoic acid and docosahexaenoic acid on cardiovascular risk factors in humans. *Lipid Metab.* **2006,** *9,* 95–104.

Mozaffarian, D. *Trans* fatty acids—Effects on systemic inflammation and endothelial function. *Atherosclerosis* **2006,** *7,* 29–32.

Mozaffarian, D.; T. Pischon; S.E. Hankinson; N. Rifai; K. Joshipura; W.C. Willett; E.B. Rimm. Dietary intake of *trans* fatty acids and systemic inflammation in women. *Am. J. Clin. Nutr.* **2004a,** *79,* 606–612.

Mozaffarian, D.; E.B. Rimm; D.M. Herrington. Dietary fats, carbohydrate, and progression of coronary atherosclerosis in postmenopausal women. *Am. J. Clin. Nutr.* **2004b**, *80,* 1175–1184.

Mozaffarian,D.; E.B. Rimm; I.B. King; R.L. Lawler; G.B. McDonald; W.C. Levy. *Trans* fatty acids and systemic inflammation in heart failure. *Am. J. Clin. Nutr.* **2004c,** *80,* 1521–1525.

Mozaffarian, D.; W.C. Willett. *Trans* Fatty Acids and Cardiovascular Risk: A Unique Cardiometabolic Imprint. *Curr. Atheroscler. Rep.* **2007,** *9,* 486–493.

Mutanen, M.; R. Freese. Fats, lipids and blood coagulation. *Curr. Opin. Lipidol.* **2001,** *12,* 25–29.

Nestel, P.J.; S.E. Pomeroy; T. Sasahara; T. Yamashita; Y.L. Liang; A.M. Dart; G.L. Jennings; M. Abbey; J.D. Cameron. Arterial compliance in obese subjects is improved with dietary plant n-3 fatty acid from flaxseed oil despite increased LDL oxidizability. *Arterioscler. Thromb. Vasc. Biol.* **1997,** *17,* 1163–1170.

Nestel, P.; H. Shiges; S. Pomeroy; M. Cehun; M. Abbey; D. Raederstorff. The n-3 fatty acids eicosapentaenoic acid and docosahexaenoic acid increase systemic arterial compliance in humans. *Am. J. Clin. Nutr.* **2002,** *76,* 326–330.

Nicholls, S.J.; P. Lundman; J.A. Harmer; B. Cutri; K.A. Griffiths; K.A. Rye; P.J. Barter; D.S. Celermajer. Consumption of Saturated Fat Impairs the Anti-Inflammatory Properties of High-Density Lipoproteins and Endothelial Function. *J. Am. Coll. Cardiol.* **2006,** *48,* 715–720.

O'Connell, B.J.; J. Genest. High-Density Lipoproteins and Endothelial Functions. *Circulation* **2001,** *104,* 1978–1983.

Osterud, B.; E. Bjorklid. Role of monocytes in atherogenesis. *Physiol. Rev.* **2003**, *83,* 1069–1112.

Pegorier, J.P.; C.L. May; J. Girard. Control of gene expression by fatty acids. *J. Nutr.* **2004**, *134,* 2444s–2449s.

Perez-Jimenez, F.; P. Castro; J. Lopez-Miranda; E. Paz-Rojas; A. Blanco; F. Lopez-Segura. Circulating levels of endothelial function are modulated by dietary monounsaturated fat. *Atherosclerosis* **1999,** *145,* 351–358.

Perez-Jimenez, F.; J.L. Miranda; P. Mata. Protective effect of dietary monounsaturated fat on arteriosclerosis: beyond cholesterol. *Atherosclerosis* **2002**, *163,* 385–398.

Perona, J.S.; R.C. Moruno; V.R. Gutierrez. The role of virgin olive oil components in the modulation of endothelial function. *J. Nutr. Biochem.* **2006,** *17,* 429–445.

Pfeuffer, M.; J. Schrezenmeir. Impact of *trans* fatty acids of ruminant origin compared with those from partially hydrogenated vegetable oils on CHD risk. *Int. Dairy J.* **2006**, *16,* 1383–1388.

Psota, T.L.; S.K. Gebauer; P. Kris-Etherton. Dietary Omega-3 Fatty Acid Intake and Cardiovascular Risk. *AJC* **2006,** *98,* 3i–18i.

Ridker, P.M.; J.E. Buring; N. Rifai. Soluble P-Selectin and the Risk of Future Cardiovascular Events. *Circulation* **2001,** *103,* 491–495.

Rioux, V.; P. Legrand. Saturated fatty acids: simple molecular structures with complex cellular functions. *Curr. Opinion Clin. Nutr. Metab.Care* **2007**, *10,* 752–758.

Robinson, J.G.; N.J. Stone. Antiatherosclerotic and Antithrombotic Effects of Omega-Fatty Acids. *AJC* **2006,** *98,* 39i–49i.

Rodríguez-Lee, M.; G. O. stergren-Lunden; B. Wallin; J. Moses; G. Bondjers; G. Camejo. Fatty Acids Cause Alterations of Human Arterial Smooth Muscle Cell Proteoglycans That Increase the Affinity for Low-Density Lipoprotein. *Arterioscler Thromb Vasc Biol* **2006,** *26,* 130–135

Ros, E. Dietary cis-monounsaturated fatty acids and metabolic control in type 2 diabetes. *Am. J. Clin. Nutr.* **2003,** *78,* 617S–625S.

Ros, E.; J. Mataix. Fatty acid composition of nuts- implications for cardiovascular health. *Br. J. Nutr.* **2006**, S29–S35.

Sadeghi, S.; F.A. Wallace; P.C. Calder. Dietary lipids modify the cytokine response to bacterial lipopolysaccharide in mice, *Immunology* **1999,** *96,* 404–410.

Samuelson, G.; L.E. Bratteby; R. Mohsen; B. Vessby. Dietary fat intake in healthy adolescents: inverse relationships between the estimated intake of saturated fatty acids and serum cholesterol. *Br. J. Nutr.* **2001**, *85,* 333–341.

Satoh, N.; A. Shimatsu; K. Kotani; N. Sakane; K. Yamada; T. Suganami; H. Kuzuya; Y. Ogawa. Purified Eicosapentaenoic Acid Reduces Small Dense LDL, Remnant Lipoprotein Particles, and C-Reactive Protein in Metabolic Syndrome. *Diabet. Care* **2007**, *30,* 144–146.

Savoia, C.; E.L. Schiffrin. Vascular inflammation in hypertension and diabetes: molecular mechanisms and therapeutic interventions. *Clin. Sci.* **2007,** *112,* 375–384.

Schwab, U.S.; E.S. Sarkkinen; A.H. Lichtenstein; Z. Li; J.M. Ordovas; E.J. Schaefer; M.I. Uusitupa. The effect of quality and amount of dietary fat on the susceptibility of low density lipoprotein to oxidation in subjects with impaired glucose tolerance. *Eur. J. Clin. Nutr.* **1998**, *52,* 452–458.

Shimokawa, H. Endothelial Dysfunction: a Novel Therapeutic Target Primary Endothelial Dysfunction: Atherosclerosis. *J. Mol. Cell Cardiol.* **1999**, *31,* 23–37.

Stocker, R.; J.F. Keaney. Role of Oxidative Modifications in Atherosclerosis. *Physiol. Rev.* **2004**, *84,* 1381–1478.

Temme, E.H.; R.P. Mensink; G. Hornstra. Effects of diets enriched in lauric, palmitic or oleic acids on blood coagulation and fibrinolysis. *Thromb. Haem.* **1999**, *81,* 259–263.

Thies, F.; E.A. Miles; G. Nebe-von-Caron; T.L.Hurst; E.A. Newsholme; P.C. Calder. Influence of dietary supplementation with long chain n-3 or n-6 polyunsaturated fatty acids on blood inflammatory cell populations and functions and on plasma soluble adhesion molecules in healthy adults. *Lipids* **2001**, *36,* 1183–1193.

Tholstrup, T. Influence of Stearic Acid on Hemostatic Risk Factors in Humans. *Lipids* **2005**, *40,* 1229–1235.

Toborek, M.; B. Hennig. Fatty acid-mediated effects on the glutathione redox cycle in cultured endothelial cells. *Am. J. Clin. Nutr.* **1994,** *59,* 60–65.

Tousoulis, D.; M. Charakida; C. Stefanadis. Endothelial function and inflammation in coronary artery disease. *Heart* **2006**, *92,* 441–444.

Trebble, T.; N.K. Arden; M.A. Stroud; S.A. Wootton; G.C. Burdge; E.A. Miles; A.B. Ballinger; R.L. Thompson; P.C. Calder. Inhibition of tumor necrosis factor-a and interleukin-6 production by mononuclear cells following dietary fish-oil supplementation in healthy men and response to antioxidant co- supplementation. *Br. J. Nutr.* **2003,** *90,* 405–412.

Tsimikas, S.; A. Philis-Tsimikas; S. Alexopoulos; F. Sigari; C. Lee; P.D. Reaven. LDL isolated from Greek subjects on a typical diet or from American subjects on an oleate-supplemented diet induces less monocyte chemotaxis and adhesion when exposed to oxidative stress. *Arterioscler. Thromb. Vasc. Biol* .**1999**, *19,* 122–130.

Turpeinen, A.M.; M. Mutanen. Similar effects of diets high oleic or linoleic acids on coagulation and fibrinolytic factors in healthy humans. *Nutr. Metab. Cardiovasc. Dis.* **1999,** *9,* 65–72.

Vallet, B.; E. Wiel. Endothelial cell dysfunction and coagulation. *Crit. Care Med.* **2001,** *29,* S–6–S41.

Wilke, M.S.; M.T. Clandinin. Influence of dietary saturated fatty acids on the regulation of plasma cholesterol concentration. *Lipids* **2005**, *40,* 1207–1213.

Vermunt, S.H.F.; B. Beaufrere; R.A. Riemersma; J.L. Sebedio; J.M. Chardigny; R.P. Mensink. Dietary *trans* α-Linolenic acid from deodorized rapeseed oil and plasma lipids and lipoproteins in healthy men: the *Trans* Line study. *Br. J.Nutr.* **2001,** *85,* 387–392.

Volk, M.G. An Examination of the Evidence Supporting the Association of Dietary Cholesterol and Saturated Fats with Serum Cholesterol and Development of Coronary Heart Disease. *Altern. Med. Rev.* **2007,** *12,* 228–245.

Wallace, F.A.; E.A. Miles; P.C. Calder. Comparison of the effects of linseed oil and different doses of fish oil on mononuclear cell function in healthy human subjects. *Br. J. Nutr.* **2003**, *89,* 679–689.

Wallenfeldt, K.; B. Fagerberg; J. Wikstrand; J. Hulthe. Oxidized low density lipoprotein in plasma is a prognostic marker of subclinical atherosclerosis development in clinically healthy men. *J. Intern. Med.* **2004**, *256,* 413–420.

Wang, C.; W.S. Harris; M. Chung; A.H. Lichtenstein; E.M. Balk; B. Kupelnick; H.S. Jordan; J. Lau. n-3 Fatty acids from fish or fish-oil supplements, but not α-linolenic acid, benefit cardio-vascular disease outcomes in primary- and secondary-prevention studies: a systematic review. *Am. J. Clin. Nutr.* **2006,** *84,* 5–17.

Warkentin, T.E.; W.C. Aird; J.H. Rand. Platelet-Endothelial Interactions: Sepsis, HIT, and Antiphospholipid Syndrome. *Hematology Am Soc Hematol Educ Program* **2003**, 497–519.

Waterman, E.; B. Lockwood. Active Components and Clinical Applications of Olive Oil. *Altern. Med. Rev.* **2007**, *12,* 331–342.

Whigham, L.D.; A.C. Watras; D.A. Schoeller. Efficacy of conjugated linoleic acid for reducing fat mass: a meta-analysis in humans. *Am. J. Clin. Nutr.* **2007,** *85,* 1203–1211.

Wijendran, V.; K.C. Hayes. Dietary n-6 and n-3 fatty acid balance and cardiovascular health. *Annu. Rev. Nutr.* **2004,** *24,* 597– 615.

Wilke, M.S.; M.T. Clandinin. Influence of Dietary Saturated Fatty Acids on the Regulation of Plasma Cholesterol Concentration. *Lipids* **2005,** *40,* 1207–1213.

Willett, W.C. The Mediterranean diet: science and practice. *Public Health Nutr.* **2006a,** *9,* 105–110.

Willett, W.C. *Trans* fatty acids and cardiovascular disease, epidemiological data. *Atherosclerosis* **2006b,** *7,* 5–8.

Yang, Z.; X.F. Ming. Recent advances in understanding endothelial dysfunction in atherosclerosis. *Clin. Med. Res.* **2006,** *4,* 53–65.

Yetik-Anacak, G.; J.D. Catravas. Nitric oxide and the endothelium: History and impact on cardiovascular disease**.** *Vasc. Pharmacol.* **2006,** *45,* 268–276.

Zambon, A.; G. Sartore; D. Passera; Francini-Pesenti; A. Bassi; C.Z. Basso; S. Zambon; E. Manzato; G. Crepaldi. Effects of hypocaloric dietary treatment enriched in oleic acid on LDL and HDL subclass distribution in mildly obese women. *J. Intern. Med.* **1999,** *246,* 191–201.

# 2

# Nutrition and Cardiovascular Disease in American Indians and Alaska Natives

**Sigal Eilat-Adar[1,2,3], Jiaqiong Xu[4], Ellie Zephier[5], Elizabeth D. Nobmann[6], Claudia Z. Mattil[1], Veronica O'Leary[7], Barbara V. Howard[1]**

*[1] Medstar Research Institute, Hyattsville, MD, USA; [2] Zinman College for Physical Education & Sports, Wingate Institute, Netanya, Israel; [3] Department of Epidemiology and Preventive Medicine, Sackler Medical Faculty, Tel Aviv University, Tel Aviv, Israel; [4] Center for Biostatistics, The Methodist Hospital Research Institute, Houston, TX, USA; [5] Aberdeen Area Indian Health Service, Aberdeen, SD, USA; [6] IDM Consulting, Anchorage, AK, USA; [7] Wagner Indian Health Service, Diabetes Prevention Project, Wagner, SD, USA.*

## Introduction

American Indians and Alaska Natives, as defined in this chapter, are diverse tribes of indigenous people living throughout the contiguous United States and in Alaska.

American Indians were long thought to have inherent protection from cardiovascular disease (CVD) (Sievers & Fisher, 1981). Indian Health Service (IHS) records from the 1960s show low rates (Howard et al., 1995), and coronary heart disease (CHD) mortality rates in Pima Indians from 1965 to 1980 were lower than those in Framingham Study participants (Nelson et al., 1990). However, by the 1980s, IHS data indicate that CVD was the leading cause of death among American Indians (IHS, 1984). American Indians have been undergoing a rapid change in lifestyle, with alterations in traditional patterns of activity and diet that might be expected to increase their risk for CVD. Additionally, diabetes prevalence, a strong determinant of CVD, is rising among American Indians.

Diabetes prevalence has increased among both American Indians and Alaska Natives. From 1990 to 1997, diabetes prevalence increased by 29% (Burrows et al., 2000; Howard et al., 1999).

Several reports on diabetes prevalence and incidence come from the Strong Heart Study (SHS), a study of American Indians in three clinical centers in Arizona, southwestern Oklahoma, and the Dakotas (Lee et al., 1990). Lee et al. (1995) showed that the age-adjusted diabetes prevalence rates in American Indians ages 45–74 years from the three centers of the SHS ranged from 33%–72%. Recent data show that diabetes incidence rates in this population are several times higher than those of other ethnic groups (Lee et al., 2002). Diabetes-associated complications decrease the quality of life and cost billions in health-care dollars (American Diabetes Association, 2003).

Obesity in adults is defined by the National Institutes of Health as having a body mass index (BMI) ≥30 kg/m², whereas overweight is defined as having a BMI ≥25 and <30 kg/m² (Clinical guidelines, 1998). The Racial Ethnic Approaches to Community Health (REACH) 2010 Risk Factor Survey found that American Indian residents of Oklahoma and North Carolina had a greater obesity prevalence (32.9%) than Hispanics, Blacks, or Asian Americans (Liau et al., 2004).

## Nutrition Transition

In addition to benefiting from public health programs for all Americans, American Indians and Alaska Natives are eligible for health services from the IHS. The IHS provides comprehensive health services, including nutrition counseling, to American Indians living on or near federal Indian communities or in traditional Native American territories, such as Oklahoma, and to Alaska Natives, through contracts with Alaska Native health organizations. Dramatic improvements have occurred in the health of American Indians since the IHS was transferred to the Public Health Service in 1955. Infant mortality rate, maternal deaths, and deaths related to infectious diseases have all decreased. As in other U.S. populations, chronic diseases are now the major cause of death for Native Americans. Nutritional factors can contribute to at least three (heart disease, cancer, and cirrhosis) of the 10 leading causes of American Indian and Alaska Native deaths, and nutrition also plays a role in diabetes, obesity, hypertension, and dental caries (Jackson, 1986).

The nutrition transition is defined as a shift in nutritional concern, from malnutrition and/or starvation to overweight and obesity, related to changing economic and social factors (Popkin & Gordon-Larson, 2004). The typical pattern associated with this nutrition transition is increased energy intake as traditional foods are replaced by processed, energy-dense convenience foods, and physical activity is reduced (Compher, 2006).

Historically, American Indians depended on food growing in the wild, such as nuts, fruits, berries, roots, and wild game (which is considerably lower in fat than purchased meat). Many American Indians were farmers, spending considerable energy to grow crops, such as beans, squash, and whole grains that are richer in nutrients and lower in calories than purchased food (Compher, 2006). Alaska Natives depended on fish and sea mammals, as well as wild game, berries, roots, and wild greens (Nobmann et al., 2005).

## Dietary Intake Among Native American Adults

Dietary changes among American Indians have been characterized for only a few communities. Table 2.1 summarizes some studies among adult American Indians published from the 1960s to 1996. The data available indicate that intakes of vitamins

**Table 2.1. Summary of Studies Addressing Dietary Change Among Adult American Indians, 1963–1996.**

| Study | Population | Method | Sampling | Low intake | Comments |
|---|---|---|---|---|---|
| Mayberry & Lindeman, 1963 | Seminole, OK (n=54) | 24-h recall | Convenience | Not reported | 44–45% energy from fat |
| Reid et al., 1971 | Pima, AZ (n=277) | 1-d record and food | Census frequency | Minerals adequate, vitamins not reported | 44% energy from fat |
| Bass & Wakefield, 1974 | Sioux, ND, SD (n=94) | 24-h recall | Convenience | Vitamins A and C, calcium, iron | Low-energy intake, traditional foods rarely used |
| Kuhnlein & Galloway, 1977 | Hopi, AZ (n=66) | Food frequency | Convenience | Vitamins A, C, B6; folacin, calcium, iron, zinc | Reduced agriculture and use of traditional foods |
| Wolfe & Sanjur, 1988 | Navajo, AZ, NM, UT (n=107) | 24-h recall | Convenience | Vitamin C, calcium, iron | High saturated fat, low- energy intake, high use of commodity foods, 21% energy from fat |
| Teufel & Dufour, 1990 | Hualapai, AZ (n=28) | 7-d 24-h recall | Convenience | Not reported | Compared obese vs. nonobese; total energy and carbohydrate higher in obese; energy per kilogram similar; 35-37% energy from fat; low use of traditional foods |
| Harland et al., 1992 | Siouan, NC (n=56) | Eating habits questionnaire | Convenience | Calcium, iron, fiber | 47% energy from fat |
| Bell et al., 1995 | Lumbee, NC (n=107) | 3-day record | Convenience | Vitamin C, calcium, iron, zinc, fiber | Low-energy intake, 36% energy from fat |
| Smith et al., 1996 | Pima, AZ (n=575) | 24-h recall, quantitative food frequency questionnaire | Stratified, random | Vitamins A and D | 37% energy from fat |

Adapted with permission from B. deGonzague, O. Receveur, D. Wedll, H.V. Kuhnlein. Dietary intake and body mass index of adults in two Ojibwe communities. *J. Am. Diet. Assoc.* 1999 Jun;99(6):710–716.

A and C, iron, zinc, and calcium are low, despite energy intakes high enough to promote or sustain excess weight. Most studies used 24-hour recalls, with convenience sampling, and sample sizes generally were small (deGonzague et al., 1999).

Taylor et al. (2005), with a convenience sample of 81 American Indian women living in Oklahoma, collected four-day weighed-food records. The women were ages 18–65 years. The food records included more than 3,300 individual foods. Soda and coffee were the foods consumed most often by these women. White bread, butter/margarine, and tea completed the top five core foods, respectively. Diet soda, chips, candies, sugar, and sugar substitutes completed the list of the 10 most commonly consumed foods. These foods comprised 53% of energy intake. Soft drinks and fried potatoes comprised much of the carbohydrate and fat intakes, respectively, as well as overall energy intake.

### *Navajo*

Lombard et al. (2006) described the dietary habits of the Navajo. With over 250,000 members, this is the largest federally recognized tribe within the United States. The reservation encompasses nearly 70,000 $km^2$ of land in three states: Arizona, New Mexico, and Utah and is larger than one-fifth of the United States. Most of the reservation is remote and rural, and many Navajo live in isolated family clusters. The median age of the inhabitants is 22.5 years. Access to quality foods on the reservation, including fresh fruits and vegetables, is limited by the remoteness of the region. Long distances between communities require long drives for food shopping. The isolated trading posts that bridge the gap between full-service grocery stores often stock foods of minimal nutrition and limited selections of produce. Many Navajo homes are without electricity and thus refrigeration.

Ballew et al. (1997) analyzed 24-hour recall data from Navajo adults. Similar to the Taylor et al. (2005) study, the core foods were found to be Navajo tortillas and fry bread; home-fried potatoes; soft drinks; coffee and tea; mutton; mixed dishes containing mutton, bacon, and sausage; and lunch and canned meats. These foods provided 41% of the total energy intake among the Navajo. Furthermore, soft drinks and fried potatoes contributed considerably to the carbohydrate and fat intakes, respectively, as well as to overall energy intake.

### *Ojibwe*

Although traditional hunting, fishing, and gathering activities are fundamental to Ojibwe culture, and food (especially wild rice) is considered a gift from the Creator, traditional, locally available food is now only consumed on special occasions or in ceremonies. In a study of 104 adult Ojibwe Indians from Minnesota and Wisconsin, fat intake was 37% and saturated fat was 13% of daily caloric intake. Ratio of polyunsaturated to saturated fat was 0.48 (deGonzague et al., 1999).

### *Pima*

Ravussin et al. (1994) studied members of a population with Pima ancestry (separation 700–1,000 years ago) living in a remote mountainous location in northwestern

Mexico, with a lifestyle markedly differing from that of Pima in Arizona. Nineteen women and 16 men were compared with sex-, age-, and diabetes status-matched Pimas living in Arizona. The results showed that obesity and possibly type 2 diabetes were less prevalent among people of Pima heritage living a traditional lifestyle than among people of Pima heritage living in an affluent environment. These findings suggest that, despite a similar possible genetic predisposition to these conditions, a traditional lifestyle, characterized by a diet including less animal fat and more complex carbohydrates and by greater energy expenditure in physical labor, may protect against the development of CVD risk factors, obesity, and type 2 diabetes.

Williams et al. (2001) examined the long-term effects of a self-reported preference for a traditional versus mixed versus nontraditional dietary pattern on the development of diabetes in 165 (77 men and 88 women) nondiabetic Pima Indians from the Gila River (AZ) Indian Community. The participants were examined periodically between June 1988 and June 1999. Women who followed the traditional diet had significantly higher intakes ($P < 0.05$) of complex carbohydrates, dietary fiber, insoluble fiber, vegetable proteins, and proportion of total calories from complex carbohydrate and vegetable proteins compared with women who followed the nontraditional diet. Women who followed a mixed diet (partly traditional and partly not) had intermediate intakes in of all these constituents. Fat intake did not differ between the traditional, nontraditional, and mixed diets and ranged between 32% and 37% of energy. Men who followed the traditional diet instead of the nontraditional diet also had higher intakes of these nutrients, but the difference was not significant. Thirty-six participants (8 men and 28 women) developed diabetes during 6.2 years of follow-up (range 0.9–10.9). After adjustment for age, sex, BMI, and total energy intake in a proportional hazards model, those who consumed the nontraditional diet had a risk of developing diabetes that was 2.5 times as high (95% CI 0.9–7.2) as those who consumed a traditional diet. Those who consumed a mixed diet had a risk 1.3 times as high (0.6–3.3) as those who consumed the traditional diet.

## *Alaska Natives*

Nutrition patterns among Alaska Natives differ from those among American Indian tribes, and information on the former is only briefly addressed in this chapter. Alaska Natives rely more on traditional foods and exhibit differences among subgroups in rates of CVD mortality (Nobmann et al., 1992).

Genetics of Coronary Artery Disease in Alaska Natives (GOCADAN) is a study of the contribution of genetics and environment to CVD in several villages in the Norton Sound area. This study is one of the largest dietary surveys of Alaskan Eskimos. Dietary intakes of Alaska Natives (Eskimos) differ from those of non-Natives (Nobmann et al., 1992). In the 1980s, Alaska Natives consumed more energy, protein, fat, carbohydrate, iron, vitamin A, and vitamin C but less calcium and six times more fish than other U.S. populations (Nobmann et al., 1992). Nobmann et al. (1999) in a later smaller investigation revealed associations between the diets of Alaska Natives and blood lipid levels. Much of the variation in the low-density lipoprotein cholesterol (LDL C)/high density lipoprotein cholesterol (HDL C) ratio was explained by negative coefficients for α-tocopherol, wild bird, evaporated milk, and cheese and positive coefficients for BMI, syrup, and pizza.

Nobmann et al. (2005) surveyed a population-based sample of 850 Eskimo men and women, ages 17–92, from the Norton Sound area, using a quantitative food-frequency questionnaire (FFQ). The leading sources of energy, saturated fat, carbohydrate, and sugars were store-bought foods (Table 2.2). Although Native foods accounted for 15% of the energy consumed, they contributed disproportionately more protein, fat, monounsaturated fat, polyunsaturated fat, omega-3 fatty acids (FAs), vitamin B-12, and iron than did the store-bought foods (Table 2.3). Generational differences were observed in the proportion of nutrients consumed from Native foods (Table 2.3). Although younger adults consumed smaller proportions of Native foods (men <13%, women 10% of energy), young adults obtained 16–64% of these same nutrients from Native foods. Among all participants, 64% reported that they ate fried foods more than once a week, most commonly fried in partially hydrogenated vegetable oil (39%) or vegetable oil (27%). Intake of omega-3 FA was high, averaging 4.9 g/day (Nobmann et al., 2005). The upper boundary for alpha-linolenic acid (1.2%) intake in this population represents the highest level consumed in the form of food by individuals in North America (Nobmann et al., 2005). The authors concluded that Alaska Native nutrient-dense foods are valued for their role in defining and maintaining Eskimo culture and for their economic value in communities where purchased foods are expensive. Of concern are the lower consumption of Native foods among young adults and their greater carbohydrate consumption, of which 40–60% are simple sugars. In another analysis from this population-based sample (Ebbesson et al., 2007a), 686 Alaskan Eskimos younger than age 35 underwent ultrasound assessment of carotid atherosclerosis. Intimal-medial thickness (IMT) of the far wall of the distal common carotid arteries and plaque score (number of segments containing plaque) were assessed. Mean consumption of total omega-3 FAs was 4.76 g/day in those without and 5.07 g/day in those with plaque. In models adjusting for relevant risk factors, the presence and extent of plaque were unrelated to the intake of C20–22 or total omega-3. In contrast, the odds of plaque rose significantly with quartiles of palmitic ($P = 0.02$) and stearic acid intake ($P = 0.04$). The extent of plaque (or plaque score) was also associated with a higher percentage intake of palmitic acid ($P = 0.01$). IMT was negatively associated with grams of C20–22 omega-3 FAs ($P = 0.05$), total omega-3 ($P = 0.05$), palmitate ($P = 0.03$), and stearate ($P = 0.03$) consumed. The authors concluded that dietary intake of omega-3 FAs in a moderate-to-high range does not appear to be associated with reduced plaque, but is negatively associated with IMT. The presence and extent of carotid atherosclerosis among Eskimos are higher with an increasing consumption of saturated fatty acid (SFA). The emerging question is whether Eskimos who develop atherosclerotic CVD consume less omega-3 FA than those without CHD or other forms of atherosclerosis, or whether high burdens of other risk factors in individuals with atherosclerosis outweigh the effects of the

**Table 2.2. Selected Nutrients Contributed by Key Foods Consumed by Alaskan Eskimo Adults in Northwest Alaska, 2000–2003,[1] the GOCADAN Study**

| Energy | % | Total Fat | % | Carbohydrate | % | Protein | % |
|---|---|---|---|---|---|---|---|
| Soda | 5.9 | Butter | 6.4 | Soda | 11.4 | Chicken | 9.4 |
| Rice | 3.9 | Beef | 5.2 | Rice | 7.1 | Caribou[2] | 6.3 |
| Pilot bread[3] | 3.9 | Chicken | 4.4 | Tang[4] | 6.6 | Beef | 6.1 |
| Pancake | 3.7 | Crisco[5] | 4.3 | Pilot bread | 6.0 | Salmon[2] | 4.7 |
| Tang | 3.5 | Evaporated milk | 4.2 | Sugar | 6.0 | Evaporated milk | 4.4 |
| Evaporated milk | 3.2 | Berry agutuk[2] | 3.9 | Kool-aid[4] | 5.4 | Chicken eggs | 4.2 |
| **SFA** | **%** | **MUFA** | **%** | **PUFA** | **%** | **(n-3) Fatty Acids** | **%** |
| Butter | 11.0 | Beef | 6.0 | Mayonnaise | 8.0 | Seal oil[2] | 20.0 |
| Evaporated milk | 6.9 | Seal oil[2] | 5.1 | Vegetable oil | 7.4 | Salmon[2] | 7.8 |
| Beef | 6.1 | Butter | 5.0 | Berry agutuk[2] | 6.1 | Mayonnaise | 6.4 |
| Cheese | 5.6 | Crisco | 5.0 | Crisco | 5.8 | Muktuk[2] | 4.7 |
| Creamer | 4.0 | Chicken | 4.5 | Chicken | 5.4 | Smoked king salmon[2] | 4.2 |
| Chicken | 3.6 | Berry agutuk[2] | 4.1 | Chips | 5.2 | Other fresh fish[2] | 3.9 |
| ***Trans*-fatty Acids** | **%** | **Total Sugars** | **%** | **Dietary Fiber** | **%** | **Iron** | **%** |
| Crisco | 11.7 | Soda | 20.4 | Pilot bread | 8.0 | Tang | 8.4 |
| Berry agutuk[2] | 10.0 | Tang | 11.1 | Hot cereal | 5.2 | Cold cereal | 7.4 |
| Margarine, stick | 8.8 | Sugar | 10.8 | Dark bread | 5.1 | Pilot bread | 6.6 |
| Pancake | 8.6 | Kool-aid | 9.1 | White bread | 4.8 | Caribou[2] | 6.1 |
| Butter | 8.0 | Evaporated milk | 4.1 | Blueberries[2] | 4.6 | Rice | 5.0 |
| French fried potatoes | 6.2 | Cake | 3.0 | Apples | 4.5 | White bread | 4.8 |

[1] Only the six leading sources are shown.
[2] Native food.
[3] Interbake Foods, Richmond, VA.
[4] Kraft Foods, Rye Brook, NY.
[5] J.M. Smucker, Orville, OH.
Reprinted with permission from E.D. Nobmann, R. Ponce, C. Mattil, R. Devereux, B. Dyke, S.O. Ebbesson, S. Laston, J. MacCluer, D. Robbins, T. Romenesko, G. Ruotolo, C.R. Wenger, B.V. Howard; GOCADAN study, 2000–2003. Dietary intakes vary with age among Eskimo adults of Northwest Alaska in the GOCADAN study, 2000–2003. *J Nutr.* 2005 Apr;135(4):856–862.

high dietary omega-3 FA intake. The authors suggested that the lack of association between omega-3 FA consumption and the presence of carotid plaque suggests that the increasing prevalence of atherosclerotic CVD in Eskimos is attributable to adverse trends in other risk factors.

## *Strong Heart Study*

The SHS was initiated in 1988 to investigate CVD and its risk factors in geographically diverse groups of American Indians. It is the first large, standardized, longitudinal

**Table 2.3. Median Percentage of Energy and Selected Nutrients From Native Foods Consumed by Alaskan Eskimos by Age Group in Northwest Alaska, 2000–2003[1]**

| | Men | | | Women | | |
|---|---|---|---|---|---|---|
| Age range, y | 17–39 | 40–60 | 61–92 | 17–39 | 40–60 | 61–92 |
| | % of energy and nutrients from native foods | | | | | |
| Nutrient | | | | | | |
| Energy | 12.5[b] | 14.1[a] | 16.0[ab] | 10.3[b] | 15.0[a] | 13.8[a] |
| Protein | 29.1 | 32.3 | 34.0 | 23.0[b] | 29.8[a] | 29.7[a] |
| Carbohydrate | 2.7[b] | 3.7[a] | 4.6[a] | 2.8[b] | 4.4[a] | 4.4[a] |
| Fat | 17.4 | 20.0 | 21.4 | 15.5[b] | 20.9[a] | 19.1[a] |
| Saturated fat | 12.0[b] | 13.4[ab] | 14.8[a] | 10.6[b] | 14.1[a] | 12.5[ab] |
| Monounsaturated fat | 20.9[b] | 24.6[a] | 23.6[ab] | 18.0[b] | 24.6[a] | 23.3[a] |
| Polyunsaturated fat | 19.5[b] | 22.5[a] | 21.7[ab] | 16.8[b] | 22.8[a] | 23.0[a] |
| (n-3) Fatty acids | 55.9[b] | 60.4[a] | 64.0[a] | 52.7[b] | 63.3[a] | 64.5[a] |
| Trans Fatty acids | 8.9 | 11.2 | 6.8 | 8.7 | 9.4 | 10.9 |
| Vitamin B-12 | 63.7 | 70.9 | 71.1 | 54.8[b] | 68.7[a] | 69.8[a] |
| Iron | 21.9 | 22.3 | 24.2 | 16.4[b] | 23.9[a] | 23.6[a] |

[1] Medians in a row for a gender with superscripts without a common letter differ, $P < 0.05$. Reprinted with permission from E.D. Nobmann, R. Ponce, C. Mattil, R. Devereux, B. Dyke, S.O. Ebbesson, S. Laston, J. MacCluer, D. Robbins,T. Romenesko, G. Ruotolo, C.R. Wenger, B.V. Howard; GOCADAN study, 2000–2003. Dietary intakes vary with age among Eskimo adults of Northwest Alaska in the GOCADAN study, 2000–2003. *J. Nutr.* 2005 Apr;135(4):856–862.

study devoted specifically to American Indian health. The sample was designed to represent the populations, ages 45–74, residing in southwestern Arizona, southwestern Oklahoma, and the Dakotas (Lee et al., 1990). Clinical examinations and interviews provided data on an array of health issues. Initially conducted in 1989–1991, the SHS baseline exam (SHS-I) was followed four years later in 1993–1995 by a second exam (SHS-II). With cooperation of the tribal nations and the IHS, 88% of the surviving cohort was re-examined at the second exam, which included 3,638 of the 4,549 original participants. A 1984–1988 mortality survey showed fewer differences in CVD mortality rates among the three geographic areas of the SHS. CVD mortality rates in these tribal groups were somewhat higher than the respective state rates in Arizona and Oklahoma and almost twice as high as the state rates in South/North Dakota (Lee et al., 1998). After five years of follow-up, cardiovascular morbidity and mortality were similar across geographic areas, and CHD incidence rates in American Indians in the SHS were almost twice as high as in U.S. whites and blacks in the ARIC study (Howard et al., 1999).

Dietary data were collected from 892 people in the first examination (Zephier et al., 1997). The SHS-II dietary component included 3,482 or 96% of the total SHS-II participants (Zephier et al., 1997), and 3,450 participants had complete nutrition data (Xu et al., 2006). The high participation rate makes the results of this study particularly valuable for the American Indian community. Nutritional information was obtained by means of a single 24-hour dietary recall. The interviews were conducted by the local field staff, trained and supervised by IHS dietitians and the principal investigator according to standardized methods (SHS operational manual, 1993).

Dietary intake data were collected and analyzed with the Minnesota Nutrition Data System (NDS version 2.1) developed by the Nutrition Coordinating Center (NCC), University of Minnesota (Minneapolis, MN; Food Database version 4A; Nutrient Database version 18 (Schakel et al., 1988, 1997). Trans fatty acids (TFA) were not available in NDS version 2.1; therefore, to include them in the nutrient data, final calculations were completed with the NCC Nutrient Database Version 36 (NDS-R 2005). The NDS-R time-related database updates analytic data while retaining nutrient profiles true to the version used for data collection (Schakel, 2001). Results from the first SHS examination showed a higher fat and cholesterol intake than among participants in the Third National Health and Nutrition Examination Survey (NHANES) (Zephier et al., 1997). Mean (SD) cholesterol intake in American Indian men from Arizona (n = 137) was 447 (331) mg/day. American Indian men from Oklahoma (n = 143) consumed a mean (SD) of 37 (8) % of energy from fat, and 13 (3) % from SFA. American Indian men from North and South Dakota (n = 118) consumed a mean (SD) of 37 (10) % of energy from fat, and 383 (232) mg/day cholesterol. All values were significantly higher than in NHANES III Phase 1 men who consumed a mean (SD) of 34 (20) % of energy from fat, 12 (8) % SFA, and 313 (326) % mg/day cholesterol. Mean (SD) SFA as a percentage of caloric intake in American Indian women from Arizona (n = 160) was 13 (4) %. Their cholesterol intake was 404 (344) mg/day. American Indian women from Oklahoma (n = 173) consumed a mean (SD) of 36 (9) % of energy from fat and 13 (5) % from SFA. American Indian women from North and South Dakota (n = 118) consumed a mean (SD) of 36 (29) % of energy from fat, 13 (3) % from SFA, and 276 (170) mg/day from cholesterol. All values were significantly higher than in NHANES III Phase 1 women who consumed a mean (SD) of 33 (15) % of energy from fat, 11(4) % from SFA, and 211 (212) mg cholesterol per day. Figure 2.1. describes the proportion of participants who achieved the 1987–1991 dietary recommendations for chronic disease prevention. These recommendations included total fat intake of <30% of total energy, SFA <10% of total energy, cholesterol intake <300 mg/day, sodium intake <2,400 mg/day, and fiber intake >20 g/day. Overall, less than half of the participants in this survey met the guidelines (Zephier et al., 1997).

Xu et al. (2006) compared data from 2,938 participants who returned for the second SHS examination with 2,344 participants from NHANES III. The Xu et al. (2006) analysis excluded adults who had definite myocardial infarction (MI) or CHD (definite CHD, definite MI, definite ECG with evident MI) before or at the second SHS examination (n = 233). Mean dietary intakes stratified by age group (<60 and ≥60) from SHS and NHANES III are presented in Table 2.4. In both SHS and NHANES

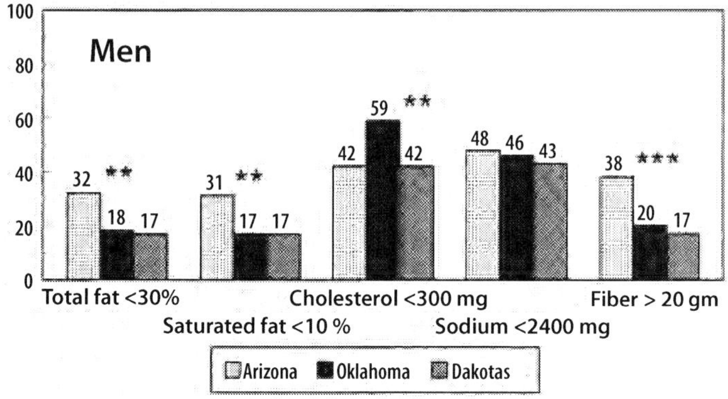


Groups significantly different, $P < 0.01$.

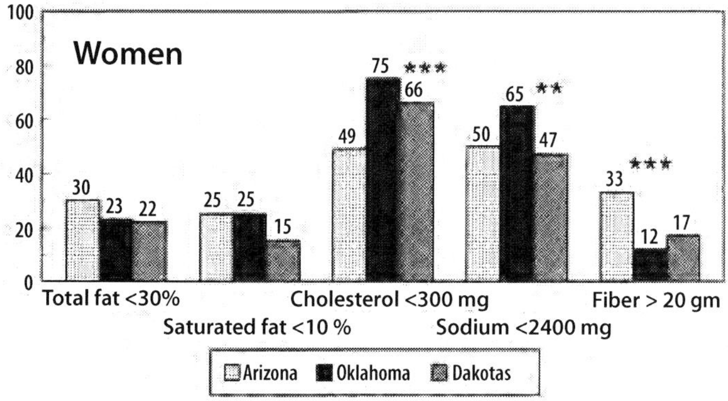


Groups significantly different, $P < 0.001$.

**Fig. 2.1.** Proportion of participants who achieve dietary recommendations for the reduction of CVD and other chronic diseases. Reprinted with permission from Zephier et al. Intake of nutrients related to cardiovascular disease risk among three groups of American Indians: the Strong Heart Dietary Study. Prev. Med. 1997 Jul–Aug;26(4):508–15.

III, dietary intakes followed a similar pattern in each age group. In the SHS, mean energy intake was lower, but cholesterol intake was higher than in the NHANES III participants in both age groups. Mean total fat intake, SFA intake, and MUFA intake (all % of energy) were also higher in the SHS participants. Polyunsaturated fatty acid (PUFA) intake was higher in the NHANES III participants than in the SHS participants in both age groups. All differences were significant ($P < 0.01$). Stang et al. (2005) also showed age-related decreases in energy and total and saturated fat intakes among SHS participants. This decreased intake is similar to findings from the overall U.S. population found in other surveys, such as NHANES III (Stang et al., 2005).

## *Summary*

Data from differing American Indian communities are consistent: American Indians are consuming less traditional food and more processed food. Although Alaska

**Table 2.4. Macronutrients and Cholesterol Intake of the SHS Sample[1] and NHANES III Study Sample by Age Groups[2]**

| | 47–59 years | | 60–79 years | |
|---|---|---|---|---|
| | SHS (n = 1659) | NHANES III (n = 934) | SHS (n = 1279) | NHANES III (n = 1410) |
| Energy (kcal) | 1938 ± 830 | 2061 ± 36.5 | 1711 ± 683 | 1820 ± 25.6 |
| Total (% of energy) | 35.7 ± 9.6 | 34.8 ± 0.6 | 33.9 ± 9.4 | 32.6 ± 0.4 |
| SFA (% of energy) | 12.2 ± 4.0 | 11.7 ± 0.2 | 11.7 ± 3.9 | 11.1 ± 0.1 |
| MUFA (% of energy) | 14.3 ± 4.3 | 13.4 ± 0.3 | 13.5 ± 4.2 | 12.5 ± 0.2 |
| PUFA (% of energy) | 6.0 ± 2.7 | 7.0 ± 0.1 | 5.6 ± 2.5 | 6.5 ± 0.1 |
| Cholesterol (mg) | 344 ± 272 | 264 ± 7.4 | 310 ± 236 | 232 ± 6.7 |

Abbreviations: SHS, Strong Heart Study; NHANES III, National Health and Nutrition Examination Survey phase III; SFA: saturated fatty acids; MUFA: monounsaturated fatty acids; PUFA: polyunsaturated fatty acids.

[1] Dietary intake data set for the SHS was obtained from the University of Minnesota Nutrition Coordinating Center Nutrient Database Version 18.

[2] All data presented as mean ± SD for the SHS and as mean ± SEM for NHANES III. The difference in dietary intake between SHS and NHANES III, as well as the difference between age groups in both studies were significant.

Reprinted with permission from Xu et al. Dietary fat intake and risk of coronary heart disease: the Strong Heart Study. Am. J. Clin. Nutr. 2006, 84, 894–902.

Natives still consume traditional food, young adults are consuming less than their elders. This shift in nutritional sources from traditional foods to the standard U.S. diet promotes coronary risk factors as well as CHD. A healthy food pyramid was developed by the California Adolescent Nutrition and Fitness (CANFit) program, which promotes programs providing culturally appropriate nutrition and physical activity assistance and resources to organizations across the country (Fig. 2.2). An Alaska Native Food Guide Pyramid (Fig. 2.3) was developed that includes traditional Alaska foods. Both pyramids are examples of nutrition education materials that were developed to recognize cultural differences; however, current recommendations of the number of servings vary based on the individual's height, weight, age, gender, and physical activity.

## Nutritional Intake Among American Indian Children

Few studies have examined food sources of nutrients among rural or urban American Indian children ages 6 years and younger. One analysis was based on data collected as part of a community-based intervention study conducted in collaboration with eight tribes and nations in northeastern Oklahoma: Eastern Shawnee, Miami, Modoc, Ottawa, Peoria, Quapaw, Seneca-Cayuga, and Wyandotte (Kegler et al., 2000). Nutritional data were gathered in 1997 from a representative cross-sectional sample of caregivers of 329 rural Native American and non-Hispanic white children ages 1–6 years living in northeastern Oklahoma (Stroehla et al., 2005). Information on

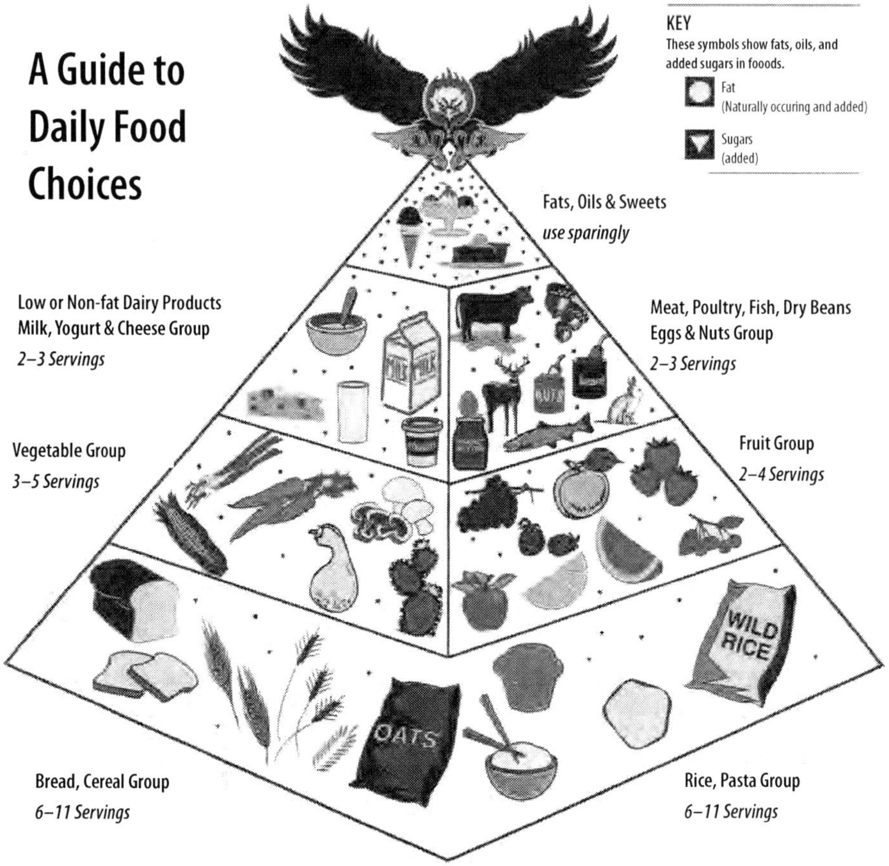


**Fig. 2.2.** Recommended Native American food pyramid. Reprinted with permission: California Adolescent Nutrition and Fitness, Berkeley, CA.

mean daily dietary nutrient and food group intake was obtained using a modified Full Block/National Cancer Institute (NCI) FFQ adapted to Native Americans and to the key informants (parents and dietitians). Food sources of energy, macronutrients, and fiber were similar for American Indian and white children. Milk and cheese were children's primary energy sources, but low-nutrient-dense foods (e.g., white breads, salty snacks, soft drinks, sweetened fruit drinks, processed meats, candy, and cake/cookies) accounted for 31% of energy intake. Whole milk contributed more to energy intake of 1- to 2-year-olds than of children ages 3–6 years ($P = 0.03$). Depending on the child's age, milk and cheese accounted for 33–41% of protein intake. Lean meats were absent from top-protein food sources. Instead, meat protein sources were dominated by hamburger and processed high-fat meats. Primary sources of children's dietary fat were foods high in saturated fats. Whole fruits accounted for only 6% of children's fiber intake, and only two vegetables (dried beans and corn) were in the top 14 fiber sources.

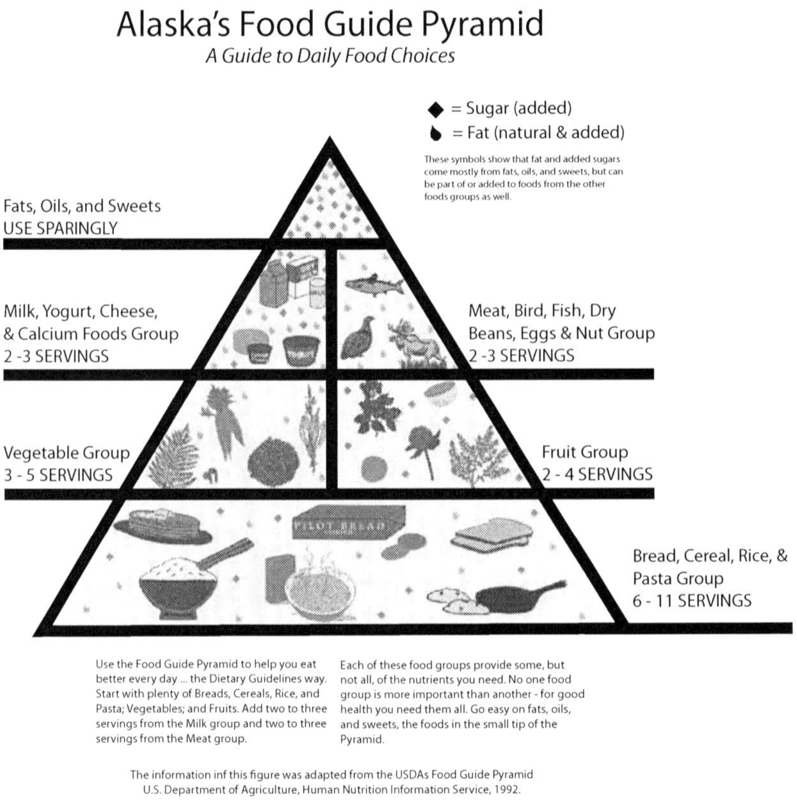


**Fig. 2.3.** Alaska's Food Guide Pyramid. Reprinted with permission from Bristol Bay Health Corporation, Food and Nutrition Services, Alaska Department of Health and Social Services.

Overall, micronutrient food sources were similar for American Indian and white children. Milk and cheese accounted for three-fourths of children's calcium intake. Cold cereals were children's primary food sources of iron, accounting for 20% of iron intake. Cheese, whole milk (especially among 1- to 2-year-olds), and cold cereals were the top sources of children's dietary zinc intake, but processed and fatty meats accounted for more than 20% of dietary zinc intake. Cold cereals and orange juice contributed more than 30% of children's dietary folate intake. Oranges were the only solid fruit to contribute at least 2% to children's vitamin C intake.

The authors concluded that in general, although there are similarities, food sources of these American Indian rural children appear less healthful than national samples. These results were confirmed by Di Noia et al. (2005) in 191 self-identified American Indian parents of children ages 8–14 years from urban American Indian centers and tribal and reservation settings in New York, Massachusetts, Connecticut, Vermont, and Maine. Data from the 1989–1991 Continuing Survey of Food Intakes by Individuals showed that beef, ready-to-eat cereals, and poultry were among the top 10 energy sources for 2- to 5-year-olds nationally (Subar et al., 1998), whereas none of these foods appeared among the primary energy sources of American Indian children in that analysis. In addition, high-fat salty snacks, such as potato chips and corn chips, contributed to 2% of children's energy intake nationally, but accounted for more than 8% of the Subar et al. (1998) sample's energy intake.

These observational data suggest that health professionals working with families of preschool-age rural children should encourage caregivers to replace high-fat processed foods, sweets, and refined carbohydrates with nutrient-dense alternatives, particularly fruits and vegetables, lean meats, and whole grains, as is recommended for all U.S. children. Milk, 100% juices (in moderation), and water should replace sweetened drinks. Because food choices and diet quality are also influenced by food costs, national programs are needed to address the higher costs of fresh fruits and vegetables and the reduced availability of healthful foods, especially in rural areas.

## Nutrition and CVD in Native Americans

The classic diet-heart hypothesis posits that diets high in SFAs and cholesterol and low in PUFAs raise serum total and LDL cholesterol, which in turn increase the risk of CHD (Grundy et al., 1982). Despite decades of intensive interest and research in the diet-heart hypothesis, however, investigations of dietary fat and CHD incidence from prospective epidemiologic studies have resulted in inconsistent findings (Xu et al., 2006).

### *Nutrition and Metabolic Syndrome (MS)*

The National Cholesterol Education Program's Adult Treatment Panel III definition of MS includes the presence of three or more of the following characteristics: (i) waist circumference >102 cm in men or >88 cm in women; (ii) triglycerides >1.69 mmol/L (150 mg/dL); (iii) HDL-C <1.04 mmol/L (40 mg/dL) in men and <1.29 mmol/L (50 mg/dL) in women; (iv) blood pressure ≥130/85 mm Hg; and (v) fasting glucose between 6.1 and 6.9 mmol/L (110–125 mg/dL). The characteristics that define MS are also associated with insulin resistance (IR) (NCEP, 2002).

Ebbesson et al. (2005) measured plasma FA concentrations in 447 Norton Sound Eskimos (35–74 years of age) and screened for type 2 diabetes, CHD, and associated risk factors. A dietary assessment (24-hour recall) was obtained for the day before the blood sampling. Plasma omega-3 FA concentrations were highly correlated with dietary omega-3 FAs and HDL-C levels and inversely correlated with plasma levels of insulin, 2-hour insulin oral glucose tolerance test (OGTT), homeostasis model assessment of insulin resistance (HOMA-IR), 2-hour glucose (OGTT), triglyceride levels, and diastolic blood pressure (Ebbesson et al., 2005).

In a later GOCADAN investigation among 691 Inupiat Eskimos ages 34–75 years, consumption of individual FAs as determined by FFQ showed associations with risk factors (Ebbesson et al., 2007b). One or more long-chain omega-3 FAs from fish and sea mammals (3–4 g/day total) were associated with lower blood pressure

(2–3 mm Hg lower from Tertile 1 compared with Tertile 3), serum triglycerides (15–17 mg/dL lower), 2-hour glucose (8 mg/dL lower), and higher HDL-C (3 mg/dL higher), fasting insulin (1μU/mL higher), and HOMA score (3 units higher). SFA consumption (34–47 g/day) was associated with higher triglyceride levels (15 mg/dL higher) and diastolic blood pressure (2 mm Hg higher). *Trans*-FA consumption (8–10 g/d) was associated with higher average blood pressure (3 mm Hg difference). The authors concluded that consumption of long-chain omega-3 FAs from marine sources may improve certain MS components, and thus may reduce the risk for CVD, while high consumption of saturated FAs and trans-FAs may have an adverse effect on MS.

In the second SHS examination (Eilat-Adar et al., 2008), PUFA intake was associated with less MS and lower HOMA scores in women [OR and 95% CI for MS in the 3rd tertile: 0.69 (0.50–0.96)], but not men. Higher simple carbohydrate intake was associated with more MS in men [OR and 95% CI in the 3rd tertile: 1.72 (1.10–2.69)] but not in women. The authors concluded that PUFA may protect against, and simple carbohydrates may increase, MS and IR in American Indians, and gender may modify the association between dietary intake and MS and IR in this population (Eilat-Adar et al., 2008).

## *Nutrition and Diabetes*

Murphy et al. (1995) investigated the frequency of food intake, excess body weight, and glucose intolerance in 1,124 Alaska Natives. Residents ≥20 years old from 15 villages along the Yukon and Kuskokwim rivers were screened at village-based health fairs and in village clinics in the winter months from January 1987 to February 1988. The self-administered FFQ inquired about intake frequency (daily, weekly, monthly, yearly, or never). Field testing confirmed that the FFQ encompassed selected foods appropriate to the region. Athabascan Indians of the interior region of Alaska had twice the rate of type 2 diabetes as Yup'ik Eskimos who live nearer the coast, with a significantly higher frequency of nonindigenous food intake, plus lower frequency of indigenous carbohydrate and fat intake. Subjects ≤30 years old consumed significantly more nonindigenous protein and fat and low-nutrient-dense carbohydrates than those ≥60 years old. Persons who had glucose intolerance reported significantly greater consumption of nonindigenous protein and less seal oil.

Xu et al. (2007) conducted an analysis in 1,284 participants ages 47–80 years who had diabetes for ≥1 year at the second SHS examination (1993–1995). Higher total fat (>25–30% of energy), SFA (>13% of energy) and MUFA (>10% of energy), and lower carbohydrate intake (<35–40% of energy) were associated with poor glycemic control (HbA1c ≥7%). Lower fiber intake and higher protein intake were marginally associated with poor glycemic control ($P$ for trend = 0.06 and 0.09, respectively). No significant association was found between PUFA or TFA and glycemic control in this population. The authors suggested that although the main MUFA sources of the SHS population were unknown, the high correlation between MUFA and SFA (r = 0.79) suggests that the MUFA may be obtained from animal sources. Therefore, this may explain the positive association found between MUFA intake and poor glycemic control. The lack of association with TFA may have resulted from the small range of TFA intake in this population. Table 2.5 shows the dietary intake of 420 diabetic men and 864 diabetic women by HbA1c status.

A study by Schulz et al. (2006) provides evidence that changes in lifestyle associated with Westernization play a major role in the global epidemic of type 2 diabetes. Adult Pima-Indian (n = 224) and non-Pima populations (n = 270) in the Sierra Madre mountains of Mexico were examined using oral glucose tolerance tests and assessments for obesity, physical activity, and other risk factors for diabetes. Results were compared with those from Pima Indians in Arizona. Both Pima populations were typed for DNA polymorphisms to establish their genetic similarity. The age- and sex-adjusted prevalence of type 2 diabetes in the Mexican Pima Indians (6.9%) was less than one-fifth that in the U.S. Pima Indians (38%) and similar to that of non-Pima Mexicans (2.6%). The prevalence of obesity was similar in the Mexican Pima Indians (7% in men and 20% in women) and non-Pima Mexicans (9% in men and 27% in women) but was much lower than in the U.S. Pima Indians. Levels of physical activity were much higher in both Mexican groups than in the U.S. Pima Indians. The two Pima groups share considerable genetic similarity relative to other Native Americans. The lower prevalence of type 2 diabetes and obesity among the Pima Indians in Mexico than in the United States indicates that even in populations genetically prone to these conditions, development is determined mostly by environmental circumstances, including nutrition.

The rise in CVD since the 1980s among American Indians may be the outcome of better health management programs that reduced morbidity and mortality from diabetes-related disorders, such as renal disease, gangrene, and others. With these disorders under better control, the survivors may be exhibiting other chronic conditions and less fatal diabetes-related complications, resulting in the increased prevalence of CVD (Wiedman, 2005). In contrast, the mortality rates from CVD, specifically ischemic heart disease, among Alaska Natives were fairly steady during the 1980s (Nobmann et al., 2005). Diabetes prevalence rates were comparatively low but have been increasing (Schraer et al., 1997 ).

From 1992 to 1994, the Centers for Disease Control and Prevention (CDC), the IHS, and three Native American communities conducted the Inter-Tribal Heart Project (ITHP) to examine the prevalence of CVD risk factors among community members. In those communities, persons diagnosed with diabetes receive standard nutrition education through the IHS and tribal clinics when they are diagnosed. To assess the effectiveness of such nutrition counseling, Archer et al. (2004) examined whether persons with diabetes (n = 294) reported different (healthier) food habits than persons without diabetes (n = 990) or with undiagnosed diabetes (n = 80) and fasting glucose ≥7 mmol/L (≥126 mg/dL). Persons with prior diabetes diagnosis were less likely than those without diabetes to report eating fast-food meals two or more times per week, visible fat on meat, or skin on poultry, fried chicken or fried fish; adding fat

**Table 2.5. Dietary Intake of 420 Diabetic Men and 864 Diabetic Women by HbA1c Status[1]**

| | Men | | Women | | |
|---|---|---|---|---|---|
| | HbA1c <7% | HbA1c ≥7% | HbA1c <7% | HbA1c ≥7% | *P*-value2 |
| Reported dietary intake | | | | | |
| Total energy (kcal)[5, 6] | 1776 (1283-2600) | 1828 (1278-2465) | 1521 (1163-1942) | 1584 (1184-2035) | NS |
| Total fat (% kcal)[3, 4] | 34.2 ± 9.4 | 37.4 ± 8.9 | 33.8 ± 10.1 | 35.0 ± 10.1 | 0.06 |
| SFA (% kcal)[3, 4] | 11.2 ± 3.6 | 12.7 ± 3.8 | 11.5 ± 4.0 | 11.8 ± 4.1 | 0.02 |
| MUFA (% kcal)[3, 5] | 13.1 ± 4.2 | 14.5 ± 4.0 | 12.8 ± 4.4 | 13.5 ± 4.4 | 0.10 |
| PUFA (% kcal) | 6.6 ± 3.1 | 6.8 ± 3.1 | 6.4 ± 3.2 | 6.4 ± 3.3 | NS |
| TFA (% kcal)[3, 5] | 2.3 ± 1.4 | 2.6 ± 1.4 | 2.3 ± 1.3 | 2.3 ± 1.3 | NS |
| Carbohydrates (% kcal)[3,4, 5] | 49.2 ± 12.3 | 45.6 ± 11.6 | 51.3 ± 12.3 | 48.9 ± 12.3 | NS |
| Sucrose (% kcal)[4] | 4.0 (1.1-8.2) | 4.1 (1.4-8.3) | 5.8 (2.8-10.4) | 4.4 (1.9-8.1) | NS |
| Protein (% kcal)[4] | 16.8 ± 4.2 | 17.2 ± 4.8 | 15.9 ± 4.2 | 16.8 ± 4.4 | NS |
| Fiber (g/1000 kcal)[3,5] | 9.7 (6.7-14.8) | 8.4 (5.5-12.2) | 8.4 (6.0-12.7) | 9.3 (6.2-13.1) | 0.001 |

Abbreviations: SFA: saturated fatty acids; MUFA: monounsaturated fatty acids; PUFA: polyunsaturated fatty acids; TFA: trans fatty acids; NS: not significant ($P > 0.10$).

[1]Data were presented as mean ± SD for continuous variables, median (first quartile– third quartile) if continuous variables were not normally distributed, and numbers (percentages) for categorical variables. *P* value was based on chi-square test for categorical variables and t-test for continuous variables (duration of diabetes, physical activity, and reported energy and fiber were normalized prior to the test) for comparing differences between $HbA_{1c}$ status and sex.

[2]*P* for interaction between sex and each variable.

[3]$P < 0.05$ for the comparison between men participants with $HbA_{1c}$ <7% and men participants with $HbA_{1c}$ ≥7%.

[4]$P < 0.05$ for the comparison between women participants with $HbA_{1c}$ <7% and women participants with $HbA_{1c}$ ≥7%.

[5]$P < 0.05$ for the comparison between men and women within participants with $HbA_{1c}$ ≥7%.

[6]$P < 0.05$ for the comparison between men and women within participants with $HbA_{1c}$ <7%.

Reprinted with permission from J. Xu, S. Eilat-Adar, C.M. Loria, B.V. Howard, R.R. Fabsitz, M.Begum, E.M. Zephier, E.T. Lee. Macronutrient intake and glycemic control in a population based sample of American Indians with diabetes: The Strong Heart Study. Am. J. Clin. Nutr. 2007, 86, 480–487.

to cooked vegetables; or drinking whole milk. Persons with undiagnosed diabetes were more likely than diagnosed persons to report eating fast-food meals twice or more per week; eating visible fat on meat, skin on poultry, fried fish; or drinking whole milk, and were less likely to drink low-fat milk. Previously undiagnosed persons were more likely than either diagnosed persons or persons without diabetes to consume lard from cooked foods and to use lard when cooking.

The authors concluded that persons with diagnosed diabetes showed healthier eating patterns than those without diabetes, while undiagnosed persons showed less favorable patterns. Because virtually all persons with diabetes in these communities receive nutrition education, the results suggest that nutrition education programs for people with diabetes may be associated with healthier eating patterns.

## Nutrition and Hypertension

Welty et al. (1986) conducted a survey in 342 Papago Indians and 375 non-Indians in Gila Bend, Arizona, from July to September 1983, where a high level of sodium (440 mg/L) was in the water supply. Participants ≥ age 25 were interviewed for health-risk factors, water consumption, and dietary sodium and calcium intake, and had height, weight, blood pressure, and urinary sodium and potassium levels measured. No consistent associations were found between any of the sodium values and systolic or diastolic blood pressure. The prevalence rates of hypertension in Gila Bend were not significantly higher than national rates.

Venkat Narayan et al. (1998) reported results from a cross-sectional study of 404 adult Pima Indians in Arizona. Dietary variables were assessed by a 24-hour recall. Hypertension (HTN) was defined as systolic blood pressure (SBP) ≥140 mmHg or diastolic blood pressure (DBP) ≥90 mmHg or treatment with antihypertensive medication. The median calcium intake was 760 mg (25th and 75th percentiles, 486 mg and 1079 mg, respectively). Multiple regression analyses controlling for age, sex, BMI, sodium, potassium, and alcohol showed that calcium intake was consistently and positively associated with SBP and DBP. However, the association was significant only for DBP, which was approximately 0.3 mmHg higher for every 100 mg/day difference in dietary calcium, an association that was stronger at higher glucose concentrations ($P < 0.01$ for the calcium–glucose interaction). These results could not be repeated in the SHS (data not published).

## Nutrition and BMI

Eilat-Adar et al. (2007) conducted an analysis from the second SHS examination (1992–1995). Calcium intake was significantly lower in SHS participants than in age-matched NHANES III participants. Mean dietary calcium intake in the SHS was 680 mg/day (range: 103–4574 mg/day) for men and 610 mg/day (range: 71–4093 mg/day) for women ($P < 0.001$ for gender). After an adjustment for potential confounders, BMI and percentage of body fat (PBF) were lower by 0.80 kg/m$^2$ (95% CI: –1.53 to –0.08, $P = 0.046$) and 1.28% (95% CI: –2.10 to –0.47, $P = 0.011$) in SHS participants with higher (≥873 mg/day in the 5th quintile) versus lower calcium intake (<313 mg/day in the 1st quintile). No relationship between calcium intake and BMI or PBF was observed among NHANES III participants.

## Nutrition and Cardiovascular Morbidity

Epidemiologic studies of the association between dietary fat and CHD incidence have been inconsistent (Table 2.6) (Xu et al., 2006). To the best of our knowledge, only one study analyzed the association between nutrition and morbidity in American Indians. Xu et al. (2006) examined the association between dietary fat intake and CHD incidence in American Indians in the SHS. A total of 2,938 participants ages 47–79 and free of CHD at the second SHS examination (1993–1995) was examined and followed for CHD, nonfatal CHD, and fatal CHD events to December 31,

2002. The mean percentages of energy from dietary fat, SFAs, MUFAs, PUFAs, and TFAs were 35.1%, 11.9%, 13.4%, 6.5%, and 2.4%, respectively. Specific types of fat intake were positively correlated with one another, with the highest correlation between SFAs and MUFAs ($r = 0.77$, $P < 0.0001$). As in the previous analysis on the association with poor glycemic control (Murphy et al., 1995), those in the highest quartile of intake of total fat, SFA, or MUFA had higher rates of CHD mortality than did those in the lowest quartile [hazard ratio (95% CI): 3.57 (1.21, 10.49), 5.17 (1.64, 16.36), and 3.43 (1.17, 10.04), respectively]. Substituting 5% of energy from either MUFA or SFA with the same amount of energy from carbohydrate was associated with a 62–68% higher rate of CHD mortality. In this population, the main sources of MUFA were meat, poultry, and fish (46%), and these same food groups provided almost the same contributions of SFA (45%). These mutual food sources for both FAs may explain the high correlation between SFA and MUFA and their lack of independent associations with CHD death. Olive oil and olives as a source for MUFA comprised only 0.3% of MUFA intake. This suggests that in other studies the beneficial effects of MUFA may have been related to other components in the olive oil rather than MUFA, and that the source of MUFA may be important in determining CHD risk. The higher intake of total fat, SFA, and MUFA and the lower intake of PUFA in the SHS than in the general U.S. population suggest a less healthy eating pattern among American Indians that contributes to higher rates of CHD death.

In the GOCADAN population, seal oil was the second major source of MUFA, contributing 5% of total MUFA intake (beef was first, contributing 6%) (Nobmann et al., 2005). The previously stable rate of CVD mortality supports the hypothesis that the source of MUFA may be important in determining CHD risk, and among Alaska Natives, MUFA may be associated with more positive heart health because it is derived from sea mammals rather than grain-fed animals. In a small study, MUFA was negatively correlated with LDL-C among Alaska Native men although not among women (Nobmann et al., 1999). These findings suggest that the role of MUFA in CVD among Alaska Natives and American Indians is unclear.

Ebbesson et al. (2007) investigated the association between omega-3 fatty acid intake and carotid atherosclerosis as measured by IMT and plaque score. Among the GOCADAN participants, the presence and extent of plaque were unrelated to intake of C20–22 omega-3 FAs or to total omega-3 FAs. The IMT was negatively associated with both. However, the odds of plaque rose significantly with quartiles of palmitic (C16 SFA) and stearic acid intakes (C18 SFA). IMT was negatively associated with palmitic and stearic acid.

## Intervention Programs

Over the past 20 years, aggressive intervention programs have been implemented in IHS clinics. Large portions of their budgets go to diabetes-related programs, such as nutrition education (Wiedman, 2005). Only a few intervention programs have been tested in controlled, randomized trials.

**Table 2.6. Major Prospective Studies of Dietary Fat Intake and Risk of CHD**

| Study | Sex | Age | Follow-up (years) | Dietary assessment method | Association |
|---|---|---|---|---|---|
| Honolulu Heart Program (McGee et al.. 1984) | 8006 men | 45-68 | 10 | 24-h recall | Positive association between total fat and CHD incidence |
| Framingham Study (Posner et al., 1991) | 859 men | 45-65 | 16 | 24-h recall | Positive association between total fat and MUFA and CHD incidence among 45–55 years old |
| Denmark (Jakobsen et al., 2004) | 3686 men and women | 30-71 | 16 | 7-day food record | Positive association between total fat, SFA and MUFA and CHD incidence among women aged less than 60 years old |
| Lipid Research Clinics Prevalence Follow-up Study (Esrey et al., 1996) | 4546 men and women | 30-79 | 12 | 24-h recall | Positive association between total fat, SFA, MUFA and CHD death among 30 to 59 years old |
| Health and Lifestyle Survey (Boniface & Tefft, 2002) | 2676 men and women | 40-75 | 16 | FFQ | Positive association between total fat and SFA and CHD death in women |
| Puerto Rico Heart Health Program (Garcia-Palmierie et al., 1980) | 8218 men | 45-64 | 6 | 24-h recall | No association |
| Health Professionals' Study (Ascherio et al., 1996) | 43757 men | 40-75 | 6 | FFQ | No association |
| Alpha-Tocopherol, Beta-Carotene Cancer Prevention Study (Pietinen et al., 1997) | 21930 men | 50-69 | 6 | FFQ | Positive association between TFA and CHD death |
| Nurses' Health Study (Oh et al., 2005) | 78778 women | 30-55 | 20 | FFQ | Inverse association between PUFA and CHD incidence, positive association between TFA and CHD incidence, more evident among women younger than age 65 years |
| Seven Countries Study (Keys et al., 1986) | 11579 men | 40-59 | 15 | 7 day food record | Positive association between SFA, inverse association between MUFA and CHD incidence |

**Table 2.6., cont. Major Prospective Studies of Dietary Fat Intake and Risk of CHD**

| Study | Sex | Age | Follow-up (years) | Dietary assessment method | Association |
|---|---|---|---|---|---|
| Ireland-Boston Diet-Heart Study (Kushi et al., 1985) | 1001 men | 30-69 | 20 | FFQ | Positive association between SFA and CHD death |
| Israeli Ischemic Heart Disease Study (Goldbourt et al., 1993) | 10059 men | 40 and over | 23 | FFQ | Positive association between SFA and CHD death, inverse association between PUFA and CHD death |
| Western Electric Study (Shekelle et al., 1981) | 1900 men | 40-55 | 20 | FFQ | Inverse association between PUFA and CHD death |
| Nurses' Health Study (Hu, 1997) | 80082 women | 30-55 | 14 | FFQ | Inverse association between MUFA and PUFA, positive association between TFA and CHD incidence |
| Zutphen Study (Kromhout et al., 1984) | 871 men | 40-59 | 10 | FFQ | No association |
| Zutphen Elderly Study (Oomen et al., 2001) | 667 men | 64-84 | 10 | FFQ | Positive association between TFA and CHD incidence |

Abbreviations: CHD: coronary heart disease; FFQ: food frequency questionnaire; SFA: saturated fatty acid; MUFA: monounsaturated fatty acid; PUFA: polyunsaturated fatty acid; TFA: trans fatty acid.

Reprinted with permission from J. Xu, S. Eilat-Adar, C. Loria, U. Goldbourt, B.V. Howard, R.R. Fabsitz, E.M. Zephier, C. Mattil, E.T. Lee. Dietary fat intake and risk of coronary heart disease: the Strong Heart Study. *Am. J. Clin. Nutr.* 2006 Oct;84(4):894–902.

Narayan et al. (1998) conducted a pilot trial to test adherence to specific lifestyle interventions among Pima Indians of Arizona and to compare them for changes in risk factors for type 2 diabetes. Ninety-five obese, normoglycemic men and women, ages 25–54, were randomized to either an "Action group," which involved structured activity and nutrition interventions, or a "Pride" group, which included unstructured activities emphasizing Pima history and culture. After 12 months of intervention, members of both intervention groups reported increased levels of physical activity (median: Action 7.3 hours/month, Pride 6.3 hours/month, $P < 0.001$ for each), and Pride members reported decreased starch intake (28 g, $P = 0.008$) compared to the control group. "Action" members gained more weight than "Pride" members (2.5 kg versus 0.8 kg, $P = 0.06$), and had a greater increase in 2-hour glucose (1.33 mM versus 0.03 mM, $P = 0.007$). The authors concluded that sustaining adherence to behavioral interventions over a long term is challenging. Pima Indians may find a less direct, less structured, and more participative intervention more acceptable than a direct and highly structured approach.

Witmer et al. (2004) conducted a pilot randomized controlled trial of a heart disease prevention program tailored for Alaska Native women. The pilot program was intended to assess feasibility and cultural acceptability and to develop enrollment procedures. The intervention included 12 weekly sessions on lifestyle change and goal setting. At 12 weeks (n = 23), significant improvements were noted in moderate walking and physical activity self-efficacy. In addition, substantial movement from the contemplation and preparation stages to the action stages of physical activity and heart-healthy eating was observed.

Pathways was the first multicenter American-Indian school-based study to test the effectiveness of an obesity prevention program promoting healthy eating and physical activity. It employed a nested cohort design in 41 schools, for a total of 1,704 third graders at baseline (Stone et al., 2003). The study's primary endpoint was percent of body fat. Secondary endpoints were levels of fat in school lunches; time spent in physical activity; and knowledge, attitudes, and behaviors regarding diet and exercise. No difference in mean percent of body fat at fifth grade was found between the intervention and control schools. Percentage of calories from fat and saturated fat in school lunches was significantly reduced in the intervention schools, as was total energy intake from 24-hour recalls. Significant increases in self-reported physical activity levels and knowledge of healthy behaviors were found for the intervention school students.

## Conclusion

The information about the association between nutrition and coronary risk factors or CHD in American Indians comes from sporadic studies in different communities. Most of the information comes from the SHS. Analyses suggest that some unique associations in American Indians may exist between diet and CVD, such as the positive associations among MUFA, poor glycemic control, and CHD mortality.

The association between nutrition and coronary risk factors among Alaska Natives may be influenced by the high consumption of long-chain FAs from fish and sea mammals. High intakes of C20–C22 FAs derived from fish and sea mammals among the GOCADAN participants were associated with reduced IMT, lower blood pressure, serum triglycerides, and 2-hour glucose levels and with higher HDL-C, fasting insulin, and HOMA. At the same time higher intakes of saturated fats were associated with increased odds and extent of plaque, as well as higher blood pressure and serum triglycerides. TFA intake was also associated with higher blood pressure.

Only a few intervention programs have been tested in controlled, randomized trials in differing geographic locations, as well as differing age groups. Future intervention programs should focus on increasing physical activity as well as on changing the Western diet patterns adopted by Native Americans. The cultural and dietary preferences of these communities should be considered while planning intervention programs.

## Acknowledgments

The Strong Heart Study was supported by cooperative agreement grants (Nos. U01HL-41642, U01HL-41652, and U01HL-41654) from the National Heart, Lung, and Blood Institute (NHLBI); support for GOCADAN came from grant no. HL64244. The authors acknowledge the assistance and cooperation of the Indian and Alaska Native communities, without whose support this study would not have been possible. We thank the Indian Health Service hospitals and clinics at each center: the directors and their staffs. We also acknowledge the contributions of the Norton Sound Health Corporation, Alaska, the participants and funding agency for the Genetics of Coronary Artery Disease in Alaska Natives (GOCADAN) Study, NHLBI grant no. HL64244. We gratefully acknowledge Rachel Schaperow, MedStar Research Institute, Hyattsville, MD, for editing the manuscript. The opinions expressed in this paper are those of the author(s) and do not necessarily reflect the views of the Indian Health Service.

### References

American Diabetes Association. Economic costs of diabetes in the United States in 2002. *Diabetes Care* **2003,** *26*, 917–932.

Archer, S.L.; K.J. Greenlund; R. Valdez; M.L. Casper; S. Rith-Najarian; J.B. Croft. Differences in food habits and cardiovascular disease risk factors among Native Americans with and without diabetes: the Inter-Tribal Heart Project. *Public Health Nutr.* **2004,** *7*, 1025–1032.

Ascherio, A.; E.B. Rimm; E.L. Giovannucci; D. Spiegelman; M. Stampfer; W.C. Willett. Dietary fat and risk of coronary heart disease in men: cohort follow up study in the United States. BMJ 1996, 313: 84–90.

Ballew, C.; L.L. White; K.F. Strauss; L.J. Benson; J.M. Mendlein; A.H. Mokdad. Intake of nutrients and food sources of nutrients among the Navajo, findings from the Navajo Health and Nutrition Survey. *J. Nutr.* **1997,***127*, S2085–S2093.

Bass, M.; L. Wakefield. Nutrient intake and food patterns of Indians on Standing Rock Reservation. *J. Am. Diet. Assoc.* **1974,** *64,* 36–41.

Bell, R.A.; H.A. Shaw; M.B. Dignan. Dietary intake of Lumbee Indian women in Robeson County, North Carolina. *J. Am. Diet. Assoc.* **1995,** *95,* 1426–1428.

Boniface, D.R.; M.E. Tefft. Dietary fats and 16-year coronary heart disease mortality in a cohort of men and women in Great Britain. *Eur. J. Clin. Nutr.* **2002,** *56,* 786–792.

Burrows, N.R.; L.S. Geiss; M.M. Engelgau; K.J. Acton. Prevalence of diabetes among Native Americans and Alaska Natives, 1990–1997: an increasing burden. *Diabetes Care* **2000,** *23,* 1786–1790.

California Adolescent Nutrition and Fitness. http://www.canfit.org/about_us.html [accessed January 21, 2008].

Clinical guidelines on the identification, evaluation and treatment of overweight and obesity in adults. Executive summary. *Am. J.Clin. Nutr.* **1998,** *63,* 899–917.

Compher, C. The nutrition transition in American Indians. *J. Transcult. Nurs.* **2006,** *17,* 217–223.

deGonzague, B.; O. Receveur; D. Wedll; H.V. Kuhnlein. Dietary intake and body mass index of adults in 2 Ojibwe communities. *J. Am. Diet. Assoc.* **1999,** *99,* 710–716.

Di Noia, J.; S.P. Schinke; I.R. Contento. Dietary patterns of reservation and non-reservation Native American youths. *Ethn. Dis.* **2005,** *15,* 705–712.

Ebbesson , S.O.; P.M. Risica; L.O. Ebbesson; J.M. Kennish; M.E. Tejero. Omega-3 fatty acids improve glucose tolerance and components of the metabolic syndrome in Alaskan Eskimos: the Alaska-Siberia project. *Int. J. Circumpolar Health* **2005,** *64,* 396–408.

Ebbesson, S.O.; M.J. Roman; R.B. Devereux; D. Kaufman; R.R. Fabsitz; J.W. Maccluer; B. Dyke; S. Laston; C.R. Wenger; A.G. Comuzzie; T. Romenesko; L.O. Ebbesson; E.D. Nobmann; B.V. Howard. Consumption of omega-3 fatty acids is not associated with a reduction in carotid atherosclerosis: The Genetics of Coronary Artery Disease in Alaska Natives Study. *Atherosclerosis.* **2007a,** Dec 3 [Epub ahead of print]

Ebbesson, S.O.; M.E. Tejero; E.D. Nobmann; J.C. Lopez-Alvarenga; L. Ebbesson; T. Romenesko; E.A. Carter; H.E. Resnick; R.B. Devereux; J.W. MacCluer; B. Dyke; S.L. Laston; C.R. Wenger; R.R. Fabsitz; A.G. Comuzzie; B.V. Howard. Fatty acid consumption and metabolic syndrome components: the GOCADAN study. *JCMS* **2007b,** *2,* 244–249.

Eilat-Adar, S.;, J. Xu; U. Goldbourt; E.M. Zephier. B.V. Howard; H.E. Resnick. Gender may modify the effects of macronutrient intake on metabolic syndrome and insulin resistance in American Indians: The Strong Heart Study. *J. Am. Diet. Assoc.* **2008,** in press.

Eilat-Adar, S.; J. Xu; C. Loria; C. Mattil; U. Goldbourt; B.V. Howard; H.E. Resnick. Dietary calcium is associated with body mass index and body fat in American Indians. *J. Nutr.* **2007,** *137,* 1955–1960.

Esrey, K.L.; L. Joseph; S.A. Grover. Relationship between dietary intake and coronary heart disease mortality: Lipid research clinics prevalence follow-up study. *J. Clin. Epidemiol.* **1996,** *49,* 211–216.

Garcia-Palmieri, M.R.; P. Sorlie; J. Tillotson; et al. Relationship of dietary intake to subsequent coronary heart disease incidence: The Puerto Rico Heart Health Program. *Am. J. Clin. Nutr.* **1980,** *33,* 1818–1827.

Goldbourt, U.; S. Yaari; J.H. Medalie. Factors predictive of long-term coronary heart disease mortality among 10,059 male Israeli civil servants and municipal employees: a 23-year mortality follow-up in the Israeli Ischemic Heart Disease Study. *Cardiology* **1993,** *82*, 100–121.

Grundy, S.M.; D. Bilheimer; H. Blackburn. Rationale of the diet-heart statement of the American Heart Association. Report of the Nutrition Committee. *Circulation* **1982,** *65*, 839A–854A.

Harland, B.F.; S.A. Smith; R. Ellis; R. O'Brien; E.R. Morris. Comparison of nutrient intakes of blacks, Siouan indians, and whites in Columbus County, North Carolina. *J. Am. Diet. Assoc.* **1992,** 348–350.

Howard, B.V.; E.T. Lee; L.D. Cowan; R.B. Devereaux; J.M. Galloway;O.T. Go. Rising tide of cardiovascular disease in American Indians. The Strong Heart Study. *Circulation* **1999,** *99*, 2389—2395.

Howard, B.V., E.T. Lee; L.B. Cowan; R.R. Fabsitz; W.J. Howard; A.J. Oopik; D.C. Robbins; P.J. Savage; J.L. Yeh; T.K. Welty.Coronary heart disease prevalence and its relation to risk factors in American Indians: The Strong Heart Study. *Am. J. Epidemiol.* **1995,** *142*, 254–268.

Hu, F.B.; M.J. Stampfer; J.E. Manson; et al. Dietary fat intake and the risk of coronary heart disease in women. *N. Engl. J. Med.* **1997,** *337*, 1491–1499.

Indian Health Service. IHS Chart Series Book, U.S. Government Printing Office, U.S. Department of Health and Human Services: Washington, DC, June 1984.

Jackson, M.Y. Nutrition in American Indian health: past, present, and future. *J. Am. Diet Assoc.* **1986,** *86*, 1561–1565.

Jakobsen, M.U.; K. Overvad; J. Dyerberg; M. Schroll; B.L. Heitmann.Dietary fat and risk of coronary heart disease: possible effect modification by gender and age. *Am. J. Epidemiol.* **2004,** *160*, 141–149.

Kegler, M.K.; L.H. Malcoe; R. Lynch; S. Whitecrow-Ollis. A community intervention to reduce lead exposure among Native American children., *Environ. Epidemiol. Toxicol.* **2000,** *2*, 121–132.

Keys, A.; A. Menotti; M.J. Karvonen; et al. The diet and 15-year death rate in the Seven Countries Study. *Am. J. Epidemiol.* **1986,** *124*, 903–915.

Kromhout, D., C. De Lezenne Coulander. Diet, prevalence and 10-year mortality from coronary heart disease in 871 middle-aged men: the Zutphen study. *Am. J. Epidemiol.* **1984,** *119*, 733–741.

Kuhnlein, H.V.; D.H. Galloway. Contemporary Hopi food intake patterns. *Ecol. Food.Nutr.* **1977,** *6*, 159–173.

Kushi, L.H.; R.A. Lew; F.J. Stare; et al. Diet and 20-year mortality from coronary heart disease: the Ireland-Boston Diet-Heart Study. *N. Engl. J. Med.* **1985,** *312*, 811–818.

Lee, E.T.; L.D. Cowan; W.J. Howard; M. Sievers; T.K. Welty; W. Wang; J.L. Yeh; E.R. Rhoades; R.B. Devereux; R.R. Fabsitz; O. Go; B.V. Howard. All-cause mortality and cardiovascular disease mortality in 3 American Indian populations aged 45 to 74 years, 1984 to 88: the Strong Heart Study. *Am. J. Epidemiol.* **1998,** *147*, 995–1008.

Lee, E.T.; B.V. Howard; P.J. Savage; L.D. Cowan; R. Fabsitz; A.J. Oopik; J.L. Yeh; O. Go; D.C. Robbins; T.K. Welty. Diabetes and impaired glucose tolerance in three American Indian populations aged 45–74 years: the Strong Heart Study. *Diabetes Care* **1995,** *18*, 599–610.

Lee, E.T.; T.K. Welty; L.D. Cowan; W.Y. Wang; D.A. Rhoades;R. Devereux; O. Go;R. Fabsitz;

B.V. Howard. Incidence of diabetes in American Indians of three geographic areas: the Strong Heart Study. *Diabetes Care* **2002,** *25*, 49–54.

Lee, E.T.; T.K. Welty; R. Fabsitz; L.D. Cowan; N.A. Le; A.J. Oopik;A.J. Cucchiara; P.J. Savage; B.V. Howard. A study of cardiovascular disease in American Indians: design and methods. The Strong Heart Study. *Am. J. Epidemiol.* **1990,** *132*, 1141–1155.

Liau,Y.; P. Tucker; C.A. Okoroa; W.H. Giles; A.H. Mokdad; B.V. Harris. REACH 2010 surveillance for health status in minority communities—United States, 2001–2002. *MMWR* **2004,** *53*(SS06),1–36.

Lombard, K.A.; S. Forster-Cox; D. Smeal; M.K. O'Neill. Diabetes on the Navajo Nation: what role can gardening and agriculture extension play to reduce it? *Rural Remote Health.* **2006,** *6*, 640.

Mayberry, R.H.; R. Lindeman. A survey of chronic disease and diet in Seminole Indians in Oklahoma. *Am. J. Clin. Nutr.* **1963,** *13*, 127–134.

McGee, D.L.; D.M. Reed; K. Yano; A. Kagan; J. Tillotson. Ten-year incidence of coronary heart disease in the Honolulu Heart Program. Relationship to nutrient intake. *Am. J. Epidemiol.* **1984,** *119*, 667–676.

Murphy, N.J.; C.D. Schraer; M.C. Thiele; E.J. Boyko; L.R. Bulkow;B.J. Doty; A.P. Lanier. Dietary change and obesity associated with glucose intolerance in Alaska Natives. *J. Am. Diet. Assoc.* **1995,** *95*, 676–682.

Narayan, K.M.; M. Hoskin; D. Kozak; A.M. Kriska; R.L. Hanson; D.J. Pettitt; D.K. Nagi; P.H. Bennett; W.C. Knowler. Randomized clinical trial of lifestyle interventions in Pima Indians: a pilot study. *Diabet. Med.* **1998,** *15*, 166–172.

National Cholesterol Education Program (NCEP). Expert Panel On Detection, Evaluation, and Treatment of High Blood Cholesterol In Adults (Adult Treatment Panel III): Third report of the National Cholesterol Education Program (NCEP) expert panel on detection, evaluation, and treatment of high blood cholesterol in adults (Adult Treatment Panel III) final report. *Circulation* **2002,** *106*, 3143–3421.

Nelson, R.G.; M.L. Sievers; W.C. Knowler; B.A. Swinburn; D.J. Pettitt; M.F. Saad; I.M. Liebow; B.V. Howard; P.H. Bennett. Low incidence of fatal coronary heart disease in Pima Indians despite high prevalence of non–insulin-dependent diabetes. *Circulation* **1990,** *81*, 987–995.

Nobmann, E.D.; T. Byers; A.P. Lanier; J.H. Hankin; M.Y. Jackson. The diet of Alaska Native adults in 1987–1988. *Am. J. Clin. Nutr.* **1992,** *55*, 1024–1032.

Nobmann, E.D.; S.O.E. Ebbesson; R.G. White; L.R. Bulkow; C.D. Schraer. Associations between dietary factors and plasma lipids related to cardiovascular disease among Siberian Yupiks of Alaska. *Int. J. Circumpolar Health* **1999,** *58*, 254–271.

Nobmann, E.D.; R. Ponce; C. Mattil; R. Devereux; B. Dyke; S.O. Ebbesson; S. Laston; J. MacCluer; D. Robbins; T. Romenesko; G. Ruotolo;C.R. Wenger; B.V. Howard GOCADAN study, 2000–2003. Dietary intakes vary with age among eskimo adults of northwest Alaska in the GOCADAN study, 2000–2003. *J. Nutr.* **2005,** *135*, 856–862.

Oh, K.; F.B. Hu; J.E. Manson; M.J. Stampfer; W.C. Willett. Dietary fat intake and risk of coronary heart disease in women: 20 years of follow-up of the Nurses' Health Study. *Am. J. Epidemiol.* **2005,** *161*, 672–679.

Oomen, C.M.; M.C. Ocke; E.J. Feskens; et al. Association between *trans* fatty acid intake and 10-year risk of coronary heart disease in the Zutphen Elderly Study: a prospective population based study. *Lancet* **2001,** *357*, 746–751.

Pietinen, P.; A. Ascherio; P. Korhonen; et al. Intake of fatty acids and risk of coronary heart disease in a cohort of Finnish men: The Alpha-tocopherol, Beta-carotene Cancer Prevention Study. *Am. J. Epidemiol.* **1997,** *145*, 876–887.

Popkin, B.M.; P. Gordon-Larson. The nutrition transition: Worldwide obesity dynamics and their determinants. *Int. J. Obes.* **2004,** *28*, S2–S9.

Posner, B.M.; J.L. Cobb; A.J. Belanger; et al. Dietary lipid predictors of coronary heart disease in men. The Framingham Study. *Arch. Intern. Med.* **1991,** *151*, 1181–1187.

Ravussin, E.; M.E. Valencia; J. Esparza; P.H. Bennett; L.O. Schulz. Effects of a traditional lifestyle on obesity in Pima Indians. *Diabetes Care,* **1994,** *17*, 1067–1074.

Reid, J.M.; S.D. Fullmer; K.D. Pettigrew; T.A. Burch; P.H. Bennett;M. Miller; G.D. Whedon. Nutrient intake of Pima Indian women: relationships to diabetes mellitus and gallbladder disease. *Am. J. Clin. Nutr. 24,* **1971,** 1281–1289.

Schakel, S.F. Procedures for estimating nutrient values for food composition databases. *J. Food Comp. Anal.* **1997,** *10*, 102–114.

Schakel, S.F. Maintaining a nutrient database in a changing marketplace: keeping pace with changing food products—a research perspective. *J. Food Comp. Anal.* **2001,** *14*, 315–322.

Schakel, S.F.; Y.A. Sievert; L.M. Buzzard. Sources of data for developing and maintaining a nutrient database. *J. Am. Diet. Assoc.* **1988,** *88*, 1268–1271.

Schraer, C.D.; A.I. Adler; A.M. Mayer; K.R. Halderson; B.A. Trimble. Diabetes complications and mortality among Alaska Natives: 8 years of observation. *Diabetes Care* **1997,** *20*, 314–321.

Schulz, L.O.; P.H. Bennett; E. Ravussin; J.R. Kidd; K.K. Kidd; J. Esparza; M.E. Valencia. Effects of traditional and western environments on prevalence of type 2 diabetes in Pima Indians in Mexico and the U.S. *Diabetes Care* **2006,** *29*, 1866–1871.

Shekelle, R.B.; A.M. Shryock; O. Paul; et al. Diet, serum cholesterol, and death from coronary heart disease: the Western Electric Study. *N. Engl. J. Med.* **1981,** *304*, 65–70.

Sievers, M.L.; J.R. Fisher. Diseases of North American Indians. Biocultural Aspects of Disease; H.R. Rothschild, Ed.; Academic Press: New York, NY, 1981; 191–252.

Smith, C.J.; R.G. Nelson; S.A. Hardy; E.M. Manahan; P.H. Bennett; W.C. Knowler. Survey of the diet of Pima Indians using quantitative food frequency assessment and 24-hour recall. *J. Am. Diet. Assoc.* **1996,** *96*, 778–784.

Stang, J.; E.M. Zephier; M. Story; J.H. Himes; J.L. Yeh; T. Welty; B.V. Howard. Dietary intakes of nutrients thought to modify cardiovascular risk from three groups of American Indians: The Strong Heart Dietary Study, phase II. *J. Am. Diet. Assoc.* **2005,** *105*, 1895–1903.

Stone, E.J.; J.E. Norman; S.M. Davis; D. Stewart; T.E. Clay; B. Caballero; T.G. Lohman; D.M. Murray. Design, implementation, and quality control in the Pathways American-Indian Multicenter Trial. *Prev. Med.* **2003,** *37*, S13–S23.

Stroehla, B.C.; L.H. Malcoe; E.M. Velie. Dietary sources of nutrients among rural Native American and white children. *J. Am. Diet Assoc.* **2005,** *105*(12), 1908–16.

Strong Heart Study Operational Manual Volume V: Dietary and Psychosocial Studies. The Strong Heart Study Coordinating Center, University of Oklahoma Health Sciences Center: Oklahoma City, OK, 1993.

Subar, A.F.; S.M. Krebs-Smith; A. Cook; L.L. Kahle. Dietary sources of nutrients among US children, 1989–1991, *Pediatrics* **1998,** *102*, 913–923.

Taylor, C.A.; K.S. Keim; A.C. Gilmore. Impact of core and secondary foods on nutritional composition of diets in native-american women. *J. Am. Diet Assoc.* **2005,** *105*, 413–419.

Teufel, N.I.; D.L. Dufour. Patterns of food use and nutrient intake of obese and nonobese Hualapai Indian women of Arizona. *J. Am. Diet Assoc.* **1990,** *90,* 1229–1235.

Venkat Narayan, K.M.; R.L. Hanson; C.J. Smith; R.G. Nelson; S.B. Gyenizse; D.J. Pettitt; W.C. Knowler. Dietary calcium and blood pressure in a Native American population. *J. Am. Coll. Nutr.* **1998,** *17*, 59–64.

Welty, T.K.; L. Freni-Titulaer; M.M. Zack; P. Weber; J. Sippel; N. Huete; J. Justice; D. Dever; M.A. Murphy. Effects of exposure to salty drinking water in an Arizona community. Cardiovascular mortality, hypertension prevalence, and relationships between blood pressure and sodium intake. *JAMA* **1986,** *255*, 622–626.

Wiedman D. American Indian diets and nutritional research: implications of the Strong Heart Dietary Study, Phase II, for cardiovascular disease and diabetes. *J. Am. J. Diet Assoc.* **2005,** *105*, 1874–1880.

Williams, D.E.; W.C. Knowler; C.J. Smith; R.L. Hanson; J. Roumain; A. Saremi; A.M. Kriska; P.H. Bennett; R.G. Nelson. The effect of Indian or Anglo dietary preference on the incidence of diabetes in Pima Indians. *Diabetes Care* **2001,** *24*, 811–816.

Witmer, J.M.; M.R. Hensel; P.S. Holck; A.S. Ammerman; A.C. Will. Heart disease prevention for Alaska Native women: a review of pilot study findings. *J. Womens Health* **2004,** *13*, 569–578.

Wolfe, W.S.; D. Sanjur. Contemporary diet and body weight of Navajo women receiving food assistance: an ethnographic and nutritional investigation. *J. Am. Diet. Assoc.* **1988,** *88,* 822–827.

Xu, J.; S. Eilat-Adar; C. Loria; U. Goldbourt; B.V. Howard; R.R. Fabsitz; E.M. Zephier; C. Mattil; E.T. Lee. Dietary fat intake and risk of coronary heart disease: the Strong Heart Study. *Am. J. Clin. Nutr.* **2006,** *84*, 894–902.

Xu, J.; S. Eilat-Adar; C.M. Loria; B.V. Howard; R.R. Fabsitz; M. Begum; E.M. Zephier; E.T. Lee. Macronutrient intake and glycemic control in a population based sample of American Indians with diabetes: the Strong Heart Study. *Am. J. Clin. Nutr.* **2007,** *86*, 480–487.

Zephier, E.M.; C. Ballew; A. Mokdad; J. Mendlein; C. Smith; J.L. Yeh; E. Lee; T.K. Welty; B.V. Howard. Intake of nutrients related to cardiovascular disease risk among three groups of American Indians: The Strong Heart Dietary Study. *Prev. Med.* **1997,** *26*, 508–815.

# 3

# Fish Oils and Stroke

**Charles H. Hennekens[1,2,3], Wendy R. Schneider[1], and Ricky M. Schneider[4]**
*Charles E. Schmidt College of Biomedical Science, Department of Clinical Science and Medical Education and Center of Excellence, Florida Atlantic University, Boca Raton, Florida [1] the Departments of Medicine & Epidemiology and Public Health, University of Miami Miller School of Medicine, Miami, Florida [2] and the Departments of Preventive Medicine [3] and Medicine [4], Nova Southeastern University College of Medicine, Ft. Lauderdale, Florida*

## Introduction

Cardiovascular disease (CVD) includes coronary heart disease (CHD), stroke, and peripheral artery disease. With respect to percentages of deaths from CVD, CHD accounts for 52% and stroke for 17% (Rosamond et al., 2008) as shown in Fig. 3.1 (Hennekens & Schneider, 2008).

Despite remarkable declines in mortality from stroke and CHD over the last several decades, CVD remains the leading cause of death in the United States and in most developed Western countries; it will remain so during the twenty-first century (Mackay & Mensah, 2004). This is mainly due to the alarming trends among

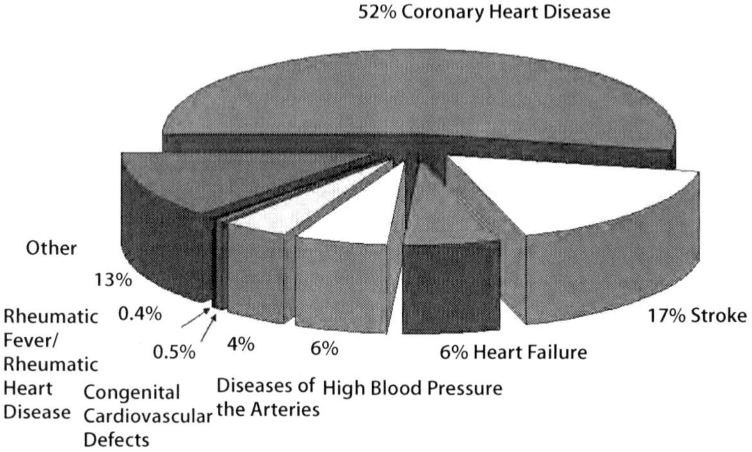


**Fig. 3.1.** Percentage breakdown of deaths from cardiovascular disease in the United States: 2004.

adolescents in increased cigarette smoking, obesity, physical inactivity, type 2 diabetes mellitus, dyslipidemia, and hypertension (Hennekens & Schneider, 2008). All of these factors contribute to the risk of stroke.

According to the World Health Organization (WHO), malnutrition and infection are declining as leading causes of death in developing countries, while increases mainly in cigarette smoking and obesity, both major risk factors for stroke, are rising at alarming rates (Hennekens, 1998; Mackay & Mensah, 2004).

For all of these reasons, CVD is the leading cause of death in the world (Mackay & Mensah, 2004). As shown in Fig. 3.2 (Hennekens & Schneider, 2008), CVD caused about 1 in 4 deaths worldwide in 1990, and is projected to cause about 1 in 3 deaths worldwide by 2020 (Murray & Lopez, 1996).

With respect to the increasing worldwide burden of CVD, 17.1 million people died from this cause in 2004, and it is projected by the WHO that 23.4 million people will die from this disease in 2030 (WHO, 2008).

In the United States in 2004, stroke ranked third among all causes of mortality, accounting for approximately 1 of every 16 total deaths. Of 780,000 annual stroke victims, 150,074 died (Rosamond et al., 2008). Globally, the relative frequency of stroke appears to be increasing in comparison with CHD. The population-based Oxford Vascular Study showed a higher incidence of stroke than of CHD, and concluded that the brain vasculature is more frequently affected than any other arterial site (Rothwell et al., 2005). Similar findings were recorded in China and Japan, where the incidence of stroke is higher than that of CHD (Bernal-Pacheco & Roman, 2007).

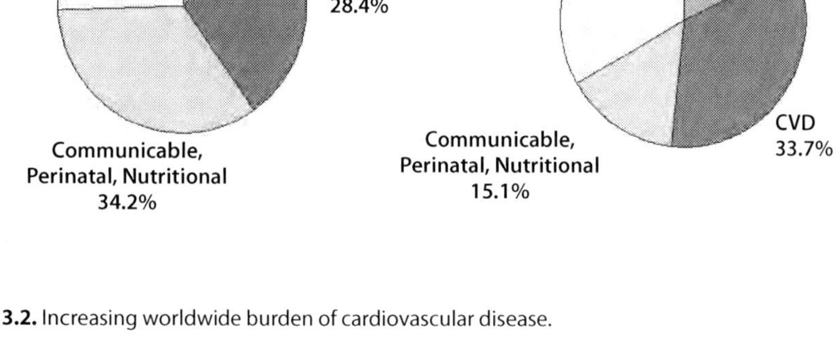


**Fig. 3.2.** Increasing worldwide burden of cardiovascular disease.

Of total strokes in the United States, 70% are first cardiovascular events, and 30% of survivors will have another stroke within 5 years, 15% within the first year. Of deaths from stroke, 60% occur in women (Rosamond et al., 2008).

Although stroke is uncommon, especially in men under age 40, (Mackay & Mensah, 2004), over 33% occur in individuals who are under 65 years of age. Of those 65 years and older, more than 25% of stroke survivors remain disabled 6 months later (Goldstein, 2008).

## Stroke

### *Risk Factors*

During the past 50 years, several major modifiable risk factors for stroke were identified, and include hypertension, diabetes mellitus, dyslipidemia, atrial fibrillation, carotid stenosis, and cigarette smoking. Atrial fibrillation is an independent risk factor for stroke, increasing the risk approximately fivefold (Rosamond et al., 2008). Nontraditional vascular risk factors emerged more recently, including inflammation and alterations of coagulation (Bernal-Pacheco & Roman, 2007). One can divide vascular risk factors into three descriptive groups: nonmodifiable (race, age, sex, low-birth weight, and genetic factors); modifiable (hypertension, dyslipidemia, diabetes, tobacco smoking, atrial fibrillation, other cardiac disorders, post-menopausal hormone therapy, diet, physical inactivity, and obesity, particularly central obesity as in the metabolic syndrome); and potentially modifiable (metabolic syndrome, alcohol or drug abuse, oral contraceptive use, sleep apnea, migraine, hypercoagulability, inflammation—C-reactive protein, and infection) (Bernal-Pacheco & Roman, 2007).

### *Relation to Transient Ischemic Attack*

Of all strokes, 87% are ischemic, 10% are intracerebral hemorrhage, and 3% are subarachnoid hemorrhage (Rosamond et al., 2008).

Approximately 15% of strokes are preceded by a transient ischemic attack (TIA), a reversible neurologic deficit that persists less than 24 hours. TIAs are associated with a substantial short-term risk of stroke, other cardiovascular events, and death. A risk of stroke is highest within the first 30 days following TIA. In population-based studies, the age and gender-adjusted incidence rates for TIA range from 68 – 83 per 100,000. Males and blacks have inordinately high rates of TIA. Within one year of TIA, up to one-fourth of patients will die. Those who have a TIA have a 10-year stroke risk of 18.8% and a combined 10-year stroke, myocardial infarction (MI), or a vascular death risk of 42.8% (Rosamond et al., 2008). These data emphasize the importance of stroke prevention.

### *Dietary Factors*

Despite decades of research, the relationship of fat intake with stroke is not yet clear. In previous decades, the recommendations from several authoritative U.S.

organizations emphasized decreasing the total amount of fat in the diet. More recent research, however, indicates that the type of fat is more important than the amount of fat. Specifically, *trans* fats are emerging as harmful, and fish oil as beneficial (Gillman, 2007).

Although the evidence from intervention studies is less inconsistent, observational epidemiologic data indicate that individuals who consume fish-oil-derived n-3 (omega-3) polyunsaturated fatty acids have a lower risk of stroke. In a large-scale population-based cohort study in Japan, individuals who consumed egg, dairy products, and fish had a significantly lower risk of mortality from stroke. Individuals who consumed animal products had lower risks of mortality from intracerebral hemorrhage, but not from cerebral infarction (Sauvaget et al., 2003).

In 1988, dietary recommendations were made to lower total fat, especially saturated fat, in the diet (AHA, 1988). More recently, both the 2002 Adult Treatment Panel III of the National Cholesterol Education Program Expert Panel (NCEP ATP III, 2002) and the 2005 Dietary Guidelines for Americans Advisory Committee (King et al., 2005) recommended dietary modifications that include the types of fat. In addition, many other pathways are available by which diet may affect not only atherosclerosis, but also thrombosis: both major contributors to the risk of stroke.

Most physicians and some health providers were limited in their expertise to provide detailed dietary advice to their patients regarding fat intake. Despite these recommendations from federal authorities, the American Heart Association (AHA) Heart Disease and Stroke Statistics—2008 Update states that The Economic Research Service of the U.S. Department of Agriculture (USDA) found that between 1970 and 2003 the average daily calorie consumption in the United States increased 16%, or by 523 calories, of which fats and oils accounted for 63%. According to USDA data, in 2002, total meat consumption (red meat, poultry, and fish) amounted to 200 lbs per person, 23 lbs higher than the level in 1970. Each American consumed an average of 18 lbs of less red meat (mostly beef), 37 lbs of more poultry, and 4 lbs of more fish than in 1970. The AHA update also cites the Minnesota Heart Survey findings that while age-adjusted, mean Heart Disease Prevention Eating Index scores increased in both sexes during the past two decades, energy balance, sodium intake, and fish intake changed unfavorably or remained at a low compliance level (Rosamond et al., 2008).

Data on the relationship of dietary fats with stroke are sparse and inconsistent. In the Framingham Heart Study, of a prospective population-based cohort of 5,207 men and women, those who consumed polyunsaturated fats (combined n-3 and n-6 fatty acids) had no decreased or increased risk of stroke. In a subgroup analysis, those who consumed saturated and monounsaturated fats had a lower risk of ischemic stroke (Gillman et al., 1997; Mozaffarian et al., 2005).

In contrast, the Health Professionals Follow-Up Study (HPFS), a prospective cohort study of 43,732 men, found that those who consumed saturated fat, monounsaturated fat, polyunsaturated fat, *trans* fat, or dietary cholesterol had no increased or decreased risk of stroke. Further, those who consumed n-3 and n-6 polyunsaturated fatty acids had no increased or decreased risk of ischemic or hemorrhagic stroke (He et al., 2003).

Both the Nurses' Health Study (NHS) in women and the HPFS in men reported that participants with higher intakes of fish and n-3 fatty acids had a reduced risk of ischemic stroke in comparison to those who consumed fish less than once a month (He et al., 2002; Iso et al., 2001)). In the HPFS, men eating fish once a month or more had a reduced risk of ischemic stroke in comparison to those who consumed fish less than once a month. (He et al., 2002). In a subgroup analysis in women, those who ate fish regularly and did not take daily aspirin had the lowest risk of ischemic stroke (Iso et al., 2001). In a prospective observational cohort study of 4775 elderly adults, those with increased fish consumption had a reduced risk of stroke (He et al., 2004).

## *Pharmacologic Therapies*

The increasing burden of CVD in developed as well as developing countries underscores the need for a more widespread and appropriate use of available pharmacologic therapies of proven benefit in the primary and secondary preventions of occlusive vascular events, including stroke. In the treatment and prevention of CVD, the major drug therapies of proven benefit include anti-platelet agents, principally aspirin; antihypertensive agents; and lipid-lowering agents, principally statins.

### *Anti-platelet*

While the principal underlying cause of CVD is atherosclerosis, in virtually all cases the proximate cause is thrombosis. Platelets are involved in the development of acute occlusive vascular events, including MI and ischemic stroke. Platelets do not adhere to healthy vascular endothelium, but do attach to foreign substances and subcollagenous fibers or damaged endothelium. Once platelets adhere to the damaged area, they secrete substances that promote aggregation, resulting in thrombus (Williams & Hennekens, 2004).

In secondary prevention, anti-platelet therapy, principally with aspirin, produces statistically significant and clinically important reductions in total stroke of about 20%, ischemic stroke of about 25%, MI of about 33%, and vascular deaths of about 15% (Anti-Thrombotic Trialist Collaboration, 2002). In the primary prevention of occlusive vascular events, the benefits of aspirin on occlusions outweigh the risks of major bleeding in those with a 10-year risk of a first CHD event of 6–10% (Hennekens et al., 2006). The possible benefits of aspirin in the primary prevention of stroke are limited to one trial in women, The Women's Health Study (Ridker et al., 2005). For all patients requiring aspirin but who are intolerant, clopidogrel is certainly an effective alternative (Gorelick et al., 2006).

***Anti-hypertensive***

Hypertension, defined as a systolic blood pressure greater than or equal to 140 mm of Hg, or a diastolic blood pressure greater than or equal to 90 mm of Hg, is a major and modifiable risk factor for stroke. In a comprehensive, worldwide meta-analysis of randomized trials, pharmacologic therapy produced a 4–5-mm reduction in blood pressure. Over three to five years of treatment and follow-up, stroke was reduced by 42% and MI by 14% (Collins et al., 1990).

The achievement of an optimal blood pressure level is more important than the particular agent used to reach the accepted goal. Thus, similar stroke-risk reductions were found in a meta-analysis of randomized trials for angiotensin-converting enzyme inhibitors (28%), beta blockers or diuretics (35%), and calcium channel blockers (39%) (Lawes et al., 2004). Clearly, for many patients, multiple drug therapies are needed to achieve the federally mandated goals (Chobanian et al., 2003) for the treatment of hypertension. Nonetheless, undiagnosed, untreated, and suboptimally treated hypertension is a leading public-health problem throughout the world.

***Lipid-lowering***

Numerous pharmacologic therapies are available to achieve lipid-lowering, including statins, niacin, fish oils, fibrates, and ezetimibe. The totality of randomized evidence is far greater for the statins than for any other therapy. In a 2005 meta-analysis of 90,056 patients who participated in large-scale randomized trials in the treatment and prevention of CVD, HMG-CoA reductase inhibitors (statins) produced statistically significant and clinically important reductions in the risks of MI, stroke, cardiovascular deaths, and total mortality (Baigent et al., 2005).

Numerous fixed-dose drug combinations that include a statin are approved by the FDA to achieve the established lipid targets. The totality of evidence on lipid modification for reducing CVD, however, is far less for the nonstatin component, leading to possible overutilization of two drugs when single-agent efficacy will suffice. The evidence of the benefits from statins is considerable as demonstrated by the meta-analysis (Baigent et al., 2005).

The results of this meta-analysis are summarized in Table 3.1 and Table 3.2 (Hennekens, 2008). Specifically, statins confer statistically significant and clinically important benefits on MI, stroke, CVD death, and total death, with no increases in non-CVD or cancer deaths. The meta-analysis also provides reassuring evidence of the safety of statins. The totality of evidence for adjunctive therapies in reducing the risk of CVD is less than that for statins (Table 3.3) (Hennekens, 2008). Healthcare providers were advised to use adjunctive therapies only after achieving goal low-density lipoprotein-cholesterol (LDL-C) levels with statin therapy (Hennekens, 2008).

Niacin (nicotinic acid) produced significant clinical benefits in 2,835 randomized patients (Berge & Canner, 1991). In the GISSI trial, omega-3 fatty acids also produced clinical benefits in 11,324 randomized patients (GISSI-Prevenzione Investigators, 1999). However, since both of these findings preceded the use of statins, it is unclear whether these benefits are additive. The fibrate gemfibrozil produced clinical benefits in 2531 patients in the VA-HIT (Veterans Affairs–High-Density Lipoprotein Intervention Trial) study, but this drug, according to the FDA database, was responsible for 38% of all cases of rhabdomyolysis, either alone or in combination with statins (Robins et al., 2001). Among diabetic patients in the FIELD (Fenofibrate Intervention and Event Lowering in Diabetes) trial, fenofibrates showed no overall benefit in the reduction of CVD, but significant benefits were seen in the subgroup of patients who were not treated with statins (Keech et al., 2005). Finally, ezetimibe has no clinical outcome data either alone or in combination with statins (Hennekens et al., 2006).

## *Carotid Artery Surgery and Stenting*

A carotid endarterectomy (CEA) is the most frequently performed surgical procedure to prevent stroke, with an estimated 103,000 in-patient CEA operations performed in the United States in 2005 (Rosamond et al., 2008). Randomized trials demonstrated a reduced stroke risk for CEA relative to medical therapy in both symptomatic and asymptomatic patients. The American Heart Association (AHA) expert consensus panel recommends CEA for symptomatic patients with good surgical risk and at least 50% stenosis in an extracranial carotid artery as well as in asymptomatic patients with at least 80% stenosis (Biller et al., 1998).

**Table 3.1. Effect of LDL-Cholesterol Level Reduction on Vascular Events.**

| Endpoint | Treatment-arm events [*n*=45,054 (%)] | Control-arm events [*n*= 45,002 (%)] | Relative risk (95% CI) |
|---|---|---|---|
| Any major vascular event | 14.1 | 17.8 | 0.79 (0.77, 0.81) |
| Any major coronary event | 7.4 | 9.8 | 0.77 (0.74m 0.80) |
| nonfatal MI | 4.4 | 6.2 | 0.74 (0.70, 0.79) |
| CHD death | 3.4 | 4.4 | 0.81 (0.75, 0.87) |
| Any coronary revascularization | 5.8 | 7.6 | 0.76 (0.73, 0.80) |
| CABG | 1.6 | 2.2 | 0.75 (0.69, 0.82) |
| PTCA | 1.1 | 1.5 | 0.79 (0.69, 0.90) |
| unspecified | 3.1 | 3.9 | 0.76 (0.69, 0.84) |
| Any stroke | 3.0 | 3.7 | 0.83 (0.78, 0.88) |

Proportional effects on major vascular events per 1 mmol/L reduction in the low-density lipoprotein-cholesterol level in 90,056 participants in 14 randomized trials utilizing HMG-CoA reductase inhibitors (statins) for the secondary prevention of cardiovascular disease.
CABG = coronary artery bypass graft; CHD = coronary heart disease; MI = myocardial infarction; PTCA = percutaneous transluminal coronary angioplasty.

**Table 3.2. Effect of LDL-Cholesterol Level Reduction on CVD Mortality.**

| Cause of death | Treatment-arm events [$n$=45,054 (%)] | Control-arm events [$n$=45,054 (%)] | Relative risk (95% CI) |
|---|---|---|---|
| All-cause mortality | 8.5 | 9.7 | 0.88 (0.84, 0.91) |
| CHD | 3.4 | 4.4 | 0.81 (0.76, 0.85) |
| Any non-CHD | 1.2 | 1.3 | 0.93 (0.83, 10.03) |
| Stroke | 0.6 | 0.6 | 0.91 (0.74, 1.11) |
| Other vascular | 0.6 | 0.7 | 0.95 (0.78, 1.16) |
| Any vascular | 4.7 | 5.7 | 0.83 (0.79, 0.87) |
| Any nonvascular | 3.8 | 4.0 | 0.95 (0.90, 1.01) |
| Cancer | 2.4 | 2.4 | 1.01 (0.91, 1.12) |

Proportional effects on total and cause-specific mortality per 1 mmol/L reduction in the low-density lipoprotein-cholesterol level in 90,056 participants in 14 randomized trails utilizing HMG-CoA reductatse inhibitors (statins) for the secondary prevention of cardiovascular disease.
CHD = coronary heart disease.

**Table 3.3. Effect of Lipid-Lowering Therapy on CVD Clinical Outcomes.**

| Treatment | No. patients |
|---|---|
| HMG-CoA reductase inhibitors (statins) | 90,056 |
| Niacin (nicotinic acid) | 2,835 |
| Fibrates | |
| gemfibrozil | 2,531 |
| fenofibrate | 9,795 |
| Omega-3 fatty acid | 11,324 |
| Ezetimibe | 0 |

Effect of lipid modifying drugs on clinical outcomes in patients randomized to lipid-lowering therapy for the secondary prevention of cardiovascular disease.

Catheter-based carotid artery stent placement is currently recommended principally in patients who are at inordinate surgical risk and who are anatomically good candidates for stenting. Patients who are not at a high surgical risk should be considered for CEA (Coward et al., 2005).

## Evidence for Fish Oil and Stroke Prevention

The hypothesis that individuals who consume high amounts of fish oils have a decreased risk of CVD was formulated about 50 years ago. Greenlandic Inuits, who consumed a traditional diet rich in fish oils, particularly omega-3 fatty acids, such as eicosapentaenoic and docosahexaenoic acids, had very low rates of CVD. Since then, a growing body of evidence suggests that the consumption of fish oils is associated with lower risks of CHD and sudden cardiac death (Skerrett & Hennekens, 2003). Now we will review the totality of evidence on fish oil and stroke. The clinical relevance of such therapy is derived from the totality of evidence, particularly randomized trial data.

## *Types of Evidence*

Advances in medical knowledge proceed along several fronts, optimally in a simultaneous fashion. Basic research provides plausible biological mechanisms to explain why an agent affects outcomes and has a high degree of precision, but has questionable relevance to free living humans. Epidemiology explains whether an agent affects outcomes and has a high degree of imprecision, but has clear relevance to free living humans. Epidemiology is crude and inexact, as observations on free living humans can never take place under the controlled conditions of basic research. The strategies of epidemiology include descriptive studies, useful to formulate hypotheses, and analytical studies, useful to test hypotheses. Analytical epidemiology can be observational, including either case-control or cohort studies, or experimental, comprising randomized trials. For large effects (i.e., a doubling or more of risk or benefit), observational studies in the context of basic research can provide a sufficient totality of evidence for rational clinical decision making and public policy. When the effect sizes are small to moderate (i.e., less than a doubling of risk or benefit), however, the amount of uncontrolled and uncontrollable confounding inherent in all observational designs can be about as big as the effect sizes. In all observational study designs, even the availability of the most precise and complete information still cannot adequately control confounding since some variables are unknown. Meta-analyses of observational studies decrease the role of chance as a plausible alternative explanation. Since individual observational studies are not randomized, each has its own unique set of confounders, so meta-analyses may even increase the amount of uncontrolled and uncontrollable confounding. Thus, meta-analyses of observational studies cannot be used to confirm or refute findings from randomized trials (Hennekens & Buring, 1987).

For all these reasons, to assess small-to-moderate effects, randomized trials of sufficient size, dose, and duration represent the most reliable design strategy. The statistical power of a trial is the probability of rejecting the null hypothesis when it is false. (Hennekens & Borzak, 2008; Hennekens & Buring, 1987). Statistical power is proportional to the number of endpoints, not the sample size. Thus, an overview or meta-analysis of individual randomized trials, giving proportionately more weight to those of larger sample size, may provide a totality of evidence upon which more rational clinical decision making for individual patients or policy decisions for the health of the general public can safely be based (Hennekens & Buring, 1987).

Randomized trials are optimally informative when conducted for their scheduled duration. Statistical stopping guidelines are usually asymmetric for benefit and risk, but should always be viewed as one component of the totality of evidence upon which early termination is based (Hennekens & Buring, 1987).

Subgroup analyses can be particularly misleading even in randomized trials since the sample size is reduced and the comparisons are no longer randomized. Thus, chance as well as uncontrolled confounding factors are always plausible alternative explanations. In general, one should view subgroup analyses as hypothesis-formulating, not hypothesis-testing (Hennekens & Buring, 1987).

***Basic Research***

The available evidence suggests that saturated and *trans* fats are associated with increased risks of CHD while monounsaturated and polyunsaturated fats are associated with decreased risks. One can classify polyunsaturated fatty acids on the basis of their chemical structure into two groups: omega-6 (n-6) fatty acids and omega-3 (n-3) fatty acids. Parent fatty acids of both the n-6 family of polyunsaturated fatty acids (linoleic acid) and the n-3 family (α-linoleic acid) are essential nutrients for humans. Meat is the primary food source of long-chain omega-6 fatty acid, arachidonic acid (AA), while fish is the primary food source of the omega-3 fatty acid, eicosapentaenoic acid (EPA). The specific biological functions of fatty acids depend on the number and position of double bonds and the length of the acyl chain. Both AA and EPA are 20-carbon fatty acids and are precursors for the formation of prostaglandins, thromboxane, and leukotrienes—hormone-like agents that are members of a larger family of substances called eicosanoids. Eicosanoids are localized tissue hormones that seem to be one of the fundamental regulatory classes of molecules in most higher forms of life. They do not travel in the blood, but are created in the cells to regulate a large number of processes, including the movement of calcium and other substances into and out of cells, dilation and contraction of muscles, inhibition and promotion of clotting, regulation of secretions including digestive juices and hormones, and control of fertility, cell division, and growth (Balk et al., 2004).

AA is the precursor of a group of eicosanoids that includes series-2 prostaglandins and series-4 leukotrienes. EPA is the precursor to a group of eicosanoids including series-3 prostaglandins and series-5 leukotrienes. The series-2 prostaglandins and series-4 leukotrienes derived from AA are involved in intense actions, such as accelerating platelet aggregation, enhancing vasoconstriction, and synthesizing inflammatory mediators in response to physiological stressors. The series-3 prostaglandins and series-5 leukotrienes that are derived from EPA are less potent physiologically than those derived from AA. More specifically, the series-3 prostaglandins are formed at a slower rate and work to attenuate excessive series-2 prostaglandins. Thus, the adequate production of the series-3 prostaglandins, which are derived from EPA, may protect against heart attack and stroke as well as inflammatory diseases such as arthritis, lupus, and asthma. In addition, animal studies demonstrate that omega-3 fatty acids, such as EPA and docosahexaenoic acid (DHA), engage in multiple cytoprotective activities that may contribute to antiarrhythmic properties (Balk et al., 2004).

Several biological mechanisms of fish oils were identified that might explain why they may decrease the risk of stroke in humans. These effects include a reduction in the production of thromboxane, an increase in prostacyclin production by endothelial cells, a decrease in blood viscosity, a reduction in the vasospastic response to catecholamines, an increased fibrinolysis, a beneficial effect on the concentration of blood lipids consistent with a reduction of cardiovascular risk, and a decrease in blood pressure (Vanschoonbeek et al., 2003).

**Lipids**

Compared with saturated fats, n-6 fatty acids from oils such as safflower, sunflower, and corn oils tend to lower the serum LDL- and high-density lipoprotein (HDL)-C as well as triglycerides, providing plausible mechanisms for beneficial effects on CHD. The n-3 fatty acids have a smaller effect on cholesterol than the n-6 fatty acids, but have a larger effect on lowering triglycerides (Skerrett & Hennekens, 2003). One of the first demonstrated effects of fish oil, this (n-3) polyunsaturated fatty acid (PUFA) effect is particularly prominent in hypertriglyceridemic patients and is explained by a reduced secretion of very low density lipoprotein (VLDL) from the liver. Fish oil only partially improves the lipid profile in blood, so no consistent effect exists of (n-3) PUFA on total cholesterol level or cholesterol in LDL (Vanschoonbeek et al., 2003).

**Ventricular Arrhythmias**

Cardiac arrhythmias can be fatal, causing sudden death, or can result in stroke, MI, congestive heart failure, and peripheral emboli, among other types of CVD. As demonstrated in animal models, the ingestion of high-levels of omega-3 fatty acids could essentially abolish fatal ventricular fibrillation. Several plausible mechanisms can explain why omega-3 fatty acids decrease the development of arrhythmias. Various animal and in vitro experiments show that omega-3 fatty acids directly modulate sodium, potassium, and calcium channels. By incorporating phospholipids into the cell membrane, the excitation–contraction coupling that can result in arrhythmia is reduced. Omega-3 fatty acids also modulate various intracellular enzymes involved in controlling the contraction and relaxation cycles of myocytes. Fish oil (EPA and DHA acids) also affects adrenergic receptors, membrane proteins whose function in the heart is to transmit the neuroendocrine message of the catecholamines (adrenaline and its derivatives). This action is similar in principle to that of beta-blockers, a group of key cardiovascular drugs used to decrease the cardiac effects of catecholamines. Omega-3 long-chain PUFA also simulate the actions of calcium channel blockers by increasing intracellular calcium sequestration and interfering with receptor-operated calcium channels, thus lowering calcium influx. The effect of omega-3 fatty acids on prostanoids and leukotrienes also theoretically reduces the arrhythmia potential of cardiac myocytes (Balk et al., 2004).

**Atrial Arrhythmias**

The incidence of atrial fibrillation increases dramatically with age (lifetime risk after age 40 is 1 in 4) and results in fatigue, reduced exercise tolerance, and increased risk and severity of stroke. Once atrial fibrillation develops, anticoagulation with coumadin reduces the risk of stroke with increased risks of bleeding. Aspirin is of less benefit, but confers less risk of bleeding and is recommended for low-to-moderate-risk patients, but other treatment options are limited (Antithrombotic Trialists' Collaboration, 2002; Fuster et al., 2006). Thus, the prevention of atrial fibrillation should be the paramount goal (Mozaffarian, 2007). Sarrazin et al. (2007) evaluated the effect of fish oil in a canine model of vagally induced atrial fibrillation. Adult dogs were fed regular chow or chow plus fish oil (1.2 g/day, containing 480 mg/day of EPA and DHA) for 14 days. Atrial fibrillation was induced by both extra stimulus (premature atrial complex, or PAC) and burst-pacing techniques. In the fish-oil-fed dogs, the risk of sustained atrial fibrillation was 70% to 80% lower for that induced by PAC and 42% lower for that induced by burst-pacing ($P < 0.05$ for each comparison). Myocardial biopsies revealed a 100% rise in atrial n-3 fatty acid levels and a 50% fall in atrial connexin levels with fish oil consumption. In a substudy, control dogs with inducible atrial fibrillation were re-evaluated after an intravenous infusion of fish oil (1.4 g); induction of sustained atrial fibrillation by PAC was less frequent than before the infusion. The fish oil treatments were neither randomized nor blinded, raising the possibility of bias due to differences in the experimental groups or in the investigators' induction or ascertainment of arrhythmia. The intravenous substudy lacked an appropriate control group, since dogs with inducible atrial fibrillation in the first attempt were simply re-examined after an intravenous infusion. Thus, one might see the decreased frequency of atrial fibrillation during the second attempt in any group of dogs in which the arrhythmia was inducible in a first attempt, reflecting a type of regression toward the mean (Mozaffarian, 2007).

The generalizability of these findings to spontaneously occurring atrial fibrillation in humans is unclear. In a randomized trial in dogs, fish oil consumption has clear anti-fibrillatory effects as well as effects on connexins. Taken together, these findings suggest a novel potential mechanism for the antiarrhythmic effects of n-3 fatty acids (Sarrazin et al., 2007). These results raise the possibility that a simple, low-risk, and low-cost dietary intervention could reduce the incidence of atrial fibrillation, the most common early complication of cardiac surgery and the most common cardiac arrhythmia in the general population (Mozaffarian, 2007). Recent findings show that fish consumption is also associated with a reduction in the incidence of atrial fibrillation in the elderly (Mozaffarian et al., 2004) and in patients undergoing coronary bypass surgery (Calo et al., 2005).

**Blood Pressure**

Randomized trials of omega-3 fatty acids in fish oils or dietary fish provide cogent evidence for a blood pressure-lowering effect. A meta-analysis of 31 placebo-controlled trials revealed an overall reduction of –3.0/–1.5 mmHg with a significant dose–response effect estimated at –0.66/–0.35 mmHg/g omega-3 fatty acid (Morris et al., 1993). The blood pressure-lowering effect was strongest in hypertensives (treated and untreated; –3.4/–2.0 mmHg). A meta-analysis of 36 trials showed that blood pressure was reduced by –2.1/–1.6 mmHg following omega-3 fatty acids. Furthermore, the blood pressure-lowering effects were greater in older (>45 years; –3.5/–2.4) and in hypertensive (≥140/90 mmHg; –4.0/–2.5) subjects (Geleijnse et al., 2002). Several double-blind placebo-controlled trials demonstrate the significant benefits of omega-3 fatty acids on blood pressure in hypertensives. The hypotensive effects of omega-3 fatty acids are potentiated by sodium restriction and the concurrent usage of antihypertensive drugs. Fish oils amplified the hypotensive effects of propranolol, a beta-adrenoceptor antagonist, but not angiotensin-converting enzyme inhibitors, in hypertensive patients. Others reported that blood pressure was reduced by –3.1/–1.8 mmHg in treated hypertensives who were taking either beta-blockers or diuretics alone, or a combination of the two. The data also suggest that EPA and DHA have differing hemodynamic and anti-atherogenic properties. DHA may be more favorable in lowering blood pressure and heart rate and in improving vascular function.

The AHA advises that a healthy eating pattern for the management of blood pressure and blood lipids should include, among other nutrients, an increased fish consumption of at least two servings a week. On the basis of the currently available, although incomplete, totality of evidence, the use of omega-3 fatty acids in conjunction with pharmacological agents for the treatment of hypertension was suggested (Mori, 2006).

**Thrombosis**

The n-3 fatty acids lower fibrinogen, reduce the production of thromboxane, and decrease platelet aggregation without increasing the risk of hemorrhagic stroke (Skerrett & Hennekens, 2003; Vanschoonbeek et al., 2003).

A high-dose supplementation of omega-3 fatty acids (e.g., 15 g/day of EPA) reduces platelet aggregation without an adverse effect on vasodilation by inhibiting the formation of thromboxane $A_2$ in platelets without substantially reducing the synthesis of prostaglandin $I_2$ in vascular endothelial cells. Furthermore, EPA (in part, converted from DHA) is transformed into a nonaggregatory agent, thromboxane $A_3$, which increases the synthesis of prostaglandin $I_3$, a vasodilator, leading to further reductions in platelet aggregation and increases in vasodilation. These alterations become apparent 3–4 days after the intake of a fish oil supplement and persist for up to 10 weeks after supplement use ceases (Skerrett & Hennekens, 2003). In addition, a high-dose omega-3 fatty acid supplement also lowers blood pressure levels in hypertensive persons (Morris et al., 1993) and reduces plasma fibrinogen concentrations in healthy volunteers, effects that may contribute to the prevention of atherosclerosis and thrombosis (Skerrett & Hennekens, 2003).

**Inflammation**

Fish oil is believed to suppress the inflammatory response through a reduction of proinflammatory cytokines. A small randomized trial in healthy elderly adults demonstrated that taking fish oil inhibited the production of pro-inflammatory cytokines (Wu et al., 2004). In vitro studies suggest that omega-3 fatty acids inhibit the 5-lipoxygenase pathway in neutrophils and monocytes, as well as the leukotriene B4-mediated functions of neutrophils, and thus may have anti-inflammatory properties which decrease the risk of stroke. Inflammation is a precursor to atherosclerosis, and C-reactive protein (CRP), an inflammatory marker, predicts the future risk of CVD, including stroke (Bernal-Pacheco & Roman, 2007). Inflammation is an important predictor of CHD and stroke, particularly in patients with hypertension and diabetes. A recent meta-analysis of five population-based prospective observational cohort studies involving almost ten thousand subjects with a long-term follow-up showed that apparently healthy individuals with the highest CRP levels had a 70% increased risk of stroke compared to those with the lowest levels. CRP is an accurate predictor of vascular disease in general and stroke in particular (Bernal-Pacheco & Roman, 2007; Ridker et al., 1997).

**Other Possible Mechanisms**

These fatty acids also reduce the production of platelet-derived growth factor-like protein from vascular endothelial cells, which may attenuate the proliferation of endothelial cells and the development of atherosclerosis (Skerrett & Hennekens, 2003).

In addition to these potentially beneficial changes, which could explain a reduced risk of ischemic stroke, omega-3 fatty acid-associated decreases in whole-blood viscosity and increases in capillary blood flow may play a role in the prevention of lacunar infarction, the pathogenesis of which involves occlusion of small cerebral arteries (Skerrett & Hennekens, 2003).

Basic research suggests beneficial effects on the cardiovascular system through mechanisms that modulate enzymatic activities, directly interacting with calcium channels, enzymes on eicosanoid pathways, and protein kinases to provide protective effects. The n-3 PUFAs can also be incorporated into phospholipids, alter signaling processes, and generate cardioprotective eicosanoids. However, most of the studies that elucidated these mechanisms of action were performed in cell culture and animal models, which may not be directly applicable to humans. Possibly, n-3 PUFAs may not be able to affect all the cellular pathways simultaneously, and individual variation may exist based on the health status (Siddiqui et el., 2008).

***Descriptive Studies***

Descriptive studies are useful to formulate hypotheses (Hennekens & Buring, 1987). One of the earliest observations regarding fish oil and stroke emerged from the decades-long assessment of diet and health among a case series of Greenlandic

Inuits. In this population with a very high intake of fatty fish, and thus omega-3 fatty acids, an excess risk existed of mortality from hemorrhagic stroke, compared with Danish whites (Skerrett & Hennekens, 2003). An ecologic study demonstrated an inverse association between fish consumption and stroke mortality in 36 countries. Using countrywide data from the Food and Agriculture Organization and the WHO, Zhang and colleagues (1999) found that the logarithm of fish consumption was significantly and inversely associated with both log all-cause ischemic heart disease and stroke mortality in both sexes across three time periods, 1961–1963, 1979–1981, and 1989–1991, after adjustment for confounding factors (Skerrett & Hennekens, 2003).

### *Observational Analytic Studies*

#### Case Control

In a population-based, case-control study in Perth, Western Australia, 536 individuals who met the WHO criteria for stroke drawn from a population-based register of acute cerebrovascular events were matched for age and sex with up to five control subjects drawn from the same geographic area (Jamrozik et al., 1994). Apparently, healthy individuals who ate fish more than two times a month had a lower risk of first-ever stroke, with a relative risk (RR) of 0.60 [95% confidence interval (CI), 0.36–0.99], and primary intracerebral hemorrhage, with an RR of 0.43 (95% CI, 0.20–0.96). No significant association was observed for ischemic stroke (RR, 0.90; 95% CI, 0.60–1.36) (Skerrett & Hennekens, 2003).

#### Cohort

Several prospective cohort studies examined the association between individuals who consume high amounts of fish and a stroke, with inconsistent results (Tables 3.4 [a–e]) (Wang et al., 2004). Observational data from the Physicians' Health Study showed a possible but not statistically significant association between apparently healthy men who ate fish and total stroke (Morris et al., 1995). Among 21,185 initially healthy physicians followed for 4 years, 173 incident cases of stroke were recorded. The RRs of total stroke for categories of fish intake were 1.0 for fewer than one meal/week, 0.9 (95% CI, 0.5–1.2) for one fish meal/week; 0.8 (95% CI, 0.5–1.2) for two to four fish meals a week; and 0.6 (95% CI, 0.3–1.6) for five or more fish meals a week ($P = 0.13$ for trend) after an adjustment for age and a randomized treatment assignment (Morris et al., 1995). The RRs were similar for quintiles of omega-3 fatty acid intake, and did not change after an adjustment for the history of hypertension, hypercholesterolemia, diabetes mellitus, or angina pectoris, parental history of MI before age 60 years, obesity, exercise, smoking, alcohol use, saturated fat intake, and vitamin supplement use. Notably, one-half of the men in the Physicians' Health Study were also taking aspirin, so any beneficial effect of fish intake may have been attenuated.

The Chicago Western Electric study, which compared the baseline assessment of fish consumption and a 30-year risk of fatal and nonfatal stroke among 1,847 men ages 40–55 years who were initially free of CHD and stroke showed no association (Orencia et al., 1996). Men consuming ≥35 g/day of fish had a higher age-adjusted death rate from stroke (23.5 per 10,000 person-years) than men consuming less fish (Orencia et al., 1996). Compared with men who reported consuming no fish, hazard ratios were 1.34 (95% CI, 0.53–3.41) for those consuming ≥ 35 g/day, 0.96 (95% CI, 0.41–2.21) for those consuming 18–34 g/day, and 1.00 (95% CI, 0.43–2.33) for those consuming 1–17 g/day. This study relied only on death certificates and information from the Health Care Financing Administration for stroke ascertainment, so random misclassification would have obscured any inverse association (Skerrett & Hennekens, 2003).

Three studies demonstrated a significant inverse association between fish consumption and stroke. In the Zutphen Study, dietary histories were obtained in 1960, 1965, and 1970 from 552 men living in the town of Zutphen, The Netherlands, who were ages 50–69 years in 1970 (Keli et al., 1994). Among men who consumed more than 20 g of fish a day in 1970, the hazard ratio for stroke in the period 1970–1985 was 0.49 (95% CI, 0.24–0.99), which did not change after an adjustment for potential confounders, including age, systolic blood pressure, cigarette smoking, serum total cholesterol, energy intake, alcohol consumption, and prescribed diet (Keli et al., 1994).

The First National Health and Nutrition Examination Survey (NHANES I) Epidemiologic Followup Study was a prospective cohort study of a national sample of white and black women and men ages 45–74 years at baseline in 1971–1975 who did not report a history of stroke at that time (Gillum et al., 1996). White women who consumed fish more than once a week had an age-adjusted RR of 0.55 (95% CI, 0.32–0.93) compared with women who never consumed fish; no association was seen among white men. Among black women and men, the age-adjusted RR of stroke was 0.51 (95% CI, 0.30–0.88) for those who reported any fish consumption compared with those reporting never consuming fish (Gillum et al., 1996).

In the largest of these studies, the NHS, 79,839 initially healthy women ages 34–59 years in 1980 completed a detailed food frequency questionnaire at a baseline that included fish and other frequently eaten foods (Iso et al., 2001). After 14 years of follow-up, 574 incident strokes were documented, including 119 subarachnoid hemorrhages, 62 intraparenchymal hemorrhages, 303 ischemic strokes (264 thrombotic and 39 embolic infarctions), and 90 strokes of an undetermined type. Among thrombotic infarctions, 90 large-artery occlusive infarctions and 142 lacunar infarctions were identified. After an adjustment for age, smoking, and other cardiovascular risk factors, the multivariate RRs of total stroke were 0.93 (95% CI, 0.65–1.34) for individuals who ate fish one to three times a week, 0.73 (95% CI, 0.47–1.14) for two to four times a week, and 0.48 (95% CI, 0.21–1.06) for five or more times a week ($P = 0.06$ for trend), compared with women who ate fish less than once a month.(Iso et al., 2001). Women in the highest quintile of the intake of long-chain omega-3 PUFAs had a significantly reduced risk of total stroke (RR, 0.72; 95% CI, 0.53–0.99) (Skerrett & Hennekens, 2003).

Regarding stroke subtypes in the NHS, a significantly reduced risk of thrombotic infarction was observed among women who ate fish two or more times a week (RR, 0.49; 95% CI, 0.26–0.93), while a nonsignificantly decreased risk (RR, 0.67; 95% CI, 0.42–1.07) was observed among women in the highest quintile of omega-3 PUFA intake. No association was observed between the consumption of fish or omega-3 PUFA intake and the risk of hemorrhagic stroke. When stratified by aspirin use, fish and omega-3 PUFA intake was significantly and inversely associated with the risk of thrombotic infarction among the subgroup of women who did not regularly take aspirin. Chance, bias, or uncontrolled, but not uncontrollable, confounding are unlikely to be plausible alternative explanations for these findings, given the large size and high follow-up rates in this cohort, and the adjustments made for age, smoking, and other cardiovascular risk factors. These data are compatible with clinical studies demonstrating that the prolongation of bleeding time is associated with an intake of omega-3 fatty acids of more than 3 g/day (Skerrett & Hennekens, 2003).

In summary, the NHS reported that the relative risk of total stroke was lower, although not significantly so, among women who regularly ate fish than among those who did not. A significant decrease in the risk of thrombotic stroke (relative risk, 0.49; 95% CI, 0.26–0.93) was observed among women who ate fish at least two times a week compared with women who ate fish less than once a month, after an adjustment for age, smoking, and other cardiovascular risk factors; a nonsignificant decrease was observed among women in the highest quintile of long-chain omega-3 PUFA intake. No association was observed between the consumption of fish or fish oil and hemorrhagic stroke (Iso et al., 2001). These data support the hypothesis that the consumption of fish several times a week reduces the risk of thrombotic stroke but does not increase the risk of hemorrhagic stroke. Despite the limitations of these observational study data, it is tempting to speculate that the reduction in lacunar infarction observed in the NHS could be due to the ability of dietary omega-3 fatty acids to reduce insulin resistance and glucose intolerance, both of which are risk factors for this event. That no excess risk of either subarachnoid or intraparenchymal hemorrhage with an intake of fish or omega-3 fatty acids was observed among women in the NHS was not surprising. While bleeding time is prolonged when the intake of omega-3 fatty acids exceeds 3 g/day, this level of intake corresponds approximately to the ingestion of fish three times or more a day, a level of consumption attained by less than 0.1% of the women in this population (Skerrett & Hennekens, 2003).

Among the published cohort studies, considerable differences existed among the populations studied, as well as in the estimates of fish or omega-3 fatty acids consumed. Most of the large cohort studies found fish consumption was associated with lower rates of all cause mortality and CVD outcomes, but several studies reported no significant or negative results for the CVD outcomes. A significant benefit for stroke was reported in only one study (He et al., 2002).

Five of the cohort studies estimated the amount of fish oil consumed, and eight studies estimated fish intake. These studies included the large U.S. cohorts of the

NHS (Iso et al., 2001), the HPFS (He et al., 2002), and the Physicians' Health Study (Morris et al., 1995), which followed subjects for 14, 12, and 4 years, respectively. Together, these three studies were comprised of a total of about 145,000 men and women. Only the HPFS reported a significant reduction of ischemic strokes with any level of fish consumption above the lowest quintile. In the NHS, a nonsignificant trend existed of decreased strokes with increasing fish consumption. Other studies showed a weak stroke-risk reduction, no effect, or a stroke-risk increase. The fish oil estimates and fish estimates gave similar results (Wang et al., 2004).

Only one study addressed the potential confounding effect of a specific variable (i.e., aspirin treatment). Iso et al. (2001) analyzed subgroups of women in the NHS who took aspirin regularly versus those who did not. Stroke events were reduced in both groups at most levels of fish intake, and a statistically significant trend with increasing fish consumption was found in women who did not take aspirin regularly (Wang et al., 2004).

A report based on NHANES I that separately analyzed data for men and women found a trend of decreased stroke with increasing fish consumption for women between ages 45 and 74, but not for men (Wang et al., 2004).

**Meta-analysis of Cohort Studies**

Differences in study populations, sample size, assessment of fish intake, and stroke endpoint, as well as an adjustment for confounding variables, and the misclassification from failure to separate ischemic from hemorrhagic stroke may have contributed to the inconsistency of the results from individual cohort studies. To provide a more reliable assessment of whether individuals who self-select for higher intakes of fish have a decreased risk of stroke, a meta-analysis of all published prospective studies was done (He et al., 2004).

In this meta-analysis, individuals who consumed high amounts of fish in their diets had a decreased risk of a stroke, particularly ischemic, although a strong dose-response relationship was not observed, there was no significant effect on hemorrhagic stroke. The findings also suggested that individuals who eat fish as seldom as 1 – 3 times a month may have a reduced risk of ischemic stroke (He et al., 2004).

### *Randomized Trials*

Randomized trials of sufficient size, dose, and duration provide the most reliable design strategy to test the most plausible small-to-moderate benefits (or harm) of interventions (Table 3.4) (Wang et al., 2004). In the randomized Gruppo Italiano per lo Studio della Sopravvivenza nell'Infarto Miocardico Prevenzione (GISSI Prevention) trial, 11,324 Italian men and women who had experienced an MI in the preceding 3 months were assigned to 850 mg/day of omega-3 fatty acids, 300 mg/day of vitamin E, both, or neither in an open-label design (GISSI-Prevenzione Investigators, 1999). After 3.5 years, those receiving omega-3 fatty acids had a 10%–15% decreased risk of the primary endpoint, a combination of all-cause death, nonfatal MI, and nonfatal stroke. This benefit was largely attributed to a decrease in the risk of CVD (Table 3.5) (GISSI-Prevenzione Investigators, 1999).

Secondary analyses of fatal and nonfatal stroke showed no significant increase or decrease in risk among those randomized to omega-3 fatty acids (Skerrett & Hennekens, 2003).

**Meta-analysis of Randomized Trials**

A meta-analysis of trials regarding the efficacy of omega-3 fatty acids in preventing cardiovascular mortality and morbidity in patients with CHD was undertaken to assess whether the same pattern of results was present in the trials preceding GISSI or whether a benefit on nonfatal events would become apparent after grouping the trials. The following endpoints were assessed: (i) fatal MI, (ii) death from all causes, (iii) nonfatal acute MI, (iv) nonfatal stroke, and (v) unstable angina. RRs of outcomes are presented with their 95% CIs (Yzebe & Lievre, 2004).

A search of the MEDLINE (1966–2003), EMBASE databases, proceedings abstracts, and references of reviewed articles was performed. Randomized controlled trials of the efficacy of omega-3 fatty acids among adults with recent or acute MI or angina were selected and are summarized in Yzebe & Lievre, 2004.

Outcomes measured included: mortality from all causes, fatal and nonfatal MI, nonfatal stroke, and angina. Ten trials with 14,727 patients were included. The mean age in each group was 59 years. The daily intake of omega-3 fatty acids for a mean duration of 37 months decreased all causes of mortality by 16% [RR 0.84, 95% CI (0.76; 0.94)] and the incidence of death due to MI by 24% [0.76, (0.66; 0.88)]. No significant effect was found for the other outcomes. Because of the suboptimal quality of the studies included in the meta-analysis and the absence of data in patients receiving statins, these results do not justify adding fish oils systematically in CHD patients (Yzebe & Lievre, 2004).

Cholesterol-lowering drugs were used in <5% of patients at the baseline in GISSI, but the proportion increased to 46% at 42 months. Apparently no patients received lipid-lowering drugs in DART. Information regarding lipid-lowering therapy was not available in the other trials (Yzebe & Lievre, 2004).

No statistically significant effect of omega-3 fatty acids was found for the other outcomes, with a 1% benefit for angina pectoris to a 36% adverse effect for a nonfatal stroke (Yzebe & Lievre, 2004).

## Conclusion

At present, the totality of evidence, while incomplete, provides intriguing, although inconsistent evidence to support the hypothesis that fish oil reduces the risk of stroke, principally thrombotic, and does not increase the risk of hemorrhagic stroke. Basic research provides plausible mechanisms for benefit. Not surprisingly, some, but not all observational studies suggest that individuals who self-select for high intakes of fish oil through diet or supplements have reduced risks of stroke. Some conclude harm,

**Table 3.4a. Observational Studies of Effects of Omega-3 Fatty Acids and Fish Consumption on Mortality and CVD Outcomes**

| Author, year | Outcome definition | Results | Funding source |
|---|---|---|---|
| Caicoya, 2002 | Stroke was defined, according to WHO criteria, as rapidly developing clinical symptoms and/or signs of local and at times global loss of cerebral function with symptoms lasting >24 h or leading to death, with no apparent cause other than vascular. | OR of stroke (all categories combined) with increasing fish consumption (multivariate)<br>1–22.5 g/d: 0.30 (0.12–0.7); 23–45 g/d: 0.44 (0.18–1.41); 46–90 g/d: 0.59 (0.24–1.47); 91–250g/d: 0.76 (0.27–2.10)<br>Adjusted for HTN, alcohol, AF, PAD<br><br>OR of ischemic stroke with increasing fish consumption (multivariate)<br>11.3–28.7 g/d: 1.05 (0.64–1.65; 28.8–46.5 g/d: 0.90 (0.55–1.48); >46.5 g/d: 1.98 (1.08–3.45)<br>OR of stroke (all categories combined) with increasing omega-3 intake (multivariate)<br>116–319 mg/d: 1.14 (0.60–1.88); 320–659 mg/d: 1.37 (0.91–2.20); >659 mg/d: 1.76 (0.96–3.26)<br>Adjusted for age, sex, HTN, alcohol, CAD, AF, PAD, energy intake | Spanish Ministry of Education, local and regional hospitals |
| Gillum, 1996 (NHANES 1 Epidemiologic Follow-up Study) | Incident stroke cases met the following criteria: death certificate with underlying or nonunderlying cause of death coded according to ICD-9, and/or hospital or nursing-home stay during the flow-up period with any discharge diagnosis according to ICD-9. Nonhemorrhagic stroke was defined by underlying or nonunderlying cause of death or hospital discharge diagnosis from ICD-9. | RR for stroke (both bleeds and ischemic stroke) and fish-consumption frequency<br>Women aged 45–74 <1/wk: 0.78 (0.54–1.12)<br>Women aged 45–74 1/wk: 0.77 (0.53–1.13)<br>Women aged 45–74 >1/wk: 0.55* (0.32–0.93)<br>Men aged 45–74 <1wk: 1.27 (0.83–1.96)<br>Men aged 45–74 1wk: 1.23 (0.79–1.91)<br>Men aged 45–74 >1wk: 0.85 (0.49–1.46)<br><br>RR for stroke incidence, stroke death, and fish-consumption frequency<br>Never: Stroke incidence 1.00; Stroke death 1.00<br>Any: Stroke incidence 0.51 (0.30–0.88) (*P*<0.05); Stroke death 0.26 (0.11–0.64) (*P*<0.01)<br>Adjusted for age, smoking, diabetes, heart disease, education, SBP, serum albumin, serum cholesterol, BMI, alcohol, physical activity.<br>*statistically significant | NIH, NCI, NHLBI |

Table 3.4b. Observational Studies of Effects of Omega-3 Fatty Acids and Fish Consumption on Mortality and CVD Outcomes

| Author, year | Outcome definition | Results | Funding source |
|---|---|---|---|
| He, 2002 (Health Professional Follow-up Study) | Stroke was defined as sudden or rapid onset of typical neurological defect of >24 h duration or leading to death attributable to CV event. Strokes were classified as ischemic (embolism or thrombosis), hemorrhagic (subarachnoid and intracerebral), unknown according to National Survey of Stroke | RR of total stroke based on fish consumption (multivariate)<br>1–3 servings/mo 1/mo 2–4/wk >5/wk<br>0.73 (0.48–1.10) 0.74 (0.52–1.04) 0.67 (0.46–0.96) 0.83 (0.53–1.29)<br>RR of ischemic stroke based on fish consumption (multivariate analysis)<br>0.57 (0.35–0.95) 0.56 (0.37–0.84) 0.55 (0.36–0.85) 0.54 (0.31–0.94)<br>RR of hemorrhagic stroke based on fish consumption (multivariate analysis)<br>1.81 (0.57–5.66) 1.40 (0.49–3.99) 0.96 (0.32–2.89) 1.55 (0.45–5.35)<br>RR of total stroke based on omega-3 intake (multivariate)<br>0.05–<0.2g/d 0.2–0.4g/d 0.4–<0.6g/d >0.6g/d<br>0.77 (0.52–1.14) 0.77 (0.52–1.14) 0.71 (0.46–1.10) 0.87 (0.56–1.37)<br>RR of ischemic stroke based on omega-3 intake (multivariate analysis)<br>0.56 (0.35–0.88) 0.63 (0.40–0.98) 0.54 (0.32–0.91) 0.73 (0.43–1.25)<br>RR of hemorrhagic stroke based on omega-3 intake (multivariate analysis)<br>1.29 (0.45–3.75) 1.02 (0.35–3.00) 0.89 (0.27–2.87) 1.14 (0.34–3.84)<br>Adjusted for BMI, physical activity, history of HTN, smoking, aspirin use, fish oil, total calories, total fat, saturated fat, *trans*-unsaturated fat, K, Mg, servings of fruits and vegetables, hypercholesterolemia. No significant associations were found between fish or omega-3 intake and risk of hemorrhagic stroke. Inverse association between fish intake and risk of ischemic stroke was not materially modified by use of aspirin or vitamin E intake. Tests for interaction were not statistically significant. | NIH |
| Iso, 2001 (Nurses' Health Study) 14 y follow-up | Stroke was confirmed according to the criteria of the National Survey of Stroke. Ischemic stroke included cerebral infarction caused by thrombi or by emboli from extracranial sources. | RR of total stroke and average frequency of fish intake (multivariate)<br>1–3/mo 1/wk 2–4/wk >5/wk<br>Total Stroke 0.93 (0.65–1.34) 0.78 (0.55–1.12) 0.73 (0.47–1.14) 0.48 (0.21–1.06)<br>Ischemic stroke 0.83 (0.50–1.38) 0.69 (0.42–1.14) 0.63 (0.34–1.15) 0.38 (0.12–1.19)<br>Hemorrhagic 1.36 (0.67–2.76) 1.13 (0.56–2.30) 0.93 (0.39–2.21) 1.02 (0.26–4.09)<br>RR of total stroke according to quintiles of EPA+DHA median intake g/d (multivariate)<br>0.118 0.171 0.221 0.481<br>Total stroke 0.87 (0.66–1.11) 0.69 (0.53–0.89) 0.83 (0.63–1.08) 0.72 (0.53–0.99)<br>Ischemic stroke 0.83 (0.59–1.18) 0.67 (0.47–0.98) 0.82 (0.57–1.18) 0.71 (0.46–1.10)<br>Hemorrhagic 0.94 (0.61–1.43) 0.66 (0.41–1.05) 0.93 (0.58–1.49) 0.76 (0.43–1.37)<br>Adjusted for joules, BMI, alcohol intake, menopause and HRT, exercise, aspirin use, vitamin use, history of HTN, frequency of fruits and vegetables, saturated fat, *trans*-unsaturated fat, linoleic acid, animal protein, Ca. | NIH |

**Table 3.4c. Observational Studies of Effects of Omega-3 Fatty Acids and Fish Consumption on Mortality and CVD Outcomes**

| Author, year | Outcome definition | Results | Funding source |
|---|---|---|---|
| Keli, 1994 8303739 (Zutphen Study) | Stroke was defined as sudden onset of neurological paralysis of >24 h duration or leading to death. Fatal strokes were coded according to ICD-8 | Hazard rations for stroke incidence (bleeds and ischemic stroke) for fish estimates<br>Fish consumption >20 g/d vs <20 0.49 (0.24–1.01)<br>Fish consumption, Always vs Never 0.71 (0.38–1.33)<br>Adjusted for age SBP, serum cholesterol, smoking, intake of energy, alcohol, prescribed diet. | Netherlands Preventive Funds, and Public Health Service Curacao |
| Kinjo, Y., 1999 | Causes of death coded according to ICD-7: 330–334 | Mortality risk of cerebrovascular disease for fish intake<br>All cerebrovasic Dis. (Death, RR) / Hemorrhagic stroke (Death, RR) / Ischemic stroke (Death, RR)<br><1 time/wk: 713 1.00 / 304 1.00 / 236 1.00<br>1–3 / wk: 6369 0.98 (0.90-1.06) / 2825 1.02 (0.90-1.15) / 2266 1.05 (0.91-1.20)<br>>4/wk: 3948 0.86 (0.79-0.94) / 1644 0.87 (0.76-0.98) / 1582 0.99 (0.86-1.14)<br>Risk of mortality from cerebrovascular disease was inversely associated with fish consumption. | Promotion of Cancer Research in Japan |
| Morris, 1995 (Physicians Health Study) | Cases of nonfatal MI were confirmed on the basis of WHO criteria. Nonfatal stroke was defined as a typical and sudden neurologic deficit, lasting >24 h and attributable to CV event. CV deaths include AMI, ischemic heart disease, sudden death, stroke, other CV disease (ICD-10) | RR of CVD outcomes and level of fish consumption meals/wk (multivariate)<br>fish/meals-wk: <1 / 1 / 2–4 / >5 / trend<br>Total MI: 1.0 / 1.5 (1.1-2.1) / 1.3 (0.9-1.9) / 0.9 (0.4-1.8) / P=0.72<br>Nonfatal MI: 1.0 / 1.4 (0.9-2.0) / 1.2 (0.8-1.8) / 0.8 (0.4-1.7) / P=0.79<br>Stroke: 1.0 / 0.9 (0.6-1.3) / 0.8 (0.5-1.2) / 0.6 (0.3-1.6) / P=0.13<br>CV deaths: 1.0 / 2.6 (1.4-4.8) / 1.7 (0.9-3.4) / 2.2 (0.8-5.9) / P=0.35<br>Total CV events: 1.0 / 1.3 (1.0-1.6) / 1.1 (0.81.4) / 0.9 (0.6-1.5) / P=0.65<br><br>RR of CVD outcomes and quintiles of omega-3 intake g/wk (multivariate)<br>omega-3 intake g/wk: 0.5–<1.0 / 1.0–<1.7 / 1.7–<2.3 / >2.3 / trend<br>Total MI: 1.6 (1.1-2.4) / 1.4 (1.0-2.2) / 1.2 (0.8-1.8) / 1.2 (0.8-1.8) / P=0.98<br>Nonfatal MI: 1.5 (1.0-2.3) / 1.3 (0.9-2.0) / 1.2 (0.8-1.9) / 1.1 (0.7-1.8) / P=0.99<br>Stroke: 0.9 (0.6-1.6) / 1.1 (0.7-1.8) / 0.7 (04-1.2) / 1.0 (0.6-1.6) / P=0.49<br>CV deaths: 1.6 (0.8-3.0) / 1.6 (0.9-3.0) / 0.9 (0.5-1.9) / 1.5 (0.8-2.9) / P=0.80<br>Total CV events: 1.3 (1.0-1.8) / 1.3 (1.0-1.7) / 0.9 (0.7-1.3) / 1.1 (0.8-1.5) / P=0.63<br>Total CV events include nonfatal MI, nonfatal stroke, CV death<br>Adjusted for age, aspirin and beta-carotene, smoking, alcohol, obesity, diabetes, vigorous exercise, parental history of MI, history of HTN, history of hpyercholesterolemia, vitamin use, saturated fat intake | NIH, National Institute of Environ Health Sciences |

Table 3.4d. Observational Studies of Effects of Omega-3 Fatty Acids and Fish Consumption on Mortality and CVD Outcomes

| Author, year | Outcome definition | Results | Funding source |
|---|---|---|---|
| Orencia, 1996 (Western Electric Study) | Only causes of death in Part I of death certificate were considered definitive endpoints. Stroke was defined as any mention of CVD (ICD-9) with exception of TIA. (There are too few ICH to stratify by stroke subtype.) | Hazards ration for fatal stroke (bleeds and ischemic stroke) and fish consumption<br>1–17 gd 0.98 (0.42–2.27)<br>18–34 g/d 0.95 (0.42–2.27)<br>>35g/d 1.47 (0.60–3.61)<br>Hazards ratio for fatal stroke and nonfatal and fish consumption<br>1–17 g/d 0.94 (0.58–1.51)<br>18–34 g/d 0.89 (0.56–1.43)<br>>35 g/d 1.28 (0.762–2.14)<br>Adjusted for age, SBP, smoking, cholesterol, diabetes, ECG abnormalities, salt, alcohol, vitamin C | NHLBI, Chicago Health Research Foundation, Otho Sprague Foundation, St. Luke's Hospital, Illini Foundation |
| Seino, 1997 9151243 | Stroke refers to a case where rapidly developing focal disturbance (or global disturbance in the case of subarachnoid hemorrhage) of the brain due to vascular lesion and its signs and symptoms lasted more than 24 h or until death. Includes cerebral hemorrhage, cerebral infarction, subarachnoid hemorrhage. TIA is excluded. | RR for cerebral infarction by quartile of n-3 intake (multivariate)<br>2.3 g/d 2.7 3.2<br>0.99 (0.52–1.90) 1.57 (0.77–3.21) 1.37 (0.54–3.47) *P*=0.23<br>Adjusted for sex and age. DBP and AF were adjusted by Cox proportional hazard model. The intake of n-3 was positively associated with development of cerebral infarction but did not reach statistical significance. The lowest risk was seen in the Q4 quartile. | Department of Health Promotion, Shibata, Japan, and regional and local hospitals |

**Table 3.4e. Observational Studies of Effects of Omega-3 Fatty Acids and Fish Consumption on Mortality and CVD Outcomes**

| Author, Year | Outcome Definition | Results | | | | | | Funding Source |
|---|---|---|---|---|---|---|---|---|
| Yuan, 2001 Shanghai Cohort Study | Causes of death coded according to ICD-9, 410, 411–414, 430–438. Specific endpoints were deaths from AMI that included sudden and nonsudden cardiac death within 28 d, ischemic heart disease other than AMI, and stroke. | RR of CVD mortality, according to dietary seafood intake (multivariate) | | | | | | — |
| | | Seafood g/wk | Person-yrs | AMI | | Stroke | | |
| | | Fish/shellfish | | Deaths | RR | Deaths | RR | |
| | | <50 | 36892 | 33 | 1.0 | 101 | 1.00 | |
| | | 50–<100 | 55115 | 28 | 0.55 (0.33–0.91) | 141 | 0.93 (0.72–1.21) | |
| | | 100–<150 | 32499 | 21 | 0.65 (0.38–1.14) | 70 | 0.79 (0.58–1.07) | |
| | | 150–<200 | 25767 | 17 | 0.66 (0.36–1.19) | 71 | 1.01 (0.74–1.37) | |
| | | ≥200 | 29194 | 14 | 0.41 (0.22–0.78) | 97 | 1.11 (0.83–1.47) | |
| | | Fish only | | | | | | |
| | | <50 | 32550 | 29 | 1.00 | 91 | 1.00 | |
| | | 50–<100 | 39355 | 30 | 0.54 (0.32–0.90) | 142 | 0.84 (0.64–1.09) | |
| | | 100–<150 | 39992 | 28 | 0.72 (0.42–1.21) | 99 | 0.87 (0.65–1.15) | |
| | | 150–<200 | 24293 | 16 | 0.63 (0.34–1.17) | 68 | 0.95 (0.69–1.31) | |
| | | ≥200 | 23277 | 10 | 0.35 (0.17–0.72) | 80 | 1.05 (0.77–1.43) | |
| | | Shellfish Only | | | | | | |
| | | <50 | 63301 | 52 | 1.00 | 183 | 1.00 | |
| | | 50–<100 | 34519 | 18 | 0.65 (0.38–1.11) | 80 | 0.86 (0.66–1.12) | |
| | | 100–<150 | 50210 | 28 | 0.66 (0.42–1.05) | 128 | 0.96 (0.77–1.21) | |
| | | 150–<200 | 20505 | 11 | 0.64 (0.33–1.23) | 59 | 1.08 (0.81–1.46) | |
| | | ≥200 | 10932 | 4 | 0.40 (0.14–1.12) | 30 | 1.02 (0.69–1.51) | |
| | | RR of CVD disease mortality, according to dietary intake from seafood (multivariate) | | | | | | |
| | | Intake | Person-yrs | AMI | | Stroke | | |
| | | | | Deaths | RR | Deaths | RR | |
| | | <27 g/wk | 35583 | 33 | 1.0 | 106 | 1.0 | |
| | | 0.27–0.43 | 32076 | 12 | 0.39* (0.20–0.75) | 75 | 0.76 (0.57–1.03) | |
| | | 0.44–0.72 | 54769 | 37 | 0.67 (0.42–1.08) | 124 | 0.76* (0.58–0.98) | |
| | | 0.73–1.1 | 28613 | 16 | 0.53* (0.29–0.97) | 81 | 0.93 (0.69–1.24) | |
| | | >1.1 | 28425 | 15 | 0.43* (0.23–0.81) | 94 | 1.00 (0.75 1.33) | |

**Table 3.4a–e abbreviations:**

WHO = World Health Organization, OR = Odds Ration, HTN = Hypertension, AF = Atrial Fibrillation, PAD = Peripheral Arterial Disease, CAD = Coronary Artery Disease, RR = Relative Risk, BMI = Body Mass Index, SBP = Systolic Blood Pressure, CV = Cardiovascular, HRT = Hormone Replacement Therapy, MI=Myocardial Infarction, AMI=Acute Myocardial Infarction, CVD=Cardiovascular Disease, TIA=Transient Ischemic Attack, ICH=Intracerebral Hemorrage, ECG=Electrocardiogram, DBP=Diastolic Blood Pressure, AF=Atrial Fibrillation.

others show no effect, while still others suggest benefit. This is because, for small-to-moderate effects (i.e., 10–50%), the amount of uncontrolled and uncontrollable confounding inherent in all observational studies is about as big as the effect sizes. In addition, individuals who self-select for high amounts of fish oil also change other characteristics, leading to confounding by indication. For example, fish is high in protein and low in saturated fat, and may be replacing red meat in the diet, thus possibly contributing to a lower stroke risk (Skerrett & Hennekens, 2003).

With respect to randomized evidence, the GISSI results were unexpected since it was difficult to reconcile a decrease in death from all causes with no benefit on nonfatal MI or stroke, since the totality of available evidence indicates several plausible mechanisms for decreasing cardiovascular risk (Yzebe & Lievre, 2004). The lack of evidence of benefit on the atherosclerotic-thrombotic events, despite the well-documented activity of n-3 PUFA on eicosanoid metabolism, inflammation, tissue factor, β-oxidation, endothelial dysfunction, cytokine growth factors, and gene expression of adhesion molecules, is difficult to explain. In GISSI, the intensive preventive interventions that were documented for the whole duration of the trial may explain, at least in part, the observed findings (GISSI-Prevenzione Investigators, 1999). Further randomized trial data from testing fish oils in stroke are necessary to supplement the present evidence.

Meanwhile, the American Dietetic Association (ADA) and the Dietitians of Canada (DC) recommend an increase in n-3 PUFAs. ADA and DC recommend a food-based approach for achieving these fatty acid recommendations: that is, a dietary pattern high in fruits and vegetables, whole grains, legumes, nuts and seeds, lean protein (lean meats, poultry and fish, especially fatty fish high in n-3 fatty acids), low-fat dairy products, and nonhydrogenated margarines and oils. Implicit to these recommendations for dietary fatty acids is that unsaturated fatty acids are the predominant fat source in the diet. These fatty acid recommendations are made in the context of a diet consistent with energy needs to promote a healthful body weight. ADA and DC recognize that scientific knowledge about the effects of dietary fats on human health is incomplete, and take a prudent approach in recommending a reduction in those fatty acids that increase the risk of disease, while promoting the intake of those fatty acids that benefit health (American Dietetic Association, 2007).

With respect to fish oil supplements, the United States Food and Drug Administration (FDA) approved a prescription formulation to treat hypertriglyceridemia. The National Heart, Lung and Blood Institute recommends

**Table 3.5. Randomized Controlled Trial of Effects of Omega-3 Fatty Acids on Mortality and CVD Outcomes**

| Author, year | Outcome, definition | Results | | | | | Funding source |
|---|---|---|---|---|---|---|---|
| Marchioli, 2002<br>GISSI-Prevenzione Trial<br>GISSI, 1999 | The causes of death were classified according to codes (ICD-9). Sudden death was defined as natural death, instantaneous or within 1 h of the onset of acute symptoms, and unexpected as to the time and mode of death. | Overall Efficacy Profile of n-3 PUFAs During GISSI-Prevenzione Follow-up (42 months) 38,418 person years) | | | | | Briston-Myers Squibb, Pharmacia-Upjohn, Society Prodotti Antibiotici, Pfizer, Bracco |
| | | | T (%) | C (%) | RR (95% CI) | *P*-value | |
| | | Death, nonfatal MI+stroke: | 718 (12.7%) | 795 (14.1%) | 0.85 (0.74–0.98) | <0.05 | |
| | | CVD death, nonfatal MI+stroke: | 556 (9.8%) | 621 (11.0%) | 0.80 (0.68–0.94) | <0.01 | |
| | | All fatal events: | 310 (5.5%) | 370 (6.5%) | 0.70 (0.56–0.86) | <0.001 | |
| | | Cardiac death: | 247 (4.4%) | 306 (6.5%) | 0.65 (0.51–0.82) | <0.001 | |
| | | Coronary death: | 209 (3.7%) | 258 (4.6%) | 0.68 (0.53–0.88) | <0.01 | |
| | | Sudden death: | 111 (2.0%) | 154 (2.7%) | 0.55 (0.39–0.77) | <0.001 | |
| | | Nonfatal MI: | 223 (3.9%) | 233 (4.1%) | 0.91 (0.70–1.18) | NS | |
| | | Nonfatal stroke: | 62 (1.1%) | 57 (1.0%) | 1.22 (0.75–1.97) | NS | |
| | | CHD death and nonfatal MI: | 418 (7.4%) | 475 (8.4%) | 0.78 (0.65–0.94) | <0.01 | |
| | | Fatal and nonfatal stroke: | 92 (1.6%) | 77 (1.4%) | 122 (0.81–1.85) | NS | |

T=Treatment, C=Control, RR=Relative Risk, CVD=Cardiovascular Disease, MI=Myocardial Infarction, CHD, Coronary Heart Disease.

fish oil as an adjunct to statins in achieving accepted goals for lipid modification (Hennekens et al., 2006; Iso et al., 2001; NCEP ATP III, 2002).

At present, we should not let the perfect be the enemy of the possible. With respect to the perfect, clear research challenges exist to discover newer and better agents and interventions to decrease stroke, including fish oil, which is promising but unproven. Regarding the possible, clear clinical and public health challenges exist that one can meet by the adoption of therapeutic lifestyle changes and drug therapies of proven benefit for stroke.

## Acknowledgments

Dr. Hennekens reports that he receives salary support from two investigator-initiated research grants funded to Florida Atlantic University by Bayer testing the effects of aspirin dose on platelet biomarkers, inflammatory markers, nitric oxide formation, and endothelial function; serves as consultant, including as Chair or Member on Data and Safety Monitoring Boards for Actelion, Agatston Research Institute (ARI), Amgen, AstraZeneca, Bayer, Biovail, Bristol-Myers Squibb, Chattem, Delaco, Food and Drug Administration, GlaxoSmithKline, Keryx, McNeil, Merck, National Institutes of Health, Novartis, Pfizer, Reliant, TAP, United BioSource Corporation and UpToDate; has received royalties for authorship or editorship of three textbooks; receives royalties as co-inventor on patents concerning inflammatory markers and cardiovascular disease which are held by Brigham and Women's Hospital and has an investment management relationship with SunTrust Bank who has sole discretionary investment authority.

### References

American Dietetic Association. Position of the american dietetic association and dietitians of canada: dietary fatty acids. *J. Am. Diet. Assoc.* **2007,** *107,* 1599–1611.

American Heart Association (AHA). Dietary guidelines for healthy american adults. A statement for physicians and health professionals by the nutrition committee, american heart association. *Circulation* **1988**, *77*, 721A.

Antithrombotic Trialists' Collaboration. Collaborative meta-analysis of randomised trials of antiplatelet therapy for prevention of death, myocardial infarction, and stroke in high risk patients. *BMJ* **2002,** *324*, 71–86.

Baigent, C.; A. Keech; P.M. Kearney; L. Blackwell; G. Buck; C. Pollicino; A. Kirby; T. Sourjina; R. Peto; R. Collins; R. Simes. For the Cholesterol Treatment Trialists' (CTT) collaborators. Efficacy and safety of cholesterol-lowering treatment: prospective meta-analysis of data from 90,056 participants in 14 randomised trials of statins. *Lancet* **2005,** *366(9493)*, 1267–1278.

Balk, E.; M. Chung; A. Lichtenstein; P. Chew; B. Kupelnick; A. Lawrence; D. DeVine; J. Lau. *Effects of Omega-3 Fatty Acids on Cardiovascular Risk Factors and Intermediate Markers of Cardiovascular Disease.* Evidence Report/Technology Assessment No. 93 (Prepared by Tufts- New England Medical Center Evidence-Based Practice Center under Contract No. 290-02-0022). AHRQ Publication No. 04-E010-2. Agency for Healthcare Research and Quality: Rockville, MD, March 2004.

Berge, K.G.; P.L. Canner. Coronary drug project: experience with niacin: coronary drug project research group. *Eur. J. Clin. Pharmacol.* **1991,** *40 (Suppl.1)*, S49–51.

Bernal-Pacheco, O.B.; G.C. Roman. Environmental vascular risk factors: new perspectives for stroke prevention. *J. Neurol. Sci.* **2007,** *262*, 60–70.

Biller, J.; W.M. Feinberg; J.E. Castaldo; A.D. Whittemore; R.E. Harbaugh; R.J. Dempsey; L.R. Caplan; T.F. Kresowik; D.B. Matchar; J.F. Tool; et al. Guidelines for carotid endarterectomy: a statement for healthcare professionals from a special writing group of the stroke council, American Heart Association. *Circulation* **1998,** *97*, 501–509.

Calo, L.; L. Bianconi; F. Colivicchi; F. Lamberti; M.L. Loricchio; E. de Ruvo; A. Meo; C. Pandozi; M. Staibano; M. Santini. N-3 fatty acids for the prevention of atrial fibrillation after coronary artery bypass surgery: a randomized, controlled trial. *J. Am. Coll. Cardiol.* **2005,** *45*, 1723–1728.

Chobanian, A.V.; G.L. Bakris; H.R. Black; W.C. Cushman; L.A. Green; J.L. Izzo, Jr; D.W. Jones; B.J. Materson; S. Oparil; J.T. Wright, Jr; et al; National Heart, Lung, and Blood Institute Joint National Committee on Prevention, Detection, Evaluation, and Treatment of High Blood Pressure, National High Blood Pressure Education Program Coordinating Committee. The seventh report of the joint national committee on prevention, detection, evaluation, and treatment of high blood pressure: the JNC 7 report. *JAMA* **2003,** *289(19)*, 2560–2572.

Collins, R.; R. Peto; S. MacMahon; P. Hebert; N.H. Fiebach; K.A. Eberlein, J. Godwin; N. Qizilbash; J.O. Taylor; C.H. Hennekens; et al. Blood pressure, stroke and coronary heart disease. II. Short term reductions in blood pressure: overview of randomised drug trials in their epidemiological context. *Lancet* **1990,** *335*, 827–838.

Coward, L.J.; R.L. Featherstone; M.M. Brown. Safety and efficacy of endovascular treatment of carotid artery stenosis compared with carotid endarterectomy: A cochrane systematic review of the randomized evidence. *Stroke* **2005,** *36*, 905–911.

Fuster, V.; L.E. Rydén; D.S. Cannom; H.J. Crijns; A.B. Curtis; K.A. Ellenbogen; J.L. Halperin; J.Le Heuzey; G.N. Kay; J.E. Lowe; et al; ACC/AHA Task Force Members; ESC Committee For Practice Guidelines; European Heart Rhythm Association; Heart Rhythm Society. ACC/AHA/ESC 2006 Guidelines for the Management of Patients with Atrial Fibrillation: A Report of the American College of Cardiology/American Heart Association Task Force on Practice Guidelines and the European Society of Cardiology Committee for Practice Guidelines (Writing Committee to Revise the 2001 Guidelines for the Management of Patients With Atrial Fibrillation): Developed in collaboration with the European Heart Rhythm Association and the Heart Rhythm Society. *Circulation* **2006,** *114*, e257–e354.

Geleijnse J.M., E.J. Giltay; D.E. Grobbee; A.R. Donders; F.J. Kok. Blood pressure response to fish oil supplementation: meta-regression analysis of randomized trials. *J. Hypertens.* **2002,** *20*, 1493–1499.

Gillman, M.W. Dietary Fat. *UpToDate.* 2007, pp. 1–18. Downloaded 10/8/2007 from http://www.utdol.com/utd/content/topic.do?topicKey=lipiddis/4418&view=print.

Gillman, M.W.; L.A. Cupples; B.E. Millen; R.C. Ellison; P.A. Wolf. Inverse association of dietary fat with development of ischemic stroke in men. *JAMA* **1997,** *278*, 2145–2150.

Gillum, R.F.; M.E. Mussolino; J.H. Madans. The relationship between fish consumption and stroke incidence. The NHANES I Epidemiologic Follow-up Study (National Health and Nutrition Examination Survey). *Arch. Intern. Med.* **1996,** *156*, 537–542.

GISSI-Prevenzione Investigators (Gruppo Italiano per lo Studio della Sopravvivenza nell'Infarto miocardico). Dietary supplementation with n-3 polyunsaturated fatty acids and vitamin e after MI: Results of the GISSI-Prevenzione Trial. *Lancet* **1999,** *354*, 447–455.

Goldstein L. Prevention and management of stroke. *Braunwald's Heart Disease, A Textbook of Cardiovascular Medicine, Eighth Edition*; P. Libby, R.O. Bonow, D.L. Mann, D.P. Zipes, Eds.; Saunders Elsevier: Philadelphia, PA, 2008; Vol. 2, pp. 1515–1522.

Gorelick, P.; O. Sechenova; C.H. Hennekens. evolving perspectives on clopidogrel in the treatment of ischemic stroke. *J. Cardiovasc. Pharmacol. Ther.* **2006,** *11*, 245–248.

He, K.; A. Merchant; E.B. Rimm; B.A. Rosner; M.J. Stampfer; A. Ascherio. Dietary fat intake and risk of stroke in male us healthcare professionals: 14 year prospective cohort study. *BMJ* **2003,** *327*, 777–782.

He, K.; E.B. Rimm; A. Merchant; B.A. Rosner; M.J. Stampfer; W.C. Willett; A. Ascherio. Fish consumption and risk of stroke in men. *JAMA* **2002**, *288*, 3130–3136.

He, K.; Y. Song; M.L. Daviglus; K. Liu; L. Van Horn; A.R. Dyer; U. Goldbourt; P. Greenland. Fish consumption and incidence of stroke: a meta-analysis of cohort studies. *Stroke* **2004,** *35*, 1538–1542.

Hennekens, C.H. increasing burden of cardiovascular disease: current knowledge and future directions for research on risk factors. *Circulation* **1998,** *97*, 1095–1102.

Hennekens, C.H. Fixed-dose combination therapy with statins strengths, limitations, and clinical and regulatory considerations. *Am. J. Cardiovasc. Drugs* **2008;** *8(3)*, 155–160.

Hennekens, C.H.; S. Borzak. Cyclooxygenase-2 inhibitors and most traditional nonsteroidal anti-inflammatory drugs cause similar moderately increased risks of cardiovascular disease. *J. Cardiovasc. Pharmacol. Ther.* **2008,** *13(1)*, 41–50.

Hennekens, C.H.; J.E. Buring. *Epidemiology in Medicine.* Little, Brown, & Co: Boston, MA, 1987.

Hennekens, C.H.; D. Hollar; C. Baigent. Sex-related differences in response to aspirin in cardiovascular disease: an untested hypothesis. *Nature Clinical Practice Cardiovasc. Med.* **2006,** *3*, 4–5.

Hennekens, C.H.; D. Hollar; R.S. Eidelman; A.S. Agatston. Update for primary healthcare providers: recent statin trials and revised national cholesterol education program iii guidelines. *Medscape General Med.* **2006,** *8(1)*, 54.

Hennekens, C.H.; W.R. Schneider. Statins and aspirin produce additive benefits in the treatment of cardiovascular disease. *Expert Rev. Cardiovasc. Ther.* **2008,** *6(1)*,109–121.

Iso, H.; K.M. Rexrode; M.J. Stampfer; J.E. Manson; G.A. Colditz; F.E. Speizer; C.H. Hennekens; W.C. Willett. Intake of fish and omega-3 fatty acids and risk of stroke in women. *JAMA* **2001,** *285*, 304–312.

Jamrozik, K.; R.J. Broadhurst; C.S. Anderson; E.G. Stewart-Wynne. The role of lifestyle factors in the etiology of stroke. A population-based case-control study in perth, western australia. *Stroke.* **1994,** *25*, 51–59.

Keech, A.; R.J. Simes; P. Barter; J. Best; R. Scott; M.R. Taskinen; P. Forder; A. Pillai; T. Davis; P. Glasziou; et al. FIELD study investigators. Effects of long-term fenofibrate therapy on cardiovascular events in 9795 people with type 2 diabetes mellitus (the field study): randomised controlled trial. *Lancet* **2005,** *366(9500)*, 1849–1861.

Keli, S.O.; E.J. Feskens; D. Kromhout. Fish consumption and risk of stroke. The zutphen study. *Stroke* **1994,** *25(2)*, 328–332.

King, J.C.; L.J. Appel; B. Caballero; F.M. Clydesdale; P.M. Kris-Etherton; T.A. Nicklas; F.X. Pi-Sunyer; Y.L. Bronner; C.A. Camargo; V.L.W. Go; et al. The Dietary Guidelines Advisory Committee for U.S. Department of Health and Human Services and U.S. Department of Agriculture. Dietary Guidelines for Americans 2005. downloaded from: http://www.health.gov/dietaryguidelines/.

Lawes, C.M.M.; D.A. Bennet; V.L. Feigin; A. Rodgers. Blood pressure and stroke: an overview of published reviews. *Stroke* **2004,** *35*, 776–785.

Mackay, J.; G. Mensah. *The Atlas of Heart Disease and Stroke*. World Health Organization, 2004. www.who.int/cardiovascular_diseases/resources/atlas/en/.

Mori, T.A. Omega-3 fatty acids and hypertension in humans. *Clin. Exp. Pharmacol. Physiol.* **2006,** *33*, 842–846.

Morris, M.C.; J.E. Manson; B. Rosner; J.E. Buring; W.C. Willett; C.H. Hennekens. Fish consumption and cardiovascular disease in the physicians' health study: a prospective study. *Am. J. Epidemiol.* **1995,** *142*, 166–175.

Morris, M.C.; F. Sacks; B. Rosner. Does fish oil lower blood pressure? A meta-analysis of controlled trials. *Circulation* **1993,** *88*, 523–533.

Mozaffarian, D. Fish oil and prevention of atrial fibrillation. *J. Am. Coll. Cardiol.* **2007,** *50*, 1513–1514.

Mozaffarian, D.; W.T. Longstreth, Jr; R.N. Lemaitre; T.A. Manolio; L.H. Kuller; G.L. Burke; D.S. Siscovick. Fish consumption and stroke risk in elderly individuals: the cardiovascular health study. *Arch. Intern. Med.* **2005,** *165*, 200–206.

Mozaffarian, D.; B.M. Psaty; E.B. Rimm; R.N. Lemaitre; G.L. Burke; M.F. Lyles; D. Lefkowitz; D.S. Siscovick. Fish intake and risk of incident atrial fibrillation. *Circulation* **2004,** *110*, 368–373.

Murray, C.J.L.; A.D. Lopez. *The Global Burden of Disease: A Comprehensive Assessment of Mortality and Disability from Diseases, Injuries and Risk Factors in 1990 and Projected to 2020.* Harvard University Press: Boston, MA, 1996.

National Cholesterol Education Program (NCEP) Expert Panel on Detection, Evaluation, and Treatment of High Blood Cholesterol in Adults (Adult Treatment Panel III). Third report of the national cholesterol education program (ncep) expert panel on detection, evaluation, and treatment of high blood cholesterol in adults (adult treatment panel iii). *Circulation* **2002,** *106*, 3143.

Orencia, A.J.; M.L. Daviglus; A.R. Dyer; R.B. Shekelle; J. Stamler. Fish consumption and stroke in men. 30-year findings of the chicago western electric study. *Stroke* **1996,** *27*, 204–209.

Ridker, P.M.; N.R. Cook; I-M. Lee; D. Gordon; J.M. Gaziano; J.E. Manson; C.H. Hennekens; J.E. Buring. A randomized trial of low-dose aspirin in the primary prevention of cardiovascular disease in women. *N. Engl. J. Med.* **2005,** *352*, 1293–1304.

Ridker, P.M.; M. Cushman; M.J. Stampfer; R.P. Tracy; C.H. Hennekens. Inflammation, aspirin, and the risk of cardiovascular disease in apparently healthy men. *NEJM* **1997,** *336*, 973–979.

Robins, S.J.; D. Collins; J.T. Wittes; V. Papademetriou; P.C. Deedwania; E.J. Schaefer; J.R.

McNamara; M.L. Kashyap; J.M. Hershman; L.F. Wexler; et al. for the VA-HIT Study Group. Veterans affairs high-density lipoprotein intervention trial: relation of gemfibrozil treatment and lipid levels with major coronary events. va-hit: a randomized controlled trial. *JAMA* **2001,** *285(12)*, 1585–1591.

Rosamond, W.; K. Flegal; K. Furie; A. Go; K. Greenlund; N. Haase; S.M. Hailpern; M. Ho; V. Howard; B. Kissela; et al. for the American Heart Association Statistics Committee and Stroke Statistics Subcommittee. AHA statistical update, heart disease and stroke statistics—2008 update. A report from the American Heart Association statistics committee and stroke statistics subcommittee. *Circulation* **2008,** *117*, e25–e146.

Rothwell, P.; A.J. Coull; E. Silver. Population-based study of event-rate, incidence, case fatality, and mortality for all acute vascular events in all arterial territories (oxford vascular study). *Lancet* **2005,** *366*, 1773–1783.

Sarrazin, J.F.; G. Comeau; P. Daleau; J. Kingma; I. Plante; D. Fournier; F. Molin. Reduced incidence of vagally induced atrial fibrillation and expression levels of connexins by n-3 polyunsaturated fatty acids in dogs. *J. Am. Coll. Cardiol.* **2007,** *50*, 1505–1512.

Sauvaget, C.; J. Nagano; N. Allen; E.J. Grant; V. Beral. Intake of animal products and stroke mortality in the hiroshima/nagasaki life span study. *Int. J. Epidemiol.* **2003,** *32*, 536–543.

Siddiqui, R.A.; K.A. Harvey; G.P. Zaloga. Modulation of enzymatic activities by n-3 polyunsaturated fatty acids to support cardiovascular health. *J. Nutr. Biochem.* **2008,** *19(7)*, 417–437.

Skerrett, P.J.; C.H. Hennekens. Consumption of fish and fish oils and decreased risk of stroke. *Prev. Cardiol.* **2003,** *6*, 38–41.

Vanschoonbeek, K.; M.P.M. de Maat; W.M. Heemskerk. Fish oil consumption and reduction of arterial disease. *J. Nutr.* **2003,** *133*, 657–660.

Wang, C.; M. Chung; E. Balk; B. Kupelnick; D. DeVine; A. Lawrence; A. Lichtenstein; J. Lau. *Effects of Omega-3 Fatty Acids on Cardiovascular Disease.* Evidence Report/Technology Assessment No. 94 (Prepared by Tufts-New England Medical Center Evidence-based Practice Center, under Contract No. 290-02-0022). AHRQ Publication No. 04-E009-2. Rockville, MD: Agency for Healthcare Research and Quality. March 2004.

Williams, A.; C.H. Hennekens. The role of aspirin in cardiovascular diseases— forgotten benefits? *Expert Opin. Pharmacother.* **2004,** *5(1)*, 109–115.

World Health Organization (WHO). Future trends in global mortality: major shifts in cause of death patterns. *World Health Statistics 2008*, 4th ed.; World Health Organization: France, 2008; pp. 29–31.

Wu, D.; S. Han; M. Meydani; S.N. Meydani. Effect of concomitant consumption of fish oil and vitamin e on production of inflammatory cytokines in healthy elderly humans. *Ann. NY Acad. Sci.* **2004,** *1031*, 422–424.

Yzebe, D.; M. Lievre. Fish oils in the care of coronary heart disease patients: a meta-analysis of randomized controlled trials. *Fundam. Clin. Pharmacol.* **2004,** *18*, 581–592.

Zhang, J.; S. Sasaki; K. Amano; H. Kesteloot. Fish consumption and mortality from all causes, ischemic heart disease, and stroke: an ecological study. *Prev. Med.* **1999,** *28(5)*, 520–529.

4

# Fatty Acids and Cardiac Ischemia-reperfusion Injury

**Sri Nagarjun Batchu, Ketul Chaudhary, Jasmine Pawa, and John M. Seubert**
*Faculty of Pharmacy and Pharmaceutical Sciences, University of Alberta, Edmonton, AB, Canada*

## Introduction

Cardiovascular diseases (CVDs) are a major cause of illness, disability, and death in both Western societies and developing nations. As populations age and co-morbidities such as obesity and diabetes become more prevalent, both the human cost and economic burden of these conditions will increase. Ischemic heart disease (IHD), also known as coronary artery disease (CAD) or coronary heart disease (CHD), results from damage incurred after severe impairment of the arteries that feed the heart muscle when both blood flow and oxygen supply are restricted. In contrast, an anoxic event occurs when perfusion to the myocardium is maintained but lacks oxygen. This allows for a washout of metabolic waste products, and limits the mechanical and energetic injury to the heart compared to ischemia. Myocardial ischemic injury occurs when ischemia exceeds a critical threshold and overwhelms the cellular repair mechanisms that are designed to maintain normal operating function and homeostasis. It is at this critical threshold level that ischemia results in irreversible myocardial cell damage or death (See Fig. 4.1). Such injury contributes to the pathogenesis of heart failure (HF), acute myocardial infarction (AMI), and sudden death.

Considerable knowledge about the anatomical and biochemical responses to ischemic injury has produced much insight into the corresponding pathobiology. Advances in early reperfusion therapy, such as thromobolytic drugs, coronary angioplasty, or bypass graft surgery, have reduced morbidity, heart failure, and infarct-associated ventricular arrhythmias. Acute cardioprotective mechanisms, concurrently, are primarily mediated by the activation of signaling pathways and the posttranslational modification of proteins, whereas delayed or late protective mechanisms are primarily mediated by gene induction and protein synthesis.

Fatty acids are carboxylic acids consisting of a long aliphatic hydrocarbon tail (chain), which is either saturated (no double bonds between carbon atoms) or unsaturated (double bonds are present). Fatty acids are the building blocks of phospholipids and glycolipids found within the body, notably in cell membranes. For several years, many have recognized the importance of dietary polyunsaturated fatty

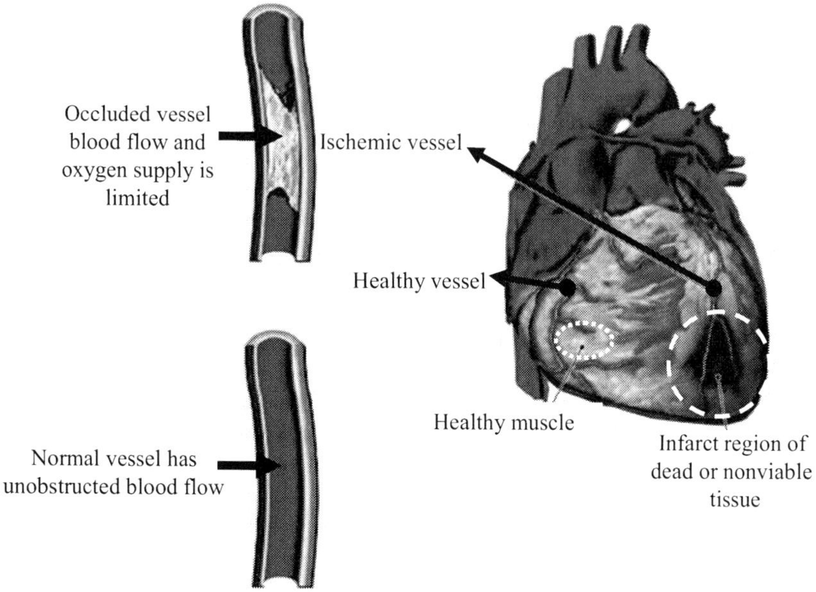


**Fig. 4.1.** Cardiac blood vessel in ischemic and nonischemic condition. Ischemia results when tissue is deprived of oxygen and metabolic substrates because of a lack of perfusion. Cells switch from aerobic to anaerobic metabolism during which time toxic substances begin to accumulate. While initial damage may be reversible, the changes ultimately lead to pathological effects such as myocardial stiffness, contractile dysfunction, arrhythmias, and reduced cardiac output leading to heart failure and death.

acids (PUFAs) in the reduction of CVD (Erkkila et al., 2008; Kritchevsky, 1998). The early studies of dietary fat and atherosclerosis investigating the association of serum cholesterol with CHD suggested that unsaturated fatty acids lower serum-cholesterol levels (Keys et al., 1957; Mensink & Katan, 1992; Mensink et al., 2003; Page, 1954) . The beneficial results were attributed to the opposite effects of saturated fatty acids (SFAs) and PUFAs on the lipid profile. However, recent literature demonstrates that dietary fat quality may also influence CVD through the effects on thrombosis, endothelial function, inflammation, abdominal obesity, insulin sensitivity, development of diabetes, and arrhythmias (Erkkila et al., 2008). Beneficial and detrimental outcomes ultimately depend on the type of fatty acid. Evidence demonstrates the adverse effects of both *trans* fatty acids (TFAs) and SFAs, whereas PUFAs are associated with a lower incidence of CVD (von Schacky, 2006, 2007; Willett, 2007). These latter studies showed a lower incidence of cardiac death, as well as decreases in blood pressure, blood viscosity, plasma triglycerides, ventricular fibrillation, arrhythmia, and MI (Harris, 2007; Simopoulos, 2008; von Schacky, 2006, 2007).

Although the molecular mechanisms of fatty acid-mediated cardioprotection are not fully defined, clearly, fatty acids are pleiotropic. For example, they alter membrane microdomain structure and function, eicosanoid metabolism, the formation and mobilization of reactive oxygen products, signaling molecules, and intracellular $Ca^{2+}$ levels. The challenge for research is to determine the extent by which PUFA influences physical properties and biochemical processes to provide protection toward contractile dysfunction, energetics, and infarction. This chapter discusses the role that fatty acids play in cardiac ischemia–reperfusion injury.

## *Membrane Organization*

Biological membranes are lined by charged hydrophilic head groups, and contain a hydrophic core, made of cholesterol and fatty-acyl chains. Fatty acids are an integral part of the cell plasma membrane and mitochondria. They play a role in maintaining the fluidity and stability of the membrane structure as well as acting as secondary signaling molecules in response to stress conditions. Biological membranes are not homogenous mixtures of lipid and protein, but consist of patches of differing composition called domains (Shaikh et al., 2004). Depending on the affinities between differing lipid species or between lipids and membrane proteins, domains can be limited to a relatively small number of molecules (microdomains) to regions in the μm range (macrodomains). Fatty acid structure also comes into play with saturated and monosaturated acyl chains being more ordered than polyunsaturated acyl chains (Shaikh & Edidin, 2008). PUFAs have high conformational flexibility despite the rigidity of the double bonds. This flexibility is dependent on acyl chain length and the number of double bonds (Feller & Gawrisch, 2005). The polyunsaturation of fatty acids sterically impedes association with some membrane components, such as cholesterol and sphingolipids, thereby influencing lipid-domain behavior and protein function (Chapkin et al., 2008). PUFAs may directly affect physical properties such as microviscosity, curvature, permeability, cytosolic protein trafficking, and microdomain formation (Chapkin et al., 2008; Shaikh & Edidin, 2008; Soni et al., 2008). They may also influence downstream signaling cascades by displacing acylated and prenylated signaling proteins found in lipid rafts (Seo et al., 2006; Stulnig et al., 2001).

Cell-surface organization of lipids, receptors, and proteins has been an area of study for a long time. One can compartmentalize specific regions of plasma membranes into microdomains referred to as membrane rafts (previously known as lipid rafts), which contain a variety of signaling and transport proteins. These discrete microdomains play an important role in facilitating specific cellular events. Subtypes of microdomains can differ in both lipid and protein composition, such as a microdomain enriched in cholesterol and sphingomyelin or one containing proteins such as caveolin-1 and caveolin-3. Caveolae are, in fact, one subset of membrane rafts that appear as flask-like (<100 nm diameter) invaginations enriched with lipids (e.g., cholesterol, glycosphingolipids) and scaffolding proteins called caveolin (caveolin-1, -2, and -3) (Patel et al., 2008b). Caveolin proteins can differ in expression patterns and their ability to regulate intracellular signaling (Ballard-Croft et al., 2006; Das et al., 2008; Der et al., 2006). As such, caveolar composition can selectively sequester membrane-targeted proteins that make a unique signaling microdomain controlling cellular function and response. Recent evidence demonstrates that caveolin-1 is critical in controlling protective signaling after ischemia–reperfusion injury (Patel et al., 2007). Indeed, fatty acid composition plays an important role in modulating caveolar lipid composition, signaling microdomain localization and function (Fig. 4.2) (Ma et al., 2004b). Alterations in n-3 PUFAs will influence fatty- acyl composition, and reduce both cholesterol and caveolin-1 content (Ma et al., 2004b). As such, fatty acid composition significantly affects plasma membrane composition, which, in turn, influences important cellular events and function.

## *Ischemia–reperfusion Injury*

Ischemic injury is an important clinical problem that depends on the site and extent of occlusion, duration between occlusion and reperfusion, and the presence of

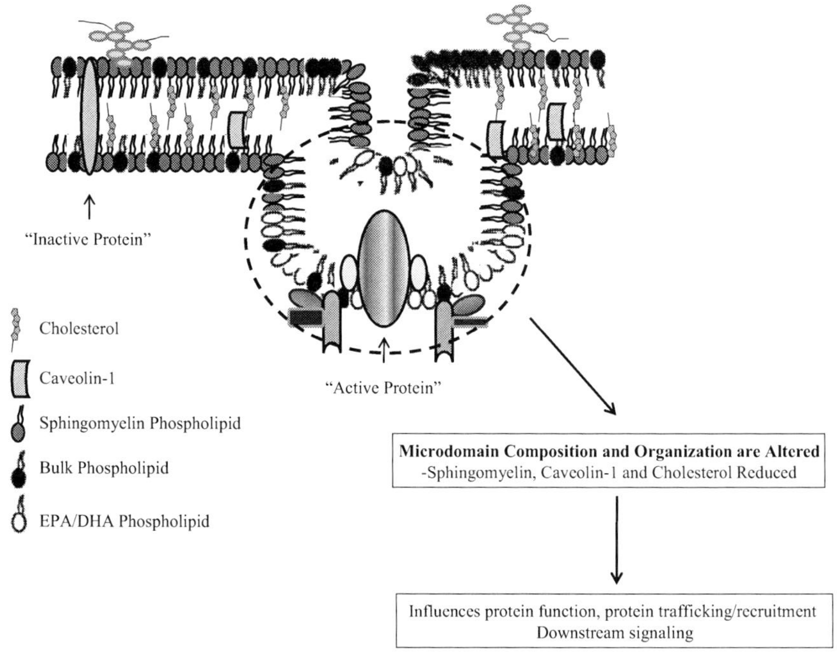


**Fig. 4.2.** Membrane function and microdomain locality is affected by phospholipid composition and protein content. Membranes are organized into various domains that differ in lipid and protein composition. Incorporation of EPA or DHA polyunsaturated fatty acids into the membrane can affect its properties and function. Alteration to membrane composition can influence protein activation and recruitment which, in turn, affects cellular signaling events. Adapted from (Harris, 2008; Patel et al., 2008a).

collateral circulation. Significant metabolic imbalances and functional changes are initiated within seconds of the onset of ischemia. The effects are initially reversible; however, if oxygen is deprived for an extended period of time, they become more severe, leading to irreversible damage. Paradoxically, the process of restoring blood flow can itself cause myocardial injury. Reperfusion injury was first postulated in 1960 when Jennings et al. (1960) reported histological features of reperfused ischemic canine myocardium. Cardiac dysfunction can take several forms: (i) stunning—where mechanical dysfunction persists after reperfusion despite the absence of irreversible injury and normal coronary flow; (ii) no-flow phenomenon—the inability to reperfuse a previous ischemic region; (iii) arrhythmias; and (iv) lethal injury (Hausenloy & Yellon, 2008). Whether irreversible cardiomyocyte damage occurs during ischemia or upon reperfusion is a matter of debate. Importantly, therapeutic interventions that reduce or salvage injured tissue are most successful when initiated as soon as possible after the ischemic event. Following the ischemia–reperfusion event, adaptive processes that alter myocardial shape, size, and function begin to take hold. These adverse adaptations include the formation of scar tissue, fibrosis, and myofibroblast proliferation which lead to pathological hypertrophy. These changes contribute to increased myocardial stiffness, contractile dysfunction, and reduced cardiac output which eventually leads to ventricular dilatation, heart failure, and death.

The brain and heart are undeniably vital systems, and an insult to either leads to death or major impairment of the individual. In the brain, 50–60% of the weight is made up of lipid, and although it appears delicate, it is thought to resist ischemia for a longer period as compared to other tissues (Plum, 1983; Rehncrona et al., 1980). On the other hand, the heart is composed primarily of much stronger muscular tissue, but is very prone to ischemic injury. Major cellular events occur following ischemia–reperfusion that result in a series of reactions leading to irreversible forms of injury. The series of events during ischemia can be generally characterized as follows: (i) reduced availability of molecular oxygen and metabolic substrates results in a decrease in ATP following inhibition of the respiratory chain and oxidative phosphorylation; (ii) cell switches from aerobic to anaerobic metabolism, accumulating inorganic phosphate, lactate, and $H^+$ protons, which subsequently inhibit glycolysis; (iii) the activation of the sodium–hydrogen exchanger (NHE) by intracellular acidosis leads to increased $Na^+$; (iv) ATP-dependent ion pumps begin to fail, causing the cell to become depolarized, and allowing ions, including $Ca^{2+}$, to flow into the cell. The ion pumps can no longer transport calcium out of the cell, resulting in increased intracellular calcium levels that inhibit contraction (reversible); (v) increased intracellular solute concentrations result in osmotic swelling and induce membrane depolarization, which, in turn, increases membrane permeability and causes a loss of membrane phospholipids; (vi) the activation of $Ca^{2+}$-dependent proteases and phospholipases begins to break down cellular components; and (vii) mitochondrial dysfunction and breakdown initiate the release of toxins and apoptotic factors (Delozier et al., 2007; Ferdinandy et al., 2007; Halestrap, 2004; Hausenloy & Yellon, 2008; Murphy & Steenbergen, 2008; O'Rourke, 2004; Yellon & Downey, 2003).

While reperfusion therapy greatly enhances survivability, reperfusion itself may lead to further complications. A balance exists between the benefits of reducing infarct and potentiating injury upon reperfusion. Reperfusion injury is an expansion or worsening of the events initiated during an ischemic event. Oxygen radicals, $Ca^{2+}$ overload, and neutrophils are thought to be the major mediators of reperfusion injury. The sudden re-introduction of oxygen causes a re-energization of the mitochondria and a reactivation of the electron- transport chain. The electrons swiftly flow into the mitochondria, but cannot be used for oxidative phosphorylation because of a loss of cytochrome oxidase and dismutase enzymatic activity. This leads to the ultimate formation of free radicals like $O_2^-$ and $H_2O_2$. The free radicals generated during reperfusion from injured mitochondria (after an ischemic insult) lead to cytoskeleton damage, increased lipid peroxidation, increased cell permeability, and altered membrane potential. An alteration in membrane potential by free radicals and increased levels of calcium lead to further injury and swelling of the inner mitochondrial membrane. This damage ultimately triggers the opening of the mitochondrial permeable transition pore (mPTP) (Crompton et al., 1998; Halestrap, 2004; Halestrap et al., 1998). The opening of the mPTP is associated with irreversible necrotic cell death in cells that sustained significant injury during ischemia; however, some cells display hallmarks of apoptosis after reperfusion injury (Ferdinandy et al., 2007). Several hours after the onset of myocardial reperfusion, an innate immune response is initiated. A complex response involving the activation of endothelial cells, complement, and increased vascular permeability results in the rapid accumulation of neutrophils and monocytes in the infracted tissue (Frangogiannis et al., 2002; Piper et al., 2003). However, the physiology and anatomy of the heart limit its capacity to tolerate inflammatory responses (Taqueti et al., 2006). As such, the degree of the inflammatory response is critical. If it exceeds the heart's capacity, the innate immune response will contribute to cardiomyocyte injury and death by causing vascular plugging, the release of degradative enzymes, and the generation of reactive oxygen species (ROS ) (Hausenloy & Yellon, 2008; Taqueti et al., 2006).

## *Cardioprotection*

Limiting ischemia–reperfusion injury has been an important concept for over three decades. Preventing cardiomyocyte death, arrhythmias, and contractile dysfunction to improve the outcome of patients following an ischemic event is the main goal (Braunwald & Maroko, 1974; Maroko et al., 1971). Interestingly, although prone to injury, the molecular plasticity of the heart provides a remarkable ability for it to adapt to ischemia–reperfusion stress (Ferdinandy et al., 2007). Numerous pharmacological and nonpharmacological interventions were investigated and reported to protect the heart in experimental animals; however, none have successfully translated into clinical practice with the exception of early reperfusion (Bolli et al., 2004). The continued development of new cardioprotective agents, strategies, and/or paradigms that can reduce this gap between experimental models and clinical practice is required (Bolli et al., 2004).

Cardioprotection aims at reducing the acute and chronic loss of myocardium, thereby limiting subsequent arrhythmias and contractile dysfunction. The discovery of ischemic preconditioning (IPC) as a powerful cardioprotective strategy that renders the heart resistant to injury set the stage for multiple investigations (Murry et al., 1986). Brief nondetrimental episodes of ischemia or pharmacological mimetics given prior to a prolonged ischemic event can initiate signaling pathways that protect the myocardium. Moreover, brief cycles of ischemia–reperfusion applied after a prolonged event, termed "postconditioning," also confer a cardioprotective response. This diverse and complex response is orchestrated by a wide range of mediators from enzymes, receptors, carriers, pumps, and ion channels to lipids, fatty acids, ROS, and peptides (Murphy & Steenbergen, 2008; Piper et al., 2003). Specific cardioprotective responses can involve activating protein kinases and adenosine triphosphate (ATP)-sensitive potassium channels, preserving mitochondrial function, and producing arachidonic-acid metabolites. The specifics of many of these cardioprotective signals were extensively covered in depth by numerous excellent reviews (Fig. 4.3) (Delozier et al., 2007; Ferdinandy et al., 2007; Murphy & Steenbergen, 2008; Piper et al., 2003; Yellon & Downey, 2003). Many of the beneficial and detrimental effects of fatty acids, however, specifically involve interactions with biological membranes, whether acting as potent signaling moieties, sources of energy, or interacting with hydrophobic regions of membrane proteins.

## *Myocardial Energetics*

The heart's high-energy demand during normal function is supplied by ATP, which is produced mainly by mitochondria (>95%) through oxidative phosphorylation, glycolysis, and the citric-acid cycle (Stanley et al., 2005; Ussher & Lopaschuk, 2008). Of the total energy produced, 60–70% is used for the contractile function, and the remaining 30–40% is used for the other channel and pump functions. Under normal aerobic conditions, over 70–80% of energy needed to produce ATP is derived from fatty acids, with the remainder coming from the oxidation of pyruvate formed from glycolysis and lactate oxidation (Burke & Virmani, 2007). Fatty acids are not as oxygen-efficient as carbohydrates, requiring approximately 10% more oxygen to produce an equivalent amount of ATP (Stanley et al., 2005).

Fatty acids can enter cardiomyocytes by passive diffusion or protein-mediated transport as well as a release from the sarcolemma. They are then esterified to acyl coenzyme A (CoA) by fatty-acyl CoA synthase, becoming available for further esterification to intracellular lipids or conversion to long-chain fatty-acyl carnitine by carnitine palmitoyltransferase I (CPT-I) (van der Lee et al., 2000). Subsequent mitochondrial uptake occurs via a carnitine-dependent transport system in which CPT-I, carnitine acyltranslocase, and CPT-II move fatty acids inside. Mitochondrial β-oxidation repeatedly cleaves off two carbon acetyl CoA units that enter the Kreb's cycle to produce reduced nicotinamide adenine dinucleotide (NADH) and the reduced flavin adenine dinucleotide (FAD) required for ATP production. Acetyl

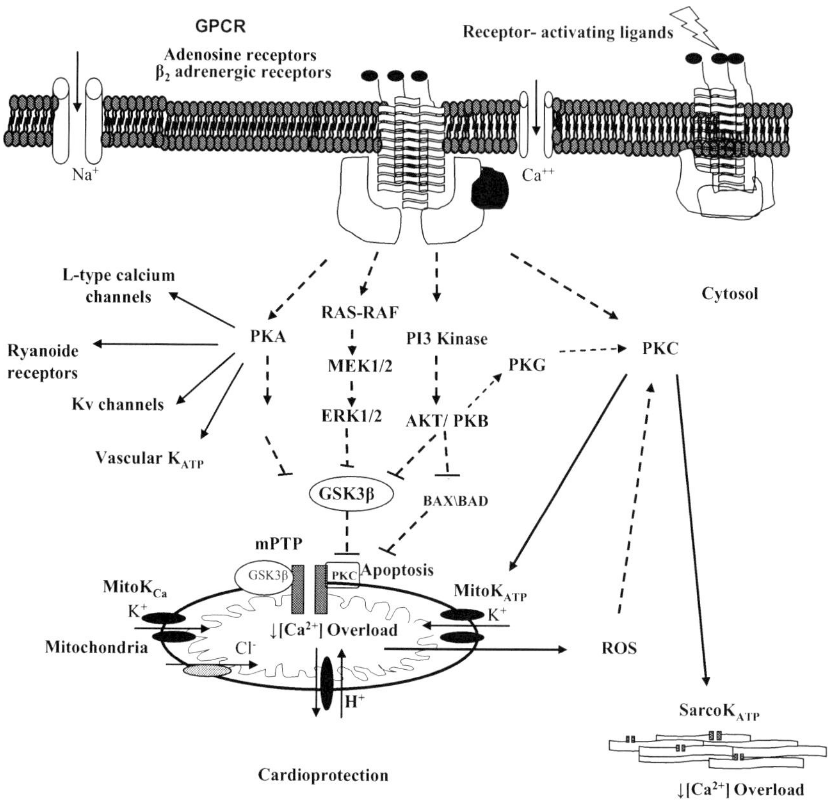


**Fig. 4.3.** Signaling pathways mediating cardioprotection after ischemia-reperfusion. Schematic representation of various proteins and pathways involved in cardioprotective responses to ischemia-reperfusion injury.

CoA can be regenerated to supply the citric-acid cycle (Ussher & Lopaschuk, 2008). Importantly, the oxidation of fatty acids increases the acetyl CoA:CoA ratio, which inhibits pyruvate dehydrogenase (PDH) and glucose oxidation via a phenomenon termed the "Randle Cycle" (Randle et al., 1963).

Ischemia–reperfusion dramatically alters cardiac energy metabolism, thereby decreasing cardiac efficiency (Fig. 4.4). Ischemic events will shift the aerobic metabolism to anaerobic within seconds, thereby triggering glycolysis, glycogen breakdown, and reduced ATP. Pyruvate is not readily oxidized in the mitochondria, and results in the production of lactate, a drop in pH, a reduction in contractile function, and a greater demand for ATP. Fatty acids become the dominate substrate for oxidative metabolism at the expense of glucose oxidation (Ussher & Lopaschuk, 2008; Whitmer et al., 1978). This triggers an uncoupling between glycolysis and

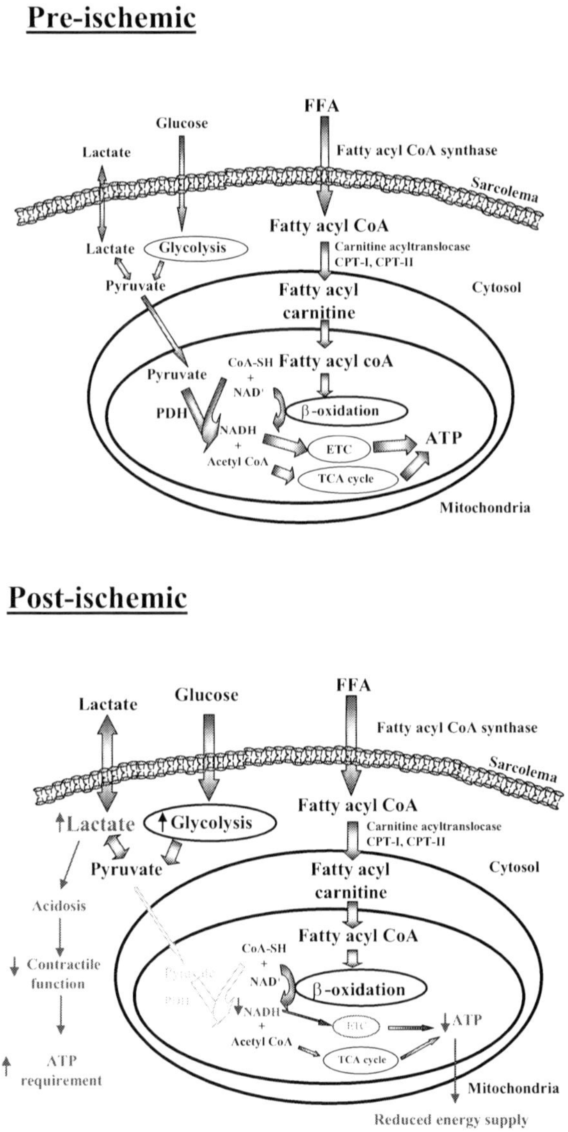


**Fig. 4.4.** Overview of myocardial energetics in pre-ischemic and post-ischemic conditions. In the pre-ischemic condition, fatty acids provide most of the energy (in the form of adenosine triphosphate or ATP) required for normal heart function, with the remainder supplied by glycolysis and lactate oxidation. Fatty-acid β-oxidation and pyruvate dehydrogenation use nicotinamide adenine dinucleotide ($NAD^+$) and Coenzyme A (CoA) to produce NADH and acetyl CoA. NADH is used in the electron transport chain (ETC) to generate ATP, while the Krebs cycle makes use of acetyl CoA. In the post-ischemic condition, however, a metabolic shift from aerobic to anaerobic metabolism occurs which causes an increase in glycogen breakdown and a concomitant reduction in pyruvate oxidation. This mitochondrial shift ultimately causes an increase in lactate production, a decrease in pH, and a reduction contractile function. As a result of the decreased NADH due to the anaerobic metabolism of fatty acids, less ATP is produced and an energy imbalance occurs.

glucose oxidation, contributing to the intracellular acidosis observed in ischemic hearts (Ferdinandy et al., 2007; Halestrap et al., 1998; Piper et al., 2003; Ussher & Lopaschuk, 2008). Indeed, decreased fatty acid oxidation and increased glucose oxidation are associated with an improved functional recovery, following ischemia–reperfusion injury in experimental animal models (Dyck et al., 2006). During reperfusion, fatty acids remain the dominate source for oxidative energy metabolism, further inhibiting glucose oxidation (Dyck & Lopaschuk, 2002; Liu et al., 1996). Ischemia–reperfusion injury results in increased plasma fatty acid levels and subcellular changes to the heart which decrease the control of fatty acid oxidation (Kurien & Oliver, 1971). For example, decreased levels of malonyl CoA, an inhibitor of CPT-I, result in an increased mitochondrial uptake of fatty acids and a subsequent oxidation (Kudo et al., 1996; Ussher & Lopaschuk, 2008). Initially, elevated energy is beneficial for the activation of different compensatory mechanisms that aid in the recovery or prevention of further injury. However, fatty acid oxidation is not an optimal energy source for heart function compared to glucose which improves cardiac efficiency (Ussher & Lopaschuk, 2008).

## n-3 Polyunsaturated Fatty Acids

An increased consumption of n-3 PUFAs is linked with the reduced risk of CVD, MI, cardiac arrhythmias, sudden cardiac death, atherosclerosis, and hypertension (Wang et al., 2006). The n-3 PUFAs are a family of unsaturated fatty acids that exist as 18–22 carbon chains with a double bond at the third carbon atom from the terminal methyl group (Jump, 2002). The α-linolenic acid (ALA, 18:3n-3), ecosapentaenoic acid (EPA, 20:5n-3), and docosahexaenoic acid (DHA, 22:6n-3) are the most important n-3 PUFAs that are not synthesized in the human body. ALA, the primary essential source of n-3 PUFA, is converted to EPA and DHA by increasing the chain length and the desaturation of the carboxyl end (Haag, 2003; Harris, 2007). ALA is a plant-derived PUFA that cannot be synthesized in mammals, and is the precursor for the synthesis of long-chain n-3 PUFAs (Burdge & Calder, 2005; Gebauer et al., 2006; Jump, 2002). Other members of this family include ecosatrienoic acid, ecosatetraenoic acid, stearidonic acid, docosapentaenoic acid, tetracosapentaenoic acid, and tetracosahexaenoic acid (Gebauer et al., 2006; Jump, 2002). Green leaves, rapeseed oil, soybean oil, flaxseed, nuts, and oily fish are the main sources of ALA in the diet. By the action of desaturase and elongase enzymes, ALA gets converted to EPA or DHA in endoplasmic reticulum (Burdge & Calder, 2005; Jump, 2002). Dietary composition of n-3 PUFAs has a profound effect on the progression of CVD. The American Heart Association (AHA) recommends 1 g/day of EPA + DHA for individuals with known CHD and the consumption of 2 meals/week of oily fish plus oils rich in ALA for persons without known CHD (Kris-Etherton et al., 2002). Recent recommendations suggest that the consumption of an EPA and a DHA intake of at least 250 mg/day should be part of a management program for the prevention of CVD (Deckelbaum et al., 2008).

Experimental studies demonstrate a broad range of overlapping cardiovascular effects attributed to n-3 PUFAs that account for an improved outcome. Several mechanisms were proposed to explain the cardioprotective effects of n-3 PUFAs, most notably for EPA and DHA. These include effects on the resting heart rate, eicosanoid signaling and gene expression, anti-arrhythmic properties, anti-atherogenic effects, reduced blood pressure, increased blood- clotting factor (fibrin), lowering plasma triacylglycerol, and the alteration of membrane microdomains and arterial cholesterol levels (Das, 2000; Dewailly et al., 2001; Jung et al., 2008; Kris-Etherton et al., 2002; Qi et al., 2008; Stillwell & Wassall, 2003). Although, the exact mechanism(s) by which n-3 PUFAs protect the heart from ischemia–reperfusion injury remains unknown; the regulation of the heart rate, a reduced myocardial oxygen consumption, and an increased coronary reserve contribute to a preconditioning-like effect that provides cardioprotective response to injury (McLennan et al., 2007).

## *n-3 PUFAs in Cardiovascular Disease*

Early evidence of the protective role of n-3 PUFAs in CVD resulted from studies suggesting that the lower risk and mortality observed in Greenland Inuits as compared to Americans and Danes were due to a diet higher in fish oil (Bang et al., 1980). Similarly, a lower incidence of thrombotic events for people living in Japan and Nunavik correlates with greater amounts of marine oil and fish in their diet (Dewailly et al., 2001; Dyerberg et al., 1978; Yamori et al., 1985). Fish-oil consumption in the diet is therefore inversely related to CHD mortality. An intake of 20 g/day of fish correlates with a ≈7% reduction in CHD mortality (Breslow, 2006; von Schacky, 2007; Xiao et al., 2008). More recently, data from a large, prospective, randomized clinical trial— "Dietary supplementation with n-3 polyunsaturated fatty acids and vitamin E after a myocardial infarction: results of the GISSI-Prevensione Trial"— demonstrated that n-3 PUFA supplementation reduced death, nonfatal MI, and stroke in individuals who had a recent MI (GISSI, 1999). More profound effects of n-3 PUFAs are observed when DHA and EPA are supplemented as ethyl esters rather than fish intake or fish-oil supplements (Hooper et al., 2004; von Schacky, 2006). These findings motivated numerous subsequent studies investigating the cardioprotective effects of n-3 PUFAs.

Some of the epidemiological studies show an ineffectiveness of n-3 PUFA in preventing myocardial ischemia and an overall risk of cardiac events. No significance was observed in any CHD including nonfatal MI, sudden cardiac death, coronary artery bypass grafting, and angioplasty in the Health Professionals' Follow-up Study (Ascherio et al., 1995). Another study also shows that no correlation exists between fish intake and a reduced risk of fatal MI, nonsudden cardiac death, and total cardiovascular mortality (Albert et al., 1998). No correlation was observed between fish intake and CHD mortality in the Seven Country Study data (Kromhout et al., 1996). Also no association was observed between n-3 PUFA intake and the risk of MI in the EURAMIC study (Guallar et al., 1999). These differences may be partially attributed to study design since some were performed in populations with a high baseline intake of n-3 PUFAs, and others utilized lower doses of EPA and DHA (Akabas & Deckelbaum, 2006; von Schacky, 2007). Many additional confounding factors include alcohol consumption, exercise habits, and a misclassification of dietary SFAs or n-6 PUFAs (Jung et al., 2008). Whether n-3 PUFAs are beneficial in preventing MI or not is still being debated; however, the majority of the literature strongly indicates that n-3 PUFAs are cardioprotective (Wang et al., 2006).

## *n-3 PUFA Anti-arrhythmic Effects*

An AMI is damage and/or death of heart muscle as a result of ischemia–reperfusion injury. Two of the adverse consequences and common predictors of mortality following myocardial ischemia are low heart-rate variability and arrhythmias. A reduction in mortality in AMI patients was observed in individuals whose fish intake was two times a week (Burr et al., 1989) or who had taken n-3 fatty acid supplements ($\approx$1 g/day) (Marchioli et al., 2002). More recently, a population-based cohort study assessing atrial fibrillation incidents over a 12-year follow-up demonstrated that an increased consumption of fish was associated with a reduction in incidents (Mozaffarian et al., 2004). Various other studies demonstrated a strong correlation between a high dietary intake (fish or supplementation) of n-3 fatty acids and an improved heart rate and reduced MI mortality (Christensen et al., 1997; Macchia et al., 2008). In addition, animal models of myocardial ischemia support the anti-arrhythmic action of n-3 PUFAs, demonstrating reduced infarction size and reduced susceptibility to arrhythmias (McLennan et al., 1985, 1988).

The exact mechanisms by which n-3 PUFAs exert anti-arrhythmic properties remain unclear. The cardioprotective effects of n-3 fatty acids may result from a direct effect on the myocardium or by incorporation into the membrane and alteration of protein function. The simple structure and unsaturated nature of n-3 PUFAs allow for easy incorporation into lipid membranes and mitochondria. In the plasma membrane, DHA binds to the *sn*-2 position of the phospholipid acyl chain while, in comparison, SFAs are found in the *sn*-1 position (Harris, 2007; Stillwell & Wassall, 2003). An alteration in membrane structure by the incorporation of n-3 fatty acids can cause secondary effects on receptors and transmembrane proteins which lead to changes in receptor–ligand interactions and downstream signals (Diniz et al., 2004). Proper ion-channel function is of the utmost importance to contractility in the heart following ischemia–reperfusion injury. Evidence demonstrates that n-3 fatty acids can affect ion channels such as voltage-gated $Na^+$ channels ($I_{Na}$), voltage-gated L-type $Ca^{2+}$ channels ($I_{Ca,L}$), human ether-a-go-go-related-gene (HERG) channels, and Kv 1.5 channels (Guizy et al., 2005, 2008; Xiao et al., 1995, 1997, 1998). The n-3 fatty acids enhance the long-activated delayed-rectifier $K^+$ current ($I_{K,1}$) and the slow-activated delayed-rectifier $K^+$ current ($I_{Ks}$). Following ischemia–reperfusion injury, the development of a gradient of depolarization can elicit action potentials to occur at inappropriate periods of the cardiac electrical cycle, thus initiating arrhythmias

(Leaf et al., 2003). Additionally, $I_{Ca,L}$ and $Ca^+$ sparks ($Ca^+$ release from sarcoplasmic reticulum) are detrimental to the heart, and partially responsible for the arrhythmic event that occurs after ischemia. The hyperpolarization of the resting-membrane potential, the increased threshold for the opening of $Na^+$ channels, the inhibition of $I_{Ca,L}$ and $Ca^+$ sparks, and prolonged refractory periods were shown to occur following n-3 PUFA treatment. Together, these effects lead to the stabilization of the heart rate and a reduced risk of arrhythmic events (Xiao et al., 1997, 1998).

Apart from the channels in the ventricles, n-3 fatty acids can block the atrial-specific Kv 1.5 channels, and play a role in the prevention of supraventricular arrhythmias (Guizy et al., 2008). Studies using cell models show that both n-3 and n-6 PUFAs block the HERG channels at physiological concentrations (Guizy et al., 2005). The blockage was time-, voltage-, and state-dependent which suggests a blockage of the channel during an open state. However, arachidonic acid is reported to block the channel in the inactive state as well. A blockage of the HERG channel with other channels ($Na^+$, $Ca^{2+}$, and several $K^+$ channels) would result in the lengthening of the refractory period and a decreased excitability of the cardiac muscle which may contribute to the anti-arrhythmic effect of n-3 PUFAs (Guizy et al., 2005). Overall, n-3 PUFAs directly affect various ion channels, and protect the heart from fatal arrhythmias after ischemic events.

## *n-3 PUFA Alteration to Membrane Microdomain*

The plasma membrane is comprised of a mosaic of functional microdomains that facilitate interactions between resident proteins and lipids (Hancock, 2006; Laude & Prior, 2004). Increasing evidence suggests that n-3 PUFAs, notably DHA, are unique because they alter cell-membrane function, particularly acyl chain order and fluidity, phase behavior, elasticity, ion permeability, and protein function (Stillwell et al., 2005). For example, the n-3 PUFA composition of membrane phospholipids modifies the activities and the function of proteins. This includes ion channels like the $Ca^{2+}$-$Mg^{2+}$-ATPase and $Na^+$-$Ca^{2+}$ exchanger, which regulate events such as $Ca^{2+}$ uptake by sarcoplasmic reticulum (SR) and cellular $Na^+$ currents (Pepe, 2005). DHA's *cis* double bonds render it sterically incompatible with cholesterol and sphingolipids; therefore, incorporation into the plasma membrane leads to a reduction in the cholesterol content of microdomains (Stillwell et al., 2005). The reduction in cholesterol levels in the plasma membrane will impact fluidity and function which can affect downstream signaling. Notably, cardiac levels of DHA are concentrated in membranes (well above circulating levels) which is functionally significant because DHA is thought to be the key n-3 PUFA found in the heart (McLennan et al., 2007). One can observe the importance of membrane-bound n-3 PUFAs in isolated heart experiments where many of the functional changes occur in the absence of circulating PUFAs (McLennan & Abeywardena, 2005).

The effect of DHA on the cholesterol content of microdomains is only one example of membrane interactions. Caveolae, another subset of membrane rafts, appear as small flask-shaped invaginations of the plasma membrane that contain the structural proteins caveolin and cavin (Patel et al., 2008a). Caveolae play an important role in intracellular signal transduction. Interestingly, the incorporation of n-3 fatty acids into the plasma membrane leads to a reduction in caveolin-1 and caveolin-3 (Ma et al., 2004a; Seo et al., 2006). These data suggest another modality by which n-3 PUFA remodeling of membrane microdomains can influence protein localization and subcellular signaling (Ma et al., 2004a). A majority of the findings suggest a positive correlation between a high n-3 PUFA diet and the protective signaling following an ischemic event (Das et al., 2008).

## *n-3 PUFA Effects on Cardiac Function*

Experimental data demonstrate that dietary fish oil can improve contractile function in hearts "stunned" from an ischemia–reperfusion injury (Pepe & McLennan, 1996). These effects may be partially attributed to lower heart rates observed in hearts treated with n-3 PUFAs, which would allow for increased diastolic filling time and increased coronary perfusion (McLennan & Abeywardena, 2005). Additionally, n-3 PUFAs can reduce myocardial oxygen consumption ($MVO_2$) and enhance oxygen utilization while maintaining cardiac output (Pepe & McLennan, 2002). This is reflected by a lower coronary flow at rest and an increased capacity to deliver greater blood flow following demand (McLennan et al., 2007). Conversely, increased SFA uptake results in increased $MVO_2$ and reduced cardiac output. Low $MVO_2$ is important to cardiac function because it will lead to reduced lactic-acid production, thereby preventing $H^+$ buildup and systemic acidosis after an ischemic event (Pepe & McLennan, 2002). The improved ventricular function following ischemia–reperfusion attributed to increased n-3 PUFA incorporation in myocardial membranes suggests direct cardioprotective effects beyond antiatherogenic and antithrombotic actions (McLennan et al., 2007; Pepe & McLennan, 2002).

## *n-3 PUFA Effects on Mitochondrial Function*

Heart function is extremely vulnerable to mitochondrial damage in light of its strict dependence on aerobic metabolism. Indeed, mitochondrial dysfunction, leading to alterations in metabolism and bioenergetics, plays a crucial role in myocardial injury. Ischemia–reperfusion injury causes extensive damage to mitochondria, such as the uncoupling of oxidative respiration, increased $Ca^{2+}$ levels, an overproduction of ROS, and increased apoptosis. Cardioprotective strategies are aimed at reducing the consequences of mitochondrial impairment in the ischemic heart. Experimental studies in rats fed a diet rich in n-3 PUFA demonstrated an increased incorporation into the mitochondrial membrane (Pepe et al., 1999). The increased mitochondrial n-3 PUFA content correlated with the lower mitochondrial $Ca^{2+}$ levels, and improved recovery compared to n-6 PUFA-rich hearts. The hyperpolarization of mitochondrial membrane potential ($\Delta\Psi m$), moreover, causes damage to mitochondria and leads to the release of mitochondrial apoptotic protein from the mitochondria (Stillwell et al., 1997). Evidence suggests that increased mitochondrial membrane n-3 PUFA content will influence $H^+$ transport, causing a depolarization of $\Delta\Psi m$. While the current understanding of the functional importance of n-3 PUFA in mitochondrial function is limited, new research investigating the beneficial aspects to energetics and cardioprotection is emerging.

### *n-3 PUFA Metabolites*

Much of the evidence suggests that n-3 PUFAs, such as EPA and DHA, play important roles in limiting ischemic injury. However, some of these effects may be mediated through the active metabolites of EPA and DHA. The n-3 PUFAs get metabolized by cyclooxygenases (COXs) and lipoxygenases (LOXs) to prostanoids and leukotrienes, respectively. A third pathway, which generates eicosanoids of n-3 PUFAs, is cytochrome P450 (CYP) monooxygenase enzymes (Barbosa-Sicard et al., 2005; Oliw et al., 1996). In humans, CYP2C subfamily enzymes are responsible for the production of EPA/DHA eicosanoids. Human CYP2C and CYP2J enzymes metabolize arachidonic acid (AA) to four regioisomeric epoxyeicosatrienoic acids (5,6-, 8,9-, 11,12-, and 14,15-EET). CYP2C8 metabolizes EPA to analogous eicosanoids 11,12- and 14,15-epoxyeicosatetraenoic acids (EETeTrs). The major eicosanoid product of EPA is 17,18-EETeTrs, which is generated when CYP2C8 acts on the 17,18-double bond to add an epoxide group. CYP2C9 is another enzyme from the CYP2C subfamily that causes the epoxidation of EPA to form eicosanoids. In contrast with CYP2C8, CYP2C9 produces more 11,12- and 14,15-EETeTrs rather than 17,18-EETeTrs (Barbosa-Sicard et al., 2005). These metabolites are important not only for the inflammatory response but also in maintaining cardiovascular function. For example, 17,18-EETeTrs activate the large-conductance $Ca^{2+}$-activated $K^+$ channels ($BK_{Ca}$ channels), and cause the relaxation of vascular smooth muscle cells (SMCs) (Lauterbach et al., 2002).

$BK_{Ca}$ channels are voltage-sensitive $K^+$ selective proteins expressed in various tissues including heart mitochondria (Xu et al., 2002). The elevations in intracellular $Ca^{2+}$ and membrane depolarization can activate $K_{Ca}$ channels (Brayden & Nelson, 1992; Calderone, 2002). The opening of $BK_{Ca}$ channels prevents ischemic injury by modulating cAMP-dependent protein kinases, preventing a loss of mitochondrial membrane potential and limiting a $Ca^{2+}$ overload in mitochondria (Ohya et al., 2005; Sato et al., 2005). As discussed previously in this chapter, the activation of $BK_{Ca}$ channels is one of the protective mechanisms of n-3 PUFAs; however, whether it is a direct effect of metabolites or an effect caused by altered membrane organization remains to be elucidated.

## n-6 Polyunsaturated Fatty Acids

The n-6 PUFAs are a family of unsaturated fatty acids that exist as 18–22 carbon chains with a double bond at the sixth carbon atom from the terminal methyl group (Jump, 2002). Linoleic acid (LA, 18:2n-6), the primary source of the essential n-6

PUFAs, is converted to AA (20:4n-6) by desaturation and elongation via enzyme systems within the body (Haag, 2003; Harris, 2007). Animals cannot convert n-6 PUFAs to n-3 PUFAs because they lack the converting enzyme, ω-3 desaturase. Both n-3 and n-6 PUFAs are essential fatty acids, and greater intakes of both are related to lower risks (Willett, 2007). Not surprisingly, n-6 PUFAs are metabolically and functionally distinct from n-3 PUFAs (Simopoulos, 2008). Importantly, both n-3 and n-6 PUFAs compete for the activity of the rate-limiting Δ6-desaturase for the conversion to longer chain PUFAs. Therefore, an overabundance of LA will limit the conversion of ALA to EPA or DHA, thus, influencing physiological events (Griffin, 2008). Indeed, a higher intake of LA is associated with a high risk of heart disease by shifting the physiological state to a more pathogenic state. This is partially attributed to the metabolism of n-6 PUFAs by COX and LOX enzymes which produce proinflammatory, prothrombotic, and proconstrictive eicosanoids (Haag, 2003). These eicosanoid products are biologically active in very small amounts, and contribute to effects such as increased blood viscosity, thrombosis, vasospasm, vasoconstriction, and decreased bleeding time, which increase the risk of CVD (Simopoulos, 2008). Contrary to the adverse effects of n-6 PUFAs, recent data suggest that some n-6 PUFAs produced from CYP epoxygenases are cardioprotective in animal models (Gross et al., 2008; Lee et al., 2006; Node et al., 1999; Seubert et al., 2007). A polymorphism in CYP2J2 epoxygenase, which metabolizes AA, is positively associated with the risk of numerous cardiac diseases in humans (Lee et al., 2007). New investigation into the beneficial effects of specific n-6 PUFAs will help resolve the inconsistencies regarding the role of n-3 and n-6 PUFAs in ischemic injury (Fig. 4.5).

## n-6 PUFA in Cardiovascular Disease

Both n-3 and n-6 PUFAs are essential nutrients that exert important effects on membranes and cellular function which ultimately impact CVD outcomes. However, the determination of the absolute intake and the n-3/n-6 ratio to achieve optimal cardiovascular health remain unknown (Wijendran & Hayes, 2004). Early epidemiological studies demonstrated that a higher intake of LA reduces the risk of CHDs, where lower dietary intake of LA predisposed individuals to MI (Ascherio, 2002; Ascherio et al., 1999; Riemersma et al., 1986; Simpson et al., 1982). In the 1960s and 1980s, the United States and other Western countries recommended replacing SFAs with unsaturated fatty acids (Stephen & Wald, 1990). As a result of this high intake of LA, a reduction occurred in the mortality rates of cardiac disease by approximately 19% during this period (Willett, 2007). The analysis of an n-6 PUFA intake with a CHD risk in the "Nurses' Health Study Cohort" also showed that increasing LA consumption was associated with a lower risk of CHD (Hu et al., 1997, 1999). In addition, the ratio of ALA to LA was not associated with a risk of fatal CHD because both were found to be beneficial. Numerous prospective cohort studies support data suggesting that a high n-6 PUFA intake is cardioprotective (Erkkila et al., 2008; Hu et al., 1997).

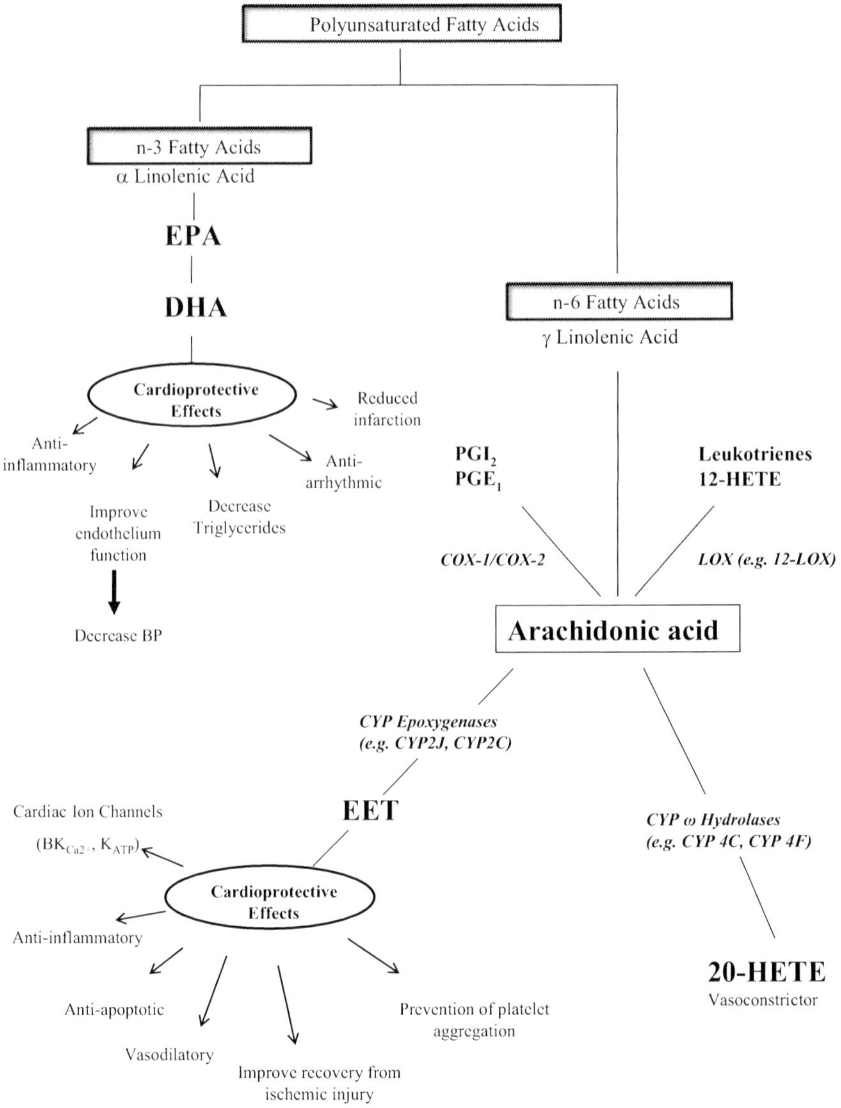


**Fig. 4.5.** An overview of n-3 and n-6 fatty-acid metabolism and cardioprotective action. Simplified overview of the cardioprotective effects of n-3 and n-6 PUFA involved in ischemia-reperfusion injury.

## n-6 PUFA CYP-Derived Metabolites of Arachidonic Acid

AA is found esterified to the *sn*-2 position of the glycophospholipids of the cell membrane. In response to various stress stimuli, the activation of phospholipase $A_2$ causes the hydrolysis of the ester linkage between phosphatidycholine (PC) and phosphatidylethanolamine (PE) to release free AA (Morisseau & Hammock, 2005). The released AA is metabolized by LOXs to lipoxins and leukotrienes, and by COXs to prostaglandins , prostacyclins , and thromboxanes. Apart from these two pathways, AA is also metabolized by CYP monoxygenase enzymes to a different class of biologically active metabolites called epoxyeicosatrienoic acids (EETs) and hydroxyeicosatetraenoic acids (HETEs) (Fang et al., 2004; Morisseau & Hammock, 2005). Various CYPs and corresponding isoforms are expressed in the liver, kidney, heart, gastrointestinal tract, lungs, and vasculature. CYP2B, CYP2C8, CYP2C9, CYP2C10, and CYP2J2 families are expressed in the human heart and vasculature, and are involved in AA metabolism (Delozier et al., 2007; Zeldin et al., 1995). Among all these CYPs, CYP2J2 is highly expressed in human cardiomyocytes, and is the predominant enzyme for the synthesis of all four reigoisomers of EETs (Spiecker & Liao, 2006). These epoxygenases replace one of the four double bonds of AA with an epoxide group that leads to the formation of four different regioisomers, 5,6-, 8,9-, 11,12-, and 14,15-EET (Fang et al., 2004). EETs are esterified to cellular membranes, metabolized by β-oxidation to shorter carbon chain molecules, and converted to corresponding dihydroxyeicosatrienoic acids (5,6-, 8,9-, 11,12-, and 14,15-DHET) by soluble epoxide hydrolase (sEH), which reduces their biological activity (Morisseau & Hammock, 2005). Although EETs incorporation into membrane lipids might alter lipid environments, their rapid release upon agonist stimulation suggests this might occur in a transient manner (Gauthier et al., 2007).

EETs are important components of many intracellular signaling pathways in both cardiac and extracardiac tissues. For example, EETs activate $Ca^{2+}$-sensitive $K^+$ channels (BKca) in vascular SMCs, resulting in the hyperpolarization of the resting-membrane potential and the vasodilation of the coronary circulation, as well as the activation of vascular and cardiac ATP-sensitive potassium channels ($K_{ATP}$ channels) (Campbell et al., 1996; Fisslthaler et al., 1999; Fleming, 2004; Ke et al., 2007; Lu et al., 2002, 2006; Ye et al., 2006). EETs have anti-inflammatory, thrombolytic, and angiogenic properties within the vasculature (Node et al., 1999). They activate mitogen-activated protein kinase (MAPK) and phosphatidylinositol-3 kinase (PI3K) signaling pathways, and increase intracellular cAMP levels (Node et al., 1999; Wang et al., 2003, 2005). Indeed, as EETs can activate many signaling pathways, the manipulation of production or metabolism can have wide-ranging consequences.

During an ischemic insult, AA is released from plasma membranes and metabolized by CYP epoxygenases to EETs, which have beneficial effects to the heart. Animal models of an ischemia–reperfusion injury in mice, rats, rabbits, and dogs demonstrated that EETs play an important role in the recovery of contractile function and the reduction of infarct development (Gross et al., 2007, 2008; Nithipatikom et al., 2006; Seubert et al., 2004, 2006). Mechanistic studies demonstrated that the improved recovery was partially due to the activation of sarcolemma ATP-sensitive potassium channels ($K_{ATP}$ channels) (Gross et al., 2007; Nithipatikom et al., 2006; Seubert et al., 2004, 2006). The activation of signaling pathways like PI3 kinase, which inhibits glycogen synthase kinase-3β, and initial bursts of ROS are involved in EET-induced cardioprotective responses (Gross et al., 2007; Nithipatikom et al., 2006; Seubert et al., 2006). 20-HETE is an example of a CYP ω-hydroxylase product of AA to make products that have vastly different physiologic effects. For example, 20-HETE has potent vasoconstrictive effects (Roman et al., 2000). Therefore, changes in the expression and/or activity of specific CYP epoxygenase and hydroxylase enzymes can alter the delicate balance between EETs and 20-HETE. For instance, recent data demonstrated that the inhibition of CYP ω-hydroxylases results in the reduction of the infarction size in rats and dogs following ischemic injury, which suggests that 20-HETE has detrimental effects in the heart (Granville et al., 2004; Gross et al., 2004; Nithipatikom et al., 2004). These results suggest that the major effect of inhibiting ω-hydroxylase in rats occurs during reperfusion, and is associated with a decrease in reperfusion injury.

Recent human epidemiological evidence identified associations between CYP2J2 polymorphisms and CAD as well as EPHX2 polymorphisms and CHD (Fornage et al., 2004; Lee, 2006; Przybyla-Zawislak et al., 2003; Spiecker et al., 2004). These findings provide strong evidence supporting the notion that EETs are cardioprotective (Seubert et al., 2004; Wu et al., 1996, 1997; Xiao et al., 2004). Studies have only begun to understand the cellular mechanisms of EET-mediated cardioprotection. They highlight the potential for this endogenous system as a therapeutic target for CVD, and may be a potent combination in alleviating the sequelae of ischemia and/or reperfusion injury in a clinical setting such as coronary-artery bypass-graft surgery.

## n-6 PUFA CYP-Derived Metabolites of Linoleic Acid

CYP epoxygenases metabolize LA to leukotoxins, (±)9(10)-epoxy-12*Z*- and (±)12(13)-epoxy-9*Z*-octadecenoic acid and 9,10-, and 12,13-EpOME (Ozawa et al., 1988). Elevated levels of leukotoxins are associated with acute respiratory burst syndrome (ARDS) and trauma. The administration of exogenous EpOME to different animal models results in ARDS-related signs of toxicity like vasodilatation, pulmonary edema, and cardiac failure (Sisemore et al., 2001; Thompson & Hammock, 2007). Epoxide hydrolase metabolizes 9,10-, and 12,13-EpOME to dihydrometabolites (9,10-, and 12,13-DiHOME, respectively) (Thompson & Hammock, 2007). Several studies demonstrate leukotoxins as protoxins because their epoxide hydrolase metabolites are responsible for ARDS and other toxic effects (Moghaddam et al., 1997; Zheng et al., 2001). Toxic effects of EpOMEs may be the result of DiHOME-mediated toxicity. DiHOMEs are reported to affect the sodium channels in cardiac cells, and trigger mitochondrial dysfunction (Thompson & Hammock, 2007). DiHOMEs depress $Na^+$ channels, and $K^+$ channels (while EpOMEs failed) exert such effects (Harrell

& Stimers, 2002; Stimers et al., 1999; Xiao et al., 1995). In experimental models of myocardial ischemia, leukotoxin levels rise from undetectable levels to 1 μg/g of tissue, while leukotriene metabolites (DiHOME) increase from 1–3 μg/g of tissue to 4–22 μg/g of tissue (Dudda et al., 1996). An intravenous administration of leukotoxins and LA in dogs resulted in the depression of cardiac functions, but more depression of cardiac functions was observed in leukotoxins as compared to LA (Fukushima et al., 1988). Leukotoxins are responsible for a massive burst of ROS, a blockage of cardiac ion channels, and mitochondrial dysfunctions, suggesting that EpOME or DiHOME may play a role in myocardial ischemia as well.

## n-6 PUFA Metabolism by Cyclooxygenase

COXs can convert AA to prostaglandins (PGs) and thromboxanes (TXs) in both the heart itself as well as coronary blood vessels. Two predominant COX isozymes are COX-1 and COX-2, which differ in expression and tissue localization. COX-1 is constitutively expressed, while the COX-2 expression is inducible by varied stimuli. The roles of COX metabolites and the effects of COX inhibition in ischemia–reperfusion injury were studied extensively. Several drug treatments are available that are based on these principles, but further study has even led to the withdrawal of certain drugs from clinical use, most notably rofecoxib and valdecoxib (FitzGerald, 2007; Funk & FitzGerald, 2007; Grosser et al., 2006; Salinas et al., 2007). COX-1 metabolites, $PGI_2$ and $PGE_1$, possess important roles in acute ischemia–reperfusion injury (Camitta et al., 2001; Farber et al., 1988; van Bilsen et al., 1989). Early studies in animal models demonstrated that COX-1 metabolite, $PGI_2$, attenuated post-ischemic contractile dysfunction in stunned myocardium, attenuated metabolic derangements, improved mitochondrial respiration, and improved regional-wall function (Farber et al., 1988; Ichihara et al., 1993).

The cardioprotective effect of COX-2 involving production of $PGI_2$ and $PGE_1$, plays a more important role in late or delayed IPC (Guo et al., 2000; Shinmura et al., 2000). The late phase of IPC is the result of the simultaneous activation of multiple stress–response pathways that initiate changes in protein expression. This results in an overall protective cardiac phenotype. Experimental models revealed that both IPC and opioid-mediated cardioprotection in rabbit and rat require the COX-2 production of $PGI_2$ and $PGE_1$ (Shinmura et al., 2000). The δ-opioid receptor agonist induces a preconditioning effect 24 hours after treatment in a rabbit model of occlusion–reperfusion. However, COX-2 inhibitors abolish this effect (Kodani et al., 2002). Further evidence, moreover, demonstrated that atorvastatin-mediated cardioprotection was attenuated when co-administered with valdecoxib (Birnbaum et al., 2005). However, valdecoxib did not affect infarction size when given alone. These data confirmed early studies in COX-1 and COX-2 knockout mice in which long-term inhibition or genetic disruption enhanced cardiac injury following ischemia–reperfusion (Camitta et al., 2001). The acute administration of indomethacin (COX inhibitor) was not detrimental, suggesting that the cardioprotective effects require an altered expression or an up-regulation of COX to generate the beneficial metabolites. Together, the data demonstrate that the protective effects of COX-2 occur in a preconditioned setting, and highlight the risk posed by COX-2 inhibitors in increased cardiovascular morbidity and mortality. COX isozymes are involved in numerous complex intracellular signaling pathways that are tissue- and cell-dependent. As such, the increased risk of adverse outcomes is much more complex than described above; however, the inhibition of intrinsic cardioprotective mechanisms by COX-2 inhibitors plays an important role in enhancing ischemia–reperfusion injury.

### *n-6 PUFA Metabolism by Lipooxygenase*

LOXs are the third main class of enzymes that can metabolize AA to generate bioactive metabolites such as leukotrienes, lipoxins, and hepoxilins (Kulkarni, 2001). The different LOX isozymes (5-,8-, 12-, and 15-LOX) metabolize AA to the corresponding 5-, 8-, 12-, 15-HPETE by dioxygenation. The reduction of these metabolites leads to the production of corresponding hydroxyl derivatives (5-, 8-, 12-, 15-HETE). Studies done on 12-LOX, 12-HpETE, and 12-HETE clearly suggest that 12-HpETE and 12-HETE are important for ischemic/pharmacological preconditioning. Early experimental data suggest that 12-HETE and 12-HpETE play a role in reducing ischemia–reperfusion injury by activating protective pathways similar to those observed in IPC (Chen et al., 1999; Gabel et al., 2001). Mice with a targeted disruption of leukocyte-type 12-LOX have a low production of 12-HETE, and have shown a reduction in post-ischemic functional recovery (Gabel et al., 2001). Elevated levels of 12-LOX-derived metabolites are important for both ischemic preconditioning and PKC-activated protection. Notably, experimental data suggest that the production of the 12-LOX metabolite, 12-HETE, is associated with an improved functional recovery in opioid or volatile anesthetic-induced delayed cardioprotection (Patel et al., 2003; Tsutsumi et al., 2006). The protective mechanism(s) of LOX metabolites is thought to be partially attributed to the activation of mitochondrial $K_{ATP}$ channels by 12-HETE or 12-HpETE (Chen et al., 1999). 12-HpETE is known to activate $K^+$ channels but inhibit $Ca^{2+}$ channels (Murphy et al., 1995). Interestingly, no effect on ischemia–reperfusion injury was observed in mice with a targeted deletion of 5-LOX. Apparently, 5-LOX does not play any role in an ischemia–reperfusion injury, but is important for the inflammatory response that occurs in response to the ischemic event (Adamek et al., 2007). Overall, published data indicate that 12-LOX and its major metabolite, 12-HETE, are important in both acute and delayed IPC.

## ***Trans* Fatty Acids**

Most naturally occurring unsaturated fatty acids have a *cis* conformation surrounding the double bond (Fig. 4.6). Isomeric *trans* forms, however, are produced by bacteria in the rumen of cattle and also by the industrial hydrogenation of unsaturated fatty acids to develop commercial products (Ascherio et al., 1994). In the early 1950s, naturally produced *trans*-unsaturated fatty acids were characterized in ruminant animals (Hartman & Shorland, 1959). The commercial process conversely, begun in the early twentieth century, involves household products such as margarine, and resulted in the prevalence of TFAs in the human dietary supply (Ascherio et al., 1999). In this process, *cis* polyunsaturated vegetable and fish oils are subjected to partial hydrogenation using a metal catalyst to produce *trans* isomeric monounsaturated and polyunsaturated compounds. As shown in Fig. 4.6, *trans* isomers result in carbon chains extending on the opposite sides of the double bond as opposed to *cis* isomers on the same side. The altered conformation allows the fatty acid chains to pack tightly together similar to the way saturated fatty acids do, and results in a semi-solid product (such as margarine).

In recent years, the association of TFAs and CVD has garnered a great deal of media attention. In humans, the primary sources of TFAs are processed foods such as margarine (Ascherio, 2002). Numerous clinical trials were conducted to elucidate the link between TFA intake and CVD. A summary of clinical trials to date finds that four distinct cohorts as well as two nested case controls found a positive correlation between TFA intake and heart disease (Booker & Mann, 2008). Other case-control studies show more variation, but a trend points toward the same positive association (Booker & Mann, 2008). Results from the Cardiovascular Health Study suggest that while increased levels of *trans*-18:2 (an isomer of oleic acid) are associated with a greater risk of fatal IHD, *trans*-16:1 (from palmitoleic acid) shows no such association, and *trans*-18:1 (from LA) levels are actually inversely associated with a cardiovascular risk (Lemaitre et al., 2006).

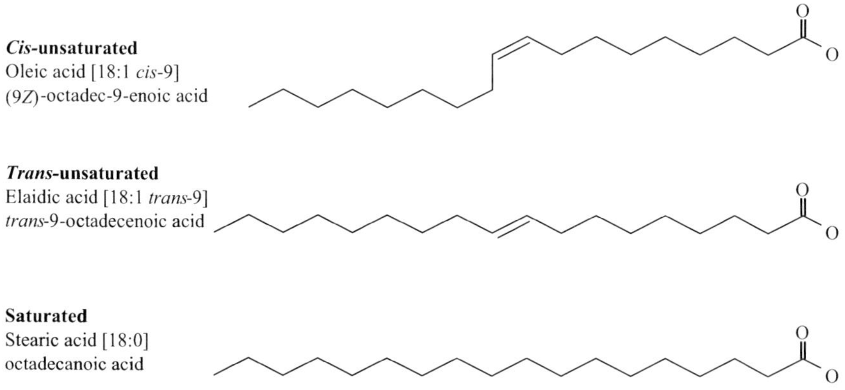


**Fig. 4.6.** Fatty-acid saturation and double-bond conformation. Fatty acids are aliphatic monocarboxylic acids that can be saturated or unsaturated. Unsaturated fatty acids contain carbon double bonds within the hydrocarbon chain that occur in a *cis* or *trans* configuration. A *cis* configuration results in "kinks or bends" in the fatty acid due to adjacent hydrogen atoms occurring on the same side of the double bond. In a *trans* configuration, hydrogen atoms are bound to opposite sides of the double bond and do not cause the chain to bend, resembling the straight shape of saturated fatty acids. Saturated fatty acids contain no double bonds or other functional groups along the hydrocarbon chain, allowing molecules to pack very tightly in a geometric fashion.

Ultimately, replacing TFAs (which account for only a small percentage of the daily intake of calories) with an identical amount of natural *cis* fatty acids confers a 50% reduction of CHD risk (Ascherio, 2002). One can compare this to the replacement of saturated fat with carbohydrates which, interestingly, decreases the risk by only 10% (Ascherio, 2002). The convincing nature of the scientific data led the United States Food and Drug Administration (FDA) to add TFA as a required component of nutrition labels at the beginning of 2006 (Moss, 2006). Note that *trans* fats produced by bacteria in ruminants are not conclusively associated with an increased risk of CVD (Lemaitre et al., 2006). While this may be attributed to the relatively low levels in the human diet, ruminant TFAs are not a primary health concern when compared to industrially produced *trans* fats (Lemaitre et al., 2006).

The mechanisms behind the deleterious effects of industrial TFAs are less well-established. Numerous papers suggest an unfavorable dose-dependent relationship between the TFA levels and the ratio of LDL to HDL (Ascherio, 2006). By lowering the LDL:HDL ratio and increasing triglyceride concentration, TFAs adversely affect the risk for a cardiac event (Ascherio, 2006). A meta-analysis of 60 trials, in fact, looked at several groups of fatty acids, and concluded that TFAs represent the most detrimental macronutrient with respect to the lipid profile (Mensink et al., 2003). The altered lipid profile, however, does not entirely account for the association of TFA intake with heart disease, and possibly, pro-inflammatory actions and endothelial dysfunction may represent part of the link (Lemaitre et al., 2006; Lopez-Garcia et al., 2005). TFAs were consistently associated with higher levels of tumor necrosis factor (TNF) activity as well as higher levels of plasma interleukin (IL)-6 and c-reactive protein (CRP) (Lemaitre et al., 2006). These substances are all associated with systemic inflammation, and CRP was, in fact, recently proposed as a biomarker for heart disease itself (Abi-Saleh et al., 2008). TFAs are positively associated with greater levels of soluble adhesion molecules (SICAM-1 and sVCAM-1) as well as E-selectin which, similarly, are accepted markers for endothelial dysfunction. This could account for the functional deficiencies in endothelial-dependent vascular reactions that were observed in randomized trials (Lemaitre et al., 2006).

In addition, dietary fat intake was shown to directly alter membrane composition in endothelial cells (Kummerow et al., 1999). Likely, TFAs are also incorporated into the membranes of other tissues proportionally to the amount ingested, and could directly affect signaling pathways (Lemaitre et al., 2006). Membrane-associated enzymes, such as $Na^+/K^+$ ATPase and adenylate cyclase, are unsurprisingly influenced by membrane composition, and their activity was lowered in the rat heart by a diet rich in TFAs (Alam et al., 1989). The same group also showed that the cardiac-membrane density of the β-adrenergic receptor was lowest in the *trans*-treated animals, suggesting another possible mechanism for TFA action (Alam et al., 1989). In addition to these proposed mechanisms, fatty acids function as ligands for several nuclear receptors such as PPAR and liver X receptor, which may mediate pathways associated with heart disease (Vanden Heuvel, 2004). Possibly, TFAs function by a similar mechanism, but the involved pathways require further study (Lemaitre et al., 2006).

Further study of not only the clinical implications of TFAs but also the molecular mechanisms responsible is required for a better understanding of the link to CVD. Preliminary investigation implicated alterations in the lipid profile, inflammation, endothelial function, and nuclear receptors. When considering TFAs, moreover, one must account for the actions of different isomers and chain lengths. While the commercial value of TFA products is undeniable, the health risks were also clearly defined. By successfully reducing TFA consumption, individuals could avoid 10 to 19% of heart-disease events (upwards of 200,000 events) in the United States (Lemaitre et al., 2006). The task now is to elucidate the mechanism, with the end goal of reducing cardiac events.

## Saturated Fatty Acids

SFAs are those that contain no double bonds within the hydrocarbon chain and have uniform fatty acid chains that allow the molecules to pack tightly together. Similar to TFAs, however, they raise numerous health concerns. Several epidemiological studies showed a positive association between dietary SFA intake and MI (Kabagambe et al., 2003; Kromhout et al., 1995). One study conducted among 12,763 men in seven countries concluded that the intake of lauric and myristic SFAs was strongly correlated with serum-cholesterol levels and heart disease over 25 years (Kromhout et al., 1995). In a more recent contrasting study done in a developing country with patients who had already survived an acute MI, an identical conclusion was reached. A higher dietary intake of SFAs, particularly lauric, myristic, and stearic as opposed to palmitic, was associated with a higher risk of MI (Kabagambe et al., 2003). Moreover, a large range of dietary intake of total SFAs exists from 3.8% of energy in Japan to 22.7% in Finland, according to one of the above studies (Kromhout et al., 1995). This discrepancy highlights only one of the considerations that must be taken into account when considering the effects of fatty acids—proportion of intake, source, isomeric activity, and chain length all play a role in mediating the action of fatty acids.

The molecular mechanisms of action for an SFA effect are limited and lag far behind those of PUFAs. Some basic understanding implies that the adverse effects of SFAs can result from a variety of mechanisms similar to TFAs. For example, studies show that replacing dietary SFAs with PUFAs can minimize arrhythmias and reduce oxidative stress in heart tissue (Diniz et al., 2004). Further, ex vivo heart studies in rats demonstrate that altered diets rich in SFAs cause a maladaptive increased coronary flow as compared to PUFA diets (Pepe & McLennan, 2002). An increased intake of SFAs may contribute to what is known as metabolic syndrome, which, in turn, is linked to obesity and diabetes—both risk factors for MI. This could occur by a direct effect on metabolic activity through a decreased membrane polyunsaturation, an alteration of insulin receptor activity, or as metabolic products or signals themselves (Hulbert et al., 2005). One group showed that the increased activation of the $K_{ATP}$ channel, leading to an impaired glucose-stimulated insulin secretion and diabetes, corresponds to an increased fatty acid side-chain length and saturation (Riedel &

Light, 2005). However, the activation of the $K_{ATP}$ channel may be protective against myocardial ischemia injury. The action of the reverse mode of the cardiac $Na^{+}/Ca^{++}$ exchanger (NCX) may contribute to reperfusion injury by increasing intracellular calcium levels which leads to contractile dysfunction (Schafer et al., 2001). Studies show, moreover, that acyl CoAs are endogenous activators of the reverse-mode NCX and that longer, saturated chains are the most effective activators—similar to the $K_{ATP}$ channels discussed above (Riedel et al., 2006). While studies show that an SFA intake is associated with the risk of an ischemic event, the mechanism(s) has not been fully elucidated.

## Conclusion

Fatty acids are essential components of the body that help maintain a normal physiological function and a protective response to pathological stimuli. Small changes in the dietary intake of fatty acids can influence membrane integrity and cellular signaling which can affect CVD outcomes. Myocardial damage resulting from ischemia–reperfusion injury has a profound effect in both the short- and long-term survivability of the individual. Relatively little mechanistic information is available regarding a molecular basis for the cardioprotective and cardiotoxic effects of fatty acids on ischemia–reperfusion injury. However, clearly, based on experimental data, the beneficial effects of PUFAs include the prevention of cardiac arrhythmias, an increased oxygen efficiency, the preservation of mitochondrial function, an altered membrane lipid composition, and a membrane-domain functionality. Thus, PUFAs can favorably modulate intracellular-signaling events in response to extracellular stress stimuli. Further mechanistic studies are needed to clarify the role of fatty acids in ischemia–reperfusion injury. However, while SFAs and TFAs tend to be detrimental, both n-3 and n-6 PUFAs play distinct roles in mediating ischemic injury. As such, maintaining the balance between n-3 and n-6 PUFAs is a critical factor influencing a CVD outcome.

### References

Abi-Saleh, B.; S.B. Iskandar; N. Elgharib; M.V. Cohen. C-reactive protein: the harbinger of cardiovascular diseases. *South Med. J.* **2008,** *101*, 525--533.

Adamek, A.; S. Jung; C. Dienesch; M. Laser; G. Ertl; J. Bauersachs; S. Frantz. Role of 5-lipoxygenase in myocardial ischemia-reperfusion injury in mice. *Eur. J. Pharmacol.* **2007,** *571*, 51–54.

Akabas, S.; R.R.J. Deckelbaum. Summary of a workshop on n-3 fatty acids: current status of recommendations and future directions. *Am. J. Clin. Nutr.* **2006,** *83*, 1536S–1538S.

Alam, S.Q.; Y.F. Ren; B.S. Alam. Effect of dietary trans fatty acids on some membrane-associated enzymes and receptors in rat heart. *Lipids* **1989,** *24*, 39–44.

Albert, C.M.; C.H. Hennekens; C.J. O'Donnell; U.A. Ajani; V.J. Carey; W.C. Willett; J.N. Ruskin; J.E. Manson. Fish consumption and risk of sudden cardiac death. *Jama* **1998,** *279*, 23–28.

Ascherio, A. Epidemiologic studies on dietary fats and coronary heart disease. *Am. J. Med.* **2002,**

*113 (Suppl. 9B)*, 9S–12S.

Ascherio, A. Trans fatty acids and blood lipids. *Atheroscler. Suppl.* **2006,** *7*, 25–27.

Ascherio, A.; C.H. Hennekens; J.E. Buring; C. Master; M.J. Stampfer; W.C. Willett. Trans-fatty acids intake and risk of myocardial infarction. *Circulation* **1994,** *89*, 94–101.

Ascherio, A.; M.B. Katan; P.L. Zock; M.J. Stampfer; W.C. Willett. Trans fatty acids and coronary heart disease. *N. Engl. J. Med.* **1999,** *340*, 1994–1998.

Ascherio, A.; E.B. Rimm; M.J. Stampfer; E.L. Giovannucci; W.C. Willett. Dietary intake of marine n-3 fatty acids, fish intake, and the risk of coronary disease among men. *N. Engl. J. Med.* **1995,** *332*, 977–982.

Ballard-Croft, C.; A.C. Locklar; G. Kristo; R.D. Lasley. Regional myocardial ischemia-induced activation of MAPKs is associated with subcellular redistribution of caveolin and cholesterol. *Am. J. Physiol. Heart Circ. Physiol.* **2006,** *291*, H658–667.

Bang, H.O.; J. Dyerberg; H.M. Sinclair. The composition of the Eskimo food in north western Greenland. *Am. J. Clin. Nutr.* **1980,** *33*, 2657–2661.

Barbosa-Sicard, E.; M. Markovic; H. Honeck; B. Christ; D.N. Muller; W.H. Schunck. Eicosapentaenoic acid metabolism by cytochrome P450 enzymes of the CYP2C subfamily. *Biochem. Biophys. Res. Commun.* **2005,** *329*, 1275–1281.

Birnbaum, Y.; Y. Ye; S. Rosanio; S. Tavackoli; Z.Y. Hu; E.R. Schwarz; B.F. Uretsky. Prostaglandins mediate the cardioprotective effects of atorvastatin against ischemia-reperfusion injury. *Cardiovasc. Res.* **2005,** *65*, 345–355.

Bolli, R.; L. Becker; G. Gross; R. Mentzer, Jr.; D. Balshaw; D.A. Lathrop. Myocardial protection at a crossroads: the need for translation into clinical therapy. *Circ. Res.* **2004,** *95*, 125–134.

Booker, C.; S.J.I. Mann. Trans fatty acids and cardiovascular health: Translation of the evidence base. *Nutr. Metab. Cardiovasc. Dis.* **2008,** *18*(6), 448–456.

Braunwald, E.P.; R. Maroko. The reduction of infarct size—an idea whose time (for testing) has come. *Circulation* **1974,** *50*, 206–209.

Brayden, J.E.M.; T. Nelson. Regulation of arterial tone by activation of calcium-dependent potassium channels. *Science* **1992,** *256*, 532–535.

Breslow, J.L. n-3 fatty acids and cardiovascular disease. *Am. J. Clin. Nutr.* **2006,** *83*, 1477S–1482S.

Burdge, G.C.P.; C. Calder. Conversion of alpha-linolenic acid to longer-chain polyunsaturated fatty acids in human adults. *Reprod. Nutr. Dev.* **2005,** *45*, 581–597.

Burke, A.P.R. Virmani. Pathophysiology of acute myocardial infarction. *Med. Clin. North Am.* **2007,** *91*, 553–572; ix.

Burr, M.L.; A.M. Fehily; J.F. Gilbert; S. Rogers; R.M. Holliday; P.M. Sweetnam; P.C. Elwood; N.M. Deadman. Effects of changes in fat, fish, and fibre intakes on death and myocardial reinfarction: diet and reinfarction trial (DART). *Lancet* **1989,** *2*, 757–761.

Calderone, V. Large-conductance, ca(2+)-activated k(+) channels: function, pharmacology and drugs. *Curr. Med. Chem.* **2002,** *9*, 1385–1395.

Camitta, M.G.; S.A. Gabel; P. Chulada; J.A. Bradbury; R. Langenbach; D.C. Zeldin; E. Murphy. Cyclooxygenase-1 and -2 knockout mice demonstrate increased cardiac ischemia/reperfusion injury but are protected by acute preconditioning. *Circulation* **2001,** *104,* 2453–2458.

Campbell, W.B.; D. Gebremedhin; P.F. Pratt; D.R. Harder. Identification of epoxyeicosatrienoic acids as endothelium-derived hyperpolarizing factors. *Circ. Res.* **1996,** *78,* 415–423.

Chapkin, R.S.; J. Seo; D.N. McMurray; J.R. Lupton. Mechanisms by which docosahexaenoic acid and related fatty acids reduce colon cancer risk and inflammatory disorders of the intestine. *Chem. Phys. Lipids* **2008,** *153,* 14–23.

Chen, W.; W. Glasgow; E. Murphy; C. Steenbergen. Lipoxygenase metabolism of arachidonic acid in ischemic preconditioning and PKC-induced protection in heart. *Am. J. Physiol.* **1999,** *276,* H2094–H2101.

Christensen, J.H.; P. Gustenhoff; E. Korup; J. Aaroe; E. Toft; J.M. Moller; K. Rasmussen; J. Dyerberg; E.B. Schmidt. [n-3 polyunsaturated fatty acids, heart rate variability and ventricular arrhythmias in post-AMI-patients. A clinical controlled trial]. *Ugeskr Laeger* **1997,** *159,* 5525–5529.

Crompton, M.; S. Virji; J.M. Ward. Cyclophilin-D binds strongly to complexes of the voltage-dependent anion channel and the adenine nucleotide translocase to form the permeability transition pore. *Eur. J. Biochem.* **1998,** *258,* 729–735.

Das, U.N. Beneficial effect(s) of n-3 fatty acids in cardiovascular diseases: but, why and how? *Prostaglandins, Leukotrienes Essent. Fatty Acids* **2000,** *63,* 351–362.

Das, M.; M. Gherghiceanu; I. Lekli; S. Mukherjee; L.M. Popescu; D. K. Das. Essential role of lipid raft in ischemic preconditioning. *Cell Physiol. Biochem.* **2008,** *21,* 325–334.

Deckelbaum, R.J.; A. Leaf; D. Mozaffarian; T.A. Jacobson; W.S. Harris; S.R. Akabas. Conclusions and recommendations from the symposium, Beyond Cholesterol: Prevention and Treatment of Coronary Heart Disease with n-3 Fatty Acids. *Am. J. Clin. Nutr.* **2008,** *87,* 2010S–2012S.

Delozier, T.C.; G.E. Kissling; S.J. Coulter; D. Dai; J.F. Foley; J.A. Bradbury; E. Murphy; C. Steenbergen; D.C. Zeldin; J.A. Goldstein. Detection of human CYP2C8, CYP2C9, and CYP2J2 in cardiovascular tissues. *Drug Metab. Dispos.* **2007,** *35,* 682–688.

Der, P.; J. Cui; D.K. Das. Role of lipid rafts in ceramide and nitric oxide signaling in the ischemic and preconditioned hearts. *J. Mol. Cell Cardiol.* **2006,** *40,* 313–320.

Dewailly, E.; C. Blanchet; S. Lemieux; L. Sauve; S. Gingras; P. Ayotte; B.J. Holub. n-3 Fatty acids and cardiovascular disease risk factors among the Inuit of Nunavik. *Am. J. Clin. Nutr.* **2001,** *74,* 464–473.

Diniz, Y.S.; A.C. Cicogna; C.R. Padovani; L.S. Santana; L.A. Faine; E.L. Novelli. Diets rich in saturated and polyunsaturated fatty acids: metabolic shifting and cardiac health. *Nutrition* **2004,** *20,* 230–234.

Dudda, A.; G. Spiteller; F. Kobelt. Lipid oxidation products in ischemic porcine heart tissue. *Chem. Phys. Lipids* **1996,** *82,* 39–51.

Dyck, J.R.; T.A. Hopkins; S. Bonnet; E.D. Michelakis; M.E. Young; M. Watanabe; Y. Kawase; K. Jishage; G.D. Lopaschuk. Absence of malonyl coenzyme A decarboxylase in mice increases cardiac glucose oxidation and protects the heart from ischemic injury. *Circulation* **2006,** *114,* 1721–1728.

Dyck, J.R.; G.D. Lopaschuk. Malonyl CoA control of fatty acid oxidation in the ischemic heart. *J. Mol. Cell Cardiol.* **2002,** *34,* 1099–1109.

Dyerberg, J.; H.O. Bang; E. Stoffersen; S. Moncada; J.R. Vane. Eicosapentaenoic acid and prevention of thrombosis and atherosclerosis? *Lancet* **1978,** *2*, 117–119.

Erkkila, A.; V.D. de Mello; U. Riserus; D.E. Laaksonen. Dietary fatty acids and cardiovascular disease: an epidemiological approach. *Prog. Lipid Res.* **2008,** *47*, 172–187.

Fang, X.; N.L. Weintraub; R.B. McCaw; S. Hu; S.D. Harmon; J.B. Rice; B.D. Hammock; A.A. Spector. Effect of soluble epoxide hydrolase inhibition on epoxyeicosatrienoic acid metabolism in human blood vessels. *Am. J. Physiol. Heart Circ. Physiol.* **2004,** *287*, H2412–2420.

Farber, N.E.; G.M. Pieper; J.P. Thomas; G.J. Gross. Beneficial effects of iloprost in the stunned canine myocardium. *Circ. Res.* **1988,** *62*, 204–215.

Feller, S.; E.K. Gawrisch. Properties of docosahexaenoic-acid-containing lipids and their influence on the function of rhodopsin. *Curr. Opin. Struct. Biol.* **2005,** *15*, 416–422.

Ferdinandy, P.; R. Schulz; G.F. Baxter. Interaction of cardiovascular risk factors with myocardial ischemia/reperfusion injury, preconditioning, and postconditioning. *Pharmacol. Rev.* **2007,** *59*, 418–458.

Fisslthaler, B.; R. Popp; L. Kiss; M. Potente; D.R. Harder; I. Fleming; R. Busse. Cytochrome P450 2C is an EDHF synthase in coronary arteries. *Nature* **1999,** *401*, 493–497.

FitzGerald, G.A. COX-2 in play at the AHA and the FDA. *Trends Pharmacol. Sci.* **2007,** *28*, 303–307.

Fleming, I. Cytochrome P450 epoxygenases as EDHF synthase(s). *Pharmacol. Res.* **2004,** *49*, 525–533.

Fornage, M.; E. Boerwinkle; P.A. Doris; D. Jacobs; K. Liu; N.D. Wong. Polymorphism of the soluble epoxide hydrolase is associated with coronary artery calcification in African-American subjects. The Coronary Artery Risk Development In Young Adults (CARDIA) Study. *Circulation* **2004,** *11*(5), 421–426.

Frangogiannis, N.G.; C.W. Smith; M.L. Entman. The inflammatory response in myocardial infarction. *Cardiovasc. Res.* **2002,** *53*, 31–47.

Fukushima, A.; M. Hayakawa; S. Sugiyama; M. Ajioka; T. Ito; T. Satake; T. Ozawa. Cardiovascular effects of leukotoxin (9, 10-epoxy-12-octadecenoate) and free fatty acids in dogs. *Cardiovasc. Res.* **1988,** *22*, 213–218.

Funk, C.D.; G.A. FitzGerald. COX-2 inhibitors and cardiovascular risk. *J. Cardiovasc. Pharmacol.* **2007,** *50*, 470–479.

Gabel, S.A.; R.E. London; C.D. Funk; C. Steenbergen; E. Murphy. Leukocyte-type 12-lipoxygenase-deficient mice show impaired ischemic preconditioning-induced cardioprotection. *Am. J. Physiol. Heart Circ. Physiol.* **2001,** *280*, H1963–1969.

Gauthier, K.M.; W. Yang; G.J. Gross; W.B. Campbell. Roles of epoxyeicosatrienoic acids in vascular regulation and cardiac preconditioning. *J. Cardiovasc. Pharmacol.* **2007,** *50*, 601–608.

Gebauer, S.K.; T.L. Psota; W.S. Harris; P.M. Kris-Etherton. n-3 fatty acid dietary recommendations and food sources to achieve essentiality and cardiovascular benefits. *Am. J. Clin. Nutr.* **2006,** *83*, 1526S–1535S.

GISSI. Dietary supplementation with n-3 polyunsaturated fatty acids and vitamin E after myocardial infarction: results of the GISSI-Prevenzione trial. Gruppo Italiano per lo Studio della Sopravvivenza nell'Infarto miocardico. *Lancet* **1999,** *354*, 447–455.

Granville, D.J.; B. Tashakkor; C. Takeuchi; A.B. Gustafsson; C. Huang; M.R. Sayen; P. Wentworth, Jr.; M. Yeager; R.A. Gottlieb. Reduction of ischemia and reperfusion-induced myocardial damage by cytochrome P450 inhibitors. *Proc. Natl. Acad. Sci. U.S.A.* **2004,** *101*, 1321–1326.

Griffin, B.A. How relevant is the ratio of dietary n-6 to n-3 polyunsaturated fatty acids to cardiovascular disease risk? Evidence from the OPTILIP study. *Curr. Opin. Lipidol.* **2008,** *19*, 57–62.

Gross, G.J.; K.M. Gauthier; J. Moore; J.R. Falck; B.D. Hammock; W. B. Campbell; K. Nithipatikom. Effects of the selective EET antagonist, 14,15-EEZE, on cardioprotection produced by exogenous or endogenous EETs in the canine heart. *Am. J. Physiol. Heart Circ. Physiol.* **2008,** *294*, H2838–2844.

Gross, G.J.; A. Hsu; J.R. Falck; K. Nithipatikom. Mechanisms by which epoxyeicosatrienoic acids (EETs) elicit cardioprotection in rat hearts. *J. Mol. Cell. Cardiol.* **2007,** *42*, 687–691.

Gross, E.R.; K. Nithipatikom; A.K. Hsu; J.N. Peart; J.R. Falck; W.B. Campbell; G.J. Gross. Cytochrome P450 omega-hydroxylase inhibition reduces infarct size during reperfusion via the sarcolemmal $K_{ATP}$ channel. *J. Mol. Cell. Cardiol.* **2004,** *37*, 1245–1249.

Grosser, T.; S. Fries; G.A. FitzGerald. Biological basis for the cardiovascular consequences of COX-2 inhibition: therapeutic challenges and opportunities. *J. Clin. Invest.* **2006,** *116*, 4–15.

Guallar, E.; A. Aro; F.J. Jimenez; J.M. Martin-Moreno; I. Salminen; P. van't Veer; A.F. Kardinaal; J. Gomez-Aracena; B.C. Martin; L. Kohlmeier; et al. Omega-3 fatty acids in adipose tissue and risk of myocardial infarction: the EURAMIC study. *Arterioscler. Thromb. Vasc. Biol.* **1999,** *19*, 1111–1118.

Guizy, M.; C. Arias; M. David; T. Gonzalez; C. Valenzuela. {Omega}-3 and {omega}-6 polyunsaturated fatty acids block HERG channels. *Am. J. Physiol. Cell. Physiol.* **2005,** *289*, C1251–1260.

Guizy, M.; M. David; C. Arias; L. Zhang; M. Cofan; V. Ruiz-Gutierrez; E. Ros; M.P. Lillo; J.R. Martens; C. Valenzuela. Modulation of the atrial specific Kv1.5 channel by the n-3 polyunsaturated fatty acid, alpha-linolenic acid. *J. Mol. Cell. Cardiol.* **2008,** *44*, 323–335.

Guo, Y.; W. Bao; W.J. Wu; K. Shinmura; X.L. Tang; R. Bolli. Evidence for an essential role of cyclooxygenase-2 as a mediator of the late phase of ischemic preconditioning in mice. *Basic Res. Cardiol.* **2000,** *95*, 479–484.

Haag, M. Essential fatty acids and the brain. *Can. J. Psychiatry* **2003,** *48*, 195–203.

Halestrap, A.P. Mitochondrial permeability: dual role for the ADP/ATP translocator? *Nature* **2004,** *430*, 1 p following 983.

Halestrap, A.P.; P.M. Kerr; S. Javadov; K.Y. Woodfield. Elucidating the molecular mechanism of the permeability transition pore and its role in reperfusion injury of the heart. *Biochim. Biophys. Acta* **1998,** *1366*, 79–94.

Hancock, J.F. Lipid rafts: contentious only from simplistic standpoints. *Nat. Rev. Mol. Cell. Biol.* **2006,** *7*, 456–462.

Harrell, M.D.; J.R. Stimers. Differential effects of linoleic Acid metabolites on cardiac sodium current. *J. Pharmacol. Exp. Ther.* **2002,** *303*, 347–355.

Harris, W.S. Omega-3 fatty acids and cardiovascular disease: a case for omega-3 index as a new risk factor. *Pharmacol. Res.* **2007,** *55*, 217–223.

Harris, W.S. The omega-3 index as a risk factor for coronary heart disease. *Am. J. Clin. Nutr.* **2008,** *87*, 1997S–2002S.

Hartman, L.; F.B. Shorland. Trans-unsaturated acids in the depot fats of ruminants and non-ruminants. *Nature* **1959,** *184(Suppl. 26)*, 2024.

Hausenloy, D.J.; D.M. Yellon. Preconditioning and postconditioning: new strategies for cardio-protection. *Diabetes Obes. Metab.* **2008,** *10*, 451–459.

Hooper, L.; R.L. Thompson; R.A. Harrison; C.D. Summerbell; H. Moore; H.V. Worthington; P.N. Durrington; A.R. Ness; N.E. Capps; G. Davey Smith; R.A. Riemersma; S.B. Ebrahim. Omega 3 fatty acids for prevention and treatment of cardiovascular disease. *Cochrane Database Syst. Rev.* **2004**, CD003177.

Hu, F.B.; M.J. Stampfer; J.E. Manson; A. Ascherio; G.A. Colditz; F. E. Speizer; C.H. Hennekens; W.C. Willett. Dietary saturated fats and their food sources in relation to the risk of coronary heart disease in women. *Am. J. Clin. Nutr.* **1999,** *70*, 1001–1008.

Hu, F.B.; M.J. Stampfer; J.E. Manson; E. Rimm; G.A. Colditz; B.A. Rosner; C.H. Hennekens; W.C. Willett. Dietary fat intake and the risk of coronary heart disease in women. *N. Engl. J. Med.* **1997,** *337*, 1491–1499.

Hulbert, A.J.; N. Turner; L.H. Storlien; P.L. Else. Dietary fats and membrane function: implications for metabolism and disease. *Biol. Rev. Camb. Philos. Soc.* **2005,** *80*, 155–169.

Ichihara, K.; K. Yamamoto; Y. Abiko. Effects of iloprost, a PGI2 derivative, on ischemic myocardial energy and carbohydrate metabolism in dogs. *Mol. Cell. Biochem.* **1993,** *119*, 133–141.

Jennings, R.B.; H.M. Sommers; G.A. Smyth; H.A. Flack; H. Linn. Myocardial necrosis induced by temporary occlusion of a coronary artery in the dog. *Arch. Pathol.* **1960,** *70*, 68–78.

Jump, D.B. The biochemistry of n-3 polyunsaturated fatty acids. *J. Biol. Chem.* **2002,** *277*, 8755–8758.

Jung, U.J.; C. Torrejon; A.P. Tighe; R.J. Deckelbaum. n-3 Fatty acids and cardiovascular disease: mechanisms underlying beneficial effects. *Am. J. Clin. Nutr.* **2008,** *87*, 2003S–2009S.

Kabagambe, E.K.; A. Baylin; X. Siles; H. Campos. Individual saturated fatty acids and nonfatal acute myocardial infarction in Costa Rica. *Eur. J. Clin. Nutr.* **2003,** *57*, 1447–1457.

Ke, Q.; Y.F. Xiao; J.A. Bradbury; J.P. Graves; L.M. Degraff; J.M. Seubert; D.C. Zeldin. Electrophysiological properties of cardiomyocytes isolated from CYP2J2 transgenic mice. *Mol. Pharmacol.* **2007,** *72*, 1063–1073.

Keys, A.; J.T. Anderson; F. Grande. Prediction of serum-cholesterol responses of man to changes in fats in the diet. *Lancet* **1957,** *273*, 959–966.

Kodani, E.; Y.T. Xuan; K. Shinmura; H. Takano; X.L. Tang; R. Bolli. Delta-opioid receptor-induced late preconditioning is mediated by cyclooxygenase-2 in conscious rabbits. *Am. J. Physiol. Heart Circ. Physiol.* **2002,** *283*, H1943–H1957.

Kris-Etherton, P.M.; W.S. Harris; L.J. Appel. Fish consumption, fish oil, omega-3 fatty acids, and cardiovascular disease. *Circulation* **2002,** *106*, 2747–2757.

Kritchevsky, D. History of recommendations to the public about dietary fat. *J. Nutr.* **1998,** *128*, 449S–452S.

Kromhout, D.; B.P. Bloemberg; E.J. Feskens; M.G. Hertog; A. Menotti; H. Blackburn. Alcohol, fish, fibre and antioxidant vitamins intake do not explain population differences in coronary heart disease mortality. *Int. J. Epidemiol.* **1996,** *25*, 753–759.

Kromhout, D.; A. Menotti; B. Bloemberg; C. Aravanis; H. Blackburn; R. Buzina; A.S Dontas; F. Fidanza; S. Giampaoli; A. Jansen, et al. Dietary saturated and trans fatty acids and cholesterol and 25-year mortality from coronary heart disease: the Seven Countries Study. *Prev. Med.* **1995,** *24,* 308–315.

Kudo, N.; J.G. Gillespie; L. Kung; L.A. Witters; R. Schulz; A.S. Clanachan; G.D. Lopaschuk. Characterization of 5'AMP-activated protein kinase activity in the heart and its role in inhibiting acetyl-CoA carboxylase during reperfusion following ischemia. *Biochim. Biophys. Acta* **1996,** *1301,* 67–75.

Kulkarni, A.P. Lipoxygenase—a versatile biocatalyst for biotransformation of endobiotics and xenobiotics. *Cell. Mol. Life Sci.* **2001,** *58,* 1805–1825.

Kummerow, F.A.; Q. Zhou; M.M. Mahfouz. Effect of trans fatty acids on calcium influx into human arterial endothelial cells. *Am. J. Clin. Nutr.* **1999,** *70,* 832–838.

Kurien, V.A.; M.F. Oliver. Free fatty acids during acute myocardial infarction. *Prog. Cardiovasc. Dis.* **1971,** *13,* 361–373.

Laude, A.J.; I.A. Prior. Plasma membrane microdomains: organization, function and trafficking. *Mol. Membr. Biol.* **2004,** *21,* 193–205.

Lauterbach, B.; E. Barbosa-Sicard; M.H. Wang; H. Honeck; E. Kargel; J. Theuer; M.L. Schwartzman; H. Haller; F.C. Luft; M. Gollasch; W. H. Schunck. Cytochrome P450-dependent eicosapentaenoic acid metabolites are novel BK channel activators. *Hypertension* **2002,** *39,* 609–613.

Leaf, A.; J.X. Kang; Y.F. Xiao; G.E. Billman. Clinical prevention of sudden cardiac death by n-3 polyunsaturated fatty acids and mechanism of prevention of arrhythmias by n-3 fish oils. *Circulation* **2003,** *107,* 2646–2652.

Lee, C.R.; K.E. North; M.S. Bray; D.J. Couper; G. Heiss; D.C. Zeldin. CYP2J2 and CYP2C8 polymorphisms and coronary heart disease risk: the Atherosclerosis Risk in Communities (ARIC) study. *Pharmacogenet. Genomics* **2007,** *17,* 349–358.

Lee, C.R.; K.E. North; M.S. Bray; M. Fornage; J.M. Seubert; J.W. Newman; B.D. Hammock; D.J. Couper; G. Heiss; D.C. Zeldin. Genetic variation in soluble epoxide hydrolase (EPHX2) and risk of coronary heart disease: The Atherosclerosis Risk in Communities (ARIC) study. *Hum. Mol. Genet.* **2006,** *15,* 1640–1649.

Lemaitre, R.N.; I.B. King; D. Mozaffarian; N. Sotoodehnia; T.D. Rea; L.H. Kuller; R.P. Tracy; D.S. Siscovick. Plasma phospholipid trans fatty acids, fatal ischemic heart disease, and sudden cardiac death in older adults: the cardiovascular health study. *Circulation* **2006,** *114,* 209–215.

Liu, B.; A.S. Clanachan; R. Schulz; G.D. Lopaschuk. Cardiac efficiency is improved after ischemia by altering both the source and fate of protons. *Circ. Res.* **1996,** *79,* 940–948.

Lopez-Garcia, E.; M.B. Schulze; J.B. Meigs; J.E. Manson; N. Rifai; M.J. Stampfer; W.C. Willett; F.B. Hu. Consumption of trans fatty acids is related to plasma biomarkers of inflammation and endothelial dysfunction. *J. Nutr.* **2005,** *135,* 562–566.

Lu, T.; M. VanRollins; H.C. Lee. Stereospecific activation of cardiac ATP-sensitive K(+) channels by epoxyeicosatrienoic acids: a structural determinant study. *Mol. Pharmacol.* **2002,** *62,* 1076–1083.

Lu, T.; D. Ye; X. Wang; J.M. Seubert; J.P. Graves; J.A. Bradbury; D. C. Zeldin; H.C. Lee. Cardiac and vascular KATP channels in rats are activated by endogenous epoxyeicosatrienoic acids through different mechanisms. *J. Physiol.* **2006,** *575*, 627 644.

Ma, D.W.; J. Seo; L.A. Davidson; E.S. Callaway; Y.Y. Fan; J.R. Lupton; R.S. Chapkin. n-3 PUFA alter caveolae lipid composition and resident protein localization in mouse colon. *FASEB J.* **2004a,** *18*, 1040–1042.

Ma, D.W.; J. Seo; K.C. Switzer; Y.Y. Fan; D.N. McMurray; J.R. Lupton; R.S. Chapkin. n-3 PUFA and membrane microdomains: a new frontier in bioactive lipid research. *J. Nutr. Biochem.* **2004b,** *15*, 700–706.

Macchia, A.; S. Monte; F. Pellegrini; M. Romero; D. Ferrante; H. Doval; A. D'Ettorre; A.P. Maggioni; G. Tognoni. Omega-3 fatty acid supplementation reduces one-year risk of atrial fibrillation in patients hospitalized with myocardial infarction. *Eur. J. Clin. Pharmacol.* **2008,** *64*(6), 627–634.

Marchioli, R.; F. Barzi; E. Bomba; C. Chieffo; D. Di Gregorio; R. Di Mascio; M.G. Franzosi; E. Geraci; G. Levantesi; A.P. Maggioni; et al. Early protection against sudden death by n-3 polyunsaturated fatty acids after myocardial infarction: time-course analysis of the results of the Gruppo Italiano per lo Studio della Sopravvivenza nell'Infarto Miocardico (GISSI)-Prevenzione. *Circulation* **2002,** *105*, 1897–1903.

Maroko, P.R.; J.K. Kjekshus; B.E. Sobel; T. Watanabe; J.W. Covell; J. Ross, Jr.; E. Braunwald. Factors influencing infarct size following experimental coronary artery occlusions. *Circulation* **1971,** *43*, 67–82.

McLennan, P.L.; M.Y. Abeywardena; J.S. Charnock. Influence of dietary lipids on arrhythmias and infarction after coronary artery ligation in rats. *Can. J. Physiol. Pharmacol.* **1985,** *63*, 1411–1417.

McLennan, P.L.; M.Y. Abeywardena; J.S. Charnock. Dietary fish oil prevents ventricular fibrillation following coronary artery occlusion and reperfusion. *Am. Heart J.* **1988,** *116*, 709–717.

McLennan, P.L.; M.Y. Abeywardena. Membrane basis for fish oil effects on the heart: linking natural hibernators to prevention of human sudden cardiac death. *J. Membr. Biol.* **2005,** *206*, 85–102.

McLennan, P.L.; A.J. Owen; E.L. Slee; M.L. Theiss. Myocardial function, ischaemia and n-3 polyunsaturated fatty acids: a membrane basis. *J. Cardiovasc. Med. (Hagerstown)* **2007,** *8 (Suppl. 1)*, S15–18.

Mensink, R.P.; M.B. Katan. Effect of dietary fatty acids on serum lipids and lipoproteins. A meta-analysis of 27 trials. *Arterioscler. Thromb.* **1992,** *12*, 911–919.

Mensink, R.P.; P.L. Zock; A.D. Kester; M.B. Katan. Effects of dietary fatty acids and carbohydrates on the ratio of serum total to HDL cholesterol and on serum lipids and apolipoproteins: a meta-analysis of 60 controlled trials. *Am. J. Clin. Nutr.* **2003,** *77*, 1146–1155.

Moghaddam, M.F.; D.F. Grant; J.M. Cheek; J.F. Greene; K.C. Williamson; B.D. Hammock. Bioactivation of leukotoxins to their toxic diols by epoxide hydrolase. *Nat. Med.* **1997,** *3*, 562–566.

Morisseau, C.B.; D. Hammock. Epoxide hydrolases: mechanisms, inhibitor designs, and biological roles. *Annu. Rev. Pharmacol. Toxicol.* **2005,** *45*, 311–333.

Moss, J. Labeling of trans fatty acid content in food, regulations and limits-the FDA view. *Atheroscler. Suppl.* **2006,** *7*, 57–59.

Mozaffarian, D.; B.M. Psaty; E.B. Rimm; R.N. Lemaitre; G.L. Burke; M.F. Lyles; D. Lefkowitz; D.S. Siscovick. Fish intake and risk of incident atrial fibrillation. *Circulation* **2004,** *110,* 368–373.

Murphy, E.; W. Glasgow; T. Fralix; C. Steenbergen. Role of lipoxygenase metabolites in ischemic preconditioning. *Circ. Res.* **1995,** *76,* 457–467.

Murphy, E.; C. Steenbergen. Ion transport and energetics during cell death and protection. *Physiology (Bethesda)* **2008,** *23,* 115–123.

Murry, C.E.; R.B. Jennings; K.A. Reimer. Preconditioning with ischemia: a delay of lethal cell injury in ischemic myocardium. *Circulation* **1986,** *74,* 1124–1136.

Nithipatikom, K.; E.R. Gross; M.P. Endsley; J.M. Moore; M.A. Isbell; J.R. Falck; W.B. Campbell; G.J. Gross. Inhibition of cytochrome P450omega-hydroxylase: a novel endogenous cardioprotective pathway. *Circ. Res.* **2004,** *95,* e65–71.

Nithipatikom, K.; J.M. Moore; M.A. Isbell; J.R. Falck; G.J. Gross. Epoxyeicosatrienoic acids in cardioprotection: ischemic versus reperfusion injury. *Am. J. Physiol. Heart Circ. Physiol.* **2006,** *291,* H537–42.

Node, K.; Y. Huo; X. Ruan; B. Yang; M. Spiecker; K. Ley; D.C. Zeldin; J.K. Liao. Anti-inflammatory properties of cytochrome P450 epoxygenase-derived eicosanoids. *Science* **1999,** *285,* 1276–1279.

Ohya, S.; Y. Kuwata; K. Sakamoto; K. Muraki; Y. Imaizumi. Cardioprotective effects of estradiol include the activation of large-conductance Ca(2+)-activated K(+) channels in cardiac mitochondria. *Am. J. Physiol. Heart Circ. Physiol.* **2005,** *289,* H1635–1642.

Oliw, E.H.; J. Bylund; C. Herman. Bisallylic hydroxylation and epoxidation of polyunsaturated fatty acids by cytochrome P450. *Lipids* **1996,** *31,* 1003–1021.

O'Rourke, B. Evidence for mitochondrial K+ channels and their role in cardioprotection. *Circ. Res.* **2004,** *94,* 420–432.

Ozawa, T.; S. Sugiyama; M. Hayakawa; F. Taki; Y. Hanaki. Neutrophil microsomes biosynthesize linoleate epoxide (9,10-epoxy-12-octadecenoate), a biological active substance. *Biochem. Biophys. Res. Commun.* **1988,** *152,* 1310–1318.

Page, I.H. Atherosclerosis; an introduction. *Circulation* **1954,** *10,* 1–27.

Patel, H.H.; R.M. Fryer; E.R. Gross; R.A. Bundey; A.K. Hsu; M. Isbell; L.O. Eusebi; R.V. Jensen; S.R. Gullans; P.A. Insel; et al. 12-lipoxygenase in opioid-induced delayed cardioprotection: gene array, mass spectrometric, and pharmacological analyses. *Circ. Res.* **2003,** *92,* 676–682.

Patel, H.H.; F. Murray; P.A. Insel. Caveolae as organizers of pharmacologically relevant signal transduction molecules. *Annu. Rev. Pharmacol. Toxicol.* **2008a,** *48,* 359–391.

Patel, H.H.; F. Murray; P.A. Insel. G-protein-coupled receptor-signaling components in membrane raft and caveolae microdomains. *Handb. Exp. Pharmacol.* **2008b**, 167–184.

Patel, H.H.; Y.M. Tsutsumi; B.P. Head; I.R. Niesman; M. Jennings; Y. Horikawa; D. Huang; A.L. Moreno; P.M. Patel; P.A. Insel; D.M. Roth. Mechanisms of cardiac protection from ischemia/reperfusion injury: a role for caveolae and caveolin-1. *FASEB J.* **2007,** *21,* 1565–1574.

Pepe, S. Effect of dietary polyunsaturated fatty acids on age-related changes in cardiac mitochondrial membranes. *Exp. Gerontol.* **2005,** *40,* 369–376.

Pepe, S.; P.L. McLennan. Dietary fish oil confers direct antiarrhythmic properties on the myocardium of rats. *J. Nutr.* **1996,** *126*, 34–42.

Pepe, S.; P.L. McLennan. Cardiac membrane fatty acid composition modulates myocardial oxygen consumption and postischemic recovery of contractile function. *Circulation* **2002,** *105*, 2303–2308.

Pepe, S.; N. Tsuchiya; E.G. Lakatta; R.G. Hansford. PUFA and aging modulate cardiac mitochondrial membrane lipid composition and Ca2+ activation of PDH. *Am. J. Physiol.* **1999,** *276*, H149–158.

Piper, H.M.; K. Meuter; C. Schafer. Cellular mechanisms of ischemia-reperfusion injury. *Ann. Thorac. Surg.* **2003,** *75*, S644–648.

Plum, F. What causes infarction in ischemic brain?: The Robert Wartenberg Lecture. *Neurology* **1983,** *33*, 222–233.

Przybyla-Zawislak, B.D.; P.K. Srivastava; J. Vazquez-Matias; H.W. Mohrenweiser; J.E. Maxwell; B.D. Hammock; J.A. Bradbury; A.E. Enayetallah; D.C. Zeldin; D.F. Grant. Polymorphisms in human soluble epoxide hydrolase. *Mol. Pharmacol.* **2003,** *64*, 482–490.

Qi, K.; C. Fan; J. Jiang; H. Zhu; H. Jiao; Q. Meng; R.J. Deckelbaum. Omega-3 fatty acid containing diets decrease plasma triglyceride concentrations in mice by reducing endogenous triglyceride synthesis and enhancing the blood clearance of triglyceride-rich particles. *Clin. Nutr.* **2008,** *27*, 424–430.

Randle, P.J.; P.B. Garland; C.N. Hales; E.A. Newsholme. The glucose fatty-acid cycle. Its role in insulin sensitivity and the metabolic disturbances of diabetes mellitus. *Lancet* **1963,** *1*, 785–789.

Rehncrona, S.; I. Rosen; B.K. Siesjo. Excessive cellular acidosis: an important mechanism of neuronal damage in the brain? *Acta Physiol. Scand.* **1980,** *110*, 435–437.

Riedel, M.J.; I. Baczko; G.J. Searle; N. Webster; M. Fercho; L. Jones; J. Lang; J. Lytton; J.R. Dyck; P.E. Light. Metabolic regulation of sodium-calcium exchange by intracellular acyl CoAs. *EMBO J.* **2006,** *25*, 4605–4614.

Riedel, M.J.; P.E. Light. Saturated and cis/trans unsaturated acyl CoA esters differentially regulate wild-type and polymorphic beta-cell ATP-sensitive K+ channels. *Diabetes* **2005,** *54*, 2070–2079.

Riemersma, R.A.; D.A. Wood; S. Butler; R.A. Elton; M. Oliver; M. Salo; T. Nikkari; E. Vartiainen; P. Puska; F. Gey; et al. Linoleic acid content in adipose tissue and coronary heart disease. *Br. Med. J. (Clin. Res. Ed.)* **1986,** *292*, 1423–1427.

Roman, R.J.; K.G. Maier; C.W. Sun; D.R. Harder; M. Alonso-Galicia. Renal and cardiovascular actions of 20-hydroxyeicosatetraenoic acid and epoxyeicosatrienoic acids. *Clin. Exp. Pharmacol. Physiol.* **2000,** *27*, 855–865.

Salinas, G.; U.C. Rangasetty; B.F. Uretsky; Y. Birnbaum. The cycloxygenase 2 (COX-2) story: it's time to explain, not inflame. *J. Cardiovasc. Pharmacol. Ther.* **2007,** *12*, 98–111.

Sato, T.; T. Saito; N. Saegusa; H. Nakaya. Mitochondrial Ca2+-activated K+ channels in cardiac myocytes: a mechanism of the cardioprotective effect and modulation by protein kinase A. *Circulation* **2005,** *111*, 198–203.

Schafer, C.; Y. Ladilov; J. Inserte; M. Schafer; S. Haffner; D. Garcia-Dorado; H.M. Piper. Role of the reverse mode of the Na+/Ca2+ exchanger in reoxygenation-induced cardiomyocyte injury. *Cardiovasc. Res.* **2001,** *51*, 241–250.

Seo, J.; R. Barhoumi; A.E. Johnson; J.R. Lupton; R.S. Chapkin. Docosahexaenoic acid selectively inhibits plasma membrane targeting of lipidated proteins. *FASEB J.* **2006,** *20*, 770–772.

Seubert, J.M.; C.J. Sinal; J. Graves; L.M. DeGraff; J.A. Bradbury; C. R. Lee; K. Goralski; M.A. Carey; A. Luria; J.W. Newman; et al. Role of soluble epoxide hydrolase in postischemic recovery of heart contractile function. *Circ. Res.* **2006,** *99*, 442–450.

Seubert, J.; B. Yang; J.A. Bradbury; J. Graves; L.M. Degraff; S. Gabel; R. Gooch; J. Foley; J. Newman; L. Mao; et al. Enhanced postischemic functional recovery in CYP2J2 transgenic hearts involves mitochondrial ATP-sensitive K+ channels and p42/p44 MAPK pathway. *Circ. Res.* **2004,** *95*, 506–514.

Seubert, J.M.; D.C. Zeldin; K. Nithipatikom; G.J. Gross. Role of epoxyeicosatrienoic acids in protecting the myocardium following ischemia/reperfusion injury. *Prostaglandins Other Lipid Mediat.* **2007,** *82*, 50–59.

Shaikh, S.R.; A.C. Dumaual; A. Castillo; D. LoCascio; R.A. Siddiqui; W. Stillwell; S.R. Wassall. Oleic and docosahexaenoic acid differentially phase separate from lipid raft molecules: a comparative NMR, DSC, AFM, and detergent extraction study. *Biophys. J.* **2004,** *87*, 1752–1766.

Shaikh, S.R.; M. Edidin. Polyunsaturated fatty acids and membrane organization: elucidating mechanisms to balance immunotherapy and susceptibility to infection. *Chem. Phys. Lipids* **2008,** *153*, 24–33.

Shinmura, K.; X.L. Tang; Y. Wang; Y.T. Xuan; S.Q. Liu; H. Takano; A. Bhatnagar; R. Bolli. Cyclooxygenase-2 mediates the cardioprotective effects of the late phase of ischemic preconditioning in conscious rabbits. *Proc. Natl. Acad. Sci. U. S. A.* **2000,** *97*, 10197–101202.

Simopoulos, A.P. The omega-6/omega-3 fatty acid ratio, genetic variation, and cardiovascular disease. *Asia Pac. J. Clin. Nutr.* **2008,** *17 (Suppl. 1)*, 131–134.

Simpson, H.C.; K. Barker; R.D. Carter; E. Cassels; J.I. Mann. Low dietary intake of linoleic acid predisposes to myocardial infarction. *Br. Med. J. (Clin. Res. Ed.)* **1982,** *285*, 683–684.

Sisemore, M.F.; J. Zheng; J.C. Yang; D.A. Thompson; C.G. Plopper; G.A. Cortopassi; B.D. Hammock. Cellular characterization of leukotoxin diol-induced mitochondrial dysfunction. *Arch. Biochem. Biophys.* **2001,** *392*, 32–37.

Soni, S.P.; D.S. LoCascio; Y. Liu; J.A. Williams; R. Bittman; W. Stillwell; S.R. Wassall. Docosahexaenoic acid enhances segregation of lipids between: 2H-NMR study. *Biophys. J.* **2008,** *95*, 203–214.

Spiecker, M.; H. Darius; T. Hankeln; M. Soufi; A.M. Sattler; J.R. Schaefer; K. Node; J. Borgel; A. Mugge; K. Lindpaintner; et al. Risk of coronary artery disease associated with polymorphism of the cytochrome P450 epoxygenase CYP2J2. *Circulation* **2004,** *110*, 2132–2136.

Spiecker, M.; J. Liao. Cytochrome P450 epoxygenase CYP2J2 and the risk of coronary artery disease. *Trends Cardiovasc. Med.* **2006,** *16*, 204–208.

Stanley, W.C.; E.E. Morgan; H. Huang; T.A. McElfresh; J.P. Sterk; I.C. Okere; M.P. Chandler; J. Cheng; J.R. Dyck; G.D. Lopaschuk. Malonyl-CoA decarboxylase inhibition suppresses fatty acid oxidation and reduces lactate production during demand-induced ischemia. *Am. J. Physiol. Heart Circ. Physiol.* **2005,** *289*, H2304–2309.

Stephen, A.M.; N.J. Wald. Trends in individual consumption of dietary fat in the United States, 1920–1984. *Am. J. Clin. Nutr.* **1990,** *52*, 457–469.

Stillwell, W.; L.J. Jenski; F.T. Crump; W. Ehringer. Effect of docosahexaenoic acid on mouse mitochondrial membrane properties. *Lipids* **1997,** *32,* 497–506.

Stillwell, W.; S.R. Shaikh; M. Zerouga; R. Siddiqui; S.R. Wassall. Docosahexaenoic acid affects cell signaling by altering lipid rafts. *Reprod. Nutr. Dev.* **2005,** *45*, 559–579.

Stillwell, W.; S.R. Wassall. Docosahexaenoic acid: membrane properties of a unique fatty acid. *Chem. Phys. Lipids* **2003,** *126*, 1–27.

Stimers, J.R.; M. Dobretsov; S.L. Hastings; A.R. Jude; D.F. Grant. Effects of linoleic acid metabolites on electrical activity in adult rat ventricular myocytes. *Biochim. Biophys. Acta* **1999,** *1438*, 359–368.

Stulnig, T.M.; J. Huber; N. Leitinger; E.M. Imre; P. Angelisova; P. Nowotny; W. Waldhausl. Polyunsaturated eicosapentaenoic acid displaces proteins from membrane rafts by altering raft lipid composition. *J. Biol. Chem.* **2001,** *276*, 37335–37340.

Taqueti, V.R.; R.N. Mitchell; A.H. Lichtman. Protecting the pump: controlling myocardial inflammatory responses. *Annu. Rev. Physiol.* **2006,** *68*, 67–95.

Thompson, D.A.; B.D. Hammock. Dihydroxyoctadecamonoenoate esters inhibit the neutrophil respiratory burst. *J. Biosci.* **2007,** *32*, 279–291.

Tsutsumi, Y.M.; H.H. Patel; D. Huang; D.M. Roth. Role of 12-lipoxygenase in volatile anesthetic-induced delayed preconditioning in mice. *Am. J. Physiol. Heart Circ. Physiol.* **2006,** *291*, H979–983.

Ussher, J.R.; G.D. Lopaschuk. The malonyl CoA axis as a potential target for treating ischaemic heart disease. *Cardiovasc. Res.* **2008,** *79*, 259–268.

van Bilsen, M.; W. Engels; G.J. van der Vusse; R.S. Reneman. Significance of myocardial eicosanoid production. *Mol. Cell. Biochem.* **1989,** *88*, 113–121.

van der Lee, K.A.; M.M. Vork; J.E. De Vries; P.H. Willemsen; J.F. Glatz; R.S. Reneman; G.J. Van der Vusse; M. Van Bilsen. Long-chain fatty acid-induced changes in gene expression in neonatal cardiac myocytes. *J. Lipid Res.* **2000,** *41*, 41–47.

Vanden Heuvel, J.P. Diet, fatty acids, and regulation of genes important for heart disease. *Curr. Atheroscler. Rep.* **2004,** *6*, 432–440.

von Schacky, C. A review of omega-3 ethyl esters for cardiovascular prevention and treatment of increased blood triglyceride levels. *Vasc. Health Risk Manag.* **2006,** *2*, 251–262.

von Schacky, C. Omega-3 fatty acids and cardiovascular disease. *Curr. Opin. Clin. Nutr. Metab. Care* **2007,** *10*, 129–135.

Wang, C.; W.S. Harris; M. Chung; A.H. Lichtenstein; E.M. Balk; B. Kupelnick; H.S. Jordan; J. Lau. n-3 Fatty acids from fish or fish-oil supplements, but not alpha-linolenic acid, benefit cardiovascular disease outcomes in primary- and secondary-prevention studies: a systematic review. *Am. J. Clin. Nutr.* **2006,** *84*, 5–17.

Wang, H.; L. Lin; J. Jiang; Y. Wang; Z.Y. Lu; J.A. Bradbury; F.B. Lih; D.W. Wang; D.C. Zeldin. Up-regulation of endothelial nitric-oxide synthase by endothelium-derived hyperpolarizing factor involves mitogen-activated protein kinase and protein kinase C signaling pathways. *J. Pharmacol. Exp. Ther.* **2003,** *307*, 753–764.

Wang, Y.; X. Wei; X. Xiao; R. Hui; J.W. Card; M.A. Carey; D.W. Wang; D.C. Zeldin. Arachidonic acid epoxygenase metabolites stimulate endothelial cell growth and angiogenesis via mitogen-activated protein kinase and phosphatidylinositol 3-kinase/Akt signaling pathways. *J. Pharmacol.*

*Exp. Ther.* **2005,** *314*, 522–532.

Whitmer, J.T.; J.A. Idell-Wenger; M.J. Rovetto; J.R. Neely. Control of fatty acid metabolism in ischemic and hypoxic hearts. *J. Biol. Chem.* **1978,** *253*, 4305–4309.

Wijendran, V.; K.C. Hayes. Dietary n-6 and n-3 fatty acid balance and cardiovascular health. *Annu. Rev. Nutr.* **2004,** *24*, 597–615.

Willett, W.C. The role of dietary n-6 fatty acids in the prevention of cardiovascular disease. *J. Cardiovasc. Med. (Hagerstown)* **2007,** *8 (Suppl. 1)*, S42–45.

Wu, S.; W. Chen; E. Murphy; S. Gabel; K.B. Tomer; J. Foley; C. Steenbergen; J.R. Falck; C.R. Moomaw; D.C. Zeldin. Molecular cloning, expression, and functional significance of a cytochrome P450 highly expressed in rat heart myocytes. *J. Biol. Chem.* **1997,** *272*, 12551–12559.

Wu, S.; C.R. Moomaw; K.B. Tomer; J.R. Falck; D.C. Zeldin. Molecular cloning and expression of CYP2J2, a human cytochrome P450 arachidonic acid epoxygenase highly expressed in heart. *J. Biol. Chem.* **1996,** *271*, 3460–3468.

Xiao, Y.F.; A.M. Gomez; J.P. Morgan; W.J. Lederer; A. Leaf. Suppression of voltage-gated L-type Ca2+ currents by polyunsaturated fatty acids in adult and neonatal rat ventricular myocytes. *Proc. Natl. Acad. Sci. U. S. A.* **1997,** *94*, 4182–4187.

Xiao, Y.F.; J.X. Kang; J.P. Morgan; A. Leaf. Blocking effects of polyunsaturated fatty acids on Na+ channels of neonatal rat ventricular myocytes. *Proc. Natl. Acad. Sci. U. S. A.* **1995,** *92*, 11000–11004.

Xiao, Y.F.; Q. Ke; J.M. Seubert; J.A. Bradbury; J. Graves; L.M. Degraff; J.R. Falck; K. Krausz; H.V. Gelboin; J.P. Morgan; D.C. Zeldin. Enhancement of cardiac L-type Ca2+ currents in transgenic mice with cardiac-specific overexpression of CYP2J2. *Mol. Pharmacol.* **2004,** *66*, 1607–1616.

Xiao, Y.F.; D.C. Sigg; M.R. Ujhelyi; J.J. Wilhelm; E.S. Richardson; P.A. Iaizzo. Pericardial delivery of omega-3 fatty acid: a novel approach to reducing myocardial infarct sizes and arrhythmias. *Am. J. Physiol. Heart Circ. Physiol.* **2008,** *294*, H2212–2218.

Xiao, Y.F.; S.N. Wright; G.K. Wang; J.P. Morgan; A. Leaf. Fatty acids suppress voltage-gated Na+ currents in HEK293t cells transfected with the alpha-subunit of the human cardiac Na+ channel. *Proc. Natl. Acad. Sci. U. S. A.* **1998,** *95*, 2680–2685.

Xu, W.; Y. Liu; S. Wang; T. McDonald; J.E. Van Eyk; A. Sidor; B. O'Rourke. Cytoprotective role of Ca2+- activated K+ channels in the cardiac inner mitochondrial membrane. *Science* **2002,** *298*, 1029–1033.

Yamori, Y.; Y. Nara; N. Iritani; R.J. Workman; T. Inagami. Comparison of serum phospholipid fatty acids among fishing and farming Japanese populations and American inlanders. *J. Nutr. Sci. Vitaminol. (Tokyo)* **1985,** *31*, 417–422.

Ye, D.; W. Zhou; T. Lu; S.G. Jagadeesh; J.R. Falck; H.C. Lee. Mechanism of rat mesenteric arterial KATP channel activation by 14,15-epoxyeicosatrienoic acid. *Am. J. Physiol. Heart Circ. Physiol.* **2006,** *290*, H1326–1336.

Yellon, D.M.; J.M. Downey. Preconditioning the myocardium: from cellular physiology to clinical cardiology. *Physiol. Rev.* **2003,** *83*, 1113–1151.

Zeldin, D.C.; R.N. DuBois; J.R. Falck; J.H. Capdevila. Molecular cloning, expression and characterization of an endogenous human cytochrome P450 arachidonic acid epoxygenase isoform.

*Arch. Biochem. Biophys.* **1995,** *322*, 76–86.

Zheng, J.; C.G. Plopper; J. Lakritz; D.H. Storms; B.D. Hammock. Leukotoxin-diol: a putative toxic mediator involved in acute respiratory distress syndrome. *Am. J. Respir. Cell. Mol. Biol.* **2001,** *25*, 434–438.

5

# Fatty Acids in Corn Oil: Role in Heart Disease Prevention

**Marie-Pierre St-Onge[1,2] and Suzette Singh[2]**

*[1] New York Obesity Research Center, St. Luke's/Roosevelt Hospital, New York, NY 10025; [2] Institute of Human Nutrition, Columbia University, New York, NY 10032*

## Introduction

### *Overview of Corn Oil: Consumption and Fatty Acid Composition*

Since the 1970s, the amount of corn oil produced in the United States has steadily increased such that, currently, corn oil is only second to soybean oil as the leading vegetable oil produced in this country (http://www.corn.org/CornOil.pdf). Corn oil—along with soybean, cottonseed, and canola oils—accounted for 95% of total vegetable oils consumed in the United States in 2004 (http://www.corn.org/CornOil.pdf). However, based on a retail food report for the first quarter of 2008, the price of corn oil increased by over 20% when compared to the fourth quarter of 2007 (http://www.fb.org/index.php?fuseaction=newsroom.newsfocus&year=2008&file=nr0327.html). Although we recognize that inflation is multifactorial, this increase perhaps was due, in part, to the increased demand for vegetable oils after the recognition of the ill effects of *trans* fats.

Before 2006, American consumers were unaware of the *trans*-fat content of foods (http://www.fda.gov/FDAC/features/2003/503_fats.html). In the summer of 2003, the U.S. Food and Drug Administration (FDA) issued a regulation requiring manufacturers to list the *trans*-fat content of their products on the Nutrition Facts panel, allowing *trans*-fat contents of less than 0.5 grams to be listed as 0 grams. With the increasing awareness of the negative health effects of *trans* fat for cardiovascular disease (CVD) risk, many U.S. cities joined in the action to reduce *trans*-fat consumption by requiring restaurants and food establishments to cook with *trans*-fat-free products. Tiburon, California, was the first American city where all restaurants voluntarily decided to cook with *trans*-fat-free oils in May 2005. In July 2007, all New York City restaurants were required by law to refrain from using frying and spreading fats containing more than 0.5 grams of *trans* fats per serving. These restaurants will have met this target with all foods by July 2008. Philadelphia also followed in this trend by requiring eateries to cease frying foods in *trans* fats starting in September 2007. Beyond regulations established by major cities and states, many organizations and restaurants, such as Walt Disney (http://www.magicalmountain.net/WDWNewsDetail.asp?page=24&NewsID=1341&type=1&tag=), Girl Scouts of America (http://www.girlscouts.org/news/news_releases/2006/gs_cookies_now_have_zero_trans_fats.asp), and Burger King (http://www.physorg.com/news102934980.html) also responded by changing their products countrywide to meet the current regulations (http://www.fda.gov/FDAC/features/2003/503_fats.html). In restricting *trans* fat in their food products, these organizations and restaurants shifted toward the use of unsaturated fats. For many, the shift may be toward the increased use of corn oil. Corn oil has desirable qualities: a high smoke point and neutral taste, making it a great choice for frying and baking. Furthermore, clinical studies show that the consumption of products that are low in *trans* and saturated fats, such as corn oil and all other vegetable oils, has beneficial effects on serum- cholesterol levels (Lichtenstein et al., 1999).

The majority of the fatty acids found in corn oil are polyunsaturated fatty acids (PUFAs; 54.7% of total fatty acids; Table 5.1), but it also has a moderate amount of monounsaturated fatty acids (MUFAs; 27.6% of total fatty acids), and some saturated fatty acids (SFAs; 13.0% of total fatty acids). Corn oil's SFA content is not unlike other vegetable oils, such as olive oil and soybean oil, which also contain approximately 13% of fat as SFA (U.S. Department of Agriculture, 2005). Of note is the high level of vitamin E in corn oil: 15 mL of corn oil contains 1.9 mg of $\alpha$-tocopherol per serving, which is 10% of the daily value (DV) for vitamin E (http://ods.od.nih.gov/factsheets/vitamine.asp). Although corn oil contains more vitamin E per unit amount than soybean oil (1.3 mg of $\alpha$-tocopherol per tablespoon; 6% of DV), other edible oils can provide a greater source of vitamin E, such as wheat-germ oil (20.3 mg of $\alpha$-tocopherol per tablespoon; 100% of DV), sunflower oil (5.6 mg of $\alpha$-tocopherol per

**Table 5.1. Fatty Acid Content of Common Vegetable Oils[1]**

| Fatty acid, % | Corn oil | Soybean oil | Canola oil | Sunflower oil | Olive oil |
|---|---|---|---|---|---|
| Total saturated fatty acids | 12.95 | 15.65 | 7.37 | 9.75 | 13.8 |
| Palmitic acid, 16:0 | 10.58 | 10.46 | 4.30 | 3.68 | 11.29 |
| Margaric acid, 17:0 | 0.07 | 0.03 | 0.00 | 0.00 | 0.02 |
| Stearic acid, 18:0 | 1.85 | 4.44 | 2.09 | 4.32 | 1.95 |
| Arachidic acid, 20:0 | 0.43 | 0.36 | 0.65 | 0.00 | 0.41 |
| Docosanoic acid, 22:0 | 0.31 | 0.37 | 0.33 | 1.00 | 0.13 |
| Total monounsaturated fatty acids | 27.58 | 22.78 | 63.28 | 83.59 | 72.96 |
| Palmitoleic acid, 16:1 | 0.11 | 0.00 | 0.21 | 0.00 | 1.26 |
| Oleic acid, 18:1 | 27.33 | 22.55 | 61.74 | 82.63 | 71.30 |
| Gadoleic acid, 20:1 | 0.13 | 0.23 | 1.32 | 0.96 | 0.31 |
| Total polyunsaturated fatty acids | 54.68 | 57.74 | 28.14 | 3.80 | 10.52 |
| Linoleic acid, 18:2 | 53.52 | 50.95 | 18.64 | 3.60 | 9.76 |
| Linolenic acid, 18:3 | 1.16 | 6.79 | 9.137 | 0.19 | 0.76 |

[1] U.S. Department of Agriculture, Agricultural Research Service (2005). USDA National Nutrient Database for Standard Reference, Release 18.

tablespoon; 30% of DV), and safflower oil (4.6 mg of α-tocopherol per tablespoon; 25% of DV) (http://ods.od.nih.gov/factsheets/vitamine.asp). Nevertheless, corn oil's vitamin-E content may contribute to its overall health effects.

## *Overview of the Effects of Corn Oil Fatty Acids on Cardiovascular Disease Risk*

The objective of this chapter is to highlight the research conducted in recent years on the cardiovascular health effects of corn oil. However, much of the research that applies to corn oil and its effects on CVD has been more generic, comparing diets high in PUFA or MUFA to diets low in fat or high in SFA on CVD. Therefore, we first establish the evidence linking PUFA and MUFA consumption to CVD risk prevention, and then focus on studies specifically examining the effects of corn oil on CVD risk.

The major risk factor for CVD that is discussed throughout this chapter is the lipid profile. However, novel risk factors for CVD have emerged, such as clotting and inflammatory markers, and oxidative status. No one has extensively studied the impact of corn oil on those risk factors, but it is discussed briefly in the "Novel Uses and Health Effects of Corn Oil" section of this chapter.

The plasma lipid-profile is an essential component to assessing health status and CVD risk because it is consistently associated with CVD risk. This chapter discusses studies that have looked at the impact of dietary fat on total cholesterol (TC), low-density lipoprotein cholesterol (LDL-C), very low density lipoprotein cholesterol (VLDL-C), high-density lipoprotein cholesterol (HDL-C), and triglyceride (TG) levels. Although LDL-C receives primary attention for the clinical management of CVD and is the primary target for therapy, growing evidence indicates that VLDL-C, TG, and HDL-C also play significant roles in CVD risk (Third Report of the National Cholesterol Education Program (NCEP) Expert Panel on Detection, Evaluation, and Treatment of High Blood Cholesterol in Adults [Adult Treatment Panel III] final report, 2002). To decrease CVD risk, foods with LDL-C-lowering and HDL-C-raising abilities have desirable outcomes in terms of CVD risk. Therapeutic lifestyle changes—including changes in diet aimed at reducing LDL-C concentrations—are an integral part of a CVD risk-prevention program (2002). Many of the risk factors for CVD are modifiable, and compelling evidence indicates that a major proportion of the current CVD burden is at least partially preventable: Consuming a healthy diet is one way to moderate risk (Bonow, 2002).

The major fatty acid components of corn oil may play separate and complementary roles in the moderation of CVD risk (see Table 5.1 and Table 5.2 for corn oil constituents). As mentioned earlier, corn oil mostly consists of PUFAs, which are recommended by various health authorities, including the American Heart Association, to prevent CVD when used as substitutes for solid fats, which are mostly saturated and hydrogenated. PUFAs have anti-arrhythmic properties, mitigate the course of atherosclerosis, and stabilize artherosclerotic plaque (von Schacky, 2007).

**Table 5.2. Approximate Composition of Refined Corn Oil: Nutrient Values[1]**

| | | | |
|---|---|---|---|
| Weight (g) | 100.0 | | |
| Moisture (g) | None | | |
| Protein (g) | None | | |
| Fat, Total (g) | 100.0 | | |
| | Triglycerides | 98.8 | |
| | | Polyunsaturated, Total (g) | 59.7 |
| | | *Cis, Cis Only* (g) | 58.7 |
| | | Monounsaturated (g) | 26.0 |
| | | Saturated, Total (g) | 13.1 |
| | *Unsaponifiable* Matter (g) | 1.2 | |
| | | Cholesterol (mg) | None |
| | | Phytosterols (mg) | 1000 |
| | | Tocopherols, Total (mg) | 88 |
| | | α-Tocopherol (mg) | 19 |
| | | Γ-Tocopherol (mg) | 67 |
| | | Δ-Tocopherol (mg) | 3 |
| Carbohydrates (g) | None | | |
| Ash (g) | None | | |
| Sodium (mg) | None | | |
| Energy (calories) | 885 | | |

[1] http://www.corn.org/CornOil.pdf

Research also shows that dietary PUFAs can have an overall cardioprotective effect (Siddiqui et al., 2008). Dietary intervention studies examining the effects of PUFAs on CVD show their ability to reduce mortality from sudden cardiac death and, when consumed over long periods, to prevent atherosclerosis (Leaf et al., 2008). As a result, both the American Dietetic Association and the Dietitians of Canada support increasing dietary PUFA intakes (Kris-Etherton et al., 2007). A section of this chapter discusses the findings of studies that examine the cholesterolemic effects of diets rich in PUFAs in comparison to other fatty acids.

Corn oil also contains other fatty acids and nutrients that may have protective effects against CVD. It has a moderate amount of MUFAs, which can manage CVD risk, provided the overall diet is also low in SFAs (Kris-Etherton, 1999). The major MUFA in corn oil is oleic acid, which favorably alters LDL-C and TG (Kris-Etherton, 1999). Corn oil also contains vitamin E, which has antioxidant and anti-inflammatory effects by inhibiting the activation of endothelial cells stimulated by high levels of LDL-C and pro-inflammatory cytokines (Meydani, 2004). This effect is shown with the consumption of diets rich in plant oils (Tomasch et al., 2001).

## Effects of Dietary Fatty Acid Profile on Lipid Concentrations

### *Effects of Diets Rich in Polyunsaturated and Monounsaturated Fatty Acids on Lipid Profile*

The lipid profile is important in determining health status, and is used as a marker of CVD risk. Overall, high levels of HDL-C are protective for CVD risk because they lower circulating serum cholesterol, and high LDL-C levels are known risk factors for CVD. The contents of PUFA, MUFA, and SFA in dietary oils were compared with respect to their effects on lipid profiles, and are reviewed in this section.

The Third Report of the National Cholesterol Education Program (NCEP) Expert Panel on Detection, Evaluation, and Treatment of High Blood Cholesterol in Adults recommends the consumption of PUFAs in place of SFAs to reduce LDL-C levels (2002). Controlled clinical trials also indicate that the substitution of PUFAs for SFAs reduces the risk for CVD. However, PUFAs can also cause small reductions in HDL-C when compared with MUFAs, especially when present in high amounts in the diet (Insull et al., 1994). The proportion of total fat as PUFA and MUFA is thus an important consideration when planning a heart-healthy diet (Lichtenstein et al., 2006). Since corn oil has a moderate amount of MUFA, we could consider it as a healthy substitute for oils high in SFA, since high-MUFA oils, such as olive oil, generally have cholesterol-lowering effects. However, whether corn oil's MUFA content can be responsible for its cholesterolemic effects remains to be determined. As is discussed in a later section, more likely the combination of MUFA and PUFA in corn oil produces lipid changes.

Low-fat diets are often recommended to lower TC, but an unfavorable side effect is often a lowering of HDL-C levels along with an increase in TG, both of which can adversely affect CVD risk (Third Report of the National Cholesterol Education Program [NCEP] Expert Panel on Detection, Evaluation, and Treatment of High Blood Cholesterol in Adults [Adult Treatment Panel III], 2001). However, MUFAs, which account for 27.6% of the fatty acids in corn oil, are useful in managing CVD risk, provided the overall diet does not exceed the SFA recommendation (Kris-Etherton et al., 1999). Therefore, to compare low-fat diets to high-MUFA diets, a study examined the effects of peanut products, which are naturally rich in MUFA and PUFA on CVD risk (Kris-Etherton et al., 1999). This randomized, double-blinded, five-period crossover study compared the CVD-risk profile after the consumption of an average American diet (AAD), an American Heart Association (AHA)/National Cholesterol Education Program (NCEP) Step II diet, and three high-unsaturated-fat diets [olive oil (OO), peanut oil (PO), and peanuts and peanut butter (PPB)]. All diets but the NCEP diet were high in fat, with approximately 38% of energy from fat. These high-fat diets differed in their fatty acid profile: high in saturated and *trans* fats for the AAD diet, high in MUFA for the OO diet, and high in MUFA and PUFA for the PO and PPB diets, respectively. The NCEP diet, by definition,

**Table 5.3. Macronutrient Profile of Typical Experimental Diets[1]**

| Diet | AAD | NCEP Step I | NCEP Step II | Mediterranean diet[2] |
|---|---|---|---|---|
| Carbohydrate (% of energy) | 50 | 55 | 59 | Not specified |
| Protein (% of energy) | 16 | 15 | 16 | 16 |
| Fat (% of energy) | 34 | 30 | 25 | 30 |
| SFAs | 16 | 8-10 | 7 | 8 |
| MUFAs | 11 | 15 | 12 | 13 |
| PUFAs | 7 | 10 | 6 | 5 |
| Cholesterol (mg/d)[2] | 400 | 300 | 200 | 203 |

[1] Source: Kris-Etherton et al., 1999.
[2] Source: Kris-Etherton et al., 2001.

provided approximately 25% of energy from fat and <7% of energy from SFA. Table 5.3 shows a comparison of the various control diets that are discussed throughout the chapter, including the ones from this study. Experimental diets were consumed for 24 days each. The results of this study showed that all three high-fat, high-unsaturated fat diets lowered TC and LDL-C by approximately 10 and 14%, respectively, compared to the AAD. These reductions in TC and LDL-C were comparable to those observed with the consumption of the NCEP diet. TGs were lower by 13% with the consumption of the high-MUFA diets (OO, PO, and PPB), while they were 11% higher with the consumption of the NCEP diet than with the AAD. The consumption of the high-MUFA diets did not lower HDL-C, whereas the NCEP diet lowered it by 4% compared with the AAD. Compared to the AAD, the OO, PO, and PPB diets decreased CVD risk by an estimated 25, 16, and 21%, respectively, whereas the NCEP diet lowered CVD risk by 12%. The authors concluded that a higher consumption of unsaturated fats can lower TC without raising TG or lowering HDL-C when compared to a low-fat diet, which increased plasma TG and decreased HDL-C (Kris-Etherton et al., 1999). Therefore, consuming a high-fat diet rich in MUFA or rich in MUFA and PUFA may be more advisable for CVD risk reduction than a low-fat diet because it does not have the adverse effect of lowering HDL-C levels and raising TG. As a result, the overall lipid profile is healthier with a higher unsaturated-fat consumption than with the consumption of a low-fat diet.

Although data regarding the health benefits of MUFA consumption are available (Kris-Etherton et al., 1999), some debate arises regarding the type of unsaturated fat to include in the diet to elicit the greatest lipid-lowering effect. Therefore, Mensink and Katan (1989) conducted a controlled feeding study to compare the effects of PUFA and MUFA on plasma-lipid concentrations in healthy men and women. The study participants initially consumed a baseline diet rich in SFA for 17 days. This diet provided 19.3% of energy from SFA, 11.5% from MUFA, and 4.6% from PUFA. For the next 36 days, they received a mixed diet with the same amount of total fat but enriched with either a mix of OO and sunflower oil (MUFA) or with sunflower oil alone (PUFA). The MUFA diet provided 12.9% of energy from SFA, 15.1% from MUFA, and 7.9% from PUFA, while the PUFA diet provided 12.6% of energy from SFA, 10.8% from MUFA, and 12.7% from PUFA. The consumption of the MUFA diet caused a 17.9% reduction in LDL-C concentrations, and the PUFA diet resulted in a 12.9% reduction in LDL-C. No difference was detected between these two diets in the extent of LDL-C reduction. Furthermore, both diets caused a slight but insignificant decrease in HDL-C levels in men only compared to baseline. The authors concluded that mixed diets rich in MUFA or PUFA were equally effective in lowering LDL-C (Mensink & Katan, 1989).

However, in the Nurses' Health Study (Hu et al., 1997), MUFA intake—adjusted for age, lifestyle, and other fatty- acid intakes—did not modify the relative risk for coronary heart disease in women. In fact, the relative risk of coronary heart disease was lowest among women who consumed the lowest amount of *trans* fat and the highest amount of PUFA. Also, higher intakes of PUFA—after adjusting for age, lifestyle, and other fatty- acid intakes—reduced the risk for coronary heart disease. The authors concluded that their findings provided evidence that higher intakes of MUFA and PUFA are associated with a reduced risk for coronary heart disease, even without reducing overall fat intake.

Since both high-PUFA and high-MUFA diets can have TC- and LDL-C-lowering effects, foods that replace SFA should include a balance of unsaturated fatty acids (Lichtenstein et al., 2006). In a double-blinded, randomized, controlled feeding study, researchers found that the higher PUFA content of a sunflower-oil diet, which was also high in MUFA, was accountable for lowering TC and LDL-C in moderately hypercholesterolemic men and women (Binkoski et al., 2005). Experimental diets provided 30% of energy as fat of which 50% came from OO or NuSun sunflower oil and 8.3 or 7.9% as SFA, 17.2 or 14.2% as MUFA, and 4.3 or 7.7% as PUFA for the OO and NuSun diets, respectively. The control diet was an AAD with 34% of energy as fat, 11.2% as SFA, 14.9% as MUFA, and 7.8% as PUFA. Subjects consumed each diet for 4 weeks with a 2-week compliance break before crossing over to the other diet. The NuSun diet decreased both TC (4.7%) and LDL-C (5.8%) levels compared with the control AAD. The OO diet did not have any significant effect on the subjects' lipid profiles when compared with the AAD. No effect of the experimental diets was detected on TG levels or markers of lipid oxidation. This study noted the importance of the balance of unsaturated fatty acids in the diet, and the authors were able to show that the higher PUFA content of an oil rich in MUFA appeared to be accountable for the TC- and LDL-C-lowering effects of the sunflower-oil diet (Binkoski et al., 2005). Therefore, seemingly, PUFA and MUFA both have cholesterol-lowering effects when compared to high-SFA diets, and since corn oil contains both, it can be potentially beneficial as a substitute for other high-SFA oils in the diet.

The cholesterol-lowering effects of PUFA and MUFA were also compared as they were varied in a reciprocal dose-dependent fashion in the context of an NCEP Step I diet (Howard et al., 1995). The study participants included 63 moderately hypercholesterolemic African American and Caucasian men and women. All participants consumed a 6-week baseline diet containing 37% of energy from total fat and 15% from SFA. After baseline, participants were randomized to consume 1 of 4 diets for 6 weeks. Each diet contained 10% of energy as SFA; 3, 6, 10, or 14% of energy as PUFA; and 17, 14, 10, or 6% of energy as MUFA. The results showed a progressive decrease in TC and LDL-C concentrations with increasing PUFA intakes. Also a small but significant decrease in HDL-C from baseline was comparable between all MUFA- and PUFA-rich diets. The authors concluded that with all other known cholesterol-influencing dietary factors held constant, substituting MUFA with increasing amounts of PUFA, within the context of an NCEP Step I diet, up to a maximal PUFA level of 14% of energy intakes, resulted in a progressive decline in TC concentrations without an adverse effect on HDL-C (Howard et al., 1995).

One cannot discuss the unsaturated fats MUFA and PUFA without a brief overview of the Mediterranean diet. This diet, which signifies a diet liberal in total fat content but low in saturated fat, is often considered one of the best heart-healthy diets consumed. In fact, the Mediterranean diet has beneficial effects on CVD factors (Estruch et al., 2006). The Mediterranean diet is low in SFA, high in unsaturated fat from vegetable oils (mostly OO), and high in dietary fiber. The typical source of fat in this diet is OO and other vegetable oils. The diet is usually rich in nuts, fruits, vegetables, legumes, and plant foods, but low in red meat, poultry, and high-fat meats. One study compared the short-term effects of two Mediterranean diets versus those of a low-fat diet on intermediate markers of cardiovascular risk (Estruch et al., 2006). This was a substudy of a multi-center, randomized, primary prevention trial of CVD with 772 men and women ages 55 to 80 years at a high risk of CVD. Participants were assigned to a low-fat diet or to one of two Mediterranean diets. Those randomized to the Mediterranean diets received nutritional education and either 1 L per week of extra-virgin OO or 30 grams of nuts per day (hazelnuts, almonds, walnuts). Body weight, blood pressure, lipid profile, glucose levels, and inflammatory markers were evaluated at 3 months. Compared with the low-fat diet, the OO and nut groups had 0.39 mmol/L and 0.30 mmol/L reductions in plasma-glucose levels, respectively; reductions of 5.9 mm Hg and 7.1 mm Hg, respectively, in systolic blood pressure; and reductions of 0.38 and 0.26, respectively, in the TC:HDL-C ratio. Since the diet enriched with nuts had greater improvements than the OO diet, additional benefits are derived from consuming a diet rich in PUFA over a higher MUFA diet. The authors concluded that compared with a low-fat diet, Mediterranean diets supplemented with OO or nuts have beneficial effects on CVD risk factors (Estruch et al., 2006).

Although many have long advocated low-fat diets for CVD risk reduction, as highlighted by the NCEP Step I and Step II diets (Table 5.3), emerging evidence points toward more liberal total-fat intakes. This is advocated if the overall fat profile of the diet is low in saturated and *trans* fats. Recent recommendations for a better heart-healthy diet state that dietary fat for the adult population should provide 20 to 35% of energy (Kris-Etherton et al., 2007). Also an emphasis is placed on reducing SFAs and *trans* fats while increasing the intake of n-3 PUFAs (Kris-Etherton et al., 2007). Studies that have looked at the impact of moderate-fat diets containing approximately 30–40% of energy from fat on CVD risk showed beneficial serum-lipid changes if the overall dietary-fat profile was shifted toward unsaturated fats (Howard et al., 1995). As discussed above, studies show that dietary PUFAs reduce the LDL-C in adults, but they also either decrease (Estruch et al., 2006) or have no impact (Howard et al., 1995) on the HDL-C levels when compared to high-MUFA diets. Both high-MUFA and high-PUFA diets can lead to reductions in TC and LDL-C concentrations without adversely affecting HDL-C and TG concentrations (Binkoski et al., 2005). This is an advantage over low-fat diets which reduce HDL-C and raise TG concentrations. Some controversy remains, however, with respect to which unsaturated fats, PUFA or MUFA, can produce the most beneficial lipid profile for CVD risk reduction. Thus, at this point, to advocate an overall shift from SFAs to unsaturated fats and to consume a mix of various vegetable oils rich in MUFA and PUFA seem prudent. Corn oil, which is high in PUFA and also contains an appreciable amount of MUFA, may be advocated to have a beneficial impact for CVD risk reduction.

## *Effects of Diets Rich in Corn Oil on Lipid Profile*

Clinical trials that compared diets rich in different types of oils showed that diets rich in corn oil lower cholesterol by about 1% for each gram of corn oil they contain (USFDA-CFSAN, 2007). The trials conclude that a daily substitution of 1 tablespoon (15 mL) of corn oil for butter or other SFA-rich oil or fat could therefore lower cholesterol concentrations by approximately 15%.

One of the earliest studies to examine the effects of corn oil on plasma-lipid concentrations aimed to compare the effects of corn oil to a hydrogenated corn oil-based margarine on plasma lipids in hypercholesterolemic men and women (Lichtenstein et al., 1993). Three controlled test diets were prepared and consumed for 32 days each with a 1-week break between each diet. All subjects consumed an initial AAD followed by a corn oil-enriched diet and a corn oil-based margarine-enriched diet. The two experimental diets were designed according to the NCEP Step II diet with two-thirds of the fat, corresponding to 20% of energy intake, coming from either corn oil or the corn oil margarine. Both experimental diets significantly reduced TC concentrations by 13 and 7% for the corn oil and the corn oil margarine diets, respectively, compared to the AAD. The reduction observed with the consumption of the corn oil diet was greater than that observed with the corn oil-based margarine diet. Similarly, LDL-C was reduced by 17% with the consumption of the corn oil diet and 10% with the consumption of the corn oil- based margarine diet compared to the AAD; however, the difference in change between the two experimental diets did not quite reach statistical significance. HDL-C was also significantly reduced with the consumption of the corn oil diet (by 9%) and corn oil-based margarine diet (by 11%) compared to the AAD. TG concentrations did not change with the consumption of the experimental diets. The results of this study thus support the consumption of corn oil, in liquid form, as a means of reducing CVD risk (Lichtenstein et al., 1993).

In a study designed to compare the effects of different dietary-oil intakes in Malaysian volunteers, researchers were able to show that corn oil significantly reduced TC, LDL-C, and HDL-C concentrations compared to palm oil (Ng et al., 1991). They observed the effects on serum lipids of diets prepared with palm oil, corn oil, and coconut oil, with the test oil supplying approximately 75% of the calories from fat. They compared three groups of healthy, young male and female volunteers, ages 20–34 years. One group received the coconut–palm–coconut diet sequence, another group received the coconut–corn–coconut, and the third group received coconut oil during all three 5-week dietary periods. The greatest LDL:HDL-C ratio reduction came with the consumption of the corn oil diet. The 25% reduction in the LDL:HDL-C ratio was greater than that observed after the consumption of the coconut-oil diet, which had no effect on the LDL:HDL-C ratio and the palm-oil diet, which resulted in an 8% reduction in the LDL:HDL-C ratio (Ng et al., 1991). This study shows that when substituted for a diet rich in palm oil or coconut oil, corn oil can have beneficial lipid-lowering effects.

One clinical study compared the effects of PUFAs in three common vegetable oils on plasma-lipid levels in normolipidemic adults. Twenty-six men and 35 women were placed on reduced- fat diets for 5 weeks each. Diets were designed to maintain the subjects' weight, and contained 22–26% of energy from fat. Corn oil, soybean oil, or sunflower oil was used as the treatment oil in separate diets (Insull et al., 1994). Subjects were randomized to one of six test-diet sequences that alternated between periods of controlled, weight-maintaining test diets and self-selected habitual, ad libitum diets for 5 weeks each. Diets differed only in their fatty acid profile, which was reflective of the oil included in the diets, either corn, soybean, or sunflower oil. The corn oil diet had the highest PUFA:SFA ratio with a ratio of 1.37:1, followed by sunflower oil with a 1.22:1 ratio, and soybean oil with a 0.86:1 ratio. All three diets lowered TC, LDL-C, and HDL-C concentrations compared to baseline, and had no effect on TG concentrations. However, reductions in TC were inversely related to baseline TC concentrations, such that individuals with the highest initial cholesterol concentrations had greater TC reductions than those with the lowest initial TC concentrations. The TC:HDL-C and LDL-C:HDL-C ratios showed no significant change from baseline with any of the test diets. The authors concluded that PUFAs at a level of approximately 6% of total energy intakes result in clinically relevant plasma cholesterol-lowering, regardless of its source (Insull et al., 1994). This research shows that oils rich in PUFAs can have a beneficial cholesterol-lowering effect. In fact, the consumption of the diet rich in corn oil reduced TC by 10.8% and LDL-C by 12% compared to baseline.

OO has beneficial cholesterol-lowering effects. Oleic acid is the primary MUFA present in OO, but it is also the major MUFA in corn oil. This fatty acid has a favorable effect on the lipid profile by lowering LDL-C and TG levels (Wagner et al., 2001). Whether oleic acid in OO and oleic acid in corn oil have similar cholesterolemic effects was examined. A clinical study conducted to clarify the effects of MUFA-rich diets compared to PUFA-rich diets (as well as the effects of single oils compared to the consumption of oil mixtures) showed that a PUFA-rich corn oil diet can reduce LDL-C significantly when compared to a plant-oil mixture high in oleic acid (Wagner et al., 2001). The oils used in this study were a mix of OO and sunflower oil, providing a SFA/MUFA/PUFA ratio of 14:69:17, and corn oil, containing a SFA/MUFA/PUFA ratio of 13:33:54. Both oils were used within a normal, balanced diet. The participants in this study were 28 healthy, nonsmoking young men of the ages of 19 to 31 years. After 2 weeks of consuming a mixed, balanced diet, subjects consumed a diet with either 80 grams of corn oil per day or a mix of 68 grams of OO and 12 grams of sunflower oil per day for 2 weeks each. Each dietary period was separated by a 2-week washout period. The results showed that TC, TG, LDL-C, and VLDL-C were significantly lower after the consumption of the corn oil diet when compared to the mixed-oil diet. The levels of HDL-C remained unchanged in both diets. The authors concluded that the 2-week corn oil diet intervention had a greater influence on lipoprotein metabolism than the MUFA-rich, plant-oil-mixture diet (Wagner et al., 2001).

Corn oil was also directly compared to OO, the main oil of the Mediterranean diet, for its effects on lipid concentrations. Sirtori et al. (1992) conducted a crossover study on 12 hypercholesterolemic subjects to compare the cardiovascular health effects of corn oil and OO relative to n-3 fatty acids. Participants received a lead-in diet that followed the NCEP Step I diet recommendations for more than one month, followed by either a PUFA-rich corn oil-supplemented diet, a MUFA-rich OO-supplemented diet, or n-3 fatty acid-supplemented diet for 6 weeks. No significant reduction appeared in TC from baseline after consumption of the corn oil and the OO diets; however, the OO diet resulted in a small, but significant, reduction in LDL-C concentrations and a raise in HDL-C compared to baseline. Corn oil, on the other hand, resulted in a small, but significant, reduction in HDL-C concentrations from baseline. The changes observed with the OO diet were small, and the endpoint concentrations of all of the lipid components were not different between corn oil and OO. The diet rich in n-3 fatty acids, however, significantly reduced TC, VLDL-C, LDL-C, and increased HDL-C compared to baseline. Although the high n-3 fatty acid diet seemed to produce the best lipid profile after 6 weeks of treatment, the authors concluded that the magnitude of effects was small and that all three diets studied provided a satisfactory choice of diet for cholesterol-lowering benefits (Sirtori et al., 1992).

Most previous studies incorporated oils in foods to test the impact of corn oil compared to other oils on lipid profile. As a result, diets contained a greater proportion of the oils than would normally be consumed by individuals. Therefore, also examining the impact of single-food substitutions, as a means of introducing various oils into the diet, on CVD risk profile is important. In an attempt to do this, one study examined whether replacing snacks that are high in fat and saturated fat with low-fat or high-fat, high-PUFA snacks could alter the lipid profile (St-Onge et al., 2007). The high-fat, high-PUFA diet contained snacks fried in corn oil. Thirty-three adults participated in this randomized, crossover trial of three controlled-feeding phases of 25 days each. During a given diet period, a different type of snack was provided: low-fat, high-fat—high-PUFA, and high-fat control. The low-fat diet contained 30.8% of energy from fat and 5.2% of energy from PUFAs, whereas the high-fat diets contained 36.3% of energy from fat for the high-PUFA diet and 37.9% of energy from fat for the high-fat control diet. The major difference between the two high-fat diets was their PUFA content which was 9.7% of energy for the high- PUFA diet and 5.8% of energy for the high-fat control diet. The high-PUFA diet reduced TG concentrations by 9.4%, a change that was significantly different from what was observed with the low-fat and high-fat control diets. Each diet reduced LDL-C significantly, but reductions were greater with the low-fat and the high-PUFA diets than with the high-fat control diet (11.8 and 12.5%, respectively, versus 8.8%). This effect was also true for the reductions in TC which were greater with the low-fat and high-PUFA diets when compared to the high-fat control diet (10.5 and 10.7%, respectively, versus 7.9%). The authors concluded that, although snacks provided only 12–15% of total daily calories, the fat quality of the snacks can have a significant impact on heart health. This research supports the notion that the consumption of foods rich in PUFA from corn oil and low in SFA or *trans* fatty acids instead of high-SFA and *trans* fatty acid or low-fat snacks leads to improvements in lipid profiles concordant with reductions in CVD risk (St-Onge et al., 2007).

Studies therefore seem to show rather positive results regarding the effects of corn oil for cholesterol reductions. When compared to higher saturated and *trans*-fat diets, a diet rich in corn oil produces beneficial effects on the lipid profile (Lichtenstein et al., 1993; Ng et al., 1991; St-Onge et al., 2007). Of the two studies that compared diets rich in corn oil to a lower fat, NCEP Step I-type diet (Sirtori et al., 1992; St-Onge et al., 2007), one showed no difference in the extent of TC and LDL-C reductions compared to baseline between the two diets (St-Onge et al., 2007), and the other showed no change from the NCEP Step I baseline diet with corn oil consumption (Sirtori et al., 1992). These two studies thus show that corn oil consumption is at least as good as an NCEP Step I diet for CVD-risk reduction. In fact, one study suggests that, with respect to its effects on TG concentrations, corn oil consumption would lead to a healthier plasma-lipid profile than a low-fat diet (St-Ongeet al., 2007). Finally, when compared to other vegetable oils, corn oil has either similar (Insull et al., 1994), better (Wagner et al., 2001), or worse (Sirtori et al., 1992) lipid effects. The mix of results is due to the comparative oils: corn oil seems to have lipid effects similar to those of soybean and sunflower oils (Insull et al., 1994), better effects than a blend of OO and sunflower oil (Wagner et al., 2001), and a worse effect than OO alone (Sirtori et al., 1992). However, the extent of the difference in lipid effects in the latter study was minimal, and thus, both OO and corn oil are healthy oils for CVD risk prevention (Sirtori et al., 1992).

## Novel Uses and Health Effects of Corn Oil

The hypocholesterolemic effect of the PUFA-rich corn oil diet is at least in part attributable to the high amount of unsaponifiable substances, mainly phytosterols, found in corn oil (Wagner et al., 2001). Although supplementing the diet with 1.6–2 grams of phytosterols reduces cholesterol absorption and LDL-C concentrations (St-Onge & Jones, 2003), very little is known about the cardiovascular health effects of smaller amounts of phytosterols present naturally in food (Ostlund et al., 2002). Vegetable oils are the richest dietary sources of phytosterols, and corn oil contains 0.77% of phytosterols by weight. This level is twice as much as the phytosterol content of soybean oil. A clinical study was conducted to test the effects of phytosterols naturally present in corn oil on cholesterol (Ostlund et al., 2002). By removing phytosterols from corn oil, researchers found an increase in cholesterol absorption when measured in single-meal tests containing corn oil as a source of fat. The cholesterol-reducing properties of corn oil were restored once the phytosterols were added back to the sterol-free corn oil. The authors concluded that the phytosterols that comprise <1% of commercial corn oil can substantially reduce cholesterol absorption and may account for part of the cholesterol-lowering activity of corn oil previously attributed solely to its unsaturated fatty acid content (Ostlund et al., 2002).

Corn oil extractable from corn fiber contains ferulate esters; particularly sitostanyl ester has a cholesterol-lowering activity in a study investigating the cholesterol-lowering mechanisms in hamsters (Jain et al., 2008). The aim of this study was to determine the effects of corn-fiber oil, ferulate phytostanyl esters (FPE), and parent compounds of FPE, including sitostanol and ferulic acid, on the lipid profile. Seventy male hamsters were randomly assigned to six experimental diets for 4 weeks: (i) cornstarch–casein–sucrose-based control diet (control) and (ii) control diet plus 0.1% cholesterol (cholesterol–control). The remaining four groups were given the cholesterol–control diet with: (iii) 10% of corn fiber oil, (iv) 0.5% of sitostanol, (v) 0.23% of ferulic acid, and (vi) 0.73% of FPE. Supplementation with corn-fiber oil decreased plasma TC by 29% compared with the cholesterol–control group, while FPE and sitostanol reduced cholesterolemia by 15 and 14%, respectively. Corn-fiber oil and sitostanol decreased cholesterol absorption by 24% compared to the cholesterol–control group. Corn-fiber oil is extracted by a novel process that includes a grinding step carried out before extraction with an effective organic solvent, such as hexane. The corn-fiber oil may be combined with an ingestible and/or edible carrier for administration as a dietary supplement for cholesterol-lowering purposes (Jain et al., 2008).

A synthetic oil called functional oil and containing mono- and diacylglycerols from corn oil has anti-atherosclerotic effects (Cho et al., 2006). This effect was shown in dietary-induced hypercholesterolemic mice. Mice consumed high-fat diets rich in cholesterol. This diet was supplemented with either 5% of regular corn oil or 5% of the functional oil as the experimental diets. All diets were fed to the mice for 4 weeks. In mice consuming the functional oil, an inhibition occurred of liver acyl-

CoA:cholesterol acyltransferase activity, an enzyme involved in cholesterol metabolism, and of serum lipoprotein-associated phospholipase $A_2$ activity, an enzyme involved in inflammation. The consumption of the functional oil also resulted in enhanced lipoprotein interactions such as HDL particle rearrangement to produce larger HDL species. Larger HDL particles represent a greater protective action against CVD. The ratio of HDL:TC was higher in the functional oil-fed group, when compared to the high-fat diet control group and the corn oil group. The functional-oil-fed mice had a 38% reduction in TC compared to the high-fat diet control group and a 20% reduction in TC compared to the corn oil group. In summary, the results from this study indicate that a functional oil rich in corn oil diacylglycerol and monoacylglycerol possesses cholesterol-lowering properties in a mouse model and inhibition effects against atherogenic enzymes (Cho et al., 2006). Since the functional oil had more desirable effects on the lipid profile than complete corn oil, some benefits may result from synthesized corn oil consumption over whole-corn oil consumption. Therefore, the engineering of corn oil to increase its diacylglycerol and monoacylglycerol content may be useful in modulating corn oil's effects on CVD risk. However, clinical studies are needed to determine whether the animal data translate to humans.

In addition to new uses for corn oil, corn oil was studied for health benefits other than CVD. A corn oil- supplemented diet has beneficial effects on vitamin K-dependent proteins in a study on 26 healthy young men (Schurgers et al., 2002). When a diet enriched with corn oil was compared to a diet enriched in an OO and sunflower-oil mixture, the corn oil diet induced reductions in matrix GLA-proteins, fasting TG, and circulating phylloquinones that were not seen with the consumption of the OO- and sunflower-oil-enriched diet. The consumption of the corn oil diet was also correlated with an increased osteocalcin, which is negatively correlated to undercarboxylated prothrombin. These findings suggest that a corn oil-supplemented diet may have anti-coagulatory effects (Schurgers et al., 2002).

Dietary antioxidants are expected to reduce cancer risk by minimizing DNA damage (Elmadfa & Park, 1999). Since plant oils and fats are major sources of vitamin E, they are major contributors of antioxidants in the diet. A double-blinded, crossover study was conducted on 20 healthy, nonsmoking men to compare the effects of $\gamma$-tocopherol-rich corn oil and the $\alpha$-tocopherol-rich mixture of OO and sunflower oil on plasma concentrations of tocopherols and on the frequency of sister chromatid exchange, an indicator of DNA damage. The combination of $\gamma$- and $\alpha$-tocopherols in the corn oil diet, despite resulting in a lower $\alpha$-tocopherol equivalents/diene acid equivalents ratio, achieved better protection against DNA damage than $\alpha$-tocopherol alone in the OO and sunflower-oil diets. This study suggests that a corn oil-enriched diet can have desirable antioxidant effects due to the corn oil's tocopherol content (Elmadfa & Park, 1999).

## Qualified Health Claims

Much of the interest in corn oil in recent years may, in part, be the result of the recognition of its important health and nutritional benefits, stemming from its PUFA

**Table 5.4.** Results of Studies Examining the Impact of High-Polyunsaturated and High-Monounsaturated Fat Diets, Including Corn Oil, on Lipid Profile.

| Publication | Subject information | | Percent age of fat in diet as: PUFA | SFA | MUFA | Results/findings[1] |
|---|---|---|---|---|---|---|
| Howard et al., 1995 | African American and Caucasian hypercholesterolemic men and women | | 3, 6, 10, or 14% | 10% | 17, 14, 10, or 6% | Increasing PUFA content as a substitution for MUFA decreases TC without effect on HDL-C in a dose-dependent manner. |
| Insull et al., 1994 | Normolipidemic, free-living men and women | Soybean oil | 9.7–10.4% | 10.2–12.1% | 24.4–27.2% | All three diets showed a decrease in TG. Authors conclude that PUFAs at approximately 6% of total energy result in lower TC and that the proportion of PUFA must be an important consideration when planning reduced-fat, reduced-SFA diets. |
| | | Corn oil | 16.0–16.7% | 10.2–12.1% | 18.1–20.9% | |
| | | Sunflower oil | 16.7–17.4% | 12.3–14.2% | 15.3–18.1% | |
| Kris-Etherton et al., 1999 | Normocholesterolemic men and women | AAD | 7% | 16% | 11% | High-MUFA diets lowered TC and LDL-C compared to the AAD diet without affecting HDL-C. Higher fat diets high in MUFA have a better impact on lipid profile than a low-fat diet. |
| | | NCEP Step 2 | 6% | 7% | 12% | |
| | | Olive oil | 6% | 7% | 21% | |
| | | Peanut oil | 9% | 7% | 17% | |
| | | PPB | 10% | 8% | 18% | |
| Mensink & Katan, 1989 | Healthy men and women | MUFA-rich diet | 7.9 % | 12.9% | 15.1% | A mixed MUFA-rich diet was as effective as an n-6 PUFA- rich diet in lowering LDL-C. Both diets lowered HDL-C slightly in men but not in women. |
| | | PUFA-rich diet | 12.7% | 12.6% | 10.8% | |

*cont. on p. 156.*

**Table 5.4., cont.** **Results of Studies Examining the Impact of High-Polyunsaturated and High-Monounsaturated Fat Diets, Including Corn Oil, on Lipid Profile.**

| Publication | Subject information | | Percent age of fat in diet as: PUFA | SFA | MUFA | Results/findings[1] |
|---|---|---|---|---|---|---|
| Kabagambe et al., 2005 | Moderately hypercholesterolemic men and women | AAD | 7.8% | 11.2% | 14.9% | NuSun sunflower-oil diet decreased TC and LDL-C. The replacement of palm oil with a PUFA-rich vegetable oil would reduce the risk of MI. |
| | | Olive oil | 4.3% | 17.2% | 8.3% | |
| | | NuSun sunflower oil | 7.7% | 14.2% | 7.9% | |
| Ng et al., 1991 | Healthy young men and women | Palm olein | 11.4% | 45.6% | 42.7% | Compared with baseline, coconut oil raised TC. Subsequent feeding of palm olein or corn oil reduced TC, LDL-C, and HDL-C. TGs were unaffected during the palm-olein period but were reduced during the corn oil period. |
| | | Corn oil | 35.6% | 30.4% | 33.8% | |
| | | Coconut oil | 2.8% | 75.1% | 11.7% | |
| Sirtori et al., 1992 | Hypercholesterolemic type 2 diabetic men and women | PUFA-rich corn oil diet | 45.4% | 32.3% | 22.2% | Dietary unsaturated fatty acids are generally effective on the plasma lipid and lipoproteins in type 2 diabetics. The olive-oil and n-3 ethyl esters diets lowered TC, the n-3 ethyl esters lowered TG and raised HDL-C and TG, and the corn- oil diet lowed HDL-C slightly. |
| | | MUFA-rich olive-oil diet | 40.3% | 32.1% | 27.5% | |
| | | n-3 fatty acid diet | 45.7% | 32.0% | 21.9% | |

**Table 5.4., cont. Results of Studies Examining the Impact of High-Polyunsaturated and High-Monounsaturated Fat Diets, Including Corn Oil, on Lipid Profile.**

| Publication | Subject information | | Percent age of fat in diet as: | | | Results/findings[1] |
|---|---|---|---|---|---|---|
| | | | PUFA | SFA | MUFA | |
| St-Onge et al., 2007 | Moderately hypercholesterolemic men and women | Low fat | 5.2% | 8.5% | 14.2% | Consuming snack chips rich in PUFA and low in SFA and *trans* fats instead of high-SFA and *trans* fats or low-fat snacks leads to improvements in lipid profiles. |
| | | High PUFA | 9.7% | 8.5% | 15.3% | |
| | | High fat | 5.8% | 11.4% | 15.9% | |
| Lichtenstein et al., 1993 | Moderately hypercholesterolemic middle-aged and elderly men and women | Corn oil- enriched diet | 10% | 6% | 11% | The corn oil rich diet lowered LDL-C more than the corn oil-margarine diet. |
| | | Corn oil-margarine-enriched diet | 8% | 8% | 12% | |
| Wagner et al., 2001 | Healthy, young, free-living men | Corn oil | 12.0% | 8.8% | 10.2% | The corn oil diet led to a greater decrease in LDL-C, TC, and TG compared to the MUFA-rich, mixed-oil diet. |
| | | Sunflower-oil and olive-oil mixture | 7.2% | 8.7% | 15.1% | |

[1] Abbreviations: AAD, average American diet; HDL-C, high-density lipoprotein cholesterol; LDL-C, low-density lipoprotein cholesterol; MUFAs, monounsaturated fatty acids; NCEP, National Cholesterol Education Program; PPB, peanuts and peanut butter; PUFAs, polyunsaturated fatty acids; SFAs, saturated fatty acids; TC, total cholesterol; TGs, triglycerides; MI, myocardial infarction.

content (Table 5.4). Corn oil can substitute for other cooking oils in attempts to decrease saturated fat in the diet and to increase intakes of PUFAs, with the intent to lower TC and LDL-C and ultimately reduce the risk of CVD (Third Report of the National Cholesterol Education Program [NCEP] Expert Panel on Detection, Evaluation, and Treatment of High Blood Cholesterol in Adults [Adult Treatment Panel III] final report, 2002). As presented in this chapter, scientific evidence supports the notion that including corn oil-containing foods in a balanced diet may reduce CVD risk factors. As a result, the U.S. FDA has approved qualified health claims for various vegetable oils (Table 5.5). Qualified health claims are statements that can be made for foods, if the foods fulfill specific requirements, to highlight the food's relationship with the prevention of chronic disease. Qualified health claims, as well as significant scientific agreement (SSA) health claims, characterize a relationship between a substance and a disease or health-related condition. The distinction between those two types of health claims lies in the level of scientific agreement achieved. SSA health claims must pass established scientific standards. When the research submitted to obtain a health claim does not meet SSA standards, which may be due to shortcomings of the supporting research, a qualified health claim may be approved. Once a health claim is approved, a specific wording for the claim is established that must be adhered to by all products presenting the claim. Although all health claims must follow specific wording approved by the FDA, qualified health claims must also state the relationship between food and health conditions in such a way as to not mislead the consumer. Corn oil was granted a qualified health claim in March 2007. Since this is a qualified health claim, as opposed to a SSA health claim, the claim states that substituting corn oil for fats high in saturated fat or for solid fats may reduce the risk of heart disease (http://www.cfsan.fda.gov/~dms/qhc-sum.html). For a manufacturer to be allowed to apply the qualified health claim to a specific food product, the food must contain at least 4 grams of corn oil per serving. The approved qualified health claim for corn oil must also be stated as such:

> "Very limited and preliminary scientific evidence suggests that eating about 1 tablespoon (16 grams) of corn oil daily may reduce the risk of heart disease due to the unsaturated fat content in corn oil. FDA concludes that there is little scientific evidence supporting this claim. To achieve this possible benefit,

**Table 5.5. Approved Qualified Health Claims for Vegetable Oils[1]**

| Oil | Claim |
|---|---|
| Corn oil | 1 tbsp reduces CVD risk when in substitution for a high-saturated-fat diet. |
| | Corn oil is very high in omega-6 fatty acid, which, compared with omega-3's, is relatively pro-inflammatory. |
| Canola oil | 1.5 tbsp reduces CVD risk when in substitution for a high-saturated-fat diet. |
| Olive oil | 2 tbsp reduce CVD risk when in substitution for a high-saturated-fat diet. |

[1] http://www.cfsan.fda.gov/~dms/qhc-sum.html.

> corn oil is to replace a similar amount of saturated fat and not increase the total number of calories you eat in a day. One serving of this product contains [x] grams of corn oil" (http://www.cfsan.fda.gov/~dms/qhc-sum.html)."

Due to the high content of unsaturated fatty acids in corn oil, corn oil products can also bear an FDA Modernization Act Health Claim. This type of health claim is approved based on an authoritative statement from an appropriate scientific body of the U.S. government or the National Academy of Science or any of its subdivisions. In May 2007, the FDA allowed a health claim stating that the substitution of saturated fats in the diet with unsaturated fatty acids may help reduce the risk of heart disease based on this legislation. The approved claim is applied to vegetable oils, spreads, and shortenings that have a total unsaturated fat content of 80% or more of total fats. This claim would therefore apply to corn oil as well as canola, safflower, flaxseed, sunflower, olive, soybean, and peanut oils, and must be stated as follows: "Replacing saturated fat with similar amounts of unsaturated fats may reduce the risk of heart disease. To achieve this benefit, total daily calories should not increase" (http://www.cfsan.fda.gov/~dms/flfats2.html).

## Conclusion

The field of unsaturated fatty acid research is in constant evolution. While earlier emphasis was placed on the consumption of MUFA for heart health, as recommended in the 1999 advisory report from the AHA (Kris-Etherton, 1999), newer recommendations have focused on foods, rather than percentages of energy from fatty acids. In fact, the 1999 AHA advisory report focused mainly on the health effects of MUFA, and recommended up to 15% of energy from MUFA and approximately 7% of energy from PUFA and 8% from SFA, for CVD prevention (Kris-Etherton, 1999). It even allowed for greater intakes of MUFA above 15% of energy and total fat intakes of >30% of energy if the SFA recommendations were not exceeded. In 2001, in a report of the AHA Nutrition Committee Conference Proceedings on dietary fatty acids and cardiovascular health, the focus on MUFA was absent, and recommendations allowed up to 10% of energy from PUFA and 10% of energy or less from SFA (Kris-Etherton et al., 2001). These recommendations were made based on: (i) the growing recognition of the health benefits of unsaturated fatty acids and (ii) the finding that a mix of MUFA and PUFA will likely confer the greatest health benefits. In that same year, the AHA also published a Science Advisory regarding the Mediterranean diet (Kris-Etherton et al., 2001), recognizing the health benefits of this diet that includes, among others, foods specifically rich in $\alpha$-linolenic acid. Finally, in 2006, the AHA Scientific Statement dropped recommendations on the percentage of energy from specific unsaturated fatty acids, keeping the recommendation to limit SFA to less than 7% of energy (Lichtenstein et al., 2006). These newer recommendations emphasize the intake of fruits, vegetables, whole grains, fish and lean meats, and low-fat dairy, and minimize the intakes of partially hydrogenated fats. Likely, the inclusion of unsaturated fats, such as those contained in corn oil, fits in this new set of recommendations for CVD risk reduction. Furthermore, the approval of health claims for unsaturated fats and corn oil shows a promising future for more research and information on this oil and its health effects for CVD risk prevention.

## References

Binkoski, A.E.; P.M. Kris-Etherton; et al. Balance of unsaturated fatty acids is important to a cholesterol-lowering diet: comparison of mid-oleic sunflower oil and olive oil on cardiovascular disease risk factors. *J. Am. Diet Assoc.* **2005,** *105(7),* 1080–1086.

Bonow, R.O. Primary prevention of cardiovascular disease: a call to action. *Circulation* **2002,** *106(25),* 3140–3141.

Cho, K.H.; J.M. Han; et al. Anti-atherosclerotic effect of a new synthetic functional oil containing mono- and diacylglycerol from corn oil. *Ann. Nutr. Metab.* **2006,** *50(5),* 467–475.

Elmadfa, I.; E. Park. Impact of diets with corn oil or olive/sunflower oils on DNA damage in healthy young men. *Eur. J. Nutr.* **1999,** *38(6),* 286–292.

Estruch, R.; M.A. Martinez-Gonzalez; et al. Effects of a Mediterranean-style diet on cardiovascular risk factors: a randomized trial. *Ann. Intern. Med.* **2006,** *145(1),* 1–11.

Executive Summary of The Third Report of The National Cholesterol Education Program (NCEP) Expert Panel on Detection, Evaluation, And Treatment of High Blood Cholesterol In Adults (Adult Treatment Panel III). *JAMA* **2001,** *285(19),* 2486–2497.

Howard, B.V.; J.S. Hannah; et al. Polyunsaturated fatty acids result in greater cholesterol lowering and less triacylglycerol elevation than do monounsaturated fatty acids in a dose-response comparison in a multiracial study group. *Am. J. Clin. Nutr.* **1995,** *62(2),* 392–402.

http://ods.od.nih.gov/factsheets/vitamine.asp.

http://www.cfsan.fda.gov/~dms/flfats2.html.

http://www.cfsan.fda.gov/~dms/qhc-sum.html.

http://www.corn.org/CornOil.pdf. http://www.fb.org/index.php?fuseaction=newsroom.newsfocus&year=2008&file=nr0327.html.

http://www.fda.gov/FDAC/features/2003/503_fats.html.

http://www.girlscouts.org/news/news_releases/2006/gs_cookies_now_have_zero_trans_fats.asp.

http://www.magicalmountain.net/WDWNewsDetail.asp?page=24&NewsID=1341&type=1&tag=.

http://www.physorg.com/news102934980.html.

Hu, F.B.; M.J. Stampfer; et al. Dietary fat intake and the risk of coronary heart disease in women. *N. Engl. J. Med.* **1997,** *337(21),* 1491–1499.

Insull, W., Jr.; A. Silvers; et al. Plasma lipid effects of three common vegetable oils in reduced-fat diets of free-living adults. *Am. J. Clin. Nutr.* **1994,** *60(2),* 195–202.

Jain, D.; N. Ebine; et al. Corn fiber oil and sitostanol decrease cholesterol absorption independently of intestinal sterol transporters in hamsters. *J. Nutr. Biochem.* **2008,** *19(4),* 229–236.

Kris-Etherton, P.M. AHA Science Advisory. Monounsaturated fatty acids and risk of cardiovascular disease. American Heart Association. Nutrition Committee. *Circulation* **1999,** *100(11),*

1253–1258.

Kris-Etherton, P.M. Monounsaturated fatty acids and risk of cardiovascular disease. *Circulation* **1999,** *100(11),* 1253–1258.

Kris-Etherton, P.; S.R. Daniels; et al. Summary of the scientific conference on dietary fatty acids and cardiovascular health: conference summary from the nutrition committee of the American Heart Association. *Circulation* **2001,** *103(7),* 1034–1039.

Kris-Etherton, P.; R.H. Eckel; et al. AHA Science Advisory: Lyon Diet Heart Study. Benefits of a Mediterranean-style, National Cholesterol Education Program/American Heart Association Step I Dietary Pattern on Cardiovascular Disease. *Circulation* **2001,** *103(13),* 1823–1825.

Kris-Etherton, P.M.; S. Innis; et al. Position of the American Dietetic Association and Dietitians of Canada: dietary fatty acids. *J. Am. Diet Assoc.* **2007,** *107(9),* 1599–1611.

Kris-Etherton, P.M.; T.A. Pearson; et al. High-monounsaturated fatty acid diets lower both plasma cholesterol and triacylglycerol concentrations. *Am. J. Clin.* **1999,** *Nutrition 70(6),* 1009-1015.

Leaf, A.; J.X. Kang; et al. Fish oil fatty acids as cardiovascular drugs. *Curr. Vasc. Pharmacol.* **2008,** *6(1),* 1–12.

Lichtenstein, A.H.; L.J. Appel; et al. Diet and lifestyle recommendations revision 2006: a scientific statement from the American Heart Association Nutrition Committee. *Circulation* **2006,** *114(1),* 82–96.

Lichtenstein, A.H.; L.M. Ausman; et al. Hydrogenation impairs the hypolipidemic effect of corn oil in humans. Hydrogenation, trans fatty acids, and plasma lipids. *Arterioscler. Thromb.* **1993,** *13(2),* 154–161.

Lichtenstein, A.H.; L.M. Ausman; et al. Effects of different forms of dietary hydrogenated fats on serum lipoprotein cholesterol levels. *N. Engl. J. Med.* **1999,** *340(25),* 1933–1940.

Mensink, R.P.; M.B. Katan. Effect of a diet enriched with monounsaturated or polyunsaturated fatty acids on levels of low-density and high-density lipoprotein cholesterol in healthy women and men. *N. Engl. J. Med.* **1989,** *321(7),* 436–441.

Meydani, M. Vitamin E modulation of cardiovascular disease. *Ann. N. Y. Acad. Sci.* **2004,** *1031,* 271–279.

Ng, T.K., K. Hassan; et al. Nonhypercholesterolemic effects of a palm-oil diet in Malaysian volunteers. *Am. J. Clin. Nutr.* **1991,** *53(Suppl. 4),* 1015S–1020S.

Ostlund, R.E., Jr.; S.B. Racette; et al. Phytosterols that are naturally present in commercial corn oil significantly reduce cholesterol absorption in humans. *Am. J. Clin. Nutr.* **2002,** *75(6).* 1000–1004.

Schurgers, L.J.; M.J. Shearer; et al. Novel effects of diets enriched with corn oil or with an olive oil/sunflower oil mixture on vitamin K metabolism and vitamin K-dependent proteins in young men. *J. Lipid Res.* **2002,** *43(6),* 878–884.

Siddiqui, R.A.; K.A. Harvey; et al. Modulation of enzymatic activities by n-3 polyunsaturated fatty acids to support cardiovascular health. *J. Nutr. Biochem.* **2008,** *19(7),* 417–437.

Sirtori, C.R.; E. Gatti; et al. Olive oil, corn oil, and n-3 fatty acids differently affect lipids, lipoproteins, platelets, and superoxide formation in type II hypercholesterolemia. *Am. J. Clin. Nutr.* **1992,** *56(1),* 113–122.

St-Onge, M.P.; I. Aban; et al. Snack chips fried in corn oil alleviate cardiovascular disease risk factors when substituted for low-fat or high-fat snacks. *Am. J. Clin. Nutr.* **2007,** *85(6),* 1503–1510.

St-Onge, M.P.; P.J. Jones. Phytosterols and human lipid metabolism: efficacy, safety, and novel foods. *Lipids* **2003,** *38(4),* 367–375.

Third Report of the National Cholesterol Education Program (NCEP) Expert Panel on Detection, Evaluation, and Treatment of High Blood Cholesterol in Adults (Adult Treatment Panel III) final report. *Circulation* **2002,** *106(25),* 3143–3421.

Tomasch, R.; K.H. Wagner; et al. Antioxidative power of plant oils in humans: the influence of alpha- and gamma-tocopherol. *Ann. Nutr. Metab.* **2001,** *45(3),* 110–115.

U.S. Department of Agriculture, A.R.S. (2005). USDA National Nutrient Database for Standard Reference, Release 18. Nutrient Data Laboratory Homepage. from http:www.nal.usda.gov/fnic/foodcomp

USFDA-CFSAN (2007). Corn oil and reduced risk of heart disease. *Qualified Health Claims Subject to Enforcement Discretion.* Retrieved August 11, 2008, from http://www.cfsan.fda.gov/~dms/qhc-sum.html.

von Schacky, C. n-3 PUFA in CVD: influence of cytokine polymorphism. *Proc. Nutr. Soc.* **2007,** *66(2),* 166–170.

Wagner, K.H.; R. Tomasch; et al. Impact of diets containing corn oil or olive/sunflower oil mixture on the human plasma and lipoprotein lipid metabolism. *Eur. J. Nutr.* **2001,** *40(4),* 161–167.

# 6

# Dairy Products: Role in the Diet and Effects on Cardiovascular Health

**D. Ian Givens[1] and Anne-Marie Minihane[2]**
*Schools of [1]Agriculture, Policy, and Development and [2]Chemistry, Food Biosciences, and Pharmacy, Faculty of Life Sciences, University of Reading, Reading RG6 6AR, United Kingdom*

## Introduction

Milk is a unique and complex food that is intended to be a complete food for young mammals. Most mammals stop drinking milk soon after weaning. For the majority of the human population, this coincides with the gene for lactase becoming down-regulated which severely compromises the ability to digest lactose. However, most people of European origin possess a version of the gene that remains active. Thus, about 90% of Europeans are able to digest lactose throughout life, and consequently have a relatively high intake of milk. Evidence from archaeological studies shows that this ability to digest lactose and hence to consume large amounts of milk developed only in the last 7000 years and that this has conferred a considerable survival advantage to those concerned (Simoons, 1978).

The important role of cow's milk in the human diet as a supplier of energy, protein, and other key nutrients including calcium is well-known. Milk is essentially a complex colloidal system comprised of globules of milk fat suspended in an aqueous medium containing lactose, a range of proteins, mineral salts, and water-soluble vitamins. The milk from modern Holstein–friesian cows will typically contain about 40, 36, and 45 g/kg of fat, protein, and lactose, respectively, and has an energy content of approximately 2.8 MJ/kg. The fat and protein contents of milk vary considerably due to the breed and nutrition of the cow. The effect of breeding is particularly noticeable in milk from Channel Island breeds, which has a higher fat content of typically about 65 g/kg. Although milk is widely consumed, and a key source of certain B-vitamins and minerals, as will be described, concern has recently increased regarding the fact that a high proportion (>50%) of the energy in milk is derived from fat, about 70% of which is made up of saturated fatty acids (SFAs). For more detail on the foregoing information, refer to the review of Givens and Shingfield (2006).

## Trends in the Consumption of Milk and Dairy Foods

The demand for animal-derived foods at a global level is growing rapidly, driven by a combination of population growth, urbanization, and rising income. Table 6.1

shows the trends in milk consumption over the past 40 years for various regions of the world. Although the historical and projected world trend is upward, in the United Kingdom and other Western countries, consumption has shown considerable change over recent decades. During the years immediately following World War II, an increase occurred in whole-milk (full-fat) consumption in the United Kingdom (Fig. 6.1) up to a plateau where consumption remained at around 130 kg per capita per year for over 20 years. In the mid-70s, whole-milk consumption started to decline quickly, but was partially replaced by the then recently introduced skimmed and semi-skimmed milk (collectively termed "lower-fat milk" in Fig. 6.1). The consumption of these lower-fat milks steadily increased up to a point in the early 1990s when they began to exceed that of whole milk. Between then and 2005, the consumption of these reduced-fat milks remained relatively constant, while that of whole full-fat milk continued to decline.

The decrease in the consumption of whole milk and the increase in lower-fat milk consumption seen in the United Kingdom reflect a general trend in a number of other developed countries. Denmark, France, the United States, and Canada have

**Table 6.1. Trends in Consumption of Milk Since the 1960s (WHO/FAO, 2003)**

| | Milk intake (kg/person/year) | | |
|---|---|---|---|
| Region | 1964-66 | 1977-99 | 2030[1] |
| World | 73.9 | 78.1 | 89.5 |
| Developing countries | 28.0 | 44.6 | 65.8 |
| Transition countries | 156.7 | 159.1 | 178.7 |
| Industrialized countries | 185.5 | 212.2 | 221.0 |

[1]projected

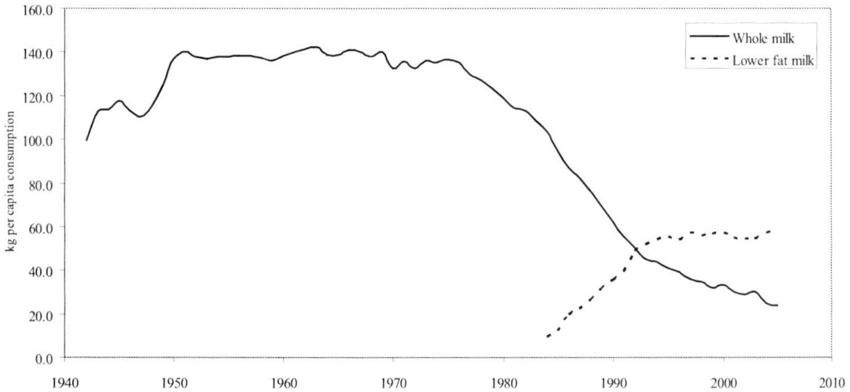


**Fig. 6.1.** Trends in UK milk consumption 1942–2005 (kg/capita/year). Sources: DEFRA (2001); DEFRA (2005).

shown similar trends since the 1970s (Figs. 6.2 and 6.3). To the contrary, Germany has maintained whole-milk consumption to a greater extent, and little change has occurred in the consumption of lower-fat milk up to 1993 although more recent data were not available. The consumption of liquid milk in Italy has always been much lower than in northern Europe, but between 1977 and 1990 this remained relatively constant for both whole- and lower-fat milk (Figs. 6.2 and 6.3).

Figure 6.4 shows the trends in cheese consumption in a number of selected countries over the period of 1977 – 2006. Of these countries, France has the highest consumption (currently about 24 kg/person/year) followed by Italy, and the United

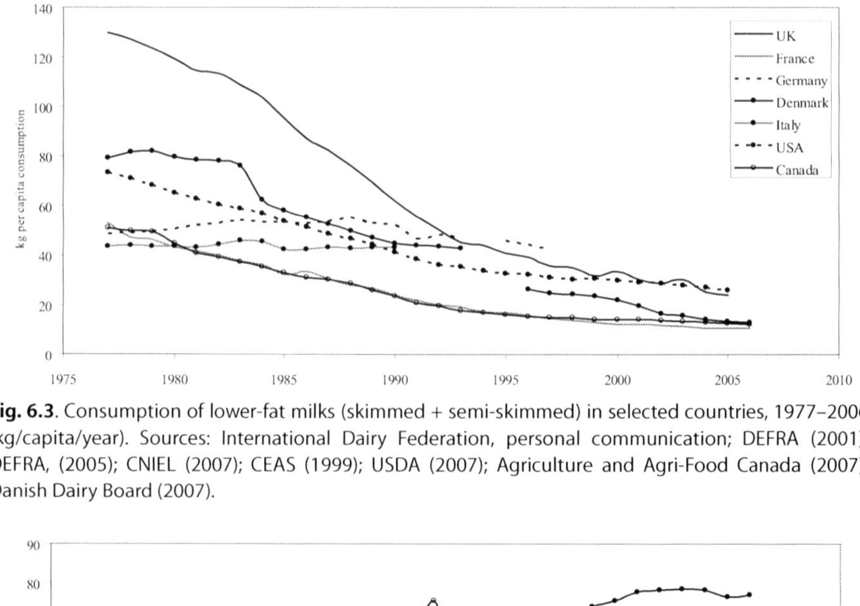


**Fig. 6.3**. Consumption of lower-fat milks (skimmed + semi-skimmed) in selected countries, 1977–2006 (kg/capita/year). Sources: International Dairy Federation, personal communication; DEFRA (2001); DEFRA, (2005); CNIEL (2007); CEAS (1999); USDA (2007); Agriculture and Agri-Food Canada (2007); Danish Dairy Board (2007).

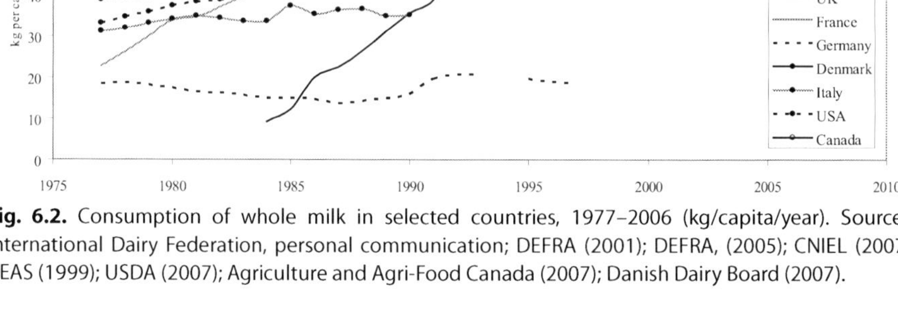


**Fig. 6.2.** Consumption of whole milk in selected countries, 1977–2006 (kg/capita/year). Sources: International Dairy Federation, personal communication; DEFRA (2001); DEFRA, (2005); CNIEL (2007); CEAS (1999); USDA (2007); Agriculture and Agri-Food Canada (2007); Danish Dairy Board (2007).

Kingdom has always had a relatively low consumption (currently about 6 kg/person/year). Most countries show a gradual increase in cheese consumption over this period, although the intake in Canada and Denmark did fluctuate during the 1990s and that of the United Kingdom post-1980s remained relatively constant. Over the same period, butter consumption in these selected countries followed several different trends, with consumption in Germany, Italy, and the United States remaining relatively constant, while in the United Kingdom and Denmark it declined. In France, a decline was also seen until the early 1990s when it recovered. Of the selected countries, France and Germany currently have the highest butter consumption at about 7.5 kg/person/year, with the United Kingdom and Denmark having the lowest at about 2 kg/person/year (International Dairy Federation, personal communication, 2007).

## Nutrients Provided by Dairy Foods

Milk and dairy-derived foods are available in the retail market in a vast array of forms. Based on data from the UK National Diet and Nutrition Survey (Henderson et al., 2003a,b) over the period from July 2000 to June 2001, Givens and Kliem (2008) summarized the contribution of the major milk-derived foods to energy and nutrient intakes and the requirements of the UK males population between the ages of 19 – 64 years (Table 6.2). Milk and dairy-food products are clearly important sources of protein, calcium (Ca), phosphorus, iodine, riboflavin, and vitamins A and $B_{12}$. Indeed milk and dairy products alone provide more than the daily recommended intake for vitamin $B_{12}$. The current nutritional importance of semi-skimmed and skimmed milk is clear, and notably, some 70% of liquid milk is now consumed as semi-skimmed milk (Milk Development Council, 2004). While milk and dairy products provide only about 13% of the recommended folate intake of 200 μg/day (Henderson et al.,

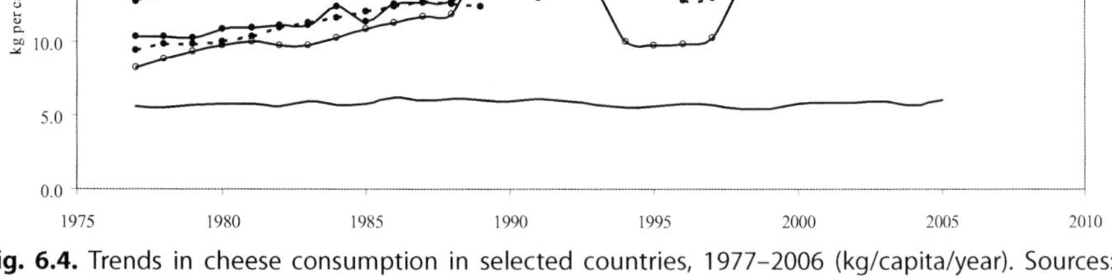


**Fig. 6.4.** Trends in cheese consumption in selected countries, 1977–2006 (kg/capita/year). Sources: International Dairy Federation, personal communication; DEFRA (2001); DEFRA, (2005); CNIEL (2007); CEAS (1999); USDA (2007); Agriculture and Agri-Food Canada (2007); Danish Dairy Board (2007).

**Table 6.2. Energy and Selected Nutrients Provided by Milk and Dairy Products to Men's Diets in the UK (Givens & Kliem, 2008)**

| Energy/ nutrient | Contribution from milk and dairy products | Liquid whole milk | Semi- and skimmed milk | Cheese | Other dairy products | Butter | Total dairy |
|---|---|---|---|---|---|---|---|
| Energy | Intake (MJ/d) | 0.49 | nas[5] | 0.29 | 0.10 | 0.10 | 0.97 |
| | % of EAR[1] | 5 | nas | 3 | 1 | 1 | 9 |
| Protein | Intake (g/d) | 1.8 | 5.3 | 4.4 | 1.8 | 0 | 13.2 |
| | % of RNI[2] | 3 | 10 | 8 | 3 | 0 | 24 |
| Fat | Intake (g/d) | 1.7 | 2.6 | 5.2 | 2.6 | 2.6 | 14.7 |
| | % of ADI[3] | 2 | 3 | 6 | 3 | 3 | 17 |
| Calcium | Intake (mg/d) | 61 | 203 | 112 | 41 | nas | 417 |
| | % of RNI | 9 | 29 | 16 | 5 | nas | 60 |
| Phosphorus | Intake (mg/d) | 45 | 165 | 90 | 30 | nas | 330 |
| | % of RNI | 8 | 30 | 16 | 6 | nas | 60 |
| Magnesium | Intake (mg/d) | 6.2 | 19 | nas | 6.2 | nas | 31 |
| | % of RNI | 2 | 6 | nas | 2 | nas | 10 |
| Zinc | Intake (mg/d) | 0.21 | 0.60 | 0.64 | 0.21 | nas | 1.7 |
| | % of RNI | 2 | 7 | 7 | 2 | nas | 18 |
| Iodine | Intake (μg/d) | 15 | 46 | 4.4 | 11 | nas | 77 |
| | % of RNI | 11 | 33 | 3 | 8 | nas | 55 |
| Vitamin A[4] | Intake (μg/d) | 20 | 31 | 61 | 31 | 41 | 183 |
| | % of RNI | 3 | 4 | 9 | 4 | 6 | 26 |
| Riboflavin | Intake (mg/d) | 0.12 | 0.40 | 0.07 | 0.09 | nas | 0.68 |
| | % of RNI | 9 | 31 | 5 | 7 | nas | 52 |
| Vitamin $B_{12}$ | Intake (μg/d) | 0.41 | 1.4 | 0.34 | 0.14 | nas | 2.2 |
| | % of RNI | 27 | 91 | 23 | 9 | nas | 150 |
| Folate | Intake (μg/d) | 25 | nas | nas | nas | nas | 25 |
| | % of RNI | 13 | nas | nas | nas | nas | 13 |

[1]EAR, estimated average requirement
[2]RNI, reference nutrient intake
[3]ADI, average daily intake
[4]retinol equivalents
[5]nas, not available separately, included in total

2003b), evidence shows that the presence of milk in the diet can increase the overall folate bioavailability compared to diets containing no milk (Wigertz et al., 1997). Also Smith et al. (1985) proposed that folate present in milk is more available than folates from other foods, at least in infants. Probably, these properties of milk are due to the fact that it uniquely contains a range of folate-binding proteins. Although their exact role is not fully understood (de Jong et al., 2005), possibly, these proteins will also increase the availability of folate in other foods consumed, and also make milk a good candidate for fortification with folate.

## Contribution of Dairy Foods to Fat and Fatty Acid Intake

In the United Kingdom, milk and dairy products, including butter, contribute almost 20% of the total fat consumed, but since the lipids in these products are rich in SFAs, they make a proportionately larger contribution to SFA intake. The National Diet and Nutrition Survey (Henderson et al., 2003a) estimated a contribution of 30% of total SFA intake although this excluded milk fats present in manufactured foods such as cakes, biscuits, etcetera. A study on fatty-acid intake across Europe (Hulshof et al., 1999) suggested a higher figure of 40% for the United Kingdom, and milk and dairy foods were consistently the largest source of SFA. The greatest contribution was seen in Germany and France, where some 60% of SFAs come from these foods (Table 6.3). Consistent with the trends identified above, the contribution of butter to SFA intake varied widely. In Greece, Spain, The Netherlands, and Norway, butter provided less than 5%, whereas high contributions were recorded in France (30%) and Germany (39%), with the United Kingdom being intermediate (10%).

Table 6.3 also shows the contribution made by milk and dairy products to the intake of *cis*-monounsaturated fatty acids (MUFAs) in the countries studied. This ranged from about 8% in Spain to 29% in Sweden. This variability partly reflects the consumption of other sources of *cis*-MUFAs, such as olive oil, but also highlights that milk and dairy products can be substantial sources.

Also noteworthy was the fact that across the countries studied, milk and milk-derived foods contributed most of the *trans* fatty acids (TFAs) consumed (Table 6.3). The contribution in Germany, Italy, and France was particularly high at approximately 72, 62, and 61%, respectively, although in the United Kingdom this was lower (25%). The high contribution in Germany arose mainly from butter consumption, while in Italy, cheese was the main source. In all countries, the predominant TFAs were *trans* C18:1, and although this study (Hulshof et al., 1999) did not report the isomeric profile, other evidence indicates that the primary isomer in foods from ruminant animals is *trans*-11

**Table 6.3. Contribution (% total intake) of Milk and Dairy Products to Intakes of Saturated (SFAs), *cis*-Monounsaturated (*cis*-MUFAs), and *Trans* Fatty Acids (TFAs) Intake in Selected European Countries (Hulshof et al., 1999)**

| Country | SFA | cis-MUFA | TFA |
|---|---|---|---|
| Belgium | 30.2 | 14.5 | 22.4 |
| Finland | 44.9 | 16.1 | 39.3 |
| France | 56.7 | 26.3 | 60.9 |
| Germany | 57.1 | 22.9 | 71.8 |
| Greece | 27.4 | 9.3 | 37.5 |
| Italy | 47.3 | 13.1 | 62.0 |
| The Netherlands | 33.9 | 14.1 | 16.7 |
| Portugal | 32.5 | 11.8 | 39.3 |
| Spain | 27.5 | 8.3 | 32.7 |
| Sweden | 48.5 | 28.6 | 40.7 |
| United Kingdom | 38.8 | 16.4 | 24.7 |

C18:1 (*trans*-vaccenic acid), unlike that from industrial hydrogenation which is usually mainly *trans*-9 C18:1, elaidic acid (Weggemans et al., 2004).

## Epidemiological Evidence of the Association Between Dairy Consumption and Cardiovascular Incidence

Because of their major contribution to SFA consumption, milk and dairy products were often considered to be a major risk factor for coronary heart disease (CHD) and cardiovascular disease (CVD) in general. Because of this, people were often advised to limit milk/dairy-product consumption. For milk, at least, however, good evidence to the contrary exists. Elwood et al. (2004) identified ten prospective cohort studies that examined the relationship between milk consumption and vascular-disease risk, and in all cases except one (with a small number of disease events) good evidence showed a reduced risk of ischemic heart disease or ischemic stroke in individuals who had the highest milk consumption relative to the lowest consumers. The authors reported a pooled relative risk of an incident of a vascular-disease event in such subjects of about 0.87 (95% CI 0.74–1.03) for ischemic heart disease, 0.70 (95% CI 0.55–0.88) for ischemic stroke, and 0.84 (95% CI 0.78–0.90) for either event. More recently, Elwood et al. (2007) examined the prevalence of the multifaceted metabolic syndrome (Nugent, 2004) in relationship to milk consumption in a cohort of 2375 men in the United Kingdom over a 20-year follow-up period. Having adjusted for age, energy intake, social class, and smoking, they found negative relationships between the consumption of both milk and dairy produce and the incidence of the syndrome. By using a food-frequency questionnaire, the adjusted relative risk in subjects who regularly drank 570 mL of milk or more daily was 0.38 (95% CI 0.18–0.78) and for dairy foods in general was 0.44 (95% CI 0.21–0.91). The data for subjects who used a seven-day weighed-intake record were similar. These data agree with an earlier shorter term study by Azadbakht et al. (2005), who linked the effect to reduced blood pressure in those consuming the greatest amounts of milk.

In addition to reduced blood pressure, increased milk consumption was associated with reduced adiposity which is a recognized significant determinant of risk for CHD and the metabolic syndrome. The impact of milk and dairy products was demonstrated in the CARDIA study, where Pereira et al. (2002) showed that the increased consumption of milk/dairy products over a 10-year period reduced the risk of obesity in subjects already overweight. Data from cross-sectional epidemiological studies reviewed by Barba and Russo (2006) support the hypothesis that the increased consumption of milk and dairy products leads to less fat accumulation in both adults and children. However, other data from intervention studies show a more complex situation; aspects are reviewed below.

## Saturated and Monounsaturated Fatty Acids from Milk and Cardiovascular Disease: Evidence from Intervention Studies

In addition to epidemiological data, an increasing body of evidence from intervention trials examined the association between increased milk and dairy intake and various components of the CVD-risk phenotype, including blood-lipid levels, markers of insulin sensitivity, and adiposity and body-weight regulation.

### *Dairy and the Blood-lipid Profile*

Over the last 40 years, numerous intervention trials, using a variety of fat sources, investigated the impact of dietary fat composition on blood cholesterol and triglyceride (TG) concentrations in humans. In 2003, Mensink and coworkers published a meta-analysis of 60 studies published between 1970 and1998, involving a total of 1672 participants, with intervention periods ranging from 13 – 91 days. Based on regression analysis, the authors derived a series of predictive equations to estimate the effect of altering the carbohydrate:saturated fat:polyunsaturated fat:monounsaturated fat (CHO:SFA:PUFA:MUFA) ratio of the diet on serum lipids and apolipoproteins. According to these equations, one would expect the replacement of 1% of dietary energy from CHO isoenergetically with SFAs to increase low-density lipoprotein cholesterol (LDLC) by 0.032 mmol/L (Mensink et al., 2003). Furthermore, the authors conclude that lauric acid (C12:0), myristic acid (C14:0), and palmitic acid (C16:0) are the major hypercholesterolemic fatty acids, although some controversy exists regarding their relative biopotency (Bonanome & Grundy, 1988; Katan et al., 1995; Temme et al., 1996;). Since much of the C12:0, C14:0, and C16:0 in the human diet is derived from milk fat (Gunstone et al., 1994), one would expect the consumption of milk and dairy foods to have adverse effects on serum LDLC levels. As is recognized, in addition to an LDLC-raising effect, SFA also increases high-density lipoprotein cholesterol (HDLC). Nevertheless, the Mensink review did predict an overall increase in the total cholesterol (TC):HDLC ratio with increased butter-fat incorporation into the diet, mainly due to the effect of C16:0.

Although the predictive equations derived from intervention trials suggest overall negative effects of dairy fats on the blood-lipid profile, the evidence from epidemiological studies described above, along with intervention studies which have specifically fed milk and other dairy fats, do not support this (Biong et al., 2004; Pfeuffer & Scherezenmeir, 2000; Poppitt et al., 2002). In a study conducted in healthy normocholesterolemic males, the provision of 20% of dietary energy as butter for 21days resulted in no significant change in the blood-lipid or apolipoprotein profile (Poppitt et al., 2002) (Table 6.4). Furthermore, evidence reveals that fermented milk products are hypocholesterolemic relative to nonfermented equivalents (Agerholm-Larsen et al., 2000; Biong et al., 2004; Nestel et al., 2005). In a meta-analysis of six relatively short-term studies, Agerholm-Larsen et al. (2000) concluded that the

**Table 6.4.** Impact of Modified Dairy Products on the Blood-lipid Profile: Evidence from Intervention Studies

| Reference | n | Subject group | Design | Dairy composition (% of total fatty acids) | Main outcomes |
|---|---|---|---|---|---|
| Noakes et al., 1996 | 33, 19M/14F | Healthy TC = 5.96 mmol/L | Sequential crossover, 2-wk low-fat diet (15% E fat) followed by 3-wk ND, (35% E fat) and 3-wk MD (35% E fat) in random order | ND- 70% SFA, 28% MUFA MD- 51% SFA, 39% MUFA | ND to MD resulted in a 0.28 (4.3%) mmol/L ↓ in TC ($P<0.001$) and 0.24 (5.3%) mmol/l ↓ in LDLC ($P<0.001$). No sign change TG, HDLC |
| Tholstrup et al., 1998 | 18M | healthy TC = 4.01 mmol/L | Crossover, 2x4 wk intervention periods, 2 mo wash-out in between, 41% E fat, ND vs. MD, vs. control | ND- 65% SFA, 21% MUFA MD- 50% SFA, 36% MUFA | ND to MD resulted in a 0.06 (2.1%) mmol/L ↓ in LDLC (P<0.05). No sign change TC, TG, HDLC |
| Poppitt et al., 2002 | 20M | Healthy TC = 4.56 mmol/L | Crossover, 2x3-wk intervention periods, 4 wk washout in between, 40% E fat residential study, ND vs. MD | ND- 71% SFA, 22% MUFA MD- 54% SFA, 32% MUFA | ND to MD resulted in a 2.8% ($P<0.05$) ↓ in TC ($P<0.05$) and 3.6% ↓ in LDLC ($P<0.01$) LDLC ($P<0.001$). No sign change TG, HDLC, apoA1 or apoB or coagulation biomarkers |
| Seidel et al., 2005 | 31, 16M/15F | 9 Hyperlipidemic, 22 healthy TC = 5.15 mmol/L | Non randomized sequential design 7-d Habitual diet, 10-d low-fat, 18-d ND 10-d low-fat, 18-d MD 10-d low-fat, 18-d Margarine | ND- 60% SFA, 26% MUFA, 3% PUFA MD- 53% SFA, 33% MUFA, 3% PUFA Margarine- (35% SFA. 28% MUFA, 37% PUFA | ND to MD resulted in a 11% ($P<0.05$) ↓ in LDLC and 19% ↓ ($P<0.05$) in LDLC:HDLC ($P<0.05$). Margarine nonsignificant effect relative to ND |
| Tholstrup et al., 2006 | 42M | Healthy TC = 4.04 mmol/L | Parallel, 5-wk intervention with ND (42% E fat) vs. MD (45% E fat) | ND- 61% SFA, 12% MUFA MD- 47% SFA, 23% MUFA | ND to MD resulted in a 0.30 (6.2%) mmol/L ↓ in TC ($P<0.05$), 0.27 (7.8%) mmol/L ↓ in LDLC (NS) and a 0.15 (9.7%) ↓ in HDLC ($P<0.01$) No sign change TG |

M- males, F= females, E-energy, ND- normal diet, MD- modified dairy diet, SFA- saturated fat, MUFA- monounsaturated fat, NS- non significant
TC- total cholesterol, LDLC- low density lipoprotein cholesterol, HDLC- high density lipoprotein cholesterol, TG- trigylceride

consumption of fermented yogurt products produced a 4 and 5% decrease in TC and LDLC, respectively. Biong and colleagues (2004) observed significantly lower LDLC ($P = 0.03$) differences of 0.15–0.26 mmol/L, following the consumption of a cheese- versus a butter-enriched standard diet for three weeks. Available data indicate modest and generally insignificant effects of dairy consumption on fasting TG and HDLC concentrations. Overall output from intervention studies suggests the presence of "protective" dairy constituents, particularly in fermented products, which negate the LDLC-raising effect of the dairy SFAs.

Nevertheless, the fat composition of dairy is approximately 70% of SFAs (mainly as C12:0, C14:0, and C16:0). Since recognized health benefits result from a reduced-SFA diet, and dairy products contribute a large proportion of the total SFA intake in most European countries (Table 6.3), the production of reduced-SFA dairy products could potentially be a major public-health benefit. Through the provision of unsaturated fat in the cow's diet, particularly in a rumen-protected form such as encapsulated or as the whole oilseed, reductions in the SFA content of milk from 70 – 50% are consistently achieved. For example, through the feeding of cracked rapeseed at concentrations up to 270 g/kg of dry matter in diets for dairy cows, we observed reductions in SFAs from 71 – 49% of total fatty acids although such diets were rather extreme (Givens et al., 2003).

A limited number of studies examined the benefits of these reduced-SFA dairy products on the blood-lipid profile in humans (Noakes et al., 1996; Poppitt et al., 2002; Seidel et al., 2005; Tholstrup et al., 1998, 2006) (Table 6.4). Noakes et al. (1996) observed a significant 4.3% ($P < 0.001$) and 5.3% ($P < 0.001$) reduction in TC and LDLC, respectively, in healthy adults, following the inclusion of modified dairy products (51% of SFA, 39% of *cis*-MUFA) versus normal dairy (70% of SFA, 28% of *cis*-MUFA) into a low-fat diet for three weeks. These changes are in the range observed by other investigators, which would be predicted to be associated with up to a 10% reduction in CHD risk (The Lipid Research Clinics Programme, 1984; Sacks & Katan, 2002). These trials demonstrate the potential of a greater production and consumption of these lower SFA dairy products to reduce population SFA intakes and potentially CHD burden.

## Dairy and Insulin Action

Although, as described above, some epidemiological evidence indicates a potential benefit of milk consumption on the incidence of the metabolic syndrome, epidemiological evidence regarding other dairy products and intervention studies with milk and other dairy products in relationship to insulin function are lacking.

As recently reviewed, the data from intervention trials which assessed the impact of dietary fatty-acid composition on insulin sensitivity and glucose disposal are equivocal, with a number of the earlier studies recognized as underpowered and too short in duration (Galgani et al., 2008; Shaw et al., 2006). No study to date has specifically explored the impact of dairy products, even though dairy is often used as part of a SFA-rich diet. In the KANWU Study, which used a relatively large sample size ($n$ = 162) and study duration (2x 12 weeks), a diet high in saturates (partly composed of butter fat) resulted in a significant reduction in insulin sensitivity relative to a *cis*-MUFA-rich diet, but only in those with a total-fat intake of <37% of total fat (Vessby et al., 2001). In the PREMIER Study, the consumption of a DASH-diet pattern, which is lower in total fat, SFAs, and cholesterol and higher in fruits and vegetables and low-fat dairy products, resulted in a 51% improvement in insulin sensitivity relative to the control group following six months of intervention (Ard et al., 2004). However, just as in the KANWU Study, this trial did not specifically examine the effects of dairy products, and "fit-for-purpose" intervention trials in this area need to be conducted.

## Dairy and Body-weight Regulation

One can broadly separate the intervention trials that examined the impact of dairy products on body-weight regulation into two groups: those with and those without energy restriction. For the studies without energy restriction, bone health rather than body weight often represented the primary outcome, and in these studies little evidence for a benefit of milk or dairy consumption on body weight or fat mass emerges (Cleghorn et al., 2001; Gunther et al., 2005; Lau et al., 2001).

Although inconsistencies exist, a more positive evidence base links milk and dairy consumption with more effective weight loss, and particularly fat-loss and lean-mass maintenance, under energy-restriction conditions (Summerbell et al., 1998; Zemel et al., 2005a,b). Furthermore, the data suggest a calcium-threshold effect with a greater impact on adiposity evidence in cohorts with a low (Zemel et al., 2005b) versus a high habitual-calcium intake (Thompson et al., 2005). In a study of obese individuals placed on an energy-restricted diet [–2.1 MJ/day (–500 kcal/day)], with (test group,1100 mg/day of Ca) or without (control group, 400–500 mg of Ca/day) a yogurt drink, fat losses of –4.4 kg and –2.8 kg ($P < 0.005$) were evident in the test versus the control group at 12 weeks, with associated reductions in waist circumferences of –4 and –1 cm ($P < 0.005$), respectively (Fig. 6.5a).

Any impact of dairy products on weight maintenance is attributed to calcium and its effect on fat absorption, lipid oxidation, and adipocyte lipid metabolism. However, the observation that calcium administered as dairy may be more efficacious in weight loss and weight maintenance relative to calcium fed in isolation as calcium supplements (Ochner & Lowe, 2007; Zemel et al., 2004) suggests that other constituents in dairy food may also regulate body weight (Fig. 6.5b).

## *Trans* Fatty Acids from Milk and Cardiovascular Disease

A comprehensive review of all available data regarding TFAs and health was published in 2007 by the Scientific Advisory Committee on Nutrition for the UK Food Standard Agency and Department of Health (SACN, 2007). Although the report detailed the available epidemiological evidence, which suggests a more consistent positive

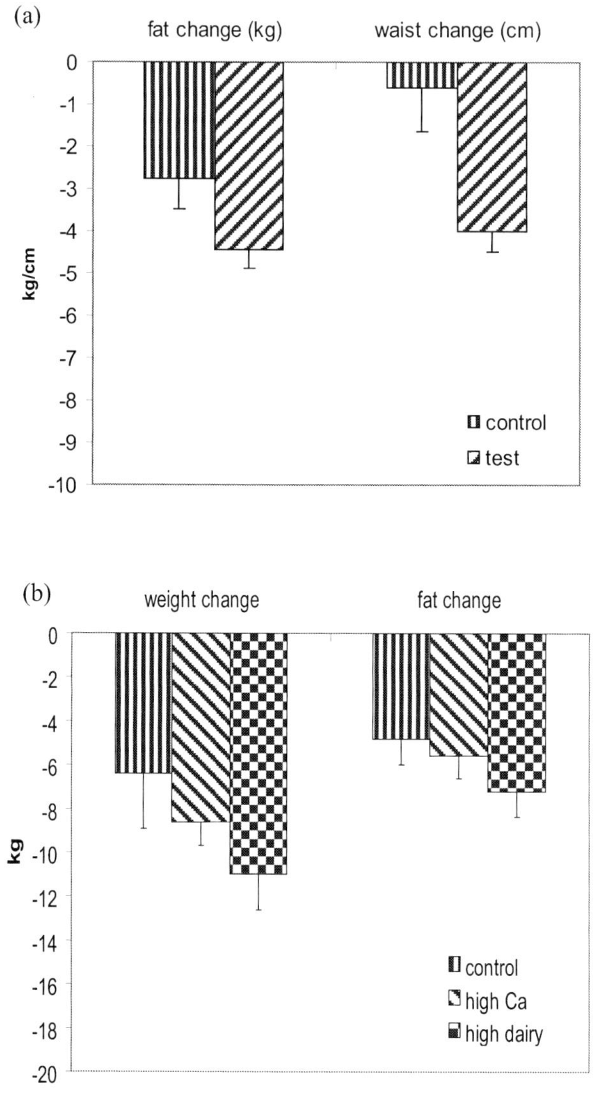


**Fig. 6.5.** The impact of dairy products and calcium on adiposity in adults. (a) Obese individuals were placed on an energy-restricted diet, with ($n = 18$, 1100 mg Ca/day) or without ($n = 16$, 400–500 mg/day) added yogurt. Test vs. control $P < 0.005$ for both fat loss and waist circumference (adapted from Zemel et al., 2005a) were observed. (b) Obese individuals were placed on an energy-restricted diet, which was unsupplemented (400–500 mg Ca/day) or supplemented with Ca as calcium supplements (1200–1300 m Ca/day) or dairy (1200–1300 mg Ca/day). For both weight change and fat change, control vs high Ca vs high dairy, $P < 0.01$, with all groups significantly different for both weight and fat change (adapted from Zemel et al., 2004).

association between biomarker levels of *trans* C18:2 (which are largely derived from biohydrogenated vegetable oils) and the risk of CHD, it concluded that "data are not sufficiently robust to enable definite conclusions to be drawn concerning the likelihood, or not, of more adverse effects of *trans* fatty acids of industrial (iTFA) rather than ruminant origin" (rTFA). At the time the SACN report was written, a general paucity of information existed from human intervention trials which directly compared industrial and ruminant TFA sources. This was in part due to the unavailability of sufficient amounts of *trans* vaccenic acid that one could include in an intervention study to avoid the introduction of substantial changes to the overall macronutrient composition of the diet.

In April 2008, the output from two such intervention studies was published. In the TRANSFACT study (Chardigny et al., 2008), the impact of rTFA and iTFA was directly compared in a crossover trial in healthy males, with TFAs constituting approximately 4.2% of total dietary-energy intake. No significant differences between TFA sources were evident in males. However, in females 15% ($P = 0.012$) and 6% ($P = 0.001$) higher serum LDLC and HDLC concentrations were evident following rTFA versus iTFA, with no overall significant treatment effect on the TC/HDLC ratio (Table 6.5). In the study of Motard-Bélanger and co-workers (2008), the impact of four individual diets, namely control (C, 0.8% of TFA), moderate-rTFA (MrTFA, 1.5% of TFA), high-rTFA (HrTFA, 3.6% of TFA), and high-iTFA (HiTFA, 3.6% of TFA) were compared. Relative to the control, comparable significant ($P = 0.002$) 6 and 5% increases in the TC/HDLC ratio were evident following both HrTFA and HiTFA interventions. Taken together, these two studies are suggestive of a greater sensitivity to TFAs in females, and are indicative of comparable deleterious effects of both rTFA and iTFA on the blood-lipid profile. However, keep in mind that the intakes of TFAs of 3.6 and 4.2% of dietary energy are three- to fourfold higher than the average UK intake of 1.2% (Henderson et al., 2003b; SACN, 2007). Furthermore, as rTFAs constitute about 25% (i.e., 0.3% of dietary energy) of total TFAs in the United Kingdom, likely, current-intake ranges represent relatively minor determinants of individuals' circulating cholesterol levels.

## Conclusion

While milk and dairy products are generally accepted as foods that provide substantial amounts of key nutrients, concern does exist that high levels of their consumption would increase the risk of CHD and other chronic health problems. This concern mainly focuses on the fact that milk-derived foods are often the largest single source of dietary SFAs. The epidemiological evidence and the evidence from dietary intervention studies do not support this contention, and indeed suggest that milk may provide some protective effects against vascular disease. Despite this, some evidence shows that one can obtain further benefits from the consumption of milk/dairy products with a reduced-SFA content. This, however, needs further evaluation in more powerful intervention studies.

**Table 6.5. Studies Directly Comparing the Impact of Industrial Versus Ruminants *Trans* Fatty Acids on Risk Factors for Cardiovascular Disease**

| Reference | n | Subject group | Design | Dairy composition (% of total fatty acids) | Main outcomes |
|---|---|---|---|---|---|
| Chardingy et al., 2008 (TRANSFACT study) | 46, 22M, 24F | Healthy TC=5.48 (M), 4.73 (F) mmol/L | crossover , 1-wk run-in, 2x 3-wk intervention periods, 1-wk washout in between | rTFA diet & iTFA diet contained ≈ 4.2% dietary E as TFA | Treatment effects only evident in females<br>rTFA vs. iTFA<br>Females, LDLC- ↑15%, P=0.012<br>Males, LDLC- ↑2%, NS<br>Females, HDLC- ↑6%, P=0.001<br>Males, LDLC- ↓ 1%, NS<br>NS effects on TC:HDLC ratio overall or in males and females |
| Motard-Bélanger et al., 2008 | 38M | Healthy TC=4.32 mmol/L | crossover, 4x 4-wk intervention periods, 3–12-wk washout in between | Control- (C, 0.8% TFA)<br>Mod-rTFA (MrTFA, 1.5% TFA)<br>High-rTFA (HrTFA, 3.6% TFA)<br>High-iTFA (HiTFA, 3.6% TFA) | End of treatment (mmol/L), * sign different vs. C<br>C MrTFA HrTFA HiTFA P<br>LDLC 3.27 3.22 3.47* 3.42 0.002<br>HDLC 1.25 1.28 1.22* 1.23 0.066<br>TC/HDLC 3.97 3.86 4.23* 4.16* 0.002<br>LDLC/HDLC 2.75 2.67 3.02* 2.94 0.003 |

M- males, F- females, E-energy, rTFA- ruminant *trans* fatty acids, MrTFA- moderate rTFA; HrTFA- high rTFA; iTFA- industrial TFA, HiTFA- high iTFA, C- control TC- total cholesterol, LDLC- low-density lipoprotein cholesterol, HDLC- high-density lipoprotein cholesterol

## References


Agerholm-Larsen, L.; M.L. Bell; G.K. Grunwald; A. Astrup. The effect of a probiotic milk product on plasma cholesterol: a meta-analysis of short-term intervention studies. *Eur. J. Clin. Nutr.* **2000,** *54*, 856–860.

Agriculture and Agri-Food Canada. *Canada Dairy Information Centre*. http://dairyinfo.gc.ca/_english/ accessed 17 September **2007**.

Ard, J.D.; S.C. Grambow; D. Liu; C.A. Slentz; W.E. Kraus; L.P. Svetkey. The effect of the PREMIER interventions on insulin sensitivity. *Diabetes Care* **2004**, *27*, 340–347.

Azadbakht, L.; P. Mirmiran; A. Esmaillzadeh; F. Azizi. Dairy consumption is inversely associated with the prevalence of the metabolic syndrome in Tehranian adults. *Am. J. Clin. Nutr.* **2005**, *82*, 523–530.

Barba, G.; P. Russo. Dairy foods, dietary calcium and obesity: A short review of the evidence. *Nutr. Metab. Cardiovasc. Dis.* **2006**, *16*, 445–451.

Biong, A.S.; H. Muller; I. Seljeflot; M.B. Veierod; J.L. Pedersen. A comparison of the effects of cheese and butter on serum lipids, haemostatic variables and homocysteine. *Br. J. Nutr.* **2004**, *92*, 791–797.

Bonanome, A.; S.M. Grundy. Effect of dietary stearic acid on plasma cholesterol and lipoprotein levels. *N. Engl. J. Med.* **1988**, *318*, 1244–1248.

CEAS. *Evaluation of the School Milk Measure*. Final Report for DGVI European Commission, submitted by CEAS Consultants (Wye) Ltd. Centre for European Agricultural Studies and Institute for the Management of Dairy Companies; Technische Universitat: München, 1999; 159 pp. Available at: http://ec.europa.eu/agriculture/eval/reports/schoolmilk/index_en.htm, Accessed 25 July 2008.

Chardigny, J.M.; F. Destaillats; C. Malpuech-Brugere; J. Moulin; D.E. Bauman; A.L. Lock; D.M. Barbano; R.P. Mensink; J.B. Bezelgues; P. Chaumont, et al. Do trans fatty acids from industrially produced sources and from natural sources have the same effect on cardiovascular disease risk factors in healthy subjects? Results of the trans Fatty Acids Collaboration (TRANSFACT) study. *Am. J. Clin. Nutr.* **2008**, *87*, 558–566.

Cleghorn, D.B.; P.D. O'Loughlin; B.J. Schroeder; B.E. Nordin. An open, crossover trial of calcium-fortified milk in prevention of early postmenopausal bone loss. *Med. J. Aust.* **2001**, *175*, 242–245.

CNIEL. http://www.maison-du-lait.com/Scripts/public/stat.asp?Language=GB. 2007.

de Jong, R.J.; M. Verwei; C.E. West; T. van Vliet; E.Siebelink; H. van der Berg; J.J. Castenmiller. Bioavailability of folic acid from fortified pasteurised and UHT-treated milk in humans. *Eur. J. Clin. Nutr.* **2005**, *59*, 906–913.

Danish Dairy Board. http://www.mejeri.dk, Accessed 17 September 2007.

DEFRA. The National Food Survey. Her Majesty's Stationary Office: London, 2001. Available at: http://statistics.defra.gov.uk/esg/, Accessed 11 September 2007.

DEFRA. Expenditure and Food Survey. Her Majesty's Stationary Office: London, 2005. Available at: http://statistics.defra.gov.uk/esg/, Accessed 11 September 2007.

Elwood, P.C.; J.E. Pickering; A.M. Fehily. Milk and dairy consumption, diabetes and the metabolic syndrome: the Caerphilly Prospective study. *J. Epidemiol. Community Health.*, **2007**, *61*,

695–698.

Elwood, P.C.; J.E. Pickering; J. Hughes; A.M. Fehily; A.R. Ness. Milk drinking, ischaemic heart disease and ischaemic stroke II. Evidence from cohort studies. *Eur. J. Clin. Nutr.* **2004,** *58*, 718–724.

Galgani, J.E.; R.D. Uauy; C.A. Aguirre; E.O Diaz. Effect of the dietary fat quality on insulin sensitivity. *Br. J. Nutr.* **2008**, in press, doi: 10.1017/S0007114508894408; Published online by Cambridge University Press 08 Apr 2008.

Givens, D.I.; R. Allison; J.S. Blake. Enhancement of oleic acid and vitamin E concentrations of bovine milk using dietary supplements of whole rapeseed and vitamin E. *Anim. Res.* **2003**, *52*, 531–542.

Givens, D.I.; K.E. Kliem. Improving the nutritional quality of milk. *Functional Beverages;* P. Paquin, Ed.; Woodhead Publishing Ltd: Cambridge, 2008 in press.

Givens, D.I.; K.J. Shingfield. Optimising dairy milk fatty acid composition. *Improving the Fat Content of Foods;* C. Williams, J. Buttriss, Eds.; Woodhead Publishing Ltd: Cambridge, 2006; pp. 252–280.

Gunstone, F.D.; J.L. Harwood; F.P. Padley. Occurrence and characteristics of oils and fats. *Lipid Handbook*; F.P. Padley, F.D Gunstone, J.L. Harwood, Eds.; Cambridge University Press: Cambridge, 1994.

Gunther, C.W.; P.A. Legowski; R.M. Lyle; G.P. McCabe; M.S. Eagan; M. Peacock; D. Teegarden. Dairy products do not lead to alterations in body weight or fat mass in young women in a 1-y intervention. *Am. J. Clin. Nutr.* **2005**, *81*, 751–756.

Henderson, L.; J. Gregory; K. Irving; G. Swan. *The National Diet and Nutrition Survey: Adults Aged 19–64 Years. Volume 2: Energy, protein, carbohydrate, fat and alcohol intake*; The Stationery Office: London, UK, 2003a; 98 pp.

Henderson, L.; K. Irving; J. Gregory; C.J. Bates; A. Prentice; J. Perks; G. Swan; M. Farron. *The National Diet and Nutrition Survey: Adults Aged 19–64 Years. Volume 3: Vitamin and Mineral Intake and Urinary Analytes;* The Stationery Office: London, UK, **2003b;** 160 pp.

Hulshof, K.F.A.M.; M.A. van Erp-Baart; M. Anttolainen; W. Becker; S.M. Church; C. Couet; E. Hermann-Kunz; H. Kesteloot; T. Leth; I. Martins, et al. Intake of fatty acids in Western Europe with emphasis on trans fatty acids: The TRANSFAIR study. *Eur. J. Clin. Nutr.* **1999**, *53*, 143–157.

Katan, M.B.; P.L. Zock; R.P. Mensink. Dietary oils, serum lipoproteins, and coronary heart disease. *Am. J. Clin. Nutr.* **1995**, *61*, 1368S–1373S.

Lau, E.M.; J. Woo; V. Lam; A. Hong. Milk supplementation of the diet of postmenopausal Chinese women on a low calcium intake retards bone loss. *J. Bone Miner Res.* **2001**, *16*, 1704–1709.

Mensink, R.P.; P.L. Zock; A.D. Kester; M.B. Katan. Effects of dietary fatty acids and carbohydrates on the ratio of serum total to HDL cholesterol and on serum lipids and apolipoproteins: a meta-analysis of 60 controlled trials. *Am. J. Clin. Nutr.* **2003**, *77*, 1146–1155.

Milk Development Council. *Dairy Facts and Figures 2003*; Milk Development Council: Cirencester, UK; **2004**; 240 pp.

Motard-Belanger, A.; A. Charest; G. Grenier; P. Paquin; Y. Chouinard; S. Lemieux; P. Couture; B. Lamarche. Study of the effect of trans fatty acids from ruminants on blood lipids and other risk factors for cardiovascular disease. *Am. J. Clin. Nutr.* **2008**, *87*, 593–599.

Nestel, P.J.; A. Chronopulos; M. Cehun. Dairy fat in cheese raises LDL cholesterol less than that in butter in mildly hypercholesterolaemic subjects. *Eur. J. Clin. Nutr.* **2005**, *59*, 1059–1063.

Noakes, M.; P.J. Nestel; P.M. Clifton. Modifying the fatty acid profile of dairy products through feedlot technology lowers plasma cholesterol of humans consuming the products. *Am. J. Clin. Nutr.* **1996**, *63*, 42–46.

Nugent, A.P. The metabolic syndrome. *Nutr. Bull.* **2004**, *29*, 36–43.

Ochner, C.N.; M.R. Lowe. Self-reported changes in dietary calcium and energy intake predict weight regain following a weight loss diet in obese women. *J. Nutr.* **2007**, *137*, 2324–2328.

Pereira, M.A.; D.R. Jacobs; L. Van Horn; M.L. Slattery; A.I. Kartashhov; D.S. Ludwig. Dairy consumption, obesity, and the insulin resistance syndrome in young adults, The CARDIA study. *J. Am. Med. Assoc.* **2002**, *287*, 2081–2089.

Pfeuffer, M.; J. Schrezenmeir. Bioactive substances in milk with properties decreasing risk of cardiovascular diseases. *Br. J. Nutr.* **2000**, *84(Suppl. 1),* S155–159.

Poppitt, S.D.; G.F. Keogh; T.B. Mulvey; B.H. McArdle; A.K. MacGibbon; G.J. Cooper. Lipid-lowering effects of a modified butter-fat: a controlled intervention trial in healthy men. *Eur. J. Clin. Nutr.* **2002**, *56*, 64–71.

Sacks, F.M.; M. Katan. Randomized clinical trials on the effects of dietary fat and carbohydrate on plasma lipoproteins and cardiovascular disease. *Am. J. Med.* **2002**, *113 (Suppl. 9B)* 13S–24S.

SACN. *Update on Trans Fatty Acids and Health;* Position statement by the Scientific Advisory Committee on Nutrition; TSO: London, 2007.

Seidel, C.; T. Deufel; G. Jahreis. Effects of fat-modified dairy products on blood lipids in humans in comparison with other fats. *Ann. Nutr. Metab.* **2005**, *49*, 42–48.

Shaw, D.I.; W.L. Hall; C.M. Williams. Dietary fatty acids, insulin resistance and diabetes. *Improving the Fat Content in Foods;* C.M. Williams; J. Buttriss, Eds.; Woodhead Publishing Ltd: Cambridge, 2006; pp. 25–38.

Simoons, F.J. The geographic hypothesis and lactose malabsorption. *Dig. Dis.* **1978**, *23*, 963–980.

Smith, A.M.; M.F. Picciano; R.H. Deering. Folate intake and blood concentrations of term infants. *Am. J. Clin. Nutr.* **1985**, *41*, 590–598.

Summerbell, C.D.; C. Watts; J.P. Higgins; J.S. Garrow. Randomised controlled trial of novel, simple, and well supervised weight reducing diets in outpatients. *BMJ* **1998**, *317*, 1487–1489.

Temme, E.H.; R.P. Mensink; G. Hornstra. Comparison of the effects of diets enriched in lauric, palmitic, or oleic acids on serum lipids and lipoproteins in healthy women and men. *Am. J. Clin. Nutr.* **1996**, *63*, 897–903.

The Lipid Research Clinics Coronary Primary Prevention Trial results. II. The relationship of reduction in incidence of coronary heart disease to cholesterol lowering. *JAMA* **1984**, *251*, 365–374.

Tholstrup, T.; M. Raff ; S. Basu; P. Nonboe; K. Sejrsen; E.M. Straarup. Effects of butter high in ruminant trans and monounsaturated fatty acids on lipoproteins, incorporation of fatty acids into lipid classes, plasma C-reactive protein, oxidative stress, hemostatic variables, and insulin in healthy young men. *Am. J. Clin. Nutr.* **2006**, *83*, 237–243.

Tholstrup, T.; B. Sandstrom; J.E. Hermansen; G. Holmer. Effect of modified dairy fat on postprandial and fasting plasma lipids and lipoproteins in healthy young men. *Lipids* **1998**, *33*, 11–21.

Thompson, W.G.; N. Rostad Holdman; D.J. Janzow; J.M. Slezak; K.L. Morris; M.B. Zemel. Effect of energy-reduced diets high in dairy products and fiber on weight loss in obese adults. *Obes. Res.* **2005**, *13*, 1344–1353.

USDA. *Food Availability (Per Capita) System.* United States Department of Agriculture/Economic Research Service. Available at: http://www.ers.usda.gov/Data/foodconsumption/ Accessed 26 September 2007.

Vessby, B.; M. Unsitupa; K. Hermansen; G. Riccardi; A.A. Rivellese; L.C. Tapsell; C. Nalsen; L. Berglund; A. Louheranta; B.M. Rasmussen. Substituting dietary saturated for monounsaturated fat impairs insulin sensitivity in healthy men and women: The KANWU Study. *Diabetologia* **2001**, *44*, 312–319.

Weggemans, R.M.; M. Rudrum; E.A.Trautwein. Intake of ruminant *versus* industrial *trans* fatty acids and risk of coronary heart disease—what is the evidence? *Eur. J. Lipid Sci. Technol.* **2004**, *106*, 390–397.

WHO/FAO. *Diet, Nutrition and the Prevention of Chronic Diseases. Report of a Joint WHO/FAO Expert Consultation;* WHO: Geneva, 2003; 148.pp.

Wigertz, K.; G. Hallmans; A.-S. Sandberg; P. Tidehag; M.I. Jägerstad. Improved apparent dietary folate absorption in ileostomy subjects with the incorporation of milk into a mixed diet. *Characterisation and Availability. Milk Folates;* (Thesis) K. Wigertz, Ed.; Lund University: Lund, Sweden, **1997;** pp. 2–19.

Zemel, M.B.; J. Richards; S. Mathis; A. Milstead; L. Gebhardt; E. Silva. Dairy augmentation of total and central fat loss in obese subjects. *Int. J. Obes. (Lond)* **2005a**, *29*, 391–397.

Zemel, M.B.; J. Richards; A. Milstead; P. Campbell. Effects of calcium and dairy on body composition and weight loss in African-American adults. *Obes. Res.* **2005b**, *13*, 1218–1225.

Zemel, M.B.; W. Thompson; A. Milstead; K. Morris; P. Campbell. Calcium and dairy acceleration of weight and fat loss during energy restriction in obese adults. *Obes. Res.* **2004**, *12*, 582–590.

# 7

# Dietary Fatty Acids in Cardiovascular Disease in Women

**Niva Shapira**
*Medical & Natural Nutrition, R&D Functional foods & diets, Stanley Steyer School of Health Professions, Tel-Aviv university, Ramat Aviv, Tel Aviv, Israel*

## Introduction: Gender-Related Perspectives on Cardiovascular Disease

Cardiovascular disease (CVD) has been the leading cause of death in both men and women in many countries since the late 1980s (Lerner & Kandel, 1986), though manifesting in somewhat different patterns between the sexes (Pilote et al., 2007). Even though initially women were thought to be inherently more protected than men, women's CVD generally occurred later in life, but with a worse prognosis. European statistics recently released by the World Health Organization (WHO) showed that women's CVD %mortality was 25% greater than men's (Fig. 7.1).

Since the first description of sex bias in treating women with suspected or diagnosed coronary artery disease (CAD, a type of CVD) in 1987 (Tobin et al., 1987), the influence of gender on the prevalence, prognosis, and manifestation of CVD is described in multiple studies, and further differences in the use of diagnostic and therapeutic measures, as well as the quality of the outcome, were also reviewed (Milcent et al., 2007).

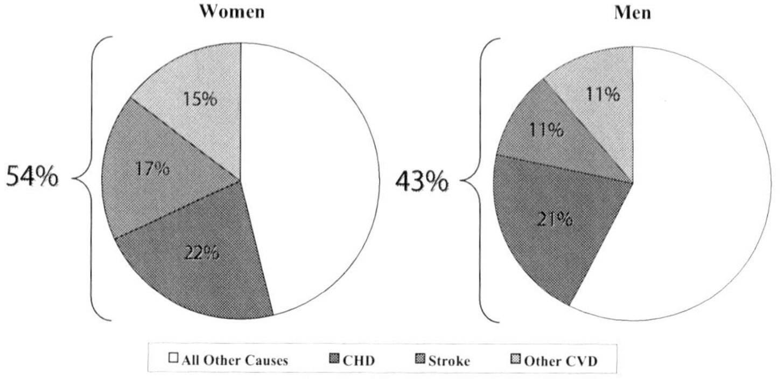


Fig. 7.1. CVD percentage (%) of all-cause mortality, Europe (WHO, 2007).

While younger men ages 35–54 have approximately twice the total incidence of CVD morbidity and mortality of women, the gender gap in morbidity tends to diminish during the later years, with a surge in female morbidity after age 45—characterized by a dramatic decrease in circulating estrogen levels (Qiao et al., 2008). Numerous observational and experimental studies demonstrated a correlation between estrogens, various biochemical markers, and CVD risk factors, morbidity, and mortality in women, most demonstrating a protective role (Cano et al., 2007). However, hormone (estrogen) replacement therapy (HRT), which was long recommended for protection against CVD, failed to provide consistent beneficial evidence, and may even increase women's risk (Mackey et al., 2005), especially after the age of 60 and/or if started 10 years or more postmenopausally, because atherogenic processes generally start around the age of menopausal transition (Rosano et al., 2006; Toles, 2007).

As serious cardiovascular events, such as acute coronary syndrome (ACS), myocardial infarction, and sudden death, occur in women later than in men, women may have more co-morbidities when diagnosed, which influence outcomes (Gottlieb et al., 2000). Despite the substantial prevalence and volume of aortic plaque in women at diagnosis (Oyama et al., 2008), as well as the rates of adverse events and death following cardiovascular interventions (Milcent et al., 2007)—independent of age (Vaccarino et al., 1999) or treatment (Redberg, 2006), women are less likely than men to be referred for invasive evaluation and procedures (Novak et al., 2008). Even when many of the risk factors for CVD and strategies for preventing disease are similar for men and women, their effects and outcomes differ depending on sex (Moriel et al., 2005; Narins et al, 2006; Reina et al., 2007 ). These data emphasize the importance of applying preventive measures in women prior to the onset of related symptoms (Oyama et al., 2008).

Characterization of CVD pathophysiology suggests several main etiologies: plasma lipids, endothelial function, inflammation, and oxidative stress. All are relevant to women's CVD (Villar et al., 2008) and are closely tied to fatty acid (FA) metabolism. However, most research was conducted in men, with the assumption that the specific mechanisms of action are similar.

In recent years, connections between specific FA and CVD—as in the Mediterranean, DASH, and "portfolio" diets—garnered increasing interest, beyond simply high- versus low-fat diets (Fung et al., 2008; Gigleux et al., 2007; Jenkins et al., 2007; Tuttle et al., 2008). Significant attention was given to the health risks of high total fat and saturated FA (SFA, mostly from animal foods and tropical oils), the benefits of both omega-3 (n-3) polyunsaturated FA (PUFA, mostly from fish oil and land-based sources such as flaxseed) and omega-9 (n-9) monounsaturated FA (MUFA, mostly from olive and canola oils), and the health impact of omega-6 (n-6) PUFA (mostly from soy, corn, and sunflower oils, as well as meat and egg)—particularly high in the typical Western diet—in relation to total dietary consumption and the n-6:n-3 PUFA ratio (Simopoulos, 2008). These dietary effects suggested the existence of gender differences (Jakobsen et al., 2004; Lapointe et al., 2006; Tappia et al., 2006,

2007; Tomàs-Moyà et al., 2007). The following chapter presents research findings regarding gender-specific effects on CVD etiologies, and explores the relationship between CVD risk and FA, with focus on gender differences in FA metabolism and possible implications for women's cardiac health.

## Etiological Factors in CVD and Gender-Specific Risks

### *Plasma Lipids*

Dyslipidemia, or impaired lipid levels in blood, was the first diet-related etiological paradigm, attributed to a Western lifestyle and obesity, and focused originally on hypercholesterolemia. What was later established as the lipid hypothesis (Davignon, 1978) postulates that an elevation in plasma cholesterol level, mostly in low-density lipoprotein (LDL) particles, results in their penetration into the arterial walls, leading to lipid accumulation in smooth muscle cells of the endothelium and in macrophages (especially when oxidized) and the creation of foam cells and fatty streaks. Here, high levels of triglycerides (or triacylglyerols, TG) interfere with cholesterol removal, and thus may enhance its levels and damaging effects, and accompanying CVD risk (Steinberg et al., 1989).

Several dyslipidemic profiles promoted atherogenesis, in particular, the tendency toward the overproduction of atherogenic and TG-rich lipoproteins, decreased concentrations of anti-atherogenic high-density lipoproteins (HDL), increased the LDL:HDL ratio, and increased the small-dense LDL (SD-LDL) and very low-density lipoprotein (VLDL). These factors therefore triggered important prevention strategies against CVD (Nicholls & Lundman, 2004).

SD-LDL particles are more atherogenic as a result of their higher penetration into the arterial wall, lower binding affinity for the LDL receptor, prolonged plasma half-life, and lower resistance to oxidative stress compared with large LDL particles (Bjornheden et al., 1998), as well as higher susceptibility to glycation, even in nondiabetics (Younis et al., 2008). Individuals with high SD-LDL had a two- to threefold increase in their risk of coronary heart disease (CHD), a type of CVD (Lamarche et al., 1999).

The best-known anti-atherogenic function of HDL is to promote the efflux of cholesterol—particularly LDL cholesterol—from the arterial wall. Where improvement in endothelial function is attained by reducing LDL levels in the studies of apheresis and statins (Nichols & Lundman, 2004), lower plasma concentrations of HDL may negatively impact endothelial function (Kuvin et al., 2002; Lupattelli et al., 2002), and HDL restoration in dyslipidemic patients is associated with improvement (Bisoendial et al., 2003; Spieker et al., 2002).

#### *Gender Perspective: Plasma Lipids*

Strong relationships between lipids, lipoproteins, and CHD development were noted among women (Carroll et al., 2005). Sexual dimorphism in lipid metabolism includes: differences in substrate kinetics, a greater rate of lipolysis and higher plasma

FA, a slower resting energy expenditure rate, a higher percentage of body fat than in men, and higher levels of circulating insulin, as well as a response to insulin's lipolytic effects not consistently accounted for by body composition (Mittendorfer, 2005; Mittendorfer et al., 2001, 2003).

Where elevated LDL, non-HDL, and TG are associated with the increased risk of CVD in both sexes (Hammoudeh et al., 2008), high TG, TG-rich VLDL, and low HDL appear to be stronger predictors in women (Bittner, 2005), possibly more than high LDL (Austin et al., 1998). Women's higher plasma clearance of VLDL–TG and VLDL–apolipoprotein B-100 accounts for their innately lower concentrations premenopausally than in men. However, differences tend to decrease with age, concurrently with estrogen levels. Specifically, the levels of total cholesterol, LDL, SD-LDL, and apoprotein B, that tend to be lower in young women than in men, increase with estrogen loss (Mersalić et al., 2008) and age in women (Carroll et al., 2005). With reduced endogenous estrogen levels, LDL receptor activity is also reduced, leading to the elevated LDL concentration in postmenopausal women. Conversely, HDL and apoprotein A-I—which tend to be higher in young women (Carroll et al., 2005) and their low levels predictive of CHD—are stronger risk factors in women than in men at ages greater than 65 (Manolio et al., 1992).

However, managing these effects may be more complex than HRT; for example postmenopausal users have higher levels of TG-rich VLDL particles without an improvement in LDL subclass distribution compared to nonusers, which may explain the inconsistent correlation of HRT to a reduction in a CHD risk in randomized clinical trials (Mackey et al., 2005).

Elevated TG concentrations were associated with an increased mortality among middle-aged women compared to men. A meta-analysis based on 17 published reports of population-based, prospective studies on the association between fasting TG levels and incident cardiovascular endpoints suggested a 1-mmol/L increase in TG to be associated with a 32% increase in the disease risk in men, compared to 76% in women, and the TG risk found to be more than double that of men (Austin et al., 1998).

## Endothelial Dysfunction

Endothelial dysfunction is now thought to be an early physiological event in the atherosclerotic process even before morphological changes are detected. It is closely related to lipid risk factors such as dyslipidemia (de Jongh et al., 2002; Vogel, 1999), inflammation, lipid oxidation, and smooth-muscle-cell permeability to LDL (DeCaterina et al., 2000), and may predict cardiac events (Schachinger et al., 2000; Schachinger & Zeiher, 2000; Suwaidi et al., 2000). It is associated with the endothelial injury hypothesis, which postulates that cumulative injury causes a loss of endothelial cells; an aggregation of platelets and their adhesion to the subendothelium; monocyte and T-cell chemotaxis; the release of platelet and monocyte-derived growth factors that induce smooth-muscle-cell migration from the media into the intima; and their collective replication and synthesis of connective tissue and proteoglycans that form plaque (DeCaterina et al., 2000; Ross & Glomset, 1976).

Newer markers of endothelial dysfunction, such as reduced postprandial endothelium-dependent vasodilation, have become broadly accepted for the assessment of risk and preventive procedures (Poredos, 2002). Interventional studies showed recovery to be associated with a reduction of lipid-related risk factors (Poredos, 2002).

***Gender Perspective: Endothelial Function***

Results from the Women's Ischemia Syndrome Evaluation (WISE) study identified gender-based differences in the vascular wall, atherosclerotic plaque deposition, and pathophysiology in CHD etiology (Quyyumi, 2006). Endothelium appears to be an important target for estradiol, since it potentiates endothelial nitric oxide (NO) and prostacyclin production, thus promoting beneficial effects such as vasorelaxation and the inhibition of platelet aggregation. Prostacyclin, an n-6 PUFA eicosanoid, appears to be involved in the atheroprotective effect of estradiol, which also accelerates endothelial regrowth, thus favoring vascular healing. The 2-methoxyestradiol form enhances the anti-atherosclerotic actions, at least in part, by preventing monocyte adhesion to the aortic endothelium (Kurokawa et al., 2007).

Recently, the potent vasoconstrictor and prothrombic eicosanoid-like TXA(2) was suggested to be estrogen-dependent and to provide significant gender-specific protection in the systemic vascular wall by increasing vascular tone and blood pressure, and thus defend against hypotension resulting from multiple estrogen-sensitive local vasodilator mechanisms (Sellers & Stallone, 2008).

## Inflammation

The concept that atherosclerosis is a specific form of a chronic inflammatory process, resulting from interactions between plasma lipoproteins, cellular components (monocytes, macrophages, T-lymphocytes, endothelial, and smooth-muscle cells), and the extracellular matrix of the arterial wall, is now well-accepted. C-reactive protein (CRP) was proposed as a key inflammatory marker, found to be predictive of CVD risk in men and women, possibly more so in women (Tonstad et al., 2007). Chronic inflammation, as indicated by a prolonged elevated CRP concentration, appears to have a greater effect on insulin resistance (IR) and on the development of other metabolic syndrome (MetS) components in women than in men (Nishida et al., 2007). Strong associations between other biochemical markers of systemic inflammation—i.e., vascular cell adhesion molecule (VCAM)-1, intercellular adhesion molecule-1 (ICAM-1), monocyte chemoattractant protein-1 (MCP-1), $\gamma$-interferon, plasminogen activator inhibitor-1 (PAI-1), tumor necrosis factor (TNF) $\alpha$ and $\beta$, interleukin (IL)-6 and IL1, serum amyloid A—and both the presence of and future risk for symptomatic CVD were also repeatedly documented (Kressel et al., 2008; Libby et al., 2002). Inflammatory interactions between lipids and cytokines and related molecules are, in turn, believed to be impacted by other physiological reactions, such as the oxidation of both dietary and serum lipids, particularly LDL (Fan & Watanabe, 2003).

The infusion of reconstituted HDL and the restoration of the HDL concentration in hypertriglyceridemic patients were associated with an improvement in the endothelial function (Bisoendial et al., 2003; Spieker et al., 2002), assumed to be related to its anti-inflammatory, antithrombotic, and antioxidant properties, including influencing the expression of cytokines, modulating recruitment and the adhesion of monocytes, and limiting lipid peroxidation (Ansell et al., 2005). Atherogenic lipoproteins, such as oxidized LDL, remnant lipoprotein (β-VLDL) and lipoprotein (a), play a critical role in the pro-inflammatory reaction (Fan & Watanabe, 2003).

### *Gender Perspective: Inflammation*

The increased cardiovascular risk associated with inflammation appears to be particularly significant in women (Reigtz-Zagrosek et al., 2006). A stronger association observed between the CRP concentration and the body mass index (BMI), obesity, and metabolic syndrome the MetS suggests that inflammatory processes may be more enhanced by adipose tissue-derived cytokines in women (Caparevic & Kostic, 2007). In research comparing premenopausal and postmenopausal women, positive correlations were also found between age, oxidized LDL, and CRP (Caparevic & Kostic, 2007).

The cardioprotection of women by estrogens may be due to a direct effect on the vasculature, through antioxidative mechanisms, the generation of NO, the prevention of apoptosis in vascular cells and the suppression of cytokines, and the renin-angiotensin system, resulting in an improvement of endothelial function and an inhibition of atherogenesis (Chakrabarti et al., 2008). Some of these markers were suggested as predictors of acute events (Mueck & Seeger, 2006). Furthermore, declines in the basal metabolic rate and FA oxidation with menopause contribute to alterations in body composition—predominantly an increase in overweight and redistribution of fat toward android-type (abdominal) obesity—and a high-risk profile (Garaulet et al., 2002).

Whereas estradiol provides an anti-inflammatory effect in vitro, eliciting an in vivo pro-inflammatory effect on vascular endothelium in response to stress could contribute to plaque destabilization (Arnal et al., 2006). Some of the postulated mechanisms include an increased expression of the pro-inflammatory receptor for advanced glycation end products—particularly relevant in diabetes mellitus—an increased tyrosine nitration of cellular proteins, and a generation of reactive oxygen species through uncoupled endothelial nitric oxide synthase (eNOS) (Chakrabarti et al., 2008).

Gender-specific differences in the metabolism of pro-inflammatory eicosanoids in females may suggest an additional mechanism of their increased tendency toward systemic inflammation and associated cardiovascular risks (Burdge & Calder, 2005; Hurtado de Catalfo & de, 2005; Marra & de Alaniz, 1989).

## Oxidative Stress

The oxidative modification hypothesis suggests that oxidized LDL is cytotoxic to endothelial cells, induces endothelial injury, and chemotactically attracts monocytes and promotes their migration, transformation, and retention in the subintimal compartment as macrophages (Steinberg et al., 1989). LDL oxidation is assumed to be an early, essential event in atherosclerosis, and may contribute to both the initiation and the progression of atherosclerosis and related disease, perhaps more than absolute LDL levels (Ansell et al., 2005; Holvoet et al., 2008; Yu-Poth et al., 2000).

Oxidative stress and decreased bioavailability of NO appear to be common denominators of risk factors that cause endothelial dysfunction. Whereas the normal redox state provides a normal oxidative metabolism in arterial walls and proper balance between superoxides versus NO anions, oxidative stress imposes high superoxide production, NO breakdown, an increased expression of adhesion molecules, and leukocyte adhesion to endothelium, which lead to an inflammatory response (Yung et al., 2006).

In contrast, HDL can reduce LDL oxidation and general vascular oxidative stress, which in turn exerts anti-inflammatory effects (Libby et al., 2002). Several components of HDL are believed to contribute to this antioxidant effect, including phospholipids in the HDL-3 fraction (Sakuma et al., 2002), apolipoprotein A-1, and key HDL enzymes, specifically paraoxanase 1 (Getz & Reardon, 2004; Thomàs-Moyà et al., 2007), which prevents the formation of lipid hydroperoxides and oxidized phospholipids and hydrolyzes them once they are formed (16) (Ansell et al., 2005).

### *Gender Perspective: Oxidative Stress*

Observations in animal trials suggest that estrogen also affects LDL oxidative processes (Makgos et al., 2007), and reduced estrogen levels in postmenopausal women could be a pathophysiologic risk factor for endothelial damage via an augmented oxidative stress. Oxidative stress is particularly increased with PUFA, and is highly facilitated by inflammation, which is observed to be higher in women compared to men (Donahue et al., 2007; van Eijk et al., 2007).The modification of the redox state of the vasculature was suggested as a therapeutic approach, targeting specific redox-dependent pathways with antioxidants (Berk, 2007). Other conditions specific to women that are associated with increased lipid peroxidation include high parity, oophorectomy, and pre-eclampsia (Castelao & Gago-Dominguez, 2008).

## Metabolic Syndrome (MetS)

Metabolic syndrome (MetS), also known as syndrome X and IR syndrome, is a plurimetabolic disease which plays a key role in the etiology of CVD. It is characterized as a combination of metabolic disturbances, generally with dysregulation of glucose and insulin metabolism at its core, and most commonly including hypertension, impaired fibrinolytic activity, a pro-inflammatory state, impaired postprandial metabolism, abdominal obesity, a pro-oxidative state, and dyslipidemia involving elevated plasma TG and low HDL (Lamarche & Desroches, 2004) with an increased number of reduced-size LDL particles (Carr, 2003; Reaven, 2002). It is related to an increased severity of atherosclerotic vascular lesions and contributes greatly to extensive and more severe vascular lesions (Lanz et al., 2006).

A fatty liver recently was recognized as another feature of MetS and a key player in the pathogenesis of dyslipidemia. It is caused by an imbalance between the influx and the production of FA and the use of FA for oxidation or secretion as VLDL triglycerides, and affects insulin disregulation of VLDL production. The result is increased concentrations of VLDL particles that further affect other lipoproteins, decreasing HDL and increasing SD-LDL (Adiels et al., 2008). An additional contributory effect to MetS is a reduced production of adiponectin, an anti-inflammatory and insulin-sensitizing cytokine (Eckel et al., 2005).

Obesity and an abundance of abdominal (visceral) adipocytes—which differ from peripheral fat cells in their lipolytic activity and their response to insulin, adrenergic and angiotensin stimulation, and sex hormones—are principal sources of free FAs and cytokines (Fig. 7.2), and therefore are related to the early development of IR, MetS, and an associated atherogenic lipid profile (Krauss et al., 1998; Marchesi et al., 2007).

Free FAs and cytokines (such as IL-6 and TNF-α secreted from visceral fat) enhance IR and lipolysis, increase hepatic glucose and VLDL production, increase muscle IR, and induce a prothrombotic state by increasing the production of fibrinogen and PAI-1 by the liver (Eckel et al., 2005).

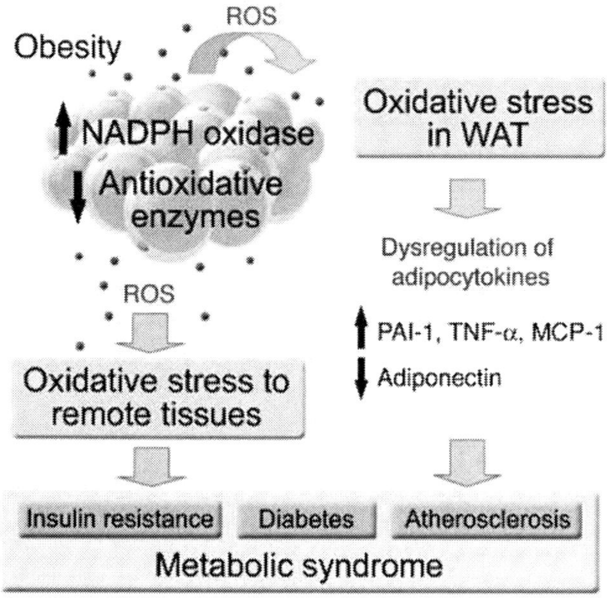


**Fig. 7.2.** Metabolic activity in adipose tissue, and the relationship to atherogenic processes in MetS (Furukawa et al., 2004).

### *Gender Perspective: MetS and Components*

The available data suggest that the pathophysiology of MetS and its contribution to the relative risk of cardiovascular events and heart failure differ with gender, and that women with MetS may be at a greater risk of developing CHD than men. In women, chronic inflammation (as indicated by an elevated CRP concentration) appears to have a greater effect on the development of MetS than in men (Regitz-Zagrosek et al., 2006). The relative risk for CHD in middle-aged participants of the Atherosclerosis Risk in Communities Study (ARIC) was higher for women than for men (2.46 versus 1.86) (Rosamond et al., 2001), especially in middle-age (McNeill et al., 2005). In NHANES III, findings supported a role for endogenous estrogen in suppressing the pro-atherosclerotic effects of MetS-related risk factors, as the prevalence of MetS-associated CHD in women aged 55–74 and in men aged of 35–74 was twofold higher than in women aged 35–54 (Tong et al., 2005).

The clustering of metabolic disorders occurs frequently in both men and women; however, respective contributions of specific disorders to the MetS are not the same. In the French MONICA study, the most significant contributors to the MetS were elevated body weight, waist girth, and low HDL in women compared to systolic and diastolic blood pressures and apolipoprotein B in men (Dallongville et al., 2004). Some of the MetS constituents—low HDL, high TG, and especially diabetes—exert a stronger effect on females than males (Austin et al., 1998), and high TG and TG-rich VLDL were also observed to be stronger predictors for CVD in women than in men (Bittner, 2005). The relative risk of CHD related to diabetes is approximately twice as high in women as in men (Gregg et al., 2007).

### *Obesity*

Females have a higher tendency to accumulate body fat, starting even before birth, with gender differences further emphasized during puberty and adolescence and progressively accumulating with age (Jousilahti et al., 1999). The greater inherent percentage of body fat and slower resting energy expenditure rate in women (Mittendorfer, 2005; Mittendorfer et al., 2003) may place them at a greater obesity risk. In recent years, a 33% increase in obesity in the United States was noted, mostly in women, and especially in women 40 years and older, with over 66% having a BMI greater than 25 (Flegal et al., 2002).

Overweight status and obesity in postmenopausal women drive MetS, which may occur in 40% of this population (Lobo, 2008). In the United States, two million more women than men are categorized as obese, and the trend for developing obesity with diabetes is increasing (Wajchenberg, 2000). This epidemic underscores the importance of defining the gender-specific characteristics for better prevention and management of MetS and related CHD risks (Steinbaum, 2004).

Fat distribution and metabolic effects are typically affected by sex, women having more femoral-gluteal and less abdominal adiposity, particularly prior to menopause. Where femoral-gluteal intermuscular adipose tissue and plasma glucose ($P < 0.05$) were positively associated as independent of visceral adipose tissue, a significant inverse association was found between femoral-gluteal subcutaneous adipose tissue and insulin ($P < 0.01$) and TG ($P < 0.05$) (Yim et al., 2008).

As the degree of obesity increases, together with visceral fat deposition (typically, android postmenopausally versus gluteal and peripheral premenopausally), a concomitant rise occurs in the accompanying IR, dyslipidemia, diabetes, and hypertension that comprise MetS, which in turn contribute to increasing rates of cardiovascular morbidity and mortality (Marchesi et al., 2007). Additionally, an inverse relationship between obesity and HDL levels is recognized (Rashid & Genest, 2007).

### *Metabolically Obese/Normal Weight (MONW)*

A condition of metabolically obese/normal weight (MONW) was identified in young women who, despite having a normal BMI, ($kg/m^2$), display metabolic characteristics that may predispose them to the development of MetS (Ruderman et al., 1981). While MONW was also observed in men (Conus et al., 2007), the greater inherent percentage of body fat and slower resting energy expenditure rate in women, possibly mediated by sex hormones, may place them at a greater risk, independent of the effects of aging and estrogen deficiency (Mittendorfer, 2005; Mittendorfer et al., 2003). The characteristic MONW body composition in women includes higher relative fat mass, lower fat-free mass, and a tendency for greater central fat mass, all of which could be related to reduced insulin sensitivity (Conus et al., 2004; Dvorak et al., 1999), even with normal glucose tolerance (Katsuki et al., 2003). MONW women were observed to have smaller LDL particles ($P < 0.01$); higher concentrations of oxidized LDL, TNF-$\alpha$, IL-6, and leptin ($P < 0.05$); and lower plasma adiponectin concentrations ($P < 0.05$) than women with normal visceral adiposity (Hyun et al., 2008). Because these findings were found in premenopausal young women, they may serve as an independent factor in women's risk, remaining largely subclinical until the levels of protective estrogen decline.

## Fatty Acid Involvement in CVD Etiology

As dyslipidemia was the first diet-related CVD etiological paradigm, attention was mostly concentrated in reducing plasma cholesterol and lipoproteins. This preferentially promoted cholesterol-lowering unsaturated FA (UFA)—MUFA and PUFA (mostly from vegetable oils)—over SFA (mostly from animal sources, which also provided cholesterol). Beyond their major role in plasma lipids, FAs also play a role in other CVD risk factors, including endothelial dysfunction, inflammation, and oxidative stress. A list of common dietary FAs and their relationship to CVD risk factors as observed in the scientific literature is presented in Table 7.1.

### *SFA and TFA*

SFAs are found in animal products and tropical oils (coconut, palm), and are solid at room temperature. *Trans* fatty acids (TFAs) are generated naturally in ruminant

**Table 7.1. Dietary FA: structure, function, and common food sources (Kris-Etherton et al., 2007).**

| Fatty Acid Classification | Structure | Biological Actions | Common Food Sources |
|---|---|---|---|
| **Saturated fatty acids** | | | |
| Lauric acid | C12:0 | Raises total LDL[a], and HDL[b] cholesterol and increases some hemostatic/thrombotic factors that promote thrombosis | Coconut oil |
| Myristic acid | C14:0 | | Butter fat, coconut oil |
| Palmitic acid | C16:0 | | Most fats and oils |
| Stearic acid | C18:0 | Does not increase total LDL and HDL cholesterol | Most fats and oils, cocoa butter, fully hydrogenated vegetable oils |
| **Monounsaturated fatty acids** | | | |
| *cis*-configuration | | | |
| Palmitoleic acid | C16:1 | Decreases total and LDL cholesterol when substituted for saturated fat and decreases total cholesterol compared with dietary carbohydrate | Some fish oils, beef fat |
| Oleic acid | C18:1 | | Most fats and oils, nuts, seeds, avocados |
| *trans*-configuration | | | |
| Elaidic acid | C18:1 | Raises total and LDL cholesterol similar to saturated fat, decreases HDL vs saturated fat, and raises the total-to-HDL ratio more so than saturated fat; induces systemic inflammation and endothelial dysfunction | Partially hydrogenated vegetable oils |
| Vaccenic acid | C18:1 | Not established | Butterfat, meat |

***Cont. on next page.***

**Table 7.1., cont. Dietary FA: structure, function, and common food sources (Kris-Etherton et al., 2007).**

| Fatty Acid Classification | Structure | Biological Actions | Common Food Sources |
|---|---|---|---|
| **Polyunsaturated fatty acids** | | | |
| **n-6 fatty acids** | | | |
| Linoleic acid | C18:2 | Decreases total and LDL cholesterol | Liquid vegetable oils, nuts, seeds |
| Arachidenic acid | C20:4 | Precursor for eicosanoids (prostaglandins, thromboxanes, leukotrienes) | Meat, poultry, fish, eggs |
| Conjugated linoleic acid | C18:2 (variants) | Anti-cancer properties, decreases body fat in growing animals | Butterfat, meat |
| **n-3 fatty acids** | | | |
| $\alpha$-linolenic acid | C18:3 | Decreases cardiovascular risk through multiple mechanisms including platelet function, inflammation, endothelial cell function, arterial compliance, arrhythmia | Flaxseed, canola oil, soybean oil, walnuts |
| Eicosapentaenoic acid | C20:5 | Decreases risk of sudden death through multiple mechanisms including platelet function, endothelial cell function, arterial compliance and arrhythmia, and has beneficial effects on nervous system development and health | Fish oil, algae |
| Docosapentaenoic acid | C22:5 | | Fish oil, algae |
| Docosahexaenoic acid | C22:6 | | Fish oil, algae |

animals (found in dairy products) and in the industrial process of hydrogenating, or solidifying, vegetable oils (found in stick margarines, vegetable shortenings, and commercial bakery products, as well as in deep-fried foods as a result of extended high heat). These two types of fat are considered to be the strongest dietary determinants of elevated LDL concentrations, and SFA is also associated with plasma TG. Strong, positive correlations between SFA intake and the risk of CHD were shown in epidemiological and prospective studies (Ford et al., 2004; Kromhout, 1999; Yusuf et al., 2004), as with high intakes of TFA—stronger even than the effect of dietary cholesterol on plasma LDL (Wilt et al., 2004). SFAs increase the level of LDL slightly more than TFAs, but can also increase HDL concentrations, whereas TFAs do not. TFAs therefore generate an overall worse LDL:HDL ratio (Hu & Willett, 2002; Lichtenstein et al., 1999).

Large prospective studies have consistently found an elevated risk of CHD with higher dietary TFA (CDC, 2005; Mosca et al., 1999; Vasan et al., 2005). Higher red-cell membrane TFA, especially from partially hydrogenated vegetable oils, is associated with an increased risk of primary cardiac arrest (Lemaitre et al., 2002), though not with sudden cardiac death (Hu & Willett 2002; Jousilahti et al., 1999).

Individual SFAs may have differential effects on CVD risks, including lipoprotein metabolism. More than 40 years ago, shorter-chain SFA lauric (C12), myristic (C14), and palmitic (C16) acids were demonstrated to be hypercholesterolemic, while the longer-chain stearic acid (C18) is no more hypercholesterolemic than high oleic acid (OA) or carbohydrate diets (Fernandez & West, 2005; Mensink, 2005), and may even lower LDL levels. Studies on individual SFA effects on HDL are less conclusive, but suggest that stearic acid may decrease slightly the total and LDL-to-HDL cholesterol ratios when compared with palmitic acid or myristic acid (Mensink, 2005).

Individual SFAs may also be differentially responsible for an increased risk of fatal ischemic heart disease as indicated by circulating prothrombotic compounds, such as plasma factor VII coagulant activity (FVII:c). The results of three controlled studies investigating a high stearic-acid diet (from shea butter) showed a 13% lower fasting plasma FVII:c than with a high palmitic-acid diet, and 18% lower than high myristic and lauric diets; a slight increase in plasma fibrinogen compared with a high myristic–lauric acid diet; and a smaller postprandial increase in FVII than with high TFA and high OA diets (Tholstrup, 2005).

SFA has unexpectedly shown sexual dimorphism in its association with CVD risk, wherein a 5% increase in SFA intake in women was associated with a 36% greater risk of CHD, with no overall effect observed in men in a 16-year follow-up study. The SFA effect on increasing coronary risk was strongest in young women (hazard ratio (HR) = 2.68), two times more than in young men (HR = 1.29), and nearly three times greater than in older men (HR = 0.94) or women (HR = 1.22) compared to a control diet (Jakobsen et al., 2004).

TFAs from "natural" dietary sources (dairy from ruminant animals) significantly increased plasma concentrations of both HDL and LDL cholesterol in women, and correspondingly apolipoproteins B and A1, but not in men. Because industrially generated TFAs do not preserve the HDL levels in women—and actually may cause a reduction—they may present a gender-specific increase in CVD risk (Chardigny et al., 2008).

## UFA: MUFA and PUFA

High intakes of PUFA and MUFA as substitutes for dietary SFA were associated with a decreased CVD risk (NCEP, 2002). Meals containing n-3 LC-PUFA EPA and DHA together with MUFA attenuated the postprandial rise in the lipoproteins that contain apolipoproteins B and C (LpB:C) and a subsequent impairment of endothelial function (Hilpert et al., 2007).

### *MUFA*

The dyslipidemia and increased lipid oxidation often associated with a high-fat diet may be attenuated by the incorporation of MUFA (Thomàs-Moyà et al., 2007). In general, a diet high in MUFA—mostly from OA (18:1)—was preferable to a low-fat diet for lowering cholesterol, improving lipid profile, and reducing CVD risk. OA lowers total and LDL cholesterol when it replaces SFA (Kris-Etherton et al., 1999; NCEP, 2002). When compared to carbohydrate replacement, MUFAs decrease TG and VLDL by approximately 20% and increase HDL modestly, without increasing LDL or total cholesterol (Garg, 1998). A high olive-oil diet was associated with: (i) a 25% decrease in CVD risk, versus 12% with a very low-fat, low-cholesterol diet ("Step II") recommended by the National Cholesterol Education Program (NCEP); (ii) a greater decrease in total (10%) and LDL (14%) cholesterol; and (iii) the preservation of plasma HDL cholesterol, compared to a 4% HDL decrease with a Step II diet. An increase in dietary OA, and subsequently increased LDL OA content at the expense of linoleic acid (LA), reduced LDL oxidation (Bonow et al., 2002; Castro et al., 2000; Yusuf et al., 2001) and LDL uptake by macrophages (National Institutes of Health, 1998). Replacing LDL PUFA with MUFA (OA) reduced LDL oxidation, monocyte-chemotaxis response, adhesion to endothelial cells, and platelet activation (Kratz et al., 2002; Stocker & Keaney, 2004). Women may benefit most from a high-MUFA diet, because it may effectively reduce total and LDL cholesterol without reducing HDL, and low HDL is a stronger predictor of CVD risk for women than for men (Kris-Etherton et al., 1999).

### *PUFA*

PUFA are divided primarily into n-6 and n-3 families and then further to intermediate-chain (C16–18) and long-chain (LC-PUFA, C20–24). The bulk of total PUFA in a typical North American diet is comprised of LA (18:2n-6) and $\alpha$-linolenic acid (ALA, 18:3n-3), with LA comprising 89% and ALA 9% (Ervin et al., 2004). LA is present in high concentrations in many commonly used grain-based oils, including safflower, sunflower, soy, and corn. ALA is present in leafy green vegetables and in some commonly used oils, primarily canola, as well as some novelty oils, such as flaxseed. Among LC-PUFA, n-6 arachidonic acid (AA, 20:4) is found primarily in meat products, and n-3 eicosapentaenoic acid (EPA, 20:5) and docosahexaenoic acid (DHA, 22:6) are found in marine algae and fish (especially cold-water marine "fatty" fish) and fish oils, as well as fortified products, such as "omega-3" eggs.

Where SFAs were found to be positively correlated to plasma total cholesterol levels, UFAs demonstrated inverse relationships; when MUFAs or PUFAs (mostly n-6) replace SFAs, levels of LDL decrease significantly, with nearly no effect on HDL. LA is the major dietary PUFA affecting LDL metabolism by down-regulating LDL production and enhancing its clearance. Further, the available mass of LA is a critical factor working against hyperlipemic and hypercholesterolemic dietary fat, such as SFA and TFA (Wijendran & Hayes, 2004). However, while high n-6 PUFA trials have long demonstrated the reduction of serum-cholesterol levels (Dayton et al., 1969; Leren, 1970), and improvements in CVD rates relative to high SFA diets (Willett, 2007), a recent systematic review suggests that the direct correlation may be weak (DeLorgeril & Salen, 2008).

Recent human and animal studies suggest that dietary FA composition may affect adiposity. High LA raises tissue AA and prostacyclin, which in turn stimulate signaling pathways and the activation of enzymes (i.e., phospholipase and/or cyclooxygenase) that may enhance adipogenesis (Alihaud et al., 2008). As women have an innately higher tendency toward adipocyte proliferation and a high capacity for desaturation, high LA intake may place them at a greater risk for increased tissue AA and associated pro-inflammatory metabolic cascades. Furthermore, increased adipose AA content from high dietary LA has itself correlated with CVD risk (Harris et al., 2007; Kark et al., 2003). The above may be more influential in women, as recently shown by a correlation between higher CHD risk and increased plasma n-6 and decreased n-3 among women, particularly postmenopausally (Rhee et al., 2008). Because PUFAs are more susceptible to oxidation than are SFAs and MUFAs, they are associated with greater LDL oxidation and inflammation, believed to be key risk factors in CVD (Lapointe et al., 2006; Sies et al., 2005).

***Essential FA (EFA) Metabolism***

Of all fats found in food, two necessary for proper physiological functioning—LA and ALA—cannot be synthesized in the human body, and are thus considered essential FAs (EFAs). EFAs are converted in the liver to LC-PUFA, LA into AA(20:4n-6), and ALA to EPA (20:5n-3) and DHA (22:6n-3). However, the conversion among n-3 PUFA occurs slowly in humans, and varies according to gender, age, and diet. Conversion is highest in young women—especially during pregnancy (Burdge & Calder, 2005)—and declines with age, along with the levels of the rate-limiting enzymes, $\Delta$-5- and $\Delta$-6-desaturase, to a greater extent in women than in men (Bolton-Smith et al., 1997). Desaturase activity was shown in humans to be inhibited in the conditions of a high-SFA diet (Warensjo et al., 2008) or a high-cholesterol intake (Brenner et al., 2002), and increased with a high n-3 PUFA and/or MUFA diet (Warensjo et al., 2008). Moreover, dietary LA and ALA share rate-limiting enzymes in their respective conversion pathways (Fig. 7.3), and thus act as competitors.

***Eicosanoid Production and Function***

LC-PUFA EPA and AA are both precursors for the formation of eicosanoids—prostaglandins (PG), thromboxane (TX), and leukotrienes—tissue hormone-like agents that regulate a large number of cellular functions, including clotting, inflammation, innervation, and immuno-modulation (Fig. 7.4) (Khanapure et al., 2007; Zamaria, 2004).

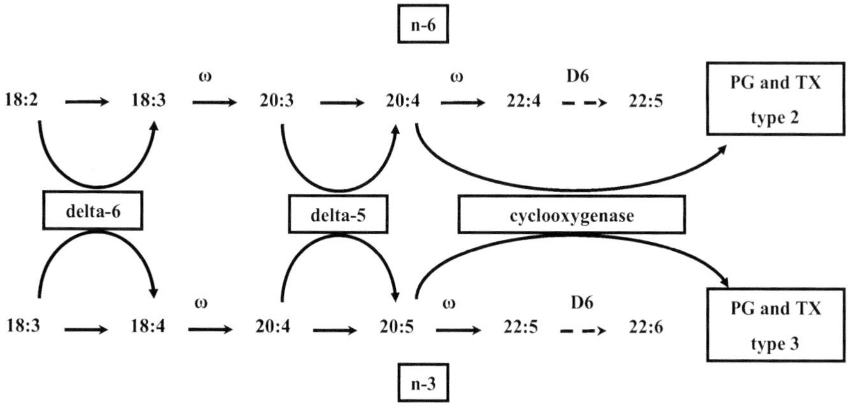


**Fig. 7.3.** The n-6 and n-3 PUFA series.

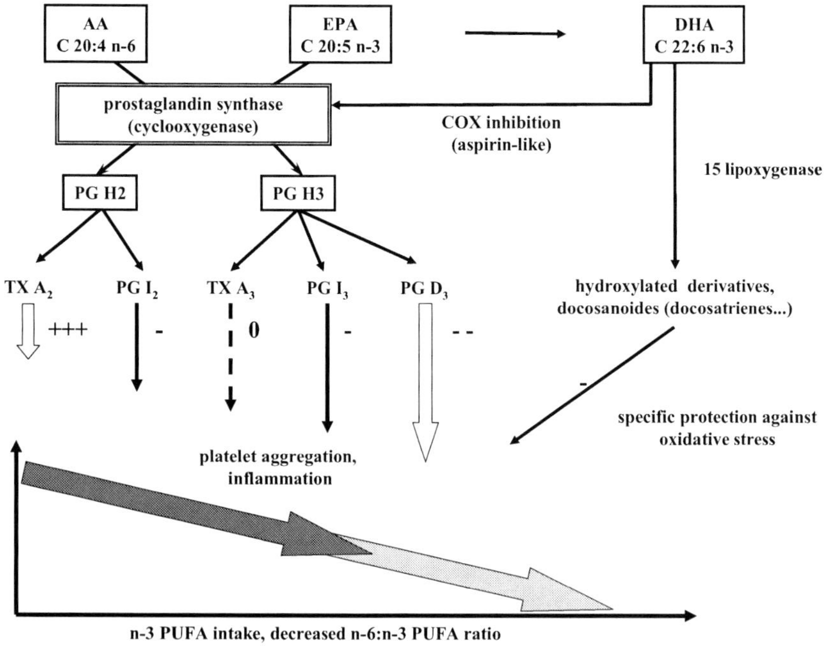


**Fig. 7.4.** Eicosanoid metabolism in pro- and anti-atherogenic processes.

The in vivo effects of sex steroids on FA metabolism show a gender-specific effect on desaturases that may influence inflammatory processes and be linked to atherosclerosis and cardiovascular pathophysiology. Testosterone significantly increased the activity of Δ-9-desaturase (responsible for the conversion of stearic acid to OA), and strongly depressed the activities of Δ-5- and Δ-6-desaturases (responsible for the conversion of EFA, LA to AA and ALA to DHA), as shown by lower male ratios of AA:LA and DHA:ALA compared to females. As a result, testosterone may drive a higher generation of 16:1 and 18:1 (OA) from 16:0 and 18:0 SFAs in males, as opposed to a greater generation of AA from LA and DHA from ALA in females (Burdge & Calder, 2005; Hurtado de Catalfo et al, 2005; Marra & de Alaniz, 1989). These mechanisms may suggest a sex-related differential predisposition to the generation of pro-inflammatory PG, a key role of EFA metabolism with strong implications for differential CVD physiopathology and clinical outcomes.

### *n-6 LC-PUFA*

AA is present only in small amounts in storage TG (0.5%); its main biological role is in membrane phospholipids, where it is a major component (14%) (Kark et al., 2003). It is the precursor of a group of eicosanoids including series-2 PGs and series-4 leukotrienes, which are involved in actions such as accelerating platelet aggregation and enhancing vasoconstriction and the synthesis of inflammatory mediators in response to physiological stressors (Fox et al., 2004). High intakes of n-6 PUFA were proposed to increase the production of proinflammatory and proaggregatory AA-derived eicosanoids (Calder & Grimble, 2002), and to increase the susceptibility of LDL and tissue lipids high in LA to oxidative modification (Tsimikas & Reaven, 1998), and thus may increase a coronary risk.

### *n-3 LC-PUFA*

Unexpected CVD protection by animal fat found in Greenland Eskimos initiated interest in n-3 LC-PUFA from marine fish as preventive (Dyerberg & Bang, 1979). The protective effects of n-3 PUFA were supported by observational (Albert et al., 2002; Erkkila et al., 2004; Mozaffarian et al., 2006) and interventional (GISSI, 1999; Kris-Etherton et al., 2002) studies.

The n-3 EPA and DHA are precursors of a group of eicosanoids including series-3 PGs and series-5 leukotrienes. The series-3 prostaglandins and series-5 leukotrienes derived from n-3 LC-PUFA work to attenuate excessive series-2 PGs and to protect against heart attack and stroke as well as certain inflammatory diseases like arthritis, lupus, and asthma, especially under high n-6 PUFA-intake conditions, as in the typical Western diet. EPA and DHA inhibited platelet aggregability, reduced pro-atherogenic cytokines, and improved endothelial function and vascular occlusion, potentially mitigating the course of coronary atherosclerosis (Das, 2008). They may also increase LDL size–thus reducing concentrations of SD–LDL (Kelly et al., 2007) —and reduce VLDL-cholesterol, VLDL–TG (Hartweg et al., 2007), and plasma TG by up to 30%

(Bays et al., 2008; Lichtenstein, 2006), by decreasing hepatic VLDL production (Lichtenstein, 2006). Further, EPA and DHA demonstrated an anti-arrhythmic effect, and are thought to be protective against sudden cardiac death (Rupp et al., 2004). The n-3 LC-PUFA incorporation into cellular phospholipids paralleled a reduction in VCAM-1 messenger RNA, indicating a pretranslational effect (DeCaterina, 2000). This could synergystically enhance conventional medications (i.e., statins) in the management of combined dyslipidemia (Skulas-Ray et al., 2008).

Though several research studies did not find the n-3 LC-PUFA precursor ALA to be anti-lipemic or to mitigate immunogenic risk for CVD, recent studies suggest that high levels of ALA may elicit cardioprotective anti-inflammatory effects by inhibiting the production, release, and activity of inflammatory cytokines (Zhao et al., 2007). Meals with MUFA and ALA attenuated the increase in lipoprotein apolipoproteins LpA-II:B:C:D:E in individuals with high blood TG (≥1.69 mmol/L) (Hilpert et al., 2007).

High n-3 PUFA consumption possibly increases insulin sensitivity, and may reduce free FA mobilization by catecholamines, inflammatory markers (Tsitouras et al., 2008) (particularly CRP and IL-6), and TG in subjects with an increased inflammatory status associated with higher BMI and with increased insulinemic response (Browning et al., 2007), which relates greatly to women's risk.

In addition to its TG-lowering effects, ALA appears to attenuate CVD risk by inhibiting vascular inflammation and endothelial activation (Zhao et al., 2007). Because chronic inflammation may have a greater effect in women, and because they have a higher innate capacity for a transformation of the n-3 intermediate-chain PUFA (ALA, 18:3) to LC-PUFA (EPA 20:5 and DHA 22:6) (Burdge & Calder, 2005), women may benefit more from ALA than men, which could translate to health advantages against CVD. Females (humans as well as rats) tend to have higher plasma DHA concentrations than males, positively associated with circulating concentrations of estradiol and progesterone but negatively associated with testosterone (Childs et al., 2008). Sex differences in EPA and DHA in phospholipids and serum cholesterol esters appear to be independent of age (Crowe et al., 2008; Stark et al., 2008).

### *n-6/n-3 PUFA Ratio*

Enzymatic competition between n-6 and n-3 PUFA in the conversion to active LC-PUFA may mean that the typical Western high-intake of n-6 PUFA could compromise the benefits of n-3 PUFA consumption. This led to a general scientific agreement supporting a reduced intake of n-6 PUFA and an increased intake of n-3 PUFA to attain the recommended dietary n-6:n-3 PUFA ratio for attenuation of CVD risk (Pilote et al., 2007; Ristić & Ristić, 2003; Simopoulos, 2008). A high dietary LA:ALA ratio was associated with an increased LDL oxidation, platelet aggregation, and an impaired incorporation of EPA and DHA into cell-membrane phospholipids (Simopoulos, 2008). Different n-6:n-3 PUFA ratios were suggested in various research studies for various conditions (Pilote et al., 2007); that is, 3:1 was associated with reduced fasting and postprandial TG concentrations and SD–LDL levels (Simopoulos, 2008), including in postmenopausal women (Griffin et al., 2006).

Fatty liver, acknowledged as a key factor in IR, was associated with a high n-6:n-3 PUFA ratio in the advanced stage of macrosteatosis (with accompanying microcirculatory dysfunction), where a dietary supplementation of n-3 PUFA in an animal model resulted in the normalization of this ratio, a reduction of intrahepatic lipids, and a decrease in the extent of disease (El Badry et al., 2007a, 2007b).

### *Conjugated Linoleic Acids (CLAs)*

Conjugated linoleic acids (CLAs) are biologically active lipid compounds exerting anti-atherogenic actions in vivo without exact knowledge of the underlying mechanisms. Recently, CLAs were shown to lower the release of vasoactive prostanoids from vascular smooth muscle cells that play a central role in atherosclerosis. The observed anti-inflammatory effect of CLA may contribute to their anti-atherogenic actions (Ringseis et al., 2006). CLA in animal models impacted mRNA expression in several key mechanisms affecting heart-muscle contractility and outcomes such as heart rate, systolic and diastolic pressures, mean arterial pressure, and left-ventricular function (Tappia et al., 2007). Different manifestations were observed in males and females regarding heart rate, systolic and diastolic pressures, mean arterial pressure, and left-ventricular systolic pressure, suggesting a sex-specific role for dietary CLA supplementation in modulating cardiac function at the molecular level (Tappia et al., 2006). However, the CVD protective hypothesis of CLA in humans is not conclusive (Badinga & Greene, 2006; Tricon et al., 2005).

## Dietary FA Application and Guidelines

The average American adult (>19 years) consumes a diet with approximately 38% of the energy as fat. Of this, just over one-third is from SFA, approximately one-fourth from PUFA, and the rest from MUFA (Ervin et al., 2004).

The main FA-related dietary approaches for modifying CVD risk have traditionally included (i) replacing SFA and/or TFA with PUFA and/or MUFA without changing total fat amount and (ii) lowering total fat. Though dietary cholesterol is a primary target in CVD risk reduction, a recent systematic review suggests that it may not be sufficient to reduce cardiac and overall mortality in the general population (DeLorgeril & Salen, 2008).

Suggested targets for the prevention of MetS-associated CVD risk include (i) the correction of an overweight status by reducing the energy density of the diet, including reducing total fat and increasing fiber, fruit, and vegetables and (ii) the improvement of insulin sensitivity and associated metabolic abnormalities through the reduction of dietary SFA, partially replaced as appropriate by MUFA and PUFA (Riccardi et al., 2004).

## Low-fat Diet

Various scientific bodies recommend reductions in dietary fat intake to treat or prevent coronary disease, including the American Heart Association (Lichtenstein et al., 2006) and the Expert Panel on Detection, Evaluation, and Treatment of High Blood Cholesterol in Adults (2001). The low-fat diet recommended by the American Heart Association yields 30% of total energy from fat, with SFA 10% of energy, along with a reduction in dietary cholesterol to ≤300 mg daily. A very low-fat regime, as specified in the NCEP Step II diet for at-risk individuals, yields 25% of energy from fat, 7% from SFA, and ≤200 mg cholesterol verified. The substitution of SFAs with carbohydrates from grains, vegetables, legumes, and fruits generally makes the diet "low-fat, high-carbohydrate," while adding protective constituents from plant sources, such as phytosterols and flavonoids. Low-fat, high-complex carbohydrate diets reduce total energy intake, increase satiation, are metabolized less efficiently than high-fat diets, and therefore were advocated to prevent obesity and promote weight loss in overweight persons, thereby reducing a major CVD risk (Yao & Roberts, 2001).

However, the effectiveness of a low-fat dietary pattern for the prevention of CHD was inconsistent, especially in women. When relationships between dietary patterns and the risk of cardiovascular mortality among free-living healthy adults were evaluated by a survey, a greater adherence to a prudent pattern (high intakes of vegetables, fruit, legumes, fish, poultry, and whole grains) correlated to reduced risk, whereas greater adherence to the Western pattern (high intakes of red meat, processed meat, refined grains, french fries, and sweets/desserts) appeared to increase the risk (Fung et al., 2001; Heidemann et al., 2008). When examined prospectively in interventional trials of the Women's Health Initiative (WHI) (Howard et al., 2006), a prudent pattern did not significantly reduce the CVD risk in postmenopausal women. However, a more targeted approach to cholesterol metabolism, as in the portfolio dietary pattern—characterized by a combination of plant sterols, soy protein, soluble fiber, and almonds—appeared to provide an additional cardiovascular benefit over the traditional low-fat NCEP Step II diet, including a pronounced reduction in cholesterol levels within the small LDL fraction comparable to a statin drug (Gigleux et al., 2007; Jenkins et al., 2007). These results support the notion that the observed benefits of fat reduction may be at least partially dependent on the modification of FA composition and other components of the whole diet, and may be further related to the specific subclinical risk factors beyond pure hypercholesterolemia.

Recent studies comparing the effects of very-low-carbohydrate/high-SFA versus high-carbohydrate/low-SFA weight-loss diets on markers of endothelial function and inflammation in adults with visceral adiposity showed no significant difference. Both diets appeared to provide equivalent benefits in managing CVD risk factors, with the exception that SFA restriction correlated to lower plasma LDL (Keogh et al., 2008; Tay et al., 2008). A cohort of women showed a higher protein:carbohydrate ratio in an energy-restricted, low-fat diet to be associated with metabolic benefits equal to and sometimes greater than those observed with high-carbohydrate diets (Noakes et al.,

2005), and the degree of improvement in blood lipids was similar to that observed with a high-MUFA/low-carbohydrate diet (Luscombe-Marsh et al., 2005).

## Low-SFA Diet

A diet restricted in SFA and cholesterol has been the general recommendation for elevated LDL, with and without drug therapy (Li et al., 2003). The reductions in LDL that may be expected with such a diet are 8–10%, an additional 3–5% with reduced cholesterol (<200 mg/day), and up to 20–30% with the incorporation of body-weight reduction and increased fiber intake (Fletcher et al., 2005).

By all estimates, the total cholesterol-raising effect of SFA is approximately twice the cholesterol-lowering effect of PUFA (Hegsted et al., 1965; Keys & Parlin, 1966). SFA also increases IR, and thus its substitution with UFA has beneficial effects on insulin sensitivity (Riserus, 2008). However, when SFA is replaced with carbohydrates, both LDL and HDL may be reduced, with little significant effect on the LDL:HDL ratio, while increasing TG. This change in diet is expected to have a minimal benefit on a CHD risk (Hu & Willett, 2002).

## PUFA Recommendations: Dietary Reference Intakes (DRI) and Ratios

The distinct functions of the n-6 and n-3 PUFA families make the balance between dietary intakes an important consideration influencing cardiovascular health. Both the absolute amounts of EFA consumed, as well as their n-6:n-3 ratio, are factors to consider when contemplating life-long dietary habits affecting cardiovascular benefit (Wijendran & Hayes, 2004). The Institute of Medicine (IOM) recommends adequate intakes (AI) for EFA and key LC-PUFA metabolites, which differ by age and gender, and for special conditions such as pregnancy and lactation (IOM, 2002).

### n-6 PUFA Recommendations

The IOM recommends the LA AI for adults to be ≥19 to be 11–17 g/day, or 6 kcal%. Unlike n-3, currently no AI exists for n-6 LC-PUFA. Though recommendations for intake in disease management were also to include proportional consumption relative to other FAs, specifically to n-3 PUFA, much debate occurred over the practical utility of the dietary n-6:n-3 PUFA ratio in cardiovascular health. Recently, a randomly controlled trial (OPTILIP) concluded that a decreased absolute intake of LA, along with an increased intake of ALA and n-3 LC-PUFA, is of greater value than the n-6:n-3 PUFA ratio in modifying CVD risk (Griffin, 2008). Epidemiological and clinical studies establishing EFAs (as well as n-3 LC-PUFA) as collectively protective against CHD and describing practical dietary intakes led to recommendations for the consumption of 6–8 kcal% from LA, similar to IOM DRI (Wijendran & Hayes, 2004; Willett, 2007).

### n-3 PUFA Recommendations

The IOM AI of ALA is 1.1–1.6 g/day. Of the ALA amount, 10% is recommended to come from LC-PUFA EPA and/or DHA. Relative to total daily dietary intake, the AI for n-3 PUFA includes 0.6–1.2 kcal% from ALA, 0.06–0.12 kcal% EPA + DHA. Recent research in CVD prevention suggests the optimal amounts to be 0.75kcal% from ALA—consistent with IOM DRI—but one-third of this, 0.25 kcal%, from EPA + DHA (Wijendran & Hayes, 2004). On the basis of available epidemiological and clinical research data, the American Heart Association recommends that the general population consume at least two servings weekly of high n-3 LC-PUFA-rich "fatty" fish, and that individuals with established CVD (including a myocardial-infarction aftermath or the prevention of a sudden cardiac death) consume 1 g of EPA + DHA daily, and hypertriglyceridemic individuals consume 2–4 g of EPA + DHA daily (vonSchacky, 2006).

The United States Food and Drug Administration (FDA) recommends limiting the total dietary intake of n-3 PUFA from fish to a maximum of 3 g/day, and no more than 2 g/day from nutritional supplements (U.S. FDA, 2004), because a perceived risk exists associated with the intake of fish and fish supplements of heavy-metal poisoning, particularly mercury, lead, nickel, arsenic, and cadmium. However, some studies show the benefits of supplementation with up to 10 g/day, including improved endothelium-dependent vasodilation (West, 2001). Moderate fish-oil supplementation (from cold-water marine fatty fish, a rich source of EPA and DHA) contributes to a reversal of lipid abnormalities in conditions of low n-3 PUFA levels, and is an important dietary step in reducing CVD pathogenesis, particularly in populations at risk (i.e., with an atherogenic lipoprotein phenotype) (Lovegrove et al., 2004). The consumption of flaxseed oil (20 g/day), a source of ALA, yields some of the benefits associated with EPA and DHA supplements, though effects depend mainly on a conversion to LC-PUFA (Balk et al., 2006; Hooper et al., 2006; Stark et al., 2008; Wang et al., 2006).

### *n-6:n-3 PUFA Ratio Recommendations*

A decreased dietary n-6:n-3 PUFA ratio yields potentially favorable CVD-related effects on the metabolic and inflammatory profiles (Guebre-Egziabher et al., 2007; Simopoulos, 2008). Published literature describing the association between absolute dietary intakes of EFA and cardiovascular health correspond to an n-6:n-3 ratio of approximately 6:1 (Wijendran & Hayes, 2004). A ratio of 4:1 was optimal in attenuating pro-atherogenic eicosanoid cascades (Ristić & Ristić, 2003).

### *FA Recommendations in CVD Prevention: Gender Perspective*

Gender differences in CVD etiology are potentially relevant for differential prevention, diagnosis, and therapy of the syndrome. The effect of dietary FA manipulation in weight loss may be particularly relevant in women's CVD risk, given their greater incidence of atherogenic obesity compared to men.

Low-fat diet, weight loss, and exercise were less effective in altering lipoprotein levels in women than in men (LaRosa, 1992), with a high degree of variability in a lipoprotein subspecies response. A low-fat diet (high in vegetables, fruits, and whole grains) in a large cohort of postmenopausal women of diverse backgrounds and ethnicities in the WHI Randomized Controlled Dietary Modification Trial did not significantly reduce the risk of CVD or individual risk factors (Howard et al., 2006). Even a very low-fat diet—consistent with the NCEP Step II diet—was shown to only partially reduce the rise in LDL observed during the transition from pre- to postmenopausal levels (Kuller et al., 2001).

Higher TFA intakes, and to a smaller extent SFA, were associated with an increased CHD risk, whereas higher intakes of nonhydrogenated PUFA and MUFA were associated with a decreased risk in a 14-year study with four repeated measures on 80,082 women in the Nurses' Health Study cohort (Hu et al., 1997; Hu & Willett, 2002). Higher SFA intake, with a lower PUFA:SFA ratio and fiber intake, was also correlated to abnormal metabolic markers in MONW women (Hyun et al., 2008).

Diets rich in or enriched with EPA and DHA—with a corresponding n-6:n-3 PUFA ratio of approximately 3:1—lowered fasting and postprandial TG concentrations and the proportion of SD-LDL, independent of insulin sensitivity or lipase activities in postmenopausal women (45–70 years of age) (Griffin et al., 2006). Higher plasma DHA was associated with the reduced progression of atherosclerosis in postmenopausal women with existing CAD (Erkillä et al., 2006). In the Nurses' Health Study I cohort, a cross-sectional study of 727 healthy middle-aged women (43–69 years of age) showed dietary n-3 PUFA to be associated with reduced biomarkers for inflammation and endothelial activation—specifically, CRP, IL-6, E-selectin, sICAM-1, and sVCAM-1—the latter two specifically related to n-3 PUFA intake. These were not responsive to HRT or other dietary components, such as fiber or vitamin E alone (Lopez-Garcia et al., 2004).

Dietary CLA supplementation was demonstrated to have a differential gender response in modulating cardiac function, though findings have not yet generated specific recommendations for humans (Tappia et al., 2006).

## Discussion

Despite the advancing awareness and accumulating knowledge regarding gender differences in epidemiology and clinical manifestations of CVD—including the differential effects of age, risk factors, response to treatments, and recovery—the question regarding a differential nutrition approach as a preventive and supporting strategy was not emphasized, mainly due to the assumption of universality in metabolic etiologies.

However, women appear to be less responsive than men to traditional approaches—such as weight loss, exercise, and low-fat or low-SFA diets (Huxley et al., 2005)—but more responsive to EFA, especially n-3 PUFA, as suggested by gender-specific etiologies and eicosanoid metabolism (Burdge & Calder, 2005; Hurtado de Catalfo et al., 2005; Marra & de Alaniz, 1989). This may suggest a role for nutritional prevention specific to women, especially important in conditions of a high n-6 PUFA consumption typical of a Western diet, which may trigger inherent metabolic cascades leading to pro-atherogenic, prothrombotic, pro-oxidative, and pro-inflammatory processes.

EFA are highly potent metabolically, playing significant roles in biochemical and physiological regulation, as well as physicochemical processes in cell membranes, plasma lipoproteins, and energy production. Additionally, they have diverse regulatory roles in cells via eicosanoid metabolism at the molecular level (Khanapure et al., 2007; Zamaria, 2004). Therefore, they could influence CVD risks in a variety of ways, and be considered a target for prevention.

Women have a significantly greater capacity for the transformation of ALA to EPA and DHA and of LA to AA than do men, especially during their reproductive years (Burdge & Calder, 2005). This suggests an even greater importance of a balance between dietary LA and ALA, given their enzymatic competition and physiologically opposing actions that may affect CVD risks. Moreover, gender differences in FA metabolism may also be related to differences in CVD etiology and risks, and thus relevant for prevention, diagnosis, and therapy. The decrease in EFA transformation capacity due to declines in Δ-5- and Δ-6-desaturase activities, concurrent with reduced estrogen (Bolton-Smith et al., 1997) and the onset of menopause, is associated with the acceleration of atherogenic processes. This may be the time for initiating nutritional prevention, including early screening and nutritional prevention, even before the onset of cardiovascular symptoms (Pilote et al., 2007). An association between higher plasma DHA and the attenuation of preexisting CVD processes in postmenopausal women (Erkkilä et al., 2006), and the advantages of a high n-3 PUFA diet—including in lowering plasma TG concentrations (Bays et al., 2008)—emphasize their potential contribution for cardiovascular protection. Women's higher risk associated with low HDL levels may also become a differential FA intervention target (i.e., with MUFA, shown to be effective in reducing LDL cholesterol, while preserving HDL).

Additionally, the effect of dietary FA manipulation in obesity may be particularly relevant in women, given their life-long greater tendency toward fat accumulation compared to men, change from premenopausal peripheral to postmenopausal abdominal (visceral) and more atherogenic obesity (Krauss et al., 1998; Marchesi et al., 2007), and recent research suggesting n-6 PUFA is associated with enhanced adipogenesis (Alihaud et al., 2008).

Overall, as women have high CVD mortality rates similar to those of men, but with different etiological factors and expression, one must determine their specific preventive measures. This chapter presents the important concept of gender differences in CVD etiologies as related to FA metabolism.

## Conclusion

As women have historically been less included than men in CVD research, studies yielding positive results with nutrition intervention in men are perceived as universal. Later findings that women may not benefit similarly from the same interventions suggested a gender effect on CVD etiology and prevention.

Among CVD risks often of greater physiological significance in women—obesity, endothelial dysfunction, inflammation, diabetes mellitus, MetS, and imbalances in TG and HDL—women appear to be less responsive to traditional low-fat and low-SFA diets, but more responsive to increased dietary EFA and MUFA. Thus, one must consider men and women separately when examining the association between disease risk and nutritional factors, specifically as related to FA. Increasing dietary n-3 PUFA and reducing the n-6:n-3 PUFA ratio may better support an anti-atherogenic and CVD-preventive metabolic cascade that is particularly relevant in a Western high n-6 PUFA dietary environment. The transition to menopause and decreased circulating estrogen levels represents a critical point of accelerated increase in CVD risk, and thus a relevant point for nutritional intervention. This warrants further research, and may have great potential for the development of a differential prevention strategy.

## References

Adiels, M.; M.R. Taskinen; J. Boren. Fatty liver, insulin resistance, and dyslipidemia. *Curr. Diab. Rep.* **2008,** *8 (1),* 60–64.

Ailhaud, G.; P. Guesnet; S.C. Cunnane. An emerging risk factor for obesity: does disequilibrium of polyunsaturated fatty acid metabolism contribute to excessive adipose tissue development? *Br. J. Nutr.* **2008,** 1–10.

Albert, C.M.; H. Campos; M.J. Stampfer; P.M. Ridker; J.E. Manson; W.C. Willett; J. Ma. Blood levels of long-chain n-3 fatty acids and the risk of sudden death. *N. Engl. J. Med.* **2002,** *346 (15),* 1113–1118.

Ansell, B.J.; K.E. Watson; A.M. Fogelman; M. Navab; G.C. Fonarow. High-density lipoprotein function recent advances. *J. Am. Coll. Cardiol.* **2005,** *46 (10),* 1792–1798.

Arnal, J.F.; H. Laurell; F. Lenfant; V. Douin-Echinard; L. Brouchet; P. Gourdy. Estradiol action in atherosclerosis and reendothelialization. *Ernst. Schering. Found. Symp. Proc.* **2006,** *1,* 69–86.

Austin, M.A.; J.E. Hokanson; K.L. Edwards. Hypertriglyceridemia as a cardiovascular risk factor. *Am. J. Cardiol.* **1998,** *81 (4A),* 7B–12B.

Badinga, L.; E.S. Greene. Physiological properties of conjugated linoleic acid and implications for human health. *Nutr. Clin. Pract.* **2006,** *21 (4),* 367–373.

Balk, E.M.; A.H. Lichtenstein; M. Chung; B. Kupelnick; P. Chew; J. Lau, Effects of omega-3 fatty acids on coronary restenosis, intima-media thickness, and exercise tolerance: a systematic review. *Atherosclerosis* **2006,** *184 (2),* 237–246.

Bays, H.E.; A.P. Tighe; R. Sadovsky; M.H. Davidson.Prescription omega-3 fatty acids and their lipid effects: physiologic mechanisms of action and clinical implications. *Expert. Rev. Cardiovasc. Ther.* **2008,** *6 (3),* 391–409.

Berk, B.C. Novel approaches to treat oxidative stress and cardiovascular diseases. Trans. *Am. Clin. Climatol. Assoc.* **2007,** *118,* 209–214.

Bisoendial, R.J.; G.K. Hovingh; J.H. Levels; P.G. Lerch; I. Andresen; M.R. Hayden; J.J. Kastelein; E.S. Stroes. Restoration of endothelial function by increasing high-density lipoprotein in subjects with isolated low high-density lipoprotein. *Circulation* **2003,** *107 (23),* 2944–2948.

Bittner, V. Perspectives on dyslipidemia and coronary heart disease in women. *J.Am. Coll. Cardiol.*

**2005,** *46,* 1628 1635.

Bjornheden, T.; G. Bondjers; O. Wiklund. Direct assessment of lipoprotein outflow from in vivo-labeled arterial tissue as determined in an in vitro perfusion system. *Arterioscler. Thromb. Vasc. Biol.* **1998,** *18 (12),* 1927–1933.

Bolton-Smith, C.; M. Woodward; R. Tavendale. Evidence for age-related differences in the fatty acid composition of human adipose tissue, independent of diet. *Eur. J. Clin. Nutr.* **1997,** *51 (9),* 619–624.

Bonow, R.O.; L.A. Smaha; S.C. Smith, Jr.; G.A. Mensah; C. Lenfant. World Heart Day 2002: the international burden of cardiovascular disease: responding to the emerging global epidemic. *Circulation* **2002,** *106 (13),* 1602–1605.

Brenner, R.R.; A.M. Bernasconi; M.S. Gonzalez; O.J. Rimoldi. Dietary cholesterol modulates delta6 and delta9 desaturase mRNAs and enzymatic activity in rats fed a low-EFA diet. *Lipids* **2002,** *37 (4),* 375–383.

Browning, L.M.; J.D. Krebs; C.S. Moore; G.D. Mishra; M.A. O'Connell; S.A. Jebb. The impact of long chain n-3 polyunsaturated fatty acid supplementation on inflammation, insulin sensitivity and CVD risk in a group of overweight women with an inflammatory phenotype. *Diabetes Obes. Metab.* **2007,** *9 (1),* 70–80.

Burdge, G.C.; P.C. Calder. Conversion of alpha-linolenic acid to longer-chain polyunsaturated fatty acids in human adults. *Reprod. Nutr. Dev.* **2005,** *45 (5),* 581–597.

Calder, P.C.; R.F. Grimble. Polyunsaturated fatty acids, inflammation and immunity. *Eur. J. Clin. Nutr.* **2002,** *56 (Suppl. 3),* S14–S19.

Cano, A.; C. Hermenegildo; P. Oviedo; J.J. Tarin. Selective estrogen receptor modulators and risk for coronary heart disease. *Climacteric.* **2007,** *10 (2),* 97–111.

Caparevic, Z.; N. Kostic. [The influence of age and the beginning of menopause on the lipid status, LDL oxidation, and CRP in healthy women]. *Srp. Arh. Celok. Lek.* **2007,** *135 (5–6),* 280–285.

Carr, M.C. The emergence of the metabolic syndrome with menopause. *J. Clin. Endocrinol. Metab.* **2003,** *88 (6),* 2404–2411.

Carroll, M.D.; D.A. Lacher; P.D. Sorlie; J.I. Cleeman; D.J. Gordon; M. Wolz; S.M. Grundy; C.L. Johnson. Trends in serum lipids and lipoproteins of adults, 1960–2002. *JAMA* **2005,** *294 (14),* 1773–1781.

Castelao, J.E.; M. Gago-Dominguez. Risk factors for cardiovascular disease in women: Relationship to lipid peroxidation and oxidative stress. *Med. Hypotheses* **2008,** *71 (1),* 39–44.

Castro, P.; J.L. Miranda; P. Gomez; D.M. Escalante; F.L. Segura; A. Martin; F. Fuentes; A. Blanco J.M. Ordovas; F.P. Jimenez. Comparison of an oleic acid enriched-diet vs NCEP-I diet on LDL susceptibility to oxidative modifications. *Eur. J. Clin. Nutr.* **2000,** *54 (1),* 61–67.

Chakrabarti, S.; O. Lekontseva; S.T. Davidge. Estrogen is a modulator of vascular inflammation. *IUBMB. Life* **2008,** *60 (6),* 376–382.

Chardigny, J.M.; F. Destaillats; C. Malpuech-Brugere; J. Moulin; D.E. Bauman; A.L. Lock; D.M. Barbano; R.P. Mensink; J.B. Bezelgues; P. Chaumont; et al. Do *trans* fatty acids from industrially produced sources and from natural sources have the same effect on cardiovascular disease risk factors in healthy subjects? Results of the trans Fatty Acids Collaboration (TRANSFACT) study.

*Am. J. Clin. Nutr.* **2008,** *87 (3),* 558–566.

Childs, C.E.; M. Romeu-Nadal; G.C. Burdge; P.C. Calder. Gender differences in the n-3 fatty acid content of tissues. *Proc. Nutr. Soc.* **2008,** *67 (1),* 19–27.

Conus, F.; D.B. Allison; R. Rabasa-Lhoret; M. St-Onge; D.H. St-Pierre; A. Tremblay-Lebeau; E.T. Poehlman. Metabolic and behavioral characteristics of metabolically obese but normal-weight women. *J. Clin. Endocrinol. Metab.* **2004,** *89 (10),* 5013.—5020.

Conus, F.; R. Rabasa-Lhoret; F. Peronnet. Characteristics of metabolically obese normal-weight (MONW) subjects. *Appl. Physiol. Nutr. Metab.* **2007,** *32 (1),* 4–12.

Crowe, F.L.; C.M. Skeaff; T.J. Green; A.R. Gray. Serum n-3 long-chain PUFA differ by sex and age in a population-based survey of New Zealand adolescents and adults. *Br. J. Nutr.* **2008,** *99 (1),* 168–174.

Dallongeville, J.; D. Cottel; D. Arveiler; J.P. Tauber; A. Bingham; A. Wagner; J. Fauvel; J. Ferrieres; P. Ducimetiere; P. Amouyel. The association of metabolic disorders with the metabolic syndrome is different in men and women. *Ann. Nutr. Metab.* **2004,** *48 (1),* 43–50.

Das, U.N. Can endogenous lipid molecules serve as predictors and prognostic markers of coronary heart disease? *Lipids Health Dis.* **2008,** *7,* 19.

Davignon, J. The lipid hypothesis. Pathophysiological basis. *Arch. Surg.* **1978,** *113 (1),* 28–34.

Dayton, S.; M. Pearce; S. Hashimoto; W. Dixon; U.A. Tomiyasu. A controlled clinical diet of a diet high in unsaturated fat in preventing complications of atherosclerosis. *Circulation* **1969,** *40 (Suppl. II),* 11–63.

DeCaterina, R. Endothelial dysfunctions: common denominators in vascular disease. *Curr. Opin. Clin. Nutr. Metab. Care* **2000,** *3 (6),* 453–467.

DeCaterina, R.; J.K. Liao; P. Libby. Fatty acid modulation of endothelial activation. *Am. J. Clin. Nutr.* **2000,** *71 (Suppl. 1),* 213S–223S.

deJongh, S.; M.R. Lilien; H.D. Bakker; B.A. Hutten; J.J. Kastelein; E.S. Stroes. Family history of cardiovascular events and endothelial dysfunction in children with familial hypercholesterolemia. *Atherosclerosis* **2002,** *163 (1),* 193–197.

DeLorgeril, M.; P. Salen. Cholesterol lowering, sudden cardiac death and mortality. *Scand. Cardiovasc. J.* **2008,** 1–4.

Donahue, R.P.; K. Rejman; L.B. Rafalson; J. Dmochowski; S. Stranges; M. Trevisan. Sex differences in endothelial function markers before conversion to pre-diabetes: does the clock start ticking earlier among women? The Western New York Study. *Diabetes Care* **2007,** *30 (2),* 354–359.

Dvorak, R.V.; W.F. DeNino; P.A. Ades; E.T. Poehlman. Phenotypic characteristics associated with insulin resistance in metabolically obese but normal-weight young women. *Diabetes* **1999,** *48 (11),* 2210–2214.

Dyerberg, J.; H.O. Bang. Lipid metabolism, atherogenesis, and haemostasis in Eskimos: the role of the prostaglandin-3 family. *Haemostasis* **1979,** *8 (3–5),* 227–233.

Eckel, R.H.; S.M. Grundy; P.Z. Zimmet. The metabolic syndrome. *Lancet* **2005,** *365 (9468),* 1415–1428.

El-Badry, A.M.; R. Graf; P.A. Clavien. Omega 3 - Omega 6: What is right for the liver? *J. Hepatol.* **2007a,** *47 (5),* 718–725.

El-Badry, A.M.; W. Moritz; C. Contaldo; Y. Tian; R. Graf; P.A. Clavien. Prevention of reperfusion injury and microcirculatory failure in macrosteatotic mouse liver by omega-3 fatty acids. *Hepatology* **2007b,** *45 (4),* 855–863.

Erkkila, A.T.; A.H. Lichtenstein; D. Mozaffarian; D.M. Herrington. Fish intake is associated with a reduced progression of coronary artery atherosclerosis in postmenopausal women with coronary artery disease. *Am. J. Clin. Nutr.* **2004,** *80 (3),* 626–632.

Erkkila, A.T.; N.R. Matthan; D.M. Herrington; A. Lichtenstein. Higher plasma docosahexaenoic acid is associated with reduced progression of coronary atherosclerosis in women with CAD. *J. Lipid Res.* **2006,** *47 (12),* 2814–2819.

Ervin, R.B.; J.D. Wright; C.Y. Wang; J. Kennedy-Stephenson. Dietary Intake of Fats and Fatty Acids for the United States Population: 1999–2000. *Centers for Disease Control* **2004,** 348; 1–7.

Expert Panel on Detection, E. a. T. o. H. B. C. i. A. Executive Summary of The Third Report of The National Cholesterol Education Program (NCEP) Expert Panel on Detection, Evaluation, and Treatment of High Blood Cholesterol in Adults (Adult Treatment Panel III). *JAMA* **2001,** *285 (19),* 2486–2497.

Fan, J.; T. Watanabe. Inflammatory reactions in the pathogenesis of atherosclerosis. *J. Atheroscler. Thromb.* **2003,** *10 (2),* 63–71.

Fernandez, M.L.; K.L. West. Mechanisms by which dietary fatty acids modulate plasma lipids. *J. Nutr.* **2005,** *135 (9),* 2075–2078.

Flegal, K.M.; M.D. Carroll; C.L. Ogden; C.L. Johnson. Prevalence and trends in obesity among US adults, 1999–2000. *JAMA* **2002,** *288 (14),* 1723–1727.

Fletcher, B.; K. Berra; P. Ades; L.T. Braun; L.E. Burke; J.L. Durstine; J.M. Fair; G.F. Fletcher; D. Goff; L.L. Hayman; et al. Managing abnormal blood lipids: a collaborative approach. *Circulation* **2005,** *112 (20),* 3184–3209.

Ford, E.S.; W.H. Giles; A.H. Mokdad. The distribution of 10-Year risk for coronary heart disease among US adults: findings from the National Health and Nutrition Examination Survey III. *J. Am. Coll. Cardiol.* **2004,** *43 (10),* 1791–1796.

Fox, C.S.; J.C. Evans; M.G. Larson, W.B. Kannel; D. Levy. Temporal trends in coronary heart disease mortality and sudden cardiac death from 1950 to 1999: the Framingham Heart Study. *Circulation* **2004,** *110 (5),* 522–527.

Fung, T.T.; S.E. Chiuve; M.L. McCullough; K.M. Rexrode; G. Logroscino; F.B. Hu. Adherence to a DASH-style diet and risk of coronary heart disease and stroke in women. *Arch. Intern. Med.* **2008,** *168 (7),* 713–720.

Fung, T.T.; W.C. Willett; M.J. Stampfer; J.E. Manson; F.B. Hu. Dietary patterns and the risk of coronary heart disease in women. *Arch. Intern. Med.* **2001,** *161 (15),* 1857–1862.

Furukawa, S.; T. Fujita; M. Shimabukuro; M. Iwaki; Y. Yamada; Y. Nakajima; O. Nakayama; M. Makishima; M. Matsuda; I. Shimomura. Increased oxidative stress in obesity and its impact on metabolic syndrome. *J. Clin. Invest.* **2004,** *114 (12),* 1752–1761.

Garaulet, M.; F. Perez-Llamas; S. Zamora; F.J. Tebar. [Comparative study of the type of obesity in pre- and postmenopausal women: Relationship with fat cell data, fatty acid composition and endocrine, metabolic, nutritional and psychological variables]. *Med. Clin. (Barc. )* **2002,** *118 (8),* 281–286.

Garg, A. High-monounsaturated-fat diets for patients with diabetes mellitus: a meta-analysis. *Am. J. Clin. Nutr.* **1998,** *67 (Suppl. 3),* 577S–582S.

Getz, G.S.; C.A. Reardon. Paraoxonase, a cardioprotective enzyme: continuing issues. *Curr. Opin. Lipidol.* **2004,** *15 (3),* 261–267.

Gigleux, I.; D.J. Jenkins; C.W. Kendall; A. Marchie; D.A. Faulkner; J.M. Wong; S.R. de; A. Emam; T.L. Parker; E.A. Trautwein; et al. Comparison of a dietary portfolio diet of cholesterol-lowering foods and a statin on LDL particle size phenotype in hypercholesterolaemic participants. *Br. J. Nutr.* **2007,** *98 (6),* 1229–1236.

GISSI. Dietary supplementation with n-3 polyunsaturated fatty acids and vitamin E after myocardial infarction: results of the GISSI-Prevenzione trial. Gruppo Italiano per lo Studio delLA Sopravvivenza nell'Infarto miocardico. *Lancet* **1999,** *354 (9177),* 447–455.

Gottlieb, S.; D. Harpaz; A. Shotan; V. Boyko; J. Leor; M. Cohen; L. Mandelzweig; B. Mazouz; S. Stern; S. Behar. Sex differences in management and outcome after acute myocardial infarction in the 1990s: A prospective observational community-based study. Israeli Thrombolytic Survey Group. *Circulation* **2000,** *102 (20),* 2484–2490.

Gregg, E.W.; Q. Gu; Y.J. Cheng; K.M. Narayan; C.C. Cowie. Mortality trends in men and women with diabetes, 1971 to 2000. *Ann. Intern. Med.* **2007,** *147 (3),* 149–155.

Griffin, B.A. How relevant is the ratio of dietary n-6 to n-3 polyunsaturated fatty acids to cardiovascular disease risk? Evidence from the OPTILIP study. *Curr. Opin. Lipidol.* **2008,** *19 (1),* 57–62.

Griffin, M.D.; T.A. Sanders; I.G. Davies; L.M. Morgan; D.J. Millward; F. Lewis; S. Slaughter; J.A. Cooper; G.J. Miller; B.A. Griffin. Effects of altering the ratio of dietary n-6 to n-3 fatty acids on insulin sensitivity, lipoprotein size, and postprandial lipemia in men and postmenopausal women aged 45–70 y: the OPTILIP Study. *Am. J. Clin. Nutr.* **2006,** *84 (6),* 1290–1298.

Guebre-Egziabher, F.; R. Rabasa-Lhoret; F. Bonnet; J.P. Bastard; M. Desage; M.R. Skilton; H. Vidal; M. Laville. Nutritional intervention to reduce the n-6/n-3 fatty acid ratio increases adiponectin concentration and fatty acid oxidation in healthy subjects. *Eur. J. Clin. Nutr.* **2007,** Aug 15 [Epub ahead of print].

Hammoudeh, A.J.; M. Izraiq; E. Al-Mousa; H. Al-Tarawneh; A. Elharassis; Z. Mahadeen; N. Badran; J. Haddad. Serum lipid profiles with and without CAD: Jordan Hyperlipidaemia and Related Targets Study (JoHARTS-1). *East Mediterr. Health J.* **2008,** *14 (1),* 24–32.

Harris, W.S.; W.C. Poston; C.K. Haddock. Tissue n-3 and n-6 fatty acids and risk for coronary heart disease events. *Atherosclerosis* **2007,** *193 (1),* 1–10.

Hartweg, J.; A.J. Farmer; R. Perera; R.R. Holman; H.A. Neil. Meta-analysis of the effects of n-3 polyunsaturated fatty acids on lipoproteins and other emerging lipid cardiovascular risk markers in patients with type 2 diabetes. *Diabetologia* **2007,** *50 (8),* 1593–1602.

Hegsted, D.M.; R.B. McGandy; M.L. Myers; F.J. Stare.Quantitative effects of dietary fat on serum cholesterol in man. *Am. J. Clin. Nutr.* **1965,** *17 (5),* 281–295.

Heidemann, C.; M.B. Schulze; O.H. Franco; R.M. van Dam; C.S. Mantzoros; F.B. Hu. Dietary Patterns and Risk of Mortality From Cardiovascular Disease, Cancer, and All Causes in a Prospective Cohort of Women. *Circulation* **2008,** *118(3),* 230–237.

Hilpert, K.F.; S.G. West; P.M. Kris-Etherton; K.D. Hecker; N.M. Simpson; P. Alaupovic. Postprandial effect of n-3 polyunsaturated fatty acids on apolipoprotein B-containing lipoproteins and vascular reactivity in type 2 diabetes. *Am. J. Clin. Nutr.* **2007,** *85 (2),* 369–376.

Holvoet, P.; D.H. Lee; M. Steffes; M. Gross; D.R. Jacobs, Jr. Association between circulating oxidized low-density lipoprotein and incidence of the metabolic syndrome. *JAMA* **2008,** *299 (19),* 2287–2293.

Hooper, L.; R.L. Thompson; R.A. Harrison; C.D. Summerbell; A.R. Ness; H.J. Moore; H.V. Worthington; P.N. Durrington; J.P. Higgins; N.E. Capps; et al. Risks and benefits of omega 3 fats for mortality, cardiovascular disease, and cancer: systematic review. *BMJ* **2006,** *332 (7544),* 752–760.

Howard, B.V.; H.L. Van; J. Hsia; J.E. Manson; M.L. Stefanick; S. Wassertheil-Smoller; L.H. Kuller; A.Z. LaCroix; R.D. Langer; N.L. Lasser; et al. Low-fat dietary pattern and risk of cardiovascular disease: the Women's Health Initiative Randomized Controlled Dietary Modification Trial. *JAMA* **2006,** *295 (6),* 655–666.

Hu, F.B.; M.J. Stampfer; J.E. Manson; E. Rimm; G.A. Colditz; B.A. Rosner; C.H. Hennekens; W.C. Willett. Dietary fat intake and the risk of coronary heart disease in women. *N. Engl. J. Med.* **1997,** *337 (21),* 1491–1499.

Hu, F.B.; W.C. Willett. Optimal diets for prevention of coronary heart disease. *JAMA* **2002,** *288 (20),* 2569–2578.

Hurtado de Catalfo, G. E.; G.D. de, I. Influence of testosterone on polyunsaturated fatty acid biosynthesis in Sertoli cells in culture. *Cell Biochem. Funct.* **2005,** *23 (3),* 175–180.

Huxley, R.; M. Woodward; F. Barzi; J.W. Wong; W.H. Pan; A. Patel. Does sex matter in the associations between classic risk factors and fatal coronary heart disease in populations from the Asia-Pacific region? *J. Womens Health (Larchmt.)* **2005,** *14 (9),* 820–828.

Hyun, Y.J.; S.J. Koh; J.S. Chae; J.Y. Kim; O.Y. Kim; H.H. Lim; Y. Jang; S. Park; J.M. Ordovas; J.H. Lee. Atherogenecity of LDL and unfavorable adipokine profile in metabolically obese, normal-weight woman. *Obesity (Silver. Spring)* **2008,** *16 (4),* 784–789.

Institute of Medicine (IOM) Dietary Reference Intakes for Energy, Carbohydrate, Fiber, Fat, Fatty Acids, Cholesterol, Protein, and Amino Acids; 2002.

Jakobsen, M.U.; K. Overvad; J. Dyerberg; M. Schroll; B.L. Heitmann. Dietary fat and risk of coronary heart disease: possible effect modification by gender and age. *Am. J. Epidemiol.* **2004,** *160 (2),* 141–149.

Jenkins, D.J.; A.R. Josse; J.M. Wong; T.H. Nguyen; C.W. Kendall. The portfolio diet for cardiovascular risk reduction. *Curr. Atheroscler. Rep.* **2007,** *9 (6),* 501–507.

Jousilahti, P.; E. Vartiainen; J. Tuomilehto; P. Puska. Sex, age, cardiovascular risk factors, and coronary heart disease: a prospective follow-up study of 14 786 middle-aged men and women in Finland. *Circulation* **1999,** *99 (9),* 1165–1172.

Kannel, W.B.; M. Feinleib; P.M. McNamara; R.J. Garrison; W.P. Castelli. An investigation of coronary heart disease in families. The Framingham offspring study. *Am. J. Epidemiol.* **1979,** *110 (3),* 281–290.

Kark, J.D.; N.A. Kaufmann; F. Binka; N. Goldberger; E.M. Berry. Adipose tissue n-6 fatty acids and acute myocardial infarction in a population consuming a diet high in polyunsaturated fatty acids. *Am. J. Clin. Nutr.* **2003,** *77 (4),* 796–802.

Katsuki, A.; Y. Sumida; H. Urakawa; E.C. Gabazza; S. Murashima; N. Maruyama; K. Morioka; K. Nakatani; Y. Yano; Y. Adachi. Increased visceral fat and serum levels of triglyceride are associated with insulin resistance in Japanese metabolically obese, normal weight subjects with normal glucose tolerance. *Diabetes Care* **2003,** *26 (8),* 2341–2344.

Kelley, D.S.; D. Siegel; M. Vemuri; B.E. Mackey. Docosahexaenoic acid supplementation improves fasting and postprandial lipid profiles in hypertriglyceridemic men. *Am. J. Clin. Nutr.* **2007,** *86 (2),* 324–333.

Keogh, J.B.; G.D. Brinkworth; M. Noakes; D.P. Belobrajdic; J.D. Buckley; P.M. Clifton. Effects of weight loss from a very-low-carbohydrate diet on endothelial function and markers of cardiovascular disease risk in subjects with abdominal obesity. *Am. J. Clin. Nutr.* **2008,** *87 (3),* 567–576.

Keys, A.; R.W. Parlin. Serum cholesterol response to changes in dietary lipids. *Am. J. Clin. Nutr.* **1966,** *19 (3),* 175–181.

Khanapure, S.P.; D.S. Garvey; D.R. Janero; L.G. Letts. Eicosanoids in inflammation: biosynthesis, pharmacology, and therapeutic frontiers. *Curr. Top. Med. Chem.* **2007,** *7 (3),* 311–340.

Kratz, M.; P. Cullen; F. Kannenberg; A. Kassner; M. Fobker; P.M. Abuja; G. Assmann; U. Wahrburg. Effects of dietary fatty acids on the composition and oxidizability of low-density lipoprotein. *Eur. J. Clin. Nutr.* **2002,** *56 (1),* 72–81.

Krauss, R.M.; M. Winston; B.J. Fletcher; S.M. Grundy. Obesity: impact on cardiovascular disease. *Circulation* **1998,** *98 (14),* 1472–1476.

Kressel, G.; B. Trunz; A. Bub; O. Hulsmann; M. Wolters; R. Lichtinghagen; D.O. Stichtenoth; A. Hahn. Systemic and vascuLAr markers of infLAmmation in reLAtion to metabolic syndrome and insulin resistance in adults with elevated atherosclerosis risk. *Atherosclerosis* **2008,** Apr 20 [Epub ahead of print].

Kris-Etherton, P.M. AHA Science Advisory. Monounsaturated fatty acids and risk of cardiovascular disease. American Heart Association. Nutrition Committee. *Circulation* **1999,** *100 (11),* 1253–1258.

Kris-Etherton, P.M.; W.S. Harris; L.J. Appel. Fish consumption, fish oil, omega-3 fatty acids, and cardiovascular disease. *Circulation* **2002,** *106 (21),* 2747–2757.

Kris-Etherton, P.M.; S. Innis; D.A. Ammerican. Dietitians of Canada Position of the American Dietetic Association and Dietitians of Canada: dietary fatty acids. *J. Am. Diet. Assoc.* **2007,** *107 (9),* 1599–1611.

Kris-Etherton, P.M.; T.A. Pearson; Y. Wan; R.L. Hargrove; K. Moriarty; V. Fishell; T.D. Etherton. High-monounsaturated fatty acid diets lower both plasma cholesterol and triacylglycerol concentrations. *Am. J. Clin. Nutr.* **1999,** *70 (6),* 1009–1015.

Kromhout, D. Serum cholesterol in cross-cultural perspective. The Seven Countries Study. *Acta Cardiol.* **1999,** *54 (3),* 155–158.

Kuller, L.H.; L.R. Simkin-Silverman; R.R. Wing; E.N. Meilahn; D.G. Ives. Women's Healthy Lifestyle Project: A randomized clinical trial: results at 54 months. *Circulation* **2001,** *103 (1),* 32–37.

Kurokawa, A.; K. Azuma; T. Mita; Y. Toyofuku; Y. Fujitani; T. Hirose; K. Iwabuchi; H. Ogawa; S. Takeda; R. Kawamori; H. Watada. 2-Methoxyestradiol reduces monocyte adhesion to aortic endothelial cells in ovariectomized rats. *Endocr. J.* **2007,** *54 (6),* 1027–1031.

Kuvin, J.T.; M.E. Ramet; A.R. Patel; N.G. Pandian; M.E. Mendelsohn; R.H. Karas. A novel mechanism for the beneficial vascular effects of high-density lipoprotein cholesterol: enhanced vasorelaxation and increased endothelial nitric oxide synthase expression. *Am. Heart. J.* **2002,** *144 (1),* 165–172.

Lamarche, B.; S. Desroches. Metabolic syndrome and effects of conjugated linoleic acid in obesity and lipoprotein disorders: the Quebec experience. *Am. J. Clin. Nutr.* **2004,** *79 ( Suppl.6),* 1149S–1152S.

Lamarche, B.; I. Lemieux; J.P. Despres. The small, dense LDL phenotype and the risk of coronary heart disease: epidemiology, patho-physiology and therapeutic aspects. *Diabetes Metab.* **1999,** *25 (3),* 199–211.

Lanz, J.R.; A.C. Pereira; E. Martinez; J.E. Krieger. Metabolic syndrome and coronary artery disease: is there a gender specific effect? *Int. J. Cardiol.* **2006,** *107 (3),* 317–321.

Lapointe, A.; E.M. Balk; A.H. Lichtenstein. Gender differences in plasma lipid response to dietary fat. *Nutr. Rev.* **2006,** *64 (5 Pt 1),* 234–249.

Lapointe, A.; C. Couillard; S. Lemieux. Effects of dietary factors on oxidation of low-density lipoprotein particles. *J. Nutr. Biochem.* **2006,** *17 (10),* 645–658.

LaRosa, J.C. Lipids and cardiovascular disease: do the findings and therapy apply equally to men and women? *Womens Health Issues* **1992,** *2 (2),* 102–111.

Lemaitre, R.N.; I.B. King; T.E. Raghunathan; R.M. Pearce; S. Weinmann; R.H. Knopp; M.K. Copass; L.A. Cobb; D.S. Siscovick. Cell membrane trans-fatty acids and the risk of primary cardiac arrest. *Circulation* **2002,** *105 (6),* 697–701.

Leren, P. The Oslo diet-heart study. Eleven-year report. *Circulation* **1970,** *42 (5),* 935–942.

Lerner, D.J.; W.B. Kannel. Patterns of coronary heart disease morbidity and mortality in the sexes: a 26-year follow-up of the Framingham population. *Am. Heart J.* **1986,** *111 (2),* 383–390.

Li, Z.; J.D. Otvos; S. Lamon-Fava; W.V. Carrasco; A.H. Lichtenstein; J.R. McNamara; J.M. Ordovas; E.J. Schaefer. Men and women differ in lipoprotein response to dietary saturated fat and cholesterol restriction. *J. Nutr.* **2003,** *133 (11),* 3428–3433.

Libby, P.; P.M. Ridker; A. Maseri. Inflammation and atherosclerosis. *Circulation* **2002,** *105(9),* 1135–1143.

Lichtenstein, A.H. Thematic review series: patient-oriented research. Dietary fat, carbohydrate, and protein: effects on plasma lipoprotein patterns. *J. Lipid Res.* **2006,** *47 (8),* 1661–1667.

Lichtenstein, A.H.; L.J. Appel; M. Brands; M. Carnethon; S. Daniels; H.A. Franch; B. Franklin; P. Kris-Etherton; W.S. Harris; B. Howard; et al. Diet and lifestyle recommendations revision 2006: a scientific statement from the American Heart Association Nutrition Committee. *Circulation* **2006,** *114 (1),* 82–96.

Lichtenstein, A.H.; L.M. Ausman; S.M. Jalbert; E.J. Schaefer. Effects of different forms of dietary hydrogenated fats on serum lipoprotein cholesterol levels. *N. Engl. J. Med.* **1999,** *340 (25),* 1933–1940.

Lobo, R.A. Metabolic syndrome after menopause and the role of hormones. *Maturitas* **2008,** *60 (1),* 10–18.

Lopez-Garcia, E.; M.B. Schulze; J.E. Manson; J.B. Meigs; C.M. Albert; N. Rifai; W.C. Willett; F.B. Hu. Consumption of (n-3) fatty acids is related to plasma biomarkers of inflammation and endothelial activation in women. *J. Nutr.* **2004,** *134 (7),* 1806–1811.

Lovegrove, J.A.; S.S. Lovegrove; S.V. Lesauvage; L.M. Brady; N. Saini; A.M. Minihane; C.M. Williams. Moderate fish-oil supplementation reverses low-platelet, long-chain n-3 polyunsaturated fatty acid status and reduces plasma triacylglycerol concentrations in British Indo-Asians. *Am. J. Clin. Nutr.* **2004,** *79 (6),* 974–982.

Lupattelli, G.; S. Marchesi; A.R. Roscini; D. Siepi; F. Gemelli; M. Pirro; H. Sinzinger; G. Schillaci; E. Mannarino. Direct association between high-density lipoprotein cholesterol and endothelial function in hyperlipemia. *Am. J. Cardiol.* **2002,** *90 (6),* 648–650.

Luscombe-Marsh, N.D.; M. Noakes; G.A. Wittert; J.B. Keogh; P. Foster; P.M. Clifton. Carbohydrate-restricted diets high in either monounsaturated fat or protein are equally effective at promoting fat loss and improving blood lipids. *Am. J. Clin. Nutr.* **2005,** *81 (4),* 762–772.

Mackey, R.H.; L.H. Kuller; K. Sutton-Tyrrell; R.W. Evans; R. Holubkov; K.A. Matthews. Hormone therapy, lipoprotein subclasses, and coronary calcification: the Healthy Women Study. *Arch. Intern. Med.* **2005,** *165 (5),* 510–515.

Magkos, F.; B.W. Patterson; B.S. Mohammed; S. Klein; B. Mittendorfer. Women produce fewer but triglyceride-richer very low-density lipoproteins than men. *J. Clin. Endocrinol. Metab.* **2007,** *92 (4),* 1311–1318.

Manolio, T.A.; T.A. Pearson; N.K. Wenger; E. Barrett-Connor; G.H. Payne; W.R. Harlan. Cholesterol and heart disease in older persons and women. Review of an NHLBI workshop. *Ann. Epidemiol.* **1992,** *2 (1–2),* 161–176.

Marchesi, S.; G. Vaudo; G. Lupattelli; R. Lombardini; A.R. Roscini; M. Brozzetti; D. Siepi; E. Mannarino. Fat distribution and endothelial function in normal-overweight menopausal women. *J. Clin. Pharm. Ther.* **2007,** *32 (5),* 477–482.

Marra, C.A.; M.J. de Alaniz. Influence of testosterone administration on the biosynthesis of unsaturated fatty acids in male and female rats. *Lipids* **1989,** *24 (12),* 1014–1019.

McNeill, A.M; W.D. Rosamond; C.J. Girman; S.H. Golden; M.I. Schmidt; H.E. East; C.M. Ballantyne; G. Heiss. The metabolic syndrome and 11-year risk of incident cardiovascular disease in the atherosclerosis risk in communities study. *Diabetes Care* **2005,** *28 (2),* 385–390.

Mensink, R.P. Effects of stearic acid on plasma lipid and lipoproteins in humans. *Lipids* **2005,** *40 (12),* 1201–1205.

Mesalic, L.; E. Tupkovic; S. Kendic; D. Balic. Correlation between hormonal and lipid status in women in menopause. *Bosn. J. Basic Med. Sci.* **2008,** *8 (2),* 188–192.

Milcent, C.; B. Dormont; I. Durand-Zaleski; P.G. Steg. Gender differences in hospital mortality and use of percutaneous coronary intervention in acute myocardial infarction: microsimulation analysis of the 1999 nationwide French hospitals database. *Circulation* **2007,** *115 (7),* 833–839.

Mittendorfer, B. Sexual dimorphism in human lipid metabolism. *J. Nutr.* **2005,** *135 (4),* 681–686.

Mittendorfer, B.; J.F. Horowitz; S. Klein. Gender differences in lipid and glucose kinetics during short-term fasting. *Am. J. Physiol. Endocrinol. Metab.* **2001,** *281 (6),* E1333–E1339.

Mittendorfer, B.; B.W. Patterson; S. Klein. Effect of sex and obesity on basal VLDL-triacylglycerol kinetics. *Am. J. Clin. Nutr.* **2003,** *77 (3),* 573–579.

Moriel, M.; S. Behar; D. Tzivoni; H. Hod; V. Boyko; S. Gottlieb. Management and outcomes of elderly women and men with acute coronary syndromes in 2000 and 2002. *Arch. Intern. Med.* **2005,** *165 (13),* 1521–1526.

Mosca, L.; S.M. Grundy; D. Judelson; K. King; M. Limacher; S. Oparil; R. Pasternak; T.A. Pearson; R.F. Redberg; S.C. Smith, Jr.; et al. Guide to Preventive Cardiology for Women.AHA/ACC Scientific Statement Consensus panel statement. *Circulation* **1999,** *99 (18),* 2480–2484.

Mozaffarian, D.; J.S. Gottdiener; D.S. Siscovick. Intake of tuna or other broiled or baked fish versus fried fish and cardiac structure, function, and hemodynamics. *Am. J. Cardiol.* **2006,** *97 (2),* 216–222.

Mueck, A.O.; H. Seeger. Biochemical markers surrogating on vascular effects of sex steroid hormones. *Gynecol. Endocrinol.* **2006,** *22 (3),* 163–173.

Narins, C.R.; F.S. Ling; M. Fischi; D.R. Peterson; J. Bausch; W. Zareba. In-hospital mortality among women undergoing contemporary elective percutaneous coronary intervention: a reexamination of the gender gap. *Clin. Cardiol.* **2006,** *29 (6),* 254–258.

National Institutes of Health. Clinical Guidelines on the Identification, Evaluation, and Treatment of Overweight and Obesity in Adults--The Evidence Report. *Obes. Res* **1998,** *6 Suppl 2,* 51S-209S.

NCEP. Expert Panel on Detection, E. a. T. o. H. B. C. i. A. Third Report of the National Cholesterol Education Program (NCEP) Expert Panel on Detection, Evaluation, and Treatment of High Blood Cholesterol in Adults (Adult Treatment Panel III) final report. *Circulation* **2002,** *106 (25),* 3143–3421.

Nicholls, S.; P. Lundman. The emerging role of lipoproteins in atherogenesis: beyond LDL cholesterol. *Semin. Vasc. Med.* **2004,** *4 (2),* 187–195.

Nishida, M.; T. Moriyama; K. Ishii; S. Takashima; K. Yoshizaki; Y. Sugita; K. Yamauchi-Takihara. Effects of IL-6, adiponectin, CRP and metabolic syndrome on subclinical atherosclerosis. *Clin Chim. Acta* **2007,** *384 (1–2),* 99–104.

Noakes, M.; J.B. Keogh; P.R. Foster; P.M. Clifton. Effect of an energy-restricted, high-protein, low-fat diet relative to a conventional high-carbohydrate, low-fat diet on weight loss, body composition, nutritional status, and markers of cardiovascular health in obese women. *Am. J. Clin. Nutr.* **2005,** *81 (6),* 1298–1306.

Novack, V.; D.E. Cutlip; A. Jotkowitz; N. Lieberman; A. Porath. Reduction in sex-based mortality difference with implementation of new cardiology guidelines. *Am. J .Med.* **2008,** *121 (7),* 597–603.

Oyama, N.; P. Gona; C.J. Salton; M.L. Chuang; R.R. Jhaveri; S.J. Blease; A.R. Manning; M. Lahiri; R.M. Botnar;D. Levy; et al. Differential impact of age, sex, and hypertension on aortic atherosclerosis: the Framingham Heart Study. *Arterioscler. Thromb. Vasc. Biol.* **2008,** *28 (1),* 155–159.

Pilote, L.; K. Dasgupta; V. Guru; K.H. Humphries; J. McGrath; C. Norris; D. Rabi; J. Tremblay; A. Alamian; T. Barnett; et al. A comprehensive view of sex-specific issues related to cardiovascular disease. *CMAJ.* **2007,** *176 (6),* S1–44.

Plan and operation of the Third National Health and Nutrition Examination Survey, 1988–94.

Series 1: programs and collection procedures. *Vital Health Stat. 1* **1994,** *(32),* 1–407.

Poredos, P. Endothelial dysfunction and cardiovascular disease. *Pathophysiol. Haemost. Thromb.* **2002,** *32 (5–6),* 274–277.

Qiao, X.; K.R. McConnell; R.A. Khalil. Sex steroids and vascular responses in hypertension and aging. *Gend. Med.* **2008,** *5 (Suppl. A),* S46–S64.

Quyyumi, A.A. Women and ischemic heart disease: pathophysiologic implications from the Women's Ischemia Syndrome Evaluation (WISE) Study and future research steps. *J. Am. Coll. Cardiol.* **2006,** *47 (Suppl. 3),* S66--S71.

Racial/ethnic and socioeconomic disparities in multiple risk factors for heart disease and stroke—United States, 2003. *MMWR Morb. Mortal. Wkly. Rep.* **2005,** *54 (5),* 113–117.

Rashid, S.; J. Genest. Effect of obesity on high-density lipoprotein metabolism. *Obesity (Silver. Spring)* **2007,** *15 (12),* 2875–2888.

Reaven, G. Metabolic syndrome: pathophysiology and implications for management of cardiovascular disease. *Circulation* **2002,** *106 (3),* 286–288.

Redberg, R.F. Gender differences in acute coronary syndrome: invasive versus conservative approach. *Cardiol. Rev.* **2006,** *14 (6),* 299–302.

Regitz-Zagrosek, V.; E. Lehmkuhl; M.O. Weickert. Gender differences in the

metabolic syndrome and their role for cardiovascular disease. *Clin. Res. Cardiol.* **2006,** *95 (3),* 136–147.

Reine, A.; M. Colmenero; E. Aguayo de Hoyos; F. Aros; H. Marti; R. Claramonte; J. Cunat. Gender differences in management and outcome of patients with acute myocardial infarction. *Int. J, Cardiol.* **2007,** *116 (3),* 389–395.

Rhee, Y.; M.J. Paik; K.R. Kim; Y.G. Ko; E.S. Kang; B.S. Cha; H.C. Lee; S.K. Lim. Plasma free fatty acid level patterns according to cardiovascular risk status in postmenopausal women. *Clin. Chim. Acta* **2008,** *392 (1-2),* 11–16.

Riccardi, G.; R. Giacco; A. Rivellese. Dietary fat, insulin sensitivity and the metabolic syndrome. *Clin. Nutr.* **2004,** *23 (4),* 447–456.

Ringseis, R.; S. Gahler; C. Herter; K. Eder. Conjugated linoleic acids exert similar actions on prostanoid release from aortic and coronary artery smooth muscle cells. *Int. J. Vitam. Nutr. Res.* **2006,** *76 (5),* 281–289.

Riserus, U. Fatty acids and insulin sensitivity. *Curr. Opin. Clin. Nutr. Metab. Care* **2008,** *11 (2),* 100–105.

Ristic, V.; G. Ristic. [Role and importance of dietary polyunsaturated fatty acids in the prevention and therapy of atherosclerosis]. *Med. Pregl.* **2003,** *56 (1–2),* 50–53.

Rosamond, W.D.; A.R. Folsom; L.E. Chambless; C.H. Wang. Coronary heart disease trends in four United States communities. The Atherosclerosis Risk in Communities (ARIC) study 1987–1996. *Int. J. Epidemiol.* **2001,** *30 (Suppl. 1),* S17–S22.

Rosano, G.M.; C. Vitale; M. Fini. Hormone replacement therapy and cardioprotection: what is good and what is bad for the cardiovascular system? *Ann. N.Y. Acad. Sci.* **2006,** *1092,* 341–348.

Ross, R.; J.A. Glomset. The pathogenesis of atherosclerosis (first of two parts). *N. Engl. J. Med.* **1976a,** *295 (7),* 369–377.

Ross, R.; J.A. Glomset. The pathogenesis of atherosclerosis (second of two parts). *N. Engl. J. Med.* **1976b,** *295 (8),* 420–425.

Ruderman, N. B.; S.H. Schneider; P. Berchtold. The "metabolically-obese," normal-weight individual. *Am. J. Clin. Nutr.* **1981,** *34 (8),* 1617–1621.

Rupp, H.; D. Wagner; T. Rupp; L.M. Schulte; B. Maisch. Risk stratification by the "EPA+DHA level" and the "EPA/AA ratio" focus on anti-inflammatory and antiarrhythmogenic effects of long-chain omega-3 fatty acids. *Herz* **2004,** *29 (7),* 673–685.

Sakuma, N.; M. Yoshikawa; T. Hibino; N. Ohte; T. Kamiya; M. Kunimatsu; G. Kimura; M. Inoue. HDL3 exerts a more powerful antiperoxidative and protective effect against peroxidative modification of LDL than HDL2 does. *J. Nutr. Sci. Vitaminol. (Tokyo)* **2002,** *48 (4),* 278–282.

Schachinger, V.; M.B. Britten; A.M. Zeiher. Prognostic impact of coronary vasodilator dysfunction on adverse long-term outcome of coronary heart disease. *Circulation* **2000,** *101 (16),* 1899–1906.

Schachinger, V.; A.M. Zeiher. Atherosclerosis-associated endothelial dysfunction. *Z. Kardiol.* **2000,** *89 (Suppl. 9),* IX/70–IX/74.

Sellers, M.M.; J.N. Stallone. Sympathy for the devil: the role of thromboxane in the regulation of vascular tone and blood pressure. *Am. J. Physiol. Heart Circ. Physiol.* **2008,** *294 (5),* H–978–H1986.

Sies, H.; W. Stahl; A. Sevanian. Nutritional, dietary and postprandial oxidative stress. *J. Nutr.* **2005,** *135 (5),* 969–972.

Simopoulos, A.P. The importance of the omega-6/omega-3 fatty acid ratio in cardiovascular disease and other chronic diseases. *Exp. Biol. Med. (Maywood.)* **2008,** *233 (6),* 674–688.

Simopoulos, A.P. The omega-6/omega-3 fatty acid ratio, genetic variation, and cardiovascular disease. Asia Pac. *J. Clin. Nutr.* **2008,** *17 (Suppl. 1),* 131–134.

Skulas-Ray, A.C.; S.G. West; M.H. Davidson; P.M. Kris-Etherton. Omega-3 fatty acid concentrates in the treatment of moderate hypertriglyceridemia. *Expert. Opin. Pharmacother.* **2008,** *9 (7),* 1237–1248.

Spieker, L.E.; I. Sudano; D. Hurlimann; P.G. Lerch; M.G. Lang; C. Binggeli; R. Corti; F. Ruschitzka; T.F. Luscher; G. Noll. High-density lipoprotein restores endothelial function in hypercholesterolemic men. *Circulation* **2002,** *105 (12),* 1399–1402.

Stark, A.H.; M.A. Crawford; R. Reifen. Update on alpha-linolenic acid. *Nutr. Rev.* **2008,** *66 (6),* 326–332.

Steinbaum, S.R. The metabolic syndrome: an emerging health epidemic in women. *Prog. Cardiovasc. Dis.* **2004,** *46 (4),* 321–336.

Steinberg, D.; S. Parthasarathy; T.E. Carew; J.C. Khoo; J.L. Witztum. Beyond cholesterol. Modifications of low-density lipoprotein that increase its atherogenicity. *N. Engl. J. Med.* **1989,** *320 (14),* 915–924.

Stocker, R.; J.F. Keaney, Jr. Role of oxidative modifications in atherosclerosis. *Physiol. Rev.* **2004,** *84 (4),* 1381–1478.

Suwaidi, J.A.; S. Hamasaki; S.T. Higano; R.A. Nishimura; D.R. Holmes, Jr.; A. Lerman. A. Long-term follow-up of patients with mild coronary artery disease and endothelial dysfunction. *Circulation* **2000,** *101 (9),* 948–954.

Tappia, P.S.; M.R. Dent; N. Aroutiounova; A.P. Babick; H. Weiler. Gender differences in the modulation of cardiac gene expression by dietary conjugated linoleic acid isomers. *Can. J. Physiol. Pharmacol.* **2007,** *85 (3-4),* 465–475.

Tappia, P.S.; R. Mangat; C. Gabriel; M.R. Dent; N. Aroutiounova; H. Weiler. Gender differences in the cardiac response to dietary conjugated linoleic acid isomers. *Can. J. Physiol. Pharmacol.* **2006,** *84 (2),* 257–264.

Tay, J.; G.D. Brinkworth; M. Noakes; J. Keogh; P.M. Clifton. Metabolic effects of weight loss on a very-low-carbohydrate diet compared with an isocaloric high-carbohydrate diet in abdominally obese subjects. *J. Am. Coll. Cardiol.* **2008,** *51 (1),* 59–67.

Tholstrup, T. Influence of stearic acid on hemostatic risk factors in humans. *Lipids* **2005,** *40 (12),* 1229–1235.

Thomas-Moya, E.; M. Gianotti; A.M. Proenza; I. Llado. Paraoxonase 1 response to a high-fat diet: gender differences in the factors involved. *Mol. Med.* **2007,** *13 (3–4),* 203–209.

Tobin, J.N.; S. Wassertheil-Smoller; J.P. Wexler; R.M. Steingart; N. Budner; L. Lense; J. Wachspress. Sex bias in considering coronary bypass surgery. *Ann. Intern. Med.* **1987,** *107 (1),* 19–25.

Toles, C.A. The incidence of cardiovascular disease in menopausal women on hormone replacement therapy: a clinical evidence-based medicine review. *J. Natl.* Black. *Nurses Assoc.* **2007,** *18 (2),* 75–80.

Tong, W.; H. Lai; C. Yang; S. Ren; S. Dai; S. Lai. Age, gender and metabolic syndrome-related coronary heart disease in U.S. adults. *Int. J. Cardiol.* **2005,** *104 (3),* 288–291.

Tonstad, S.; E. Sandvik; P.G. Larsen; D. Thelle. Gender differences in the prevalence and determinants of the metabolic syndrome in screened subjects at risk for coronary heart disease. *Metab. Syndr. Relat Disord.* **2007,** *5 (2),* 174–182.

Tricon, S.; G.C. Burdge; C.M. Williams; P.C. Calder; P. Yaqoob. The effects of conjugated linoleic acid on human health-related outcomes. *Proc. Nutr. Soc.* **2005,** *64 (2),* 171–182.

Tsimikas, S.; P.D. Reaven. The role of dietary fatty acids in lipoprotein oxidation and atherosclerosis. *Curr. Opin. Lipidol.* **1998,** *9 (4),* 301–307.

Tsitouras, P.D.; F. Gucciardo; A.D. Salbe; C. Heward; S.M. Harman. High omega-3 fat intake improves insulin sensitivity and reduces CRP and IL6, but does not affect other endocrine axes in healthy older adults. *Horm. Metab. Res.* **2008,** *40 (3),* 199–205.

Tuttle, K.R.; L.A. Shuler; D.P. Packard; J.E. Milton; K.B. Daratha; D.M. Bibus; R.A. Short. Comparison of low-fat versus Mediterranean-style dietary intervention after first myocardial infarction (from The Heart Institute of Spokane Diet Intervention and Evaluation Trial). *Am. J. Cardiol.* **2008,** *101 (11),* 1523–1530.

US Food and Drug Administration. FDA Announces Qualified Health Claims for Omega-3 Fatty Acids.; 04.

Vaccarino, V.; L. Parsons; N.R. Every; H.V. Barron; H.M. Krumholz. Sex-based differences in early mortality after myocardial infarction. National Registry of Myocardial Infarction 2 Participants. *N. Engl. J. Med.* **1999,** *341 (4),* 217–225.

van Eijk, L.T.; M.J. Dorresteijn; P. Smits; J.G. van der Hoeven; M.G. Netea; P. Pickkers. Gender differences in the innate immune response and vascular reactivity following the administration of endotoxin to human volunteers. *Crit. Care Med.* **2007,** *35 (6),* 1464–1469.

Vasan, R.S.; L.M. Sullivan; P.W. Wilson; C.T. Sempos; J. Sundstrom; W.B. Kannel; D. Levy; R.B. D'Agostino. Relative importance of borderline and elevated levels of coronary heart disease risk factors. *Ann. Intern. Med.* **2005,** *142 (6),* 393–402.

Villar, I.C.; A.J. Hobbs; A. Ahluwalia. Sex differences in vascular function: implication of endothelium-derived hyperpolarizing factor. *J. Endocrinol.* **2008,** *197 (3),* 447–462.

Vogel, R.A. Cholesterol lowering and endothelial function. *Am. J. Med.* **1999,** *107 (5),* 479–487.

vonSchacky C. A review of omega-3 ethyl esters for cardiovascular prevention and treatment of increased blood triglyceride levels. *Vasc. Health Risk Manag.* **2006,** *2 (3),* 251–262.

Wajchenberg, B.L. Subcutaneous and visceral adipose tissue: their relation to the metabolic syndrome. *Endocr. Rev.* **2000,** *21 (6),* 697–738.

Wang, C.; W.S. Harris; M. Chung; A.H. Lichtenstein; E.M. Balk; B. Kupelnick; H.S. Jordan; J. Lau. n-3 Fatty acids from fish or fish-oil supplements, but not alpha-linolenic acid, benefit cardiovascular disease outcomes in primary- and secondary-prevention studies: a systematic review. *Am. J. Clin. Nutr.* **2006,** *84 (1),* 5–17.

Warensjo, E.; U. Riserus; I.B. Gustafsson; R. Mohsen; T. Cederholm; B. Vessby. Effects of saturated and unsaturated fatty acids on estimated desaturase activities during a controlled dietary intervention. *Nutr. Metab. Cardiovasc. Dis.* **2008.**

West, S.G. Effect of diet on vascular reactivity: an emerging marker for vascular risk. *Curr. Atheroscler. Rep.* **2001,** *3 (6),* 446–455.

Wijendran, V.; K.C. Hayes. Dietary n-6 and n-3 fatty acid balance and cardiovascular health. *Annu. Rev. Nutr.* **2004,** *24,* 597–615.

Willett, W.C. The role of dietary n-6 fatty acids in the prevention of cardiovascular disease. *J. Cardiovasc. Med. (Hagerstown.)* **2007,** *8 (Suppl. 1),* S42–S45.

Wilt, T.J.; H.E. Bloomfield; R. MacDonald; D. Nelson; I. Rutks; M. Ho; G. Larsen; A. McCall; S. Pineros; A. Sales. Effectiveness of statin therapy in adults with coronary heart disease. *Arch. Intern. Med.* **2004,** *164 (13),* 1427–1436.

World Health Organization (WHO) Total number of deaths by cause and sex, latest available year; 07.

Yao, M.; S.B. Roberts. Dietary energy density and weight regulation. *Nutr. Rev.* **2001,** *59 (8 Pt 1),* 247–258.

Yim, J.E.; S. Heshka; J.B. Albu; S. Heymsfield; D. Gallagher. Femoral-gluteal subcutaneous and intermuscular adipose tissues have independent and opposing relationships with CVD risk. *J. Appl. Physiol.* **2008,** *104 (3),* 700–707.

Younis, N.; V. Charlton-Menys; R. Sharma; H. Soran; P.N. Durrington. Glycation of LDL in non-diabetic people: Small dense LDL is preferentially glycated both in vivo and in vitro. *Atherosclerosis* **2008.**

Yung, L.M.; F.P. Leung; X. Yao; Z.Y. Chen; Y. Huang. Reactive oxygen species in vascular wall. *Cardiovasc. Hematol. Disord. Drug Targets* **2006,** *6 (1),* 1–19.

Yu-Poth, S.; T.D. Etherton; C.C. Reddy; T.A. Pearson; R. Reed; G. Zhao; S. Jonnalagadda; Y. Wan; P.M. Kris-Etherton. Lowering dietary saturated fat and total fat reduces the oxidative susceptibility of LDL in healthy men and women. *J. Nutr.* **2000,** *130 (9),* 2228–2237.

Yusuf, S.; S. Hawken; S. Ounpuu; T. Dans; A. Avezum; F. Lanas; M. McQueen; A. Budaj; P. Pais; J. Varigos; L. Lisheng. Effect of potentially modifiable risk factors associated with myocardial infarction in 52 countries (the INTERHEART study): case-control study. *Lancet* **2004,** *364 (9438),* 937–952.

Yusuf, S.; S. Reddy; S. Ounpuu; S. Anand. Global burden of cardiovascular diseases: part I: general considerations, the epidemiologic transition, risk factors, and impact of urbanization. *Circulation* **2001,** *104 (22),* 2746–2753.

Zamaria, N. Alteration of polyunsaturated fatty acid status and metabolism in health and disease. *Reprod. Nutr. Dev.* **2004,** *44 (3),* 273–282.

Zhao, G.; T.D. Etherton; K.R. Martin; P.J. Gillies; S.G. West; P.M. Kris-Etherton. Dietary alpha-linolenic acid inhibits proinflammatory cytokine production by peripheral blood mononuclear cells in hypercholesterolemic subjects. *Am. J. Clin. Nutr.* **2007,** *85 (2),* 385–391.

# 8

# Free Fatty Acids: Role in Insulin Resistance, Type 2 Diabetes, and Cardiovascular Disease

**Guenther Boden**
*Division of Endocrinology/Diabetes/Metabolism and the Clinical Research Center, Temple University School of Medicine, Philadelphia, PA 19140*

## Introduction

Obesity, which has reached epidemic proportions in the United States and other industrialized nations, is now spreading out to the rest of the world (Bray, 2004; Mokdad et al., 2001). Obesity is associated with a two- to five-fold increase (depending on gender and age) in the risk for atherosclerotic vascular disease (ASVD), such as heart attacks, strokes, and peripheral arterial disease (Bray, 2004). Most, and perhaps all, of the risks for ASVD are explained by the fact that obese people are prone to have a number of serious health problems, including type 2 diabetes mellitus (T2DM), hypertension, atherogenic dyslipidemias, and disorders of coagulation and fibrinolysis. Important in understanding why obesity is associated with these disorders is the recognition that obesity causes insulin resistance and a state of low-grade chronic inflammation (Bray, 2004; Pickup & Crook, 1998; Tataranni & Ortega, 2005) (Fig. 8.1). Insulin resistance is a core pathogenetic abnormality in the development of T2DM, and also plays a role in the pathogenesis of hypertension and atherogenic dyslipidemias (Ingelsson et al., 2005; Reaven, 1988). Exactly how obesity causes insulin resistance is still not completely understood. However, inasmuch as excessive body fat is what most differentiates obese from lean people, it stands to reason that factors related to adipose tissue may cause insulin resistance. In fact, it is now recognized that fat, aside from being a storage site for unspent calories, is a metabolically active tissue that synthesizes and secretes a large number of biologically active substances that are collectively called adipokines (Kershaw & Flier, 2004). Many of these adipokines were postulated to cause insulin resistance (Tataranni & Ortega, 2005). So far, however, a major role as a physiologic link between obesity and insulin resistance in humans is established only for free fatty acids (FFAs). Therefore, this review focuses on the effects of FFAs on three major insulin targets (i.e., skeletal muscle, liver, and endothelial cells). In addition, recent data indicating a direct link between elevated plasma FFA levels, the activation of the proinflammatory nuclear

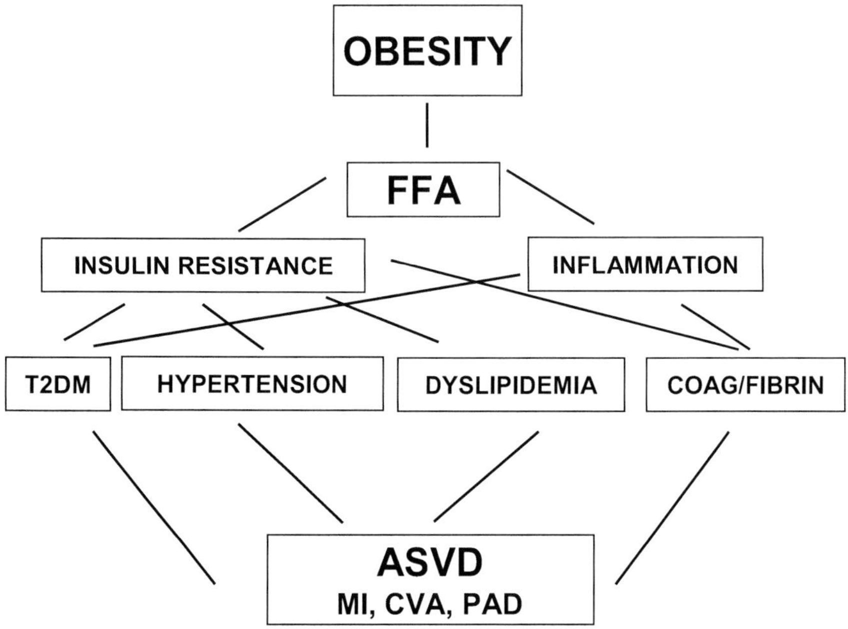


**Fig. 8.1.** Relationship between obesity, insulin resistance, inflammation, and atherosclerotic vascular disease (ASVD). Obesity causes insulin resistance and a state of low-grade inflammation. Both contribute to the development of several disorders, including type 2 diabetes mellitus (T2DM), hypertension, atherogenic dyslipidemia, and disorders of coagulation (COAG) and fibrinolysis (FIBRIN)—all of which are independent risk factors for the development of atherosclerotic vascular disease. Abbreviations: MI: Myocardial infarction; CVA: cerobrovascular accident; PAD: Peripheral arterial disease.

factor-κB (NF-κB) pathway, and the synthesis and release of inflammatory cytokines are also discussed.

## FFAs and Insulin Resistance

Several factors can lead to elevated plasma FFA levels in obese people including: the consumption of fat-rich meals, an increased release of FFAs from enlarged adipose tissue, a decreased FFA clearance (Bjorntorp et al., 1969), and, at a later stage, increased lipolysis as a result of insulin resistance (Jensen et al., 1989). Once established, acute as well as chronically elevated plasma FFA levels will dose-dependently inhibit several metabolic insulin actions, such as glucose uptake, glycogen synthesis, lipogenesis, and nitric oxide (NO) production, in all people regardless of gender and age. For instance, raising plasma FFA levels acutely decreases insulin-stimulated glucose uptake in skeletal muscle (reviewed by Boden, 1997), whereas the lowering of chronically elevated plasma FFA levels improves insulin-stimulated glucose uptake (Santomauro et al., 1999). Acute elevations of plasma FFA levels also interfere with the insulin suppression of hepatic glucose production. They do this primarily by inhibiting insulin- stimulated suppression of glycogenolysis with little acute effect on gluconeogenesis (Boden et al., 2002). Raising plasma FFA levels also decreases the insulin-induced enhancement of endothelial NO production and peripheral blood flow (Steinberg et al., 1997).

## FFAs and Insulin Secretion

The National Health and Nutrition Examination Survey 3 (NHANES 3) showed that 23% of overweight/obese individuals had impaired glucose tolerance, and 23% had T2DM. The remaining 54% (who presumably were also insulin-resistant, at least to some extent) had normal glucose tolerance (Benjamin et al., 2003). Insulin resistance will result in impaired glucose tolerance or T2DM unless compensated by an oversecretion of insulin. Thus, one assumes that the 54% of overweight/obese individuals, who maintained normal glucose tolerance despite being insulin-resistant, did so by increasing their insulin secretion appropriately, whereas the remaining 46% were unable to do so. The link between insulin resistance and compensatory insulin secretion is usually assumed to be very small and difficult to detect increments in blood glucose. No evidence supports this hypothesis, although it cannot be ruled out either. On the other hand, evidence suggests that FFAs, which are strong insulin secretagogues, may be the link between obesity-associated insulin resistance and the compensatory hypersecretion of insulin (Boden et al., 1996; Kim et al., 2007).

### *Acute Effects of FFAs on Insulin Secretion*

Elevating plasma FFA levels acutely has been shown to increase serum-insulin levels more than 40 years ago (Felber & Vanotti, 1964; Pelkonen et al., 1968). Moreover, FFAs stimulate insulin secretion when infused directly into the pancreatic artery (Crespin et al., 1973). Of interest was the recent recognition that long-chain fatty acids are ligands for the membrane- bound G-protein receptor GPR-40, which is preferentially expressed in pancreatic β-cells of rodents and humans (Brown et al., 2005). A physiologic role for GPR-40 in insulin secretion, however, is not yet established. Evidence suggests that, depending on the prevailing blood-glucose levels, the FFA-induced increase in plasma-insulin concentrations can be due to: the stimulation of insulin secretion, a decrease in insulin clearance, or a combination of both. For instance, Hennes et al. (2007) showed that, in healthy young women in whom blood-sugar concentrations were clamped at 5.5 mM, raising plasma FFAs from ≈0.5 to 1.1 mM increased insulin secretion without affecting insulin clearance. On the other hand, when blood glucose was clamped at 7 mM, the same increase in plasma FFAs raised serum insulin partly by increasing insulin secretion and partly by decreasing insulin clearance; when blood glucose was clamped at 11 mM, the increase in serum insulin was almost entirely due to an increase in insulin clearance with little change in insulin secretion (Hennes et al., 1997). Similar results were reported by others (Balent et al., 2002). The mechanisms responsible for these changes in insulin secretion and clearance are not known. However, the development of insulin resistance was frequently associated with a decrease in insulin clearance (Kim et al., 2005; Mittelman et al., 2000; Peiris et al., 1986 ). Thus, one could speculate that reducing insulin clearance may be an effort to compensate for insulin resistance in situations where compensatory additional insulin secretion is insufficient.

## *Chronic Effects of FFAs on Insulin Secretion*

On the basis of animal experiments, Unger proposed in 1995 a lipotoxicity hypothesis: plasma FFA levels of <1.5 mmol/L induce both hyperinsulinemia and insulin resistance, thereby maintaining normal glycemia, whereas more severe elevations of plasma FFA levels produce insulin resistance and β-cell dysfunction (Unger, 1995). Although very high FFA levels (>2–3 mmol/L) are likely toxic to β-cells, such high FFA levels are rarely seen in human subjects. In vitro studies in isolated rat islets and in an isolated perfused rat pancreas showing biphasic effects of FFAs on insulin secretion (an initial increase followed after ≈24 hours by a decrease in insulin secretion) (Zhou & Grill, 1994), are also apparently not applicable to the human experience. Most obese individuals have high FFA levels and are insulin-resistant (Bray, 2004; Reaven et al., 1988). If elevated FFA levels did cause β-cell dysfunction, all obese individuals with elevated FFA levels (i.e., most obese people) would have to become diabetic. This, however, is not the case (Benjamin et al., 2003). In fact, a large body of evidence shows that even chronically elevated FFA levels stimulate insulin secretion in healthy people (Boden & Chen, 1995; Jensen et al., 2003; Kashyap et al., 2003). Moreover, the lowering of chronically elevated plasma FFA levels in obese nondiabetic and diabetic subjects decreased insulin-secretion rates by 30–50% (Boden et al., 1998; Dobbins et al., 1998; Santomauro et al., 1999), indicating that the elevated plasma FFA levels had supported a large part of basal insulin secretion. Lastly, in a prospective study of 107 glucose-tolerant Pima Indians who had elevated plasma FFA levels at the start of the study, no deterioration occurred in their acute insulin responses to intravenous glucose over a 5.8-year follow-up period (Stefan et al., 2003). Together, these results indicate that in healthy individuals, long-term elevations of plasma FFA levels within the physiological range stimulate, rather than decrease, insulin secretion. Why then are some obese individuals unable to compensate for their FFA-induced insulin resistance with increased insulin secretion? The answer seems to be that these patients have an inherited β-cell defect (Boden et al., 1968; Pimenta et al., 1995). Therefore, apparently, in these individuals, elevated plasma FFA levels are unable to elicit a normal compensatory insulin secretory response and may, in fact, compound an already existing β-cell dysfunction. Compatible with this concept are reports showing (i) that raising plasma FFA levels for 72 hours in glucose-tolerant, first-degree relatives of patients with T2DM resulted in impaired insulin secretion in response to hyperglycemia (Kashyap et al., 2003) and (ii) that in patients with impaired glucose tolerance and/or overt T2DM, 24-hour elevations of plasma FFA levels resulted in subnormal glucose-stimulated insulin secretion rates (Storgaard et al., 2003). Thus, current evidence in human subjects suggests that in individuals with impaired β-cell function (i.e., in pre-diabetic individuals or in patients with impaired glucose tolerance or T2DM), a long-term elevation of plasma FFAs cannot adequately potentiate, and may even impair, glucose-stimulated insulin secretion. Supporting this concept, in vitro studies showed that basal insulin secretion from normal Wistar rat islets increased when cultured for 7 days in 2 mM of FFAs, but decreased in islets from Zucker fatty rats (who are predisposed to develop diabetes) (Hirose et al., 1996). More recently, it was proposed that the combination of increased FFAs and increased glucose may lead to β-cell insufficiency (the β-cell gluco-lipotoxicity hypothesis) (El-Assaad et al., 2003). While this may explain the continuous decline in β-cell function in patients with uncontrolled diabetes and high FFA levels, β-cell gluco-lipotoxicity obviously cannot be responsible for the initial development of T2DM.

## Mechanisms of FFA-Induced Insulin Resistance

### *Skeletal Muscle*

Based on work performed with rat heart and diaphragm muscle, Randle (Randle et al., 1963) proposed more than 40 years ago his glucose–fatty acid cycle hypothesis: FFAs inhibit insulin-stimulated glucose uptake by increasing fat oxidation, resulting in a rise in the muscle-citrate concentration. Citrate inhibits phosphofructokinase 1, the enzyme that controls flux through glycolysis. Inhibiting glycolysis will increase glucose-6-phosphate levels, and inhibit the hexokinase reaction and glucose uptake. Subsequent studies in humans, however, revealed that the FFA-induced increase in fat oxidation and the associated decrease in carbohydrate oxidation were probably not the causes of the insulin resistance because they occurred several hours before any inhibition of an insulin-stimulated glucose uptake (ISGU) occurred (Boden et al., 1994). Rather, FFAs were found to inhibit insulin action at the level of glucose transport and/or phosphorylation. This conclusion was based on two observations: (i) FFAs inhibit all intracellular pathways of glucose metabolism [i.e., ISGU, glycogen synthesis, and glycolysis equally (Boden & Chen, 1995)] and (ii) FFAs inhibit the insulin-stimulated activation of phosphatidylinositol 3 kinase (PI3K), a key enzyme in the insulin-signaling pathway (Dresner et al., 1999). Several mechanisms were proposed to explain how FFAs interfere with insulin signaling. First, an increase in plasma FFA levels resulted in an intramyocellular accumulation of triglycerides and of several lipid metabolites, including long-chain acyl-CoA and diacylglycerol (DAG) (Boden et al., 2001; Itani et al., 2002; Ravikumar et al., 2005). Of those, DAG, rather than long-chain acyl-CoA or triglycerides, was the most likely lipid metabolite responsible for the FFA-induced insulin resistance (Yu et al., 2002). DAG is a potent allosteric activator of conventional and novel protein kinase C (PKC) isoforms (Farese, 2004). Elevated plasma FFA concentrations activated PKC-β2 and -δ several-fold during 4 hours of euglycemic–hyperinsulinemic clamping in human skeletal muscle (Itani et al., 2002). PKCs are serine/threonine kinases that can cause insulin resistance by decreasing tyrosine phosphorylation of the insulin-receptor substrate-1/2 (IRS-1/2) (Yu et al., 2002) (Fig. 8.2).

Another mechanism is an FFA-mediated increase in oxidative stress, resulting in the production of reactive oxygen species (ROS) and endoplasmic reticulum (ER) stress (Gregor &Hotamisligil, 2007). Both, oxidative stress and ER stress, can trigger the activation of several serine/threonine kinases, including the c-jun N-terminal kinase (JNK) and the IκB kinase (IKK), which were involved in the development of insulin resistance (Hirosumi et al., 2002; Itani et al., 2002; Nakatani et al., 2005; Ozcan et al., 2004) as well as inflammation (Hirosumi et al., 2002) (Fig. 8.2).

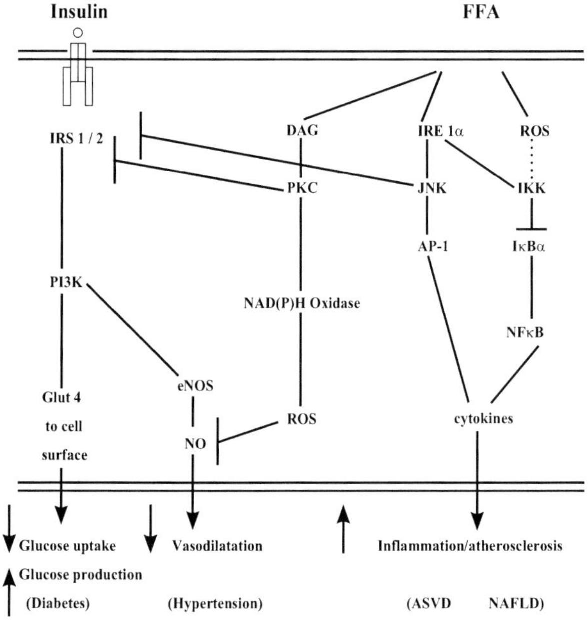


**Fig. 8.2.** Potential mechanisms of free fatty acid (FFA)-induced insulin resistance and inflammation. The key event is an increase in plasma FFA concentration. This leads to the accumulation of diacylglycerol (DAG) and the activation of protein kinase C (PKC) in skeletal muscle, liver, and vascular endothelial cells. It is assumed that the activation of PKC interrupts insulin signaling by serine phosphorylation of IRS–1/2, resulting in a decrease in tyrosine phosphorylation of IRS–1/2. In endothelial cells, PKC was shown to activate NADPH oxidase, which produces reactive oxygen species and destroys nitric oxide (NO). The elevation of plasma FFA levels also leads to the production of inflammatory and proatherogenic proteins through the activation of the IKK/IκB-α/NFκB and endoplasmic reticulum stress (IRE-1α, JNK) pathways. Increased FFA-induced insulin resistance reduces glucose uptake in muscle, and increases glucose production in the liver. Together, this results in hyperglycemia. In endothelial cells, FFA-mediated insulin resistance results in decreased NO and decreased vasodilatation, which may contribute to the development of hypertension. In muscle and liver, FFA-induced accumulation of reactive oxygen species (ROS) and the activation of the IKK/IκB-α/NFκB and JNK pathways result in chronic low-grade inflammation, which may promote atherosclerotic vascular disease (ASVD) and non-alcoholic fatty liver disease (NAFLD). Other Abbreviations: eNOS:endothelial nitric oxide synthase; Glut4: glucose transporter 4; IκBα: inhibitor of NFκB; IKK: IκB kinase; IRE-1α: inositol requiring enzyme 1 α; IRS: insulin receptor substrate; JNK: c jun N-terminal kinase; NADPH: nicotinamide adenine dinucleotide phosphate, reduced; NFκB: nuclear factor κ B; PI3 K: phosphoinositide 3 kinase.

### *Liver*

Acutely elevated plasma FFA levels also produce hepatic insulin resistance (i.e., they inhibit insulin's suppressive action on hepatic glucose production, specifically on glycogenolysis) (Boden et al., 2002). The mechanism by which FFAs cause insulin resistance in the liver appears to be similar to the mechanisms by which FFAs cause insulin resistance in skeletal muscle, consisting of the activation of several serine/threonine kinases which, by decreasing tyrosine phosphorylation of the IRS-1/2, interrupt insulin signaling (Boden et al., 2005; Lam et al., 2002).

### *Endothelial Cells*

Insulin increases peripheral vascular blood flow (Baron, 2002). In vivo and in vitro evidence suggests that this is due to the insulin-mediated stimulation of NO production via the IRS/PI3 kinase pathway in endothelial cells (Zeng et al., 2000). FFAs reduce the insulin-induced increase in peripheral venous NO and in peripheral blood flow (Steinberg et al., 1997) by interrupting insulin signaling at the IRS/PI3 kinase level. In addition, FFAs can activate nicotinamide adenine dinucleotide phosphate, reduced (NADPH) oxidase in a DAG/PKC-dependent manner, leading to the production of ROS and the destruction of NO (Inoguchi et al., 2000).

## FFAs and Inflammation

Obesity is associated with a state of low-grade inflammation and with increased synthesis and the release of a large number of cytokines and chemokines (collectively called adipokines) from the expanded adipose tissue (Kershaw & Flier, 2004). Plasma levels of many of these adipokines—including tumor necrosis factor-α (TNF-α), interleukin (IL)-1β, IL-6, monocyte chemotactic protein-1, plasminogen activator inhibitor-1, and others—are elevated in the blood taken from obese people (Tataranni & Ortega, 2005). Several of these adipokines are inflammatory and proatherogenic, whereas others inhibit insulin action. Recent studies did shed some light on the reasons for the increased synthesis and the release of adipokines from adipose tissue in obesity. The acute elevation of plasma FFA levels (by infusion of heparinized lipid emulsions) activated the NFκB pathway in human skeletal muscle (Itani et al., 2002) and in rat liver (Boden et al., 2005). Similarly, linoleic acid (C18:2) activated the NFκB, and increased IL-6 and TNF-α in cultured human adipocytes and stromal vascular cells obtained from biopsied human adipose tissue (Chung et al., 2005). NFκB is a transcription factor involved in virtually all inflammatory processes (Barnes & Karin, 1997). The IκB, the physiological inhibitor of the NFκB, is bound to the NFκB in the cytoplasm, and inhibits its entrance into the nucleus. When phosphorylated by the IKK-β or possibly other serine kinases, the IκB separates from the NFκB complex, is ubiquitinated, and degraded. This allows the NFκB to enter the nucleus, where it induces the expression of genes responsible for the synthesis of numerous inflammatory proteins (Barnes & Karin, 1997). Not surprisingly, therefore, the observed changes (a decrease in the IκB-α and the activation of the IKK and NFκB that were seen after plasma FFA levels were raised acutely) were accompanied by an increased hepatic expression of several NFκB-dependent inflammatory cytokines, including IL1-β, TNF-α, and IL-6, and by an increase in plasma MCP-1 levels (Boden et al., 2005). Other studies showed that mice fed a high-fat diet developed subacute hepatic inflammation that was accompanied by the NFκB activation and an increased production and secretion of several inflammatory cytokines (Cai et al., 2005). The effectors of the NFκB activation upstream of the IKK are not well-established. However, high-fat diets as well as FFAs resulted in an ER stress-mediated increase in several unfolded protein response (UPR) proteins (include IRE-1) and the activation of the JNK as well as the activation of the NFκB and excessive ROS production (Gregor & Hotamisligil, 2007; Ozcan et al., 2004) (Fig. 8.2). ER stress, JNK, and ROS all activated the NFκB (reviewed by Gregor & Hotamisligil, 2007).

## FFAs and Matrix Metalloproteinases (MMPs) and Tissue Inhibitors of MMPs (TIMPs)

MMPs belong to a family of enzymes with proteolytic activity for extracellular (EC) matrix proteins, including collagens, protoglycans, and elastins (Visse & Nagase, 2003). The activity of these enzymes is tightly controlled by tissue inhibitors of MMPs (TIMPs) (Visse & Nagase, 2003). The EC matrix constantly undergoes synthesis and degradation. Changes in the MMP/TIMP activity ratio, therefore, can lead to changes in EC matrix formation and can have health consequences. In fact, evidence shows that changes in MMP activities (i) play key roles in the development of unstable coronary artery disease (Galis et al., 1994; Newby, 2005), (ii) are involved in the development of vascular aneurysms (Longo et al., 2002), and (iii) (elevated plasma MMP levels) predict cardiovascular mortality in patients with coronary artery disease (Blankenberg et al., 2003). As pointed out, obese individuals are insulin-resistant and hyperinsulinemic; they frequently have elevated plasma FFA levels, and their risk to develop ASVD is several-fold higher than that of nonobese individuals. The possibility that insulin resistance, perhaps via hyperinsulinemia and/or elevated FFAs, may promote ASVD by changing the MMP/TIMP balance was recently investigated. In this study, physiological hyperinsulinemia for 4 hours increased the active forms of MMP-2, MMP-9, and MT1-MMP in the aortic tissue of normal rats, and high plasma FFA levels further augmented the stimulatory activity of hyperinsulinemia (Boden et al., 2008). Neither hyperinsulinemia nor elevated FFAs, however, changed the activities of the two major TIMPs (TIMP-1 and TIMP-2). Thus, even a brief increase in hyperinsulinemia and FFA levels, a condition which is commonly seen in obese insulin-resistant individuals, dramatically increased the MMP/TIMP balance (Fig. 8.3). Over time, this could lead to the degradation of the EC matrix, and together with other inflammatory changes, contribute to the increased risk for ASVD in obesity.

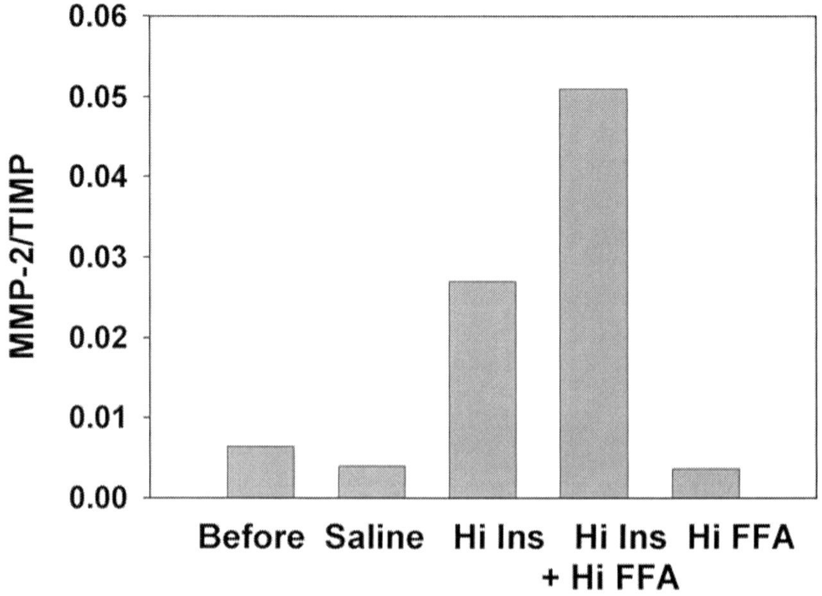


**Fig. 8.3.** Proteolytic activity of matrix metalloproteinase 2 (MMP-2) in rat aorta. Shown are ratios of MMP-2 over tissue inhibitors of MMPs (TIMPs) (the arithmetic mean of TIMP-1 and TIMP-2) before and after 4 hours of saline, high insulin (Hi Ins), high insulin plus high free fatty acid (Hi FFA), or high FFA during euglycemic clamps (n = 6).

## References


Balent, B.; G. Goswami; G. Goodloe; E. Rogatsky; O. Rauta; R. Nezami; L. Mints; R.H. Angeletti; D.T. Stein. Acute elevation of NEFA causes hyperinsulinemia without effect of insulin secretion rate in healthy human subjects. *Ann. N.Y. Acad. Sci.* **2002,** *967,* 535–543.

Barnes, P.J.; M. Karin. Nuclear factor-kappaB: a pivotal transcription factor in chronic inflammatory diseases. *N. Engl. J. Med.* **1997,** *336,* 1066–1071.

Baron, A.D. Insulin resistance and vascular function. *J. Diabetes Complications* **2002,** *16,* 92–102.

Benjamin, S.M.; R. Valdez; L.S. Geiss; D.B. Rolka; K.M. Narayan. Estimated number of adults with prediabetes in the US in 2000: opportunities for prevention. *Diabetes Care* **2003,** *26,* 645–649.

Bjorntorp, P.; H. Bergman; E. Varnauskas. Plasma free fatty acid turnover in obesity. *Acta Med. Scand.* **1969,** *185,* 351–356.

Blakenberg, S.; H.J. Rupprecht; O. Poirier; C. Bickel; M. Smieja; G. Hafner;J. Meyer; F. Cambien; L. Tiret. AtheroGene Investigators. Plasma concentrations and genetic variation of matrix metalloproteinase 9 and prognosis of patients with cardiovascular disease. *Circulation* **2003,** *107,* 1579–1585.

Boden, G. Role of fatty acids in the pathogenesis of insulin resistance and NIDDM. *Diabetes* **1997,** *46,* 3–10.

Boden, G.; X. Chen. Effects of fat on glucose uptake and utilization in patients with non-insulin-dependent diabetes. *J. Clin. Invest.* **1995,** *96,* 1261–1268.

Boden, G.; X. Chen; N. Iqbal. Acute lowering of plasma fatty acids lowers basal insulin secretion in diabetic and nondiabetic subjects. *Diabetes* **1998**, *47,* 1609–1612.

Boden, G.; X. Chen; J. Ruiz; J.V. White; Rossetti. Mechanisms of fatty acid-induced inhibition of glucose uptake. *J. Clin. Invest.* **1994,** *93,* 2438–2446.

Boden, G.; X. Chen; J.L. Urbain. Evidence for a circadian rhythm of insulin sensitivity in patients with NIDDM caused by cyclic changes in hepatic glucose production. *Diabetes* **1996,** *45,* 1044–1050.

Boden, G.; P. Cheung; T.P. Stein; K. Kresge; M. Mozzoli. FFA cause hepatic insulin resistance by inhibiting insulin suppression of glycogenolysis. *Am. J. Physiol.* **2002,** *283,* E12–E19.

Boden, G.; B. Lebed; M. Schatz; C. Homko; S. Lemieux. Effects of acute changes of plasma free fatty acids on intramyocellular fat content and insulin resistance in healthy subjects. *Diabetes* **2001,** *50,* 1612–1617.

Boden, G.; P. She; M. Mozzoli; P. Cheung; K. Gumireddy; P. Reddy; X. Xiang; Z. Luo; N. Ruderman. Free fatty acids produce insulin resistance and activate the proinflammatory nuclear factor-kappaB pathway in rat liver. *Diabetes* **2005,** *54,* 3458–3465.

Boden, G.; J.S. Soeldner; R.E. Gleason; A. Marble. Elevated serum human growth hormone and decreased serum insulin in prediabetic males after intravenous tolbutamide and glucose. *J. Clin. Invest.* **1968,** *47,* 729–739.

Boden, G.; W. Song; L. Pashko; K. Kresge. In vivo effects of insulin and free fatty acids on matrix metalloproteinases in rat aorta. *Diabetes* **2008,** *57,* 476–483.

Bray, G.A. Medical consequences of obesity. *J. Clin. Endocrinol. Metab.* **2004,** *89,* 2583–2589.

Brown, A.J.; S. Jupe; C.P. Briscoe. A family of fatty acid binding receptors. *DNA Cell Biol.* **2005,** *24,* 54–61.

Cai, D.; M. Yuan; D.F. Frantz; P.A. Melendez; L. Hansen; J. Lee; S.E. Shoelson. Local and systemic insulin resistance resulting from hepatic activation of IKK-beta and NF-kappaB. *Nat. Med.* **2005,** *11,* 183–190.

Chung, S.; J.M. Brown; J.N. Provo; R. Hopkins; M.K. McIntosh. Conjugated linoleic acid promotes human adipocyte insulin resistance through NFkappaB-dependent cytokine production. *J. Biol. Chem.* **2005,** *280,* 38445–38456.

Crespin, S.R.; W.B. Greenough; D. Steinberg. Stimulation of insulin secretion by long-chain free fatty acids. *J. Clin. Invest.* **1973,** *52,* 1979–1984.

Dobbins, R.L.; M.W. Chester; M.B. Daniels; D.J. McGarry; D.T. Stein. Circulating fatty acids are essential for efficient glucose-stimulation insulin secretion after prolonged fasting in humans. *Diabetes* **1998,** *47,* 1613–1618.

Dresner, A.; D. Laurent; M. Marcucci; M.E. Griffin; S. Dufour; G.W. Cline;L.A. Slezak; D.K. Andersen; R.S. Hundal; D.L. Rothman; K.F. Petersen;G.I. Shulman. Effects of free fatty acids on glucose transport and IRS-1 associated phosphatidylinositol 3-kinase activity. *J. Clin. Invest.* **1999, 103,** 253–259.

El-Assaad, W.; J. Buteau; M.L. Peyot; C. Noland; R. Roduit; S. Hardy; E. Joly; G. Dbaibo; L. Rosenberg; M. Prentki. Saturated fatty acids synergize with elevated glucose to cause pancreatic β-cell death. *Endocrinology* **2003,** *144,* 4154–4163.

Farese R. Protein kinase C. *Diabetes Mellitus: A Fundamental and Clinical Text;* D. LeRoith et al., Eds.; Lippincott, Williams and Wilkinson: Philadelphia, 2004; pp. 301–316.

Felber, J.P.; A. Vanotti. Effects of fat infusions on glucose tolerance and insulin plasma levels. *Med. Exp.* **1964,** *10,* 153–156.

Galis, Z.S.; G.K. Sukhova; M.W. Lark; P. Libby. Increased expression of matrix metalloproteinases and matrix degrading activity in vulnerable regions of human atherosclerotic plaques. *J. Clin. Invest.* **1994,** *94,* 2493–2503.

Gregor, M.F.; G.S. Hotamisligil. Adipocyte stress: The endoplasmic reticulum and metabolic disease. *J. Lipid Res.* **2007,** *48,* 1905–1914.

Hennes, M.M.I.; A. Dua; A.H. Kissebah. Effects of free fatty acids and glucose on splanchnic insulin dynamics. *Diabetes* **1997,** *46,* 57–62.

Hirose, H.; Y.H. Lee; L.R. Inman; Y. Nagasawa; J.H. Johnson; R.H. Unger. Defective fatty acid mediated beta-cell compensation in Zucker diabetic fatty rats. *J. Biol. Chem.* **1996,** *271,* 5633–5637.

Hirosumi, J.; G. Tuncman; L. Chang; C.Z. Gorgun; K.T. Uysal; K. Maeda;M. Karin; G.S. Hotamisligil. A central role for JNK in obesity and insulin resistance. *Nature 420,* 333–336.

Ingelsson, E.; J. Sundstrom; J. Arnlov; B. Zethelius; L. Lind. Insulin resistance and risk of congestive heart failure. *JAMA* **2005,** *294,* 334–341.

Inoguchi, T.; P. Li; F. Umeda; H.Y. Yu; M. Kakimoto; M. Imamura; T. Aoki; T. Etoh; T. Hashimoto; M. Naruse; H. Sano; H. Utsumi; H. Nawata. High glucose level and free fatty acid stimulate reactive oxygen species production through protein kinase C-dependent activation of NAD(P)H oxidase in cultured vascular cells. *Diabetes* **2000,** *49,* 1939–1945.

Itani, S.I.; N.B. Ruderman; F. Schmieder; G. Boden. Lipid-induced insulin resistance in human muscle is associated with changes in diacylglycerol, protein kinase C, and IkappaB-alpha. *Diabetes* **2002,** *51,* 2005–2011.

Jensen, M.D.; M.W. Haymond; R.A. Rizza; P.E. Cryer; J.M. Miles.Influence of body fat distribution on free fatty acid metabolism obesity. *J. Clin. Invest.* **1989**, *83,* 1168–1173.

Jensen, C.B.; H. Storgaard; J.J. Holst; F. Dela; S. Madsbad; A.A. Vaag. Insulin secretion and cellular glucose metabolism after prolonged low-grade intralipid infusion in young men. *J. Clin. Endocrinol. Metab.* **2003,** *88,* 2774–2783.

Kashyap, S.; R. Belfort; A. Gastaldelli; T. Pratipanawatr; R. Berria; W. Pratipanawatr; M. Bajaj; L. Mandarino; R. DeFronzo; K. Cusi. A sustained increase in plasma free fatty acids impairs insulin secretion in nondiabetic subjects genetically predisposed to develop type 2 diabetes. *Diabetes* **2003,** *52,* 2461–2474.

Kershaw, E.E.; J.S. Flier. Adipose tissue as an endocrine organ. *J. Clin. Endocrinol. Metab.* **2004,** *89,* 2548–2556.

Kim, S.H.; F. Abbasi; J.W. Chu; T.L. McLaughlin; C. Lamendola; K.S. Polonsky; G.M. Reaven. Rosiglitazone reduces glucose-stimulated insulin secretion rate and increases insulin clearance in nondiabetic, insulin-resistance individuals. *Diabetes* **2005,** *54,* 2447–2452.

Kim, S.P.; K.H. Catalano; I.R. Hsiu; J.D. Chiu; J.M. Richey; R.N. Bergman. Nocturnal free fatty acids are uniquely elevated in the longitudinal development of diet-induced insulin resistance and hyperinsulinemia. *Am. J. Phyisol. Endocrinol. Metab.* **2007,** *292,* E1590–E1598.

Lam, T.K.T.; H. Yoshii; C.A. Haber; E. Bogdanovic; L. Lam; I.G. Fantus;A. Giacca. Free fatty acid-induced hepatic insulin resistance: a potential role for protein kinase C-delta. *Am. J. Physiol.* **2002,** *283,* E682–E691.

Longo, G.M.; W. Xiong; T.C. Greiner; Y. Zhao; N. Fiotti; B.T. Baxter. Matrix metalloproteinases 2 and 9 work in concert to produce aortic aneurysms. *J. Clin. Invest.* **2002,** *110,* 625–632.

Mittelman, S.D.; G.W. Van Citters; S.P. Kim; D.A. Davis; M.K. Dea;M. Hamilton-Wessler; R.N. Bergman. Longitudinal compensation for fat-induced insulin resistance includes reduced insulin clearance and enhanced β-cell response. *Diabetes* **2000,** *49,* 2116–2125.

Mokdad, A.N.; B.A. Bowman; E.S. Ford. The continuing epidemics of obesity and diabetes in the United States. *JAMA* **2001,** *286,* 1195–1200.

Nakatani, Y.; H. Kaneto; D. Kawamori; K. Yoshiuchi; M. Hatazaki; T.A. Matsuoka; K. Ozawa; S. Ogawa; M. Hori; Y. Yamasaki; M. Matsuhisa. Involvement of endoplasmic reticulum stress in insulin resistance and diabetes. *J. Biol. Chem.* **2005,** *280,* 847–851.

Newby, A.C. Dual role of matrix metalloproteinases (matrixns) in intimal thickening of atherosclerotic plaque rupture. *Physiol. Rev.* **2005,** *85,* 1–31..

Ozcan, U.; Q. Cao; E. Yilmaz; A-H. Lee; N.N. Iwakoshi; E. Ozdelen;G. Tuncman; C. Gorgun; L.H. Glimcher; G.S. Hotamisligil. Endoplasmic reticulum stress links obesity, insulin action, and type 2 diabetes. *Science* **2004,** *306*, 457–461.

Peiris, A.N.; R.A. Mueller; G.A. Smith; M.F. Struve; A.H. Kissebah. Splanchnic insulin metabolism in obesity. Influence of body fat distribution. *J. Clin. Invest.* **1986,** *78,* 1648–1657.

Pelkonen, R.; A. Miettinen; M.R. Taskinen; E.A. Nikkila. Effects of acute elevation on plasma glycerol, triglyceride and FFA levels on glucose utilization and plasma insulin. *Diabetes* **1968,** *17,* 76–82.

Pickup, J.C.; M.A. Crook. Is type II diabetes mellitus a disease of the innate immune system? *Diabetologia* **1998,** *41,* 1241–1248.

Pimenta, W.; M. Korytkowski; A. Mitrakou; T. Jenssen; H. Yki-Jarvinen; W. Evron; G. Daily; J. Gerich. Pancreatic beta-cell dysfunction as the primary genetic lesion in NIDDM: evidence from studies in normal glucose-tolerant individuals with a first-degree NIDDM relative. *JAMA* **1995,** *273*, 1855–1861.

Randle, P.J.; P.B. Garland; C.N. Hales; E.A. Newsholme. The glucose-fatty acid cycle, its role in insulin sensitivity and the metabolic disturbances of diabetes mellitus. *Lancet 1* **1963,** 785–789.

Ravikumar, B.; P.E. Carey; J.E. Snaar; D.K. Deelchand; D.B. Cook; R.D. Neely; P.T. English; M.J. Firbank; P.G. Morris; R. Taylor. Real-time assessment of postprandial fat storage in liver and skeletal muscle in health and type 2 diabetes. *Am. J. Physiol. Endocrinol. Metab.* **2005,** *288,* E789–E797.

Reaven, G.M. Banting lecture 1988. Role of insulin resistance in human disease. *Diabetes* **1988,** *37,* 1595–1607.

Reaven, G.M.; C. Hollenbeck; C-Y. Jeng; M.S. Wu; Y.D. Chen. Measurement of plasma glucose, free fatty acid, lactate and insulin for 24 h in patients with NIDDM. *Diabetes* **1988,** *37,*1020–1024.

Santomauro, A.T.; G. Boden; M. Silva; D.M. Rocha; R.F. Santos; M.J. Ursich; P.G. Strassmann;

B.L. Wajchenberg. Overnight lowering of free fatty acids with acipimox improves insulin resistance and glucose tolerance in obese diabetic and nondiabetic subjects. *Diabetes* **1999,** *48,* 1836–1841.

Stefan, N.; M. Stumvoll; C. Bogardus; P.A. Tataranni. Elevated plasma nonesterified fatty acids are associated with deterioration of acute insulin response in IGT but not NGT. *Am. J. Physiol.* **2003,** *284,* E1156–E1161.

Steinberg, H.O.; M. Tarshoby; R. Monestel; G. Hook; J. Cronin; A. Johnson;B. Bayazeed; A.D. Baron. Elevated circulating free fatty acid levels impair endothelium-dependent vasodilation. *J. Clin. Invest.* **1997,** *100,* 1230–1239.

Storgaard, H.; C.B. Jensen; A.A. Vaag; A. Volund; S. Madsbad. Insulin secretion after short- and long-term low-grade free fatty acid infusion in men with increased risk of developing type 2 diabetes. *Metabolism* **2003,** *52,*885–894.

Tataranni, P.A.; E. Ortega. A burning question. Does adipokines-induced activation of the immune system mediate the effect of overnutrition on type 2 diabetes? *Diabetes* **2005,** *54,* 917–927.Unger, R.H. Lipotoxicity in the pathogenesis of obesity-dependent NIDDM. Genetic and clinical implications. *Diabetes* **1995,** *44,* 863–870.

Visse, R.; H. Nagase. Matrix metalloproteinases and tissue inhibitors of metalloproteinases. Structure, function and biochemistry. *Circ. Res.* **2003,** *92,* 827–839.

Yu, C.; Y. Chen; G.W. Cline; D. Zhang; H. Zong; Y. Wang; R. Bergeron;J.K. Kim; S.W. Cushman; G.J. Cooney; B. Atcheson; M.F. White; E.W. Kraegen; G.I. Shulman. Mechanism by which fatty acids inhibit activation of insulin receptor substrate-1 (IRS-1)-associated phosphatidylinositol 3-kinase activity in muscle. *J. Biol. Chem.* **2002,** *277,* 50230–50236.

Zeng, G.; F.H. Nystrom; L.V. Ravichandran; L.N. Cong; M. Kirby; H. Mostowski; M.J. Quon. Roles for insulin receptor, PI3-kinase and Akt in insulin-signaling pathways related to production of nitric oxide in human vascular endothelial cells. *Circulation* **2000,** *101,* L1539–L1545.

Zhou, Y.P.; V.E. Grill. Long-term exposure of rat pancreatic islets to fatty acids inhibits glucose-induced insulin secretion and biosynthesis through a glucose fatty acid cycle. *J. Clin. Invest.* **1994,** *93,* 870–876.

# 9

# Gender Differences in Gene Expression Due to Fatty Acids: Role in Atherosclerosis and Cardiovascular Disease

**Natalie P. Prairie[1] and Paramjit S. Tappia[2]**

*Institute of Cardiovascular Sciences, St. Boniface General Hospital Research Centre & Departments of [1]Human Nutritional Sciences, Faculty of Human Ecology and [2]Human Anatomy & Cell Science, Faculty of Medicine, University of Manitoba, Winnipeg, Canada*

## Introduction

Dietary interventions for human health and the prevention and treatment of disease are growing areas of interest. The n-3 polyunsaturated fatty acids (PUFAs) are essential for normal growth and development, and they may play an important role in the prevention and treatment of coronary artery disease, hypertension, diabetes, arthritis, other inflammatory and autoimmune disorders, and cancer (Simopoulos, 2000). Specifically, their beneficial effects are shown in the prevention and management of coronary heart disease, hypertension, type 2 diabetes, renal disease, rheumatoid arthritis, ulcerative colitis, and pulmonary disease (Appel et al., 1993, 1994; Arita et al., 2005; Belluzzi et al., 1994; Calder, 2002; Cawood et al., 2005; Darlington & Stone, 2001; Das, 2000, 2004; Mahmud et al., 2006). Other fatty acids, such as conjugated linoleic acid (CLA), are also linked with cardiovascular benefits (Inoue et al., 2004; Khosla & Fungwe, 2001; Kritchevsky et al., 2000; Nagao et al., 2003; Pal et al., 2005; Tappia et al., 2006).

Even though men and women share most genetic information, they exhibit significant differences in susceptibilities to complex diseases such as atherosclerosis and diabetes (Ordovas, 2007). An individual's gender and genetic background determine nutrient status, metabolic response, and predisposition to diet-related diseases. Nutrigenomics, or molecular nutrition, refers to research that investigates the interaction between the human genome and nutrient intake (H.M. Roche, 2004). This interaction determines gene expression and the metabolic response, which ultimately affect an individual's health status and/or predisposition to disease. Nutrients, including fatty acids, can also have a direct effect by interacting with transcription factors to regulate gene expression (Deckelbaum et al., 2006), which also can be influenced by gender (Fig. 9.1). In addition, fatty acid metabolites may mediate the effect of a dietary lipid interaction to alter gene expression. Furthermore, fatty acid derivatives also may alter gene expression by modifying the activities of participating signal transduction mechanisms. This chapter addresses the impact of the interaction between fatty acids and gene expression and subsequent predisposition/risk to atherosclerosis and cardiovascular disease in a gender-related manner. Accordingly, altering the expression of specific genes through nutritional interventions involving specific fatty acids could constitute an efficient therapeutic or preventative option.

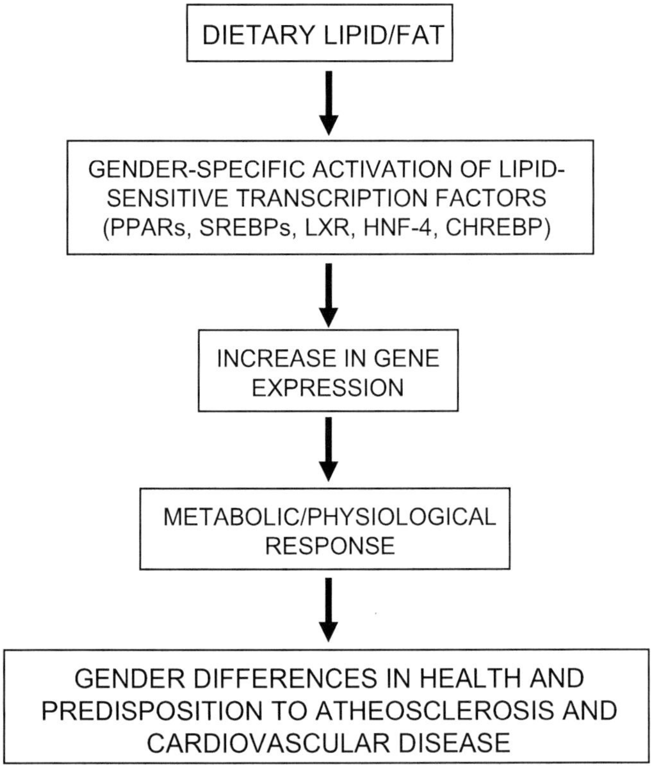


**Fig. 9.1.** Activation of lipid-sensitive transcription factors in response to dietary lipid/fat and gender differences in the predisposition to atherosclerosis and cardiovascular disease. PPARs, peroxisome proliferator-activated receptors; SREBPs, sterol regulatory element binding proteins; LXR, liver X receptor; HNF-4, hepatocytes nuclear factor-4; CHREBP, carbohydrate response element binding protein.

## Pathophysiology of Atherosclerosis

### *Stages of Plaque Development*

Discrete points of the arterial tree (mainly branching points, bifurcations, and the convex site of bending arteries) are areas in which atherosclerotic plaques originate. These plaques are characterized by low or oscillatory shear stresses that may favor the passive transport of arterial blood components into the vessel wall (Ku et al., 1985). Complex lesions are usually observed in adults and can assume different appearances and can reflect different natural histories in plaque development (Fuster et al., 1992; Stary et al., 1989). These are considered the earliest detectable lesions in hypercholesterolemic animal models of atherosclerosis in different species, and most investigators now agree that arterial fatty streaks represent the earliest stage of plaque development (Faggiotto et al., 1984a, 1984b; Gerrity, 1981; Joris et al., 1983; Masuda & Ross, 1990a, 1990b; Rosenfeld et al., 1987; Stary et al., 1989). Fatty streaks are areas of focal intimal thickening produced by the intimal accumulation of lipid-laden macrophages (foam cells) surrounded by an extracellular matrix and a variable number of lymphocytes. An autopsy study provided evidence that lesions are present in the coronary arteries of 50% of children between 10 and 14 years of age (Stary et al., 1989). The development of fatty streaks to more advanced atherosclerosis lesions has long been challenged, and their full reversibility is generally accepted (Mitchell & Schwartz, 1965; Smith et al., 1974; Smith & Slater, 1973;). Observations in various animal models, particularly in primates with low-level hypercholesterolemia (Masuda & Ross, 1990b), clarified that fatty streaks indeed precede more advanced atherosclerotic lesions, which develop at the same arterial points of the arterial vasculature.

### *Gender Differences in Atherosclerosis Development and Progression*

Gender differences exist in the risk of the development and progression of atherosclerosis (Thomas & Smart, 2007). Premenopausal women have a lower risk of developing atherosclerosis and cardiovascular disease than men (Brevetti et al., 2008; Foppa et al., 2006; Kardys et al., 2007). However, after the onset of menopause, the protection associated with gender is lost, and the risk of women developing atherosclerosis gradually approaches that of men. In an effort to treat the elevated risk of cardiovascular disease in postmenopausal women, hormone replacement therapy is used. However, the results of the randomized trials of the Women's Health Initiative indicated that hormone replacement therapy may not be cardioprotective (Collins et al., 2007).

Mouse models, along with the gender effects attributed to sex hormones, are being used to generate a more complete understanding of the development of atherosclerosis. The role of estrogen in atherosclerosis is supported by the use of mice lacking one or both of the genes for estrogen receptors. In addition to estrogen, the role of testosterone in cholesterol homeostasis was discovered through several mechanisms in many animal models. Some studies examined the role of specific fatty acids in the regulation of gene expression, as it relates to gender and the pathogenesis of atherosclerosis. Gender differences play a key role in the onset as well as in the progression of the disease. In fact, a higher mortality for cardiovascular diseases is detected in diabetic women with respect to men; thus, one should consider type 2 diabetes a gender-associated disease (Franconi et al., 2008)

## Fatty Acids, Gene Expression, and Atherosclerosis

### *Fatty Acid Regulation of Gene Transcription*

While PUFAs can modulate membrane lipid composition and affect signal transduction mechanisms by partially replacing the corresponding n-6 analogs in membrane phospholipids (Ma et al., 2004), n-3 fatty acids decrease the transcriptional activation of genes such as adhesion molecules, chemoattractants, and inflammatory cytokines, which are involved in the endothelial activation in response to inflammatory and pro-atherogenic stimuli (De Caterina et al., 2000, 2005). This regulation occurs, at least in part, through a decreased activation of the nuclear factor-kappa B (NFκB) system of transcription factors. Gender differences in the activation of NFκB may exist since males are more sensitive to dietary fatty acids. In fact, the effect of the most common oils used in human nutrition on the development of atherosclerosis in apo-E knockout mice was examined.

### *Fatty Acids and Apolipoproteins*

ApoE-knockout mice were separated by gender, and 10 diets containing different oils were administered: two types of sunflower oil (rich in linoleic acid); palm oil (rich in saturated fatty acid, palmitic acid, and monounsaturated oleic acid); and two types of olive oil (rich in monounsaturated oleic acid). Some diets caused significant reductions in the size of atherosclerotic lesions in males, whereas other diets induce this response in females; males responded most to sunflower oils and females to palm and olive oils. The lesion reduction in males consuming sunflower oils was associated with the decrease of triglycerides in triglyceride-rich lipoproteins, whereas the decrease in females consuming olive oil or palm oil was accompanied by an increase in plasma ApoA-1. The increase in plasma ApoA-1 in the olive oil or palm oil fed female mice was mainly due to the overexpression of the hepatic message elicited by a mechanism independent of the apo-E ligand. Calleja et al. (1999) concluded that the different diets modulate the lesion development in a gender-specific manner and by different mechanisms, and the development of atherosclerosis, due to genetic deficiencies, could be re-modulated by nutritional interventions. However, one should conduct a thorough analysis of the gender-dependent effects of different fatty acids on apolipoproteins, particularly since subnormal expression levels of the Apo-E gene lead to an increased susceptibility to the development of atherosclerosis (van Ree et al., 1994). In this regard, heterozygous Apo-E-deficient mice on a severe semi-synthetic atherogenic diet exhibited an increased susceptibility to atherosclerosis, which is influenced by gender (mean lesion area per section of 9524 microns 2 versus 61,388 microns 2 for males and females, respectively), whereas wild-type mice displayed far fewer lesions (354 microns 2 and 9,196 microns 2 for males and females, respectively). Interestingly, serum cholesterol levels in female heterozygotes were doubled compared to male heterozygotes (15.0 mM versus 7.5 mM). Interestingly, in this study the serum cholesterol levels in female heterozygotes were two-fold higher than in male heterozygotes.

### Gender-linked Mechanisms of Anti-atherogenic Effects of Fatty Acids

Morise et al. (2004) determined that n-3 PUFAs and estrogens are recognized as protective factors of atherosclerosis. Male and female hamsters were fed for 9 weeks diets containing 12.5% lipids, rich in either α-linolenic acid (ALA) (linseed diet) or saturated fatty acids (SFA) (butter diet). In male hamsters fed the butter diet, plasma triglycerides and VLDL concentration were two- to four-fold higher than in the females, along with 30–50% higher increases of the HDL receptor, and activities of HMG-CoA reductase and cholesterol 7-α hydroxylase indicated that gene and/or metabolic regulations by fatty acids could interact with that of sex hormones. The same group reported no gender effect on the transcription level of the peroxisome proliferator-activated receptor (PPAR) -α and sterol regulatory element binding protein (SREBP1c) in response to the butter and linseed oil diets (Morise et al., 2006).

On the other hand, the lipid-lowering effect of flax (rich in ALA) was independent of the effect on hepatic lipogenic genes such as LDL, HMG-CoA reductase, phospholipid transfer protein, cholesterol 7-α hydroxylase, fatty acid synthase, and acyl-CoA oxidase, but could be at the level of cholesterol absorption and/or bile acid re-absorption (Pellizzon et al., 2007) in both male and female mice.

PPARs are major players in the regulation of lipid metabolism, and the targeting of PPARs may be relevant for the treatment of atherosclerosis. In the liver of female mice, the PPAR reporter homogene is more than one order of magnitude less expressed, thus concluding that the signaling in females is much less activated than in males (Ciana et al., 2007). Interestingly, a high-fat diet or gonad removal and hormone replacement do not influence this low activation. The nature of the gender difference in PPAR transcriptional activity and the ineffectiveness of hormone treatments or diet to significantly elevate liver PPAR activity in females are suggestive of gender-specific susceptibility to atherosclerosis. In addition, the gender differences in the expression levels of PPAR may be tissue-specific. In this regard, the expression of PPARα mRNA in the heart or soleus muscle was independent of gender (Jalouli et al., 2003).

Evidence shows that linoleic acid plays a critical role in gene expression and vascular function as it relates to the pathogenesis of atherosclerosis (Toborek & Hennig, 1998). Linoleic acid is an atherogenic fatty acid because it activates the vascular endothelium. The mechanism for linking lipid/cytokine-mediated vessel-wall dysfunction appears to involve the modulation of the levels of activity of a select set of endothelial transcription factors and its relationship with the onset of atherosclerotic lesion formation. The influence of gender in this pathological response remains to be determined; however, since males are more sensitive to the effects of dietary fatty acids, differences according to gender may exist.

Regional arterial hemodynamics correlates with distinct endothelial phenotypes that risk factors may modify to influence focal and regional susceptibility to atherosclerosis. Male and female pigs fed a normal diet and males fed a high-fat diet for two weeks were assessed based on endothelial transcript profiles from hemodynamically distinct arterial. Preferential grouping of arrays by region over risk factor was shown in a hierarchical clustering analysis. The regions of disturbed flow from undisturbed flow were distinguished by a set of differentially expressed genes. Based on gender or diet, few differences were observed within the same region. Perhaps regional hemodynamics is a predominant epigenetic determinant of endothelial phenotypic heterogeneity underlying atherosusceptibility in vivo (Passerini et al., 2005).

A 1.5% conjugated linoleic acid (CLA) diet increased acyl-coA oxidase mRNA by three-fold in male rats, as well as caused a similar increase in liver fatty acid-binding protein mRNA. However, the effect of dietary treatments on hepatic PPAR-responsive genes in female rats was weaker than in male rats. These data indicated that CLA is able to activate PPARs in rats; the extent of activation appears to be gender-related (Moya-Camarena et al., 1999). Interestingly, the effects of short-term cafeteria (CAF) diet feeding on the expression of adipogenic transcription factors and their association with adiposity were investigated (Rodriguez et al., 2004). Male and female Wistar rats were fed either a CAF diet or a standard chow for 2 weeks. Short-term CAF diet feeding resulted in increases in body weight, adipose tissue weights, and lipid serum levels. Increased adiposity was more related to an increase in visceral fat than an increase in subcutaneous fat.

The difference in deposition of adiposity was associated with a higher expression of key adipogenic transcription factors (mainly PPARγ2 and CCAAT enhancer-binding protein-α) in gonadal white adipose tissue (gWAT), the visceral depot, when compared with inguinal white adipose tissue (iWAT), the subcutaneous depot. Males showed higher hypertrophy of iWAT, whereas females showed a higher hypertrophy of gWAT. Differential depot and gender response to the CAF diet could be explained by depot and gender differential expression of key adipogenic transcription factors, especially PPARγ2. Reduced hypertrophy of female iWAT and defective thermogenesis in interscapular brown adipose tissue in response to the CAF diet were related to decreased PPARγ2 mRNA levels, whereas increased hypertrophy in male iWAT and in female gWAT was related to a tendency toward increased PPARγ2 mRNA levels in response to overfeeding. The conclusion was that PPARγ2 is involved in the gender- and depot-specific effects of the CAF diet on the development and function in adipose tissues. Figure 9.2 summarizes a cascade of events modulated by fatty acids, and the potential sites where gender may influence this pathway.

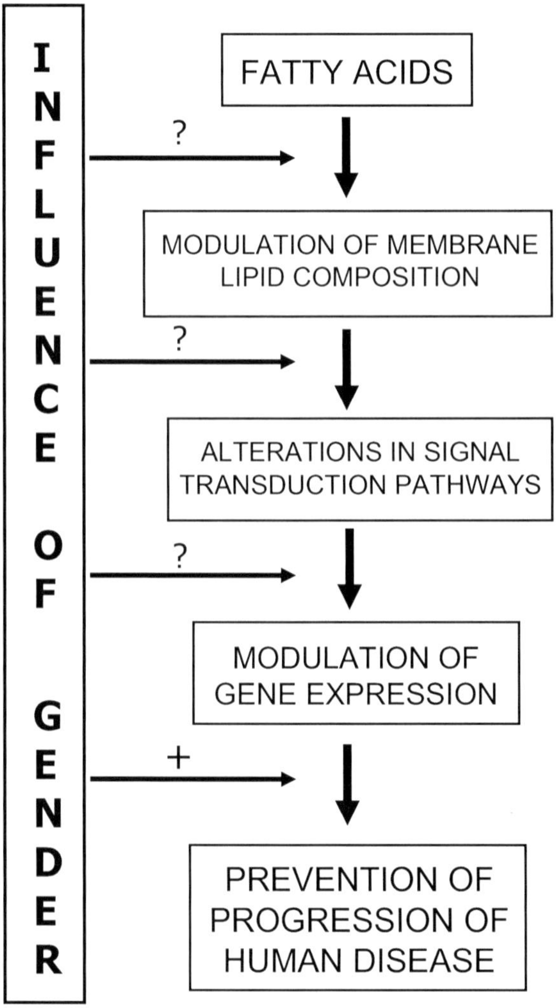


**Fig. 9.2.** Potential sites of the influence of gender in the beneficial mechanisms of fatty acids.

## *Gender-associated Nonalcoholic Fatty Liver Disease*

Nonalcoholic fatty liver disease (NAFLD) is present in up to one-third of the general population and in the majority of patients with cardio-metabolic risk factors such as abdominal obesity, type 2 diabetes, and other components of the metabolic syndrome (Choi et al., 2008). In fact, current evidence strongly suggests that NAFLD is likely associated with increased CVD and possibly considered as an early mediator of atherosclerosis (Loria et al., 2007; Targher, 2007a, Targher & Arcaro, 2007b). NAFLD defines alcohol-like hepatic histological lesions seen in the nonalcoholic (Loria et al., 2007). Some studies show gender differences in the susceptibility of male mice to a high-fat-diet-induced fatty liver. In this regard, Agellon et al. (2007) examined liver mass and hepatic TG deposition and L-FABP expression in male and female intestinal (I) -FABP-deficient mice fed a diet enriched with either PUFA or SFA in the absence of cholesterol. Male, but not female I-FABP mice, exhibited increased liver mass and hepatic TG deposition; however, no gender differences in hepatic L-FABP mRNA and protein contents were observed. The hepatic L-FABP mRNA abundance was higher in both male and female wild-type and I-FABP mice fed PUFA diet versus an SFA diet. These investigators concluded that the loss of I-FABP renders male mice sensitive to high fat-diet-induced fatty liver, independent of hepatic-L-FABP.

In contrast, an increased severity of alcohol liver injury in female versus male rats was demonstrated in male and female rats fed fish oil [rich in eicosapentaenoic acid (EPA) and docosahexaenoic acid (DHA)] and ethanol diets (Sharma et al., 2008). An up-regulation of gender involved in proteosome endopeptidase activity, catalylic activity, lipid metabolism, alcohol metabolism, mitochondrial, and oxidoreductase activity was observed in the female liver. Genes involved in oxidoreductase activity, chaperase activity, and electron transparent activity were also down-regulated in the female heart. While the direct effect of fish oil on the expression of these genes in the female liver remains to be determined, such gender differences in alcoholic liver injury may be because fatty acids can potentiate the severity of alcoholic liver injury, and differences in the responsiveness to fatty acids may be gender-related. Evidently, different dietary fatty acids can exert effects at the level of the gene, which not only can modulate cell function, but also can influence the development of atherosclerosis and cardiovascular disease in a gender-specific manner.

## Fatty Acid-induced Myocardial Gene Expression

### *Gender-related Changes in the Expression of Genes Involved in Lipid Metabolism in the Heart in Response to Fatty Acids*

Many studies have addressed the effects of PUFAs on gene expression in the liver (Jump, 2008). Other than their recognized cardioprotective effects and their ability to modulate gene expression, little is known about the effects in the heart, and virtually nothing is known about the role of gender in the cardiac gene expression in response to fatty acids. Fatty acids are the most important source of energy for the adult heart. However, the cardiac substrate preference changes during development and alters in pathophysiological states. Fatty acids were also involved in signal transduction pathways, thereby affecting gene expression in various cell systems (van Bilsen et al., 1997).

Bordoni et al. (2007) evaluated the effects of n-3 PUFA (EPA and DHA) supplementation on the global gene expression profile in cultured neonatal rat cardiomyocytes. They detected many genes related to lipid transport and metabolism among the up-regulated ones. Many of the down-regulated genes appeared related to inflammation, cell growth, extracellular and cardiac matrix remodeling, calcium movements, and ROS generation. Accordingly, perhaps the cardioprotective effect of n-3 PUFAs is related to a direct modulation of genes in the cardiac cells; however, the influence of gender in the expression of these genes remains to be determined. In addition, a prolonged exposure (48 hours) of neonatal rat cardiomyocytes with a combination of palmitic/oleic acids (C16:0/C18:1 fatty acids) resulted in a nearly four-fold increase of the H-FABP mRNA level (van Bilsen et al., 1997). On the other hand, neonatal cardiomyocytes stimulated with a hypertrophic agent (phenylephrine) mitigated the stimulatory effect of fatty acids on H-FABP expression. These findings strongly suggest that fatty acids are able to modulate gene expression in the cardiomyocyte; however; the influence of gender still remains to be explored. Most likely, gender differences in the expression levels of H-FABP might occur because, in muscle, FATP-1 mRNA levels were higher in lean women than in lean men, whereas FATP-1 mRNA expression is lower in the skeletal muscle in obese women, including both nondiabetic and type 2 diabetic patients (Binnert et al., 2000).

The chronic overutilization of fatty acids by diabetic hearts is considered to contribute to the reduced mechanical function that constitutes a diabetic cardiomyopathy (Lopaschuk, 2002; Taha & Lopaschuk, 2007). In fact, lower transcript levels of PPAR-$\alpha$, muscle-type carnitine palmitoyltransferase 1, and pyruvate dehydrogenase kinase 4 in female control hearts versus male hearts were reported (Essop et al., 2007). However, these genes were significantly higher in obese (db/db) female mice. While these changes were associated with the poor recovery of cardiac mitochondrial respiratory function, they are also seen to contribute to enhanced cardiac fatty acid utilization and to reduce the contractile function of the diabetic heart (Lopaschuk, 2002; Taha & Lopaschuk, 2007). Therefore, discovering interventions that can reduce FA utilization by diabetic hearts is an important goal for future investigations; the influence of gender is an important determinant for the design and subsequent understanding of the mechanisms of beneficial action for such types of interventions.

## *Gender Differences in the Fatty Acid-induced Alterations in Myocardial Genes Involved in Signal Transduction*

Animal and human studies reveal gender differences in myocardial function as well as in the incidence and manifestation of heart disease (Bae & Zhang, 2005; Gardner et al., 2002; Jessup & Pina, 2004; Mendelsohn, 2002; Pieretti et al., 2007; Regitz-Zagrosek & Lehmkuh, 2005; Schönfelder et al., 2004; Stromberg & Martensson, 2003). Cardiomyocyte $Ca^{2+}$ cycling regulates normal contractile function, whereas cardiac dysfunction in heart failure is associated with alterations in $Ca^{2+}$-handling proteins. The $\beta$-adrenoceptor ($\beta$-AR) signaling regulates the activity of several $Ca^{2+}$-handling proteins (Fig. 9.3), and alterations in $\beta$-AR signaling are associated with heart disease. Differences in the expression of $\beta_1$-AR, $\beta_2$-AR, and $Ca^{2+}$-handling

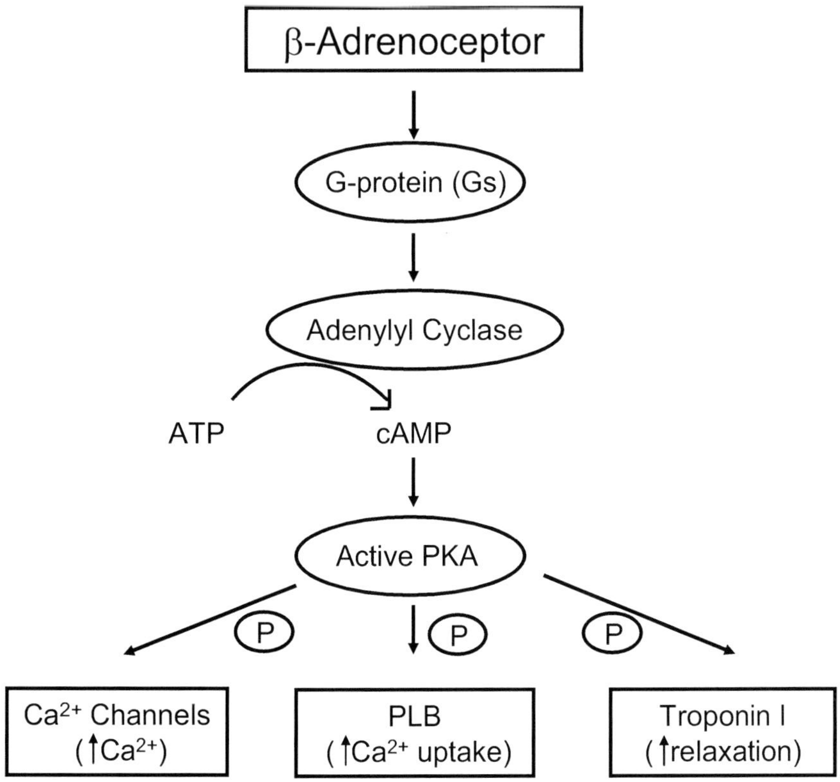


**Fig. 9.3.** Mechanisms of the β-adrenoceptor-mediated regulation of Ca2+-handling proteins. ATP, adenosine triphosphate; cAMP, cyclic adenosine monophosphate; PKA, protein kinase A; PLB, phospholamban; P, phosphorylation.

proteins including: L-type calcium channel, ryanodine calcium-release channels (RyR), sarcoplasmic reticular $Ca^{2+}$-ATPase (SERCA2), phospholamban (PLB), and $Na^{+}$-$Ca^{2+}$-exchange protein (NCX) were reported in healthy hearts from male and female Sprague-Dawley rats (Chu et al., 2005). The female ventricle had significantly higher levels of L-type calcium channel, RyR, and NCX protein compared to males. Messenger RNA abundance for RyR and NCX protein was significantly higher in females, whereas L-type calcium channel mRNA was higher in males. On the other hand, no differences were detected in β-ARs, SERCA2, or PLB. While these data demonstrate gender differences in the expression of key ventricular $Ca^{2+}$-handling proteins, small differences in the rates of contraction and relaxation were observed.

Although the effects of fatty acids on the gene expression of the components of the β-AR are yet to be determined, the effects of fatty acids, specifically CLA, on the expression of genes for $Ca^{2+}$-cycling proteins were reported. Our laboratory is the first to report that dietary CLA isomers exert differential effects on heart function in a gender-specific manner (Tappia et al., 2006). We examined some of the potential mechanisms that could contribute to these responses. We hypothesized that abnormalities in the sarcolemmal (SL)- and sarcoplasmic reticulum (SR)-mediated regulation of intracellular $Ca^{2+}$ contribute to the altered cardiac contractile function of male and female rats because of dietary CLA isomers. Significant gender differences were seen in the myocardial NCX, the L-type $Ca^{2+}$ channel, and the RyR mRNA expression levels in control male and female rats (Tappia et al., 2007). Dietary CLA isomers in the various forms induced changes in the mRNA levels of SERCA 2a, NCX, and L-type $Ca^{2+}$ channel in both male and female hearts. Whereas the protein contents of the $Ca^{2+}$ cycling proteins were altered, changes in SR $Ca^{2+}$-uptake and -release were also detected in both male and female rats in response to dietary CLA. Thus, long-term dietary supplementation can modulate cardiac gene expression and SR function in a gender-related manner and may, in part, contribute to altered cardiac contractility (Tappia et al., 2006).

Heart failure increases NCX expression and activity, contributing to both depressed contractility and ventricular arrhythmias (Wei et al., 2007), and the SERCA 2a expression is reduced in heart failure in human and mice models (Butter et al., 2008; Hovnanian, 2007). In our studies the *t*10,*c*12 CLA isomer specifically increased the SERCA 2a gene expression in male hearts, while it induced a decrease in the NCX gene expression in the female heart (Tappia et al., 2007), clearly indicating the potential therapeutic value of specific CLA isomers. In summary, while numerous studies have addressed the effects of different fatty acids on cardiomyocyte function, very little information is available in the literature on gender-specific cardiomyocyte gene expression in response to fatty acids, thus warranting further investigation. Such knowledge will provide the molecular basis of altered cardiomyocyte biology in response to different fatty acids.

## Conclusion

From the aforementioned discussion, evidently, specific fatty acids can modulate gene expression. This review also provided some information on the impact of the interaction between fatty acids and gene expression and the subsequent predisposition/risk to atherosclerosis and cardiovascular disease in a gender-related manner. However, at the time of this writing, the pathways involved in gender effects on cardiovascular disease are not completely understood.

### *Future Perspectives*

With the availability of numerous animal models, an opportunity exists to dissect the cellular and molecular mechanisms involved and to delineate the influence of gender on fatty acid-induced (as well as other nutrients) modulation of gene expression in various tissue/cell types. The gender-related differences in the incorporation of fatty acids in the cell membrane and subsequent alterations in signal transduction pathways

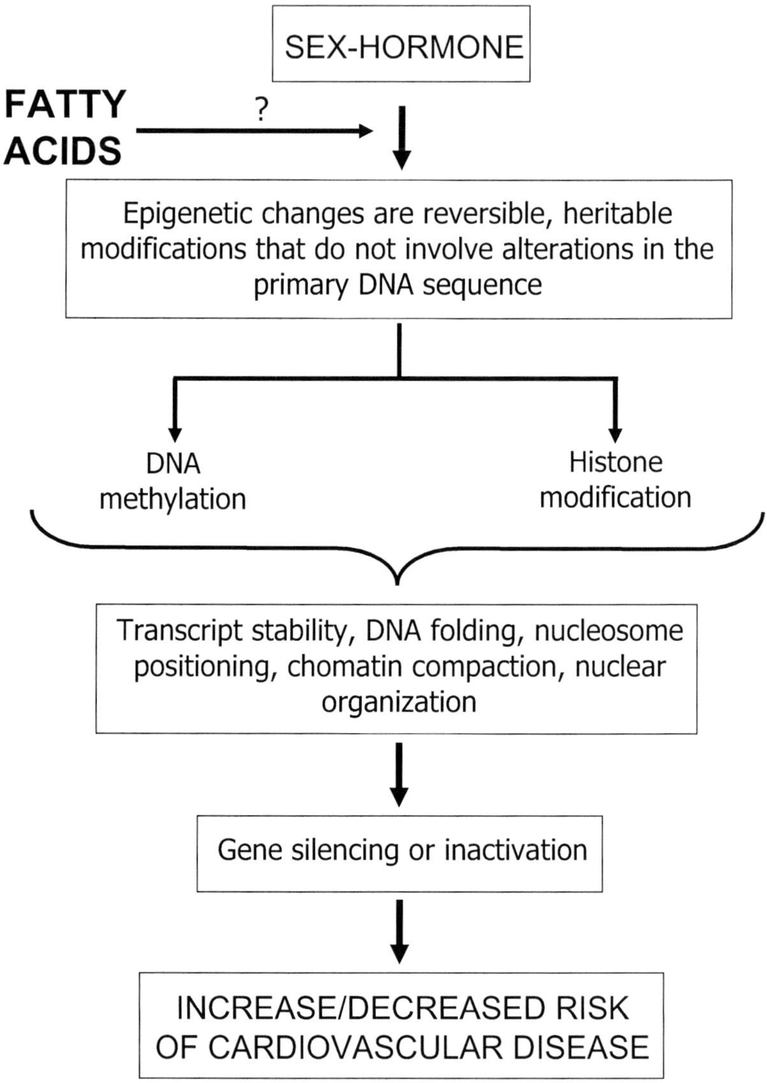


**Fig. 9.4.** Possible interaction of fatty acids in the sex-hormone- induced epigenetic changes and predisposition to cardiovascular disease.

need to be vigorously addressed. In view of the role of maternal nutrition and genetic imprinting and increased predisposition to cardiovascular disease in the offspring in later life, it would be interesting to examine the effects of maternal dietary fats on the developing fetus and the predisposition to disease in later life.

The interaction of specific fatty acids on the hormone-induced epigenetic changes, including DNA methylation and histone modification at specific gene regulatory regions, warrants investigation as it may increase or reduce the risk of atherosclerosis and cardiovascular disease (Fig. 9.4). Estrogen can modulate the distribution and function of β-adrenoceptors in the heart (Kocić et al., 2007). Thus, it would be interesting to determine the interaction of fatty acids on the estrogen-induced modulation of β-adrenoceptors in pre- and post-menopausal women. Without a doubt, a paucity of information is available on the influence of gender on the molecular response to fatty acids; a need exists to bring this field to the forefront of health research. Also consider genetic polymorphisms in the responsiveness to fatty acids. Prudently examine the role of ethnicity in the gender-associated molecular response to fatty acids. Accordingly, a complete understanding of the modulation of gene expression in a gender-specific manner by fatty acids present in human nutrition and atherogenesis may open new approaches to the dietary intervention of atherosclerosis and cardiovascular disease.

## References

Agellon, L.B.; L. Drozdowski; L. Li; C. Iordache; L. Luong; M.T. Clandinin; R.R. Uwiera; M.J. Toth; A.B. Thomson. Loss of intestinal fatty acid binding protein increases the susceptibility of male mice to high fat diet-induced fatty liver. *Biochim. Biophys. Acta.* **2007**, *1771*, 1283–1288.

Appel, L.J.; E.R. Miller; A.J. Seidler; P.K. Whelton. Diet supplementation with fish oils and blood pressure reduction: a meta-analysis. *Ann. Intern. Med.* **1994**, *120(Suppl.)*, 9.

Appel, L.J.; E.R. Miller; A.J. Seidler; P.K. Whelton. Does supplementation of diet with "fish oil' reduce blood pressure? A meta-analysis of controlled clinical trials. *Arch. Intern. Med.* **1993**, *153*, 1429–1438.

Arita, M.; M. Yoshida; S. Hong; E. Tjonahen; J.N. Glickman; N.A. Petasis; R.S. Blumberg; C.N. Serhan. Resolvin E1, an endogenous lipid mediator derived from ω-3 eicosapentaenoic acid, protects against 2, 4, 6-trinitrobenzene sulfonic acid-induced colitis. *Proc. Natl. Acad. Sci. U.S.A.* **2005**; *102*, 7671–7676.

Bae, S.; L. Zhang. Gender differences in cardioprotection against ischemia/reperfusion injury in adult rat hearts: Focus on Akt and protein kinase C signaling. *J. Pharmacol. Exp. Ther.* **2005**, *315*, 1125–1135.

Belluzzi, A.; C. Brignola; M. Campieri; A. Pera; S. Boschi; M. Miglioli. Effects of new fish oil derivative on fatty acid phospholipid-membrane pattern in a group of Crohn's disease patients. *Dig. Dis. Sci.* **1994**, *39*, 2589–2594.

Binnert, C.; H.A. Koistinen; G. Martin; F. Andreelli; P. Ebeling; V.A. Koivisto; M. Laville; J. Auwerx; H. Vidal. Fatty acid transporter protein-1 mRNA expression in skeletal muscle and in adipose tissue in humans. *Am. J. Physiol. Endocrinol. Metab.* **2000**, *279*, E1072–E1079.

Bordoni, A.; A. Astolfi; L. Morandi; A. Pession; F. Danesi; M. Di Nunzio; M. Franzoni; P. Biagi; A. Pession. n-3 PUFAs modulate global gene expression profile in cultured rat cardiomyocytes.

Implications in cardiac hypertrophy and heart failure. *FEBS Lett.* **2007**, *581*, 923–929.

Brevetti, G.; R. Bucur; A. Balbarini; E. Melillo; S. Novo; I. Muratori; M. Chiariello. Women and peripheral arterial disease: same disease, different issues. *J. Cardiovasc. Med.* **2008**, *9*, 382–388.

Butter, C.; S. Rastogi; H.H. Minden; J. Meyhöfer; S. Burkhoff; H.N. Sabbah. Cardiac contractility modulation electrical signals improve myocardial gene expression in patients with heart failure. *J. Am. Coll. Cardiol.* **2008**, *51*, 1784–1789.

Calder, P.C. Dietary modification of inflammation with lipids. *Proc. Nutr. Soc.* **2002**, *61*, 345–358.

Calleja, L.; M.A. Paris; A. Paul; E. Vilella; J. Joven; A. Jimenez; G. Beltran; M. Uceda; N. Maeda; J. Osada. Low-cholesterol and high-fat diets reduce atherosclerotic lesion development in ApoE-knockout mice. *Arterioscler. Throm. Vasc. Biol.* **1999**, *19*, 2368–2375.

Cawood, A.L.; M.P. Carroll; S.A. Wootton; P.C. Calder. Is there a case for n-3 fatty acid supplementation in cystic fibrosis? *Curr. Opin. Clin. Nutr. Metab. Care.* **2005**, *8*, 153–159.

Choi, S.Y.; D. Kim; J.H. Kang; M.J. Park; Y.S. Kim; S.H. Lim; C.H. Kim; H.S. Lee. Nonalcoholic fatty liver disease as a risk factor of cardiovascular disease: relation of non-alcoholic fatty liver disease to carotid atherosclerosis. *Korean J. Hepatol.* **2008**, *14*, 77–88.

Chu, S.H.; K. Sutherland; J. Beck; J. Kowalski; P. Goldspink; D. Schwertz. Sex differences in expression of calcium-handling proteins and β-adrenergic receptors in rat heart ventricle. *Life Sci.* **2005**, *76*, 2735–2749.

Ciana, P.; A. Biserni; L. Tatangelo; C. Tiveron; A.F. Sciarroni; L. Ottobrini; A. Maggi. A novel peroxisome proliferator-activated receptor responsive element-luciferase reporter mouse reveals gender specificity of peroxisome proliferator-activated receptor activity in liver. *Mol. Endocrinol.* **2007**, *21*, 338–400.

Collins, P.; G. Rosano; C. Casey; C. Daly; M. Gambacciani; P. Hadji; R. Kaaja; T. Mikkola; S. Palacios; R. Preston; et al. Management of cardiovascular risk in the perimenopausal women: a consensus statement of European cardiologists and gynecologists. *Climacteric.* **2007**, *10*, 508–526.

Darlington, L.G.; T.W. Stone. Antioxidants and fatty acids in the amelioration of rheumatoid arthritis and related disorders. *Br. J. Nutr.* **2001**, *85*, 251–269.

Das, U.N. Beneficial effect(s) of n-3 fatty acids in cardiovascular disease: but, why and how? *Prostaglandins Leukotrienes Essent. Fatty Acids* **2000**, *63*, 351–362.

Das, U.N. Long-chain polyunsaturated fatty acids interact with nitric oxide, superoxide anion, and transforming growth factor-β to prevent human essential hypertension. *Eur. J. Clin. Nutr.* **2004**, *58*, 195–203.

De Caterina, R.; J.K. Liao; P. Libby. Fatty acid modulation of endothelial activation. *Am. J. Clin. Nutr.* **2000**, *71*, 213S–223S.

De Caterina, R.; M. Massaro. Omega-3 fatty acids and the regulation of expression of endothelial proatherogenic and pro-inflammatory genes. *J. Membr. Biol.* **2005**, *206*, 103–116.

Decklbaum, R.J.; T.S. Worgall; T. Seo. n-3 Fatty acids and gene expression. *Am. J. Clin. Nutr.* **2006**, *83*, 1520S–1525S.

Essop, M.F.; W.Y. Chan; H. Taegtmeyer. Metabolic gene switching in the murine female heart parallels enhanced mitochondrial respiratory function in response to oxidative stress. *FEBS J.*

**2007**, *274*, 5278–5284.

Faggiotto, A.; R. Ross. Studies of hypercholesterolemia in the nonhuman primate. II. Fatty streak conversion to fibrous plaque. *Arteriosclerosis* **1984a**, *4*, 341–356.

Faggiotto, A.; R. Ross; L. Harker. Studies of hypercholesterolemia in the nonhuman primate. I. Changes that lead to fatty streak formation. *Arteriosclerosis* **1984b**, *4*, 323–340.

Foppa, M.; B.B. Duncan; D.K. Arnett; E.J. Benjamin; P.R. Liebson; T.A. Manolio; T.N. Skelton. Diabetes, gender, and left ventricular structure in African-Americans: the atherosclerosis risk in communities study. *Cardiovasc. Ultrasound.* **2006**, *4,* 43–50.

Franconi, F.; G. Seghieri; S. Canu; E. Straface; I. Campesi; W. Malorni. Are the available experimental models of type 2 diabetes appropriate for a gender perspective? *Pharmacol. Res.* **2008**, *57*, 6–18.

Fuster, V.; L. Badimon; J.J. Badimon; J.H. Chesebro. The pathogenesis of coronary artery disease and the acute coronary syndromes (first of two parts). *N. Engl. J. Med.* **1992**, *326*, 242–251.

Gardner, J.D.; G.L. Brower; J.S. Janicki. Gender differences in cardiac remodeling secondary to chronic volume overload. *J. Card. Fail.* **2002**, *8*, 101–107.

Gerrity, R.G. The role of the monocyte in atherogenesis: I. Transition of blood-borne monocytes into foam cells in fatty lesions. *Am. J. Pathol.* **1981**, *103*, 181–190.

Hovnanian, A. SERCA pumps and human disease. *Subcell. Biochem.* **2007**, *45,* 337–363.

Inoue, N.; K. Nagao; J. Hirata; Y.M. Wang; T. Yanagita. Conjugated linoleic acid prevents the development of essential hypertension in spontaneously hypertensive rats. *Biochem. Biophys. Res. Commun.* **2004**, *323*, 679–684.

Jalouli, M.; L. Carisson; C. Ameen; D. Linden; A. Ljungberg; L. Michalik; S. Eden; W. Wahli; J. Oscarsson. Sex differences in hepatic peroxisome proliferator-activated receptor α expression: influence of pituitary and gonadal hormones. *Endocrinology* **2003**, *144*, 101–109.

Jessup, M.; I.L. Piña. Is it important to examine gender differences in the epidemiology and outcome of severe heart failure? *J. Thorac. Cardiovasc. Surg.* **2004**, *127*, 1247–1252.

Joris, I.; T. Znad; J.J. Nunnari; F.J. Krolikowski; G. Majno. Adhesion and emigration of mononuclear cells in the aorta of hypercholesterolemic rats. *Am. J. Pathol.* **1983**, *113*, 341–358.

Jump, D.B. n-3 Polyunsaturated fatty acid regulation of hepatic gene transcription. *Curr. Opin. Lipidol.* **2008**, *19*, 242–247.

Kardys, I.; R. Vliegenthart; M. Oudkerk; A. Hofman; J.C. Witteman. The female advantage in cardiovascular disease: do vascular beds contribute equally? *Am. J. Epidemiol.* **2007**, *166*, 403–412.

Khosla, P.; T.V. Fungwe. Conjugated linoleic acid: effects on plasma lipids and cardiovascular function. *Curr. Opin. Lipidol.* **2001**, *12*, 31–34.

Kocić, I.; M. Gruchala; J. Petrusewicz. Pretreatment of male guinea pigs by 17-β-estradiol induces hypersensitivity of β-adrenoceptors in electrically driven left atria. *Int. J. Cardiol.* **2007,** *129,* 22–25.

Kritchevsky, D.; S.A. Tapper; S. Wright; S.K. Czarnecki. Influence of conjugated linoleic acid (CLA) on establishment and progression of atherosclerosis in rabbits. *J. Am. Coll. Nutr.* **2000**, *19*, 472S–477S.

Ku, D.N.; D.P. Giddens; C.K. Zarins; S. Glagov. Pulsatile flow and atherosclerosis in the human carotid bifurcation: positive correlation between plaque location and low and oscillating shear stress. *Arteriosclerosis.* **1985**, *5*, 293–302.

Lopaschuk, G.D. Metabolic abnormalities in the diabetic heart. *Heart Fail. Rev.* **2002**, *7*, 149–159.

Loria, P.; A. Lonardo; S. Bellentani; C.P. Day; G. Marchesini; N. Carulli. Non-alcoholic fatty liver disease (NAFLD) and cardiovascular disease: an open question. *Nutr. Metab. Cardiovasc. Dis.* **2007**, *17*, 684–698.

Ma, D.W.L.; J. Seo; K.C. Switzer; Y-Y. Fan; D.N. McMurray; J.R. Lupton; R.S. Chapkin. n-3 PUFA and membrane micodomains: a new frontier in bioactive lipid research. *J. Nutr. Biochem.* **2004**, *15,* 700–706.

Mahmud, F.H.; M.G. Earing; R.A. Lee; A.N. Lteif; D.J. Driscoll; A. Lerman. Altered endothelial function in asymptomatic male adolescents with type 1 diabetes. *Congenit. Heart Dis.* **2006**, *1*, 98–103.

Masuda, J.; R. Ross. Atherogenesis during low level hypercholesterolemia in the nonhuman primate. II. Fatty streak conversion to fibrous plaque. *Arteriosclerosis* **1990a**, *10*, 178–187.

Masuda, J; R. Ross. Atherogenesis during low level hypercholesterolemia in the nonhuman primate. I. Fatty streak formation. *Arteriosclerosis* **1990b**, *10*, 164–177.

Mendelsohn, M.E. Protective effects of estrogen on the cardiovascular system. *Am. J. Cardiol.* **2002**, *89*, 12–17.

Mitchell, J.R.A.; C.J. Schwartz. *Arterial Disease;* Blackwell Scientific Publishers: Oxford, UK, 1965.

Morise, A.; J. Mourot; C. Boue; N. Combe; G. Amsler; D. Gripois; A. Quignard-Boulange; L. Yvan-Charvet; E. Fenart; P. Weill; D. Hermier. Gender-related response of lipid metabolism to dietary fatty acids in the hamster. *Br. J. Nutr.* **2006**, *95,* 709–720.

Morise, A.; C. Serougne; D. Gripois; M.F. Blouquit; C. Lutton; D. Hermier. Effects of dietary alpha linolenic acid on cholesterol metabolism in male and female hamsters of the LPN strain. *J. Nutr. Biochem.* **2004**, *15*, 51–61.

Moya-Camarena, S.Y.; J.P. Van den Heuval; M.A. Belury. Conjugated linoleic acid activates peroxisome proliferator-activated receptor alpha and beta subtypes but does not induce hepatic peroxisome proliferation in Sprague-Dawley rats. *Biochem. Biophys. Acta* **1999**, *1436*, 331–342.

Nagao, K.; N. Inoue; Y.M. Wang; J. Hirata; Y. Shimada; T. Nagao; T. Matsui; T. Yanagita. The 10 trans, 12 cis isomer of conjugated linoleic acid suppresses the development of hypertension in Otsuka Long-Evans Tokushima fatty arts. *Biochem. Biophys. Res. Commun.* **2003**, *306*, 134–138.

Ordovas, J.M. Gender, a significant factor in the cross talk between genes, environment, and health. *Gend. Med.* **2007**, *4 (Suppl. B)*, S111–122.

Pal, S.; R. Takechi; S.S. Ho. Conjugated linoleic acid suppresses the secretion of atherogenic lipoproteins from human HepG2 liver cells. *Clin. Chem. Lab. Med.* **2005**, *22*, 266–277.

Passerini, A.G.; C. Shi; N.M. Francesco; P. Chuan; E. Manduchi; G.R. Grant; C.J. Stoeckert, Jr.; J.W. Karanian; D. Wray-Cahen; W.F. Pritchard; P.F. Davies. Regional determinants of arterial endothelial phenotype dominate the impact of gender or short-term exposure to a high-fat diet. *Biochem. Biophys. Res. Commun.* **2005**, *332*, 142–148.

Pellizzon, M.A.; J.T. Billheimer; L.T. Bloedon; P.O. Szapary; D.J. Rader. Flaxseed reduces plasma cholesterol levels in hypersholesterolemic mouse models. *J. Am. Coll. Nutr.* **2007**, *26*, 66–75.

Pieretti, J. ; M.J. Roman; R.B. Devereux; M.D. Lockshin; M.K. Crow; S.A. Paget; J.E. Schwartz; L. Sammaritano; D.M. Levine; J.E. Salmon. Systemic lupus erythematosus predicts increased left ventricular mass. *Circulation.* **2007**, *116*, 419–426.

Regitz-Zagrosek, V.; E. Lehmkuh. Heart failure and its treatment in women. Role of hypertension, diabetes, and estrogen. *Herz.* **2005**, *30*, 356–367.

Roche, H.M. Dietary lipids and gene expression. *Biochem. Soc. Transactions.* **2004**, *32*, 999–1002.

Rodriguez, E.; J. Ribot; A.M. Rodriguez; A. Palou. PPAR-γ2 expression in response to cafeteria diet: gender- and depot-specific effects. *Obes. Res.* **2004**, *12*, 1455–1463.

Rosenfeld, M.E.; T. Tsukada; A.M. Gown; R. Ross. Fatty streak initiation in Watanabe heritable hyperlipemic and comparably hypercholesterolemic fat-fed rabbits. *Arteriosclerosis* **1987**, *7*, 9–23.

Schönfelder, G. The biological impact of estrogens on gender differences in congestive heart failure. *Cardiovasc. Res.* **2005**, *67*, 573–574.

Sharma, M.R.; R. Polavarapu; D. Roseman; V. Patel; E. Eaton; P.B. Kishor; A.A. Nanji. Increased severity of alcoholic liver injury in female versus male rats: a microarray analysis. *Exp. Mol. Pathol.* **2008**, *84*, 46–58.

Simpopoulos, A.P. Human requirement for n-3 polyunsaturated fatty acids. *Poult. Sci.* **2000**, *79*, 961–970.

Smith, E.B.; R.S. Slater. Lipids and low-density lipoproteins in intima in relationship to its morphological characteristics. *Atherogenesis: Initiating Factors* (Ciba Foundation symposium no. 12)*;* D. Schletter, A. Weizel, Eds.*;* Elsevier Publishing Co.: Amsterdam, 1973; pp. 39–62.

Smith, E.B.; R.S. Slater; D.X. Crothers. Quantitative interrelationships between plasma constituents and normal and atherosclerotic human intimal tissue. *Atherosclerosis III;* D. Schletter, A. Weizel, Eds.; Springer-Verlag: Berlin, 1974, pp. 96–102.

Stary, H. Evolution and progression of atherosclerotic lesions in coronary arteries of children and young adults. *Arteriosclerosis.* **1989**, *88 (Suppl.),* 1–32.

Strömberg, A.; J. Mårtensson. Gender differences in patients with heart failure. *Eur. J. Cardiovasc. Nurs.* **2003**, *2,* 7–18.

Taha, M.; G.D. Lopaschuk. Alterations in energy metabolism in cardiomyopathies. *Ann. Med.* **2007,** *39*, 594–607.

Tappia, P.S.; M.R. Dent; N. Aroutiounova; A.P. Babick; H. Weiler. Gender differences in the modulation of cardiac gene expression by dietary conjugated linoleic acid isomers. *Can. J. Physiol. Pharmacol.* **2007**, *85*, 465–475.

Tappia, P.S.; R. Mangat; C. Gabriel; M.R. Dent; N. Aroutiounova; H. Weiler. Gender differences in the cardiac response to dietary conjugated linoleic acid isomers. *Can. J. Physiol. Pharmacol.* **2006**, *84*, 257–264.

Targher, G. Non-alcoholic fatty liver disease, the metabolic syndrome and the risk of cardiovascular disease: the plot thickens. *Diabet. Med.* **2007a**, *24*, 1–6.

Targher, G.; G. Arcaro. Non-alcoholic fatty liver disease and increased risk of cardiovascular discasc. *Atherosclerosis.* **2007b**, *191*, 235–240.

Thomas, C.M.; E.J. Smart. Gender as a regulator of atherosclerosis in murine models. *Curr. Drug. Targets.* **2007**, *8*, 1172–1180.

Toborek, M.; B. Hennig. The role of linoleic acid in endothelial cell gene expression. Relationship to atherosclerosis. *Subcell. Biochem.* **1998**, *30*, 415–436.

van Bilsen, M.; J.E. de Vries; G.J. Van der Vusse. Long-term effects of fatty acids on cell viability and gene expression of neonatal cardiac myocytes. *Prostaglandins, Leukottrienes Essent. Fatty Acids* **1997**, *57*, 39–45.

van Ree, J.H.; W.J. van den Broek; V.E. Dahlmans; P.H. Groot; M. Vidgeon-Hart; R.R. Frants; B. Wieringa; L.M. Havekes; M.H. Hofker. Diet-induced hypercholesterolemia and atherosclerosis in heterozygous apolipoprotein E-deficient mice. *Atherosclerosis.* **1994**, *111*, 25–37.

Wei, S.K.; J.M. McCurley, S.U. Hanlon; M.C. Haigney. Gender differences in Na/Ca exchanger current and β-adrenergic responsiveness in heart failure in pig myocytes. *Ann. N.Y. Acad. Sci.* **2007**, *1099*, 183–189.

# 10

# Fatty Acids in Nuts: Cardiometabolic Health Benefits

**Alison Coates[1] and Peter R.C. Howe[2]**
*[1]Nutritional Physiology Research Centre, School of Health Sciences, University of South Australia, BJ1-71, City East Campus, Adelaide, SA 5001 Australia; [2]Director, Nutritional Physiology Research Centre, School of Health Sciences, University of South Australia, GPO Box 2471, Adelaide, SA 5001*

## Introduction

Since the time of ancient civilizations, the diet has included nuts. (Dreher, 1996). The traditional Mediterranean diet is rich in nuts (Spiller & Bruce, 1997), but reports also reveal that native populations of America (Pringle, 2008) and Australia (O'Dea, 1991) regularly consumed nuts. Today the role of nuts in maintaining good health is recognized by their place in the USDA Food Guide Pyramid's Meat/Meat Alternate Group (Allen, 2008). Regular consumption of nuts is also promoted by several health authorities around the world, including the American Dietetic Association (ADA) and Dietitians of Canada (DC) (Kris-Etherton et al., 2007) several European dietary associations (Aranceta & Serra-Majem, 2001), and in the *Australian Dietary Guidelines for Adults* (2003a) and the *Australian Dietary Guidelines for Children and Adolescents* (2003b).

Some of the first evidence for the role of nuts in the prevention of chronic disease came from data collected on the diet of Mediterranean populations. The seven-countries study published in 1980 (Keys, 1980) indicated that diets rich in monounsaturated fat (MUFA) and polyunsaturated fat (PUFA), contrary to saturated fat (SFA), reduced both serum cholesterol and the incidence of coronary artery disease (CAD). The fat profile of nuts matches this recommendation, highlighting their potential role in heart health (Willett et al., 1995).

Much of the research to date has focused on those nuts more common in the Mediterranean diet, including almonds, walnuts, pecans, and pistachios—all of which are tree-derived nuts (Griel & Kris-Etherton, 2006). Although peanuts are botanically classified as legumes because they grow in the ground, the fatty acid and nutrient profiles of peanuts are very similar to other nuts (O'Byrne et al., 1997). Moreover, the peanut also has many lipid-lowering properties (O'Byrne et al., 1997; Kris-Etherton et al., 1999b) and other cardiovascular (CV) and metabolic health benefits (Alper & Mattes, 2003; Jiang et al., 2006) which are similar to tree nuts. This review addresses several aspects of health that regular nut consumption can improve.

## *Who Is Eating Nuts?*

Frequency and quantity of nut consumption are documented to be higher in vegetarian than in nonvegetarian populations (Fraser et al., 1992; Spiller & Bruce, 1997). Nuts still constitute an important part of the modern Mediterranean (Sabate et al., 1993) and Asian diets, which are typically plant-based. Nuts are regularly consumed in the diet either as a whole food, in spreads, or from hidden sources (e.g., commercial products). Total nut consumption for each country studied in the European Prospective Investigation into Cancer and Nutrition (EPIC) is shown in Fig. 10.1 (data adapted from Jenab et al., 2006; Sabate et al., 2006). These proportions are substantially lower than previous reports from large U.S. cohorts: 65% of women in The Nurses' Health Study (Jiang et al., 2002), 59% of women in the Iowa Women's Health Study (Ellsworth et al., 2001), and 80% of men in the Physicians' Health Study (Albert et al., 2002) reported eating nuts (a portion = 28 g [1 ounce]) at least once per month. However, these data should be explored further since participants in the large cohort studies in the United States were interested in health outcomes, and this is likely to have skewed their data in comparison to the whole population. In fact, data suggest that nut consumption in countries following a more Mediterranean-style diet is twice that of the American diet (Dreher et al., 1996).

A recent survey of dietary trends in Spain from 1992 to 2003 revealed that nut consumption was still an important part of the diet in both children and adults. The survey was comprised of approximately 4700 men and women (10–75 years of age) and a 2.8% increased proportion of people who ate nuts daily over that period (Ribas-Barba et al., 2007).

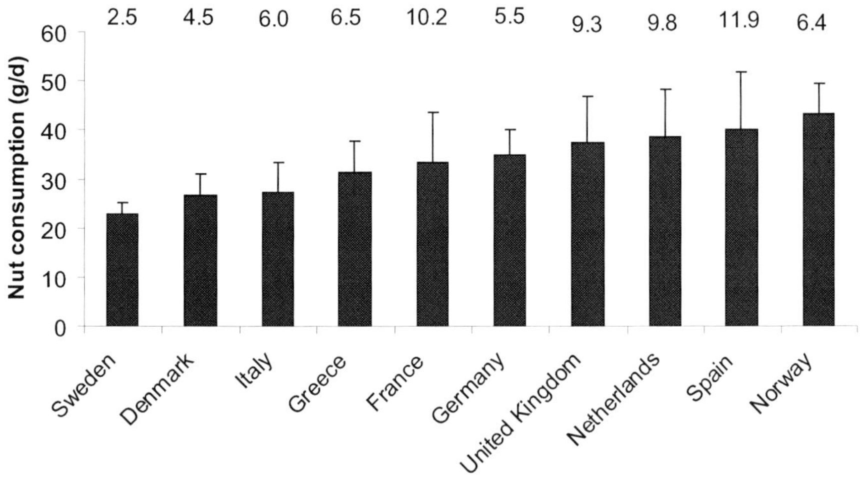


**Fig. 10.1.** Nut consumption (g/day) reported from 24-hour recall assessments in the EPIC study (Jenab et al., 2006). Data shown as mean and SEM for average portion sizes in consumers only. The numbers at the top of the figure represent the percentage of the population who consumed nuts.

Data from The National Diet and Nutrition Survey in the UK conducted in 2000/01(2003) (Henderson et al., 2003) indicated that ≈20% of the adult population consumed nuts, which was higher than indicated in the previous survey in 1986–1987. For those nut consumers, the average intake was 62 g/day for women and 81 g/day for men, whereas the overall mean for the whole population was 12 and 17 g/day, respectively. This is higher than the average intake in Australia which was 4 g/day, with only 12% of adults reporting regularly consuming nuts (Australian Bureau of Statistics, 1998).

### *What Types of Nuts Are Most Popular?*

Nuts are consumed raw, roasted, crushed (as a butter), or the oil extracted from them. A recent study also reported on an extract from peanut husks, suggesting this by-product may have further potential (Moreno et al., 2006).

Recent U.S. Department of Agriculture data show that 68% of the nuts eaten in the United States are peanuts (approximately one-third consumed as peanut butter), about 6% are almonds, 6% are coconuts, 5% are pecans, 5% are walnuts, and 10% are other nuts (USDA, 2000). These data are consistent with the data from the Nurses' Health Study that showed about one-half of the nuts eaten were peanuts. Data from the EPIC study revealed that, overall, only 4.4% of that population reported consuming tree nuts, and 2.3% reported eating peanuts (Jenab et al., 2006). The study also indicated that Spain and Italy consumed the highest amounts of walnuts, The Netherlands had the highest intake of cashew nuts, and Sweden had the greatest intake of almonds. Peanut consumption made up the highest proportional intake in Norway (63% of all nuts consumed), although this figure does not include nuts eaten as part of hidden sources or spreads (Jenab et al., 2006).

## Nutrient Profile of Nuts

Nuts are high in fat, but are also good sources of protein and high fiber. The protein content of nuts ranges from 10% in walnuts to 17% in almonds; the dietary fiber ranges from 5% in macadamia nuts to 10–14% in almonds and pistachios (USDA database). See Table 10.1 for the macronutrient profile and later Table 10.3 for the micronutrient profile of nuts.

### *Fatty Acid Profile of Nuts*

The fatty acid profiles of individual nut varieties are shown below in Table 10.2. Fat accounts for 50–75% of the macronutrient content of nuts; hence, nuts are energy-dense foods (23.7–29.3 kJ/g) with fat content ranging from 46% in cashews and pistachios to 76% in macadamia nuts. The exception to this is the chestnut which contains little fat (Kris-Etherton et al., 1999a). However, nuts are also nutrient-dense foods, where the quality of the fat, which is predominantly in the form of MUFA, is of greater significance than its energy content. Most nuts contain high levels of

**Table 10.1. Macronutrient Profile of Nuts (per 100 g of nuts)**

| | Energy (kJ) | Protein (g) | Fat total (g) | CHO by diff (g) | CHO (sugars) (g) | Dietary fiber (g) |
|---|---|---|---|---|---|---|
| Almonds | 2408 | 21.22 | 49.42 | 21.67 | 3.89 | 12.2 |
| Brazil nuts | 2743 | 14.32 | 66.43 | 12.27 | 2.33 | 7.5 |
| Cashews | 2314 | 18.22 | 43.85 | 30.19 | 5.91 | 3.3 |
| Hazelnuts | 2629 | 14.95 | 60.75 | 16.7 | 4.34 | 9.7 |
| Macadamia nuts | 3004 | 7.91 | 75.77 | 13.82 | 4.57 | 8.6 |
| Peanuts | 2220 | 25.8 | 49.24 | 16.13 | 3.97 | 8.5 |
| High-oleic peanuts | 2374 | 26.3 | 49.8 | 11.4 | 5.7 | 13.3 |
| Pecans | 2889 | 9.17 | 71.97 | 13.86 | 3.97 | 9.6 |
| Pistachios | 2332 | 20.61 | 44.44 | 27.97 | 7.64 | 10.3 |
| Walnuts | 2738 | 15.23 | 65.21 | 13.71 | 2.61 | 6.7 |

Data from U.S. Department of Agriculture, Agricultural Research Service. 2006 USDA National Nutrient Database for Standard Reference, Release 20 (U.S. Department of Agriculture) (www.ars.usda.gov/nutrientdata) and aPeanut Company of Australia (http://www.pca.com.au/index.php).

**Table 10.2. Fatty acid Composition of Nuts (per 100 g of nuts)**

| Nut | Total Fat | SFA (g) | MUFA (g) | PUFA (g) | ALA (18:3) (g) | LA (18:2) (g) | Oleic acid (18:1) (g) | Palmitic acid (16:0) (g) |
|---|---|---|---|---|---|---|---|---|
| Almonds | 49.42 | 3.73 | 30.89 | 12.07 | 0.006 | 12.061 | 30.611 | 3.044 |
| Brazil nuts | 66.43 | 15.14 | 24.55 | 20.58 | 0.04 | 20.543 | 24.223 | 9.085 |
| Cashews | 43.85 | 7.78 | 23.797 | 7.85 | 0.062 | 7.782 | 23.523 | 3.916 |
| Hazelnuts | 60.75 | 4.46 | 45.65 | 7.92 | 0.087 | 7.833 | 45.405 | 3.097 |
| Macadamia nuts | 75.77 | 12.06 | 58.88 | 1.5 | 0.21 | 1.296 | 43.755 | 6.036 |
| Peanuts | 49.24 | 6.83 | 24.43 | 15.56 | 0.003 | 15.555 | 23.756 | 5.154 |
| High-oleic peanuts | 49.8 | 5.9 | 38.3 | 21.61 | 0.019 | 2.9 | 75 | 6 |
| Pecans | 71.97 | 6.18 | 40.8 | 21.614 | .986 | 20.628 | 40.594 | 4.366 |
| Pistachios | 44.4 | 5.44 | 23.32 | 13.46 | 0.26 | 13.201 | 22.686 | 4.889 |
| Walnuts | 65.21 | 6.13 | 8.93 | 47.17 | 9.08 | 38.093 | 8.799 | 4.404 |

Abbreviations: SFAs, saturated fatty acids; MUFAs, monounsaturated fatty acids; PUFAs, polyunsaturated fatty acids ALA, alpha linolenic acid; LA, linoleic acid. Data derived from http://www.nal.usda.gov/fnic/foodcomp/search/ (accessed June 2008) and information on the high-oleic peanuts derived from the Peanut Company of Australia.

**Table 10.3.** Micronutrient Profile of Nuts

| | $Na^+$ (mg) | $K^+$ (mg) | $Mg^{2+}$ (mg) | $Ca^{2+}$ (mg) | Fe (mg) | Zn (mg) | Thia (mg) | Ribo (mg) | Niacin (mg) | Folate (µg) | Vit $B_6$ (mg) | Vit A (IU) | Vit E (mg) | Cu (mg) | Mang (mg) | Sel (µg) | Arg (g) | Phyto (mg) |
|---|---|---|---|---|---|---|---|---|---|---|---|---|---|---|---|---|---|---|
| Almonds | 1 | 705 | 268 | 264 | 4.72 | 3.08 | 0.24 | 1.01 | 3.39 | 50 | 0.14 | 0 | 26.2 | 1 | 2.29 | 2.5 | 2.45 | 31 |
| Brazil nuts | 3 | 659 | 376 | 160 | 2.43 | 4.06 | 0.62 | 0.04 | 0.3 | 22 | 0.1 | 0 | 5.73 | 1.74 | 1.22 | 1917 | 2.15 | No data |
| Cashews | 12 | 660 | 292 | 37 | 6.68 | 5.78 | 0.42 | 0.06 | 1.06 | 25 | 0.42 | 0 | 0.9 | 2.2 | 1.66 | 19.9 | 2.12 | No data |
| Hazelnuts | 0 | 680 | 163 | 114 | 4.7 | 2.45 | 0.64 | 0.11 | 1.8 | 113 | 0.56 | 1 | 15.0 | 1.73 | 6.18 | 2.4 | 2.21 | 96 |
| Macadamia nuts | 5 | 368 | 130 | 85 | 3.69 | 1.3 | 1.2 | 0.16 | 2.47 | 11 | 0.28 | 0 | 0.54 | 0.76 | 4.13 | 3.6 | 1.4 | 116 |
| Peanuts | 18 | 705 | 168 | 92 | 4.58 | 3.27 | 0.64 | 0.14 | 12.07 | 240 | 0.35 | 0 | 8.3 | 1.14 | 1.93 | 7.2 | 3.09 | 220 |
| Pecans | 0 | 410 | 121 | 70 | 2.53 | 4.53 | 0.66 | 0.13 | 1.17 | 22 | 0.21 | 56 | 1.4 | 1.2 | 4.5 | 3.8 | 1.18 | 102 |
| Pistachios | 1 | 1025 | 121 | 107 | 4.15 | 2.2 | 0.87 | 0.16 | 1.3 | 51 | 1.7 | 553 | 2.3 | 1.3 | 1.2 | 7.0 | 2.03 | 214 |
| Walnuts | 2 | 441 | 158 | 98 | 2.91 | 3.09 | 0.34 | 0.15 | 1.13 | 98 | 0.54 | 20 | 0.7 | 1.59 | 3.41 | 4.9 | 2.28 | 72 |

Data from U.S. Department of Agriculture, Agricultural Research Service. 2006 USDA National Nutrient Database for Standard Reference, Release 20 (U.S. Department of Agriculture) (www.ars.usda.gov/nutrientdata) and aPeanut Company of Australia (http://www.pca.com.au/index.php).

the 18-carbon MUFA oleic acid. In the high-oleic variety of peanuts, for example, more than 80% of fat is oleic acid (http://www.pca.com.au/index.php). Thus, peanuts deliver this beneficial fatty acid in a highly concentrated solid-food form. The macadamia nut has the highest proportion of MUFA of all nut oils (Ako et al., 1995). Nuts are low in SFA with some varieties (e.g., brazil nuts, pine nuts, and walnuts) having substantial levels of PUFA (U.S. Department of Agriculture, 2006).

## *A Role for Alpha Linolenic Acid*

Nuts are an important source of the predominant short-chain omega-3 PUFA alpha linolenic acid (ALA). Walnuts, in particular, are recognized as rich sources of ALA, although the linoleic (LA):ALA ratio is still 4:1 (Table 10.2). Diets rich in ALA, such as a Mediterranean diet, are associated with a beneficial impact on coronary heart disease (CHD), with previous reports finding ALA intakes to be associated with a 50–70% reduction of the risk of recurrence after 4 years of follow-up in the Lyon Diet Heart Study (de Lorgeril & Salen, 2006). Based on data from Table 10.2, as little as 11 g of walnuts would need to be eaten to achieve an intake of 1 g of ALA. Zhao et al. (2004) reported that the fatty acid profile of a nut in its solid form versus the extracted oil differed slightly with 100 g of walnuts containing ≈38 g of LA and 9 g of ALA, while 100 g of walnut oil provide 53 g of LA and 10 g of ALA. Nuts and nut oil can contribute significantly to omega-3 PUFA dietary intakes, especially in a vegetarian population (Li et al., 2006).

## *Low in Saturated Fat*

When nuts are substituted into the diet, not only an increase in PUFA and MUFA intake occurs, but also often an associated reduction in SFA occurs (King et al., 2008). This is usually because nuts are substituted for other high-fat foods which tend to be higher in SFA (Gilbert & Khokhar, 2008). This substitution and increase in the proportion of unsaturated fatty acids and the decrease in SFA impact favorably on a cardiovascular disease (CVD) risk. Replacing even one snack per day with nuts has a beneficial impact on a CVD risk (Lloyd-Williams et al., 2008).

The macadamia nut has the highest SFA content of all nuts; thus, it does not have as healthy a profile as other nuts. However, a recent study by Griel et al. (2008) indicates that the macadamia nut may, in fact, still be a healthy option. These authors reported significant reductions in low-density lipoprotein–cholesterol (LDL–C) and total cholesterol (TC) following the consumption of the macadamia-rich diet compared with an average American diet. While no change was noted in serum-triglyceride concentration, this still suggests that one can include macadamia nuts in a heart-healthy dietary pattern that reduces lipid/lipoprotein CVD risk factors. This study supports the handful of previous studies conducted with macadamia nuts (Colquhoun et al., 1996; Curb et al., 2000; Garg et al., 2007; Griel et al., 2008; Hiraoka-Yamamoto et al., 2004).

## Whole Nuts versus Nut Oils

Only a few studies have tested whole nuts against nut components. Much of the interest in nuts comes from the oil which one can readily extract and which can withstand oxidation (Miraliakbari & Shahidi, 2008). The fatty acid compositions of tree-nut oils were analyzed by using gas chromatography, showing that oleic acid was the predominant fatty acid in all samples except for pine-nut and walnut oils, which contained high amounts of LA. An elevated plasma concentration of LDL–C is an important risk factor for CVD (Castelli et al., 1992), and a large proportion of the Western population would probably benefit from cholesterol reduction (Grundy, 1997). Diets rich in MUFA are effective for reducing LDL–C, with the more atherogenic particles being selectively reduced (Gill et al., 2003).

Recently, reportedly, nut oils, such as hazelnut oil, can reduce lipid peroxidation, which is possibly related to the high-MUFA content (Balkan et al., 2003). The administration of hazelnut oil to hypercholesterolemic rabbits resulted in both reduced oxidative stress and cholesterol accumulation in the aortas of rabbits fed a high-cholesterol diet (Hatipoglu et al., 2004). Both walnuts and walnut oil are equally effective in enhancing vascular function through reducing the expression of aortic endothelin-1, which is an important endothelial regulator (Davis et al., 2006).

Spiller and colleagues (2003) tested whether raw almonds had the same impact on cholesterol levels as roasted, salted almonds and roasted almond butter. Thirty-eight hypercholesterolemic volunteers supplemented a heart-healthy diet with 100 g of almonds [in one of the two forms—either as a solid nut (roasted or raw) or as almond butter] for 4 weeks, and all achieved a significant reduction in LDL–C compared with baseline levels. Hyson et al. (2002) conducted a crossover study where they replaced 50% of the participants' usual dietary intake with almonds or almond oil for 6 weeks. They reported that almonds and almond oil cause similar reductions in TC (4%) and LDL (6%), and concluded that the cholesterol-lowering effect of almonds is due mainly to constituents of the lipid fraction. This should be considered with caution since other components of nuts, such as dietary fiber and arginine, may also be able to reduce cholesterol. In both of the studies highlighted above, the consumption of the whole almonds was also associated with an increase in fiber. Fiber is one of the components of nuts that is likely to also impact their satiating effects. In a study comparing peanut oil with whole peanuts on satiation, Coehlo et al. (2006) found that peanut oil was less satiating. Consider this when setting recommendations for nut consumption as part of a heart-healthy diet.

## Bioactive Nutrients in Nuts

Nuts are also rich sources of other bioactive nutrients that have the potential to deliver metabolic and CV health benefits. They are an excellent source of protein (≈25% of energy intake) and, in the case of peanuts, have an exceptionally high content of L-arginine (Alper & Mattes, 2003). Only 15% of energy is in the form of carbohydrate. However, nuts are a good source of dietary fiber, ranging from 4–11%

by weight, which in a standard serving provides 5–10% of daily-fiber requirements (U.S. Department of Agriculture, 2006) (see Table 10.1).

Nuts are also important sources of micronutrients, including folate, magnesium and calcium, and are a very rich source of potassium. Brazil nuts are a rich source of the micronutrient selenium with levels 100 times higher than any other nut (Thomson et al., 2008), and pistachios are the richest nut source of potassium. Nuts also contain other potentially cardioprotective constituents including phytosterols, such as stigmasterol, campesterol, and sitosterol (Alper & Mattes, 2003; U.S. Department of Agriculture, 2006), tocopherols, and squalene (Maguire et al., 2004; Ryan et al., 2006) (see Table 10.3). Of the tree nuts, walnuts, pecans, and chestnuts have the highest contents of antioxidants (Blomhoff et al., 2006) although studies reported that regular nut consumption can increase antioxidant capacity (ORAC) without altering the serum-antioxidant profiles of subjects (Davis et al., 2006).

Being rich sources of antioxidant vitamins (e.g., tocopherols) and flavonoids (e.g., resveratrol in peanuts) (Sanders et al., 2000; Shahidi et al., 2007), nuts can reduce oxidative stress (Kocyigit et al., 2006) and counteract any potential pro-oxidative effects of the unsaturated fatty acids in nuts (Kiokias et al., 2008). Almonds, in particular, are especially rich in many tocopherols, including α-tocopherol, the most active form of vitamin E, with potential anti-atherogenic effects (Sabate, 1999). Almonds are also rich sources of vitamin A which was first reported in the 1920s (Coward & Drummond, 1920). Evidence from cell cultures, as well as animal and human clinical and observational studies, strongly supports the contribution of dietary vitamin E to the maintenance of vascular function and health (Meydani, 2004). The vitamin-K (phylloquinone) content of a range of nuts was analyzed. Pine nuts and cashews had detectable levels, but the majority of nuts only have very low levels, and thus are not major contributors of vitamin K to the diet (Dismore et al., 2003).

Peanuts are a rich source of B-vitamins, vitamin E, and a number of micronutrients, including magnesium, copper, and phosphorus (Griel et al., 2004). In addition, they are a source of plant protein, arginine, dietary fiber, and unsaturated fatty acids. Numerous bioactive substances (i.e., flavonoids, resveratrol, and plant sterols) are also present in peanuts (Griel et al., 2004). All of these components of nuts contribute to a reduced risk of CHD (Sabate, 1999).

In addition to being rich in several vitamins and minerals, unsaturated fatty acids, and fiber, tree nuts and peanuts contain numerous phytochemicals (Ryan et al., 2006) that may contribute to promoting health and reducing the risk of chronic disease (Chen & Blumberg, 2008). Walnut polyphenolics are found in the highest concentration in the pellicle, the thin tan-brown "skin" that lines the meat of the nut. These polyphenols are effective inhibitors of LDL oxidation in vitro. An extract from a handful of walnuts, one 50 g serving (8–9 shelled walnuts), contains 802 mg of gallic-acid equivalents (GAEs) of total phenols (Anderson et al., 2001), while the equivalent amount of pecans has a total- phenol content of 500 mg of GAEs.

Polyphenolic compounds vary between nut varieties with particularly high levels seen in peanut skins (Lou et al., 2004). The skin of the peanuts contains a range of catechins and procyanidins, with the main polyphenol being resveratrol (Kris-Etherton et al., 2002). The peanut and the pistachio nut are the only types of nuts known to contain substantial levels of resveratrol (Sanders et al., 2000; Tokusoglu et al., 2005). A growing body of evidence shows that polyphenols can facilitate circulatory function through the increased production of the primary mediator of endothelial dilatation, namely, nitric oxide (NO) (Stoclet et al., 2004).

## Nuts and Heart Disease

### *Epidemiological Evidence*

Epidemiological evidence suggests an association between nut consumption and a reduced incidence of CHD. This is based on data from the Adventist Health Study (Fraser et al., 1992; Fraser, 1999), the Iowa Women's Health Study (Blomhoff et al., 2006; Ellsworth et al., 2001; Kushi et al., 1996), the Nurses' Health Study (Hu et al., 1998), and the Physicians' Health Study (Albert et al., 2002). When combined, the evidence suggests that the risk of CHD is 37% lower for people consuming nuts more than four times per week compared to those who never or seldom consume nuts, with an average reduction of 8.3% for each weekly serving of nuts (Feldman, 2002; Kelly & Sabate, 2006). Nut consumption may also increase longevity through the prevention of other conditions (Sabate, 1999).

In the Adventist Health Study, subjects who consumed nuts five or more times per week had a significantly reduced risk of both fatal CHD [relative risk (RR), 0.52] and nonfatal myocardial infarction (MI) (RR, 0.49) (Fraser et al., 1992). In the Nurses' Health Study, those who consumed nuts five or more times per week had a 35% reduced risk of total CHD among women (Hu et al., 1998). The Iowa's Women's Health Study reported a reduced risk of fatal CHD among women who consumed nuts two to four times per week. Also a weak inverse association was noted between frequent nut intake and all-cause mortality (RR, 0.88; 95% confidence interval [CI]: 0.77–0.99, $P$ for trend = 0.047) (Ellsworth et al., 2001). The Physicians' Health Study findings are consistent with the other studies, but weaker associations were found between nut consumption and CHD (Albert et al., 2002). Results of all of these studies are now discussed in more detail.

#### *Adventist Health Study*

The Adventist Health Study looked at a population of non-Hispanic Caucasian Seventh-Day Adventists in California which consisted of 10,003 men (mean age 51.3 ± 16.0 years) and 16,740 women (mean age 53 2 ± 16.6 years). Fraser et al. (1992) reported on the incidence of CHD over a 6-year period (1977 to 1982), and investigated the relationship between the incidence of MIs or nonfatal events and several diet and lifestyle factors. Of this population, 34% consumed nuts less than once per week, 42% consumed nuts one to four times per week (42%), and 24% consumed nuts more than five times per week. In this population, 346 definite CHD events occurred. Those with the highest nut consumption had the lowest incidence of CHD cases ($P < 0.001$); data are shown below in Table 10.4.

### *Iowa Women's Health Study*

The Iowa Women's Health Study is a prospective study of just over 34,000 postmenopausal women (55–69 years of age) at enrollment. Intake was assessed for 127 foods, including nuts, by using a food-frequency questionnaire, as well as lifestyle factors relevant to CHD. In comparison to the Adventist Health Study, nut consumption in this population was considerably low: 41% never ate nuts, 35% ate them one to three times per month, 15% ate them once per week, and only 9% ate nuts two or more times per week. After 7 years of follow-up in 19,411 women not using vitamin supplements, those in the highest quartile of nut consumption had a 40% reduction in the risk of fatal CHD compared to the lowest quartile that seldom or never ate nuts (RR, 0.60; 95% CI: 0.36–1.01; *P* for trend, 0.016) (Kushi et al., 1996).

Further analysis conducted after 12 years indicated that 3726 women died (657 from CHD). After multiple adjustments, an inverse relationship between nut consumption and the risk of death from CHD was still present. The highest category of nut consumption (two or more 28.5 g servings per week) had a risk reduction of 19% compared to those who ate nuts less than once per month (RR, 0.81; 95% CI: 0.60–1.11; *P* for trend, 0.30), and a 12% lower risk of all-cause mortality (Ellsworth et al., 2001).

Results after 15 years of follow-up were reported by Blomhoff et al. (Blomhoff et al., 2006). For that analysis on postmenopausal women without heart disease or diabetes at baseline, the combined frequency of consumption of nuts plus peanut butter showed strong and consistent reductions in the risk of CHD death. After adjusting for the recognized CHD risk and dietary factors, women consuming nuts/peanut butter one to four times per week and five or more times per week had, respectively, an 18 and 29% risk reduction of CHD deaths (Blomhoff et al., 2006).

### *Nurses' Health Study*

The Nurses' Health Study (Hu et al., 1998) also investigated the relationship between nut consumption and CHD. This prospective study of female nurses (30–55 years of age) from across the United States is the largest epidemiological study to examine this association. Data from the Nurses' Health Study suggest that total CHD and the frequency of nut consumption were inversely associated at baseline using age-

**Table 10.4. Adventist Health Study: Frequency of Nut Consumption and Relative Risk (Confidence Intervals) of Fatal Coronary Heart Disease (CHD), and Nonfatal Myocardial Infarction (MI) Stratified on Age, Sex, Smoking, Exercise, Relative Weight, and High Blood Pressure (Fraser et al., 1992)**

| | <1/week | 1–4 /week | >5 week |
|---|---|---|---|
| Nonfatal MI ($P < 0.05$) | 1.0 | 0.74 (0.49–1.11) | 0.52 (0.30–0.87) |
| Fatal CHD ($P < 0.01$) | 1.0 | 0.73 (0.54–0.99) | 0.62 (0.44–0.90) |

adjusted analyses. The RR in women consuming nuts more than five times per week compared with those who never ate nuts was 0.48 (0.35–0.65, *P* for trend, 0.0001). When controlling for potential confounding factors (age, cigarette smoking, body-mass index (BMI), hormones for treating menopause, alcohol, and multivitamin and vitamin-E supplements), this relationship was reduced to 0.65 (0.47–0.89, *P* for trend, 0.0009). Table 10.5 below reports the age- and multivariate-adjusted RRs associated with fatal and corresponding nonfatal CHD.

### *Physicians' Health Study*

The Physicians' Health Study was a prospective study of 22,071 male physicians between 40 and 84 years of age in 1982 with no history of MI, stroke, transient ischemic attacks, or cancer who randomly assigned participants to receive aspirin, beta carotene, both active drugs, or both placebos. Nut consumption over a 12-month period was determined via a food- frequency questionnaire, and the relationship between nut consumption and the end points of fatal and nonfatal MI and death from CHD was evaluated after 17 years of follow-up. The frequency of nut consumption was inversely associated with death from CHD only for the highest intake category (more than twice per week). Those people consuming nuts more than once a week had a 33% reduction in the risk of CHD death, although an insignificant trend existed (RR, 0.77; 95% CI: 0.59–1.0; *P* for trend, 0.06) (Albert et al., 2002). After adjusting for multiple confounders, those people who consumed nuts one to three times per week had a 20% reduction in the risk of sudden cardiac death (SCD), those consuming nuts twice per week had a 40% reduction, and those consuming nuts more than once a week had a 47% reduction in risk of SCD (*P* for trend, 0.01) (see 10.6).

## Evidence from Clinical Studies

### *How the Evidence Gets Incorporated into Dietary Guidelines*

Numerous clinical studies have assessed the effects of different tree nuts, including walnuts, almonds, hazelnuts, macadamia nuts, peanuts, pecans, and pistachios, by utilizing various experimental designs in diverse population groups (Griel & Kris-Etherton, 2006). Studies were conducted in both healthy populations and those at

**Table 10.5. Data Source from the Nurses' Health Study (Hu et al., 1998)**

| | | <1/month | 1–4 /month | 2–4/ week | >- 5/ week |
|---|---|---|---|---|---|
| Age-adjusted RR | Fatal CHD (*P* = 0.0001) | 1.0 | 0.57 (0.46– 0.70) | 0.39 (0.25– 0.61) | 0.41 (0.24– 0.70) |
| Multivariate-RR | Fatal CHD (*P* = 0.007) | 1.0 | 0.75 (0.61– 0.93) | 0.56 (0.36– 0.89) | 0.61 (0.35– 1.05) |
| Age-adjusted RR | Nonfatal MI (*P* = 0.0001) | 1.0 | 0.85 (0.73– 0.98) | 0.66 (0.50– 0.86) | 0.52 (0.36– 0.75) |
| Multivariate-RR | Nonfatal MI (*P* = 0.04) | 1.0 | 1.0 (0.87– 1.16) | 0.87 (0.66– 1.14) | 0.68 (0.47– 1.00) |

risk of CHD due to elevated cholesterol levels. The average reduction in the risk of CHD death is 8.3% for each serving of nuts (about 30 g) consumed weekly (Kelly & Sabate, 2006). Based on this evidence, nutrition organizations around the world recommend eating nuts as part of a healthy diet (Krauss et al., 2000; Lipid Management Guidelines-2001, 2001). This was translated into the following qualified health claim approved by the Food and Drug Administration (FDA) in the United States: "Scientific evidence suggests but does not prove that eating 1.5 ounces (43 g) of most nuts per day as part of a diet low in saturated fat and cholesterol may help to reduce the risk of heart disease." [Food and Drug Administration. Qualified Health Claims: Letter of Enforcement Discretion—Nuts and Coronary Heart Disease (Docket No. 02P-0505), 2003].

## Nuts Improve Risk Factors for Cardiometabolic Disease

The strongest evidence for a health role for nuts in the diet relates to lipid management, particularly the reduction of non-high-density lipoprotein–C (non-HDL–C). However, as more research continues to investigate the impact of nuts in the diet, evidently regular nut consumption is also associated with the attenuation of weight gain. Results from the SUN study indicate that participants who consume nuts at least two times per week were 30% less likely to gain weight (5 kg or more) in comparison with those who rarely ate nuts (Bes-Rastrollo et al., 2007). The next section discusses the impact of nuts on risk factors for cardiometabolic disease.

### *Impact of Nuts on Lipid Profiles*

An extensive body of literature describes the beneficial effects of nuts on lipid profiles which are covered in comprehensive systematic reviews by Mukuddem-Petersen et al. (2005) and Griel & Kris-Etherton (2006). These authors conclude that the inclusion of 50–100 g (approximately 1.5–3.5 servings) five or more times a week (in conjunction with a low-fat diet) helps to decrease TC and LDL–C and protect against

**Table 10.6. Physicians' Health Study: Frequency of Nut Consumption and Age-Adjusted (Age–adj RR) and Multivariate Relative Risk (Multi-RR) Confidence Interval (CI) of Fatal Coronary Heart Disease (CHD) and Sudden Cardiac Death (SCD) (Albert et al., 2002)**

| | | <1/month | 1–3 /month | 1/week | >2/week |
|---|---|---|---|---|---|
| Age-adj RR | Fatal CHD ($P = 0.06$) | 1.0 | 0.93 (0.75–1.15) | 0.89 (0.70–1.13) | 0.77 (0.59–1.00) |
| Multi-RR | Fatal CHD ($P = 0.06$) | 1.0 | 0.89 (0.67–1.16) | 0.90 (0.67–1.22) | 0.70 (0.50–0.98) |
| Age-adj RR | SCD ($P = 0.04$) | 1.0 | 0.98 (0.68–1.40) | 0.85 (0.57–1.28) | 0.64 (0.40–1.01) |
| Multi-RR | SCD ($P = 0.01$) | 1.0 | 0.80 (0.52–1.23) | 0.60 (0.36–1.00) | 0.53 (0.30–0.92) |

CVD. However, improved lipid profiles are noted with the consumption of as little as 20 g/day for some nuts (Chisholm et al., 2005; Tamizifar et al., 2005), and a clinically relevant improvement (1% reduction in LDL–C) was achieved with as little as 4 g of nuts per day (Griel & Kris-Etherton, 2006). However, data from two dose-response studies with almonds (Jenkins et al., 2002; Sabate et al., 2003) suggest that a lower level of enrichment (25–50 g/day accounting for 10% of energy) was insufficient to lower either LDL–C or TC, while a higher level (20% of energy from 50–100 g/day) was effective.

The beneficial effects of a high-MUFA intake from nuts were tested against The National Cholesterol Education Program (NCEP)/AHA Step I or Step II diets, which are typically recommended for lowering blood-cholesterol concentrations. The NCEP Step I and II diets are low in fat (with a particular focus on reducing SFA and cholesterol) and high in carbohydrate. Although these diets can reduce both TC and LDL–C by 5–14%, they tend to increase plasma-triacylglycerol concentrations and decrease HDL–C concentrations, which may adversely impact CVD risk. High nut consumption on the other hand is able to achieve a further 0.21-mmol/L reduction in TC and LDL–C versus the NCEP Step I diet (Griel & Kris-Etherton, 2006), while preserving HDL–C and reducing triacylglycerol levels by up to 17% (Griel & Kris-Etherton, 2006; Kris-Etherton et al., 1999). This was found for whole kernels, nut oils, and peanut butter, although the extent of benefit depends on the level and duration of intake (Hyson, 2002; Kris-Etherton, 1999; Zibaeenezhad, 2005). Thus, nuts have a broader benefit in dyslipidemia; health authorities should consider them for inclusion in lipid-lowering diets.

The cholesterol reduction observed in clinical studies of tree nuts is typically 25% greater than is expected from blood-cholesterol-predictive equations developed by Mensink and Katan (1992) that are based on dietary fatty acid profiles (Kris-Etherton, 1999). Griel et al. reported that a macadamia-rich diet, in fact, had a 48% greater reduction in TC than one could have predicted (Griel et al., 2008). Although the improvement in blood lipids is attributable primarily to the favorable fatty acid profiles of nuts, the discrepancies indicated above suggest that other components of nuts, including dietary fiber and phytosterols (Ostlund, 2004; Segura, 2006), may also contribute to blood-lipid improvements.

Several controlled feeding trials with a variety of nuts convincingly show that the daily consumption of small portions of nuts for periods of 4–8 weeks has a clear cholesterol-lowering effect (see Table 10.7 for studies reporting a significant level of reduction). In nut studies using hyperlipidemic participants, decreased TC and LDL–C were observed but were not significant in all studies (Spiller et al., 1992; Sabate et al., 1993; Colquhoun DM et al., 1996; O'Byrne et al., 1997; Chisholm et al., 1998; Spiller et al., 1998; Edwards et al., 1999; Kris-Etherton et al., 1999; Zambon et al., 2000; Almario et al., 2001; Rajaram et al., 2001; Jenkins et al., 2002; Garg et al., 2003; Ros et al., 2004; Gebauer et al., 2008). The total-fat intakes in previous studies varied considerably ranging from 20% (Morgan et al., 2000) to 42% of total energy (Colquhoun et al., 1996).

While several studies reported improvements in all lipid parameters (Sabate et al., 1993), this was not consistent. This may be related to the population studies, the extent of the enrichment of the diet, and/or the length of supplementation. Also many studies reported improvements in TC and LDL–C without changes in HDL–C or triglycerides.

Only a few studies reported improvements in triglycerides. Reductions were seen with hazelnuts (Mercanligil et al., 2007), although not consistently (Durak et al., 1999), pecans (Rajaram et al., 2001), macadamia nuts (Curb et al., 2000), and peanuts (Kris-Etherton, 1999b). The improvements ranged from a 9% reduction following 4 weeks of consuming macadamias to a 32% reduction following 8 weeks of consuming 40 g of hazelnuts per day (Mercanligil et al., 2007).

## Blood Pressure

Nuts provide a highly favorable anti-hypertensive electrolyte profile with their very high content of potassium, very low level of sodium, and additional calcium and magnesium contents. Increased intakes of potassium, calcium, and magnesium all have the potential to reduce blood pressure (Cappuccio & MacGregor, 1991). The Dietary Approaches to Stop Hypertension (DASH) study tested a diet rich in fruits, vegetables, and low-fat dairy products, including whole grains, fish, poultry, and nuts, and reduced in fats, red meats, sweets, and sugar-containing beverages. Significant reductions in blood pressure over 8 weeks were associated with regular adherence to such diets in comparison to diets which did not contain nuts (Conlin et al., 2000). Despite this and the positive impact of nuts on CHD risk, the anti-hypertensive electrolyte profile of nuts was not a primary focus of clinical trials; hence, little evidence exists of the impact of nut consumption on blood pressure (Sabate, 1993; Edwards et al., 1999; Iwamoto, 2000; Jenkins et al., 2002; Mukuddem-Petersen et al., 2007; Sheridan et al., 2007).

An impaired baroreflex function or an altered autonomic nervous control of the CV system, expressed by baroreflex sensitivity (BRS), is involved in the progression of many CVDs (Cai et al., 2005). Schutte et al. (2006) tested two nut-rich diets in an 8-week parallel-design randomized controlled trial. Subjects were randomized to a diet rich in unsalted cashew nuts (MUFA), a diet rich in unsalted walnuts (PUFA) (both providing 20% of total energy from nuts), or a control diet. The two nut diets showed the opposite effects on BRS, while subjects given a control diet did not show any significant changes in BRS. BRS in the walnut-fed study group worsened with a significant reduction ($P = 0.038$), while BRS significantly improved in the cashew-fed study group ($P = 0.036$). While this study suggests that walnuts had a detrimental impact on CV regulation, scientists should further develop this area of research given the body of evidence supporting a role for nuts in a heart-healthy diet.

## Vascular Function

Diet can influence vascular reactivity. Short-term feeding trials show the potential of food for improving endothelial vasodilator function, either as isolated nutrients—such as n-3 PUFA, L-arginine, and antioxidant vitamins—or as healthy-food patterns—such as diets rich in nuts (West, 2001).

Maintaining the functional capacity of the endothelial cells lining blood vessels is vital to vascular health, and improvements in endothelial vasodilator function occurred with high nut consumption (Ros et al., 2004). This section focuses on the ability of nuts to influence endothelial function through multiple mechanisms: (i) NO production, (ii) endothelin-1 production, and (iii) mediators of cell adhesion and inflammatory processes.

Peanuts are also a rich source of the amino acid L-arginine, the precursor of NO (Huynh & Chin-Dusting, 2006). Previous studies found an improvement in endothelial function after supplementation with L-arginine at doses of 8–21 g/day (Brown & Hu, 2001). Supplementation is particularly efficacious in subjects with impaired endothelial NO synthesis (e.g., patients with elevated cholesterol or CHD). One could readily increase the average daily consumption of L-arginine to around 8 g per day by adding approximately 70 g/day of peanuts to the average American diet (http://www.pca.com.au/index.php). The ability to deliver both the NO precursor and polyphenols to facilitate NO production in endothelial cells makes peanuts an ideal food for vascular health.

The predominant endothelial vasoconstrictor is endothelin-1 (ET-1). A recent paper by Davis et al. (2006) compared individual antioxidants found in walnuts with walnut oil and whole walnuts on aortic ET-1 expression. Only after whole-nut consumption did the significant inhibition of ET-1 mRNA expression occur. The authors did not speculate which component of the nut was responsible for this effect.

Epidemiological evidence suggests that nut consumption is inversely correlated with pro-inflammatory markers (Esposito et al., 2004; Jiang et al., 2006), with the possible exception of C-reactive protein, and positively correlated with adiponectin, a cardioprotective marker (Mantzoros et al., 2006). Normal endothelial function is impaired by inflammatory cytokines and cell-adhesion molecules. However, adiponectin enhances endothelial function by direct actions on endothelial NO synthase synthesis by inhibiting pro-inflammatory cytokines and by inhibiting the expression of cell-adhesion molecules, including vascular cell-adhesion molecule-1 (VCAM-1) and intercellular cell-adhesion molecule-1 (Ritchie et al., 2004). Recent studies by Ros et al. (2004) and Zhao et al. (2004) found that walnut consumption improved endothelium-dependent vasodilation and reduced levels of VCAM-1 without altering other mediators of vascular damage. Hence, multiple mechanisms are available by which bioactive nutrients in nuts may act, possibly synergistically, to improve circulation by enhancing endothelial function.

Furthermore, previous studies tested the effects of nuts on fibrinogen, factor VII coagulant activity, tissue plasminogen-activator activity, and plasminogen-activator inhibitor 1 activity, but found no effect after the consumption of 64 g/day of walnuts for 6 weeks in patients with borderline-high TC (Morgan et al., 2002) or when either walnuts or cashew nuts contributed 20% of total energy (63–108 g) for 8 weeks (Pieters et al., 2005).

**Table 10.7. Comparison Made Between Lipid Levels at the End of the Nut Diet versus the End of the Control Diet**

| Nut | Reference | Diet comparison | Length (wk) | Amount (g/day) | LDL | HDL | TCHOL | TG |
|---|---|---|---|---|---|---|---|---|
| Walnut | (Sabate, 1993) | Step 1 | 4 | 84 | | −4.9# | −12.4 | NS |
| Walnut | (Abbey M et al., 1994) | Control | 3 | 68 | | NS | −5.0# | NS |
| Walnut | (Zambon et al., 2000) | MED | 6 | 41–56 | | NS | | NS |
| Walnut | (Almario et al., 2001) | Habitual | 6 | 48 | −10.2# | NS | NS | NS |
| Walnut | (Almario et al., 2001) | Low-fat | 6 | 48 | −12.3# | NS | −7.7# | NS |
| Walnut | (Iwamoto, 2000) | Japanese diet | 4 | 44–58 | | NS | | NS |
| Walnut | (Ros et al., 2004) | MED | 4 | 40–65 | −6.7# | NS | −4.3^ | NS |
| Walnut | (Tapsell et al., 2004) | Baseline | 24 | 30 g | −10.1^ | 18.2^ | NS | NS |
| Almond | (Spiller et al., 1992) | Baseline | 9 | 100 | −12.4# | NS | −8.9^ | NS |
| Almond | (Abbey et al., 1994) | Control | 3 | 84 | | NS | −7.0# | NS |
| Almond | (Spiller et al.,1998) | Control | 4 | 100 | | NS | | NS |
| Almond | (Jenkins et al., 2002) | Control | 4 | 25–50 | NS | NS | −2.0^ | NS |
| Almond | (Jenkins et al., 2002) | Control | 4 | 50–100 | −7.1# | 2.2^ | −4.4# | NS |
| Almond | (Lovejoy et al., 2002) | High-fat | 4 | 57–113 | NS | −3.4# | NS | NS |
| Almond | (Lovejoy et al., 2002) | Low-fat | 4 | 57–113 | NS | −2.6# | NS | NS |
| Almond | (Sabate et al., 2003) | Step 1 | 4 | 10% energy | NS | NS | NS | NS |
| Almond | (Sabate et al., 2003) | Step 1 | 4 | 20% energy | −7.0^ | NS | −4.4^ | NS |
| Hazelnut | (Durak et al., 1999) | Baseline | 4 | 1 g/kgbw/day | | 7.2^ | −6.1# | |
| Hazelnut | (Mercanligil et al., 2007) | Low-fat | 8 | 40 | NS | 12.6^ | NS | −31.8^ |
| Macadamia | (Curb, 2000) | AAD | 4 | not recorded | −4.5^ | −4.2# | −4.8# | −9.2^ |
| Macadamia | (Garg, 2003) | Baseline | 4 | (15% Tot E) | −6^ | 6.7^ | −3.2^ | NS |
| Macadamia | (Griel, 2008) | AAD | 5 | 42.5 | −8.7^ | −7.5^ | −9.4^ | NS |
| Peanut | (O'Byrne et al., 1997) | Low-fat | 24 | 35–68 | −9.1# | −0.3# | −7.4# | NS |

**Table 10.7., cont.** Comparison Made Between Lipid Levels at the End of the Nut Diet versus the End of the Control Diet

| Nut | Reference | Diet comparison | Length (wk) | Amount (g/day) | LDL | HDL | TCHOL | TG |
|---|---|---|---|---|---|---|---|---|
| Peanut | (Kris-Etherton et al., 1999) | AAD | 3.5 | not recorded | −13.9^ | NS | −10.9^ | 12.8^ |
| Peanut | (Kris-Etherton et al., 1999) | Step II | 3.5 | not recorded | NS | NS | −2^ | −21.6^ |
| Pecan | (Morgan & Clayshulte, 2000) | Control | 8 | 68 | −16.3^ | 1.2^ | −10.7^ | NS |
| Pecan | (Rajaram et al., 2001) | Step 1 | 4 | 72 | −10.4# | 5.6# | −6.7# | −11.1# |
| Pecan | (Eastman & Clayshulte, 2005) | Control | 8 | 68 | NS | NS | NS | 38.1^ |
| Pistachio | (Edwards et al., 1999) | Baseline | 3 | 20% Tot E | NS | 8^ | −3.7^ | NS |
| Pistachio | (Gebauer et al., 2006) | Control | 4 | 20% Tot E | NS | NS | −8^ | NS |

Data shown as percentage difference. Abbreviations: AAD, average American diet; MED, Mediterranean; Step 1, American Heart Association/National Cholesterol Education Program Step I diet with 30% energy from fat; Step II, American Heart Association/National Cholesterol Education Program Step I diet with 25% energy from fat; LDL, low-density lipoprotein; HDL, high-density lipoprotein; TCHOL, total cholesterol; TG, triglycerides.
* denotes $P < 0.001$, ^ denotes $P < 0.01$, # denotes $P < 0.05$.

## *Impact of Nuts on Body Weight and Obesity*

The high-energy density of nuts caused concern that their consumption would promote weight gain. Yet data collected from over 12,000 participants in the U.S. Department of Agriculture's Continuing Survey of Food Intakes by Individuals (Sabate, 2003) revealed that BMI was lower in nut consumers compared to those who never ate nuts (23.8 ± 0.1 kg/m$^2$ versus 25.0 ± 0.1 kg/m$^2$) despite their higher energy intakes (2191 ± 20 kcal/day versus 1997 ± 9 kcal/day). Moreover, clinical interventions (Alper & Mattes, 2002; Kris-Etherton et al., 1999) indicate that including nuts in an energy-restricted diet can help promote weight loss or at least limit weight gain.

The impact of nuts on body weight was recently reviewed by Garcia Lorda et al. (2003) and St Onge (2005). These reviews concluded that, while the evidence for nut consumption facilitating weight loss is weak, support exists for the role of nuts in contributing to the maintenance of healthy weight. Very few studies have addressed, as a primary outcome, the ability of nuts to reduce weight (Alper and Mattes, 2002; Fraser et al., 2002; Wien et al., 2003; Pelkman et al., 2004; Hollis and Mattes, 2007); thus, much of the evidence is gathered from studies showing weight maintenance where weight gain was predicted based on energy-intake data.

Wien et al. (Wien et al., 2003) compared low-calorie diets (LCD) which were high in carbohydrate (CHO) or, alternatively, enriched with almonds on various metabolic parameters and markers of body composition. After 24 weeks on the diet, all subjects had lost weight. However, the almond–LCD group experienced a 62% greater reduction in weight, a 50% greater reduction in waist circumference, and a 56% greater reduction in fat mass than the CHO–LCD intervention, and showed greater improvements in glucose homeostasis. Similar findings were reported by McManus et al. (2001), who observed a twofold greater reduction in weight when a low-energy, moderate-fat diet rich in nuts was compared with a low-energy, low-fat diet. Moreover, a dramatic difference was noted in the reduction of waist circumference (6.9 cm versus 2.6 cm), representing the loss of abdominal fat.

Pelkman et al. (2004) found that the incorporation of peanuts in a low-energy diet achieved the same weight loss as a low-fat diet, but improved CVD-risk markers. However O'Byrne et al. (1997) reported a 3.6-kg reduction of body weight in a 6-month dietary trial with subjects on a low-fat diet supplemented with high-oleic peanuts compared to a low-fat diet without peanuts. These studies indicate that the incorporation of nuts in a low-energy diet plan is an effective and safe method to boost weight reduction.

Data from the SUN study indicate that regular nut consumption can help limit weight gain. In this prospective cohort of 8,865 adult men and women, data on dietary habits were collected by using a validated semi-quantitative food-frequency questionnaire after a median period of 28 months, and then compared against changes in weight. Participants with little nut consumption (never/almost never) gained an average of 424 g (95% CI: 102– 746) more than frequent nut eaters (Bes-Rastrollo et al., 2007). The group with the highest nut intake also had the highest energy intake, but the lowest intake of SFA and the highest level of dietary fiber.

## *Influence on Appetite and Energy Balance*

Appetite suppression may result from the satiating effects of the high-fiber, protein, and energy contents of nuts (see Table 10.1). As indicated in the section on whole nuts versus nut oils, Coehlo et al. (2006) found that peanut oil was less satiating than whole peanuts. The fatty acid profiles of nuts may also influence satiety (French, 2004). Although fat does not have the same satiating ability as protein or carbohydrate, fatty acid chain length and saturation influenced appetite through their differential rates of oxidation (Kamphuis et al., 2001). However, other studies did not find differential effects of fat sources on satiety (Iyer et al., 2006; MacIntosh et al., 2003). Many studies reported weight gains that were less than that predicted by the increase in energy intake following nut consumption (Alper & Mattes, 2002; Fraser et al., 2002; Coelho et al., 2006). This could be due to incomplete absorption of energy caused by the high-fiber content of nuts or, alternatively, to enhanced energy utilization, as their high unsaturated fat content may stimulate fat metabolism (Jump et al., 2005).

Moreno et al. (2006) made the interesting observation that an alcohol extract of peanut husks could inhibit intestinal fat absorption, hepatic metabolism, and lipolysis in adipocytes through dose-dependent reductions of pancreatic lipase, hormone-sensitive lipase, and lipoprotein lipase (LPL). Adding the extract (1%, w/w) to a high-fat diet fed to rats for 12 weeks also resulted in a 5% reduction in body weight, while food consumption remained unaffected (Moreno et al., 2006). The reduction in weight coincided with a twofold increase in fecal weight, attributed to the inhibition of pancreatic lipase, and reduced the digestibility of dietary fat.

## *Insulin-sensitizing Effect of Nuts*

Mechanistic explanations are available for the influence of dietary PUFA on insulin action and energy metabolism (Storlien et al., 1996). Both chain length and the degree of saturation of fat impacted glucose and insulin regulation. Large cohort studies of U.S. women demonstrated a reduced risk of developing type 2 diabetes with dietary PUFA replacing *trans* or SFAs (Meyer et al., 2001; Salmeron et al., 2001). Hu et al. (2001) reviewed a vast body of literature, and proposed that the proportion of unsaturated fat, compared with saturated- and *trans*-fat, may be beneficial for glucose homeostasis and insulin sensitivity, although this is not universally accepted (Mayer-Davis et al., 1997).

The evidence to support a beneficial effect of nuts on insulin sensitivity comes from the Nurses' Health Study. Jiang et al. (2002) reported an inverse association between nut consumption and the risk of developing type II diabetes. Data for age-adjusted RR (95% CI) are shown in Fig. 10.2. Following multivariate adjustments, women who consumed nuts at least five times per week had the greatest benefit (multivariate RR: 0.73) compared with less than one time per week intakes (Jiang et al., 2002). Moreover, the RR was 0.79 for the highest compared with the lowest quintile of peanut-butter consumption, indicating a specific benefit of peanuts. This protective effect persisted after an adjustment for possible confounders, and was maintained for all subgroup analyses. Although this benefit was attributed mainly to the fat profile of nuts, one should recognize that other components of nuts, such as fiber or magnesium, also were inversely associated with the risk of type 2 diabetes (Marlett et al., 2002).

Due to the high-fat content of nuts, these foods may be helpful in regulating glucose and insulin levels. Randomized controlled trials (RCTs) of patients with type 2 diabetes confirmed the beneficial effects of nuts on blood lipids also seen in nondiabetic subjects, but the trials did not report an improvement in HbA1c or other glycated proteins. Lovejoy et al. (2002) found that the addition of almonds to either a high-fat or low-fat background diet did not improve glycemic control in volunteers with type II diabetes (determined by fasting and postprandial glucose or insulin concentrations, or HbA1c levels). However, Garg et al. (1988) reported that a high-MUFA diet was associated with an improvement in glycemia in patients with type II diabetes. In the latter study, a 50%-fat diet was used and compared against a high-carbohydrate diet. Lovejoy et al. (2002) used a relatively lower fat diet (37% fat), but compared the effect of almonds against other MUFA sources which may explain why no benefit was observed. However, Schutte et al. (2006) reported that regular cashew-nut consumption (20% of total energy for 8 weeks) was associated with an increase in fasting blood glucose in participants with metabolic syndrome (MetS). No other determinants of MetS were significantly altered.

Tapsell et al. (2004) conducted a 6-month RCT where 30 g of walnuts were supplemented into the diet of patients with type II diabetes in comparison with two low-fat dietary regimes. Although no improvements occurred in blood-glucose control (as indicated by HbA1c levels) or body composition, the walnut group achieved a significantly greater increase in the HDL–C-to-TC ratio ($P = 0.049$) and HDL ($P = 0.046$) than low-fat diets, one which was rich in fish.

Acute feeding studies, however, demonstrate the ability of nuts, when eaten with carbohydrate (bread), to depress postprandial glycemia. Johnston & Buller (2005) used an interesting approach to determine the impact of peanuts on glycemic response. They compared the addition of either peanuts or vinegar to both a low- and high-glycemic load test meal. They found that both additions were able to significantly reduce postprandial glycemia following the high-glycemic load meal. Why peanuts might alter the glycemic response is not known, but one hypothesis is that the high level of L-arginine stimulates insulin release and glucose uptake, as L-arginine was previously found to be a potent insulin secretagogue (Ishiyama et al., 2006). The authors concluded that this benefit from nuts was yet another reason that one should include them as part of a healthy diet.

## *Influence of Nuts on Other Metabolic Complications*

A condition that is associated with MetS is gallstone disease. The prevalence of this condition is markedly elevated among subjects with MetS, increased insulin resistance, or fatty liver (even after taking BMI into account), and is associated with

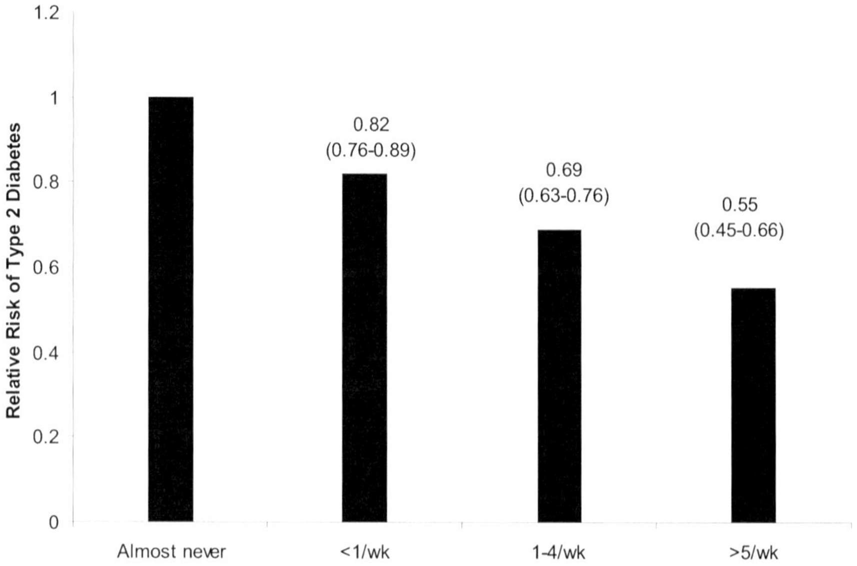


**Fig. 10.2.** Relative risks (RRs) of type 2 diabetes in women according to the frequency of nut consumption. Data shown are age-adjusted RR (95% CI) adapted from Jiang et al., 2002.

each individual component of MetS (Shaffer, 2006). Recently, nut consumption (peanuts, other nuts, and peanut butter) was studied prospectively in relation to the risk of cholecystectomy, a surrogate of symptomatic gallstone disease, in the Nurses' Health Study and Health Professionals' Follow-up. A higher consumption of nuts was associated with a lower risk of gallstone disease in both men and women (Tsai et al., 2004a,b). They reported that men consuming five or more ounces of nuts per week (frequent consumption) had a significantly lower risk of gallstone disease (RR = 0.70; 95% CI: 0.60–0.86; *P* (trend), < 0.001) than men who never ate or who ate less than 1 ounce per month. After an adjustment for age and other known or suspected risk factors, women who consumed more or at least 5 ounces of nuts per wk had a significantly lower risk of cholecystectomy (RR, 0.75; 95% CI: 0.66, 0.85; *P* for trend, < 0.0001) than women who never ate nuts or who ate <1 ounce per month.

## Conclusion

Nuts have been part of our diet for centuries. They have a long shelf life since they are: naturally protected from degradation due to their natural antioxidants, they are energy- and nutrient-dense, satisfying, have healthy lipid profiles, and are excellent sources of protein. Evidence from epidemiological studies suggests that up to 1.5 ounces (43 g) per day of nuts may help to reduce the risk of CHD, mainly by lowering LDL–C [Food and Drug Administration. Qualified Health Claims: Letter of Enforcement Discretion—Nuts and Coronary Heart Disease (Docket No. 02P-0505), 2003], but bioactive compounds in nuts may also contribute to their heart-healthy profiles. While nuts can also improve metabolic parameters, more remains to be learned about the effects of nuts on postprandial glycemic and insulin response, glycemic control, and the improvement of disease risk factors in subjects with pre-diabetes and diabetes and, as such, what role they have in combating the development of MetS and other complications. Further research is needed to establish the intakes of different varieties of nuts, alone or in combination with other foods, to deliver optimal CV and metabolic health benefits. It should be emphasized that the greatest benefit can be achieved by eating the unsalted varieties.

## References

Abbey M.; M. Noakes; G.B. Belling; P.J. Nestel. Partial replacement of saturated fatty acids with almonds or walnuts lowers total plasma cholesterol and low-density-lipoprotein cholesterol. *Am J Clin Nutr* **1994,** *59*: 995–999.

Ako, H.; D. Okuda; D. Gray. Healthful new oil from macadamia nuts. *Nutrition* **1995,** *11*(3): 286–8.

Albert, C.M.; J.M. Gaziano; W.C. Willett; J.E. Manson. Nut consumption and decreased risk of sudden cardiac death in the Physicians' Health Study. *Arch Intern Med* **2002,** *162*(12): 1382–7.

Allen, L.H. Priority areas for research on the intake, composition, and health effects of tree nuts and peanuts. *J Nutr* **2008,** *138*(9): 1763S–1765S.

Almario, R.U.; V. Vonghavaravat; R. Wong; S.E. Kasim-Karakas. Effects of walnut consumption on plasma fatty acids and lipoproteins in combined hyperlipidemia. *Am J Clin Nutr* **2001,** *74*(1): 72–9.

Alper, C.M. and R.D. Mattes. Effects of chronic peanut consumption on energy balance and hedonics. *Int J Obes Relat Metab Disord* **2002,** *26*(8): 1129–37.

Alper, C.M. and R.D. Mattes. Peanut consumption improves indices of cardiovascular disease risk in healthy adults. *J Am Coll Nutr* **2003,** *22*(2): 133–41.

Anderson, K.J.; S.S. Teuber; A. Gobeille; P. Cremin; A.L. Waterhouse; F. M. Steinberg. Walnut polyphenolics inhibit in vitro human plasma and LDL oxidation. *J Nutr* **2001,** *131*(11): 2837–42.

Aranceta, J. and L. Serra-Majem. Dietary guidelines for the Spanish population. *Public Health Nutr* **2001,** *4*(6A): 1403-8.

Balkan, J.; A. Hatipoglu; G. Aykac-Toker; and M. Uysal. Influence on hazelnut oil administration on peroxidation status of erythrocytes and apolipoprotein B 100-containing lipoproteins in rabbits fed on a high cholesterol diet. *J Agric Food Chem* **2003,** *51*(13): 3905–9.

Bes-Rastrollo, M.; J. Sabate; E. Gomez-Gracia; A. Alonso; J. A. Martinez; M.A. Martinez-Gonzalez. Nut Consumption and Weight Gain in a Mediterranean Cohort: The SUN Study. *Obesity* **2007,** *15*(1): 107–116.

Blomhoff, R.; M.H. Carlsen; L.F. Andersen; D.R. Jacobs, Jr. Health benefits of nuts: potential role of antioxidants. *Br J Nutr* **2006,** *96 Su*PP*l 2*: S52–60.

Brown, A.A. and F.B. Hu. Dietary modulation of endothelial function: implications for cardiovascular disease. *Am J Clin Nutr* **2001,** *73*(4): 673–86.

Cai, G.J.; C.Y. Miao; H.H. Xie; L.H. Lu; D.F. Su. Arterial baroreflex dysfunction promotes atherosclerosis in rats. *Atherosclerosis* **2005,** *183*(1): 41–7.

Cappuccio, F.P. and G.A. MacGregor. Does potassium supplementation lower blood pressure? A meta-analysis of published trials. *J Hypertens* **1991,** *9*(5): 465–73.

Castelli, W.P.; K. Anderson; P.W. Wilson; D. Levy. Lipids and risk of coronary heart disease. The Framingham Study. *Ann Epidemiol* **1992,** *2*(1-2): 23–8.

Chen, C.Y. and J.B. Blumberg. Phytochemical composition of nuts. *Asia Pac J Clin Nutr* **2008,** *17 SuPPl 1*: 329–32.

Chisholm, A.; J. Mann; M. Skeaff; C. Frampton; W. Sutherland; A. Duncan; S. Tiszavari. A diet rich in walnuts favourably influences plasma fatty acid profile in moderately hyperlipidaemic subjects. *Eur J Clin Nutr* **1998,** *52*(1): 12–6.

Chisholm, A.; K. Mc Auley; J. Mann; S. Williams; M. Skeaff. Cholesterol lowering effects of nuts compared with a Canola oil enriched cereal of similar fat composition. *Nutr Metab Cardiovasc Dis* **2005,** *15*(4): 284–92.

Coelho, S.B.; R.L. de Sales; S.S. Iyer; J. Bressan; N.M. Costa; P. Lokko; R. Mattes. Effects of peanut oil load on energy expenditure, body composition, lipid profile, and appetite in lean and overweight adults. *Nutrition* **2006,** *22*(6): 585–92.

Colquhoun D.M.; J.A. Humphries; D. Moores; S. SM. Effects of a macadamia nut enriched diet on serum lipids and lipoproteins compared to a low fat diet. *Food Aust.* **1996,** *48*: 216–22.

Conlin, P.R.; D. Chow; E.R. Miller, 3rd; L.P. Svetkey; P.H. Lin; D.W. Harsha; T.J. Moore; F.M. Sacks; L.J. Appel. The effect of dietary patterns on blood pressure control in hypertensive patients: results from the Dietary Approaches to Stop Hypertension (DASH) trial. *Am J Hypertens* **2000,** *13*(9): 949–55.

Coward, K.H. and J.C. Drummond. Researches on the Fat-soluble Accessory Substance. IV: Nuts as a Source of Vitamin A. *Biochem J* **1920,** *14*(5): 665–7.

Curb, J.D.; G. Wergowske; J.C. Dobbs; R.D. Abbott; B. Huang. Serum lipid effects of a high-monounsaturated fat diet based on macadamia nuts. *Arch Intern Med* **2000,** *160*(8): 1154–8.

Davis, L.; W. Stonehouse; T. Loots du; J. Mukuddem-Petersen; F. H. van der Westhuizen; S. M. Hanekom; J. C. Jerling. The effects of high walnut and cashew nut diets on the antioxidant status of subjects with metabolic syndrome. *Eur J Nutr* **2007,** *46*(3): 155–64.

Davis, P.; G. Valacchi; E. Pagnin; Q. Shao; H.B. Gross; L. Calo; W. Yokoyama. Walnuts Reduce Aortic ET-1 mRNA Levels in Hamsters Fed a High-Fat, Atherogenic Diet. *J. Nutr.* **2006,** *136*(2): 428–432.

de Lorgeril, M. and P. Salen. The Mediterranean diet in secondary prevention of coronary heart disease. *Clin Invest Med* **2006,** *29*(3): 154–8.

Dismore, M.L.; D.B. Haytowitz; S.E. Gebhardt; J.W. Peterson; S.L. Booth. Vitamin K content of nuts and fruits in the US diet. *J Am Diet Assoc* **2003,** *103*(12): 1650–2.

Dreher, M. L.; C.V. Maher; P. Kearney. The traditional and emerging role of nuts in healthful diets. *Nutrition Reviews,* **1996,** *54*, 241–5.

Durak, I.; I. Koksal; M. Kacmaz; S. Buyukkocak; B.M. Cimen, H.S. Ozturk. Hazelnut supplementation enhances plasma antioxidant potential and lowers plasma cholesterol levels. *Clin Chim Acta* **1999,** *284*(1), 113–5.

Eastman, W.A. and B.J. Clayshultc. Pecan Effects on Serum Lipoproteins and Dietary Intakes of Hyperlipidemic Individuals Consuming Self-Selected Diets. *Fam Consum Sci Res J* **2005,** *33*, 197–207.

Edwards, K.; I. Kwaw; J. Matud; I. Kurtz. Effect of pistachio nuts on serum lipid levels in patients with moderate hypercholesterolemia. *J Am Coll Nutr* **1999,** *18*(3): 229–32.

Ellsworth, J.L.; L.H. Kushi; A.R. Folsom. Frequent nut intake and risk of death from coronary heart disease and all causes in postmenopausal women: The Iowa Women's Health Study. *Nutr Metab Cardiovasc Dis* **2001,** *11*(6), 372-7.

Esposito, K.; R. Marfella; M. Ciotola; C. Di Palo; F. Giugliano; G. Giugliano; M. D'Armiento; F. D'Andrea; D. Giugliano. Effect of a mediterranean-style diet on endothelial dysfunction and markers of vascular inflammation in the metabolic syndrome: a randomized trial. *JAMA* **2004,** *292*(12), 1440–6.

Feldman, E.B. The scientific evidence for a beneficial health relationship between walnuts and coronary heart disease. *J Nutr* **2002,** *132*(5), 1062S–1101S.

Food and Drug Administration. Qualified Health Claims: Letter of Enforcement Discretion -Nuts and Coronary Heart Disease (Docket No. 02P-0505). (2003). from http://www.cfsan.fda.gov/~dms/qhcnuts2.html.

Food for Health. Dietary Guidelines for Australian Adults. Canberra: Commonwealth Department of Health and Ageing & National Health and Medical Research Council, 2003.

Food for Health. Dietary Guidelines for Children and Adolescents in Australia. Canberra: Department of Health and Ageing, 2003.

Fraser, G.E. Nut consumption, lipids, and risk of a coronary event. *Clin Cardiol* **1999,** *22*(7 Suppl), III11–5.

Fraser, G.E.; H.W. Bennett; K.B. Jaceldo; J. Sabate. Effect on body weight of a free 76 Kilojoule (320 calorie) daily supplement of almonds for six months. *J Am Coll Nutr* **2002,** *21*(3), 275–83.

Fraser, G.E.; J.Sabate; W.L.Beeson; T.M.Strahan A possible protective effect of nut consumption on risk of coronary heart disease. The Adventist Health Study. *Arch Intern Med* **1992,** *152*, 1416–1424.

French, S. Effects of dietary fat and carbohydrate on appetite vary depending upon site and structure. *Br J Nutr* **2004,** *92 SuPPl 1*, S23–6.

Garcia-Lorda, P.; I. Megias Rangil; J. Salas-Salvado. Nut consumption, body weight and insulin resistance. *Eur J Clin Nutr* **2003,** *57 SuPPl 1*, S8–11.

Garg, A.; A. Bonanome; S.M. Grundy; Z.J. Zhang; R. H. Unger. Comparison of a high-carbohydrate diet with a high-monounsaturated-fat diet in patients with non-insulin-dependent diabetes mellitus. *N Engl J Med* **1988,** *319*(13), 829–34.

Garg, M.L.; R.J. Blake; R.B. Wills. Macadamia nut consumption lowers plasma total and LDL cholesterol levels in hypercholesterolemic men. *J Nutr* **2003,** *133*(4), 1060–3.

Garg, M.L.; R.J. Blake; R.B. Wills; E.H. Clayton. Macadamia nut consumption modulates favourably risk factors for coronary artery disease in hypercholesterolemic subjects. *Lipids* **2007,** *42*(6), 583–7.

Gebauer, S.K.; T.L. Psota; W.S. Harris; P.M. Kris-Etherton. n-3 fatty acid dietary recommendations and food sources to achieve essentiality and cardiovascular benefits. *Am J Clin Nutr* **2006,**

*83*(6 Suppl), 1526S–1535S.

Gebauer, S.K.; S.G. West; C.D. Kay; P. Alaupovic; D. Bagshaw; P.M. Kris-Etherton. Effects of pistachios on cardiovascular disease risk factors and potential mechanisms of action: a dose-response study. *Am J Clin Nutr* **2008,** *88*(3), 651–9.

Gilbert, P.A. and S. Khokhar. Changing dietary habits of ethnic groups in Europe and implications for health. *Nutr Rev* **2008,** *66*(4), 203–15.

Gill, J.M.; J.C. Brown; M.J. Caslake; D.M. Wright; J. Cooney; D. Bedford; D.A. Hughes; J.C. Stanley; C.J. Packard. Effects of dietary monounsaturated fatty acids on lipoprotein concentrations, compositions, and subfraction distributions and on VLDL apolipoprotein B kinetics: dose-dependent effects on LDL. *Am J Clin Nutr* **2003,** *78*(1), 47–56.

Griel, A.E.; Y. Cao; D.D. Bagshaw; A.M. Cifelli; B. Holub; P.M. Kris-Etherton. A macadamia nut-rich diet reduces total and LDL-cholesterol in mildly hypercholesterolemic men and women. *J Nutr* **2008,** *138*(4), 761–7.

Griel, A.E.; B. Eissenstat; V. Juturu; G. Hsieh; P.M. Kris-Etherton. Improved diet quality with peanut consumption. *J Am Coll Nutr* **2004,** *23*(6), 660–8.

Griel, A.E. and P.M. Kris-Etherton. Tree nuts and the lipid profile: a review of clinical studies. *Br J Nutr* **2006,** *96 Suppl 2*, S68–78.

Grundy, S.M. Primary prevention of coronary heart disease: role of cholesterol control in the United States. *J Intern Med* **1997,** *241*(4), 295–306.

Hatipoglu, A.; O. Kanbagli; J. Balkan; M. Kucuk; U. Cevikbas; G. Aykac-Toker; H. Berkkan; M. Uysal. Hazelnut oil administration reduces aortic cholesterol accumulation and lipid peroxides in the plasma, liver, and aorta of rabbits fed a high-cholesterol diet. *Biosci Biotechnol Biochem* **2004,** *68*(10): 2050–7.

Henderson L.; J. Gregory; K. Irving K. The National Diet and Nutrition Survey: adults aged 19 to 64 years. Energy, protein, carbohydrate, fat and alcohol intake. London (2003) TSO, 2.

Hiraoka-Yamamoto, J.; K. Ikeda; H. Negishi; M. Mori; A. Hirose; S. Sawada; Y. Onobayashi; K. Kitamori; S. Kitano; M. Tashiro; et al. Serum lipid effects of a monounsaturated (palmitoleic) Fatty Acid-rich diet based on macadamia nuts in healthy, young Japanese women. *Clin Ex*P P*harmacol* P*hysiol* **2004,** *31 Suppl 2*, S37–8.

Hollis, J. and R. Mattes. Effect of chronic consumption of almonds on body weight in healthy humans. *Br J Nutr* **2007,** *98*(3), 651–6.

Hu, F.; M. Stampfer; J. Manson; E. Rimm; G. Colditz; B. Rosner; F. Speizer; C. Hennekens; W. Willett. Frequent nut consumption and risk of coronary heart disease in women: prospective cohort study. *BMJ* **1998,** *317*, 1341–1345.

Hu, F.B.; J.E. Manson; W.C. Willett. Types of dietary fat and risk of coronary heart disease: a critical review. *J Am Coll Nutr* **2001,** *20*(1), 5–19.

Huynh, N.N. and J. Chin-Dusting. Amino acids, Arginase and nitric oxide in vascular health. *Clinical and Experimental Pharmacology and Physiology* **2006,** *33*(1-2), 1–8.

Hyson, D.A.; B. O. Schneeman; P.A. Davis. Almonds and almond oil have similar effects on plasma lipids and LDL oxidation in healthy men and women. *J Nutr* **2002,** *132*(4), 703–7.

Ishiyama, N.; M.A. Ravier; J. C. Henquin. Dual mechanism of the potentiation by glucose of insulin secretion induced by arginine and tolbutamide in mouse islets. *Am J Physiol Endocrinol*

*Metab* **2006,** *290*(3), E540–9.

Iwamoto, M.; M. Sato; M. Kono; Y. Hirooka; K. Sakai; A. Takeshita; K. Imaizumi. Walnuts lower serum cholesterol in Japanese men and women. *J Nutr* **2000,** *130*: 171–176.

Iyer, S.S.; L.A. Boateng; R.L. Sales; S.B. Coelho; P. Lokko; J.B. Monteiro; N.M. Costa; R. D. Mattes. Effects of peanut oil consumption on appetite and food choice. *Int J Obes (Lond)* **2006,** *30*(4), 704–10.

Jenab, M.; J. Sabate; N. Slimani; P. Ferrari; M. Mazuir; C. Casagrande; G. Deharveng; A. Tjonneland; A. Olsen; K. Overvad; et al. Consumption and portion sizes of tree nuts, peanuts and seeds in the European Prospective Investigation into Cancer and Nutrition (EPIC) cohorts from 10 European countries. *Br J Nutr* **2006,** *96 Suppl 2*, S12–23.

Jenkins, D.J.A.; C.W.C. Kendall; A. Marchie; T.L. Parker; P.W. Connelly; W. Qian; J.S. Haight; D. Faulkner; E. Vidgen; K. G. Lapsley; et al. Dose Response of Almonds on Coronary Heart Disease Risk Factors: Blood Lipids, Oxidized Low-Density Lipoproteins, Lipoprotein(a), Homocysteine, and Pulmonary Nitric Oxide: A Randomized, Controlled, Crossover Trial. *Circulation* **2002,** *106*(11), 1327–1332.

Jiang, R.; D.R. Jacobs, Jr.; E. Mayer-Davis; M. Szklo; D. Herrington; N.S. Jenny; R. Kronmal; R. G. Barr. Nut and seed consumption and inflammatory markers in the multi-ethnic study of atherosclerosis. *Am J Epidemiol* **2006,** *163*(3), 222–31.

Jiang, R.; J. E. Manson; M. J. Stampfer; S. Liu; W.C. Willett; F.B. Hu. Nut and peanut butter consumption and risk of type 2 diabetes in women. *JAMA* **2002,** *288*(20), 2554–60.

Johnston, C.S. and A J. Buller. Vinegar and peanut products as complementary foods to reduce postprandial glycemia. *J Am Diet Assoc* **2005,** *105*(12), 1939–42.

Jump, D.B.; D. Botolin; Y. Wang; J. Xu; B. Christian; O. Demeure. Fatty acid regulation of hepatic gene transcription. *J Nutr* **2005,** *135*(11), 2503–6.

Kamphuis, M.M.; M.S. Westerterp-Plantenga; W.H. Saris. Fat-specific satiety in humans for fat high in linoleic acid vs fat high in oleic acid. *Eur J Clin Nutr* **2001,** *55*(6), 499–508.

Kelly, J.H., Jr. and J. Sabate. Nuts and coronary heart disease: an epidemiological perspective. *Br J Nutr* **2006,** *96 Suppl 2*, S61–7.

Keys, A. Seven Countries: A Multivariate Analysis of Death and Coronary Heart Disease,. Harvard University Press, Cambridge, MA, 1980, 1–381.

King, J.C.; J. Blumberg; L. Ingwersen; M. Jenab; K.L. Tucker. Tree nuts and peanuts as components of a healthy diet. *J Nutr* **2008,** *138*(9), 1736S–1740S.

Kiokias, S.; T. Varzakas; V. Oreopoulou. In vitro activity of vitamins, flavonoids, and natural phenolic antioxidants against the oxidative deterioration of oil-based systems. *Crit Rev Food Sci Nutr* **2008,** *48*(1), 78–93.

Kocyigit, A.; A.A. Koylu; H. Keles. Effects of pistachio nuts consumption on plasma lipid profile and oxidative status in healthy volunteers. *Nutrition, Metabolism and Cardiovascular Diseases* **2006,** *16*(3), 202–209.

Krauss, R.M.; R.H. Eckel; B. Howard; L.J. Appel; S.R. Daniels; R.J. Deckelbaum; J.W. Erdman, Jr.; P. Kris-Etherton; I.J. Goldberg; T.A. Kotchen; et al. AHA Dietary Guidelines: revision 2000: A statement for healthcare professionals from the Nutrition Committee of the American Heart Association. *Stroke* **2000,** *31*(11), 2751–66.

Kris-Etherton, P.M.; K.D. Hecker; A. Bonanome; S.M. Coval; A.E. Binkoski; K.F. Hilpert; A.E. Griel; T.D. Etherton. Bioactive compounds in foods: their role in the prevention of cardiovascular disease and cancer. *The American Journal of Medicine* **2002,** *113*(9, Supplement 2), 71–88.

Kris-Etherton, P.M.; S. Innis. American Dietetic and C. Dietitians of Position of the American Dietetic Association and Dietitians of Canada: dietary fatty acids. *J Am Diet Assoc* **2007,** *107*(9), 1599–611.

Kris-Etherton, P.M.; S. Yu-Poth; J. Sabate; H.E. Ratcliffe; G. Zhao; T.D. Etherton. Nuts and their bioactive constituents: effects on serum lipids and other factors that affect disease risk. *Am J Clin Nutr* **1999a,** *70*(3 Suppl), 504S–511S.

Kris-Etherton, P.M.; T.A. Pearson; Y. Wan; R.L. Hargrove; K. Moriarty; V. Fishell; T.D. Etherton. High-monounsaturated fatty acid diets lower both plasma cholesterol and triacylglycerol concentrations. *Am J Clin Nutr* **1999b,** *70*(6), 1009–15.

Kushi, L.H.; R.M. Fee; T.A. Sellers; W. Zheng; A.R. Folsom. Intake of vitamins A, C, and E and postmenopausal breast cancer. The Iowa Women's Health Study. *Am J Epidemiol* **1996,** *144*(2), 165–74.

Li, D.; T. Yao; S. Siriamornpun. Alpha-linolenic acid content of commonly available nuts in Hangzhou. *Int J Vitam Nutr Res* **2006,** *76*(1), 18–21.

Lipid management guidelines–2001. National Heart Foundation of Australia, The Cardiac Society of Australia and New Zealand. *Med J Aust* **2001,** *175 SuPPl,* S57–85.

Lloyd-Williams, F.; M. Mwatsama; R. Ireland; S. Capewell. Small changes in snacking behaviour: the potential impact on CVD mortality. *Public Health Nutr* **2008,** 1–6.

Lou, H.; H. Yuan; B. Ma; D. Ren; M. Ji; S. Oka. Polyphenols from peanut skins and their free radical-scavenging effects. *Phytochemistry* **2004,** *65*(16), 2391–9.

Lovejoy, J.C.; M.M. Most; M. Lefevre; F. L. Greenway; J. C. Rood. Effect of diets enriched in almonds on insulin action and serum lipids in adults with normal glucose tolerance or type 2 diabetes. *Am J Clin Nutr* **2002,** *76*(5), 1000–6.

MacIntosh, C.G.; S.H. Holt; J.C. Brand-Miller. The degree of fat saturation does not alter glycemic, insulinemic or satiety responses to a starchy staple in healthy men. *J Nutr* **2003,** *133*(8), 2577–80.

Maguire, L.S.; S.M. O'Sullivan; K. Galvin; T.P. O'Connor; N.M. O'Brien. Fatty acid profile, tocopherol, squalene and phytosterol content of walnuts, almonds, peanuts, hazelnuts and the macadamia nut. *Int J Food Sci Nutr* **2004,** *55*(3), 171–8.

Mantzoros, C.S.; C.J. Williams; J.E. Manson; J.B. Meigs; F.B. Hu. Adherence to the Mediterranean dietary pattern is positively associated with plasma adiponectin concentrations in diabetic women. *Am J Clin Nutr* **2006,** *84*(2), 328–35.

Marlett, J.A.; M.I. McBurney; J.L. Slavin. Position of the American Dietetic Association: health implications of dietary fiber. *J Am Diet Assoc* **2002,** *102*(7), 993–1000.

Mayer-Davis, E.J.; J.H. Monaco; H.M. Hoen; S. Carmichael; M.Z. Vitolins; M.J. Rewers; S.M. Haffner; M.F. Ayad; R.N. Bergman; A.J. Karter. Dietary fat and insulin sensitivity in a triethnic population: the role of obesity. The Insulin Resistance Atherosclerosis Study (IRAS). *Am J Clin Nutr* **1997,** *65*(1), 79–87.

McManus, K.; L. Antinoro; F. Sacks. A randomized controlled trial of a moderate-fat, low-energy diet compared with a low fat, low-energy diet for weight loss in overweight adults. *Int J Obes Relat Metab Disord* **2001,** *25*(10), 1503–11.

Mensink, R.P. and M.B. Katan. Effect of dietary fatty acids on serum lipids and lipoproteins. A meta-analysis of 27 trials. *Arterioscler Thromb* **1992,** *12*(8), 911–9.

Mercanligil, S.M.; P. Arslan; C. Alasalvar; E. Okut; E. Akgul; A. Pinar; P.O. Geyik; L. Tokgozoglu; F. Shahidi. Effects of hazelnut-enriched diet on plasma cholesterol and lipoprotein profiles in hypercholesterolemic adult men. *Eur J Clin Nutr* **2007,** *61*(2), 212–20.

Meydani, M. Vitamin E modulation of cardiovascular disease. *Ann N Y Acad Sci* **2004,** *1031*, 271–9.

Meyer, K.A.; L.H. Kushi; D.R. Jacobs, Jr.; A.R. Folsom. Dietary fat and incidence of type 2 diabetes in older Iowa women. *Diabetes Care* **2001,** *24*(9), 1528–35.

Miraliakbari, H. and F. Shahidi. Oxidative stability of tree nut oils. *J Agric Food Chem* **2008,** *56*(12), 4751–9.

Moreno, D.A.; N. Ilic; A. Poulev; I. Raskin. Effects of Arachis hypogaea nutshell extract on lipid metabolic enzymes and obesity parameters. *Life Sciences* **2006,** *78*(24), 2797–2803.

Morgan, J.M.; K. Horton; D. Reese; C. Carey; K. Walker; D.M. Capuzzi. Effects of walnut consumption as part of a low-fat, low-cholesterol diet on serum cardiovascular risk factors. *Int J Vitam Nutr Res* **2002,** *72*(5), 341–7.

Morgan, W.A. and B. J. Clayshulte. Pecans lower low-density lipoprotein cholesterol in people with normal lipid levels. *J Am Diet Assoc* **2000,** *100*(3), 312–8.

Mukuddem-Petersen, J.; W. Oosthuizen; J.C. Jerling. A Systematic Review of the Effects of Nuts on Blood Lipid Profiles in Humans. *J. Nutr.* **2005,** *135*(9), 2082–2089.

Mukuddem-Petersen, J.; W. Stonehouse Oosthuizen; J.C. Jerling; S.M. Hanekom; Z. White. Effects of a high walnut and high cashew nut diet on selected markers of the metabolic syndrome: a controlled feeding trial. *Br J Nutr* **2007,** *97*(6), 1144–53.

National nutrition survey: nutrient intakes and physical measurements, 1995. C. ABS, 1998. ABS Cat. No. 4805.0.

Nutrition Insights: The Role of Nuts in a Healthy Diet. USDA Center for Nutritional Policy and Promotion Washington DC, 2000.http://www.cnpp.usda.gov/Publications/NutritionInsights/Insight23.pdf accessed July 2008.

O'Byrne, D.J.; D.A. Knauft; R. B. Shireman. Low fat-monounsaturated rich diets containing high-oleic peanuts improve serum lipoprotein profiles. *Lipids* **1997,** *32*(7), 687–95.

O'Dea, K. Traditional diet and food preferences of Australian aboriginal hunter-gatherers. *Philos Trans R Soc Lond B Biol Sci* **1991,** *334*(1270), 233–40; discussion 240–1.

Ostlund, R. E., Jr. Phytosterols and cholesterol metabolism. *Curr Opin Lipidol* **2004,** *15*(1), 37–41.

Pelkman, C.L.; V.K. Fishell; D.H. Maddox; T.A. Pearson; D.T. Mauger; P.M. Kris-Etherton. Effects of moderate-fat (from monounsaturated fat) and low-fat weight-loss diets on the serum lipid profile in overweight and obese men and women. *Am J Clin Nutr* **2004,** *79*(2), 204–12.

Pieters, M.; W. Oosthuizen; J.C. Jerling; D.T. Loots; J. Mukuddem-Petersen; S.M. Hanekom. Clustering of haemostatic variables and the effect of high cashew and walnut diets on these variables in metabolic syndrome patients. *Blood Coagul Fibrinolysis* **2005,** *16*(6), 429–37.

Pringle, H. Society for American Archaeology meeting. Herring and nuts for the 'salmon people'. *Science* **2008,** *320*(5873), 174–5.

Rajaram, S.; K. Burke; B. Connell; T. Myint; J. Sabate. A monounsaturated fatty acid-rich pecan-enriched diet favorably alters the serum lipid profile of healthy men and women. *J Nutr* 2001, *131*(9), 2275–9.

Ribas-Barba, L.; L. Serra-Majem; G. Salvador; C. Castell; C. Cabezas; L. Salleras; A. Plasencia. Trends in dietary habits and food consumption in Catalonia, Spain (1992–2003). *Public Health Nutr* **2007,** *10*(11A), 1340–53.

Ritchie, S.A.; M.A. Ewart; C.G. Perry; J.M. Connell; I.P. Salt. The role of insulin and the adipocytokines in regulation of vascular endothelial function. *Clin Sci (Lond)* **2004,** *107*(6), 519–532.

Ros, E.; I. Nunez; A. Perez-Heras; M. Serra; R. Gilabert; E. Casals; R. Deulofeu. A Walnut Diet Improves Endothelial Function in Hypercholesterolemic Subjects: A Randomized Crossover Trial. *Circulation* **2004,** *109*, 1609–1614.

Ryan, E.; K. Galvin; T.P. O'Connor; A.R. Maguire; N.M. O'Brien. Fatty acid profile, tocopherol, squalene and phytosterol content of brazil, pecan, pine, pistachio and cashew nuts. *Int J Food Sci Nutr* **2006,** *57*(3–4), 219–28.

Sabate, J. Does nut consumption protect against ischaemic heart disease? *Eur J Clin Nutr* **1993,** *47 Suppl 1*, S71–5.

Sabate, J. Nut consumption, vegetarian diets, ischemic heart disease risk, and all-cause mortality: evidence from epidemiologic studies. *Am J Clin Nutr* **1999,** *70*(3 Suppl), 500S–503S.

Sabate, J. Nut consumption and body weight. *Am J Clin Nutr* **2003,** *78*(3 Suppl), 647S–650S.

Sabate, J.; G.E. Fraser; K. Burke; S.F. Knutsen; H. Bennett; K.D. Lindsted. Effects of walnuts on serum lipid levels and blood pressure in normal men. *N Engl J Med* **1993,** *328*(9), 603–7.

Sabate, J.; E. Haddad; J.S. Tanzman; P. Jambazian; S. Rajaram. Serum lipid response to the graduated enrichment of a Step I diet with almonds: a randomized feeding trial. *Am J Clin Nutr* **2003,** *77*(6), 1379–84.

Salmeron, J.; F.B. Hu; J.E. Manson; M. J. Stampfer; G.A. Colditz; E.B. Rimm; W.C. Willett. Dietary fat intake and risk of type 2 diabetes in women. *Am J Clin Nutr* **2001,** *73*(6), 1019–26.

Sanders, T.H.; R.W. McMichael; K.W. Hendrix. Occurrence of Resveratrol in Edible Peanuts. *J. Agric. Food Chem.* **2000,** *48*(4), 1243–1246.

Schutte, A. E.; J.M. Van Rooyen; H.W. Huisman; J. Mukuddem-Petersen; W. Oosthuizen; S.M. Hanekom; J.C. Jerling. Modulation of baroreflex sensitivity by walnuts versus cashew nuts in subjects with metabolic syndrome. *Am J Hypertens* **2006,** *19*(6), 629–36.

Segura, R.; C. Javierre; M.A. Lizarraga; E. Ros. Other relevant components of nuts: phytosterols, folate and minerals. *Br J Nutr* **2006,** *96 Suppl 2*, S36–44.

Shaffer, E.A. Gallstone disease: Epidemiology of gallbladder stone disease. *Best Pract Res Clin Gastroenterol* **2006,** *20*(6), 981–96.

Shahidi, F.; C. Alasalvar; C.M. Liyana-Pathirana. Antioxidant phytochemicals in hazelnut kernel (Corylus avellana L.) and hazelnut byproducts. *J Agric Food Chem* **2007,** *55*(4): 1212–20.

Sheridan, M.J.; J.N. Cooper; M. Erario; C.E. Cheifetz. Pistachio nut consumption and serum lipid levels. *J Am Coll Nutr* **2007,** *26*(2), 141–8.

Spiller, G. and B. Bruce. Nuts and healthy diets. *Veg Nutr Int J* **1997,** *1*, 12–16.

Spiller, G.A.; D.A. Jenkins; O. Bosello; J.E. Gates; L.N. Cragen; B. Bruce. Nuts and plasma lipids: an almond-based diet lowers LDL-C while preserving HDL-C. *J Am Coll Nutr* **1998,** *17*(3), 285–90.

Spiller, G.A.; D.J. Jenkins; L.N. Cragen; J.E. Gates; O. Bosello; K. Berra; C. Rudd; M. Stevenson; R. Superko. Effect of a diet high in monounsaturated fat from almonds on plasma cholesterol and lipoproteins. *J Am Coll Nutr* **1992,** *11*(2), 126–30.

Spiller, G.A.; A. Miller; K. Olivera; J. Reynolds; B. Miller; S.J. Morse; A. Dewell; J.W. Farquhar. Effects of plant-based diets high in raw or roasted almonds, or roasted almond butter on serum lipoproteins in humans. *J Am Coll Nutr* **2003,** *22*(3), 195–200.

St-Onge, M.P. Dietary fats, teas, dairy, and nuts: potential functional foods for weight control? *Am J Clin Nutr* **2005,** *81*(1), 7–15.

Stoclet, J.C.; T. Chataigneau; M. Ndiaye; M.H. Oak; J. El Bedoui; M. Chataigneau; V.B. Schini-Kerth. Vascular protection by dietary polyphenols. *Eur J Pharmacol* **2004,** *500*(1–3), 299–313.

Storlien, L.H.; L.A. Baur; A.D. Kriketos; D.A. Pan; G.J. Cooney; A.B. Jenkins; G.D. Calvert; L.V. Campbell. Dietary fats and insulin action. *Diabetologia* **1996,** *39*(6), 621–31.

Tamizifar, B.; M. Rismankarzadeh; A. Vosoughi; M. Rafieeyan; B. Tamizifar; A. Arastou Aminzade. A low-dose almond-based diet decreases LDL-C while preserving HDL-C. *Archives of Iranian Medicine* **2005,** *8*(1), 45–51.

Tapsell, L.C.; L.J. Gillen; C.S. Patch; M. Batterham; A. Owen; M. Bare; M. Kennedy. Including walnuts in a low-fat/modified-fat diet improves HDL cholesterol-to-total cholesterol ratios in patients with type 2 diabetes. *Diabetes Care* **2004,** *27*(12), 2777–83.

Thomson, C.D.; A. Chisholm; S.K. McLachlan; J.M. Campbell. Brazil nuts: an effective way to improve selenium status. *Am J Clin Nutr* **2008,** *87*(2), 379–84.

Tokusoglu, O.; M.K. Unal; F. Yemis. Determination of the phytoalexin resveratrol (3,5,4'-trihydroxystilbene) in peanuts and pistachios by high-performance liquid chromatographic diode array (HPLC-DAD) and gas chromatography-mass spectrometry (GC-MS). *J Agric Food Chem* **2005,** *53*(12), 5003–9.

Tsai, C.J.; M.F. Leitzmann; F.B. Hu; W.C. Willett; E.L. Giovannucci. Frequent nut consumption and decreased risk of cholecystectomy in women. *Am J Clin Nutr* **2004a,** *80*(1), 76–81.

Tsai, C.J.; M.F. Leitzmann; F.B. Hu; W.C. Willett; E.L. Giovannucci. A prospective cohort study of nut consumption and the risk of gallstone disease in men. *Am J Epidemiol* **2004b,** *160*(10), 961–8.

U.S. Department of Agriculture. "Agriculture Research Service, 2006. USDA national nutrient database for standard reference, release 19. Retrieved from the Nutrient Data Laboratory Web site http:// nal.usda.gov/fnic/foodcomp." 19. from http:// nal.usda.gov/fnic/foodcomp.

West, S.G. Effect of diet on vascular reactivity: an emerging marker for vascular risk. *Curr Atheroscler Rep* **2001,** *3*(6), 446–55.

Wien, M.A.; J.M. Sabate; D.N. Ikle; S.E. Cole; F.R. Kandeel. Almonds vs complex carbohydrates in a weight reduction program. *Int J Obes Relat Metab Disord* **2003,** *27*(11), 1365–72.

Willett, W.C.; F. Sacks; A. Trichopoulou; G. Drescher; A. Ferro-Luzzi; E. Helsing; D. Trichopoulos. Mediterranean diet pyramid: a cultural model for healthy eating. *Am J Clin Nutr* **1995,** *61*(6 Suppl), 1402S–1406S.

Zambon, D.; J. Sabate; S. Munoz; B. Campero; E. Casals; M. Merlos; J.C. Laguna; E. Ros. Substituting walnuts for monounsaturated fat improves the serum lipid profile of hypercholesterolemic men and women. A randomized crossover trial. *Ann Intern Med* **2000,** *132*(7), 538–46.

Zhao, G.; T.D. Etherton; K.R. Martin; S.G. West; P.J. Gillies; P.M. Kris-Etherton. Dietary alpha-linolenic acid reduces inflammatory and lipid cardiovascular risk factors in hypercholesterolemic men and women. *J Nutr* **2004,** *134*(11), 2991–7.

Zibaeenezhad, M.J.; S.J. Shamsnia; M. Khorasani. Walnut consumption in hyperlipidemic patients. *Angiology* **2005,** *56*(5), 581–3.

PART 2

# *Trans* Fatty Acids in Health

# 11

# *Trans* Fatty Acids and Cardiometabolic Syndrome

**Vijaya Juturu**
*Nutrition 21 Inc, Purchase NY 10522*

## Introduction

Cardiometabolic syndrome (CMS) is a progressive disorder and a better term to understand how to treat diabetes and cardiovascular disease (CVD) risk factors. In the United States, diabetes affects 20 million people, with 47 million afflicted with CMS. It consists of obesity, hypertension, dyslipidemia, impaired glucose tolerance, increase in inflammatory markers such as C-reactive protein (CRP), cytokines, tumor necrosis factor alpha (TNF$\alpha$), interleukins 6 and 10 (IL-6 and IL-10), changes in cell adhesion molecules, prothrombotic and fibrinolytic changes, and an increase in oxidative endothelial and stress dysfunction. Growing evidence suggests that aggressive, comprehensive treatment for risk-factor management will improve survival and will reduce recurring events, and several interventional procedures will improve the quality of life (Juturu, 2006). Several experts believe that treating all risk factors associated with CVD may be beneficial in reducing the cardiac events (Table 11.1). Early diagnosis and intervention of CMS risk factors can prevent or delay the serious complications associated with diabetes (e.g., nerve damage, blindness, and kidney disease) and cardiovascular disease.

Fat is a major source of energy for the body and aids in the absorption of vitamins A, D, E, K and carotenoids. Both animal- and plant-derived food products contain fat, and when eaten in moderation, fat is important for proper growth, development, and maintenance of good health. Figure 11.1 shows the molecular structure of

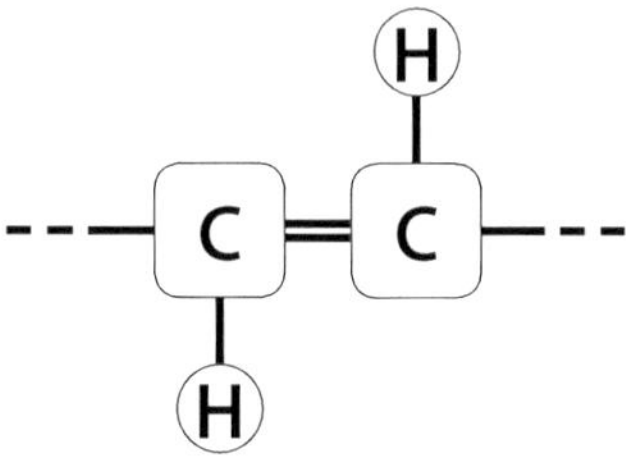


**Fig. 11.1.** Structure of *trans* fatty acid.

**Table 11.1. Target Risk Factors of Metabolic Syndrome and Cardiometabolic Syndrome**

| | *Metabolic syndrome* | | | |
|---|---|---|---|---|
| *Characteristics* | NCEP/ATP III | AACE* | WHO[#] | *Cardiometabolic syndrome*[1] |
| Plasma glucose, mg/dL | | | | IGT: 100-125 mg/dL |
| Fasting | 110-125 | >140 | >110 and <126 | HbA1c : <7% |
| 120 min post-glucose challenge [‡] | 140-200 | | ≥ 140 and < 200 | |
| Triglycerides, mg/dL | ≥ 150 | ≥ 150 | ≥ 150 | ≥ 200; Patients with very high triglycerides should not consume alcohol. The use of bile acid sequestrant is relatively contraindicated when triglycerides are >200 mg/dL. |
| HDL-C, mg/dL | | | | LDL-C: <100 mg/dL |
| Men | <40 | <40 | <35 | If triglycerides are ≥200 mg/dL, non-HDL-C should be <130 mg/dL[†] |
| Women | <50 | <50 | <39 | |
| Blood pressure, mm Hg | ≥ 130/85 | ≥ 130/85[†] | ≥ 160/90 | <140 mm Hg or <130 mm Hg if the patient has diabetes and kidney disease |
| Abdominal obesity or | | - | | Body mass index: 18.5 to 24.9 kg/m$^2$ |
| waist circumference | | | WHR | Waist circumference: <40 inches for men and <35 for women |
| Men | >102 cm (>40 in) | | Men : >0.90 | |
| Women | >88 cm ( >35 in) | | Women: >0.85 | |
| Microalbuminuria urinary albumin excretion rate, mg/g | - | - | ≥ 20 | + |
| Smoking | - | - | - | Complete cessation. No exposure to environmental tobacco smoke |
| Age, sex, family history, race | - | - | - | + |
| Inflammation and coagulation | - | - | | + |
| Physical activity | - | - | - | 30 minutes, 7 days per week (minimum 5 days per week) |

NCEP/ATP III: National Cholesterol Education Program/Adult Treatment Panel III; AACE: American Association Clinical Endocrinologists; WHO: World Health Organization; [1]CMS is defined based on ACC/AHA/ADA recommendations; [#]Syndrome present if two or more of the other components met; [†] Current use of antihypertensive medication; [‡]After a 75 g glucose load; * Absence of diabetes–fulfillment of 2 of the risk factors; [+] Non-HDL-C = total cholesterol minus HDL-C; Creatinine should be <2.5 mg/dL in men and <2.0 mg/dL in women; Potassium should be <5.0 mEq/L *trans* fatty acids (TFA)—unsaturated fatty acids with at least one double bond in the *trans* molecular configuration and are produced by the partial hydrogenation of vegetable oils. In a TFA, the carbon chain is relatively straight, so that in this respect the *trans* isomer resembles the corresponding saturated fatty acid (in this case, stearic acid, C18:0); but the chain is twisted slightly, which affects its sectional area and therefore its space requirements. The quantity and quality of the dietary fats predict coronary heart disease (CHD). Studies show a positive association between industrially produced TFA intake and the risk of CHD and an inverse association between ruminant TFA (R-TFA) intake and CHD, implying that R-TFA intake is innocuous or even protective against CHD. (Chardigny et al., 2008).

## Dietary Sources of *trans* Fatty Acid

Dietary TFA originate from commercially hydrogenated oils and from dairy and meat fats. They also occur naturally in small amounts in a few foods; however, most are formed during the partial hydrogenation of vegetable oils. This process converts vegetable oils into semi-solid fats for use in margarines, commercial cooking, and manufacturing processes. Dietary sources of TFA are given in Table 11.2.

## Dietary Intake of *trans* Fatty Acid

In 2006, Craig-Schmidt reported worldwide consumption of TFA. In North America, daily intakes were estimated by a food frequency questionnaire to be 3–4 g per person and by extrapolation of human milk data to be greater than 10 g per person. Diets in northern Europe traditionally contain more TFA than those in Mediterranean countries where olive oil is used. Intakes in Europe range from minimal values in Italy, Portugal, Greece, and Spain (1.4–2.1 g/day) to greater values in Germany, Finland, Denmark, Sweden, France, United Kingdom, Belgium, Norway, The Netherlands, and Iceland (2.1–5.4 g/day). In a meta-analysis of four prospective cohort studies involving nearly 140,000 subjects (Ascherio et al., 1996; DerSimonian & Laird, 1986; Oh et al., 2005; Oomen et al., 2001; Pietinen et al., 1997 ) including updated analyses from the two largest studies, a 2% increase in energy intake from TFA was associated with a 23% increase in the incidence of CHD (pooled relative risk, 1.23; 95% confidence interval, 1.11 to 1.37; $P<0.001$). Table 11.3 provides both the TFA intake and the risk of CHD. Among the retrospective studies, the risk of nonfatal myocardial infarction was evaluated for extreme quartiles of adipose TFA levels (approximately equal to a 1.5 to 2% difference in energy intake) in the European Community Multicenter Study on Antioxidants, Myocardial Infarction, and Cancer [EURAMIC] (Aro et al., 1995) and in the Costa Rican study (Baylin et al., 2003) or for a difference of 1 SD in adipose TFA levels in the Australian study (Clifton et al., 2004). The relative risk in EURAMIC was 1.44 (95% confidence interval, 0.94 to 2.20) after the exclusion of two Spanish centers in which adipose *trans* fat levels were extremely low ($P<0.05$ for the interaction with center) (Aro et al., 1995). The

**Table 11.2. Dietary Sources of *trans* Fatty Acids (TFA)**

| Product | Common serving size | Total fat g | Trans fat g | Combined sat. & trans fat g | %DV for cholesterol | Sources |
|---|---|---|---|---|---|---|
| French-fried potatoes± (Fast Food) | Medium (147 g) | 27 | 8 | 15 | 0% | Mainly resulting from hydrogenation |
| Butter** | 1 tbsp | 11 | 0 | 7 | 10% | Natural |
| Margarine, stick† | 1 tbsp | 11 | 3 | 5 | 0% | Mainly resulting from hydrogenation |
| Margarine, tub† | 1 tbsp | 7 | 0.5 | 1.5 | 0% | Mainly resulting from hydrogenation |
| Mayonnaise†† (Soybean Oil) | 1 tbsp | 11 | 0 | 1.5 | 2% | Mainly resulting from hydrogenation |
| Shortening± | 1 tbsp | 13 | 4 | 7.5 | 0% | Mainly resulting from hydrogenation |
| Potato chips± | Small bag (42.5 g) | 11 | 3 | 5 | 0% | Mainly resulting from hydrogenation |
| Milk, whole± | 1 cup | 7 | 0 | 4.5 | 12% | Natural |
| Milk, skim† | 1 cup | 0 | 0 | 0 | 2% | Natural |
| Doughnut± | 1 | 18 | 5 | 9.5 | 8% | Mainly resulting from hydrogenation |
| Cookies± (Cream-Filled) | 3 (30 g) | 6 | 2 | 3 | 0% | Mainly resulting from hydrogenation |
| Candy Bar± | 1 (40 g) | 10 | 3 | 7 | 1% | Mainly resulting from hydrogenation |
| Cake, pound± | 1 slice (80 g) | 16 | 4.5 | 8 | 0% | Mainly resulting from hydrogenation |

*Nutrient values rounded based on FDA's nutrition labeling regulations.
** Butter values from FDA Table of *Trans* Values, 1/30/95.
† Values derived from 2002 USDA National Nutrient Database for Standard Reference, Release 15.
†† Prerelease values derived from 2003 USDA National Nutrient Database for Standard Reference, Release 16.
± 1995 USDA Composition Data.

relative risk of CHD associated with an absolute increase of 2% in the intake of TFA was 1.36 (95% confidence interval, 1.03 to 1.81) in the Health Professionals Follow-up Study (Ascherio et al., 1996), 1.14 (95% confidence interval, 0.96 to 1.35) in the Alpha-Tocopherol Beta-Carotene Cancer Prevention Study (Pietinen et al., 1997), and 1.93 (95% confidence interval, 1.43 to 2.61) in the Nurses' Health Study (Hu et al., 1997).

## *Trans* Fatty Acid and Metabolism

In most respects, the digestion, absorption, and metabolism of TFA are the same as that of *cis* isomers. Fatty acids modulate nuclear receptors that regulate gene transcription, such as peroxisome–proliferator-activated receptors, metabolic and inflammatory responses of the endoplasmic reticulum. TFA modulate inflammatory markers and enhance the risk of CHD.

## Biological Effects of *trans* Fatty Acid

TFA are unsaturated fatty acids with at least a double *trans* configuration, resulting in a more rigid molecule close to a saturated fatty acid. Hydrogenated oils, margarines, shortenings, and baked goods are good sources of TFA. TFA from industrially produced and from natural sources have different effects on CVD risk factors in women. The HDL cholesterol-lowering property of TFA seems to be specific to industrial sources (Chardigny et al., 2008).

### *TFA and CMS*

TFA may increase the risk of sudden death from cardiac causes. In a larger, community-based case-control study (179 cases), levels of TFA in erythrocyte membranes were associated with an increase in the risk of sudden cardiac death (odds ratio for inter quintile range, 1.47; 95% confidence interval, 1.01 to 2.13), after adjustment for other risk factors (Lemaitre et al., 2002). Table 11.4 provides a summary of the effects of TFA on CMS risk factors.

#### *TFA and Diabetes*

Analysis of the Nurses' Health Study after 14 years of observation showed that the risk of the development of type-2 diabetes was associated with TFA intake. The intake of industrially produced TFA in the United States is on average 3% energy; a reduction in TFA intake of 2% energy could reduce the incidence of type-2 diabetes by 40% if the fats containing the TFA are consumed in their original unhydrogenated form (Mozaffarian et al., 2006). In the administration of a high-fat meal of variable fatty acid composition, elaidic acid (9*trans*-18:1) compared with oleic acid (9*cis*-18:1) gave rise to higher insulin levels in the blood at the same blood sugar level, which indicates that elaidic acid produces increased insulin resistance (Bray et al., 2002). TFA may also down-regulate peroxisome–proliferator-activated receptor-g (PPAR-g) in adipose tissue (Saravanan et al., 2005). Adipocytes exposed to CLA secreted more proinflammatory cytokines than controls, and an elevated increased macrophage infiltration occurred in adipose tissue treated with *trans*10*cis*12-CLA. Christiansen et al. (1997) conducted a study on an insulin-resistant group comprised of overweight patients with type-2 diabetes. A TFA diet caused a significantly elevated postprandial insulin response to a standardized meal, which was given 6 weeks after the intervention. A higher insulin response suggests increased insulin resistance, but could also involve impaired insulin clearance or stimulated insulin secretion by beta cells.

**Table 11.3. *Trans* Fatty Acid Intake and Relative Risk of Coronary Heart Disease**

| Author, Year | No. of subjects | No. of events | Relative risk | Conclusions |
|---|---|---|---|---|
| Oh et al., 2005 | 78,778 | 1766 | 1.33 | *trans*-fat intake was associated with increased risk of CHD, particularly for younger women |
| Ascherio et al., 1996 | 38.461 | 1702 | 1.26 | Intake of linolenic acid was inversely associated with risk of myocardial infarction; this association became significant only after adjustment for non-dietary risk factors and was strengthened after adjustment for total fat intake (relative risk 0.41 for a 1% increase in energy, *P* for trend < 0.01). |
| Pietinen et al.,1997 | 21,930 | 1399 | 1.14 | For men in the top quintile of *trans*-fatty acid intake (median = 6.2 g/day), the multivariate relative risk of coronary death was 1.39 (95% confidence interval (CI) 1.09-1.78) (*P* for trend = 0.004) as compared with men in the lowest quintile of intake (median = 1.3 g/day). |
| Oomen et al., 2001 | 667 | 98 | 1.28 | *Trans* fatty acid intake at baseline was positively associated with the 10-year risk of coronary heart disease. The relative risk for a difference of 2% of energy in *trans* fatty acid intake at baseline was 1.28 (95% CI 1.01-1.61). |
| Aro et al.,1995 | 1,388 | 671 | 0.97 | The risk of AMI did not differ significantly from 1.0 over quartiles of adipose C18:1 *trans* fatty acids: the multivariate odds ratio was 0.97 (95% CI 0.56-1.67) for the highest versus lowest quartile |
| Baylin et al., 2003 | 964 | 482 | 2.94 | Adipose tissue 16:1 *trans*-FA were also associated with MI; OR = 1.00, 1.57, 1.39, 1.34 and 2.58 (*P*-test for trend < 0.05). High 18:2 *trans*-FA in adipose tissue are associated with increased risk of MI. |
| Clifton et al., 2004 | 78 | 44 | 2.50 | Logistic regression showed that *trans* 18:1(n-11) (*P* = 0.03) was an independent predictor of a first MI. |

**Table 11.3., cont. *Trans* Fatty Acid Intake and Relative Risk of Coronary Heart Disease**

| Author, Year | No. of subjects | No. of events | Relative risk | Conclusions |
|---|---|---|---|---|
| Merchant et al., 2008 | 620 persons | - | - | A 1-g/d higher intake of *trans* fat was associated with a 0.03-mm higher IMT ($P = 0.02$) after multivariate adjustment. |
| Sun et al., 2007 | 32 826 | 166 incident cases | The multivariable relative risks (95% confidence intervals) of CHD from the lowest to highest quartiles of total trans fatty acid content in erythrocytes were 1.0 (reference), 1.6 (0.7 to 3.6), 1.6 (0.7 to 3.4), and 3.3 (1.5 to 7.2) (*P* for trend <0.01). | Total *trans* fatty acid content in erythrocytes was significantly correlated with dietary intake of *trans* fat (correlation coefficient =0.44, $P<0.01$) and was associated with increased plasma low-density lipoprotein cholesterol (*P* for trend =0.06), decreased plasma high-density lipoprotein cholesterol concentrations (*P* for trend <0.01), and increased plasma low-density lipoprotein to high-density lipoprotein ratio (*P* for trend <0.01). |
| Lemaitre et al., 2006 | 214 cases of fatal IHD (fatal myocardial infarction and coronary heart disease death) | - | *Trans*-18:1 levels above the 20th percentile were associated with lower risk (OR 0.34, 95% CI 0.18 to 0.63). In analyses limited to cases of sudden cardiac death (n=95), higher levels of *trans*-18:2 fatty acids were associated with higher risk (OR 2.34, 95% CI 1.27 to 4.31) and higher *trans*-18:1 with lower risk (OR 0.18, 95% CI 0.06 to 0.54). | Higher levels of plasma phospholipid *trans*-18:2 fatty acids were associated with higher risk of fatal IHD (odds ratio [OR] for interquintile range 1.68, 95% confidence interval [CI] 1.21 to 2.33) after adjustment for risk factors and *trans*-18:1 levels |

## *TFA and Blood Pressure*

High blood pressure is often associated with various metabolic abnormalities. Arterial hypertension is often a part of a larger constellation of anthropometric and metabolic abnormalities that includes abdominal (or visceral) obesity, a characteristic dyslipidemia (low high-density lipoprotein cholesterol and high triglycerides), glucose intolerance, insulin-resistance, and hyperuricemia. Dietary TFA are directly and significantly related to higher systolic and diastolic blood pressures, at least in men at high risk of CHD. Consuming 6 g of additional TFA a day—less than the amount found in a typical large order of french fries—would increase systolic blood pressure (SBP) by 1.4 mm Hg and diastolic by 1 mm Hg (Borzo, 2000).

**Table 11.4. Effect of TFA on Cardiometabolic Syndrome**

| Author, Year | Number of subjects | Study population | TFA dose/duration | Conclusion |
|---|---|---|---|---|
| **Lipids and Liproproteins** | | | | |
| Mensink and Katan, 1990 | 34 women/25 men | Healthy subjects | 10% of daily energy | Increased LDL cholesterol levels by 14 mg per deciliter (0.37 mmol per liter) and decreased HDL cholesterol levels by 7 mg per deciliter (0.17 mmol per liter). Mean HDL cholesterol level was lower; LDL cholesterol level higher on the *trans*-fatty acid diet than on the oleic acid diet |
| Chardigny et al., 2008 | 19 men and 21 women | Healthy subjects | 11–12 g/d, representing ≈5% of daily energy/3 week | TFAs from industrially produced and from natural sources have different effects on CVD risk factors in women. The HDL cholesterol-lowering property of TFAs seems to be specific to industrial sources. TFAs from natural sources significantly ($P = 0.012$) increased HDL cholesterol in women but not in men. Significant ($P = 0.001$) increases in LDL-cholesterol concentrations were observed in women, but not in men, after the consumption of TFAs from natural sources. |
| Willett et al.,1993 | 69,181 women | Healthy population (Nurses' health study) | margarine consumption over the previous 10 years had been stable; other sources are cookies [biscuits], cake, and white bread | Consumption of partially hydrogenated vegetable oils may contribute to occurrence of CHD. |
| Ascherio et al., 1994 | 239 patients | A first acute myocardial infarction | Intake of margarine | Intake of *trans*-fatty acids was directly related to risk of myocardial infarction (relative risk for highest compared with lowest quintile, 2.44; 95% confidence interval, 1.42, 4.19; for trend $P < .0001$). Intake of partially hydrogenated vegetable oils may contribute to the risk of myocardial infarction. |

**Table 11.4., cont. Effect of TFA on Cardiometabolic Syndrome**

| | | | | |
|---|---|---|---|---|
| van de Vijver et al., 2000 | 327 men and 299 women | Healthy | TFA intake was calculated with recent figures on TFA levels of foods, collected in the TRANSFAIR study | Current European intake levels of *trans* fatty acids they are not associated with an unfavorable serum lipid profile |
| Pietinen et al., 1997 | 21,930 smoking men | Smokers | median = 6.2 g/day), 6.1 year follow up | Multivariate relative risk of coronary death was 1.39 |
| **Inflammatory Markers** | | | | |
| Han et al., 2002 | 19 subjects | hyperc-holester-olemia, | 6.7% of energy from *trans* fatty acids | interleukin-6 and TNF-α elevated |
| Baer et al., 2004 | 50 men | Healthy men | 4.0% of energy from TFA | interleukin-6 and C- reactive protein |
| **Endothelial Functions** | | | | |
| Lopez-Garcia et al., 2005 | 730 women | Nurses' health study | Highest qunitile of TFA (2.1% Energy from TFA) | *Trans* fatty acid intake was positively related to plasma concentration of CRP ($P = 0.009$), sTNFR-2 ($P = 0.002$), E-selectin ($P = 0.003$), sICAM-1 ($P = 0.007$), and sVCAM-1 ($P = 0.001$) |

## *TFA and Obesity*

Abdominal obesity, due to intraabdominal adiposity, drives the progression of multiple cardiometabolic risk factors independently of body mass index (BMI). This occurs both through altered secretion of adipocyte-derived biologically active substances (adipokines), including free fatty acids, adiponectin, interleukin-6, TNF alpha, and plasminogen activator inhibitor-1 (PAI-1), and through exacerbation of IR and associated cardiometabolic risk factors. A review of 28 publications from 1999 to 2002, including animal and human studies, reveals conflicting results that do not allow for conclusions to be drawn about a positive impact on human body composition even with intakes of up to 7 grams of CLA per day. A recent Swedish study indicates that certain CLA isomers that are present only in very low levels in ruminant fat increase the insulin resistance of men with abdominal obesity (Ricerus et al., 2002).

## *TFA and Endothelial Function*

Endothelial dysfunction occurs in a wide variety of pathophysiological settings such as diabetes. It is accompanied by altered expression of adhesion molecules that affect thrombosis, as described below, and increase permeability (leakiness), which is one of the earliest manifestations of diabetic vasculopathy. Endothelial dysfunction is also noted in persons with hypertension and dyslipidemia. *Trans* fats are shown to increase circulating biomarkers of endothelial dysfunction and to impair nitric oxide-dependent arterial dilatation. Lopez-Garcia et al. (2005) observed that a greater intake of TFA was associated with increased levels of several markers of endothelial dysfunction, including soluble intercellular adhesion molecule 1, soluble vascular-cell adhesion molecule 1, and E-selectin. CRP levels were 73% higher among those in the highest quintile of *trans* fat intake, compared with the lowest quintile. IL-6 levels were 17% higher, sTNFR-2 5%, E-selectin 20%, sICAM-1 10%, and sVCAM-1 levels 10% higher. TFA intake was positively related to the plasma concentration of CRP ($P = 0.009$), sTNFR-2 ($P = 0.002$), E-selectin ($P = 0.003$), sICAM-1 ($P = 0.007$), and sVCAM-1 ($P = 0.001$). De Ross et al. (2001) reported that the replacement of dietary saturated fatty acids by TFA impaired the FMD of the brachial artery, which suggests an increased risk of CHD. Evidence from both observational and experimental studies indicates that TFA are pro-inflammatory. Limited evidence suggests that pro-inflammatory effects may be stronger for *trans* isomers of linoleic acid (*trans*-C18:2) and oleic acid (*trans*-C18:1), rather than of palmitoleic acid (*trans*-C16:1). TFA are proinflammatory. The mechanisms underlying these effects are not well-established, but may involve TFA incorporation into endothelial cell, monocyte/macrophage, or adipocyte cell membranes (affecting membrane signaling pathway relating to inflammation) or ligand-dependent effects on peroxisome–proliferator-activated receptor (PPAR) or retinoid X receptor (RXR) pathways. Activation of inflammatory responses and endothelial dysfunction may represent important mediating pathways between TFA consumption and the risk of CHD, sudden death, and diabetes (Mozaffarrian, 2006). Harvey et al. (2008) reported that TFA treatment of human aortic endothelial cell (HAEC) significantly increased the expression of endothelial adhesion molecules, including intercellular adhesion molecule-1 (CD54) and vitronectin receptor (CD51/CD61). Incorporation of TFA into membranes increased HAEC adhesion to fibronectin- or vitronectin-coated plates by 1.5- to 2-fold, respectively. Neutrophil and monocyte adhesion to HAEC monolayers was nearly proportional to adhesion molecule expression. TFA treatment also induced the release of monocyte chemoattractant protein-1 by nearly threefold in nonstimulated HAEC.

### *TFA and Blood Lipids/Lipoproteins*

Elevated plasma FFA levels can lead to increased oxidative stress, dimished NO synthesis, and impaired fibrolysis. Low-density lipoprotein (LDL) particles are smaller, denser, and more artherogenic. TFA have markedly adverse effects on serum lipids and lipoproteins. Consumption of TFA increases LDL-C (Stampfer et al., 1991), triglycerides, levels of Lp(a) lipoprotein (Ascherio et al., 1999), and reduces the particle size of LDL cholesterol (Mauger et al., 2003).

### *TFA and Microalbuminuria*

Microalbuminuria is a strong and independent indicator of increased cardiovascular risk among individuals with and without diabetes. Therefore, microalbuminuria is used for stratification of risk for cardiovascular disease. Luchi et al. (2000) reported that the increased levels of CLA in plasma and adipose tissue of end-stage chronic renal failure patients may be due either to a reduced metabolization of CLA to CD18:3 and CD20:3, or to an altered site distribution with reduced incorporation in cellular membranes and accumulation in the plasma and adipose tissue.

### *TFA and Inflammatory Markers*

Abnormalities of various adipocytokines' (particularly reduced circulating levels of adiponectin and leptin) resistance may also play a role in the genesis of insulin resistance. Inflammation not only contributes to acute cardiovascular events but is also a key player in the initiation and progression of atherosclerosis. TFA elevated inflammatory markers such as C- reactive protein (Baer et al., 2004), TNF alpha, and IL-6 (Han et al., 2002). TFA intake increases systemic inflammation in healthy persons (Mozaffarrian et al., 2004). Mozaffarian et al. (2004) observed that TFA levels were positively associated with interleukin (IL) 1ß (difference from mean: 0.38 pg/mL; percentage difference from mean: 66%; $P = 0.04$), IL-1 receptor antagonist (4033 pg/mL; $P = 0.006$), IL-6 (9.5 pg/mL; $P = 0.006$), IL-10 (241 pg/mL; $P = 0.02$), tumor necrosis factor (TNF) $\alpha$(256 pg/mL; $P = 0.02$), TNF receptor 1 (537 pg/mL; $P = 0.03$), TNF receptor 2 (39 242 pg/mL; $P = 0.001$), monocyte chemoattractant protein 1 (117 pg/mL; $P = 0.004$), and brain natriuretic peptide (40 pg/mL; $P = 0.04$).

### *TFA and Hypercoagulation*

Increases in fibrinogen, factor VII activity, and PAI-1 in both plasma and the atherosclerotic plaque; decreases in urokinase in the plaque; and increases in platelet aggregation. Hypercoagulation in diabetes appears to contribute to both the pathogenesis of progressive atherosclerosis and acute events in diabetes. Where coagulation and fibrinolysis are concerned, no need exists to differentiate between stearic acid or *trans* monoenoic fatty acids (Mutanen & Aro, 1997). Fats rich in stearic (S), palmitic (P), palmitic + myristic (M), oleic (O), *trans* 18:1 (T), and linoleic (L) acid increase FVII activation (Tholstrup et al., 2003). The administration of a fatty meal induces a postprandial procoagulant tendency, irrespective of the type of fat consumed.

### *TFA and Oxidative Stress*

The free radicals can lead to increased lipid peroxidation, including oxidation of lipoproteins. Oxidative stress can influence the expression of multiple genes in vascular cells, which may accelerate atherogenesis. These include signaling molecules such as protein kinase C, nuclear factor-κB, and extracellular signal-regulated kinase. TFA can influence the physical characteristics of bilayer microdomains, affecting membrane properties and functions. The high consumption of *trans* fat is associated with high oxidative stress in humans, which could increase the risk of the development or the acceleration of several diseases, such as atherosclerosis, cancer, and type-2 diabetes.

An increase in urinary 8-iso-PGF(2alpha) was observed, and the effects of prolonged high (i.e., >5.0 g/d) consumption of *trans* fat could be relevant to the development of diseases (Kuhnt et al., 2006).

## Nutrition Labeling Issues and Health Claims

TFA are listed on nutrition labels along with saturated fatty acids. The risk to health of consuming TFA from industrial sources is recognized and acknowledged by the Food and Drug Administration (FDA), which made it compulsory in 2006 for companies to indicate the content of TFA on nutrition labels for all conventional foods and supplements.

In addition, the Department of Agriculture made a limited intake of TFA a key recommendation of the new food-pyramid guidelines, following the recommendations of the Dietary Guidelines Advisory Committee — intake of TFA should be less than 1% of total energy. Recently, the New York City Department of Health and Mental Hygiene asked 20,000 restaurants and 14,000 food suppliers to eliminate partially hydrogenated oils from their kitchens and to provide foods free from industrially produced TFA.

The major food sources of TFA are hard margarines and shortenings used in frying and in preparing baked goods and other processed foods.

*Trans* and saturated fatty acids may not all be the same (i.e., 18:0 compared with 12, 14, and 16-carbon chains).

TFA are less significant because the U.S. diet provides a smaller proportion of TFA, and the data on their biological effects are limited. TFA must be listed separately, or be included with saturated fatty acids on nutrition labels.

### References


Aro, A,; A.F. Kardinaal; I .Salminen; et al. Adipose tissue isomeric trans fatty acids and risk of myocardial infarction in nine countries: the EURAMIC study. *Lancet* **1995,** *345,* 273–278.

Ascherio, A; C.H. Hennekens; J.E.Buring; C. Master; M.J. Stampfer; W.C. Willett. *Trans*-fatty acids intake and risk of myocardial infarction. *Circulation* **1994,** *89,* 94–101.

Ascherio, A.; M. Katan; P.L. Zock; M.J. Stampfer; W.C .Willett. Trans fatty acids and coronary heart disease. *N. Engl. J. Med.* **1999,** *340,*1994–1998.

Ascherio, A .; E.B. Rimm; E.L. Giovannucci; D. Spiegelman; M. Stampfer; W.C. Willett. Dietary fat and risk of coronary heart disease in men: cohort follow up study in the united states. *BMJ* **1996,** *313,* 84–90.

Baer, D.J.; J.T. Judd; B.A. Clevidence; R.P. Tracy. Dietary fatty acids affect plasma markers of inflammation in healthy men fed controlled diets: a randomized crossover study. *Am. J. Clin. Nutr.* **2004,** *79,* 969–973.

Baylin, A.; E.K. Kabagambe; A. Ascherio; D. Spiegelman; H. Campos. High 18:2 trans-fatty acids in adipose tissue are associated with increased risk of nonfatal acute myocardial infarction in Costa Rican adults. *J. Nutr.* **2003,** *133,* 1186–1191.

Borzo, G. “Trans-Fatty Acids Linked to High Blood Pressure.” *Family Practice News.* Oct. 15,

2000.

Bray, G.A.; J.C. Lovejoy; S.R. Smith; J.P .DeLany; M .Lefevre; D. Hwang; D.H. Ryan; D.A York. The influence of different fats and fatty acids on obesity, insulin resistance and inflammation. *J. Nutr.* **2002,** *132,* 2488–2491.

Chardigny, J.M.; F. Destaillats; C. Malpuech-Brugère; J. Moulin; D.E. Bauman; A.L. Lock; D.M Barbano; R.P. Mensink; J.B. Bezelgues; C.P. Haumont; N. Combe; I. Cristiani; F. Joffre; J.B. German; F. Dionisi; Y. Boirie; J.L. Sébédio. Do trans fatty acids from industrially produced sources and from natural sources have the same effect on cardiovascular disease risk factors in healthy subjects? Results of the trans fatty acids collaboration (TRANSFACT) study. *Am. J. Clin. Nutr.* **2008,** *87,* 558–566.

Christiansen, E.; S. Schnider; B. Palmvig; E. Tauber-Lassen; O. Pedersen. Intake of a diet high in trans monounsaturated fatty acids or saturated fatty acids. Effects on postprandial insulinemia and glycemia in obese patients with NIDDM. *Diabetes Care* **1997,** *20,* 881–887.

Clifton, P.M.; J.B. Keogh; M. Noakes. Trans fatty acids in adipose tissue and the food supply are associated with myocardial infarction. *J. Nutr.* **2004,** *134,* 874–879.

Craig-Schmidt, M.C. World-wide consumption of *trans* fatty acids. *Atherosclerosis Suppl.* **2006,** *7,*1–8.

de Roos, N.M.; M.L. Bots; M.B. Katan. Replacement of dietary saturated fatty acids by trans fatty acids lowers serum HDL cholesterol and impairs endothelial function in healthy men and women. *Arterioscler. Thromb. Vasc. Biol.* **2001,** *21,*1233–1237.

DerSimonian, R.; N. Laird. Meta-analysis in clinical trials. *Control Clin. Trials* **1986,** *7,*177–188.

Han, S.N.; L.S. Leka; A.H. Lichtenstein; L.M. Ausman; E.J. Schaefer; S.N. Meydani. Effect of hydrogenated and saturated, relative to polyunsaturated, fat on immune and inflammatory responses of adults with moderate hypercholesterolemia. *J. Lipid Res.* **2002**, *43,* 445–452.

Harvey, K.A.; T. Arnold; T. Rasool; C. Antalis; S.J. Miller; R.A. Siddiqui. Trans-fatty acids induce pro-inflammatory responses and endothelial cell dysfunction. *Br. J. Nutr.* **2008,** *99(4),* 723–731.

Hu, F.B.; M.J. Stampfer; J.E. Manson; E. Rimm; G.A. Colditz; B.A. Rosner; C.H. Hennekens, W.C. Willett. Dietary fat intake and the risk of coronary heart disease in women. *N. Engl. J. Med.* **1997,** *337,* 1491–1499.

Juturu, V. Cardiometabolic syndrome: current perspectives and challenges. *Med. Nutr. Lett.* 2007 (Spring).

Kuhnt, K.; A. Wagner; J. Kraft; S. Basu; G. Jahreis. Dietary supplementation with 11trans- and 12trans-18:1 and oxidative stress in humans. *Am. J. Clin. Nutr.* **2006,** *84(5),* 981–988.

Lemaitre, R.N.; I.B. King; D. Mozaffarian; N. Sotoodehnia; T.D. Rea; L.H. Kuller; R.P. Tracy; D.S. Siscovick. Plasma phospholipid trans fatty acids, fatal ischemic heart disease, and sudden cardiac death in older adults: the cardiovascular health study. *Circulation* **2006,** *114(3),* 209–215.

Lemaitre, R.N.; I.B. King; T.E. Raghunathan; R.M. Pearce; S. Weinmann; R.H. Knopp; M.K. Copass; L.A. Cobb; D.S. Siscovick. Cell membrane trans-fatty acids and the risk of primary cardiac arrest. *Circulation* **2002,** *105,* 697–701.

Lopez-Garcia, E.; M.B. Schulze; J.B.Meigs; J.E .Manson; N. Rifai; M.J. Stampfer; W.C. Willett; F.B. Hu. Consumption of trans fatty acids is related to plasma biomarkers of inflammation and endothelial dysfunction. *J. Nutr.* **2005,** *135,* 562–566.

Lucchi, L.; S. Banni; M.P. Melis; E. Angioni; G. Carta; V. Casu; R. Rapanà; A. Ciuffreda; F.P. Corongiu; A. Albertazzi. Changes in conjugated linoleic acid and its metabolites in patients with chronic renal failure. *Kidney Int.* **2000,** *58(4),*1695–1702.

Mauger, J.F.; A.H. Lichtenstein; L.M. Ausman; S.M. Jalbert; M. Jauhiainen; C. Ehnholm; B. Lamarche. Effect of different forms of dietary hydrogenated fats on LDL particle size. *Am. J. Clin. Nutr.* **2003,** *78,* 370–375.

Mensink, R.P.; M.B. Katan. Effect of dietary trans fatty acids on high-density and low-density lipoprotein cholesterol levels in healthy subjects. *N. Engl. J. Med.***1990,** *323,* 439–445.

Merchant, A.T.; L.E. Kelemen; L. de Koning; E. Lonn,; V. Vuksan; R. Jacobs; B. Davis; K.K. Teo; S. Yusuf; S.S. Anand; SHARE and SHARE-AP investigators. Interrelation of saturated fat, trans fat, alcohol intake, and subclinical atherosclerosis. *Am. J. Clin. Nutr.* **2008,** *87(1),* 168–174.

Mozaffarian, D. Trans fatty acids—effects on systemic inflammation and endothelial function. *Atheroscler. Suppl.* **2006,** *7(2),* 29–32.

Mozaffarian, D.; E.B. Rimm; I.B. King; R.L. Lawler; G.B. McDonald; W.C. Levy. Trans fatty acids and systemic inflammation in heart failure. *Am. J. Clin. Nutr.* **2004,** *80,* 1521–1525.

Mutanen, M.; A. Aro. Coagulation and fibrinolysis factors in healthy subjects consuming high stearic or trans fatty acid diets. *Thromb. Haemost.* **1997,** *77(1),* 99–104.

Oh, K.; F.B. Hu; J.E. Manson; M.J. Stampfer; W.C. Willett. Dietary fat intake and risk of coronary heart disease in women: 20 years of follow-up of the nurses' health study. *Am. J. Epidemiol.* **2005,** *161,* 672–679.

Oomen, C.M.; M.C. Ocke; E.J. Feskens; M.A. van Erp-Baart; F.J. Kok; D. Kromhout. Association between trans fatty acid intake and 10-year risk of coronary heart disease in the zutphen elderly study: a prospective population-based study. *Lancet* **2001,** *357,* 746–751.

Pietinen, P.; A. Ascherio; P. Korhonen; A.M. Hartman; W.C. Willett; D. Albanes; J. Virtamo. Intake of fatty acids and risk of coronary heart disease in a cohort of Finnish men: the alpha-tocopherol, beta-carotene cancer prevention study. *Am. J. Epidemiol.* **1997,** *145,* 876–887.

Ricerus, U.; P. Arner; K. Brismar; B. Vessby. Treatment with dietary *trans*10*cis*12 conjugated linoleic acid causes isomer-specific insulin resistance in obese men with the metabolic syndrome. *Diabetes Care* **2002,** *25,* 1516–1521.

Saravanan, N.; A. Haseeb; N.Z. Ehtesham; S.A. Ghafoorunissa. Differential effects of dietary saturated and transfatty acids on expression of genes associated with insulin sensitivity in rat adipose tissue. *Eur. J. Endocrinol.* **2005,** *153,* 159–165.

Stampfer, M.J.; F.M. Sacks; S. Salvini; W.C .Willett; C.H. Hennekens. A prospective study of cholesterol, apolipoproteins, and the risk of myocardial infarction. *N. Engl. J. Med.* **1991,** *325,* 373–381.

Sun, Q.; J. Ma; H. Campos; S.E. Hankinson; J.E. Manson; M.J. Stampfer; K.M. Rexrode; W.C. Willett; F.B. Hu. A prospective study of trans fatty acids in erythrocytes and risk of coronary heart disease. *Circulation* **2007,** *115(14),* 1858–1865.

van de Vijver, L.P.L.; A.F.M. Kardinaal; C. Couet; A. Aro; A. Kafatos; L. Steingrimsdottir; J.A. Amorim Cruz; O. Moreiras; W. Becker; J.M. van Amelsvoort; et al. Association between *trans* fatty acid intake and cardiovascular risk factors in Europe: the TRANSFAIR study. *Eur. J. Clin.*

*Nutr.* **2000,** *54,*126–135.

Willett, W.C.; M.J. Stampfer; J.E. Manson; G.A. Colditz; F.E. Speizer; B.A. Rosner; L.A. Sampson; C.H. Hennekens. Intake of *trans* fatty acids and risk of coronary heart disease among women. *Lancet* **1993,** *341,* 581–585.

# 12

# Effects of Fatty Acids Containing a *trans* Double Bond on Body Composition

**Lance H. Baumgard[1], Aileen F. Keating[2] and James W. Perfield II[3]**
[1]*University of Arizona, Department of Animal Sciences and Department of Nutritional Sciences, Tucson, Arizona;* [2]*University of Arizona, Department of Physiology, Tucson, Arizona;* [3]*Jean Mayer-USDA Human Nutrition Research Center on Aging at Tufts University, Boston, Massachusetts*

## Introduction

The ability to regulate changes in body composition has obvious implications for the health of humans and companion animals, as well as animal agriculture. In humans and pets, an increase in adipose tissue mass is associated with an increased risk of chronic diseases such as type 2 diabetes, cardiovascular disease, hypertension and stroke, hypercholesterolemia, and certain cancers. In addition to excessive caloric intake, a connection may exist between total and specific types of dietary fats on disease and body composition. Regarding agriculturally important animals, excess fat deposition represents inefficient nutrient utilization and impacts consumer acceptance of products; thus, it is a large economic concern. *Trans* fatty acids are receiving a lot of attention not only for their potential deleterious effects, but also for their impressive ability (of at least a few specific *trans* fatty acids) to reduce body-fat content and accretion in experimental models. However, clearly, not all *trans* fatty acids are equal, and each probably has its own biological effect. In the following chapter, we briefly discuss epidemiological data connecting *trans* fatty acids to health disorders. The main focus is *trans*-10, *cis*-12 conjugated linoleic acid (CLA), a *trans* fatty acid demonstrated to be a powerful regulator of body composition in animal models.

## *Trans* Fatty Acid Background

### *Fatty Acid Chemistry*

A fatty acid is defined as a hydrocarbon chain with a methyl group on one end and a carboxyl group on the other. The length of a fatty acid chain can vary, and carbons are connected to each other by single or double bonds. Mono- and polyunsaturated fatty acids are identified by the presence of one or more double bonds which can be positioned anywhere along the carbon chain. Double bonds may be described as being either *cis* or *trans,* depending on the orientation of the hydrogen atoms attached to the double-bonded carbons. The majority of fatty acid double bonds found in nature are *cis* in orientation, indicating the hydrogen atoms are on the same side of the carbon molecule. A fatty acid is referred to as being a *trans* fatty acid when it contains at least one double bond in the *trans* configuration, indicating the hydrogen atoms of the double bond are on opposite sides of the carbon. In *cis* double bonds, the hydrogen atoms are repelled by each other, and this places a "bend" in the molecule. However, in *trans* double bonds, the opposing forces of the hydrogen atoms are balanced, causing the fatty acid to remain relatively straight and structurally to resemble a saturated fatty acid. If more than one double bond is present, they can be positioned in either a nonconjugated or conjugated arrangement. The term "nonconjugated" indicates that two double bonds along the carbon chain are separated by one or more methylene groups ($CH_2$).

## *Industrial* trans *Fatty Acid Production*

Hydrogenation is a reductive chemical reaction resulting in the addition of hydrogen atoms to the double bonds of a molecule through the use of a catalyst (nickel, copper, etcetera). The end product of hydrogenation is rarely complete or specific, and depending on the conditions (i.e., type of catalyst, hydrogen pressure, temperature, etcetera), various *trans* fatty acids are produced (Martin et al., 2007). The most common of these industrial *trans* fatty acids are eighteen-carbon molecules with a single double bond (C18:1) along the carbon chain, with *trans*-9 18:1 (eladic acid) often being the most abundant isomer (Sommerfeld, 1983). Industrial hydrogenation of liquid vegetable oils (primarily polyunsaturated fatty acids) increases the content of saturated and *trans* fatty acids, allowing for the production of solid and semi-solid spreads, such as margarine. The original impetus for producing a butter substitute was economic and took place in Europe during the mid nineteenth century (Martin et al., 2007). This process was widely adopted by the food industry for reasons of functionality, cost, stability, and organoleptic qualities. However, a change in food-labeling laws in 2006 (discussed below) caused manufacturers to alter production procedures and identify alternative fats to replace industrial *trans* fats in foods (Hunter, 2004).

## *Natural* trans *Fatty Acid Production*

*Trans* fatty acids are also present in small quantities in the meat and milk of ruminants (cows, goats, sheep, etcetera) due to the hydrogenation of dietary unsaturated fatty acids in the rumen (first stomach of the ruminant animal). Instead of a chemically catalyzed reaction, this process is performed by populations of microorganisms present in the rumen and is termed "biohydrogenation" (Bauman et al., 2000). During the process of biohydrogenation, some intermediates, including a variety of *trans* 18:1 monoenes, escape complete hydrogenation and are intestinally absorbed and incorporated into body fat and milk lipid. As a consequence, humans have consumed *trans* fatty acids in ruminant products for thousands of years. However, the *trans* fatty acid profile of ruminant fat is quite different than that of industrially manufactured hydrogenated fats, and consequently the biological properties of these *trans* fats differ (discussed below). The major *trans* fatty acid in ruminant lipid is *trans*-11 18:1 (vaccenic acid; >60%; Kay et al., 2005) while historically the predominant isomer in margarine was eladic acid (Sommerfeld, 1983).

### Trans *Fatty Acid Labeling*

The U.S. Food and Drug Administration ruled that the *trans* fatty acid content must appear on nutrition labels starting on January 1, 2006 (Moss, 2006). The reason for this labeling change is that *trans* fatty acids, like total fat and saturated fat, are thought to adversely affect the parameters of coronary heart disease, inflammation, and indices of type II diabetes (Willet, 2006). Diets high in *trans* fatty acids increased total and low-density lipoprotein (LDL) cholesterol and decreased high-density lipoprotein (HDL) cholesterol (Mensink & Katan, 1990), and the effects of diets rich in *trans* fatty acids appear to consistently increase total blood- cholesterol levels (Eckel et al., 2007). The labeling guidelines include all fatty acids containing at least one *trans* double bond (except fatty acids containing a conjugated *trans* double bond) and do not discriminate among *trans* 18:1 isomers or between those originating from industrial or natural sources. Grouping all *trans* fatty acids under one label is bewildering, as individual *trans* 18:1 isomers almost certainly have specific biological properties (German & Dillard, 2006), and yet individual *trans* 18:1 fatty acids have not been evaluated (Aro, 2006). In fact, the *trans* profile produced from the hydrogenation of vegetable oils (primarily elaidic acid) adversely affects blood indices (Sundram et al., 1997), while growing evidence suggests that the *trans* profile in ruminant lipids (primarily vaccenic acid) either has no effect (Booker & Mann, 2008; Chardigny et al., 2008; Gebauer et al., 2007; Motard-Belanger et al., 2008) or actually improves (Sjogren et al., 2004; Wang et al., 2008) cardiovascular disease risk factors. Furthermore, epidemiological data demonstrate no connection between ruminant lipid intake and coronary heart disease (Biong et al., 2006; Hodgson et al., 2007; Iso et al., 1999; Tholstrup, 2006; Waijers et al., 2006). Clearly, recent research has identified biological differences between industrial and naturally derived *trans* fats, which are not distinguished by the current labeling guidelines. One group of *trans* fatty acids, identified to have beneficial health effects and not included under the current regulations, is CLAs (see below).

## Conjugated Linoleic Acids (CLAs)

CLAs are another form of *trans* fatty acids found in ruminant-derived fats. "Conjugated linoleic acid" is a collective term for different positional and geometric configurations of an 18-carbon fatty acid containing a pair of double bonds in a conjugated configuration (double bonds not separated by a methylene group). Numerous CLA isomers are theoretically possible with both the position (7–9, 8–10, 9–11, etcetera) and geometric configuration (*cis* or *trans*) of the double bonds varying. Similar to *trans*-18:1 monoenes, CLAs are intermediates created during biohydrogenation of linoleic and linolenic acids (Bauman et al., 2000). Also, similar to *trans* 18:1 fatty acids, some CLAs escape complete biohydrogenation and are intestinally absorbed and incorporated into meat and milk lipids. The primary (≈90% of total CLA) CLA isomer found in ruminant fats is *cis*-9, *trans*-11 18:2, and it originates via the rumen (as described above) and through vaccenic-acid desaturation by steroyl-CoA desaturase (Bauman et al., 2000). In fact, the majority (>80%) of *cis*-9, *trans*-11 CLA found in ruminant lipids originates via the desaturation of vaccenic acid (also a product of rumen biohydrogenation; Corl et al., 2001; Kay et al., 2004). Due to the unique origin, CLA is only naturally found in ruminant-derived food products (not from monogastric animals) and is not in plants.

CLA originally received considerable attention from the medical community because of its potent anticarcinogenic properties, and it is effective in a variety of in vivo and in vitro cancer models. The *cis*-9, *trans*-11 and the *trans*-10, *cis*-12 CLA isomers are both anticarcinogens (Ip et al., 2003; Kelley et al., 2007; Lee et al., 2005), and the primary human CLA source (particularly the *cis*-9, *trans*-11 isomer) is from consuming ruminant-derived food products (McGuire & McGuire, 2000). In fact, the National Academy of Sciences indicates "conjugated linoleic acid (CLA) is the only fatty acid shown unequivocally to inhibit carcinogenesis in experimental animals" (NRC, 1996).

## Body Composition, Obesity, and Health Disorders

### *Human Health*

Obesity is a health issue in industrialized countries, and targets all socioeconomic, racial, and ethnic groups; also, it does not distinguish between children and adults (Smith et al., 2005). Although some controversy surrounds the severity of the "epidemic" (Campos, 2004; Oliver, 2005), being overweight is well-documented not only to be associated with, but actually to cause, a number of human diseases such as type II diabetes and cardiovascular disease (Mokdad et al., 2003; Sullivan et al., 2005). Although not as well-covered in the media, being overweight also has profound effects on reproduction, and this is especially pertinent because obesity is more prevalent in women (Rosenberg et al., 2003). Female obesity is associated with early onset menarche (Ahemed et al., 1999), anovulation (Al-Azemi et al., 2004), oligomenorrhoea (Pettigrew & Hamilton-Fairley, 1997), and polycystic ovarian syndrome (Pettigrew & Hamilton-Fairley, 1997). Polycystic ovarian syndrome is the most common gynecological problem associated with obesity, and affects 10% of child-bearing age women (Liepa et al., 2008). In addition, puberty occurs at an earlier age in obese females (Himes, 2006; Must et al., 2005). For example, the mean age of menarche decreased in U.S. white (3- month decrease) and African American (5.5-month decrease) girls between the late 1960s and 1990, and the increased prevalence of obesity is thought to be the cause (Himes, 2006). Male obesity is associated with changes in sperm viability (Hammound et al., 2008), erectile dysfunction (Feldman et al., 1994), and alterations in hormonal profiles (Pauli et al., 2008).

### *Agricultural Implications*

Efforts to decrease the fat content of meat and milk from farm animals is important as consumers continue to request leaner food products and demand "healthier" dietary fat. In addition, excess body fat represents inefficient nutrient utilization and therefore reduced economic return for farmers/producers. This is especially true when carcasses are sold based on a grading scheme because back fat (subcutaneous fat) is unfavorable and marbling (intramuscular lipid) is valued. Furthermore, frequent situations exist (i.e., post-parturition, heat stress, poor pasture availability, etcetera) when a lactating animal's energetic state (caloric intake–caloric output) may either limit productivity and/or increase its risk of developing metabolic disorders (i.e., ketosis). By decreasing milk-fat synthesis, the energy content of the secreted milk improves an animal's energetic status: this may be a benefit to its well-being (Bauman et al., 2008).

## ***Trans*** **Fatty Acids and Body Composition**

Limited research exists that investigates the effects of *trans* 18:1 fatty acids on body composition. However, in humans, an association is reported between *trans*-fat intake and increased waist circumference (Koh-Banerjee et al., 2003), and a recent controlled experiment performed in monkeys indicates that *trans* fats increase weight gain and intra-abdominal fat accretion (Kavanagh et al., 2007).

In contrast to *trans* monoenes, dietary CLAs markedly alter body composition in growing animals. Currently CLAs are being evaluated for possible commercial use as a human and pet weight- loss management tool and a nutrient partitioning agent in domesticated animal agriculture. Dietary CLA supplements were first reported to dramatically decrease the fat content of growing and adult mice by Park et al. (1997). The following sections attempt to summarize studies investigating the potential of CLA supplementation as a tool to regulate body composition in a variety of species. In addition, we briefly discuss a range of mechanisms that are postulated for CLAs mode of action.

### *Specific CLA Isomers and Lipid Metabolism*

Most investigations evaluating the effects of CLA on lipid metabolism in growing animals used a commercial supplement containing a mixture of isomers. As a consequence, it was unclear if the physiological effects were the result of one or a combination of CLA isomers. Two of the predominant isomers in CLA supplements used in body-composition studies are *cis*-9, *trans*-11 and *trans*-10, *cis*-12 CLA. Trials with growing mice demonstrated that the reduced body fat associated with feeding dietary CLA was due to the *trans*-10, *cis*-12 isomer, whereas *cis*-9, *trans*-11 CLA had no effect (Park et al., 1999b). Another model that was employed to investigate the regulation of lipid metabolism by CLA isomers is the lactating dairy cow (discussed below). Interestingly, the identification of *trans*-10, *cis*-12 CLA as a potent inhibitor of fat synthesis in the bovine mammary gland occurred (Baumgard et al., 2000) approximately at the same time (Park et al., 1999b) as did its ability to reduce fat synthesis in a rodent growth model. Numerous other CLA isomers were investigated in this model (for their effects on lipid metabolism), and in addition to the well-established effects of *trans*-10, *cis*-12 CLA, *trans*-9, *cis*-11 CLA, and *cis*-10, *trans*-12 CLA were identified as inhibitors of milk-fat synthesis (Perfield et al., 2004, 2006, 2007; Saebo et al., 2005). Thus, three CLA isomers are now discovered to be potent inhibitors of milk-fat synthesis in dairy cows. These data suggest that additional *trans* isomers may also be effective in regulating body composition in other species.

## Animal Studies

Although the magnitude varies, subsequent research corroborated initial studies demonstrating the ability of CLA to reduce body fat in rodents, including growing mice and rats (DeLany et al., 1999; Luccia et al., 2001; Park et al., 1999a, 1999b; Stangl, 2000a; West et al., 1998), and representative data for several species are presented in Table 12.1. In addition to rodents, CLA-induced reduction in body fat was observed for growing hamsters (Matsuba et al., 2000), neonatal pigs (Corl et al., 2008), growing pigs (Ostrowska et al., 1999), mature dogs (Schoenherr & Jewell, 1999), and adult humans (Blankson et al., 2000; Gudmundsen et al., 2001). However, the effects of CLA on lipid metabolism are not consistent across studies because some observed little or no effect of CLA on the body-fat content of growing rats (Azain et al., 2000), Zucker rats (Sanders et al., 2004), growing pigs (Eggert et al., 2001), growing transgenic pigs (Mitchell & Pursel, 2001), growing bass (Twibell et al., 2000), and adult humans (Smedman & Vessby, 2001; Wosje et al., 2001; Zambell et al., 2000).

Reasons for the discrepancies among studies are not apparent, but species and/or genotypic variation may be likely contributors. In fact, even within the same species, large differences exist in the CLA effect on lipid metabolism; for example, CLA decreased the adiposity of lean Zucker rats, but actually increased fat-pad weights in the obese Zucker rats (Sisk et al., 2001). Similar inconsistencies were demonstrated in different strains of mice (Clement et al., 2002). The mechanism by which these species differences exist is not clear, but the rate of intracellular adipocyte triglyceride turnover (Pariza et al., 2001) and basal metabolic rate (Terpstra et al., 2002) were identified as probable causes.

## Human Studies

The impressive effect that CLA has on adiposity in animal models led to human experiments where CLA was hypothesized to be an anti-obesity compound. However, these studies frequently produce conflicting results, and it is difficult to analyze human results due to the differences in CLA dose and isomers, duration of supplementation, differences in age and sex, and differences in the method of body-composition detection (Tricon & Yaqoob, 2006). Relatively few studies demonstrated that CLA reduces fat mass in humans (Blankson et al., 2000; Thom et al., 2001) while many others have shown no effect (Atkinson, 1999; Benito et al., 2001; Berven et al., 2000; Zambell et al., 2000). However, a recent meta-analysis of 18 human CLA-

**Table 12.1. The Effect of CLA on Body Fat and Adipose Depots**

| Author | Species | Sex | Age | Fat depot | %Decrease |
|---|---|---|---|---|---|
| Akahoshi et al., 2002 | Mice | Male | 3 wk | Epidydimal | 80% |
| | | | | Perirenal | 60% |
| Battacharya et al., 2005 | Mice | Male | 8wk | Total | 75% |
| Clement et al., 2002 | Mice | Female | Not reported | Periuteral | 85% |
| de Deckere et al., 1999 | Hamsters | Male | 13 wk | Epidydimal | 16% |
| DeLany et al., 1999 | Mice | Male | 6 wk | Inguinal | 35% |
| | | | | Epidydimal | 21% |
| | | | | Retroperitoneal | 33% |
| | | | | Mesenteric | 46% |
| | | | | Perirenal | 47% |
| Faulconnier et al., 2004 | Rats | Male | 17 wk | Epidydimal | 47% |
| Hargrave et al., 2002 | Mice | Male & female | 12 wk | Total | 20% |
| Kang et al., 2004 | Mice | Not reported | 7 wk | Epidydimal | 40% |
| | | | | Retroperitoneal | 60% |
| Kelley et al., 2006 | Mice | Female | 8 wk | Retroperitoneal | 59% |
| Meadus et al., 2002 | Pigs | Male | Not reported | Subcutaneous | 9% |
| Miner et al., 2001 | Mice | Male | 12 wk | Brown adipose tissue | 29% |
| | | | | Epidydimal | 30% |
| | | | | Retroperitoneal | 50% |
| Nakanishi et al., 2004 | Mice | Male | Not reported | Epidydimal | 71% |
| | | | | Perirenal | 54% |
| Ostrowska et al., 2003 | Pigs | Female | Not reported | Total | 12% |
| Park et al., 1997 | Mice | Female | 6 wk | Total | 60% |
| Rahman et al., 2007 | Mice | Female | 12 mo | Total | 43% |
| Terpstra et al., 2002 | Mice | Male | 6 wk | Total | 67% |
| Tsuboyama- | Mice | Female | 7 wk | Parametrial | 73% |
| Kasaoka et al., 2000 | | | | Perirenal | 93% |
| | | | | Retroperitoneal | 100% |
| | | | | Abdominal subcutaneous | 96% |
| | | | | Dorsal subcutaneous | 97% |
| | | | | Brown adipose tissue | 100% |

supplementation studies concluded that CLA can induce a modest loss of body fat (Whigham et al., 2007).

## CLA Dose

The quantity of CLA required to reduce body fat in growing and adult animals is highly variable and appears to be largely species-dependent. Traditionally, the dose of CLA fed is reported as the percentage of the diet, and this usually ranges from 0.5 to 2.0% (Table 12.2). However, when expressed as milligrams of CLA/kg of body weight, a large difference in dose exists among species. For example, the amount of CLA required to reduce the quantity of body fat by about 30% is approximately five times more in mice than in pigs (DeLany et al., 1999; Ostrowska et al., 1999). Dose may also be part of the reason why the fat-reducing effects in humans were variable and unimpressive because the typical CLA dose fed to humans was markedly less (≈10 fold) than used in rodent studies (Table 12.2). However, logistics and acceptance (i.e., number of pills/day) probably prevent the study of humans receiving a similar dose as that used in rodent trials. Furthermore, the amount of CLA required to reduce milk-fat synthesis is considerably lower (based both on the percentage of diet and body weight) than in growth models. Therefore, in addition to differences in the sensitivity of species and genotypes to CLA, cellular differences apparently exist because the mammary-lipid-synthesizing machinery is extremely responsive to *trans*-10, *cis*-12 CLA (Bauman et al., 2008).

## Adipose Depots

Metabolic differences do exist between visceral and subcutaneous adipose depots (Perrini et al., 2008), and some indication exists that responses to CLA differ among adipose-tissue depots. West et al. (1998) were the first to illustrate this in studies with growing mice. They reported that dietary CLA supplements markedly reduced the weight of the retroperitoneal (back fat) depot, but the inguinal, epididymal, and mesenteric fat depots were less affected. In agreement, DeLany et al. (1999) reported similar differences for the same adipose depots in a study with growing mice. Additionally, Azain et al. (2000) indicated that dietary CLA reduced the weight of the retroperitoneal and parametrial fat depots, but not the inguinal fat pads in growing female rats. Although the effects of dietary CLA on specific adipose depots in pigs were not described in detail, feeding CLA was shown to significantly decrease the retroperitoneal-fat depot in growing gilts (Ostrowska et al., 1999) and barrows (Theil-Cooper et al., 2001). The subcutaneous-fat content of commercial meat cuts was also slightly reduced in growing pigs fed CLA supplements (Dugan et al., 1997). While the differences between fat depots in response to CLA are not consistently reported throughout the literature, it is an area that requires further investigation and could help provide an understanding of the mode of action.

**Table 12.2. Conjugated Linoleic Acid Dose in Growth and Lactation Models**

| Species | CLA % of diet | CLA mg/d | CLA mg/kg[1] | Duration d | Fat % decrease | Reference |
|---|---|---|---|---|---|---|
| | Growth Model | | | | | |
| Pigs | 0.125 | 1900 | 24 | 50 | NS | Ostrowska et al., 1999 |
| | 0.250 | 3900 | 47 | 50 | 15 | |
| | 0.500 | 7700 | 94 | 50 | 18 | |
| | 0.750 | 11500 | 142 | 50 | 17 | |
| | 1.000 | 15400 | 188 | 50 | 31 | |
| Humans | NR | 1950 | 31 | 94 | NS | Zambell et al., 2000 |
| Humans | NR | 1700 | 19 | 84 | 3 | Blankson et al., 2000 |
| | | 3400 | 41 | 84 | 6 | |
| | | 5100 | 59 | 84 | NS | |
| | | 6800 | 76 | 84 | 4 | |
| Mice | 0.25 | 8.6 | 266 | 39 | NS | DeLany et al., 1999 |
| | 0.50 | 16.0 | 448 | 39 | 21 | |
| | 0.50 | 22.5 | 691 | 39 | 21 | |
| | 1.00 | 32.0 | 983 | 39 | 35 | |
| Mice | 0.5 | 20.0 | 800 | 32 | 60 | Park et al., 1997 |
| Mice | 1.0 | 35.0 | 1045 | 42 | 64 | West et al., 1998 |
| | 1.2 | 42.0 | 1267 | 42 | 55 | |
| | Lactation Model | | | | | |
| Women | NR | 1,200 | 57 | 5 | 25 | Masters et al., 2002 |
| Cows | 0.014 | 3,500 | 27 | 5 | 25 | Baumgard et al., 2002 |
| Cows | 0.04 | 10,000 | 78 | 5 | 50 | Baumgard et al., 2000 |

[1]Based on mg CLA/kg body weight.

# Mechanisms for CLA action

Adipose-tissue mass reflects the net result or balance between energy intake and energy expenditure. Energy intake and energy expenditure are not distinct entities because energy balance is the key homeostatic regulator of feed intake. Energy demand depends on many variables, but mainly the physiological state (e.g., lactation), and body composition as lean tissue is energetically more expensive to maintain. Therefore, factors regulating energy demand, energy supply, lipid synthesis, lipid mobilization, fuel preference, energetic transfer efficiencies, and thermoregulation are possible points by which CLA could regulate body composition. Numerous potential mechanisms behind the fat-lowering properties of CLA were developed, including increased energy expenditure, increased adipocyte apoptosis, increased fatty acid oxidation, increased adipocyte lypolysis, decreased adipocyte lipogenesis and fatty acid uptake, and increased adipocyte differentiation (House et al., 2005); these are discussed below. Identification of the mechanism behind the ability of CLA to regulate adipose tissue accretion will help us to better understand how one can apply this nutraceutical as a therapeutic agent in humans and agricultural species.

## *Caloric Intake*

The biological mechanism(s) by which CLA or specifically *trans*-10, *cis*-12 CLA exerts its effects on lipid metabolism in growing animals is unknown, but is clearly complex and multifaceted. Reduced feed intake is a variable that might partly explain some of the reduction in body-fat accretion; however, results are inconsistent. While dietary CLA decreased feed intake in growth studies with mice (Park et al., 1999a, 1999b; West et al., 1998), hamsters (de Deckere et al., 1999), dogs (Schoenherr & Jewell, 1999), pigs (Dugan et al., 1997), and fish (Twibell et al., 2000), an even greater number of studies reported no effect on the intake during growth studies with mice (Belury & Kempa-Steczko, 1997; DeLany et al., 1999; Park et al., 1997), rats (Buison et al., 2000; Chin et al., 1994; Luccia et al., 2001; Martin et al., 2000; Sakono et al., 1999; Sisk et al., 2001; Yamasaki et al., 1999 ), and pigs (Ostrowska et al., 1999; Theil-Cooper et al., 2001) or during lactation studies with cows (Baumgard et al., 2000; Bernal-Santos et al., 2003; Perfield et al., 2002). In one study with growing hamsters, CLA treatment even increased feed intake (Gavino et al., 2000). These studies are further complicated by the fact that many researchers used mixed isomers of CLA, and isomer differences may exist in the effects on feed intake since ZDF diabetic rats fed *cis*-9, *trans*-11 CLA had increased feed intake, but those fed *trans*-10, *cis*-12 CLA had reduced feed intake (Ryder et al., 2001). Accurately determining caloric intake can be difficult (especially in rodent experiments), but regardless, apparently, reduced feed intake does not explain a significant portion of CLA effects on lipid metabolism.

## *Lipogenesis*

CLA could influence lipid metabolism through the effects on the rates of lipogenesis because fat accretion in the growing animal is a balance between lipid synthesis (both de novo synthesis and preformed fatty acid incorporation) and lipid mobilization. Consistent with in vivo data, *trans*-10, *cis*-12 reduced intracellular triglyceride synthesis in HepG2 cells while *cis*-9, *trans*-11 CLA at similar concentrations had no effect (Yotsumoto et al., 1999). Reduced activities or expression of key lipogenic enzymes and thus decreased rates of de novo lipogenesis would logically be a major component of the decreased carcass fat accretion of animals fed a high-carbohydrate/low-fat diet supplemented with CLA; this may be the mechanism in growing pigs (Ostrowska et al., 1999). This is supported by evidence indicating dietary CLA dramatically reduced the adipose-tissue mRNA abundance of Fatty Acid Synthase (FAS), Acetyl-CoA Carboxylase (ACC), and Glucose Transporter 4 (GLUT4) in growing mice

(Tsuboyama-Kasaoka et al., 2000), and decreased glucose incorporation into fatty acids in adipose tissue (ex vivo) when mice were fed CLA for only 3 to 4 days (Xu et al., 2001). In contrast, CLA supplements neither reduced FAS activity in the cultures of 3T3-L1 adipocytes nor decreased FAS activity in omental- and backfat-adipose depots of pigs (Bee, 2000; Choi et al., 2000; Park et al., 1997), and had no effect on hepatic- and adipose-tissue expression of FAS and ACC in mice and rats fed CLA-supplemented diets (Azain et al., 2000). In addition, the use of deuterium oxide to evaluate the rates of lipogenesis indicated that the rates of de novo fatty acid synthesis were not altered in mice fed CLA (West et al., 1998); although mice in that study were fed a diet that was 40% fat, and thus the amount and contribution of de novo fatty acid synthesis to body- fat accretion would undoubtedly be minimal and of little importance.

CLAs also reduced the fat content of animals consuming a high-fat diet, thereby suggesting that the uptake of preformed fatty acids must be affected (West et al., 1998). This may be the result of the ability of *trans*-10, *cis*-12 CLA to reduce lipoprotein lipase (LPL) activity in adipose tissue as suggested by the in vivo studies with mice (DeLany & West, 2000; Park et al., 1999b) and the in vitro culture studies with 3T3-L1 adipocytes (Park et al., 1997). However, results are inconsistent because other studies found that dietary CLA had no effect on adipose tissue LPL activity in mice (Tsuboyama-Kasaoka et al., 2000), and it increased adipose-tissue LPL activity in rats (Buison et al., 2000) and in cultured pig adipose cells (Ding et al., 2000).

In contrast to the variation reported in adipose-tissue studies, consistently over 80% (on a molar basis) of the decrease in the yield of milk fatty acids observed when cows are supplemented with CLA are accounted for by reductions in de novo synthesized fatty acids (Baumgard et al., 2000, 2002). The altered milk fatty acid profile is corroborated by the reduced mammary ACC and FAS mRNA abundance in *trans*-10, *cis*-12 CLA-treated cows (Baumgard et al., 2002). In addition, *trans*-10, *cis*-12 CLA also reduces the mammary mRNA abundance of LPL, stearoyl-CoA desaturase (SCD), and diacylglycerol transferase, indicating that regulation occurs at multiple lipogenic steps (Baumgard et al., 2002; Sorensen et al., 2008). In addition, *trans*-10, *cis*-12 CLA reduces the activity of the SCD gene promoter, and this is mediated through a specific response element termed the "SCD transcriptional enhancer element" (STE; Keating et al., 2006). Therefore, reduced rates of lipogenesis appear to be a major point of regulation by which CLA inhibits milk-fat synthesis, but the inconsistencies in the adipose-focused literature are difficult to explain.

## *Lipolysis*

Lipolysis and fat mobilization are of interest because these are also potential mechanisms by which CLA could affect lipid metabolism. Circulating plasma nonesterified fatty acids (NEFA) concentrations are known to be highly correlated with rates of mobilization. In the case of growing animals, basal concentrations of plasma NEFA were slightly elevated in pigs and rats fed dietary CLA supplements (Azain et al., 2000; Ostrowska et al., 1999). However, most studies observed no changes or even reduced plasma NEFA levels, and this includes studies with pigs (Tagliaferro et al., 2000) and rats (Houseknecht et al., 1998; Rahman et al., 2001; Ryder et al., 2001; Yamasaki et al., 1999). Consistent with these reports, adipose tissue obtained from mice fed CLA had similar rates of lipolysis as controls (Xu et al., 2001).

Increasing adipose sensitivity to lipolytic agents could also partially explain the effects of CLA on body composition. For example, growing pigs fed a CLA supplement had an increased lipolytic response to a β-adrenergic challenge (Ostrowska et al., 1999), as did adipocytes obtained from rats fed CLA (Pariza et al., 1997). In addition, increased glycerol release from 3T3-L1 adipocytes in response to epinephrine was reported when cells were incubated with CLA (DeLany & West, 2000; Park et al., 1997). However, CLA had no effect on the NEFA response to a β-adrenergic challenge in mice (Xu et al., 2001). Consequently, apparently, increased adipose tissue breakdown may help explain a small portion of the CLA effect in a few specific models, but it is probably not CLAs' primary point of regulation in most models.

## Glucose Homeostasis

Altering the parameters associated with glucose homeostasis could contribute to the mechanism whereby CLA affects body-fat accretion. For example, a reduction in the pancreatic release of insulin or a decrease in the response of extrahepatic tissue to insulin could result in an alteration in glucose uptake and use for fat synthesis. In addition, insulin is a potent inhibitor of fatty acid mobilization from adipose tissue, and thus, reduced plasma concentrations of insulin may allow for increased lipolysis (see previous section). The results from studies on the effects of dietary CLA on insulin-related variables are conflicting. Dietary CLA decreased both plasma insulin and glucose concentrations in the Zucker Diabetic Fatty *fa/fa* rat and thus alleviated the symptoms of type II diabetes mellitus (Houseknecht et al., 1998). Subsequent work verified these effects and attributed them to the *trans*-10, *cis*-12 CLA isomer (Ryder et al., 2001). However, in other nondiabetic models, dietary CLA had no effect on plasma insulin concentrations in mice (West et al., 2000), rats (Azain et al., 2000; Buison et al., 2000; Rahman et al., 2001; Sisk et al., 2001), pigs (Ostrowska et al., 1999), and humans (Medina et al., 2000). In addition, increased blood-insulin levels and an increase in β-cell mass and number were reported by others (Clement et al., 2002; DeLany et al., 1999; Poirier et al., 2005). Likewise, plasma-glucose levels were reported to be unchanged in studies with mice (Clement et al., 2002; DeLany et al., 1999; West et al., 2000), pigs (Ostrowska et al., 1999; Stangl et al., 1999), and humans (Medina et al., 2000), while other studies report increased plasma glucose with CLA supplementation in mice (Tsuboyama-Kasaoka et al., 2000), rats (Buison et al., 2000; Stangl, 2000a, 2000b), and humans (Riserus & Vessby, 2001). In fact, some have postulated that dietary CLA causes insulin resistance because of the tendency of dietary CLA to increase insulin and glucose concentrations (Poirier et al., 2005; Riserus & Vessby, 2001; Tsuboyama-Kasaoka et al., 2000). Clearly, model and genotype differences exist in how CLA alters glucose homeostasis, and whether or not

CLA directly affects glucose parameters or indirectly via altering body composition is currently unknown.

## *Adipocyte Maturation*

Reducing pre-adipocyte proliferation and/or the differentiation and growth of adipocytes would offer a basis to explain the effects of CLA on body-fat accretion. Adding CLA inhibited differentiation and reduced proliferation in human 3T3-L1 and porcine preadipocyte cultures (Brodie et al., 1999; Evans et al., 2000; Fischer-Posovszky et al., 2007; Satory & Smith, 1999). The mechanism for these effects may involve apoptosis stimulation. Dietary CLA is shown to cause adipocyte apoptosis in in vivo studies with mice (Hargrave et al., 2002, 2004; Miner et al., 2001; Tsuboyama-Kasaoka et al., 2000) and in cultures of human and 3T3-L1 adipocytes (Evans et al., 2000; Fischer-Posovszky et al., 2007). Decreasing adipocyte proliferation and differentiation and increasing apoptosis would decrease the total number of adipocytes. However, recent studies demonstrated that dietary CLA had no effect on adipocyte hyperplasia but decreased adipocyte size (Azain et al., 2000; Evans et al., 2000; Sisk et al., 2001). Small adipocytes are more sensitive and responsive to insulin (Spiegelman, 1998), which may explain the effect of CLA on glucose homeostasis in diabetic models (see section on glucose homeostasis).

Decreased cellular differentiation and proliferation and increased apoptosis are clearly not involved in the mechanisms whereby CLA affects milk-fat synthesis because the yields of milk, milk protein, and milk lactose are unchanged (Baumgard et al., 2000; Perfield et al., 2004). Furthermore, these studies demonstrate that milk-fat yield is quickly rescued after the removal of exogenous CLA, indicating that mammary cells remain competent. However, a clear dose-dependent effect appears to exist on mammary epithelial-cell functionality as very large quantities of *trans*-10, *cis*-12 CLA in vivo markedly reduce milk yield (Bell & Kennelly, 2003). In addition, high levels (>35 $\mu$molar) of both *cis*-9, *trans*-11 and *trans*-10, *cis*-12 CLA induced mammary cell (Mac-T cells, in vitro) apoptosis (Keating et al., 2008).

The anti-carcinogenic effects of CLA were also (in-part) mediated through apoptosis. In breast cancer MCF-7 cells, CLA (a mixture of *trans*, *trans* CLA isomers) induced an expression of the pro-apoptotic Bax while pro-survival Bcl-2 was down-regulated (Islam et al., 2008; Seo et al., 2008). Additionally, the p53 tumor-suppressor protein was also up-regulated (Islam et al., 2008). The treatment of colon-cancer cell lines with a number of CLA isomers (*cis*-9, *cis*-11; *cis*-9, *trans*-11; *trans*-9, *trans*-11; *trans*-10, *cis*-12) demonstrated a dose- and time-dependent effect (of all isomers) for inducing apoptosis, and this was mediated through a down-regulation of Bcl-2 (Beppu et al., 2006).

## *Fatty Acid Oxidation*

Increased fat oxidation could also promote reductions in body fat when animals are fed CLA. Carnitine palmitoyltransferase-1 (CPT; carnitine acyltransferase) is responsible for transporting fatty acids into the mitochondria, and is considered to be the rate-limiting step in the β-oxidation of fatty acids. Dietary CLA supplements enhanced total CPT activity in the muscle of mice and rats (Park et al., 1997; Rahman et al., 2001), in the white and brown adipose tissue of mice and rats (Martin et al., 2000; Rahman et al., 2001), and in the hepatic tissue of rats (Rahman et al., 2001). An increased preference for fatty acids as fuel in CLA-treated animals is supported by the findings that mice, rats, and pigs fed CLA had lower respiratory quotients (RQ) at specific but variable times during the period of CLA feeding (Azain et al., 2000; Tagliaferro et al., 2000; West et al., 1998). In contrast, dietary CLA had no effect on the RQ in other studies with mice (West et al., 2000), dogs (Schoenherr & Jewell, 1999), pigs (Müller et al., 1999), and humans (Zambell et al., 2000). The increased basal metabolic rate and enhanced energy expenditure were hypothesized to explain CLA's effect on the body-fat content in mice (DeLany & West 2000; West et al., 2000), but no effect of CLA on energy expenditure in humans occurred (Wosje et al., 2001). Furthermore, CLA had no effect on heat production in mice or pigs (Miner et al., 2001; Müller et al., 1999) and no effect on plasma thyroxine and triiodothryonine in rats and pigs (Sisk et al., 2001; Stangl et al., 1999). However, a dietary supplement of CLA increased the mass of brown adipose tissue in rats, and this may explain the effects on thermogenesis that are sometimes observed (Ryder et al., 2001).

Rats fed dietary CLA had increased myocardial oxygen consumption even though cardiac β-oxidation rates were unchanged, suggesting an uncoupling between oxygen consumption and cardiac activity (Demaison et al., 1999). However, data are inconsistent with dietary CLA increasing the expression of uncoupling protein-2 in liver, skeletal muscle, and white adipose tissue in mice and rats (Ryder et al., 2001; Tsuboyama-Kasaoka et al., 2000), but having no effect on the expression of uncoupling proteins in skeletal muscle in another study (West et al., 2000). In addition to these apparent inconsistencies, Terpstra et al. (2002) pointed out that interpreting the effects of CLA on bioenergetics is difficult because the large differences in metabolic rate between species have not been considered.

## CLA and Protein Metabolism

CLA effects on lean tissue metabolism are equivocal. Increased body-protein content is often reported when animals are fed CLA: Park et al. (1997, 1999b), DeLany et al. (1999), and Stangl (2000a) reported significant increases in body protein. However, unlike body fat where substantial reductions occur in the percentage and amount of lipid, our calculations indicate that the mass of lean tissue is similar between control and CLA-treated animals. Thus, the increased body-protein percentage in these studies is mainly a consequence of the marked decrease in body fat rather than an actual increase in protein accretion. In agreement, CLA is ineffective at increasing the quantity of body protein in growing mice (West et al., 1998), growing bass (Twibell et al., 2000), growing rats (Azain et al., 2000), pigs (Mitchell & Pursel, 2001), and humans (Blankson et al., 2000; Wosje et al., 2001). However, a marginal increase in the amount of lean tissue was reported for CLA-treated growing mice (DeLany et al., 1999), growing pigs (Ostrowska et al., 1999), and aged mice (Baker et al., 2005).

The results of studies on lean mass in humans produced conflicting results, similar to those results for fat mass (Salas-Salvado et al., 2006; Tricon & Yaqoob, 2006). Although few human studies indicate an increase in lean mass with CLA supplementation (Gaullier et al., 2004; Kamphuis et al., 2003), the vast majority reports no effect of CLA (Kreider et al., 2002; Malpuech-Brugere et al., 2004; Riserus et al., 2002; Salas-Salvado et al., 2006; Whigham et al., 2004). Again, these inconsistencies in the literature are likely due to the differences in the CLA dose and the length of supplementation, the differences in the age, sex, and physical condition of the subjects, and the differences in how lean mass was measured. For a thorough evaluation of the effects of CLA supplementation in humans, see the review by Salas-Salvado et al. (2006).

Evaluating the CLA effects on actual rates of tissue accretion requires body-composition data prior to the initiation and at the termination of treatment. While rodent studies were not designed this way, such a study was conducted with growing pigs (Ostrowska et al., 1999). Pigs initially weighed 57 kg and were fed six different doses of CLA for 8 weeks. CLA resulted in a linear decrease in fat accretion over the dose range while rates of lean accretion were significantly increased, demonstrating a quadratic response curve with a CLA dose of 0.5% of the diet being most effective. Carcass lean is composed of protein and water, and characteristically a reduction in fat results in a corresponding increase in water. A consistent phenomenon that occurs with feeding CLA (particularly *trans*-10, *cis*-12) is an increase in carcass water (Ostrowska et al., 1999; Sanders et al., 2004). This may be a consequence of an increase in lean mass because muscle is composed of approximately 70% water. Due to the large concentration of water in muscle, a significant change in water content may be more easily detected before a change in protein mass (Sanders et al., 2004).

## CLA and Liver Enlargement

Several studies using rodent models indicate CLA, and specifically *trans*-10, *cis*-12 induces marked hepatomegaly (Baker et al., 2005; Clement et al., 2002; de Deckere et al., 1999; Terpstra, 2002; West et al., 1998), but others report no change in liver weight (Azain et al., 2000; Sanders et al., 2004; Stangl, 2000a). The CLA effect on hepatic lipid metabolism is clearly species-dependent as dietary CLA actually decreased liver weight in the obese and lean Zucker rats (Sisk et al., 2001) and fish (Twibell et al., 2000). In addition to liver size, hepatic lipid content often increases (Clement et al., 2002; Delany et al., 1999; Sanders et al., 2004; Tsuboyama-Kasaoka et al., 2000). The mechanism by which *trans*-10, *cis*-12 CLA mediates hepatocyte lipid filling is not clear, but a reduced, very low density lipoprotein export via decreasing apo B secretion was demonstrated (Yotsumoto et al., 1999). In addition, the CLA-induced increase in plasma insulin, which is sometimes observed (Belury, 2002), is thought to increase hepatic fat synthesis via up-regulating FAS and ACC, resulting in liver fat accumulation (Clement et al., 2002). However, this hypothesis is challenged as *trans*-10, *cis*-12 CLA-treated Zucker rats had reduced insulin levels (Henriksen et al., 2003) but enhanced liver lipid content (Sanders et al., 2004), thus suggesting that the increase in hepatic fat content is insulin-independent. Regardless of the mechanism, the effects of CLA on liver enlargement and lipid filling are two potential negative side effects that may limit CLA utilization as a weight-loss tool.

## Partitioning versus Repartitioning Agent

CLA is referred to as a repartitioning agent because of its effects on the metabolism of adipose and lean tissues (Dugan et al., 1997; Stangl, 2000a). The term "repartitioning" implies that one form of nutrient (i.e., fat) is mobilized to support the synthesis of a different nutrient class (i.e., protein). In this example, protein synthesis, which previously (by definition) must have been limited by energy availability, would now be supplied with the necessary fuel (because of the increased lipolysis) to meet its anabolic capacity. Numerous β-agonists fit this example and are referred to as repartitioning agents (NRC, 1994). Although reductions in body fat are generally observed in animals fed a dietary CLA supplement, most studies observed little or no increase in protein accretion, as previously discussed. Furthermore, fat accretion still occurs in CLA-treated animals, but the rate of accretion is reduced. Therefore, these data do not support the concept that CLA is a repartitioning agent.

In contrast, dietary CLA does alter nutrient partitioning as most clearly indicated by the reduction in the rates of fat accretion observed in the studies with pigs (Ostrowska et al., 1999) and mice (DeLany et al., 1999). Overall, studies on carcass composition demonstrate that CLA reduces fat deposition, but effects on protein accretion are minor, and the calculated increase in body-protein percentage of CLA-treated animals is predominately a consequence of the reduced quantity of body fat.

## The Mammary Gland as a Model to Study Lipid Metabolism

The lactating ruminant mammary gland synthesizes easily measurable quantities of both lipid and protein daily. Consequently, it offers a unique model to noninvasively study the acute and temporal changes of fat and protein synthesis. This is a distinct advantage to a growth model where several weeks are often necessary to quantify treatment differences in tissue accretion (Bauman et al., 2008). In addition, the size of the mammary gland allows for serial biopsies from the same animal for mechanistic-focused research. As mentioned previously, this model was validated when *trans*-10, *cis*-12 CLA was identified as a potent inhibitor of fat synthesis in the bovine mammary gland (Baumgard et al., 2000) similar to its ability to reduce fat synthesis in a rodent-growth model (Park et al., 1999a). Utilizing the mammary model has identified *trans*-9, *cis*-11 CLA and *cis*-10, *trans*-12 CLA as inhibitors of fat synthesis (Perfield et al., 2007; Saebo et al., 2005), and just as importantly, it also allowed for the ruling out of CLA isomers (*trans*-8, *cis*-10; *cis*-9, *trans*-11; *trans*-9, *trans*-11; *trans*-10, *trans*-12; *cis*-11, *trans*-13; Bauman et al., 2008) and *trans* monoene isomers (*trans*-10 18:1; Lock et al., 2007) that do not affect lipid synthesis. Logically, the aforementioned CLA and *trans* monoene isomers will similarly affect body-fat synthesis and accretion.

## Conclusion

The *trans* fatty acid family is large, and some isomers appear to have deleterious effects on health (i.e., elaidic acid), while others appear to have beneficial effects on health and body composition (i.e., *trans*-10, *cis*-12 CLA) in animal models. In a wide variety of experiments, *trans*-10, *cis*-12 CLA markedly reduces the fat content in animal models, but the effects vary; this probably, in large part, depends on dose. The mechanism by which CLA decreases body-fat accretion and mammary lipid synthesis is clearly multifaceted and includes numerous points of regulation. Nonetheless, results are exciting, and an opportunity may exist for CLA to be utilized as an important component of a human and pet weight-loss plan and as a nutrient partitioning agent in agriculturally important animals. Thus, despite the negative press associated with *trans* fatty acids and human health, CLA is an example of a fatty acid that is the exception rather than the rule, underlining the fact that all *trans* fatty acids are not created equal.

### References


Ahemed, M.L.; K. Ong; D. Morrel; L. Cox; N. Drayer; L. Perry; M.A. Preece; D.B. Dunger. Longitudinal study of leptin concentrations during puberty: sex differences and relationship to changes in body composition. *J. Clin. Endocrinol. Metab.* **1999,** *84,*899–905.

Akahoshi, A.; Y. Goto; K. Murao; T. Miyazaki; M. Yamasaki; M. Nonaka; K. Yamada; M. Sugano. Conjugated linoleic acid reduces body fats and cytokine levels of mice. *Biosci. Biotechnol. Biochem.* **2002,** 66, 916–920.

Al-Azemi, M.; F.E. Omu; A.E. Omu. The effect of obesity on the outcome of infertility management in women with polycystic ovary syndrome. *Arch. Gynecol. Obstet.* **2004,** *270,* 205–210.

Aro, A. The scientific basis for trans fatty acid regulations—Is it sufficient? A European perspective. *Atheroscler. Suppl.* **2006,** *7,* 67–68.

Atkinson, R. Conjugated linoleic acid for altering body composition and treating obesity. *Advances in Conjugated Linoleic Acid Research;* M.P. Yurawecz, M.M. Mossoba, J.K.G. Kramer, M.W. Pariza, G.J. Nelson, Eds.; AOCS Press: Champaign, IL, 1999; Vol. I, pp. 348–353.

Azain, M.J.; D.B. Hausman; M.B. Sisk; W.P. Flatt; D.E. Jewell. Dietary conjugated linoleic acid reduces rat adipose tissue cell size rather than cell number. *J. Nutr.* **2000,** *130,* 1548–1554.

Baker, S.H.; S.R. Sanders; S. Zibadi; R.R. Watson; L.H. Baumgard. Effects of conjugated linoleic acid (CLA) on whole animal body composition parameters in geriatric mice. *FASEB J.* **2005,** *19,* A45–46.

Bauman, D.E.; L.H. Baumgard; B.A. Corl; J.M. Griinari. Biosynthesis of CLA in ruminants. *Proc. Am. Soc. Anim. Sci.,* **2000**. Available at htpp://www.asas.org/jas/symposia/proceedings/0937.pdf.

Bauman, D.E.; J.M. Perfield; K.J. Harvatine; L.H. Baumgard. Regulation of fat synthesis by CLA:

Lactation and the ruminant model. *J. Nutr.* **2008,** *38,* 403–409.

Baumgard, L.H.; B.A. Corl; D.A. Dwyer; A. Saebo; D.E. Bauman. Identification of the conjugated linoleic acid isomer that inhibits milk fat synthesis. *Am. J. Physiol.* **2000,** *278,* R179–R184.

Baumgard, L.H.; E. Matitashvili; B.A. Corl; D.A. Dwyer; D.E. Bauman. *Trans*-10, *cis*-12 CLA decreases mRNA expression of key mammary lipogenic enzymes in lactating dairy cattle. *J. Dairy Sci.* **2002,** *85,* 2155–2163.

Bee, G. Dietary conjugated linoleic acid consumption during pregnancy and lactation influences growth and tissue composition in weaned pigs. *J. Nutr.* **2000,** *130,* 2981–2989.

Bell, J.A.; J.J. Kennelly. Short communication: Postruminal infusion of conjugated linoleic acid negatively impacts milk synthesis in Holstein cows. *J. Dairy Sci.* **2003,** ***86,*** 1321–1324.

Belury, M.A. Dietary conjugated linoleic acid in health: physiological effects and mechanisms of action. *Annu. Rev. Nutr.* **2002,** *22,* 505–531.

Belury, M.A.; A. Kempa-Steczko. Conjugated linoleic acid modulates hepatic lipid composition in mice. *Lipids* **1997,** *32,* 199–204.

Benito, P.; G. Nelson; D. Kelley; G. Bartolini; P. Schmidt; and V. Simon. The effect of conjugated linoleic acid on plasma lipoproteins and tissue fatty acid composition in humans. *Lipids* **2001,** *36,* 229–236.

Beppu, F.; M. Hosokawa; L. Tanaka; H. Kohno; T. Tanaka; K. Miyashita. Potent inhibitory effect of trans9, trans11 isomer of conjugated linoleic acid on the growth of human colon cancer cells. *J. Nutr. Biochem.* **2006,** *17,* 830–836.

Bernal-Santos, G.; J.W. Perfield II; T.R. Overton; D.E. Bauman. Production responses of dairy cows to dietary supplementation with conjugated linoleic acid (CLA) during the transition period and early lactation. *J. Dairy Sci.* 2003, *86,* 3218–3228.

Berven, G.; A. Bye; O. Hals; H. Blankson; H. Fagertun; E. Thom; J. Wadstein; O. Gudmundsen. Safety of conjugated linoleic acid (CLA) in overweight or obese human volunteers. *Eur. J. Lipid. Sci. Technol.* **2000,** *102,* 455–462.

Bhattacharya, A.; M. Rahman; D. Sun; R. Lawrence; W. Mejia; R. McCarter; M. O'Shea; G. Fernandes. The combination of dietary conjugated linoleic acid and treadmill exercise lowers gain in body fat mass and enhances lean body mass in high fat-fed male Balb/C mice. *J. Nutr.* **2005,** *135,* 1124–1130.

Biong, A.S.; M.B. Veierod; J. Ringstad; D.S. Thelle; J.I. Pedersen. Intake of milk fat, reflected in adipose tissue fatty acids and risk of myocardial infarction: a case-control study. *Eur. J. Clin. Nutr.* **2006,** *60,* 236–244.

Blankson, H.; J.A. Stakkestad; H. Fagertun; E. Thom; J. Wadstein; O. Gudmundsen. Conjugated linoleic acid reduces body fat mass in overweight and obese humans. *J. Nutr.* **2000,** *130,* 2943–2948.

Booker, C.S.; J.I. Mann. Trans fatty acids and cardiovascular health: translation of the evidence base. *Nutr. Metab. Cardiovasc. Dis.* **2008,** *18,* 448–456.

Brodie, A.E.; V.A. Manning; K.R. Ferguson; D.E. Jewell; C.Y. Hu. Conjugated linoleic acid inhibits differentiation of pre- and post- confluent 3T3-L1 preadipocytes but inhibits cell proliferation only in preconfluent cells. *J. Nutr.* **1999,** *129,* 602–626.

Buison A.; F. Ordiz, Jr.; M. Pellizzon; K.L.C. Jen. Conjugated linoleic acid does not impair fat regain but alters IGF-I levels in weight-reduced rats. *Nutr. Res.* **2000,** *20,* 1591–1601.

Campos. P.F. *The Obesity Myth: Why American's Obsession With Weight Is Hazardous To Your Health;* Gotham Books: New York, NY, 2004.

Chardigny, J.M.; F. Destaillats; C. Malpuech-Brugere; J. Moulin; D.E. Bauman; A.L. Lock; D.M. Barbano; R.P. Mensink; J.P. Bezelgues; P. Chaumont; et al. Do *trans* fatty acids from industrially produced sources and from natural sources have the same effect on cardiovascular disease risk factors in healthy subjects? Results of the trans Fatty Acids Collaboration (TRANSFACT) study. *Am. J. Clin. Nutr.* **2008,** *87,* 558– 566.

Chin, S.F.; J.M. Storkson; K.J. Albright; M.E. Cook; M.W. Pariza. Conjugated linoleic acid is a growth factor for rats as shown by enhance weight gain and improved feed efficiency. *J. Nutr.* **1994,** *124,* 2344–2349.

Choi, Y.J.; Y.C. Kim; Y.B. Han; Y. Park; M.W. Pariza; J.M. Ntambi. The *trans*-10, *cis*-12 isomer of conjugated linoleic acid down regulates stearoyl-CoA desaturase 1 gene expression in 3T3-L1 adipocytes. *J. Nutr.* **2000,** ***130,*** 1920–1924.

Clement, L.; H. Poirier; I. Niot; V. Bocher; M. Guerre-Millo; S. Krief; B. Staels; P. Besnard. Dietary trans-10,cis-12 conjugated linoleic acid induces hyperinsulinemia and fatty liver in the mouse. *J. Lipid Res.* **2002,** *43,* 1400–1409.

Corl, B.A.; L.H. Baumgard; D.A. Dwyer; J.M. Griinari; B.S. Phillips; D.E. Bauman. The role of $\Delta^9$-desaturase in the production of *cis*-9, *trans*-11 CLA. *J. Nutr. Biochem.* **2001,** *12,* 622–630.

Corl, B.A.; S.A. Matthews Oliver; X. Lin; W.T. Oliver; Y. Ma; R.J. Harrell; J. Odle. Conjugated linoleic acid reduced body fat accretion and lipogenic gene expression in neonatal pigs fed low- or high-fat formulas. *J. Nutr.* **2008,** *138,* 449–454.

de Deckere, E.A.M.; J.M.M. van Amelsvoort; G.P. McNeill; P. Jones. Effects of conjugated linoleic acid (CLA) isomers on lipid levels and peroxisome proliferation in the hamster. *Br. J. Nutr.* **1999,** *82,* 309–317.

DeLany, J.P.; F.Y. Blohm; A.A. Truett; J.A. Scimeca; D.B. West. Conjugated linoleic acid rapidly reduces body fat content in mice without affecting energy intake. *Am. J. Physiol.* **1999,** *276,* R1172–R1179.

DeLany, J.P.; D.B. West. Changes in body composition with conjugated linoleic acid. *J. Am. Coll. Nutr.* **2000,** *19,* 487S–493S.

Demaison, L.; S. Gregoire; P Juaneda; J.M. Chardigny; J.L. Sebedio. Dietary conjugated linoleic acid isomers and myocardial function. *Chem. Phys. Lipids* **1999,** *101,* 141 (abs.).

Ding, S.T.; R.L. McNeel; H.J. Mersmann. Conjugated linoleic acid increases the differentiation of porcine adipocytes in vitro. *Nutr. Res.* **2000,** *20,* 1569–1580.

Dugan, M.E.R.; J.L. Aalhus; A.L. Schaefer; J.K.G. Kramer. The effect of conjugated linoleic acid on fat to lean repartitioning and feed conversion in pigs. *Can. J. Anim. Sci.* **1997,** *77,* 723–725.

Eckel, R.H.; S. Borra; A.H. Lichtenstein; S.Y. Yin-Piazza. Understanding the complexity of the trans fatty acid reduction in the American diet. *Circulation* **2007,** *115,* 2231–2246.

Eggert, J.M.; M.A. Belury; A. Kempa-Steczko; S.E. Mills; A.P. Schinckel. Effects of conjugated linoleic acid on the belly firmness and fatty acid composition in genetically lean pigs. *J. Anim. Sci.* **2001,** *79,* 2866–2872.

Evans, M.; C. Geigerman; J. Cook; L. Curtis; B. Kuebler; M. McIntosh. Conjugated linoleic acid suppresses triglyceride accumulation and induces apoptosis in 3T3-L1 preadipocytes. *Lipids* **2000,** *35,* 899–910.

Faulconnier, Y.; M.A. Arnal; P. Patureau Mirand; J.M. Chardigny; Y. Chillard. Isomers of conjugated linoleic acid decrease plasma lipids and stimulate adipose tissue lipogenesis without changing adipose weight in post-prandial adult sedentary or trained Wistar rat. *J. Nutr. Biochem.* **2004,** *15,* 741–748.

Feldman, H.A.; I. Goldstein; D.G. Hatzichkristou; R.J. Krane; J.B. McKinley. Impotence and its medical and psychosocial correlates: results of the Massachusetts male aging study. *J. Urol.* **1994,** *151,* 54–61.

Fischer-Posovszky, P.; V. Kukulus; M.A. Zulet; K.M. Debatin; M. Wabitsch. Conjugated linoleic acids promote human fat cell apoptosis. *Horm. Metab. Res.* **2007,** *39,* 186–191.

Gaullier, J.; J. Halse; K. Hoye; K. Kristiansen; H. Fagertun; H. Vik; O. Gudmundsen. Conjugated linoleic acid supplementation for 1 y reduces body fat mass in healthy overweight humans. *J. Nutr.* **2004,** *79,* 1118–1125.

Gavino, V.C.; G. Gavino; M.J. Leblanc; B. Tuchweber. An isomeric mixture of conjugated linoleic acids but no pure *cis*-9, *trans*-11-octadecadienoic acid affects body weight gain and plasma lipids in hamsters. *J. Nutr.* **2000,** *130,* 27–29.

Gebauer, S.K.; T.L. Psota; P.M. Kris-Etherton. The diversity of health effects of individual trans fatty acid isomers. *Lipids* **2007,** *42,* 787–799.

German, J.B.; C.J. Dillard. Composition, Structure and Absorption of milk lipids: A source of energy, fat-soluble nutrients and bioactive molecules. *Crit. Rev. Food Sci. Nutr.* **2006,** *46,* 57–92.

Gudmunsen, G.; J. Wadstein; E. Thom. *Human Studies with CLA in Norway.* 1st International Conference on Conjugated Linoleic Acid (CLA); pp. 21; Alesund, Norway, June 10–13.

Hammoud, A.O.; N. Wilde; M. Gibson; A. Parks; D.T. Carrell; A.W. Meikle. 2008. Male obesity and alteration in sperm parameters. *Fert. Sterl. 90.*

Hargrave, K.M.; C. Li; B.J. Meyer; S.D. Kachman; D.L. Hartzell; M.A. Della-Fera; J.L. Miner; C.A. Baile. Adipose depletion and apoptosis induced by trans-10, cis-12 conjugated linoleic acid in mice. *Obes. Res.* **2002,** *10,* 1284–1290.

Hargrave, K.M.; B.J. Meyer; C. Li; M.J. Azain; C.A. Baile; J.L. Miner. Influence of dietary conjugated linoleic Acid and fat source on body fat and apoptosis in mice. *Obes. Res.* **2004,** *12,* 1435–1444.

Henriksen, E.J.; M.K. Teachey; Z.C. Taylor; S. Jacob; A. Ptock; K. Kramer; O. Hasselwander. Isomer-specific actions of conjugated linoleic acid on insulin action in the obese Zucker rat. *Am. J. Physiol. Endocrin. Metab.* **2003,** *285,* E98–E105.

Himes, J.H. Examining the evidence for recent secular changes in the timing of puberty in U.S. children in light of increases in the prevalence of obesity. *Mol. Cell. Endocrinol.* **2006,** *254–255* 12–13.

Hodgson, J.M.; N.C. Ward; V. Burke; L.J. Beilin; I.B. Puddy. Increased lean red meat intake does not elevate markers of oxidative stress and inflammation in humans. *J. Nutr.* **2007,** *137,* 363–367.

House, R.L.; J.P. Cassady; E.J. Eisen; M.K. McIntosh; J. Odle. Conjugated linoleic acid evokes de-lipidation through the regulation of genes controlling lipid metabolism in adipose and liver tissue. *Obes Rev.* **2005,** *6,* 247–258.

Houseknecht, K.L.; J.P. Vanden Heuvel; S.Y. Moya-Camarena; C.P. Portocarrero; L.W. Peck; K.P. Nickel; M.A. Belury. Dietary conjugated linoleic acid normalizes impaired glucose tolerance in the Zucker diabetic fatty *fa/fa* rat. *Biochem. Biophys. Res. Comm.* **1998,** *248,* 678–682.

Hunter, J.E. Alternatives to *trans* fatty acids in foods. *Inform* **2004,** *15,* 510–512.

Ip, M.M.; P.A. Masso-Welch; C. Ip. Prevention of mammary cancer with conjugated linoleic acid: role of the stroma and the epithelium. *J. Mammary Gland Biol. Neoplasia* **2003,** *8,* 103–118.

Islam, M.A.; Y.S. Kim; W.J. Jang; S.M. Lee; H.G. Kim; S.Y. Kim; J.O. Kim; Y.L. Ha. A mixture of trans, trans conjugated linoleic acid induces apoptosis in MCF-7 human breast cancer cells with reciprocal expression of Bax and Bcl-2. *J. Agric. Food Chem.* **2008,** *5614,* 5970–5976.

Iso, H.; T. Shimamoto; A. Kitamura; M. Iida; Y. Komachi. Trends of cardiovascular risk factors and diseases in Japan: Implications for primordial prevention. *Prevent. Med.* **1999,** *29,* S–02–S105.

Kamphuis, M.; M. Lejeune; W. Saris; M.S. Westertep-Plantega. The effect of conjugated linoleic acid supplementation after weight loss on body weight regain, body composition, and resting metabolic rate in overweight subject. *Int. J. Obes. Relat. Metabol. Disord.* **2003,** *25,* 1516–1521.

Kang, K.; M. Miyazaki; J.M. Ntambi; M.W. Pariza. Evidence that the anti-obesity effect of conjugated linoleic acid is independent of effects on stearoyl-CoA desaturase1 expression and enzyme activity. *Biochem. Biophys. Res. Comm.* **2004,** *315,* 532–537.

Kavanagh, K.; K.L. Jones; J. Sawyer; K. Kelley; J.J. Carr; J.D. Wagner; L.L Rudel. Trans fat induces abdominal obesity and changes in insulin sensitivity in monkeys. *Obesity.* **2007,** *15,* 1675–1684.

Kay, J.K.; T.R. Mackle; M.J. Auldist; N.A. Thomson; D.E. Bauman. Endogenous synthesis of cis-9, trans-11 conjugated linoleic acid in dairy cows fed fresh pasture. *J. Dairy Sci.* **2004,** *87,* 369–378.

Kay, J.K.; E.S. Kolver; N.A. Thomson; J.R. Roche; L.H. Baumgard. The effect of vitamin E supplementation on production and fatty acid profiles. *J. Dairy Res.***2005,** *72,* 322–332.

Keating, A.F.; F.Q. Zhao; K.A. Finucane; D.R. Glimm; J.J. Kennelly. Effect of conjugated linoleic acid on bovine mammary cell growth, apoptosis and Stearoyl Co-A desaturase gene expression. *Dom. Anim. Endocrinol.* **2008,** *34,* 284–292.

Keating, A.F.; F.Q. Zhao; J.J. Kennelly. Characterization and regulation of the bovine Stearoyl-CoA desaturase gene promoter. Biochem. *Biophys. Res. Comm.* **2006,** *344,* 233–240.

Kelley, D.S.; G.L. Bartolini; J.W. Newman; M. Vemuri; B.E. Mackey. Fatty acid composition of liver, adipose tissue, spleen, and heart of mice fed diets containing t10, c12-, and c9, t11-conjugated linoleic acid. *Prostaglandins Leukotrienes Essent. Fatty Acids* **2006,** *74,* 331–338.

Kelley, N.S.; N.E. Hubbard; K.L. Erickson. Conjugated linoleic acid isomers and cancer. *J. Nutr.* **2007,** *137,* 2599–2607.

Koh-Banerjee, P.; N.F. Chu; D. Spiegelman; B. Rosner; G. Colditz; W. Willet; E. Rimm. Prospective study of the association of changes in dietary intake, physical activity, alcohol consumption, and smoking with 9-y gain in waist circumference among 16587 US men. *Am. J. Clin. Nutr.* **2003,** *78,* 719–727.

Kreider, R.; M. Ferreira; M. Greenwood; M. Wilson; A. Almada. Effects of conjugated linoleic acid supplementation during resistance training on body composition, bone density, strength, and selected hematological markers. *J. Strength Cond. Res.* **2002,** *16,* 325–334.

Lee, K.W.; H.J. Lee; H.Y. Cho; Y.J. Kim. Role of the conjugated linoleic acid in the prevention of cancer. *Crit. Rev. Food Sci. Nutr.* **2005,** *45,* 135–144.

Liepa, G.U.; A. Sengupta; D. Karsies. Polycystic ovary syndrome (PCOS) and other androgen excess-related conditions: can changes in dietary intake make a difference? *Nutr. Clin. Pract.* **2008,** *23,* 63–71.

Lock, A.L.; C. Tyburczy; D.A. Dwyer; K.J. Harvatine; F. Destaillats; Z. Mouloungui; L. Candy; D.E. Bauman. Trans-10 octadecenoic acid does not reduce milk fat synthesis in dairy cows. *J. Nutr.* **2007,** *137,* 2559–2566.

Luccia, B.H.D.; T.C. Jenkins; M.E. Kunkel. Assessment of conjugated linoleic acid bioavailability in rats. *FASEB J.* **2001,** *15,* A987 (abs.).

Malpuech-Brugere, C.; W.P. Verboeket-van de Venne; R.P. Mensink; M.A. Arnal; B. Morio; M. Brandolini; A. Saebo; T.S. Lassel; J. Chardigny; et al. Effects of two conjugated linoleic acid isomers on body fat mass in overweight humans. *Obes. Res.* **2004,** *12,* 591–598.

Martin, J.G.; S. Gregoire; M.H. Siess; M. Genty; J.M. Chardigny; O. Berdeaux; P. Juaneda; J.L. Sebedio. Effects of conjugated linoleic acid isomers on lipid-metabolizing enzymes in male rats. *Lipids* **2000,** *35,* 91–98.

Martin, C.A.; M.C. Milinsk; J.V. Visentainer; M. Matsushita; N.E. De-Souza. Trans fatty acid-forming process in foods: A review. *An Acad. Bras. Cienc* **2007,** *79,* 343–350.

Masters, N.; M.A. McGuire; K.A. Beerman; N. Dasgupta; M.K. McGuire. Maternal supplementation with CLA decreases milk fat in humans. *Lipids* **2002,** *37,* 133–138.

Matsuba, K.; G. Gavino; B. Tuchweber; V. Gavino. Pure dietary cis-9, trans-11-octadecadienoic and an isomeric mixture of conjugated linoleic acids have different effects in hamsters. *FASEB J.* **2000,** *14,* A726. (abs.).

McGuire, M.A.; and M.K. McGuire. 2000. Conjugated linoleic acid (CLA): A ruminant fatty acid with beneficial effects on human health. Proceedings, American Society of Animal Science (1999) available at: http://www.asas.org/jas/symposia/proceedings/0938.pdf

Meadus, W.J.; R. MacInnis; M.E.R. Dugan. Prolonged dietary treatment with conjugated linoleic acid stimulates porcine muscle peroxisome proliferator activated receptor γ and glutamine-fructose aminotransferase gene expression *in vivo*. *J. Mol. Endocrinology***2002,** *28,* 79–86.

Medina, E.A.; W.F. Horn; N.L. Keim; P.J. Havel; P. Benito; D.S. Kelley; G.J. Nelson; K.L. Erickson. Conjugated linoleic acid supplementation in humans: effects on circulating leptin concentrations and appetite. *Lipids* **2000,** *35,* 783–788.

Mensink, R.P.; M.B. Katan. Effect of dietary trans fatty acids on high-density and low-density lipoprotein cholesterol levels in healthy subjects. *N. Engl. J. Med.* **1990,** *323,* 439–445.

Miner, J.L.; C.A. Cederberg; M.K. Nielson; X. Chen; C.A. Baile. Conjugated linoleic acid (CLA), body fat, and apoptosis. *Obes. Res.* **2001,** *9,* 129–134.

Mitchell, A.D.; V.G. Pursel. Effects of dietary conjugated linoleic acid on growth and body composition of control and IGF-I transgenic pigs. *FASEB J.* **2001,** *15,* A961 (abs.).

Mokdad, A.H.; E.S. Ford; B.A. Bowman; W.H. Dietz; F. Vinicor; V.S. Bales; J.S. Marks. Prevalence of obesity, diabetes and obesity-related health risk factors, 2001. *J. Am. Med. Assoc.* **2003,**

*289,* 76–79.

Moss, J. Labeling of trans fatty acid content in food, regulations and limits—The FDA view. *Atheroscler. Suppl.* **2006,** *7,* 57–59.

Motard-Belanger, A.; A Charest; G. Greinier; P. Paquin; Y. Chouinard; S. Lemieux; P. Couture; B. Lamarche. Study of the effect of trans fatty acids from ruminants on blood lipids and other risk factors for cardiovascular disease. *Am. J. Clin. Nutr.* **2008,** *87,* 515–516.

Müller, H.L.; G.S. Stangl; M. Kirchgessner. Energy balance of conjugated linoleic acid-treated pigs. *J. Anim. Physiol. Anim. Nutr.* **1999,** *81,* 150–156.

Must, A.; E.N. Naumova; S.M. Phillips; M. Blum; B. Dawson-Hughes; W.M.Rand. Childhood overweight and the maturational timing in the development of adult overweight and fatness: the Newton Girls Study and its follow-up. *Pediatrics* **2005,** *116,* 620–627.

Nakanishi, T.; D. Oikawa; T. Koutoku; H. Hirakawa; Y. Kido; T. Tachibana; M.Furuse. γ-Linoleic acid prevents conjugated linoleic acid-induced fatty liver in mice. *Nutrition* **2004,** *20,* 390–393.

NRC. *Metabolic Modifiers: Effects on the Nutrient Requirements of Food-Producing Animals;* National Academy Press: Washington, DC, 1994.

NRC. *Carcinogens and Anticarcinogens in the Human Diet.* National Academy Press: Washington, DC, 1996.

Oliver, E.J. *Fat Politics. The Real Story Behind America's Obesity Epidemic;* Oxford University Press: New York, NY, 2005.

Ostrowska, E.; M. Muralitharan; R.F. Cross; D.E. Bauman; F.R. Dunshea. Dietary conjugated linoleic acids increase lean tissue and decrease fat deposition in growing pigs. *J. Nutr.* **1999,** *129,* 2037–2042.

Ostrowska, E.; D. Suster; M. Muralitharan; R.F. Cross; B.J. Leury; D.E. Bauman; F.R. Dunshea. Conjugated linoleic acid decreases fat accretion in pigs: evaluation by dual-energy X-ray absorptiometry. *Br. J. Nutr.* **2003,** *89,* 219–229.

Pariza, M.; Y. Park; S. Kim; K. Sugimoto; K. Albright; W. Liu; J. Storkson; M.Cook. Mechanism of body fat reduction by conjugated linoleic acid. *FASEB J.* **1997,** *11,* A139 (abs.).

Pariza, M.W.; Y. Park; M.E. Cook. The biologically active isomers of conjugated linoleic acid. *Progr. Lipid Res.* **2001,** *40,* 283–298.

Park, Y.; K.J. Albright; W. Liu; J.M. Storkson; M.E. Cook; M.W. Pariza. Effect of conjugated linoleic acid on body composition in mice. *Lipids* **1997,** *32,* 853–858.

Park, Y.; K.J. Albright; J.M. Storkson; W. Liu; M. Cook; M.W. Pariza. Changes in body composition in mice during feeding and with drawl of conjugated linoleic acid. *Lipids* **1999a,** *34,* 243–248.

Park, Y.; J.M. Storkson; K.J. Albright; W. Liu; M.W. Pariza. Evidence that the *trans*-10, *cis*-12 isomer of conjugated linoleic acid induces body composition changes in mice. *Lipids* **1999b,** *34,* 235–241.

Pauli, E.M.; R.S. Legro; L.M. Demers; A.R. Kunselman; W.C. Dodson; P.A. Lee.Diminished paternity and gonadal function with increasing obesity in men. *Fertil. Steril.* 2008. (in press)

Perfield, II, J.W.; G. Bernal-Santos; T.R. Overton; D.E. Bauman. Effects of dietary supplementation of rumen-protected conjugated linoleic acid in dairy cows during established lactation. *J.*

*Dairy Sci.* 2002, *85,* 2609–2617.

Perfield, J.W., II; P. Delmonte; A.L. Lock; M.P. Yurawecz; D.E. Bauman. Trans-10, trans-12 conjugated linoleic acid does not affect milk fat yield but reduces delta-9-desaturase index in dairy cows. *J. Dairy Sci.* **2006,** *89,* 2559–2566.

Perfield, J.W., II; A.L. Lock; J.M. Griinari; A. Saebo; P. Delmonte; D.A. Dwyer; D.E. Bauman. *Trans*-9, *cis*-11 conjugated linoleic acid reduces milk fat synthesis in lactating dairy cows. *J. Dairy Sci.* **2007,** *90,* 2211–2218.

Perfield J.W., II; A. Saebo; D.E. Bauman. Use of conjugated linoleic acid (CLA) enrichments to examine the effects of *trans*-8, *cis*-10 CLA, and *cis*-11, *trans*-13 CLA on milk-fat synthesis. *J. Dairy Sci.* **2004,** *87,* 1196–1202.

Perrini, S.; L. Laviola; A. Cignarelli; M. Melchiorre; F. De Stefano; C. Caccioppoli; A. Natalicchio; M.R. Orlando; G. Garruti; M. De Fazio; G. Catalano; V. Memeo; R. Giorgino; F. Giorgino. Fat depot-related differences in gene expression, adiponectin secretion, and insulin action and signaling in human adipocytes differentiated in vitro from precursor stromal cells. *Dibetologia* **2008,** *51,* 155–164.

Pettigrew, R.; D. Hamilton-Fairley. Obesity and female reproductive function. *Brit. Medical Bull.* **1997,** *53,* 341–358.

Poirier, H.; I. Niot; L. Clement; M. Guerre-Millo; P. Besnard. Development of conjugated linoleic acid (CLA)-mediated lipoatrophic syndrome in the mouse. *Biochimie* **2005,** *87,* 73–79.

Rahman, M.M.; A. Bhattacharya; J. Banu; G. Fernandes. Conjugated linoleic acid protects against age-associated bone loss in C57BL/6 female mice. *J. Nutr. Biochem.* **2007,** *18,* :467–474.

Rahman, S.M.; Y.M. Wang; H. Yotsumoto; J.Y. Cha; S.Y. Han; S. Inoue; T. Yanagita. Effects of conjugated linoleic acid on serum leptin concentration, body-fat accumulation, and β-oxidation of fatty acid in OLETF rats. *Nutrition* **2001,** *17,* 385–390.

Riserus, U.; P. Arner; K. Brismar; B. Vessby. Treatment with dietary *trans*-10 *cis*-12 conjugated linoleic acid causes isomer specific insulin resistance in obese men with the metabolic syndrome. *Diabetes Care* **2002,** *25,* 840–847.

Riserus, U.; B. Vessby. 2001. Diverging effect of CLA isomers on insulin resistance and lipid metabolism in obese men with the metabolic syndrome. 1st International Conference on Conjugated Linoleic Acid (CLA); pp. 20. Alesund, Norway, June 10–13.

Rosenberg, T.J.; S. Garbers; W. Chavkin; M.A. Chiasson. Prepregnancy weight and adverse perinatal outcomes in an ethnically diverse population *Obstet. Gynecol.* **2003,** *102,* 1022–1027.

Ryder, J.W.; C.P. Portocarrero; X.M. Song; L. Cui; M. Yu; T. Combatsiaris; D. Galuska; D.E. Bauman; D.M. Barbano; M.J. Charron; J.R. Zierath; K.L. Houseknecht. Isomer-specific antidiabetic properties of conjugated linoleic acid. *Diabetes* **2001,** *50,* 1149–1157.

Saebo, A.; P.C. Saebo; J.M. Griinari; K.J. Shingfield. Effect of abomasal infusions of geometric isomers of 10,12 conjugated linoleic acid on milk fat synthesis in dairy cows. *Lipids* **2005,** *40,* 823–832.

Sakono, M.; F. Miyanaga; S. Kawahara; K. Yamauchi; N. Fukuda; K. Watanabe; T. Iwata; M. Sugano. Dietary conjugated linoleic acid reciprocally modifies ketogenesis and lipid secretion by the rat liver. *Lipids* **1999,** *34* 997–1000.

Salas-Salvado, J.; F. Marquez-Sandoval; M. Bullo. Conjugated linoleic acid intake in humans: A systematic review focusing on its effect on body composition, glucose and lipid metabolism. *Crit. Rev. Food Sci. Nutr.* **2006,** *46,* 479–488.

Sanders, S.R.; M.K. Teachey; A. Ptock; K. Kraemer; O. Hasselwander; E.J. Henriksen; L.H. Baumgard. Effects of specific conjugated linoleic acid (CLA) isomers on growth characteristics in obese Zucker rats. *Lipids* **2004,** *39,* 537–543.

Satory, D.L.; S.B. Smith. Conjugated linoleic acid inhibits proliferation but stimulates lipid filling of murine 3T3-L1 preadipocytes. *J. Nutr.* **1999,** *129,* 92–97.

Schoenherr, W.; D. Jewell. Effect of conjugated linoleic acid on body composition of mature obese beagles. *FASEB J.* **1999,** *13,* A262 (abs.).

Seo, J.H.; H.S. Moon; I.Y. Kim; D.D. Guo; H.G. Lee; Y.J. Choi; C.S. Cho. PEGylated conjugated linoleic acid stimulation of apoptosis via a p53-mediated pathway in MCF-7 breast cancer cells. *Eur. J. Pharm. Biopharm.* **2008.** (in press)

Sisk, M.B.; D.B. Hausman; R.J. Martin; M.J. Azain. Dietary conjugated linoleic acid reduces adiposity in lean but not obese Zucker rats. *J. Nutr.* **2001,** *131,* 1668–1678.

Sjogren, P.; M. Rosell; C. Skoglund-Anderson; S. Zdravkovic; B. Vessby; U. De Faire; A. Hamsten; M.L. Hellenius; R.M. Fisher. Milk-derived fatty acids are associated with a more favorable LDL particle size distribution in healthy men. *J. Nutr.* **2004,** *134,* 1729–1735.

Smedman, A.; B. Vessby. 2001. Conjugated linoleic acid (CLA) supplementation in humans—effects on anthropometric variables and lipid metabolism. 1st International Conference on Conjugated Linoleic Acid (CLA); pp. 60. Alesund, Norway, June 10–13.

Smith, S.C.; L.T. Clark; R.S. Cooper; S.R. Daniels; S.K. Kumanyika; E. Ofili. Discovering the full spectrum of cardiovascular disease. *Minority Health Summit 2003: Report of the Obesity, Metabolic Syndrome, and Hypertension Writing Group, Circulation, E134–E139.*

Sommerfeld, M. Trans unsaturated fatty acids in natural products and processed foods. *Prog. Lipid Res.* **1983,** *22,* 221–233.

Sørensen, B.M.; E.C. Kazala; G.K. Murdoch; A.F. Keating; C. Cruz-Hernandez; J. Wegner; J.J. Kennelly; E.K. Okine; R.J. Weselake. Effect of CLA on diacylglycerol acyltranferase expression and activity in bovine mammary gland. *Lipids* **2008.** (in press)

Spiegelman, B. PPAR-γ: Adipogenic regulator and thiazolidinedione receptor. Diabetes **1998,** *47,* 507–514.

Stangl, G.I. 2000a. Conjugated linoleic acids exhibit a strong fat-to-lean partitioning effect, reduce serum VLDL lipids and redistribute tissue lipids in food-restricted rats. *J. Nutrition* **2000a,** *130,* 1140–1146.

Stangl, G.I. High dietary levels of a conjugated linoleic acid mixture alter hepatic glycerophospholipid class profile and cholesterol-carrying serum lipoproteins of rats. *J. Nutr. Biochem.* **2000b,** *11,* 184–191.

Stangl, G.I.; H. Müller; M. Kirchgessner. Conjugated linoleic acid effects on circulating hormones, metabolites and lipoproteins, and its proportion in fasting serum and erythrocyte membranes of swine. *Eur. J. Nutr.* **1999,** *38,* 271–277.

Sullivan, P.W.; E.H. Morrato; V. Ghushchyan; H.R. Wyatt; J.O. Hill. Obesity, inactivity, and the prevalence of diabetes and diabetes-related cardiovascular comorbidities in the U.S., 2000–2002. *Diabetes Care* **2005,** *28,* 15999–15603.

Sundram, K.; A. Ismail; K.C. Hayes; R. Jeyamalar; R. Pathmanathan. Trans-elaidic fatty acids adversely affect the lipoprotein profile relative to specific saturated fatty acids in humans. *J. Nutr.* **1997,** *127,* 514S–520S.

Tagliaferro, A.R.; A. Rivera; A. Ronan; J. Allen. Dietary conjugated linoleic acid promotes greater utilization of lipids for energy in miniature swine. *FASEB J.* **2000,** *14,* A565 (abs.).

Terpstra, A.H.M.; A.C. Beynen; H. Everts; S. Kocsis; M.B. Katan; P.L. Zock. The decrease in body fat in mice fed conjugated linoleic acid is due to increases in energy expenditure and energy loss in the excreta. *J. Nutr.* **2002,** *132,* 940–945.

Theil-Cooper, R.L.; F.C. Parish, Jr.; J.C. Sparks; B.R. Weigand; R.C. Ewan. Conjugated linoleic acid changes swine performance and carcass. *J. Anim. Sci.* **2001,** *79,* 1821–1828.

Tholstrup, T. Dairy products and cardiovascular disease. *Curr. Opin. Lipodol.* **2006,** *17,* 1–10.

Thom, E.; J. Wadstein; O. Gudmundsen. Conjugated linoleic acid reduces body fat in healthy exercising humans. *J. Ent. Med. Res.* **2001,** *29,* 392–396.

Tricon, S.; P. Yaqoob. Conjugated linoleic acid and human health: a critical evaluation of the evidence. *Curr. Opin. Clin. Nutr. Metab. Care* **2006,** *9,* 105–110.

Tsuboyama-Kasaoka, N.; M. Takahashi; K. Tanemura; H.J. Kim; T. Tange; H. Okuyama; M. Kasai; S. Ikemoto; O. Ezaki. Conjugated linoleic acid supplementation reduces adipose by apoptosis and develops lipodystrophy in mice. *Diabetes* **2000,** *49,* 1534–1542.

Twibell, R.G.; B.A. Watkins; L. Rogers; P.B. Brown. Effects of dietary conjugated linoleic acids on hepatic and muscle lipids in hybrid striped bass. *Lipids* **2000,** *35,* 155–161.

Waijers, P.M.; M.C. Ocke; C.T. van Rossum; P.H. Peeters; C. Bamia; Y. Chloptsios; Y.T. van der Schouw; N. Slimani; H.B Bueno-de-Mesquita. Dietary patterns and survival in older Dutch women. *Am. J. Clin. Nutr.* **2006,** *83,* 1170–1176.

Wang, Y.; J. Lu; M.R. Ruth; S.D. Goruk; M.J. Reaney; D.R. Glimm; D.F. Vine; C.J. Field; S.D. Proctor. Trans-11 vaccenic acid dietary supplementation induces hypolipidemic effects in an animal model of dyslipidemia and the metabolic syndrome. *J. Nutr.* **2008.** (in press)

West, D.B.; F.Y. Blohm; A.A. Truett; J.P. DeLany. Conjugated linoleic acid persistently increases total energy expenditure in AKR/J mice without increasing uncoupling protein gene expression. *J. Nutr.* **2000,** *130,* 2471–2477.

West, D.B.; J.P. DeLany; P.M. Camet; F. Blohm; A.A. Truett; J. Scimeca. Effects of conjugated linoleic acid on body fat and energy metabolism in the mouse. *Am. J. Physiol.* **1998,** *275,* R–67–R672.

Whigham, L.D.; M. O'Shea; I.C. Mohede; H.P. Walaski; R.L. Atkinson. Safety profile of conjugated linoleic acid in a 12-month trial in obese humans. *Food Chem. Toxicol.* **2004,** *42,* 1701–1709.

Whigham, L.D.; A.C. Watras; D.A. Schoeller. Efficacy of conjugated linoleic acid for reducing fat mass: a meta-analysis in humans. *Am. J. Clin. Nutr.* **2007,** *85,* 1203–1211.

Willet, W.C. The scientific basis for TFA regulations-Is it sufficient? Comments from the USA. *Atheroscler. Suppl.* **2006,** *7,* 69–71.

Wosje, K.S.; V.L. Englert; B.R. Mair; B.L. Specker. No benefit of CLA supplementation on body composition in overweight females. *FASEB J.* **2001,** *15,* A252. (abs.).

Xu, X.; J. Storkson; M. Pariza. Effects of conjugated linoleic acid on lipid metabolism in mouse adipose tissue. *FASEB J.* **2001,** *15,* A997. (abs.).

Yamasaki, M.; K. Mansho; H. Mishima; M. Kasai; M. Sugano; H. Tachibana; K. Yamada. Dietary effect of conjugated linoleic acid on lipid levels in white adipose tissue of sprague-dawley rats. *Biosci. Biotechnol. Biochem.* **1999,** *63,* 110–1106.

Yotsumoto, H.; E. Hara; S. Naka; R.O. Adlof; E.A. Emken; T. Yanagita. 10*trans,* 12*cis*-linoleic acid reduces apolipoprotein B secretion in HepG2 cells. *Food Res. Internat.* **1999,** *31,* 403–409.

Zambell, K.L.; N.L. Keim; M.D. Van Loan; B. Gale; P. Benito; D.S. Kelley; G.J. Nelson. Conjugated linoleic acid supplementation in humans: effects on body composition and energy expenditure. *Lipids* **2000,** *35,* 777–782.

# 13

# *Trans* and Other Fatty Acids: Role in Diabetic Disease and Health

**Andrew Odegaard**

*Department of Epidemiology and Community Health, School of Public Health, University of Minnesota, 1300 S. 2nd St. suite 300, Minneapolis, MN 55454*

## Introduction

The focus of this chapter is a summary and review of the peer-reviewed scientific literature pertaining to *trans* fatty acids (TFAs) and their potential role in insulin resistance and type 2 diabetes. Additionally, this chapter aims to touch on other fatty acids such as conjugated linoleic acid (CLA), omega-3 fatty acids, and the omega-6/omega-3 fatty acid ratio and their potential roles in insulin/glucose metabolism and type 2 diabetes. A brief overview of the epidemiology and pathophysiology of type 2 diabetes and insulin resistance is presented. The chapter proceeds with a detailed section on TFAs, and is followed by shorter descriptions and a review of the other aforementioned fatty acids.

## Overview of Type 2 Diabetes and Insulin Resistance

Type 2 diabetes accounts for 90–95% of prevalent cases of diabetes (ADA, 2004). The disease is characterized by insulin resistance and relative insulin deficiency due to impaired pancreas ß-cell function (ADA, 2004; DeFronzo, 2004; Wild et al., 2004). The prevalence of the disease was estimated at 171 million people worldwide in the year 2000 (Wild et al., 2004), and appears to be increasing due to population growth, aging, urbanization, the increasing prevalence of obesity, and physical inactivity (Narayan et al., 2003; Wild et al., 2004). The number of people with type 2 diabetes is projected to rise to 366 million in 2030 (Wild et al., 2004). For this reason, type 2 diabetes is considered to be a pandemic of the twenty-first century. The estimated lifetime risks of developing type 2 diabetes for individuals born in the United States in the year 2000 are estimated at 1 in 3 for males and 2 in 5 for females (Narayan et al., 2003). The costs of the epidemic are felt both in the loss of the quality of life and the number of deaths (Engelgau et al., 2004). Medical costs in the management of diabetes and its complications in micro- and macrovascular diseases such as cardiovascular disease, renal failure, amputation, and blindness pose an enormous strain on health-care systems (Engelgau et al., 2004).

Insulin resistance is central to the pathogenesis of type 2 diabetes and helps maintain the diabetic state (DeFronzo, 2004). Insulin resistance precedes the development of diabetes and increases the risk of future diabetes (DeFronzo, 2004). Insulin resistance is associated with multiple clinical and anthropometric traits such as obesity, hypertension, dyslipidemia, glucose intolerance, high triglycerides, and low high-density lipoprotein (HDL) cholesterol, among other related traits (Haffner & Taegtmeyer, 2003; Reaven, 1994). However, the underlying pathophysiology of this constellation of risk factors remains unclear in relationship to insulin resistance and obesity. Insulin resistance is the underlying abnormality in most people who develop type 2 diabetes (DeFronzo, 2004). Insulin resistance appears to stem from interactions between environmental factors such as obesity (especially central of visceral body fat), physical inactivity, dietary attributes, and many poorly understood genetic factors (DeFronzo, 2004; Haffner & Taegtmeyer, 2003). As compensation for insulin resistance, ß cells of the pancreas increase insulin secretion to maintain normal blood-glucose levels (DeFronzo, 2004). If the compensatory insulin secretion is insufficient, blood-glucose concentration increases in the fasting [impaired fasting glucose (IFG)] and postprandial state [impaired glucose tolerance (IGT)]. Individuals with IFG and/or IGT are at high risk for proceeding to type 2 diabetes, although diabetes may not be inevitable in this group (DeFronzo, 2004).

Irreversible risk factors for type 2 diabetes, because of their strong associations with insulin resistance and/or β-cell function, include age, race/ethnicity, family history, many genetic factors, and possibly gender (higher in women) (DeFronzo, 2004; Steyn et al., 2004). Modifiable risk factors for the disease include obesity, physical inactivity, numerous dietary components, and cigarette smoking (Steyn et al., 2004; Willi et al., 2007). Independent of high-energy intake, which may lead to obesity, the composition of the diet, from overall dietary patterns (e.g., Western versus vegetarian) to specific macro- and micronutrients (e.g., magnesium), has received a great deal of research investigation with respect to diabetes risk.

Much is now understood from a wealth of clinical studies on the role of saturated fatty acids (SFAs), monounsaturated fatty acids (MUFAs), and certain polyunsaturated acids (PUFAs) in modulating insulin sensitivity. However, much less is known on the developing topics of the possible effects of dietary TFAs, CLAs, omega-3 fatty acids, and if the ratio of omega-6/omega-3 fatty acids has any role in insulin resistance and type 2 diabetes. Generally, dietary fatty acids appear to be involved in diabetes pathophysiology through their incorporation into structural lipids in skeletal muscle and adipose tissue that may lead to the altered function of insulin receptors (Ibrahim et al., 2005; Lichtenstein & Schwab, 2000; Natarajan & Ibrahim, 2005).

## ***Trans*** **Fatty Acids**

TFAs come from two major sources—industrial production (partial hydrogenation) and from ruminant animals. Industrial TFAs are produced artificially by heating liquid vegetable oils in the presence of metal catalysts and hydrogen (Ascherio et al., 1999). The partial hydrogenation causes the carbon atoms to bond in a straight configuration and remain in a solid state at room temperature (Ascherio et al., 1999). TFAs are produced in large quantities industrially to harden margarine, to turn vegetable oils into shortening, to lengthen shelf life by replacing fatty acids that would oxidize more quickly, and to give a certain "mouth feel" or flavor to deep-fried foods or other processed foods with added fats (Ascherio et al., 1999; Mensink & Katan, 1990). TFAs are primarily consumed in bakery products, fast and fried foods, packaged snacks, and margarines. The main TFA isomers from industrial sources, which make up approximately more than 90% of TFA consumption (Gebauer et al., 2007), include elaidic acid (C18:1Δ9*t*) and linolelaidic acid (C18:2-*t*9*t*12).

Metabolic studies show that the effects of industrial TFAs on risk factors for cardiovascular disease may be more detrimental than the effects of SFAs. Whereas SFAs are known to increase low-density lipoprotein (LDL) cholesterol, with little or no effect on HDL-cholesterol and triglycerides, TFAs appear to increase LDL-cholesterol similarly or perhaps more so than SFAs (Ascherio et al., 1999; Mensink & Katan, 1990; Lichtenstein et al., 1999). Additionally, TFAs decrease HDL-cholesterol and possibly increase triglycerides as supported by both controlled feeding studies as well as by large-scale epidemiological studies (Ascherio et al., 1999; Lichtenstein et al., 1999; Mensink & Katan 1990, 1992). Therefore, gram for gram, TFAs may increase the risk of cardiovascular disease more so than SFAs. As such, the replacement of TFAs with unhydrogenated oils in the U.S. diet was estimated to prevent 100,000 coronary deaths each year (Ascherio et al., 1999). More recently, TFAs were found to be associated with systemic inflammation as reflected by higher tumor necrosis factor-α (TNF-α) receptor concentrations (Mozaffarian et al., 2004) and higher interleukin-6 (IL-6) and C-reactive protein (CRP) concentrations in women (Mozaffarian et al., 2004).

In light of this recent research on the adverse effects of TFAs, legislative initiatives to reduce TFAs in the food supply were put forth by multiple countries spread across the globe as well as major cities in the United States (EURODIET, 2000; Lichtenstein et al., 2006; WHO/FAO, 2003). Additionally, numerous expert committees have put forth statements about keeping TFA-consumption levels as low as possible (USDA-HHS, 2005; Lichtenstein et al., 2006). Furthermore, in the United States, labeling regulations have been in effect since January 1, 2006, so consumers are able to make more informed decisions (DHHS/FDA, 2003). However, a gray area in the labeling is that TFA content greater than or equal to 0.5 g per serving must be listed, and anything less, but not necessarily 0 g, may be listed as 0 g.

## Trans *Fatty Acids, Insulin Resistance, and Type 2 Diabetes*

TFAs may reduce insulin sensitivity through their effects on increasing the concentrations of IL-6, TNF-α, and prostaglandins (Prentice, 2001). Although the precise biochemical mechanisms that may link dietary TFAs to insulin resistance and glucose homeostasis need further study several biologically plausible pathways are available to support the hypothesis that high intakes of dietary TFAs increase the risk of type 2 diabetes. The following subsections highlight the research related to TFAs, insulin resistance, and diabetes, and include animal, clinical, and population studies.

## Animal Studies

Animal studies are important in delineating the potential biological mechanisms to disease etiology in humans. Axen et al. (2003) examined the effects of high-TFA intake on the development of the metabolic syndrome in rats. Lean rats fed a high-fat diet for 9 weeks [60% of fat, 15% of carbohydrate (CHO), and 25% of protein] with 17% of the total energy coming from TFAs showed impaired glucose tolerance and insulin resistance compared to lean rats fed a low-fat diet (12% of fat, 60% of CHO, 28% of protein, and no TFAs) (Axen et al., 2003). The TFA group also had increased visceral fat mass and elevated liver-lipid content in the rats (Axen et al., 2003).

Alstrup et al. (1999) examined the impact of *cis* and TFAs on insulin release and glucose oxidation in isolated mouse islets. Both elicited a dose- dependent increase in glucose-stimulated (16.7 mmol/L) insulin secretion during static islet incubations; however, the TFAs produced a significantly higher insulin output (Alstrup et al., 1999). Also, *cis*fatty acids significantly inhibited glucose oxidation at 16.7 mmol/L when compared to TFAs (Alstrup et al., 1999). Investigators hypothesized that the differential effect on glucose oxidation was responsible for the differential effect on insulin action. The study concluded that fatty acid spatial configuration modulates glucose oxidation and insulin secretion in mouse ß cells.

Ibrahim and colleagues (2005) investigated the effects of replacing 2% of energy from SFAs and 1% from MUFAs with TFAs (3% energy) on adipocyte plasma-membrane fatty acid composition, fluidity, and insulin action in rats. They found a significant increase in fasting insulin levels and triglycerides on the SFA and TFA diets compared to the control (Ibrahim et al., 2005). Additionally, TFAs produced nearly 17% higher fasting-insulin levels than SFAs (Ibrahim, et al. 2005). TFAs also significantly lowered HDL-cholesterol, and decreased membrane fluidity compared to the control group (Ibrahim et al., 2005).

Natarajan & Ibrahim, 2005 examined the effect of TFAs as compared to SFAs on diaphragm phospholipid fatty acid composition, intramyocellular triacylglycerol content, and insulin-stimulated glucose uptake in a study of male WNIN rats. Compared to rats fed 10% of their energy from SFAs for three months, those on the 10% TFA diet experienced increased intramyocellular triacylglycerols, decreased long-chain PUFAs in phospholipids, and significantly decreased (approximately 30%) insulin-stimulated glucose transport (Natarajan & Ibrahim, 2005).

Kavanagh et al. (2007) looked at the effects of two isocaloric, equivalent diets: one supplemented with 8% of energy from MUFAs and one with 8% of energy from TFAs for six years in monkeys. The TFA-fed monkeys gained significantly more weight, intra-abdominal fat, and had elevated postprandial hyperinsulinemia compared to the control group. This is the first long-term controlled look at TFAs that shows a direct association with risk factors for type 2 diabetes as well as insulin resistance.

Hypothesis-driven animal models such as these are important in supporting a theory to the mechanism of TFAs on insulin resistance and the development of type 2 diabetes.

## *Epidemiological Studies*

Relative to animal studies, observational studies have provided mixed conclusions on the topic. Lovejoy and colleagues (2002) examined the association between self-reported dietary intake, fatty acid composition and insulin resistance, and glucose metabolism in a small cross-sectional study. Subjects were 38 adults, 19 male and 19 female, with a range of ages, body mass index (BMI), and glucose tolerance (5 with type 2 diabetes). All participants completed a three-day diet record after a session with a dietitian. The analysis of the TFA content of foods was computed by using three different nutrient databases. Fasting and two-hour oral glucose-tolerance tests were used to assess insulin and glucose metabolism in the study. Multiple linear regression models were used to examine the independent associations between the various energy-adjusted dietary fatty acids and the insulin-resistance parameters. Dietary TFAs were not significantly associated with the markers of insulin resistance. Consistent with other studies, SFAs were positively associated with fasting (or postprandial) insulin concentrations ($r = 0.44$, $P < 0.01$). In addition, MUFA was found to have positive associations with concentrations of insulin and glucose. Results for glucose concentrations were similar. The cross-sectional design of this study precludes any conclusions about causation. Also, self-reported data on food habits are prone to a great deal of measurement error, including both nondifferential misclassifications as well as certain systematic biases as an underestimation of total intake (Willett, 1998). Obese individuals appear to be more prone to underreporting diet, and this population is, of course, more insulin-resistant than leaner groups (Willett, 1998). Possibly, TFA, which comprises much less energy in the typical diet as compared to SFA and MUFA fat, may have been particularly poorly measured in this study.

Salmeron and colleagues (2001) investigated dietary-fat intake and the risk of type 2 diabetes in the Nurses' Health Study. The intake of energy-adjusted TFAs was positively associated with type 2 diabetes, with an adjustment for age and BMI. This association became stronger upon further adjustment for other types of dietary fat. A 2% increase in energy consumption from TFAs was associated with a 39% increase in risk (Relative Risk (RR) =1.39, 95% CI; 1.15, 1.67) of type 2 diabetes in this study. Additionally, replacing 2% of energy from TFAs with PUFAs was associated with a 40% decrease in risk (RR = 0.60, 95% CI: 0.48, 0.75). A strength of this study was that the food-frequency questionnaire was repeated over time, allowing the investigators to compute updated averages of the participants' dietary habits, thereby reducing measurement error. Additionally, this appears to be the only study to adjust for other types of fat in their analysis, and this study may be the only observational study that has considered TFA trends as well as had an a priori hypothesis on the role of TFAs in chronic disease (Willett, 2006).

The Health Professionals Follow-up Study also included in their analysis an association of TFAs and type 2 diabetes (van Dam et al., 2002). In analyses adjusted for age and energy intake, TFAs were associated with the increased risk of type 2 diabetes in the highest three quintiles compared to the lowest: RR 1.24 (1.04–1.49), 1.33 (1.11–1.59), and 1.39 (1.16–1.67), corresponding to 1.3%, 1.5%, and 2.0% of total energy from TFAs, respectively. These results were not materially altered after further adjustment for physical activity, smoking, alcohol consumption, hypercholesterolemia, hypertension, and family history. However, the finding for TFAs was attenuated after further adjustment for cereal fiber, magnesium, and BMI. A potential limitation of this paper was the lack of adjustment for other types of fatty acids in the diet. A strength of the study was the repeated administering of an extensive food-frequency questionnaire over time (1986, 1990, and 1994).

The Iowa Women's Health Study also investigated the association between TFA and a type 2 diabetes risk (Meyer et al., 2001). In contrast to the Nurses Health Study (Salmeron et al., 2001), this study observed a weak inverse association between the intake of dietary TFA and the risk of type 2 diabetes. Relative risks among quintiles of TFA intake were 1.0, 0.93, 0.90, 0.84, and 0.87 ($P = 0.03$). Limitations of this study include potential misclassification of dietary habits relative to the Nurses' Health Study because TFAs and adverse outcomes did not appear to be an a priori hypothesis, and the Health Professionals Follow-Up, as the food-frequency questionnaire, was only administered at baseline. However, one-time assessment of dietary data is the norm rather than the exception in large epidemiological studies and has shown to accurately predict chronic disease risk in a number of areas. Also, in contrast to the Nurses' Health Study, this study did not appear to adjust the TFA relative-risk estimates for other types of dietary fat, particularly vegetable-fat intake. This is an important omission because PUFA is hypothesized to decrease insulin resistance and type 2 diabetes.

In summary, the available human observational literature illustrates inconsistencies in the associations between TFAs and insulin resistance and the risk of type 2 diabetes. This area showed much more ambiguity than the relationship of SFAs, PUFAs, and MUFAs fats to type 2 diabetes. SFAs are associated with the increasing risk of type 2 diabetes in numerous studies, just as the potential benefits of MUFAs and PUFAs fats also were researched to some depth (Hu et al., 2001a, b). Possible alternative explanations exist for the results obtained in the prospective studies mentioned. Possible differences in the amount of *trans*fat consumed in these studies may explain the difference in results: The median intake at baseline was 1.2% of energy in the Health Professionals Study compared to 2.2% in the Nurses' Health Study (van Dam et al., 2002). Additionally, TFAs have a strong potential to be misclassified. This confusion was due to temporal changes in consumption and manufacturing patterns in the United States during the 1980s when the consumption of hard, *trans*-fat laden margarines, cooking oils, and salad oils decreased, and softer margarines and oils were used with less TFAs (Meyer et al., 2001). However, this is likely not an issue in the

Nurses' Health Study and Health Professionals Study (Willett, 2006). Strengths of the studies mentioned include their large sample sizes and the scope of dietary and lifestyle information to account for potential confounding.

## *Experimental Studies in Humans*

Lovejoy et al. (2002) examined the effects of diets enriched with SFAs, MUFAs, or TFAs on insulin sensitivity in healthy, young adults. The study design was a randomized, double-blind, crossover feeding study comparing three controlled four-week diets (57% of CHO, 28% of fat, and 15% of protein) enriched with 9% of total energy from MUFAs, 9% of SFAs, and 9% of TFAs in each respective diet. The study was conducted in 25 men and women whose body weight was kept constant throughout the study. After each four-week diet period, insulin pulsatile secretion, insulin-sensitivity index, serum lipids, and fat oxidation by indirect calorimetry were measured. The mean age at randomization was 28 years, and the mean BMI was 23.5 $kg/m^2$. Of the 25 subjects, 18 were lean (BMI <25 $kg/m^2$), and 7 were overweight (BMI 25–30 $kg/m^2$). Overall, the study found no main effects on any of the insulin parameters (Lovejoy et al., 2002). When subjects were stratified by weight status, in comparison to the MUFA diet, overweight participants experienced a drop in insulin sensitivity of 24% in response to the SFA diet, and 11% in response to the TFA diet (Lovejoy et al., 2002). However, with limited statistical power, these estimates were not statistically significant. As one may expect, the young, lean, healthy subjects showed no change in insulin sensitivity on any of the diets. Of the data pertaining to TFA, the study did show some possible effects on insulin resistance in the overweight group, but the only significant results reported were in fat oxidation compared to the MUFA group. Of note, and in contrast to other studies and data examined, also no effect existed of a high SFA diet on insulin action (Folsom et al., 1996; Lovejoy et al., 2001). A possible limitation of this study was that the diets were low-fat, and therefore the specific fatty acid doses may have been the level needed to impact insulin resistance. As discussed by the authors, another reason why no clear findings were found in this study could be that the sample included insulin-sensitive healthy, lean, young adults, in whom even the analyses stratified on BMI were not particularly helpful.

Louheranta et al. (1999) also investigated the effects of TFA on insulin sensitivity. The study design was a randomized crossover feeding study comparing a high-TFA diet with a high-oleic acid or MUFA diet in 14 healthy, lean, young women with an average age of 23 and an average BMI of 20.8 $kg/m^2$ (Louheranta et al., 1999). Each diet lasted four weeks with a two-week run in the period for each diet. TFAs and MUFAs were substituted for 5% of SFAs at baseline. The total fat consumption was set at 36–37% of energy in the diet. The results produced no significant results in fasting plasma glucose, acute insulin response, insulin sensitivity, or levels of insulin between the two diets. Fasting insulin levels were slightly higher after the consumption of the TFA diet, 8.1 ± 0.6, compared to 7.4 ± 0.5 (mU/L) in the MUFA diet, but this was not statistically significant ($P = .09$) (Louheranta et al., 1999). The study's strengths include a significant, high level of compliance and the strict regulation and design of the diets. As with the study discussed above, a major limitation included studying lean, young, healthy females who were presumably quite insulin-sensitive, as well as a small sample size ($n = 14$).

Christiansen et al. (1997) investigated the effects of a diet high in TFA on insulin and glucose in obese people with type 2 diabetes. Sixteen people participated in the randomized crossover study, and were fed three different diets that consisted of 50% of CHO, 30% of fat, and 20% of protein as percentages of energy intake. Each of the three respective diets was isocaloric, lasted six weeks, and had 20% of total energy intake as either SFA, MUFA, or TFA. No washout or run-in periods existed. The levels of insulin and plasma glucose were determined by fasting and mixed-meal blood samples. Postprandial insulin levels were significantly elevated in participants after consuming the TFA diet (17.4 nmol/L per 240 min, $P < .05$) (Christiansen et al., 1997). This diet was 59% higher than the MUFA diet ($P < .05$), and 26% higher than the baseline diet ($P < .05$) (Christiansen et al., 1997). The same pattern was observed when evaluating C-peptide concentrations as a marker of insulin secretion. The postprandial serum C-peptide response was, respectively, 42% and 32% higher after the TFA diet than after the MUFA and baseline diets ($P < .05$) (Christiansen et al., 1997). The SFA diet also produced similar results as the TFA diet. Strengths of this study included the experimental nature, controlled diets, length of time, and biological plausibility. However, note that the very high amount of TFAs fed in this study raises concern about generalizability.

Recently, Lefevre and colleagues (2005) conducted an experimental investigation on the single-meal acute effects of C18:1*cis* versus *trans* on postprandial glycemia, insulinemia, and lipemia. Twenty-two moderately overweight men and women were fed a basal 24% fat diet for 16 days. On days 10 and 16, they were fed a large (40% of daily energy needs) high-fat (50% of energy) meal in a randomized crossover design. This meal included 15% of energy as C18:1*cis* fatty acid on one day, while on the other day 10% of the C18:1*cis* was replaced with C18:1TFA. From this study, the absolute amount of C18:1TFA that was fed to the subjects is unclear. Nonetheless, the results support the hypothesis that replacing *cis* with TFA may acutely exacerbate insulin resistance after only a single high-fat meal, as indicated by high-postprandial insulinemia and C-peptide concentrations following the TFA treatment. Future studies are needed to clarify the potential acute impact of the types and amounts of TFAs on insulin resistance, and more sophisticated clinical methods are necessary to partition out effects on peripheral insulin resistance versus insulin secretion.

### *Summary of the Clinical Studies*

The few clinical studies on this topic are largely equivocal. In a group of people where insulin sensitivity is of great concern (Christiansen et al., 1997), TFAs exacerbated the markers of the diabetic state. In the other studies, only hints of possible mal-effects were elucidated, but no significant positive or negative associations were observed. One should question the necessity and biologic plausibility of studying young, healthy, lean adults because this population is of extremely low general risk for developing type 2 diabetes. Additionally, possible limitations and definite inconsistencies are present in the study designs and methods employed in these studies. Thus, comparing them is a moot question. One example was that insulin sensitivity was not measured directly. The findings from these studies leave open the possibility of future research in numerous areas, especially where investigating the effects of TFAs is considered in at-risk populations: obese children, obese adults, elder persons, and certain minority groups.

Considering the labeling initiatives put forth, the efforts to limit TFAs in U.S. cities and different countries, and the wide expert agreement of the harmful effects for heart disease, clearly, a trend of limiting consumption among populations exists. Yet, the question remains whether TFAs will be removed from the food supply. Despite this publicity and the initial action on the potential health hazards of TFAs, they remain ubiquitous in the U.S. food supply, particularly in processed foods and in meals eaten at fast-food and other chain restaurants. Scientifically, gaining insight and knowledge of the effects of TFAs for diabetes risk and insulin resistance is of high interest. This is especially true considering the diabetes pandemic. However, the hard evidence from numerous clinical trials, epidemiological studies, and animal studies on the pernicious effects of TFAs on cardiovascular disease risk, and the fact that studies on TFAs showed no evidence of any health benefits may make this question more of a secondary point of interest rather than a hot topic of scientific investigation. Simply put, continued efforts, independent and governmental, on reducing and limiting TFA content in foods will likely have an important public-health impact on cardiovascular diseases. Whether these changes contribute to reduced rates of type 2 diabetes remains to be seen. That said, a well-designed trial looking at parameters directly related to type 2 diabetes by using an appropriate sample population has a strong potential to contribute scientifically and on the policy level.

## Conjugated Linoleic Acid

CLAs are a group of conjugated isomers of linoleic acids. They are typified as PUFAs and have a single pair of conjugated double bonds. CLA is mainly derived from ruminant meat and milk products (>90%) in the form of rumenic acid (18:2 *cis*-9, *trans*-11) (Tricon & Yaqoob, 2006). Chemically produced, CLAs are usually composed of a 50:50 mixture of rumenic acid and 18:2 *trans*-10, *cis*-12 (Bauman et al., 2006; Gebauer et al., 2007). The estimated habitual intake levels are 0.1–0.3 g/day (Whigham et al., 2007). Recent interest has arisen in CLAs due to the beneficial effects related to carcinogenesis, immune function, obesity, atherogenesis, and diabetes in animal studies (Tricon & Yaqoob, 2006; Yaqoob et al., 2006). However, the relationship between CLA, insulin sensitivity, and diabetes is unclear at the current time. The brief discussion that follows focuses specifically on human studies that included diabetes-related endpoints.

Riserus et al. (2002) examined the effect of 1% of energy from *trans*-10, *cis*-12 CLA on insulin sensitivity in abdominally obese men with risk factors for the metabolic syndrome, and found significantly decreased insulin sensitivity compared to a placebo. A similar study by Riserus et al. (2004) using the same design and a similar population tested the effect of 1% of energy from *cis*-9, *trans*-11 against a placebo, and found that this isomer of CLA also induced a significant decline in insulin sensitivity. A 50:50 mix of the two isomers did not produce any statistically significant results compared to the placebo intake.

Moloney et al. (2004) examined the effects of 3 g/day of a 50:50 mix of the two CLA isomers compared to a placebo in stable, diet-controlled type 2 diabetics. This study provided mixed results among the different measures of insulin sensitivity and glucose metabolism. In some measures, CLA appeared to be pernicious on insulin sensitivity, whereas no effect was seen in other indices. Additionally, the control and experimental groups had significant differences in response to insulin/glucose tests at baseline. The consideration of these differences at baseline actually shows that no significant effect of the CLA treatment occurred. One should interpret the metabolic effect of this CLA mixture in type 2 diabetics with caution regarding this study.

Lambert et al. (2007) tested the effect of a CLA-isomer mixture along with other fatty acids versus sunflower oil on glucose homeostasis and insulin sensitivity in a group of men and women who were of normal weight as defined by BMI and were participating in an exercise routine. Their interest lay in the effect of this CLA mixture and the potential interaction with exercise. Participants received a high dose (3.9 g/day) of the mixture or sunflower oil. Women in the CLA group had significantly reduced plasma insulin levels compared to the control group, showing a beneficial effect. Again, interpret this study with caution because findings were in a subgroup who exercised at a high level and also experienced a significant weight loss over the course of the study, both established factors in improving insulin sensitivity.

One other study that was likely statistically underpowered ($n$ = 6) found that young, sedentary individuals who received a CLA isomer also had a slight improvement in insulin sensitivity independent of body composition (Eyjolfson et al., 2004).

Indeed, the literature from human studies, CLA and insulin sensitivity, and diabetes provides equivocal results with some negative, some mixed, and some uninterpretable effects due to study design. However, the results in animals studies showed highly positive effects of CLA (Taylor & Zahradka, 2004). Additionally, CLA isomers comprise only a small percentage of the habitual diet of most populations where data are available (Bauman et al., 2006), and the studies to date have generally tested the extreme levels of CLA intake to isolate any potential effects over a reasonable period of time. Not enough data exist to make any conclusions on the biological effects of CLA on insulin sensitivity and type 2 diabetes. Consequently, any effects possibly observed in the future will likely be due to supplementation rather than the normal-intake levels: a factor that differs from industrial TFAs.

## Omega-3 Fatty Acids

Omega-3 fatty acids have received increasing attention for the potential health benefits they may portend. Omega-3 fatty acids are essential fatty acids for humans since they are not able to synthesize them in the body. α-Linolenic acid (ALA, 18:3n-3) is an abundant omega-3 fatty acid found in plant foods such as nuts, legumes, and green leafy vegetables (Gebauer et al., 2006). ALA is the precursor to three other important omega-3 fatty acids, which are found mainly in fish oils. Specifically, they are eicosapentaenoic acid (EPA, 20:5n-3), docosapentaenoic acid (DPA, 22:5n-3), and docosahexaenoic acid (DHA, 22:6n-3). Numerous different studies and systematic reviews show that omega-3 fatty acids, especially those derived from fish oil, have potential benefits related to cardiovascular function, inflammatory responses and diseases, and central nervous system function, behavior, and even certain autoimmune diseases (Stark et al., 2008). However, the research and evidence specifically related to insulin and glucose metabolism and type 2 diabetes are comparatively lacking and equivocal in nature. What follows is a brief overview of population and human studies related to the topic.

Increased insulin sensitivity was seen in humans with a higher proportion of omega-3 fatty acids in their skeletal muscle membrane (Borkman et al., 1993; Pan et al., 1995). However, these studies did not directly assess the effect of omega-3 fatty acids, so this may be a marker of a more prudent diet for a diabetes risk rather than a direct effect. In two smaller prospective cohort studies, an inverse association with a diabetes risk was observed with high fish consumption, a marker for omega-3 consumption (Feskens et al., 1991, 1995). However, in another small prospective study, no association was observed (Vessby et al., 1994). In the Nurses' Health Study, the largest prospective study on the topic, a suggestive moderate inverse association with a diabetes risk was found (Salmeron et al., 2001).

Tsitouras et al. (2008) investigated the effects of high omega-3-rich fish consumption and oil supplementation versus a diet essentially lacking in fish oil in a small sample of healthy, elderly participants, and found an improvement in insulin sensitivity after the omega-3-rich diet, but no change in any measures of glucose levels. The dietary periods were likely long enough to test the hypothesis; however, the sample size ($n$ = 12), lack of randomization, and the finding being in a secondary aim suggest that one should interpret these results with caution.

Ramel et al. (2008) investigated the effects of the regular consumption of lean fish, fatty fish, or fish oil versus a control group of no seafood over eight weeks in young, overweight Europeans consuming an energy-restricted diet. Their main reported finding was that the fish-oil group had positive effects on insulin levels and a measure of insulin resistance compared to the control group. The study measured the biological endpoints completely and thoroughly, and likely had enough statistical power to test their hypothesis; however, these results should be interpreted with caution. First, a significantly greater weight loss was experienced in the fish-oil capsule group compared to the control group; also this weight-loss group had a better baseline profile of insulin and glucose measures. Second, while the participants received thorough counseling and recommendations related to their assigned diets, they were responsible for the food preparation and the foods they ate beyond the fish or capsule supplements. This may explain why the fatty-fish group, which was assigned a higher level of omega-3 intake, did not have any significant statistical findings or trends compared to the control group. Lastly, since weight loss was a major outcome and is also a major predictor of insulin sensitivity, this may confound the results.

Another recent study by Mostad et al. (2006) investigated the effects of fish-oil supplements versus corn-oil supplements on metabolic measures related to type 2 diabetes in persons with type 2 diabetes. This double-blind randomized controlled trial employed strong outcome measurements, and was rigorously conducted since participants' weights were stable and diets were continuous through the study. Their main finding was that omega-3 supplementation slightly, but significantly, impaired insulin action in the participants. Contrary to this study, Popp-Snijders et al. (1987) found that omega-3 fatty acids improved insulin sensitivity in a very small pilot study of persons with type 2 diabetes.

Numerous other clinical studies have investigated this question in one way or another; they found no direct findings between omega-3 fatty acids and insulin and glucose measures. Krebs et al. (2006) examined the joint effect of weight loss and fish consumption on a number of cardiovascular and metabolic-disease measures, and found no evidence that omega-3 fatty acids have any effect on insulin sensitivity or measures of glucose metabolism. Brady et al. (2004) found no effects of omega-3 supplementation on insulin sensitivity in Indian Asians. A large intervention study looking at dietary fat and weight maintenance also found no impact of fish-oil supplementation on insulin sensitivity (Vessby et al., 2001). Mori et al. (1999) conducted a study similar to Krebs et al.(2006), and also found no evidence that omega-3 fatty acids directly affect glucose or insulin parameters. Indeed, all of these studies (Brady et al., 2004; Krebs, 2006; Mori et al., 1999; Vessby et al., 2001) found potentially beneficial effects of omega-3 fatty acids that may effect hypothesized pathways to blood glucose and insulin metabolism, but no direct effects were found.

In short, omega-3 fatty acids are essential fatty acids, and demonstrate an extensive promise of health benefits in multiple areas. Unfortunately, the research directly examining their effects related to type 2 diabetes is nebulous. The few positive studies have a number of study design and analysis issues that cloud their results. The studies finding null results were much larger and generally better designed, but none of the completed studies in this area are considered a benchmark study. Lastly, the negative findings were not replicated in a nondiabetic population. A well-designed trial and further reporting of large, well-done epidemiologic studies would help to further elucidate any potential effects that omega-3 fatty acids might have.

## Omega-6/Omega-3 Fatty Acid Ratio

The omega-6/omega-3 fatty acid ratio is a ratio that estimates the intake proportions of omega-6 fatty acids (linoleic and arachidonic acids) to omega-3 fatty acids (ALA, EPA,

DPA, DHA). Omega-6 fatty acid intake generally occurs through the consumption of seeds from most plants, with the largest portions in the form of oil from these seeds, or through industrially produced animals for meat which consume these seeds/grains for feed (Simopoulos, 2008). This ratio is proposed to be important in chronic disease, especially cardiovascular-disease risk, and a high ratio is a potential marker of a Western-type diet. One rationale for the importance of this ratio is that a high ratio differs from the nutritional environment from which humans' genetic selection took place (low ratio), and this may lead to physiological problems when exposed to a high level of omega-6 intake (Simopoulos, 2008).

Furthermore, the ratio is of interest because the fatty acids compete in metabolic pathways that impact cellular responses to physiologic stresses (Harris, 2006). Increasing the intake of one fatty acid changes the membrane phospholipid composition as well as the potential to change the physiological response to stress. Populations with higher omega-3 intake have less inflammatory, aggregatory, and vasodilatory physiological responses to stress (Harris, 2006). The underlying hypothesis for the importance of this fatty acid ratio is intriguing; however, the research related to insulin and glucose metabolism as well as type 2 diabetes is sparse. In a related topic, a paper examining a number of trials and studies looking at the ratio and using cardiovascular-disease-related endpoints, Harris et al. (2006) concluded that the ratio had little prognostic value and that the total level of omega-3 consumption should be the preferred marker.

A few studies have tried to assess the effect of the ratio on insulin and glucose parameters. Griffin et al. (2006) tested an n-6/n-3 ratio of 3:1/5:1 compared to a ratio of 10:1 in a parallel-arm dietary intervention of those of the ages of 45–70 years in the United Kingdom in general good health. One goal of the study was to test the indexes of insulin sensitivity between the two groups; however, no evidence was found of any effects of the lower ratio or overall omega-3 fatty acid intake on any measures of insulin sensitivity. The study was likely well-powered, and did base the intervention on foods, rather than on supplements, and a fairly rigid design was imposed on other parameters. The greater majority of participants (60%) were also insulin-resistant, making it an ideal population to assess an improvement in insulin sensitivity. Note that a large proportion of the study population was also taking medications; how these were considered in the analysis was not clear. Questions on this study relate to the length (6 months) and if this is appropriate or if this topic is better suited to a longer term study. Furthermore, this wasn't a complete feeding study, and was relying, to an extent, on the report of individuals. Lastly, one should consider whether the ratios were sufficiently different.

Giacco et al. (2007) also considered the n-6/n-3 ratio in a subanalysis of the KANWU Study (Vessby et al., 2001), and also found no evidence of any contribution to the improvement of insulin sensitivity or glucose parameters. This held even when considering the omega-3 supplementation while taking into account the ratio. Minihane et al. (2005) examined the question in a population susceptible to diabetes, and found no effect of a high n-6/n-3 ratio on insulin sensitivity or any related parameters in Indian Asians in the United Kingdom. Thus, no evidence suggests that the n-6/n-3 ratio plays a role in insulin sensitivity or glucose metabolism to date. Further studies may help differentiate whether this ratio is important in the pathophysiology of type 2 diabetes.

# Conclusion

In summary, mixed evidence exists on the extent that TFAs are harmful for diabetes risk. Indeed, strong evidence exists that TFAs are pernicious for cardiovascular- disease risk, which is the force behind many of the policy and regulation initiatives currently underway. The limited data on CLA suggest that they impair insulin sensitivity in their pure isomer forms, but other studies of mixed and pure isomers suggest that they may have positive or negative effects on insulin and glucose metabolism. More research on CLA is needed because numerous limitations in the current literature and animal models suggest potential beneficial effects in a number of chronic-disease areas in addition to diabetes. Thus, if and how these animal mechanisms are relevant to human populations are the overarching questions on this topic. Data from studies looking at omega-3 fatty acids and their relationship to type 2 diabetes, insulin, and glucose metabolism contain mixed results. Observational studies have generally been null, and clinical studies on the topic generally showed null results also, with some showing positive effects of omega-3 fatty acids, and one in a diabetic population showed potential negative effects. The n-6/n-3 ratio is an intriguing hypothesis for its involvement in a chronic-disease risk, but no data currently link this ratio to a diabetes risk in a beneficial or harmful manner.

## References


Alstrup, K.K.; S. Gregersen, et al. Differential effects of cis and trans fatty acids on insulin release from isolated mouse islets.*Metabolism* **1999,** *48(1),* 22–29.

Ascherio, A.; M.B. Katan, et al. Trans fatty acids and coronary heart disease. *N. Engl. J. Med.* **1999,** *340(25),* 1994–1998.

Axen, K.V.; A. Dikeakos, et al. High dietary fat promotes syndrome X in nonobese rats. *J. Nutr.* **2003,** *133(7),* 2244–2249.

Bauman, D.; A.L. Lock; B.A. Corl, et al. *Milk Fatty Acids and Human Health: Potential Role of Conjugated Linoleic Acid and Trans Fatty Acids;* Academic Publishers: Wageningen, The Netherlands, 2006.Borkman, M.; L.H. Storlien; D.A. Pan, et al. The relation between insulin sensitivity and the fatty-acid composition of skeletal muscle phospholipids. *N. Engl. J. Med.* **1993,** *328,* 238–244).

Brady, L.; S.S. Lovegrove; S.V. Lesauvage, et al. Increased n-6 polyunsaturated fatty acids do not attenuate the effects of long-chain n-3 polyunsaturated fatty acids on insulin sensitivity or triacylglycerol reduction in Indian Asians. *Am. J. Clin. Nutr.* **2004,** *79,* 983–991.

Christiansen, E.; S. Schnider, et al. Intake of a diet high in trans monounsaturated fatty acids or saturated fatty acids. Effects on postprandial insulinemia and glycemia in obese patients with NIDDM. *Diabetes Care* **1997,** ***20****(5),* 881–887.

DeFronzo, R.A. Pathogenesis of type 2 diabetes mellitus. *Med. Clin. North Am.* **2004,** *88(4),* 787–835, ix.

DHHS/FDA. Food labeling: *Trans* fatty acids in nutrition labeling: nutrient content claims, and health claims: finale rule. *Fed. Regist.* **2003,** *68,* 41433–41506.

Diagnosis and classification of diabetes mellitus. *Diabetes Care* **2004,** *27(Suppl.1)* S5–S10.

Engelgau, M.M.; L.S. Geiss, et al. The evolving diabetes burden in the United States. *Ann. Intern. Med.* **2004,** *140(11),* 945–950.

EURODIET. Nutrition & diet for healthy lifestyles in Europe. *Sci. Policy Implications* **2000,** *Crete,* 1–17.

Eyjolfson, V.; L.L. Spriet; D.J. Dyck. Conjugated linoleic acid improves insulin sensitivity in young, sedentary humans. *Med. Sci. Sports Exer.* **2004,** *36(5),* 814–820.

Feskens, E.; C.H. Bowles; D. Kromhout. Inverse association between fish intake and risk of glucose intolerance in normoglycemic elderly men and women. *Diabetes Care* **1991,** *14,* 935–941.

Feskens, E.; S.M. Virtanen; L. Rasanen, et al. Dietary factors determining diabetes and impaired glucose tolerance. A 20-year follow-up of the Finnish and Dutch cohorts of the Seven Countries. *Diabetes Care* **1995,** *18,* 1104–1112.

Folsom, A.R.; J. Ma, et al. Relation between plasma phospholipid saturated fatty acids and hyperinsulinemia. *Metabolism* **1996,** *45(2),* 223–228.

Gebauer, S.; T.L. Psota; W.S. Harris; P.M. Kris-Etherton. n-3 fatty acid dietary recommendations and food sources to achieve essentiality and cardiovascular benefits. *Am. J. Clin. Nutr.* **2006,** *83 (6),* 1526S–1535S.

Gebauer, S.; T.L. Psota; P.M. Kris-Etherton. The diversity of health effects of individual trans fatty acid isomers. *Lipids* **2007,** *42,* 787–799.

Giacco, R.; V. Cuomo; V. Vessby, et al. Fish oil, insulin sensitivity, insulin secretion and glucose tolerance in healthy people: is there any effect of fish oil supplementation in relation to the type of background diet and habitual dietary intake of n-6 and n-3 fatty acids? *Nutr. Metab. Cardiovasc. Dis.* **2007,** *8,* 572–580.

Griffin, M.; T.A.B. Sanders; I.G. Davies, et al. Effects of altering the ratio of n-6 to n-3 fatty acids on insulin sensitivity, lipoprotein size, and postprandial lipemia in men and postmenopausal women aged 45–70 y: the OPTILIP study. *Am. J. Clin. Nutr.* **2006,** *84,* 1290–1298.

Haffner, S.; H. Taegtmeyer. Epidemic obesity and the metabolic syndrome. *Circulation* **2003,** *108(13),* 1541–1545.

Harris, W.; B. Assaad; W.C. Poston. Tissue omega-6/omega-3 fatty acid ratio and risk for coronary artery disease. *Am. J. Cardiol.* **2006,** *98(Suppl.),* 19i–26i.

Hu, F.B.; J.E. Manson, et al. Diet, lifestyle, and the risk of type 2 diabetes mellitus in women. *N. Engl. J. Med.* **2001a,** *345(11),* 790–797.

Hu, F.B.; R.M. van Dam, et al. Diet and risk of Type II diabetes: the role of types of fat and carbohydrate. *Diabetologia* **2001b,** *44(7),* 805–817.

Ibrahim, A.; S. Natrajan, et al. Dietary trans-fatty acids alter adipocyte plasma membrane fatty acid composition and insulin sensitivity in rats. *Metabolism* **2005,** *54(2),* 240–246.

Kavanagh, K.; K.L. Jones; J. Sawyer, et al. Trans fat diet induces abdominal obesity and changes in insulin sensitivity in monkeys. *Obesity (Silver Spring)* **2007,** *15(7),* 1675–1684.

Krebs, J.; L.M. Browning; N.K. McLean, et al. Additive benefits of long-chain n-3 polyunsaturated fatty acids and weight-loss in the management of cardiovascular disease risk in overweight hyperinsulinaemic women. *Int. J. Obes.* **2006,** *30(10),* 1535–1544.

Lambert, E.; J.H. Goedecke; K. Bluett, et al. Conjugated linoleic acid versus high-oleic acid sunflower oil: effects on energy metabolism, glucose tolerance, blood lipids, appetite and body composition in regularly exercising individuals. *Br.J. Nutr.* **2007,** *97,* 1001–1011.

Lefevre, M.; J.C. Lovejoy; et al. Comparison of the acute response to meals enriched with cis- or trans-fatty acids on glucose and lipids in overweight individuals with differing FABP2 genotypes. *Metabolism* **2005,** *54(12),* 1652–1658.

Lichtenstein, A.; L.J. Appel; M. Brands, et al. Diet and lifestyle recommendations revision 2006: a scientific statement from the American Heart Association Nutrition Committee. *Circulation* **2006,** *114,* 82–96.

Lichtenstein, A.H.; L.M. Ausman, et al. Effects of different forms of dietary hydrogenated fats on serum lipoprotein cholesterol levels. *N. Engl. J. Med.* **1999,** *340(25),* 1933–1940.

Lichtenstein, A.H.; U.S. Schwab. Relationship of dietary fat to glucose metabolism. *Atherosclerosis* **2000,** *150(2),* 227–243.

Louheranta, A.M.; A.K. Turpeinen, et al. A high-trans fatty acid diet and insulin sensitivity in young healthy women. *Metabolism* **1999,** *48(7),* 870–875.

Lovejoy, J.C.; C.M. Champagne, et al. Relationship of dietary fat and serum cholesterol ester and phospholipid fatty acids to markers of insulin resistance in men and women with a range of glucose tolerance. *Metabolism* **2001,** *50(1),* 86–92.

Lovejoy, J.C.; S.R. Smith, et al. Effects of diets enriched in saturated (palmitic), monounsaturated (oleic), or trans (elaidic) fatty acids on insulin sensitivity and substrate oxidation in healthy adults. *Diabetes Care* **2002,** *25(8),* 1283–1288.

Mensink, R.P.; M.B. Katan. Effect of dietary trans fatty acids on high-density and low-density lipoprotein cholesterol levels in healthy subjects. *N. Engl. J. Med.* **1990,** *323(7),* 439–445.

Mensink, R.P.; M.B. Katan. Effect of dietary fatty acids on serum lipids and lipoproteins. A meta-analysis of 27 trials. *Arterioscler. Thromb.* **1992,** *12(8),* 911–919.

Meyer, K.A.; L.H. Kushi, et al. Dietary fat and incidence of type 2 diabetes in older Iowa women. *Diabetes Care* **2001,** *24(9),* 1528–1535.

Minihane, A.; L.M. Brady; S.S. Lovegrove, et al. (2005). Lack of effect of dietary n-6:n-3 PUFA ratio on plasma lipids and markers of insulin responses in Indian Asians living in the UK. *Eur. J. Nutr.* **2005,** *44(1),* 26–32.

Moloney, F.; T.P. Yeow; A. Mullen, et al. Conjugated linoleic acid supplementation, insulin sensitivity, and lipoprotein metabolism in patients with type 2 diabetes mellitus. *Am. J. Clin. Nutr.* **2004,** *80,* 887–895.

Mori, T.; D.Q. Bao; V. Burke, et al. Dietary fish as a major component of a weight-loss diet: effect on serum lipids, glucose, and insulin metabolism in overweight hypertensive subjects. *Am. J. Clin. Nutr.* **1999,** *70,* 817–825.

Mostad, I.; K.S. Bjerve; M.R. Bjorgaas, et al. Effects of n-3 fatty acids in subjects with type 2 diabetes: Reduction of insulin sensitivity and time-dependent alteration from carbohydrate to fat oxidation. *Am. J. Clin. Nutr.* **2006,** *84,* 540–550.

Mozaffarian, D.; T. Pischon, et al. Dietary intake of trans fatty acids and systemic inflammation in women. *Am. J. Clin. Nutr.* **2004,** *79(4),* 606–612.

Mozaffarian, D.; E.B. Rimm, et al. Trans fatty acids and systemic inflammation in heart failure. *Am. J. Clin. Nutr.* **2004,** *80(6),* 1521–1525.

Narayan, K.M.; J.P. Boyle, et al. Lifetime risk for diabetes mellitus in the United States. *Jama* **2003,** *290(14),* 1884–1890.

Natarajan, S.; A. Ibrahim. Dietary trans fatty acids alter diaphragm phospholipid fatty acid composition, triacylglycerol content and glucose transport in rats. *Br. J. Nutr.* **2005,** *93(6),* 829–833.

Nutrition and Your Health: Dietary Guidelines for Americans. (2005) http://www.health.gov/dietaryguidelines/dga2005/report/, U.S. Departments of Agriculture and Health and Human Services**: Washington, DC.** (In press)

Pan, D.; S. Lillioja; M.R. Milner, et al. Skeletal muscle membrane lipid composition is related to adiposity and insulin action. *J. Clin. Invest.* **1995,** *96,* 2802–2808.

Popp-Snijders, C.; J.A. Schouten; R.J. Heine, et al. Dietary supplementation of omega-3 polyunsaturated fatty acids improves insulin sensitivity in non-insulin-dependent diabetes. *Diabetes Res.* **1987,** *4(3),* 141–147.

Prentice, A.M. Overeating: The health risks. *Obes. Res.* **2001,** *9(Suppl. 4),* 234S–238S.

Ramel, A.; A. Martinéz; M. Kiely, et al. Beneficial effects of long-chain n-3 fatty acids included in an energy-restricted diet on insulin resistance in overweight and obese European young adults. *Diabetologia* **2008,** *51(7),* 1261–1268.

Reaven, G.M. Syndrome X: 6 years later. *J. Intern. Med. Suppl.* **1994,** *736,* 13–22.

Riserus, U.; P. Arner; K. Brismar, et al. Treatment with dietary trans10cis12 conjugated linoleic acid causes isomer-specific insulin resistance in obese men with the metabolic syndrome. *Diabetes Care* **2002,** *25,* 1516–1521.

Riserus, U.; B. Vessby; J. Arnlov; S. Basu. Effects of cis-9,trans-11 conjugated linoleic acid supplementation on insulin sensitivity, lipid peroxidation, and proinflammatory markers in obese men. *Am. J. Clin. Nutr.* **2004,** *80,* 279–283.

Salmeron, J.; F.B. Hu, et al. Dietary fat intake and risk of type 2 diabetes in women. *Am. J. Clin. Nutr.* **2001,** *73(6),* 1019–1026.

Simopoulos, A. The importance of the omega-6/omega-3 fatty acid ratio in cardiovascular disease and other chronic diseases. *Exp. Biol. Med.* **2008,** *233,* 674–688.

Stark, A.; M.A. Crawford; R. Reifen. Update on alpha-linolenic acid. *Nutr. Rev.* **2008,** *66(6),* 326–332.

Steyn, N.P.; J. Mann, et al. Diet, nutrition and the prevention of type 2 diabetes. *Public Health Nutr.* **2004,** *7(1A),* 147–165.

Taylor, C.; P. Zahradka. Dietary conjugated linoleic acid and insulin sensitivity and resistance in rodent models. *Am. J. Clin. Nutr.* **2004,** *79 (Suppl.),* 1164–1168S.

Tricon, S.; P. Yaqoob. Conjugated linoleic acid and human health: A critical evaluation of the evidence. *Curr. Opin. Clin. Nutr. Metab. Care* **2006,** *9,* 105–110.

Tsitouras, P.; F. Gucciardo; A.D. Salbe, et al. High omega-3 fat intake improves insulin sensitivity and reduces CRP and IL6, but does not affect other endocrine axes in healthy older adults. *Horm. Metab. Res.* **2008,** *40(3),* 199–205.

van Dam, R.M.; W.C. Willett, et al. Dietary fat and meat intake in relation to risk of type 2 diabetes in men. *Diabetes Care* **2002,** *25(3),* 417–424.

Vessby, B.; A. Aro; E. Skarfors, et al. The risk to develop NIDDM is related to the fatty acid composition of the serum cholesterol esters. *Diabetes* **1994,** *43,* 1353–1357.

Vessby, B.; M. Unsitupa; K. Hermansen, et al. Substituting dietary saturated for monounsaturated fat impairs insulin sensitivity in healthy men and women: The KANWU Study. *Diabetologia* **2001,** *44,* 312–319.

Whigham, L.; A.C. Watras; D.A. Schoeller. Efficacy of conjugated linoleic acid for reducing fat mass: a meta-analysis in humans. *Am. J. Clin. Nutr.* **2007,** *85,* 1203–1211.

WHO/FAO, e., consultation. Diet, nutrition and the prevention of chronic diseases. *WHO Technical Report Series;* WHO: Geneva, 2003; pp. 86–90.

Wild, S.; G. Roglic, et al. Global prevalence of diabetes: estimates for the year 2000 and projections for 2030. *Diabetes Care* **2004,** *27(5),* 1047–1053.

Willett, W. *Nutritional Epidemiology,* Oxford University Press, 1998.

Willett, W.C. *Trans* fatty acids and cardiovascular disease-epidemiological data. *Atherosclerosis* **2006,** *7(Suppl.),* 5–8.

Willi, C.; P. Bondenmann; W.A. Ghali, et al. Active smoking and the risk of type 2 diabetes: a systematic review and meta-analysis. *Jama* **2007,** *298(22),* 2654–2664.

Yaqoob, P.; S. Tricon; C.M. Williams, et al. Conjugated linoleic acid and human health-related outcomes. *Br. Nutr. Foundation Nutr. Bull.* **2006,** *31,* 93–99.

# 14

# Effect of Dietary Long-chain Polyunsaturated Fatty Acids in Infancy on Both Visual and Neural Development

**Lisa G Smithers[1-3] and Maria Makrides[1,2]**

[1] *Women's and Children's Health Research Institute at the Children Youth and Women's Health Service, 72 King William Road, North Adelaide 5006 and Flinders Medical Centre, Flinders Drive, Bedford Park, 5042 Australia;* [2] *School of Paediatrics and Reproductive Health, University of Adelaide, Adelaide 5005 Australia;* [3] *Department of Paediatrics and Child Health, Flinders University, GPO Box 2100 Adelaide 5001 Australia*

## Introduction

The development of visual and neural tissues begins before birth and continues well into the postnatal period. The brain grows at its greatest velocity in late pregnancy, and is near adult size by 2 years. Diet plays a key role in early development because many nutrients are needed to construct rapidly growing tissues. Human milk is the feed-of-choice during infancy (World Health Organization, 2003) because it provides the infant with essential nutrients as well as a range of nonnutritive bioactive molecules to support growth, development, and protection from infection. One group of nutrients naturally present in human milk that has inspired much research activity is the long-chain polyunsaturated fatty acids (LCPUFAs).

LCPUFAs are present in all human tissues, but particularly high quantities are located in neural and retinal tissues. Nearly one-third of the neural tissues are composed of the n-3 LCPUFA docosahexaenoic acid (DHA) (Cotman et al., 1968), whereas the predominant n-6 LCPUFA is arachidonic acid (AA). Both DHA and AA are distributed throughout the phospholipid membranes of neurons; however, a substantial quantity of DHA is located in the neuronal synaptosome, which is the area of the nerve cell responsible for the transmission of signals. The tissue with the highest concentration of DHA is the tiny, but extremely important, area of the retina called the "fovea" (Anderson, 1970; Anderson & Sperling, 1971). The fovea contains tightly packed photoreceptor cells, which convert light from our central field of view into electrical signals that are sent to the brain. The fovea is responsible for the high degree of visual acuity that humans enjoy. Overall, the high concentration of DHA in the membranes of retinal photoreceptors and neurons is indicative of the importance of DHA in membrane-associated functions including signal transduction, neurotransmission, and neurogenesis (Innis, 2007).

Retinal and neural tissues begin accumulating LCPUFA during fetal development (Martinez, 1992). The placenta preferentially transfers n-3 LCPUFA from the maternal circulation to the developing fetus (Haggarty et al., 1997). By the end of gestation, retinal tissues apparently complete DHA accretion; however, neural tissues continue to accumulate LCPUFA well into the postnatal period (Martinez & Mougan, 1998).

The high concentration of LCPUFA in retinal and neural tissues, as well as the early accretion of fatty acids in these tissues, led many investigators to studying the effects of the dietary supply of LCPUFA on both visual and cognitive development. This chapter contains a summary of the evidence from clinical trials that assessed the dietary supply of LCPUFA in infancy and visual or cognitive development. The main focus is on randomized controlled trials (RCTs) because this methodology offers the most rigorous scientific design by minimizing the bias associated with other research methodologies. The chapter is separated into sections covering the development of full-term and preterm infants because preterm infants are potentially more vulnerable to low-LCPUFA status since they are denied the full gestational period to accrue LCPUFA. Before presenting the evidence on the effects of dietary LCPUFA and infant development, we briefly describe the laboratory methods used for assessing infant LCPUFA status, and present an overview of the techniques used to measure both visual and cognitive function.

## Measuring Fatty Acid Status of Infants

The phospholipid bilayer of all cell membranes contains some LCPUFA, which means that one can observe the effect of a dietary intervention by studying the fatty-acid composition of many tissues. The most direct measure of fatty-acid status is to analyze a sample of tissue, but this is neither practical nor acceptable for trials conducted in infants. Assessing the fatty-acid status from blood samples is far less invasive. In LCPUFA-supplementation trials, plasma and erythrocyte membrane phospholipids are used to describe fatty-acid status and to demonstrate the success of dietary intervention. Plasma phospholipids are a major transporter of LCPUFA in circulation (Clandinin et al., 1999), and therefore plasma-phospholipid fatty acids can provide a simple, reliable indicator of circulating fatty acids. A further advantage of using plasma samples in a clinical trial setting is that one can collect the specimens and store them at –20°C for later batch testing of all trial samples. Not surprisingly, erythrocyte-membrane phospholipids are slower to respond to changes in fatty-acid status than plasma phospholipids, and may therefore be indicative of a longer term fatty-acid status (Cao et al., 2006; Harris et al., 2007; Katan et al., 1997). Trials in infants show that both erythrocyte-membrane and plasma-phospholipid LCPUFA concentrations are strongly related to the LCPUFA concentration of human milk or formula in the infant diet (Clandinin et al., 1997, 1999; Gibson et al., 1997). Presumably, plasma-

and erythrocyte-membrane phospholipid LCPUFA concentrations are indicative of the LCPUFA supply to the tissues. Therefore, circulating fatty acids are considered useful surrogate markers of tissue fatty-acid status; this assumption is supported by studies conducted in primates (Hsieh et al., 2007). As yet, no specific concentration of circulating LCPUFA is defined as optimal for infant development.

## Measuring Visual or Cognitive Function of Infants and Young Children

### *Methods of Assessing Visual Function*

The techniques predominantly used in LCPUFA trials to assess the development of the visual system in pre-verbal infants or young children include the measurement of retinal sensitivity by using the electroretinogram (ERG) and visual acuity. Acuity is the smallest-sized element that the visual system can discriminate, and both electrophysiological methods (using visual-evoked potentials, VEPs) and behavioral methods (e.g., Teller acuity cards) were used to measure the acuity of infants enrolled in the LCPUFA trials. Few trials have assessed visual abilities during childhood, and therefore, the techniques appropriate for older children (including acuity charts and stereo-acuity) were used less frequently.

The ERG involves the placement of a small, sensitive electrode on the outer surface of the eye (cornea), which measures the entire electrical signal released from the retina in response to a series of flashes of light. Specific information is gleaned from the sequences of light, including the measurements of rod-and-cone-photoreceptor function. The ERG provides a measurement of the sensitivity of the retina to light. VEP acuity is an electrophysiological technique, where electrodes are placed on the infant's scalp over the visual cortex, which is the primary area of the brain for processing visual information. The electrodes detect changes in the electrical response of neurons to a visual stimulus of a known size (Fig. 14.1). VEP acuity is the largest-visual stimulus that does not result in any detectable electrical response, and is thought to be the limit of an infant's visual ability. In adults, VEP acuity correlates well with acuity measured using the common Snellen (letter) chart (Ohn et al., 1994; Xu et al., 2001). Behavioral measurements of acuity capitalize on an infant's innate preference to look at a striped pattern rather than a homogeneous gray color. Infants are simultaneously shown two cards in a series: one has a different-sized striped pattern; the other card is matte gray. An observer hidden behind the cards watches the infant's eye movements in response to the cards to determine which card the infant prefers (Teller et al., 1986). Acuity is estimated to be the largest-sized pattern that the infant no longer exhibits a preference over the plain gray card. Behavioral measurements of acuity are less invasive and cheaper to use, but have a higher variation and require larger sample sizes than electrophysiological measurements of acuity.

HOTV acuity is used to measure acuity in young (verbal) children using a vision chart. Before the testing, the child must be able to correctly identify the letters H, O, T, and V verbally or by pointing to the matching letter on a hand-held response card

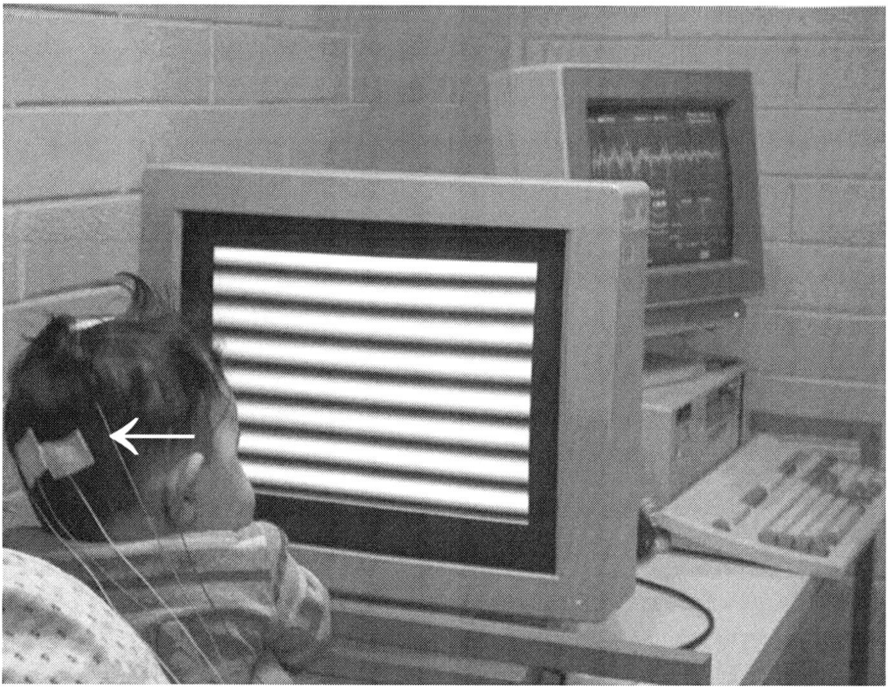

**Fig. 14.1.** Visual-evoked potential acuity assessment of a 4-month-old infant. The infant is seated at a standard distance from the display monitor. In this test the infant is presented a horizontal grating pattern for measuring visual acuity. Electrodes placed over the visual cortex (white arrow) detect the electrical signals released by neurons in response to the grating pattern. The electrical signals are amplified and sent to a computer (in background) which records the infant's response. The grating pattern reduces in size during the test. The limit of acuity is the point at which no detectable response to the grating pattern is noted.

(Duckman 2006; Holmes et al., 2001). The HOTV-acuity wall chart is adapted for computer use. Stereo-acuity techniques measure "depth-perception," which requires information from both eyes to correctly discern the location of a letter or symbol with a three-dimensional appearance (Han & Duckman, 2006). Both wall charts and cards were used to assess stereo-acuity.

## Methods of Assessing Development and Cognition

Many different techniques are used to assess infant development in response to LCPUFA-supplementation trials. The most frequently used methods include those that assess global development, such as Bayley Scales of Infant Development (BSID) (Bayley 1993, 2006). Such techniques measure performance across a number of developmental domains (such as gross and fine-motor function, problem solving, behavior). Global-development tools are usually designed to compare an individual's performance to a population norm to identify infants with developmental delay.

Developmental tests are generally used in early childhood, whereas tests that focus on intelligence are used at older ages. Like developmental tests, intelligence quotient (IQ) tests measure cognitive abilities across a range of areas. The focus of the assessment, as well as the administration and scoring procedures, differs with each test. For example, the Stanford-Binét test measures reasoning, knowledge, visual–spatial processing, and memory abilities, while the Weschler Preschool and Primary School Intelligence test focuses on verbal function and cognitive performance. Scoring of both global-development and intelligence tests is usually based on combining performances across a range of skills to produce a total composite score. Arguably, tests that use composite scores may be unsuitable for measuring specific domains of neural function, such as memory or attention (Cheatham et al., 2006; Wainwright & Colombo, 2006), and this could result in differences in neural function as a result of LCPUFA interventions passing unnoticed. Some advantages of the widely used global-development and intelligence tests are that most are extensively validated and are standardized for age and sex. All tests have well-documented, systematic procedures for administration and scoring which improve the reliability of the tests and enable the tests to be administered at many sites. Furthermore, most are accepted and understood by health-care workers, and many developmental or intelligence tests have clinical relevance.

Some of the other assessment techniques occasionally used in LCPUFA trials include the Fagan Infantest, MacArthur Communicative Development Inventory (MCDI), and problem-solving tests. The Fagan Infantest capitalizes on an infant's preference for a novel visual stimulus. The infant is shown a picture of a face, and after a short period of time, the infant's attention to the face usually wanes; this period is called the "familiarization" phase. The infant is then shown a picture of a different face, and the infant usually shows a renewed interest in the picture. The number and duration of looks to the new stimulus are determined. This test shows that the infant has formed a memory of the familiar face, and the behavior in looking at the new face indicates the speed of processing new information. These measurements are modestly predictive of intelligence in childhood (Thompson et al., 1991). The MCDI is a comprehensive questionnaire exploring various language and communication skills including gestures, receptive vocabulary (what is understood), and expressive vocabulary (the number of words used and the structure of sentences). The MCDI was validated for use in infants and young children, and is standardized for age and sex. Problem-solving tests that assess an infant's ability to retrieve and construct a two- or three-step task were also used in LCPUFA trials. Although some data describing the development of problem-solving ability in infancy were described (Slater, 1995), these tests were not validated, and gender-standardized norms were not published.

## Visual and Neural Functions of Infants Born at Full Term

In the first six months of life, an infant depends solely on milk as the single food to supply the entire nutritional needs for rapid growth and development. Human milk provides a wide range of LCPUFAs (Kneebone et al., 1985; Yuhas et al., 2006).

However, infant formulas contained no LCPUFAs until relatively recently. Research showing that breast-fed infants exhibited better development than formula- fed infants generated an interest in the role of LCPUFAs in infant development (Anderson et al., 1999; Mortensen et al., 2002). Presumably, the LCPUFAs in human milk enhanced neural function and this culminated in improved performance in intelligence tests.

In addition to population studies, other research supports the role of LCPUFA in improving development. The post-mortem analysis of neural tissues showed that infants fed human milk had higher neural cortex DHA compared to infants fed a formula devoid of LCPUFAs (Makrides et al., 1994). Further supporting evidence from biochemical studies shows that infants fed a standard (nonsupplemented) formula have lower concentrations of DHA circulating in plasma and red-blood-cell phospholipids than breast-fed infants, and that feeding an infant a DHA-enriched formula normalizes the circulating DHA concentrations to those of the breast-fed infants (Clandinin et al., 1997). Observational studies also linked higher concentrations of DHA in plasma and erythrocyte phospholipids with better visual and cognitive outcomes (Innis et al., 2001; Jorgensen et al., 2001; Lauritzen et al., 2004). Although the n-6 LCPUFA AA is also accumulated in neural tissues during postnatal development, no differences in tissue AA composition were noted between breast-fed and formula-fed infants, which suggests that AA accrual does not depend on diet (Makrides et al., 1994). Hence, observational evidence indicates that a postnatal supply of DHA may be necessary for infants born at term to achieve high tissue DHA status. However, to establish physiological and clinical significance, one must demonstrate that higher DHA is causally linked with a developmental advantage. RCTs best provide this evidence. By a random, concealed allocation of infants to an LCPUFA-enriched formula or a standard nonsupplemented formula, many of the factors that may influence child development—such as socioeconomic status, maternal education, exposure to smoking, birth order, sex—are balanced across diets. In a simplistic sense, one may attribute any differences in development between the groups to the intervention. By comparison, observational studies are subject to increased risks of bias because they cannot address all of the possible confounding influences. In the following sections, LCPUFA trials conducted in breast-fed infants are considered separately from formula-fed infants because one can not ethically randomly allocate infants to breast-feeding or formula-feeding, and the dietary intervention strategies clearly differ.

## *Term Infants Fed Human Milk*

International studies of human-milk composition show that the concentration of AA is relatively stable (at approximately 0.4–0.5% of total fatty acids), whereas DHA concentration varies widely between 0.15 and 1.0% of fatty acids (Kneebone et al., 1985; Yuhas et al., 2006). The concentration of DHA in human milk is strongly influenced by the DHA content of the maternal diet (Yuhas et al., 2006). Fish is a rich source of DHA; therefore, lactating women from communities that eat large quantities of fish have high concentrations of DHA in their milk.

Trials that manipulate the concentration of DHA in human milk take advantage of the relationship between maternal fatty-acid intake and the release into milk. Three randomized trials supplemented lactating mothers with fish or algal oil, or foods fortified with fish oil, to increase human-milk DHA, and then measured some aspect of infant development (Table 14.1). Although all trials were successful in raising milk-DHA concentrations, none showed the benefits of increased milk-DHA on infant visual acuity. This finding is surprising considering that other data support the relationship between DHA in milk and infant visual acuity (Jorgensen et al., 2001; Lauritzen et al., 2004). The absence of any effect of DHA on visual acuity may indicate that the lower amount of DHA present in the breast milk (0.2–0.4%) of the control group is adequate to support visual development. Although, other design issues—including small sample sizes (Gibson et al., 1997), a relatively high concentration of DHA in milk of the control group (Lauritzen et al., 2004), or a small difference in milk-DHA between supplemented and control groups (Jensen et al., 2005)—may have contributed to the inability to detect an effect of increased milk-DHA on infant visual acuity.

Neurodevelopmental assessments of children whose lactating mothers were supplemented with DHA yielded mixed findings. The global development of human-milk-fed infants did not differ between those infants whose mothers were supplemented with DHA and those infants whose mothers were not supplemented with DHA (Gibson et al., 1997; Jensen et al., 2005). Although differences in language and motor skills between the supplemented and the control infants were noted, these effects were not consistently observed in all three trials. Further research on the effects of increasing human-milk DHA is warranted since the trials reported here demonstrate that a paucity of evidence is available describing the effects of a relationship between human-milk DHA and specific areas of neurodevelopment such as memory and attention. The push for evidence is particularly pressing because the dietary-supplement industry is including DHA in formulations for lactating women based on the current evidence.

### *Term Infants Fed Formula*

The formula industry commissioned most trials examining LCPUFA and infant development with the aim of preparing infant formulas that mimic the advantageous outcomes of infants fed human milk. Over the last decade, LCPUFA-supplemented formulas for full-term infants were introduced into the Asian, European, and U.S. markets. Although scientists attempted to arrive at a consensus regarding formula enrichment with LCPUFA (Koletzko et al., 2001), disagreement remains regarding the benefits of LCPUFA-supplemented formulas for infants born full term (Simmer et al., 2008a).

**Table 14.1. Randomized Controlled Trials Investigating the Visual or Cognitive Function of Term Infants Fed Human Milk**

| | Intervention | | | Assessment details | | | |
|---|---|---|---|---|---|---|---|
| References | DHA dose (mg/day) and duration of supplementation | *Human milk DHA concentration (% total fat)* | *Sample size* | *Technique* | *Age* | *Findings (treatment group relative to control)* | *Comments* |
| (Gibson et al., 1997) | C: no DHA | C 0.21 | 12 | VEP acuity | 12 and 16 wk | No difference | Small sample sizes |
| | Treatment groups: | | | | | | |
| | $T_A$: 200 mg | $T_A$ 0.35 | 10 | BSID | 1 and 2 yr | No difference | |
| | $T_B$: 400 mg | $T_B$ 0.46 | 12 | | | | |
| | $T_C$: 900 mg | $T_C$ 0.86 | 10 | | | | |
| | $T_D$: 1300 mg | $T_D$ 1.13 | 8 | | | | |
| | Duration: to 12 wk postpartum | | | | | | |
| (Lauritzen et al., 2004; Lauritzen et al., 2005) | C: no DHA | 0.3–0.7 | 60 | VEP acuity | 2 and 4 mo | No difference | Milk DHA in control group is higher than average of American women. |
| | T ≈860 mg | 0.7–1.3 | 62 | | | | |
| | | | | Problem solving | 9 mo | No difference | |
| | Duration: to 4 mo of age | | | MCDI | 1 and 2 yr | Lower vocabulary comprehension at 1 yr, ND at 2 yr | |
| (Jensen et al., 2005) | C no DHA | 0.2 | 115 | VEP and Teller acuity | 4 and 8 mo | No difference | Visual acuity of both groups was lower than expected at 8 months of age. |
| | T≈200 mg | 0.35 | 115 | | | | |
| | Duration: to 4 mo of age | | | GDI<br>CLAMS<br>CAT | 12 and 30 mo | No difference | |
| | | | | BSID | 30 mo | 8-point improvement in BSID MDI | |

Abbreviations: BSID, Bayley Scales of Infant Development; C, control group; CAT, Clinical Adaptive Test; CLAMS, Clinical linguistic and auditory milestone scale; DHA, docosahexaenoic acid; GDI, Gesell Development Inventory; MCDI, MacArthur Communicative Development Inventory; T, treatment group; MDI, mental development index; ND, no difference; VEP, visual-evoked potential.

The disparate opinions in the scientific literature may arise from the small number of RCTs reporting the beneficial effects of LCPUFA supplementation, and, in part, one could attribute this to the low dose of DHA tested in infant formulas. Despite wide variations in human-milk DHA, most infant-formula trials tested relatively low-DHA concentrations within a limited range (0.1–0.4%), and many tested a level of DHA comparable to the "worldwide average" of 0.3% of total fatty acids (Table 14.2). Even though human-milk AA concentrations are fairly consistent across different populations (at ≈0.4%), formulas containing 0–0.7% of AA were tested in term infants. An unclear concern is whether one should base an LCPUFA fortification of formula on concentrations present in human milk, particularly since "optimal" concentrations in human milk are not established.

While the issue of a DHA dose remains controversial, the current evidence from LCPUFA trials examining a broad range of visual and neurodevelopmental outcomes is presented in Table 14.2. The extensive list of trials in Table 14.2 is a testament to the interest in improving formula composition and the outcomes for formula-fed infants.

Trials measuring the visual development of infants either reported positive effects or no difference between infants fed LCPUFA-supplemented formula or nonsupplemented control formula. Of the eight trials using electrophysiological methods to assess visual acuity, five reported an improved acuity in infants fed an LCPUFA-supplemented formula. Only one of the three trials that utilized behavioral techniques reported improved acuity at 2 months of age in infants fed LCPUFA-supplemented formula compared with the control. Uauy et al. (2003) combined data from several trials in a "meta-regression" analysis, and demonstrated that the supply of n-3 fatty acids was strongly related to visual acuity in infancy ($r^2 = 0.68$, $P < 0.001$). Other visual outcome data from LCPUFA-formula trials are consistent with the VEP and behavioral acuity data. An improved stereo-acuity of infants fed LCPUFA-supplemented formulas was reported at 4 months, but no differences are observed by 1 year (Birch et al., 2002, 2005). Interestingly, trials measuring visual outcomes reported the effects of LCPUFA early in infancy, but not at later ages. Do not dismiss these observations as transient effects of LCPUFA because infants learn about their environment through visual experience. In severe cases, a poorer visual input while the visual system is developing can lead to lasting visual impairment (Neuringer, 1996). Nevertheless, it is unknown whether the more subtle differences in infant visual acuity are related to a long-term visual ability or affect other developmental domains.

Summarizing the literature surrounding the effect of LCPUFA-supplemented formula on visual ability raises numerous important issues. One issue is related to trial-sample size, and this is raised again in relationship to developmental assessments. Few trials have had adequate sample sizes to detect a modest effect of DHA-supplemented formulas on behavioral acuity (Tolley & Carlson, 2000), and therefore the trials have an increased risk of a type II error (alternatively called a "false-negative

**Table 14.2. Randomized Controlled Trials Evaluating the Development of Term Infants Fed LCPUFA-supplemented Compared with Standard Formulas**

| | Intervention | | | Outcome assessment[1] |
|---|---|---|---|---|
| References | LCPUFA (% total fat) | Duration | Sample size enrolled | Visual |
| (Makrides et al., 1995) | C: no LCPUFA<br>T: DHA 0.4<br>EPA 0.6<br>GLA 0.3 | Birth to 30 wk | C 19<br>T 13 | VEP acuity at 16 and 30 wk; enhanced in T group |
| (Carlson et al., 1996a) | C: no LCPUFA<br>T: DHA 0.1<br>AA 0.4 | Not stated | C 31<br>T 28 | Teller Acuity at 2, 4, 6, 9, and 12 mo; 0.8 cpd higher in T at 2 mo, ND other times |
| (Auestad et al., 1997; Auestad et al., 2003; Scott et al., 1998) | C: no LCPUFA<br>$T_A$: DHA 0.23<br>$T_B$: DHA 0.12<br>AA 0.43 | Birth to 1 yr | C 65<br>$T_A$ 68<br>$T_B$ 65 | VEP & Teller acuity at 2, 4, 6, 9, 12, and 39 mo; ND |
| (Auestad et al., 2001) | C: no LCPUFA<br>$T_A$: DHA 0.14<br>AA 0.45<br>$T_B$: DHA 0.13<br>AA 0.46 | Birth to 1yr | 77<br>80<br>82 | Behavioral acuity at 2, 4, 6, and 12 mo: ND |
| (Agostoni et al.; 1995; Agostoni et al., 1997) | C: no LCPUFA<br>T: DHA 0.3<br>EPA 0.05<br>GLA 0.3<br>AA 0.44 | Birth to 4 mo | C 31<br>T29 | |
| (Jorgensen et al., 1998) | C: no LCPUFA<br>$T_A$: DHA 0.32<br>AA 0.06<br>$T_B$: DHA 0.32<br>GLA 0.54<br>AA 0.06 | From 1 to 4 mo | C 11<br>$T_A$ 12<br>$T_B$ 14 | sVEP at 4 mo; ND |
| (Willats et al., 1998a; Willatts et al., 1998b) | C: no LCPUFA<br>T: DHA 0.15–0.25<br>AA 0.30–0.40 | Birth to 4 mo | C 38<br>T 34 | |
| (Birch et al., 1998; Birch et al., 2000; Birch et al., 2007; Hoffman et al., 2000) | C: no LCPUFA<br>$T_A$: DHA 0.35<br>$T_B$: DHA 0.36<br>AA 0.72 | Birth to 4 mo | C 26<br>$T_A$ 26<br>$T_B$ 27 | ERG in subset at 6 wk and 4 mo: $T_B$ more mature than $T_A$ and control at 6wk, ND at 4 mo<br>Teller acuity at 6 wk, 4, 6, and 12 mo; ND<br>sVEP acuity: $T_A$ and $T_B$ better than C at 6 wk, 4 and 12 mo<br>HOTV acuity at 4 yr; higher in T (in right eye but not left) |

| Outcome assessment[1] | | |
|---|---|---|
| Global development and intelligence tests | Other outcomes | Comments |
| | | Small SS, dropouts unclear |
| | | 38% dropouts from 4 mo |
| BSID at 12 mo; ND<br>S-B IQ at 39 mo; ND | MCDI at 14 mo; $T_A$ lower than $T_B$ & C in subscales<br>PPVT-R, MLU & Beery-VM at 39 mo; ND | 26–48% dropouts 1997–2003 |
| BSID at 6 and 12 mo: ND | Fagan Infantest at 6 and 9 mo: ND<br>MCDI at 9 and 14 mo: ND | 27% loss to follow up |
| B-L DQ at 4 and 24 mo; ≈9 point higher in T at 4 mo, ND at 24 mo | | 4 mo data NS after adjusting for parent occupation and education |
| | | LCPUFA-supplemented formula groups combined for sVEP analysis |
| | 2-step problem-solving test at 9 mo; ND<br>3-step problem-solving test at 10 mo: T showed greater intention to complete test | Test not standardized or validated for infants |
| BSID at 18 mo; 7-point higher MDI in $T_B$ compared with C. ND between T groups.<br>WPPSI-R at 4 yr; ND | | 24% loss to follow up by 1 yr, 34% at 4 yr |

***Cont. on p. 360.***

**Table 14.2., cont. Randomized Controlled Trials Evaluating the Development of Term Infants Fed LCPUFA-supplemented Compared with Standard Formulas**

| | Intervention | | | Outcome assessment[1] |
|---|---|---|---|---|
| References | LCPUFA (% total fat) | Duration | Sample size enrolled | Visual |
| (Makrides et al., 2000) | C: no LCPUFA<br>$T_A$: DHA 0.35<br>EPA 0.1<br>$T_B$: DHA 0.34<br>AA 0.34 | Birth to 1 yr | C 28<br>$T_A$ 27<br>$T_B$ 28 | VEP acuity at 16 and 34 wk; ND |
| (Lucas et al., 1999; Singhal et al., 2007) | C: no LCPUFA<br>T: DHA 0.32<br>AA 0.30 | Birth to 6 mo | C 155<br>T 154 | Stereo acuity at 4–6 yr: ND<br><br>Visual acuity at 4–6 yr: ND |
| (Birch et al., 2002) | C: no LCPUFA<br>T: DHA 0.36<br>AA 0.72 | BF from birth, then trial formula from 6 wk to 12 mo | C 33<br>T 32 | sVEP at 6 wk, 4, 6, and 12 mo; higher in T at 4, 6, and 12 mo, ND at 6 wk<br><br>Stereo-acuity at 4, 6, 9, and 12 mo: higher in T at 4 mo but ND at other ages |
| (Hoffman et al., 2003) | C: no LCPUFA<br>T: DHA 0.36<br>AA 0.72 | BF 4-6 mo, then trial formula 4 mo to 12 mo | C 35<br>T 33 | VEP acuity at 4, 6, and 12 mo; ND at 4 and 6 mo, T higher than C at 12 mo<br><br>Stereo-acuity at 4, 6, 9, and 12 mo: ND |
| (Bouwstra et al., 2003; Bouwstra et al., 2005) | C: no LCPUFA<br>T: DHA 0.23<br>AA 0.39 | Birth to 2 mo | C 167<br>T 145 | |
| (Unay et al., 2004) | C: no LCPUFA<br>T: DHA 0.5 | Birth to 16 wk | C 26<br>T 28 | |
| (Ben et al., 2004) | C: no LCPUFA<br>$T_A$: DHA 6.9 mg/dm³<br>AA 6.9 mg/dm³<br>$T_B$: mixed BM and $T_A$ | 1 wk to 6 mo | C 52<br>$T_A$ 69<br>$T_B$ 124 | |
| (Birch et al., 2005) | C: no LCPUFA<br>T: DHA 0.36<br>AA 0.72 | Birth to 1 yr | C 52<br>T 51 | VEP acuity at 6 wk, 4 mo, 9 mo and 1 yr; T better than C<br><br>Random-dot stereo-acuity at 4 mo, 9 mo, and 1 yr: higher in T at 4 mo, ND at 9 mo or 1 yr |

Abbreviations: AA, arachidonic acid; BAEP, brainstem auditory-evoked potential; BF, breast-fed; Beery-VM, Beery visuo-motor Index; BSID, Bayley Scales of Infant Development; B-L DQ, Brunet-Lézine Developmental Quotient; C, control group; DHA, docosahexaenoic acid; EPA, eicosapentaenoic acid; ERG, electroretinogram; GLA, gamma linolenic acid; ITT, intention-to-treat; KPS, Knobloch Passamanick and Sherrards test; LCPUFA, long-chain polyunsaturated fatty acids; MCDI, MacArthur Communicative Development Inventory; MDI, Mental Development Index; MLU, mean length of utterance; mo, months; ND, no difference in treatment compared with control group; NS, not significant; PPVT-R, Peabody Picture Vocabulary Test Revised edition; PDI, Psychomotor Development Index; QGM, quality of

| Outcome assessment[1] | | |
|---|---|---|
| Global development and intelligence tests | Other outcomes | Comments |
| BSID at 1 and 2 yr: ND | | |
| BSID at 18 mo: ND<br><br>KPS at 9 mo: ND | | Large SS, well-powered for studying BSID outcomes. 40% loss to follow up at 4–6 yr. |
| | | Low losses to follow-up at 12 mo (only 11%) |
| | | Not ITT analysis |
| BSID at 18 mo: ND | QGM at 3 mo: C group had more infants with mildly abnormal QGM compared with T<br>Hempel classification of motor function at 18 mo: ND | |
| | BAEP at 1wk and 16 wk: maturation was faster in T | Not ITT |
| BSID at 3 and 6 mo: ND | | Unclear loss to follow up and whether ITT. |
| | | 17% loss to follow up at 12 months |

general movements; S-B IQ, Stanford-Binet Intelligence Test; SS, sample size; sVEP, sweep Visual evoked potential; T, treatment group; VEP, visual-evoked potential; wk, week; WPPSI-R, Wechsler preschool and primary scale of intelligence revised; yr, year

[1]Technique, age at assessment, findings in treatment group relative to control.

error," which is accepting the null hypothesis of no effect of DHA when actually a difference does exist). Another issue is that numerous perinatal characteristics and environmental factors were identified as influencing the development of acuity, including birth weight, gender, LCPUFA status at trial entry, and exposure to passive smoking (Makrides et al., 2001). Many trials inadequately reported these variables, and their influence on visual development may have confounded the effects of DHA on infant visual function. Overall, the available trials suggest that supplementing formula with LCPUFA may improve the visual acuity of term infants, but the extent of improvement is not clear.

Seven trials tested the effect of feeding infants LCPUFA-enriched formula on global development. For these trials, the period of supplementation ranged between 2 and 12 months, with follow-up assessments conducted between 3 months to 4 years of age. Sample sizes for trials vary between 11 and over 150 participants per group (Jorgensen et al., 1998; Lucas et al., 1999). Although the majority of trials reported no effect of LCPUFA-supplemented formula on development, a closer examination of the trials shows that few have had an adequate sample size to detect realistic differences in global development. The largest trial showed that infants fed LCPUFA-supplemented formula from birth to 6 months of age exhibited an insignificant 0.5-point improvement in the motor and mental development at 18 months of age (Lucas et al., 1999). Large differences in development between infants fed LCPUFA-supplemented and control formulas are unlikely, considering that the intervention involves a single nutrient in an otherwise well-nourished, healthy population of infants born at term. To demonstrate this point further, observational studies comparing infants fed breast milk and formula show a difference in development of ≈3 points (Anderson et al., 1999; Horwood & Fergusson, 1998). A sample size of 395 per group is needed to demonstrate a 3-point improvement in mental development between infants fed LCPUFA-supplemented and control formulas with 80% power and 95% significance. No trials conducted in term infants have had such a large sample size, and are therefore underpowered for detecting the modest differences in quotients of global development.

Interestingly, the field of LCPUFA research is beginning to move away from measuring child development by using global developmental techniques in favor of more specific measures of cognitive ability, such as the control of attention, memory, as well as social or emotional regulation. This is because these skills contribute, and are important for schooling, learning ability, and socio–emotional interactions. Performance in tests of specific neural functions may also aid in locating any precise effects of DHA supplementation, and prevent any potential blunting when scores across many skills are combined, as is the procedure for assessing global development. We can draw on the knowledge of developmental neuroscientists to create new models for studying the influence of dietary fatty acids on development. Broadly speaking, two general approaches are used to study early development. The first and preferred approach is to conduct a series of assessments of a particular skill, with the assessments growing in complexity as the child's development matures. One can use these data to determine whether the trajectory of the developing skill is influenced by LCPUFA (i.e., whether LCPUFA results in accelerated or delayed maturation). However, for clinical trials, this approach can be time-consuming, expensive, and burdensome to participants with multiple assessments that may limit a successful follow-up. An alternative approach is to assess children at the emergence of a skill, and determine whether LCPUFA accelerates maturation. Colombo et al. (2004) used this approach to study the development of attention in young infants, and noted that those fed LCPUFA-supplemented formulas had more mature-looking behavior than those fed an nonsupplemented formula. The multiple-assessment approach was used by Auestad et al. (1997, 2001, 2003) to examine the effect of LCPUFA-supplemented formula on emerging language skills. Although no differences in language abilities were reported between infants fed the LCPUFA-supplemented formula and the control between 14 and 39 months of age, the study was comprehensive because numerous standardized, age-appropriate techniques were used to assess language abilities.

Exploring the effects of LCPUFA-supplemented formulas on outcomes other than global techniques—such as measuring visual–motor performance, problem-solving abilities, and auditory function (Table 14.2)—provides important information for understanding the full benefits of dietary LCPUFA. Trials reported improved brain-stem auditory responses and problem-solving abilities in infants fed LCPUFA-supplemented formulas compared to the control. A reduction in the incidence of abnormal motor movements after feeding LCPUFA-supplemented formulas also was noted early in infancy; however, these findings were not supported by motor assessments at 18 months of age.

Overall, most of the trials conducted to date describe small advantages or no effect of LCPUFA-supplemented formula on various aspects of both visual and neural development. In examining the evidence from these trials, determining the impact of methodological or trial-design issues on the results (e.g., trials involving a low dose, a short period of supplementation, or small sample sizes) is difficult. Particularly important is to consider whether the trials were designed to detect a realistic difference in development. For future research, the impetus is to examine the long-term effects of LCPUFA-supplemented formulas (i.e., into childhood) because these findings will be more strongly associated with adult outcomes. Long-term effects of LCPUFA need to be addressed by high-quality, adequately powered, randomized controlled trials.

## Visual and Neural Functions of Preterm Infants

Although DHA is accumulated in neural tissues throughout development, the most rapid phase of DHA accretion occurs during the brain-growth spurt in the last trimester of pregnancy (Clandinin et al., 1980). Preterm infants are denied the usual gestational period to accrue DHA in retinal and neural tissues. Since DHA is concentrated in retinal and neural tissues, possibly the supply of DHA may contribute to the poorer visual and cognitive outcomes that preterm infants exhibit compared with infants born at full term.

Feeding preterm infants can be problematic due to their high requirement for nutrients to support rapid growth, minimal nutrient stores, and also their immaturity. In most cases, very preterm infants are fed intravenously while they are stabilized, after which they are cautiously introduced to enteral feeds through a nasogastric feeding tube (Jones Wessel, 2000). Very preterm infants are too immature to commence sucking feeds, and mothers of preterm infants invest considerable energy in expressing milk to initiate and maintain lactation. One can introduce sucking feeds only when the infant is medically stable and mature enough to coordinate the breathe–suck–swallow reflex, which usually occurs around 32–34 weeks post-menstrual age (Gryboski, 1969; Mizuno & Ueda, 2003; Nyqvist et al., 1999).

As with term infants, LCPUFA trials involving preterm infants were predominantly conducted on those fed formula. As a result of this research effort, DHA-enriched preterm formulas are now widely used in neonatal nurseries. Although optimizing the DHA content of formula is important, until recently, few trials had investigated human-milk DHA. This is surprising because studies involving preterm infants fed human milk are important for two reasons. First, most preterm infants are fed human milk during the neonatal period (Furman et al., 1998; Yip et al., 1996), and therefore this research has relevance for a large number of preterm infants. Second, human milk offers the immunologically immature, vulnerable preterm infant crucial protection from disease (Oddy, 2002).

## *Preterm Infants Fed Human Milk*

Using different approaches to supplementation, two RCTs involved the DHA supplementation of human milk fed to preterm infants (Table 14.3). Smithers et al. (2008b) incorporated both human milk and formula feeding into their intervention by supplementing lactating mothers with tuna-oil capsules to increase human-milk DHA and by supplying a preterm formula with a matching DHA composition if complementary milk was required. By comparison, Henriksen et al. (2008) examined the addition of LCPUFA (both DHA and AA) as algal and fungal oil or placebo oil directly to expressed human milk, and then sonicated the milk to emulsify the oil. Both trials reported improved outcomes in LCPUFA-supplemented infants compared to the control, which included higher visual acuity at 4 months and problem solving and recognition-memory ability at 6 months.

Clearly, the consistency in the size, direction, and benefits of feeding preterm infants higher concentrations of DHA than usually present in human milk of Western women provides important evidence to support changes in clinical practice. These data also raise questions about formula-DHA composition because both trials supplemented human milk with DHA concentrations higher than current preterm formulas that are currently enriched with 0.35%. Both groups are planning further follow-up of the preterm infants in their trials that will provide evidence of the long-term effects of high-dose DHA.

**Table 14.3. Randomized Controlled Trials Involving LCPUFA Supplementation of Human Milk to Fed Preterm Infants**

| | Intervention | | | Outcome assessment (technique, age at assessment, findings in treatment group relative to control) | | | |
|---|---|---|---|---|---|---|---|
| References | LCPUFA (% total fat) | Duration | Sample size enrolled | Visual | Global development and intelligence tests | Other outcomes | Comments |
| (Smithers et al., 2008b) | C: DHA 0.2– 0.35 AA 0.5<br>T: DHA 1.0 AA 0.5 | ≤ 5 days from commencement of enteral feeds to EDD | 74<br>69 | VEP acuity at 2 and 4 moCA; ND at 2 moCA but 1.4 cpd improvement in acuity at 4 moCA | | | 8% loss to follow up |
| (Henriksen et al., 2008) | C: DHA 0.7 AA 0.5<br>T: DHA 1.4 AA 1.2 | When EI >100 mL/kg/day to discharge or completion of 100-mL bottle of study oil | 73<br>68 | | Ages and Stages Q'naire at 6 mo; improved problem-solving subscore in T group | ERPs at 6 mo; lower amplitudes in T group indicating better recognition memory processing | ≈ 25% infants received some formula 26% loss to follow up |

Abbreviations: AA, arachidonic acid; C, control group; cpd, cycles per degree; DHA, docosahexaenoic acid; EDD, estimated due date; EI, enteral intake; ERP, event related potentials; moCA, months corrected age; ND, no difference; Q'nnaire, questionnaire; T, treatment group; VEP, visual-evoked potential.

**Table 14.4.** **Randomized Controlled Trials Involving LCPUFA Supplementation of Formula Fed to Preterm Infants**

| | Intervention | | | Outcome assessment[1] |
|---|---|---|---|---|
| References | LCPUFA (% total fat) | Duration | Sample size enrolled | Visual |
| (Birch et al., 1992) | C: no LCPUFA<br>T: DHA 0.4 | <d 11 to 4 moCA | Total *n* = 73 (unclear which group) | ERG: improved rod responses at 37 wk PMA but not at 4 moCA<br>VEP acuity: improved acuity at 37 wk PMA and 4 moCA<br>Teller acuity: no difference |
| (Faldella et al., 1996) | C: no LCPUFA<br>T: DHA 0.3<br>AA 0.4 | To 3 moCA | 26<br>23 | Flash VEP latencies at 3 moCA; more mature latency in T group<br>Flash ERG at 3 moCA: ND |
| (Bougle et al., 1999) | C: no LCPUFA<br>T: DHA 0.6<br>AA 0.1 | d 2 for at least 30 days | 11<br>14 | Flash VEP latency at d 30: ND |
| (O'Connor et al., 2001) | C: no LCPUFA<br>$T_A$: DHA 0.27<br>AA 0.43<br>$T_B$: DHA 0.24<br>AA 0.41 | d 4 until 12 moCA | <br>144<br><br>140 | VEP acuity at 4 and 6 moCA: ≈4 cpd improvement in subset of infants (*n* = 126) at 6 moCA.<br>Behavioral acuity at 2, 4, and 6 moCA: ND |
| (Innis et al., 2002) | C: no LCPUFA<br>$T_A$: DHA 0.3<br>AA 0<br>$T_B$: DHA 0.3<br>AA 0.6 | >28 days | 62<br>66<br><br>66 | Behavioral acuity at 2 and 4 moCA: ND |
| (van Wezel-Meijler et al., 2002) | C: no LCPUFA<br>T: DHA 0.3<br>AA 0.7 | <d 14 to 6 moCA | 26<br>29 | Behavioral acuity at 3, 6, 12, and 24 moCA: ND<br>Flash VEP latency at 3 and 12 moCA: ND |
| (Carlson, 1993; Carlson et al., 1993; Werkman & Carlson, 1996) | C: no LCPUFA<br>T: DHA 0.2<br>AA 0 | From ≈d 25 (≈32 wk PMA) to 9 moCA | 33<br>39<br>Number completed trial | Behavioral acuity at 2, 4, 6.5, 9,and 12 moCA; improved acuity at 2 and 4 mo CA but ND at other ages |

| Outcome assessment[1] | | |
|---|---|---|
| Global development and intelligence tests | Other outcomes | Comments |
| | | Randomization and follow-up of participants unclear |
| | BAEP at 3 mo: ND | ERG method deviated from standard protocol which may have reduced test sensitivity |
| | BAEP at d 30: ND<br>Motor NCV at d 30: longer latency indicating slower maturation | |
| BSID at 12 moCA; overall ND, but infants born <1250 g had 9-point improvement in PDI | Fagan Infantest at 6 and 9 moCA: $T_A$ better than $T_B$ and C at 6 but not 9 moCA MCDI at 9 and 14 moCA: ND, but removal of twins or non-native English speakers from analysis showed higher vocabulary comprehension | |
| | | |
| BSID at 3, 6, 12, and 24 mo CA: ND | Cerebral myelination at 3 and 12 moCA by MRI: ND | Infants excluded after randomization if developed neurological symptoms |
| BSID at 12 mo: ND in MDI , 10-point lower PDI | Fagan Infantest at 6.5, 9, and 12 moCA: increased number of looks but decreased overall look duration | |

***Cont. on p. 368.***

**Table 14.4., cont. Randomized Controlled Trials Involving LCPUFA Supplementation of Formula Fed to Preterm Infants**

| | Intervention | | | Outcome assessment[1] |
|---|---|---|---|---|
| References | LCPUFA (% total fat) | Duration | Sample size enrolled | Visual |
| (Carlson et al., 1994; Carlson & Werkman, 1996; Carlson et al., 1996b) | C: no LCPUFA<br>T: DHA 0.2<br>AA 0 | From ≈d 3 to 2 moCA | 33<br>26<br>Number completed trial | Behavioral acuity at 2, 4, 6, 9, and 12 moCA: improved acuity at 2 moCA, ND at other ages |
| (Fewtrell et al., 2002) | C: no LCPUFA<br>T: DHA 0.17<br>AA 0.31 | d 10 to discharge | 100<br>95 | |
| (Fewtrell et al., 2004) | C: no LCPUFA<br>T: DHA 0.5<br>GLA 0.9<br>AA 0.04 | To 9 moCA | 116<br>122 | |
| (Clandinin et al., 2005) | C: no LCPUFA<br>$T_A$: DHA 0.3<br>AA 0.7<br>$T_B$: DHA 0.3<br>AA 0.7 | From start of enteral feeds to 12 moCA | 119<br>112<br>130 | |
| (Fang et al., 2005) | C: no LCPUFA<br>T: DHA 0.2<br>AA 0.4 | To 6 moCA | 11<br>16 | VEP acuity at 4 and 6 moCA; ND<br>Lea behavioral acuity cards at 4 and 6 moCA: ND<br>Hiding Heidi contrast cards at 4 and 6 moCA: ND |

Abbreviations: AA, arachidonic acid; BAEP, brainstem auditory-evoked potential; BSID, Bayley scales of infant development; C, control group; DHA, docosahexaenoic acid; ERG, electroretinogram; ITT, intention to treat analysis; LCPUFA, long-chain polyunsaturated fatty acid; MCDI, MacArthur communicative development inventory; MDI, mental development index; moCA, months Corrected Age; NCV, nerve conduction velocity; MRI, magnetic resonance imaging; ND, no difference between treatment and control groups; PDI, psychomotor development index; PMA, post-menstrual age; T, treatment group; VEP, visual-evoked potential.

[1] Technique, age at assessment, findings in treatment group relative to control.

| Outcome assessment[1] | | |
|---|---|---|
| Global development and intelligence tests | Other outcomes | Comments |
| BSID at 12 moCA: 11-point higher MDI | Fagan Infantest at 12 moCA; increased number and shorter duration of looks | Large number of dropouts after 2 moCA |
| KPS at 9 moCA: ND<br>BSID at 18 moCA: ND | | |
| KPS at 9 moCA: ND<br>BSID at 18 moCA: ND overall but ≈6-point increase in MDI in the boys subgroup | | |
| BSID at 18 moCA: ≈8-point improvement in MDI and PDI | | $T_A$ fatty acids sourced from algal and fungal oils, $T_B$ from fish oil. Not ITT as only part of cohort that complied with protocol followed to 18 moCA |
| BSID at 6 and 12 moCA: approximately 5-point improvement in MDI and PDI at 6 mo and 8- to 11- point improvement at 12 moCA | | LCPUFA in formula estimated from published data. Not ITT |

### *Preterm Infants Fed Formula*

Trials conducted in exclusively or predominantly formula-fed preterm infants generally demonstrated improved visual and cognitive functions (Table 14.4), and these data supported the widespread use of LCPUFA-supplemented formulas in this population.

Improved ERG responses, indicating an enhanced sensitivity of the retina to light, show that visual function of preterm infants could be increased after only 3 weeks of feeding them LCPUFA-supplemented formulas (Birch et al., 1992). By 4 months of age, differences in retinal function were no longer present; however, improved VEP acuity was observed in infants fed the LCPUFA-supplemented formula compared to the control (Birch et al., 1992). Further work confirmed that the visual acuity of preterm infants fed LCPUFA-supplemented formulas is improved, with most trials observing improvements around 2 and 4 months of age (Carlson et al., 1993, 1996b; O'Connor et al., 2001). Although three trials reported no differences between infants fed LCPUFA-supplemented formula and the control, the potential to detect a difference in acuity may have been impeded by the fact that these trials had small sample sizes, a low dose, or a short duration of DHA supplementation (Fang et al., 2005; Innis et al., 2002; van Wezel-Meijler et al., 2002).

Improved global development was observed in some of the LCPUFA-supplementation trials (Table 14.4). We recently conducted a systematic review and meta-analysis to quantitate the extent of the benefit of LCPUFA-supplemented formulas on the global development of preterm infants (Smithers et al., 2008a). We found that infants fed LCPUFA-supplemented formulas had a 2-point improvement in mental development compared with those fed a nonsupplemented formula, but motor development did not differ. These findings were in contrast to the Cochrane review (Simmer et al., 2008b), but were consistent with recommendations made by international working groups (Koletzko et al., 2008) and learned scientific societies (International Society for the Study of Fatty Acids and Lipids, 2008).

Other neurodevelopmental data show that preterm infants fed LCPUFA-supplemented formulas display differences in visual attention, as measured by recognition-memory testing (using the Fagan Infantest). Possibly, changes in visual-looking behavior associated with LCPUFA-enriched formulas may be indicative of faster or more mature processing of visual information (Cheatham et al., 2006).

Any improvement in visual or neural functions of preterm infants is important because these infants are at an increased risk of poorer long-term development compared with term-born infants. Trials conducted in preterm infants indicate improved visual and global development with LCPUFA fortification of human milk and formula. However, the recent publication of trials in preterm infants fed high doses of DHA in human milk raises questions about formula-DHA composition, and highlights that further work is needed to elucidate the dietary supply of DHA that results in optimal development.

## Conclusion

The n-3 LCPUFA DHA was implicated as a factor influencing both visual and neural development of infants. In general, the enrichment of formula with LCPUFA appears to be safe in terms of child development; this resulted in widespread acceptance and use of these formulas. The evidence of efficacy of LCPUFA is strongest for preterm infants, yet recent studies highlight that further work is necessary to optimize the amount of DHA in human milk; this may inevitably lead to changes in preterm-formula composition. For infants born full-term, current evidence indicates small benefits to visual development in infancy, and while the potential for improved global development is plausible, findings from clinical trials are less clear. Future research should focus on the dose of DHA, a variety of outcome measures linked with long-term development, and the determination of whether any benefits of an early dietary supply of LCPUFA are sustained into childhood. One should also emphasize the study of breast-milk DHA for further research. Clearly establishing the concentration of DHA required in breast milk for optimal visual and neural development is a fundamental issue, which will ultimately support breastfeeding and the wider benefits that human-milk feeding can provide to both mother and infant.

### References

Agostoni, C.; S. Trojan; R. Bellu; E. Riva; M.G. Bruzzese; M. Giovannini. Developmental quotient at 24 months and fatty acid composition of diet in early infancy: a follow up study. *Arch. Dis. Child.* **1997,** *76(5),* 421–424.

Agostoni, C.; S. Trojan; R. Bellu; E. Riva; M. Giovannini. Neurodevelopmental quotient of healthy term infants at 4 months and feeding practice: the role of long-chain polyunsaturated fatty acids. *Pediatr. Res.* **1995,** *38(2),* 262–266.

Anderson, R.E. Lipids of ocular tissues. IV. A comparison of the phospholipids from the retina of six mammalian species. *Exp. Eye Res.* **1970,** *10,* 339–344.

Anderson, J.W.; B.M. Johnstone; D.T. Remley. Breast-feeding and cognitive development: a meta-analysis. *Am. J. Clin. Nutr.* **1999,** *70(4),* 525–535.

Anderson, R.E.; L. Sperling. Positional distribution of the fatty acids in the phospholipids of bovine retina rod outer segments. *Arch. Biochem. Biophys.* **1971,** *144(2),* 673–677.

Auestad, N.; R. Halter; R.T. Hall; M. Blatter; M.L.G. Bogle; W. Burks; J.R. Erickson; K.M. Fitzgerald; V. Dobson; S.M. Innis; et al. Growth and development in term infants fed long-chain polyunsaturated fatty acids: A double-masked, randomized, parallel, prospective, multivariate study. *Pediatrics* **2001,** *108(2),* 372–381.

Auestad, N.; M.B. Montalto; R.T. Hall; K.M. Fitzgerald; R.E. Wheeler; W.E. Connor; M. Neuringer; S.L. Connor; J.A. Taylor; E.E. Hartmann. Visual acuity, erythrocyte fatty acid composition, and growth in term infants fed formulas with long chain polyunsaturated fatty acids for one year. *Pediatr. Res.* **1997,** *41(1),* 1–10.

Auestad, N.; D.T. Scott; J. Janowsky; C. Jacobsen; R. E. Carroll; M.B. Montalto; R. Halter; W. Qiu; J. Jacobs; W.E. Connor; et al. Visual, cognitive and language assessments at 39 months. A follow-up study of children fed formulas containing long-chain polyunsaturated fatty acids to 1 year of age. *Pediatrics* **2003,** *112(3),* e177 e183.

Bayley, N. *Bayley Scales of Infant Development,* 2nd ed.; The Psychological Corporation, Harcourt Brace & Company: San Antonio, TX, 1993.

Bayley, N. *Bayley Scales of Infant and Toddler Development Administration Manual,* 3rd ed.; Harcourt Assessment: San Antonio, TX, 2006.

Ben, X.-m.; X.-y. Zhou; W.-h. Zhao; W.-l. Yu; W. Pan; W.-l. Zhang; S.-m. Wu; C.M. Van Beusekom; A. Schaafsma. Growth and development of term infants fed with milk with long-chain polyunsaturated fatty acid supplementation. *Chin. Med. J.* **2004,** *117(8),* 1268–1270.

Birch, D.; E. Birch; D.R. Hoffman; R. Uauy. Retinal development of very low birthweight infants fed diets differing in n-3 fatty acids. *Invest. Ophthalmol. Vis. Sci.* **1992,** *33,* 2365–2376.

Birch, E.E.; Y.S. Castaneda; D.H. Wheaton; D.G. Birch; R.D. Uauy; D.R. Hoffman. Visual maturation of term infants fed long-chain polyunsaturated fatty acid-supplemented or control formula for 12 mo. *Am. J. Clin. Nutr.* **2005,** *81(4),* 871–879.

Birch, E.; S. Garfield; Y.S. Castaneda; D. Hughbanks-Wheaton; R. Uauy; D.R. Hoffman. Visual acuity and cognitive outcomes at 4 years of age in a double-blind, randomized trial of long-chain polyunsaturated fatty acid-supplemented infant formula. *Early Hum. Dev.* **2007,** *83(5),* 279–283.

Birch, E.; S. Garfield; D.R. Hoffman; R. Uauy; D. Birch. A randomized controlled trial of early dietary supply of long-chain polyunsaturated fatty acids and mental development in term infants. *Dev. Med. Child Neurol.* **2000,** *42,* 174–181.

Birch, E.E.; D.R. Hoffman; Y.S. Castaneda; S.L. Fawcett; D.G. Birch; R.D. Uauy. A randomized controlled trial of long-chain polyunsaturated fatty acid supplementation of formula in term infants after weaning at 6 wk of age. *Am. J. Clin. Nutr.* **2002,** *75(3),* 570–580.

Birch, E.; D.R. Hoffman; R. Uauy; D. Birch; C. Prestidge. Visual acuity and the essentiality of docosahexaenoic acid and arachidonic acid in the diet of term infants. *Pediatr. Res.* **1998,** *44(2),* 201–209.

Bougle, D.; P. Denise; F. Vimard; A. Biyvekit; M.J. Penniello; B. Guillois. Early neurological and neurophysiological development of the preterm infant and polyunsaturated fatty acids supply. *Clin. Neurophysiol.* **1999,** *110,* 1363–1370.

Bouwstra, H.; A.J. Dijck-Brouwer; G. Boehm; E.R. Boersma; F.A.J. Muskiet; M. Hadders-Algra. Long-chain polyunsaturated fatty acids and neurological developmental outcome at 18 months in healthy term infants. *Acta Paediatr.* **2005,** *94,* 26–32.

Bouwstra, H.; D.A.J. Dijck-Brouwer; J.A.L. Wildeman; H.M. Tjoonk; J.C. van der Heide; E.R. Boersma; F.A.J. Muskiet; M. Huadders-Algra. Long-chain polyunsaturated fatty acids have a positive effect on the quality of general movements of healthy term infants. *Am. J. Clin. Nutr.* **2003,** *78,* 313–318.

Cao, J.; K.A. Schwichtenberg; N.Q. Hanson; M.Y. Tsai. Incorporation and clearance of omega-3 fatty acids in erythrocyte membranes and plasma phospholipids. *Clin. Chem.* **2006,** *52(12),* 2265–2272.

Carlson, S.E. Lipid requirements of very-low-birth-weight infants for optimal growth and development. *Lipids, Learning, and the Brain: Fats in Infant Formulas*; J. Dobbing; Ed Ross Laboratories: Columbus, Ohio, 1993; pp. 188–207.

Carlson, S.E.; A.J. Ford; S.H. Werkman; J.M. Peeples; W.W. Koo. Visual acuity and fatty acid status of term infants fed human milk and formulas with and without docosahexaenoate and arachidonate from egg yolk lecithin. *Pediatr. Res.* **1996a,** *39(5),* 882–888.

Carlson, S.E.; S.H. Werkman. A randomized trial of visual attention of preterm infants fed docosahexaenoic acid until two months. *Lipids* **1996,** *31(1),* 85–90.

Carlson, S.E.; S.H. Werkeman; J.M. Peeples; W.M. Wilson. *Growth and Development of Premature InfantsiIn Relation to ω3 and ω6 Fatty Acid Status,* 1994; C. Galli, A.P. Simopoulos, E. Tremoli, Eds.; Karger: 1994; pp. 63–69.

Carlson, S.E.; S.H. Werkman; P.G. Rhodes; E.A. Tolley. Visual-acuity development in healthy preterm infants: effect of marine-oil supplementation. *Am. J. Clin. Nutr.* **1993,** *58,* 35–42.

Carlson, S.E.; S.H. Werkman; E.A. Tolley. Effect of long-chain n-3 fatty acid supplementation on visual acuity and growth of preterm infants with and without bronchopulmonary dysplasia. *Am. J. Clin. Nutr.* **1996b,** *63,* 687–697.

Cheatham, C.L.; J. Colombo; S.E. Carlson. n-3 Fatty acids and cognitive and visual acuity development: methodologic and conceptual considerations. *Am. J. Clin. Nutr.* **2006,** *83 (Suppl.),* 1458S–1466S.

Clandinin, M.T.; J.E. Chappell; S. Leong; T. Heim; P.R. Sawyer; G.W. Chance. Intrauterine fatty acid accretion rates in human brain: implications for fatty acid requirements. *Early Hum. Dev.* **1980,** *4(2),* 121–129.

Clandinin, M.T.; J.E. Van Aerde; K.L. Merkel; C.L. Harris; M.A. Springer; J.W. Hansen; D.A. Diersen-Schade. Growth and development of preterm infants fed infant formulas containing docosahexaenoic acid and arachidonic acid. *J. Pediatr.* **2005,** *146,* 461–468.

Clandinin, M.T.; J.E. Van Aerde; A. Parrott; C.J. Field; A.R. Euler; E.L. Lien. Assessment of the efficacious dose of arachidonic and docosahexaenoic acids in preterm infant formulas: Fatty acid composition of erythrocyte membrane lipids. *Pediatr. Res.* **1997,** *42,* 819–825.

Clandinin, M.T.; J.E. Van Aerde; A. Parrott; C.J. Field; A.R. Euler; E. Lien. Assessment of feeding different amounts of arachidonic and docosahexaenoic acids in preterm infant formulas on the fatty acid content of lipoprotein lipids. *Acta Paediatr.* **1999,** *88,* 890–896.

Colombo, J.; K.N. Kannass; J. Shaddy; S. Kundurthi; J.M. Maikranz; C.J. Anderson; O.M. Blaga; S.E. Carlson. Maternal DHA and the development of attention in infancy and toddlerhood. *Child Dev.* **2004,** *75(4),* 1254–1267.

Cotman, C.; M.L. Blank; A. Moehl; F. Synder. Lipid composition of synaptic plasma membranes isolated from rat brain by zonal centrifugation. *Biochemistry* **1968,** *8(11),* 4606–4611.

Duckman, R.H. Infant, toddler, and children's visual acuity—practical aspects. *Visual Development, Diagnosis, and Treatment of the Pediatric Patient;* R.H. Duckman, Ed.; Lippincott Williams & Wilkins: 2006; pp. 190–204.

Faldella, G.; M. Govoni; R. Alessangroni; E. Marchiani; G.P. Salvioli; P.L. Biagi; C. Spano. Visual evoked potentials and dietary long chain polyunsaturated fatty acids in preterm infants. *Arch. Dis. Child Fetal Neonatal Ed.* **1996,** *75,* F108–F112.

Fang, P.-C.; H.-K. Kuo; C.-B. Huang; T.-Y. Ko; C.-C. Chen; M.-Y. Chung. The effect of supplementation of docosahexaenoic acid and arachidonic acid on visual acuity and neurodevelopment in larger preterm infants. *Chang Gung Med. J.* **2005,** *28,* 708–715.

Fewtrell, M.S.; R.A. Abbott; K. Kennedy; A. Singhal; R. Morley; E. Caine; C. Jamieson; F. Cockburn; A. Lucas. Randomized, double-blind trial of long-chain polyunsaturated fatty acid supplementation with fish oil and borage oil in preterm infants. *J. Pediatr.* **2004,** *144*, 471–479.

Fewtrell, M.S.; R. Morley; R.A. Abbott; A. Singhal; E.B. Isaacs; T. Stephenson; U. MacFadyen; A. Lucas. Double-blind, randomized trial of long-chain polyunsaturated fatty acid supplementation in formula fed to preterm infants. *Pediatrics* **2002,** *110(1),* 73–82.

Furman, L.; N. Minich; M. Hack. Breastfeeding of very low birth weight infants. *J. Hum. Lact.* **1998,** *14(1),* 29–34.

Gibson, R.A.; M.A. Neumann; M. Makrides. Effect of increasing breast milk docosahexaenoic acid on plasma and erythrocyte phospholipid fatty acids and neural indices of exclusively breast fed infants. *Eur. J. Clin. Nutr.* **1997,** *51,* 578–584.

Gryboski, J.D. Suck and swallow in the premature infant. *Pediatrics* **1969,** *43(1),* 96–102.

Haggarty, P.; K. Page; D.R. Abramovich; J. Ashton; D. Brown. Long-chain polyunsaturated fatty acid transport across the perfused human placenta. *Placenta* **1997,** *18,* 635–642.

Han, M.H.E.; R.H. Duckman. Clinical tests of fusion and stereopsis. *Visual Development, Diagnosis, and Treatment of the Pediatric Patient;* R.H. Duckman, Ed.; Lippincott, Williams and Wilkins: 2006.

Harris, W.S.; J.V. Pottala; S.A. Sands; P.G. Jones. Comparison of the effects of fish and fish-oil capsules on the n-3 fatty acid content of blood cells and plasma phospholipids. *Am. J. Clin. Nutr.* **2007,** *86(6),* 1621–1625.

Henriksen, C.; K. Haugholt; M. Lindgren; A.K. Aurvag; A. Ronnestad; M. Gronn; R. Solberg; A. Moen; B. Nakstad; R.K. Berge; et al. Improved cognitive development among preterm infants attributable to early supplementation of human milk with docosahexaenoic acid and arachidonic acid. *Pediatrics* **2008,** *121(6),* 1137–1145.

Hoffman, D.R.; E.E. Birch; D.G. Birch; R. Uauy; Y.S. Castaneda; M.G. Lapus; D.H. Wheaton. Impact of early dietary intake and blood lipid composition of long-chain polyunsaturated fatty acids on later visual development. *J. Pediatr. Gastroenterol. Nutr.* **2000,** *31(5),* 540–553.

Hoffman, D. R.; E. E. Birch; Y. S. Castaneda; S. L. Fawcett; D. H. Wheaton; D. G. Birch; R. Uauy. Visual function in breast-fed term infants weaned to formula with or without long-chain polyunsaturates at 4 to 6 months: a randomized clinical trial. *J Pediatr* **2003,** *142*, 669-677.

Holmes, J.M.; R.W. Beck; M.X. Repka; D.A. Leske; R.T. Kraker; C.R. Blair; P. S. Moke; E.E. Birch; R.A. Saunders; R.W. Hertle; et al. The amblyopia treatment study visual acuity testing protocol. *Arch. Ophthal.* **2001,** *119(9),* 1345–1353.

Horwood, L.J.; D.M. Fergusson. Breastfeeding and later cognitive and academic outcomes. *Pediatrics* **1998,** *101(1)*, e9–e16.

Hsieh, A.T.; J.C. Anthony; D.A. Diersen-Schade; S.C. Rumsey; P. Lawrence; C. Li; P.W. Nathanielsz; J.T. Brenna. The influence of moderate and high dietary long chain polyunsaturated fatty acids (LCPUFA) on baboon neonate tissue fatty acids. *Pediatr. Res.* **2007,** *61(5),* 1–9.

Innis, S.M. Dietary (n-3) fatty acids and brain development. *J. Nutr.* **2007,** *137(4)*, 855–859.

Innis, S.M.; D.H. Adamkin; R.T. Hall; S.C. Kalban; C. Lair; M. Lim; D.C. Stevens; P.F. Twist; D.A. Diersen-Schade; C.L. Harris; et al. Docosahexaenoic acid and arachidonic acid enhance growth with no adverse effects in preterm infants fed formula. *J. Pediatr.* **2002,** *140*, 547–554.

Innis, S.M.; J. Gilley; J. Werker. Are human milk long-chain polyunsaturated fatty acids related to visual and neural development in breast-fed term infants? *J. Pediatr.* **2001,** *139*, 532–538.

International Society for the Study of Fatty Acids and Lipids. Policy Statement 2: ISSFAL Statement on dietary fats in infant nutrition; *International Society for the Study of Fatty Acids and Lipids;* Kansas City, MO, 2008.

Jensen, C.L.; R.G. Voight; T.C. Prager; Y.L. Zou; K. Fraley; J.C. Rozelle; M.R. Turcich; A.M. Llorente; R.E. Anderson; W.C. Heird. Effects of maternal docosahexaenoic acid intake on visual function and neurodevelopment in breastfed term infants. *Am. J. Clin. Nutr.* **2005,** *82*, 125–132.

Jones Wessel, J. Feeding methodologies. *Nutritional Care for High-risk Newborns*, 3rd ed.; S. Groh-Wargo, M. Thompson, J. Hovasi Cox, Eds.; Precept Press: Chicago, Illinois, 2000.

Jorgensen, M.H.; O. Hernell; E.L. Hughes; K.F. Michaelsen. Is there a relation between docosahexaenoic acid concentration in mothers' milk and visual development in term infants? *J. Pediatr. Gastroenterol. Nutr.* **2001,** *32*, 293–296.

Jorgensen, M.H.; G. Holmer; P. Lund; O. Hernell; K.F. Michaelsen. Effect of formula supplemented with docosahexaenoic acid and gamma-linolenic acid on fatty acid status and visual acuity in term infants. *J. Pediatr. Gastroenterol. Nutr.* **1998,** *26*, 412–421.

Katan, M.B.; J.P. Deslypere; A.P. van Birgelen; M. Penders; M. Zegwaard. Kinetics of the incorporation of dietary fatty acids into serum cholesteryl esters, erythrocyte membranes, and adipose tissue: an 18-month controlled study. *J. Lipid Res.* **1997,** *38(10)*, 2012–2022.

Kneebone, G.M.; R. Kneebone; R.A. Gibson. Fatty acid composition of breast milk form three racial groups from Penang, Malaysia. *Am. J. Clin. Nutr.* **1985,** *41*, 765–769.

Koletzko, B.; C. Agostini; S.E. Carlson; M.T. Clandinin; G. Horntsra; M. Neuringer; R. Uauy; Y. Yamashiro; P. Willats. Long chain polyunsaturated fatty acids (LC-PUFA) and perinatal development. *Acta Paediatr.* **2001,** *90*, 460–464.

Koletzko, B.; E. Lien; C. Agostoni; H. Bohles; C. Campoy; I. Cetin; T. Decsi; J.W. Dudenhausen; C. Dupont; S. Forsythe; I. Hoesli; W. Holzgreve; A. Lapillone; G. Putet; N.J. Secher; M. Symonds; H. Szajewska; P. Willats; R. Uauy. The roles of long-chain polyunsaturated fatty acids in pregnancy, lactation and infancy: review of current knowledge and consensus recommendations. *J. Perinat. Med.* **2008,** *36(1),* 5–14.

Lauritzen, L.; M.H. Jorgensen; T.B. Mikkelsen; I.M. Skovgaard; E.-M. Straarup; S.F. Olsen; C.-E. Hoy; K.F. Michaelsen. Maternal fish oil supplementation in lactation: Effect on visual acuity and n-3 fatty acid content of infant erythrocytes. *Lipids* **2004,** *39(3),* 195–206.

Lauritzen, L.; M.H. Jorgensen; S.F. Olsen; E.M. Straarup; K.F. Michaelsen. Maternal fish oil supplementation in lactation: effect on developmental outcome in breast-fed infants. *Reprod. Nutr. Dev.* **2005,** *45(5),* 535–547.

Lucas, A.; M. Stafford; R. Morley; R.A. Abbott; T. Stephenson; U. MacFadyen; A. Elias-Jones; H. Clements. Efficacy and safety of long-chain polyunsaturated fatty acid supplementation of infant-formula milk: a randomised trial. *Lancet* **1999,** *354(4),* 1948–1954.

Makrides, M.; M.A. Neumann; R.W. Byard; K. Simmer; R.A. Gibson. Fatty acid composition of brain, retina, and erythrocytes in breast- and formula-fed infants. *Am. J. Clin. Nutr.* **1994,** *60*, 189–194.

Makrides, M.; M.A. Neumann; R.A. Gibson. Perinatal characteristics may influence the outcome of visual acuity. *Lipids* **2001,** *36(9),* 897–900.

Makrides, M.; M.A. Neumann; K. Simmer; R.A. Gibson. A critical appraisal of the role of dietary long-chain polyunsaturated fatty acids on neural indices of term infants: A randomized controlled trial. *Pediatrics* **2000,** *105,* 32–38.

Makrides, M.; M.A. Neumann; K. Simmer; J. Pater; R.A. Gibson. Are long-chain polyunsaturated fatty acids essential nutrients in infancy? *Lancet* **1995,** *345,* 1463–1468.

Martinez, M. Tissue levels of polyunsaturated fatty acids during early human development. *J. Pediatr.* **1992,** *120(Suppl.),* S129–S138.

Martinez, M.; I. Mougan. Fatty acid composition of human brain phospholipids during normal development. *J. Neurochem.* **1998,** *71,* 2528–2533.

Mizuno, K.; A. Ueda. The maturation and coordination of sucking, swallowing, and respiration in preterm infants. *J. Pediatr.* **2003,** *142(1),* 36–40.

Mortensen, E.L.; K.F. Michaelsen; S.A. Sanders; J.M. Reinisch. The association between duration of breastfeeding and adult intelligence. *JAMA* **2002,** *287(18),* 2365–2371.

Neuringer, M. Assessment of retinal function and vision in infants. *Assessment of Infant Visual and Cognitive Function in Relation to Long Chain Polyunsaturated Fatty Acids;* S.E. Carlson, M. Neuringer, S. Reisbick, Eds.; Roche: Basel, Switzerland, 1996; pp. 19–48.

Nyqvist, K.H.; P.-O. Sjoden; U. Ewald. The development of preterm infants' breastfeeding behavior. *Early Hum. Dev.* **1999,** *55(3),* 247–264.

O'Connor, D.L.; R. Hall; D. Adamkin; N. Auestad; M. Castillo; W.E. Connor; S.L. Connor; K.M. Fitzgerald; S. Groh-Wargo; E.E. Hartmann; et al. Growth and development in preterm infants fed long-chain polyunsaturated fatty acids: A prospective randomized controlled trial. *Pediatrics* **2001,** *108(2),* 359–371.

Oddy, W.H. The impact of breast milk on infant and child health. *Breastfeed Rev.* **2002,** *10(3),* 5–18.

Ohn, Y.H.; O. Katsumi; Y. Matsui; H. Tetsuka; T. Hirose. Snellen visual acuity versus pattern reversal visual-evoked response acuity in clinical applications. *Ophthalmic Res.* **1994,** *26(4),* 240–252.

Scott, D.T.; J. Janowsky; R.E. Carroll; J.A. Taylor; N. Auestad; M.B. Montalto. Formula supplementation with long-chain polyunsaturated fatty acids: are there developmental benefits? *Pediatrics* **1998,** *102(5),* e59.

Simmer, K.N.; S.K. Patole; S.C. Rao. Long-chain polyunsaturated fatty acid supplementation in infants born at term. *Cochrane Database Syst. Rev.* **2008a,** *1.*

Simmer, K.N.; S.M. Schulzke; S. Patole. Long-chain polyunsaturated fatty acid supplementation in preterm infants. *Cochrane Database Syst. Rev.* **2008b,** *2008*:1.

Singhal, A.; R. Morley; T.J. Cole; K. Kennedy; P. Sonksen; E. Isaacs; M. Fewtrell; A. Elias-Jones; T. Stephenson; A. Lucas. Infant nutrition and stereoacuity at age 4–6 y. *Am. J. Clin. Nutr.* **2007,** *85(1),* 152–159.

Slater, A. Individual differences in infancy and later IQ. *J. Child Psychol. Psychiatry* **1995,** *36(1),* 69–112.

Smithers, L.G.; R.A. Gibson; A. McPhee; M. Makrides. Effect of long-chain polyunsaturated fatty acid supplementation of preterm infants on disease risk and neurodevelopment: a systematic review of randomized controlled trials. *Am. J. Clin. Nutr.* **2008a,** *87(4),* 912–920.

Smithers, L.G.; R.A. Gibson; A. McPhee; M. Makrides. Higher dose of DHA in the neonatal period improves visual acuity of preterm infants: The results of a randomized controlled trial. *Am. J. Clin. Nutr.* **2008b** (In press).

Teller, D.Y.; M. McDonald; K. Preston; S.L. Sebris; V. Dobson. Assessment of visual acuity in infants and children: the acuity card procedure. *Dev. Med. Child Neurol.* **1986,** *28,* 779–789.

Thompson, L.A.; J.F.I. Fagan; D.W. Fulker. Longitudinal prediction of specific cognitive abilities from infant novelty preference. *Child Dev.* **1991,** *62(3),* 530538.

Tolley, E.A.; S.E. Carlson. Considerations of statistical power in infant studies of visual acuity development and docosahexaenoic acid status. *Am. J. Clin. Nutr.* **2000,** *71(1),* 1–2.

Uauy, R.; D.R. Hoffman; P. Mena; A. Llanos; E. Birch. Term infants studies of DHA and ARA supplementation on neurodevelopment: results of randomized controlled trials. *J. Pediatr.* **2003,** *143,* s17–s25.

Unay, B.; S.U. Sarici; U.H. Ulas; R. Akin; F. Alpay; E. Gokcay. Nutritional effects on auditory brainstem maturation in healthy term infants. *Arch. Dis. Child Fetal Neonatal Ed.* **2004,** *89(2),* F177–179.

van Wezel-Meijler, G.; M.S. van der Knapp; J. Huisman; E.J. Jonkman; J. Valk; H.N. Lafeber. Dietary supplementation of long-chain polyunsaturated fatty acids in preterm infants: effects on cerebral maturation. *Acta Paediatr.* **2002,** *91*:942–950.

Wainwright, P.E.; J. Colombo. Nutrition and the development of cognitive functions: interpretation of behavioral studies in animals and human infants. *Am. J. Clin. Nutr.* **2006,** *84,* 961–970.

Werkman, S.H.; S.E. Carlson. A randomized trial of visual attention of preterm infants fed docosahexaenoic acid until nine months. *Lipids* **1996,** *31(1),* 91–97.

Willats, P.; J.S. Forsythe; M.K. DiModugno; S. Varma; M. Colvin. Influence of long-chain polyunsaturated fatty acids on infant cognitive function. *Lipids* **1998a,** *33(10),* 973–980.

Willatts, P.; J.S. Forsyth; M.K. DiModugno; S. Varma; M. Colvin. Effect of long-chain polyunsaturated fatty acids in infant formula on problem solving at 10 months of age. *The Lancet* **1998b,** *352(9129),* 688–691.

World Health Organization. *Global Strategy for Infant and Young Child Feeding*; World Health Organization: Geneva, 2003.

Xu, S.; D. Meyer; S. Yoser; D. Mathews; J.L. Elfervig. Pattern visual evoked potential in the diagnosis of functional visual loss. *Ophthalmology* **2001,** *108(1),* 76–81.

Yip, E.; J. Lee; Y. Sheehy. Breast-feeding in neonatal intensive care. *J. Paediatr. Child Health* **1996,** *32,* 296–298.

Yuhas, R.; K. Pramuk; E. Lien. Human milk fatty acid composition from nine countries varies most in DHA. *Lipids* **2006,** *41(9),* 851–858.

15

# *Trans* Fatty Acids and Oxidative Transformations by Free Radicals: The Role in Health

**Carla Ferreri**
*I.S.O.F. —BioFreeRadicals, Consiglio Nazionale delle Ricerche, Via P. Gobetti 101, 40129 Bologna, Italy*

## Introduction

The hydrophobic part of the majority of lipid molecules consists of fatty acid residues that are carboxylic acids with a long hydrocarbon chain (up to 26 carbon atoms), saturated or unsaturated with up to six double bonds. The naturally occurring mono- and polyunsaturated fatty acid (MUFA and PUFA) residues of glycerol-based phospholipids in eukaryotes generally have the *cis* double-bond geometry, and PUFA double bonds have the characteristic methylene-interrupted motif. Examples of MUFA and PUFA structures and also of some *trans* isomers are shown in Fig. 15.1, with the common names and the abbreviations describing the position and geometry of the double bonds (e.g., 9*cis* or 9*trans*), as well as the notation of the carbon chain length and the total number of unsaturations (e.g., C18:1) (Vance & Vance, 2002).

Moreover, because the *cis* geometry is connected with biological activities, this feature is strictly controlled during MUFA and PUFA biosynthesis by the regiospecific and stereoselective enzymatic activities of desaturases (Fox et al., 2004).

Having double bonds and bis-allylic positions as reactive centers, the transformation of lipid molecules can occur either by enzymatic or chemical pathways (the former makes part of the lipid metabolism; the latter is involved in degradation processes that play roles in pathological processes and aging). One of the most relevant groups of reactions occurring to unsaturated fatty acids is represented by free radical processes.

This chapter does not intend to give an exhaustive review of lipid free radical transformations that were extensively treated elsewhere (Halliwell & Gutteridge, 2007). The aim is to highlight results derived from research in a multidisciplinary context, therefore connecting chemical reactivity and molecular transformations with their biological significance that ultimately indicates medical applications.

Products and mechanisms of free radical reactions on lipids were thoroughly investigated from the chemical point of view. Various products are formed that include either modifications of the original fatty acid structures that leave the chain

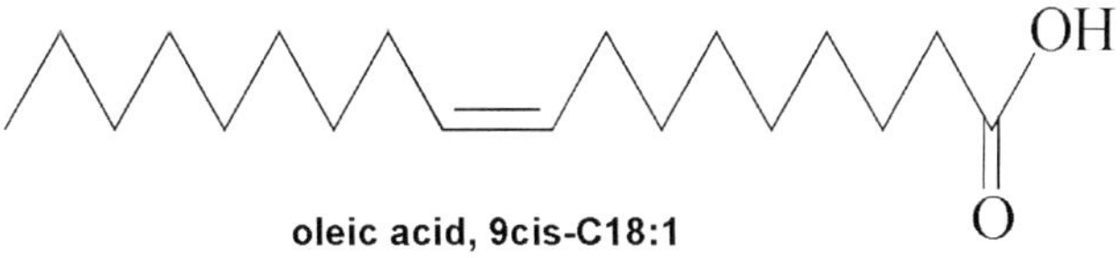


**oleic acid, 9cis-C18:1**

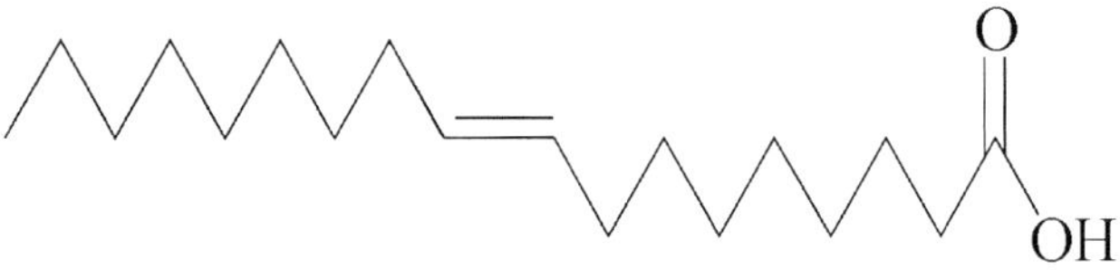


**elaidic acid, 9trans-C18:1**

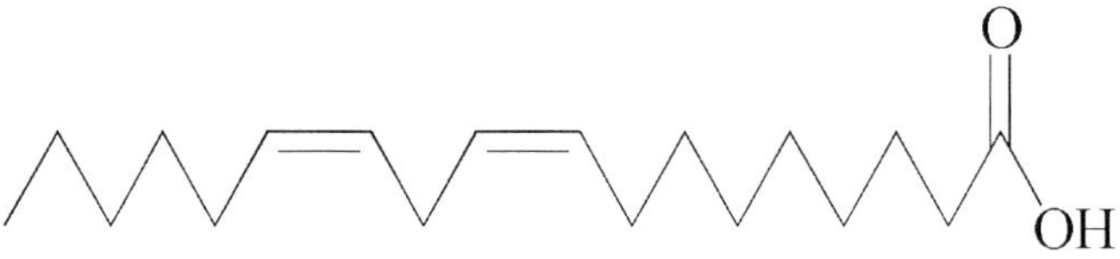


**linoleic acid, 9cis,12cis-C18:2**

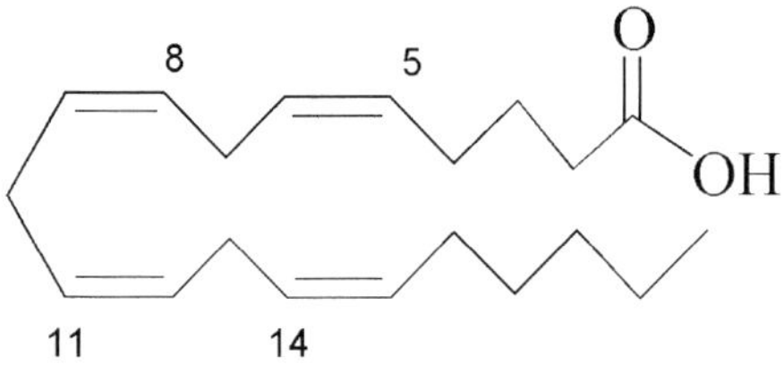


**arachidonic acid, 5cis,8cis,11cis,14cis-C20:4**

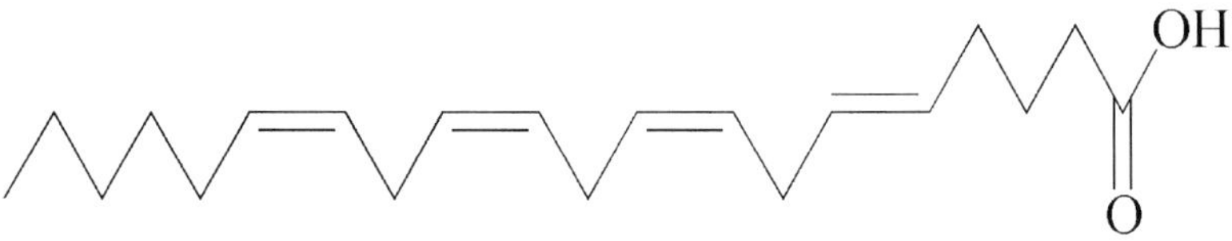


**mono-trans arachidonic acid isomer, 5trans,8cis,11cis,14cis-C20:4**

**Fig. 15.1.** Examples of mono- and polyunsaturated fatty acids.

length intact or progressive carbon chain degradation that forms low molecular weight products (Dianzani, 1998; Marathe et al., 2000). One can apply molecular libraries derived from chemical studies in biochemical and biological investigations, therefore allowing the free radical chemistry of lipids to be successfully extrapolated to life science research. As shown in this chapter, studies of radical-based lipid transformations not only disclosed the molecular basis of physiological and pathological conditions, but also indicated strategies of intervention, either by replacing the damaged lipids or, upstream, by stopping the radical chain processes by convenient inhibitors or radical trapping agents.

A few years ago, the field of lipid research in a multidisciplinary context motivated the birth of the discipline of lipidomics (Watson, 2006; Wenk, 2005; Wilson, 2003). The novelty brought about by the approach of lipidomics consisted of a dynamic vision of lipid structures existing in living organisms, following up their transformations both quantitatively and qualitatively and providing a useful comparison between physiological and pathological conditions.

One can perform research in lipidomics by using different kinds of models, such as liposomes, microorganisms, and cell cultures, to extrapolate and apply the results to more complex metabolic situations of animals and humans.

The approach of lipidomics in evaluating the fatty acid families has different targets: membrane lipidomics focuses on this cell compartment, which is governed by the type and quantity of phospholipids as structural and functional units, whereas mediator lipidomics studies the biological roles of lipids as signaling molecules and primers of metabolic cascades (Serhan, 2005). In this chapter, lipidomics focuses on unsaturated fatty acids affected by free radical transformations, in particular by peroxidation and geometrical isomerization, highlighting some recent perspectives of their roles in the biological environment. The health effects of isomerization and peroxidation processes are also considered, giving some hints for preventive and repair strategies derived from the lipidomic studies.

## Membranes and the Geometry of Fatty Acids in Living Systems

A large amount of data confirmed that the broad spectrum of lipid mixtures has a crucial role in the adaptability and flexibility of the cell membrane to environment necessities. The cell membrane is also a supporting matrix for proteins involved in many cellular processes; therefore, its physical and chemical properties can directly or indirectly affect cell metabolism. In this respect, unsaturated fatty acid residues of membrane phospholipids are recognized for their contribution to permeability and fluidity (Cevc, 1993). The change of the saturated/unsaturated ratio and of phospholipid polar headgroups, as well as of the chain length or branching of the fatty acid residues, has a strict correlation with the physical properties of biological membranes, going from a highly ordered to a fluid liquid crystalline phase. Noteworthy at this point is that the molecular shapes of saturated and *cis* unsaturated lipids are quite different, since the *cis* geometry confers a kink in the lipid hydrocarbon chain with an angle of ca. 30°. The molecular shape of the saturated fatty acyl chain is instead straight, and the *cis* to *trans* isomerization can partially correspond to a "cancellation" of the bending, because *trans* isomers also have a straight molecular shape, more similar to that of saturated compounds (Fig. 15.2).

The existence of double bonds in living systems with the ubiquitous *cis* geometry of eukaryotes and the meaning of a change to *trans* lipids were not addressed in a unifying manner until a few years ago. Here some results on membrane lipid geometry in different fields of life science are summarized.

## *Unsaturated Lipids in Different Organisms*

Differences of lipid composition among organisms are well-known. Many prokaryotes have saturated fatty acids [hexadecanoic (C16:0), heptadecanoic (C17:0), and octadecanoic (C18:0)] and MUFA [hexadecenoic (C16:1), heptadecenoic (C17:1), and octadecenoic (C18:1)] as the main components of their membranes and lipid deposits (Wältermann & Steinbüchel, 2005). Most of microorganisms, such as *Escherichia coli* and the yeast *Saccharomyces cerevisiae*, can synthesize only saturated fatty acids and MUFA, whereas a few others, as well as most plants, are able to synthesize PUFA starting from saturated fatty acid precursors. In this pathway, the interplay of elongase and desaturase enzymes works with the elongation of the hydrocarbon chain and the creation of double bonds, respectively. For completeness, recent studies revealed a novel PUFA biosynthetic pathway found in prokaryotic and eukaryotic microorganisms that does not require the elongase/desaturase system, and instead uses a polyketide synthase (PKS) to produce long-chain PUFA (20:5 and 22:6 in the omega-3 series) (Metz et al., 2001). The free-living nematode *Caenorhabditis elegans* possesses all of the enzymes required for the synthesis of omega-6 and omega-3 fatty acids, and actually is used as a model, both to study the effects of mutation in

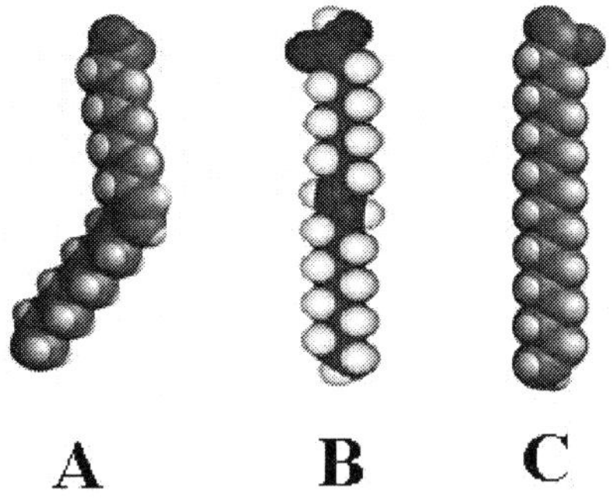


**Fig. 15.2.** Molecular models of *cis* (A), *trans* (B), and saturated (C) fatty acids.

the gene expression that regulates the levels of desaturase and elongase enzymes and to evaluate the influence of different fatty acid production on membrane characteristics (Brock et al., 2007).

Angiosperm plants convert oleic acid (C18:1) into linoleic acid (9*c*,12*c*-C18:2; omega-6 series) and α-linolenic acid (9*c*,12*c*,15*c*-C18:3; omega-3 series), which are essential fatty acids for mammals. Seed oils are the main source of essential PUFA in the human diet; therefore some double bonds are of "exogenous" origin. This implies that the *cis* geometry in humans can be "contaminated" when the diet introduces unnatural fatty acids. As a matter of fact, the chemical manipulation of oils and fats of natural origins by partial hydrogenation or deodorization processes, which are largely employed in food industries, is responsible for this contamination, because it converts the naturally occurring *cis* isomers to *trans* fatty acids (Sèbèdio & Christie, 1998). An important note is that the structures of *trans* isomers coming from hydrogenation or deodorization processes are, to a minor extent, those of the geometrical isomers (the major products are isomers with a shifted position of the double bonds that are called positional isomers). This positional shift is particularly relevant for linoleic acid that is converted into its conjugated isomers (CLA) (Evans et al., 2002). This structural observation is connected to another important question: whether knowing the total *trans* fatty acid content is relevant, or instead, ascertaining each type and quantity of *trans* isomers. In the last decade, nutritional and epidemiological studies addressed the dietary issue, and revealed the harmful effects of *trans* lipids for human health. This topic is mentioned further and treated in other chapters of this book.

In considering the adaptation responses, when a stress is applied to cells, the first consequence is a specific injury to the membranes. In fact, the greatest adaptive response is keeping the fluidity of membranes at a constant value, despite the changing environmental conditions. This is known as "homeoviscous adaptation" (Sinensky, 1974), which is effected through the variation of the fatty acid composition of membrane lipids. In particular, the regulation of the degree of phospholipid saturation/unsaturation occurs in animals and plants, where the higher fluidity is obtained by the increase of the double-bond content (Murakami et al., 2000; Sakamoto & Murata, 2002). For example, at low temperatures, adaptation is afforded by the enrichment of polyunsaturated lipids, whereas at high temperatures saturated fatty acid residues play the most important role for keeping the right properties of the lipid assembly. In this scenario, the *cis* double bond of unsaturated fatty acid structures is a constant and important feature ensuring growth under different conditions.

## Geometrical Isomerization in Bacteria

The first observation of the existence of *trans* geometry in vivo came from microbiological research, toppling the certainty of the *cis* geometry as a ubiquitous feature of unsaturated lipids in living organisms. In the early 1990s, some papers reported the presence of *trans* lipids in the membranes of the psychrophilic bacterium *Vibrio* sp. strain ABE-1 (Okuyama et al., 1991) and in *Pseudomonas Putida* P8

(Heipieper et al., 1992), having undergone a chemical or environmental stress. *Trans* isomer formation was not dependent on growth, so that it did not derive from a de novo synthesis of lipids. In particular, geometrical isomers (9*trans*-C16:1) were found in anaerobic bacteria *Pseudomonas* sp.strain E-3, *P. Putida,* and *Vibrio* sp. strain ABE-1, as determined by gas chromatographic (GC) analyses. Also observed was that by adding a MUFA, such as 9*cis*-C18:1 that is not present in *P. Putida* P8, it can be incorporated into the membrane, and with the addition of toxic compounds, it was also converted to the corresponding *trans* isomer (Diefenbach & Keweloh, 1994). The total amount of MUFA remained constant, but the *cis/trans* ratio changed according to the stress conditions. (Heipieper et al., 2003). This was the proof of a biological path carried out by a specific enzyme that worked on the naturally occurring *cis* unsaturated lipid without changing the position of the double bond but only its geometry, thus, forming the *trans* isomer. The existence of a *cis–trans* isomerase (Cti) was first hypothesized and then proved by cloning the Cti gene from *Pseudomonas* strains, followed by the purification and characterization of the enzyme. The optimal pH of isomerases is 7–8. The Cti in the solvent-tolerant bacterium *P. putida* S12 mainly works for the transformation of palmitoleic acid (9*cis*-C16:1) to its geometrical isomer, palmitelaidic acid (9*trans*-C16:1), and in the case of the addition of 3-nitrotoluene, it gives a final *cis/trans* ratio of 32:68. No enzyme inhibition was detected under anoxic conditions as well as in the presence of chelating agents, but the activity was strongly inhibited by 1 mM of cathecolic antioxidants, such as α-tocopherol and nordihydroguaretic acid. Several other stress elicitors were tested so that osmotic stress (caused by NaCl and sucrose), heavy metals, heat shock, and membrane-active antibiotics are all able to activate the *cis–trans* conversion (Isken et al., 1997; Neumann et al., 2003).

Why do bacteria choose the *cis–trans* conversion as an adaptive response? Consider two main factors: (i) In the case of high temperature, salt stress or the presence of toxic compounds, the membrane fluidity and permeability have to decrease as a protective response, and this is achieved in conditions of growth by increasing the saturated/unsaturated ratio, as previously described. On the other hand, having a mechanism independent of the biosynthesis and directly effective on *cis* compounds allows rapid modifications of membranes to occur. In this way, the organism can rapidly cope with the emerging environmental stress. After this response, acting on a time scale of minutes, other mid- and long-term mechanisms come into play, finally leading to a complete adaptation. (ii) Despite the similarity of the straight molecular shape between saturated and *trans* lipids, the modifications induced in membrane properties are not completely similar. *Trans* lipid-packing has a more ordered state compared to the *cis* isomers, and a substantial effect on the rigidity of the membrane is obtained. Several studies showed that the change from *cis* to *trans* unsaturated double bonds does not have the same decreasing effect on membrane fluidity and other properties, also in comparison to the change from *cis* to saturated fatty acids (Ferreri et al., 2006, 2006a, 2006b; Roach et al., 2004). The microorganisms having such an isomerizing system are those of wide occurrence in all niches of a great number of ecosystems, comprising soil, human skin, and water.

Thus, the enzymatic isomerization mechanism, active in prokaryotic cells, is unknown for eukaryotes where unsaturated fatty acids are provided during the biosynthesis only with *cis* double bonds, regio- and stereospecifically. Such diversity still has unexplored meanings related to the role of geometry during the life evolution of different organisms. It can certainly inspire scientific curiosity in asking the existence of unknown surveillance systems on the integrity of the thermodynamically less stable *cis* isomers in eukaryotes, therefore in humans. Geometric isomerism is a subject worthy of further investigations, considering its interdisciplinary applications.

## *Geometrical Isomerization by Radical Stress*

Starting from the assumption that the enzymatic *cis–trans* isomerization in eukaryotic cells is unknown, the presence of lipid isomers is largely attributed to exogenous sources from foods, as previously mentioned. The level of *trans* isomers of the main fatty acid residues in human adipose tissue was also found in the range of 0.5–3.8%, and correlations with dietary intakes in different countries were determined (van de Vijver et al., 2000). Moreover, a microbial biohydrogenation occurring in the first stomach of ruminants contributes to the 2–8% *trans* fatty acid content of dairy products (Schwarz, 2000). Detailed information came from nutritional studies (Hu et al., 1997; Larquè et al., 2001; Roberts et al., 1995; Stender et al., 1995) and is summarized in other chapters of this book.

Together with the exogenous contribution given by foods, some years ago another source of *trans* lipids was envisaged due to free radical stress. Chemical researchers found that many free radicals (e.g., $RS^\bullet$, $RSe^\bullet$, $RSO_2^\bullet$, $NO_2^\bullet$, $R_3Sn^\bullet$, $(Me_3Si)_3Si^\bullet$, etcetera) and atoms (e.g., $Br^\bullet$, $I^\bullet$, etcetera) can induce the *cis–trans* isomerization of double bonds by addition–elimination steps (Chatgilialoglu et al., 2000, 2005). The efficiency of the isomerization process strongly depends on the characteristics of the attacking radicals, and notably, the thiyl radical ($RS^\bullet$) is very effective in this transformation. The isomerization occurs via the mechanism shown in Fig. 15.3, starting from the thiyl radical addition to the double bond with the formation of a radical intermediate, where the carbon-carbon bond can rotate. Upon fragmentation of this intermediate, the *cis* or *trans* double bond is generated together with the ejection of the thiyl radical, which continues the catalytic cycle. The final *cis/trans* isomeric mixture is in favor of the most stable *trans* structure (>80%).

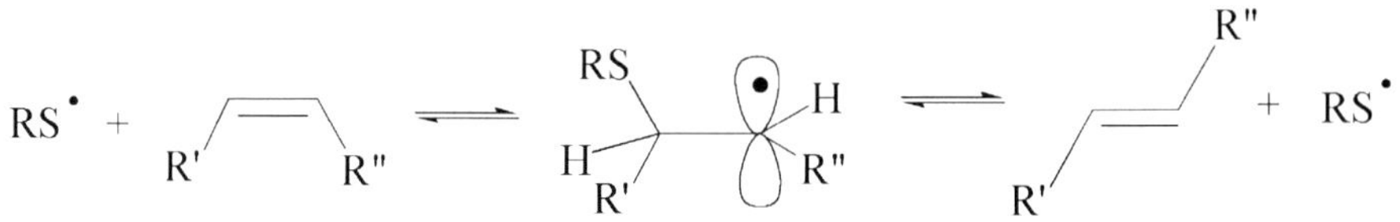


**Fig. 15.3.** Thiyl radical catalyzed isomerization of a double bond.

Considering the prevalence of *cis* double bonds in living systems, it is remarkable how different the two configurational isomers of a double bond are considered by chemistry and biology.

In the last years, free radical research addressed the *trans* lipid formation of membrane phospholipids in several interdisciplinary fields (Chatgilialoglu & Ferreri, 2005, 2006):

i. in biomimetic chemistry with the design of models, such as liposomes as membrane models, to study the conditions of the *trans* lipid formation in the presence of biologically meaningful sulfur-containing compounds and to examine different radical precursors; these studies also addressed the setting-up of molecular libraries of *trans* lipids useful to to extend studies in biology;

ii. in biology, using cell cultures or animal models for the investigation of (a) the factors influencing the membrane lipid composition under *trans*-free conditions and (b) the role of sulfur-containing compounds responsible for the isomerization of *cis* lipids; and

iii. in lipidomics, studying several human physiological and pathological conditions to envisage the conditions of radical stress that can be linked to a change of the membrane lipids asset and the geometrical configuration.

These studies address the general questions on what the conditions are of free radical stress acting on membrane lipid isomerization. A related task is to have markers to distinguish the exogenous origin of *trans* fatty acids from the radical-based endogenous isomerization. Actually, the membrane compartment was found to be very significant to provide such markers. In fact, by using biomimetic models of vesicles made of egg yolk lecithin, researchers demonstrated that the double bonds located closest to the membrane polar region are the most reactive toward the attack of diffusing isomerizing radicals (Ferreri et al., 2002, 2004). In the case of the linoleic acid residues in vesicles, the double bond in position 9 resulted as more reactive than that in position 12. Moreover, arachidonic acid residues were more reactive than oleic and linoleic acid residues, and two positions (i.e., the double bonds in 5 and 8) over the four unsaturations present in this PUFA structure were transformed preferentially. The arachidonate mono-*trans* isomers were characterized by using gas chromatography/mass spectrometry (GC/MS) and $^{13}$C nuclear magnetic resonance (NMR) (see Fig. 15.1 for the 5-mono-*trans* isomer). This observation is crucially important because the desaturase enzymes intervene to provide two *cis* unsaturations during the arachidonic biosynthesis, as depicted in Fig. 15.4. The double bonds in 5 and 8 positions can only exhibit the *cis* configuration, unless they are transformed into *trans* isomers by an endogenous radical attack.

The library of PUFA mono-*trans* isomers can be very useful in the complex approach to the lipid analysis of biological samples, and particularly, arachidonic acid isomers were significant for detecting radical stress conditions associated with human pathologies and aging, as mentioned later.

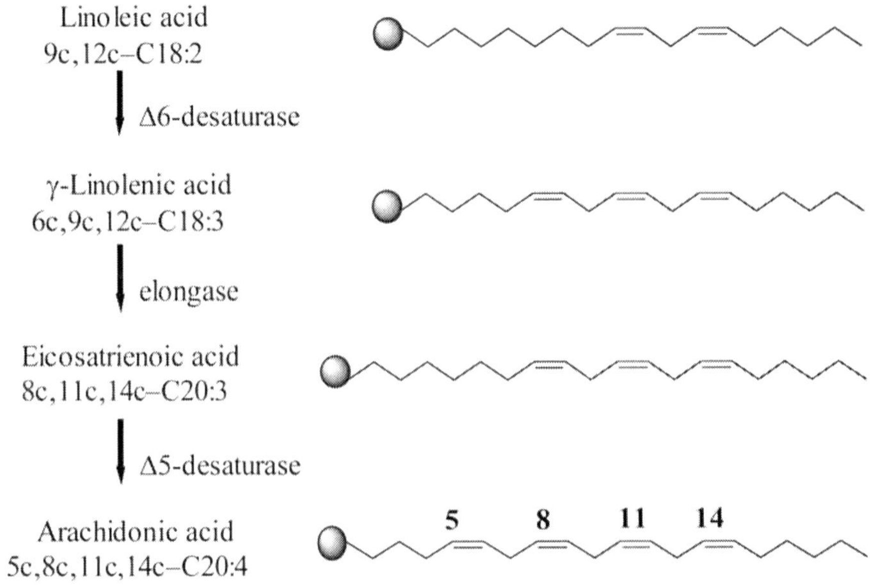


**Fig. 15.4.** The interplay of desaturase and elongase enzymes in the biosynthesis of arachidonic acid.

## *The Biological Effects of Trans Geometry*

The effects of *trans* fatty acids can be first evaluated on membrane properties due to the different contribution given by the molecular shape of these isomers, compared with the bent structures of the natural *cis* counterparts. As previously noted, the membrane properties of fluidity and permeability are influenced by the more rigid lipid packing; this can be correlated to other membrane functions governed by the phospholipid organization, such as the proper assistance to the ion channel formation or to protein interaction. *Trans* fatty acid residues in membranes have an influence on calcium channels in human arterial endothelial cells (Kummerow et al., 1999) that was even pronounced by the decrease of magnesium in the medium. The molecular interaction with membrane receptor rhodopsin, a prototypical member of the G-protein coupled receptor family, is also affected. The level of rhodopsin activation was lowered, and it was accompanied by a higher membrane cholesterol affinity (Niu et al., 2005). The interaction of *trans* acyl chains in membranes was evaluated with elaidic acid (9*trans*-C18:1) as *trans* residues in the phosphatidylcholine and sphingomyelin portion of membrane lipids. This caused the enrichment of cholesterol in lateral domains with a higher order, suggesting a possible contribution to the organization of lipid rafts (Bjorkbom et al., 2007).

Another interesting effect of *trans* fatty acids was studied on protein folding, where fatty acids can form complexes that maintain the interactions required for the biological activity. In the case of C18 fatty acid conformations that bind apo α-lactalbumin and form HAMLET (a human α-lactalbumin made lethal to tumor cells), elaidic acid was found, similarly to stearic acid, to not be able to produce stable complexes, whereas the *cis* counterpart does (Svensson et al., 2003).

Since the first biological investigations, the fact was evident that *cis* and *trans* isomers can interact in common enzymatic pathways but with different behavior. In the case of the geometrical isomers of linoleic acid (9*cis*,12*cis*-C18:2), the effects on ketogenesis and lipid secretion were studied. The hepatic uptake of two different isomers was similar, and *trans* residues were actively incorporated into hepatic lipids and secreted at the expense of the *cis* fatty acids. *Trans* isomers also stimulated ketogenesis; however, some differences were found in the position and number of the *trans* double bonds in the 18:2 structure, thus evidencing the need for the determination of each type of *trans* isomer (Fukuda et al., 1993). The transformation of the two mono-*trans* isomers of linoleic acid by rat liver microsomes showed that the 9*cis*,12*trans*-isomer is better desaturated, whereas the 9*trans*,12*cis*-isomer (Scheme 15.1) is better elongated (Berdeaux et al., 1998).

A *trans* fatty acid diet influenced the membrane composition of liver microsomes and mitochondria in pregnant rats, together with the decrease of the activity of desaturase and glucose-6-phosphate enzymes (Larquè et al., 2003). Similar results are expected in the essential fatty acid metabolism, as determined in the arterial cells of piglets born from pregnant porcine fed during gestation and lactation with hydrogenated fats (Kummerow et al., 2004).

The effects of *trans*-18:1 and 18:2 isomers were also evaluated on the arachidonic acid metabolism, particularly showing that they can inhibit the $PGI_2$ release by the cells through controlling the level of arachidonic acid as substrate, either inhibiting the conversion of linoleic acid or shunting the activity of phospholipase enzymes ($PLA_2$), leaving less substrate available for the prostaglandin synthesis (Kummerow et al., 2007).

In platelets, 18:1 and 18:2 *trans* fatty acids were incorporated at the membrane level and produced perturbation in specific lipid domains. They interacted with membrane and transmembrane proteins similarly to the *cis* isomers; however, they modified the activity of receptors and changed the membrane surface activities, thus propagating the effects to the cell. As a result, the activity of cytoplasmic enzymes, such as 12-P-LOX and cyclooxygenase/thromboxane synthase, was affected (Stachowska et al., 2004).

A mono-*trans* isomer of arachidonic acid with the *trans* double bond in position 14 is able to react with cytochrome P450 epoxygenase, a monooxygenase enzyme present in rat liver microsomes, and to give the corresponding epoxide, which is an unnatural compound (Roy et al., 2004). The previously reported mono-14*trans* isomer of arachidonic acid is also an inhibitor of the synthesis of thromboxane $B_2$ and, therefore, can prevent rat platelet aggregation (Berdeaux et al., 1996).

The specific roles of *trans* fatty acids in the activation of lipid signalling cascades were checked. The effects of elaidic acid (9*trans*-C18:1) were evaluated in the hepatic cell line (HepG2) by treating with 100 μM concentration and showing that already after 1 hour the signal of externalization of phosphatidylserine was obtained. (Kondoh et al., 2007). Other apoptotic effects were reported on human endothelial cells by similar activation together with the increase of reactive oxygen species (ROS) production (Zapolska-Downar et al., 2005).

The involvement of elaidic acid in apoptosis suggests possible synergism with other biological or pharmacological activities. The report of the activity of a 5'-elaidic derivative of cytarabine in solid tumors (P-4055) gives some support to this hypothesis. Cytarabine is used in the therapy of hematological malignancies, but not in solid tumors, due to the rapid inactivation by an enzymatic deamination. The association with fatty acids at the 5' OH position of this nucleoside was designed to increase the cellular uptake or to delay the metabolic clearance. The best results were obtained by association with elaidic acid, that enabled the formation of natural aggregates of the compounds driven by the organization of the fatty acid tail (Breistøl et al., 1999). However, the results with the *cis* analog were poor. Esters of elaidic acid were prepared also with other tumoral drugs, such as ganciclovir, gemcitabicine, and others. In these studies, the possibility of a synergism resulting from the intrinsic biological activity of the *trans* fatty acid isomer was not considered, perhaps because of an incorporation of the *trans* fatty acid residues at the membrane level. In these last years, several fatty acid-based compounds were tested, leading to the discovery of potent anticancer effects of natural structures. This is an important indication in medicinal chemistry for the development of "membrane-lipid therapy" drugs that will represent an important approach to treat several pathologies (Escribà, 2006).

## Oxidative Processes Involving Lipids

The main oxidative paths of transformation occurring to lipids in the biological environment are caused by enzymatic or chemical processes. The chemical path mainly consists of free radical-based processes such as lipid peroxidation, the well-known degradation process that occurs mostly at the expense of fatty acids containing bisallylic positions, therefore concerning PUFA. This field was first approached by chemists (Porter et al., 1995), and then it involved, and still does, research in life sciences (Niki et al., 2005). This topic is certainly a successful example of the fruitful relationship between chemical and biological investigations.

The enzymatic path consists of oxidative processes that occur in biological systems to generate specific oxidized lipids, which belong to very relevant cascades of lipid signaling and mediator synthesis. Again, PUFA are the substrates, and several of these enzymatic processes were discovered to have a free radical-based mechanism. The fact that free radical intermediates are involved in natural processes has to be carefully evaluated for considering the free radical activity either as a damaging or as a functioning mode in cell metabolism. The consequences of this evaluation have a practical application to the choice of the correct therapeutic strategies to control, but not suppress, the level of free radicals in living organisms, as pointed out in the section dedicated to health.

The rapidly expanding field of oxidative lipidomics is at the interface of the traditional membrane/lipid biochemistry and biophysics with free radical chemistry and cell biology, following up the formation and effects of oxidatively modified lipid molecules, for example in the apoptosis or the regulation of inflammatory response (Kagan & Quinn, 2004). Lipidomic analysis of signaling pathways focuses on the follow-up of certain lipids and the evaluation of related parameters, such as protein binding or activation (Wakeldm et al., 2007). Due to the development of analytical techniques, such as mass spectrometry, the mapping of the lipidome of living systems under different conditions seems more feasible. Notably, the perfect recognition of fatty acids, including *trans* isomers, can be very complicated, especially in the category of PUFA, to be done directly on a whole biological sample. Assistance for investigation and recognition tasks in biology comes from the use of biomimetic models to study different free radical conditions, such as the influence of the supramolecular arrangement of membranes, to gain knowledge on the scenario of the transformations, as well as to characterize the most feasible variations of the lipid structures to be used as markers.

## Radical-based Oxidation Processes

Several different enzymes can precipitate the oxygenation of PUFA. Epoxidation involves the activity of cytochrome-based enzymes, such as cytochrome P450, and the epoxy lipids belong to the fatty acid diversity, especially in plants (Broun et al., 1998). In animals, the activity of lipoxygenase (LOX) and cyclooxygenase (COX) enzymes is found as the initial step in the formation of a diverse array of lipid mediators (Funk, 2001). The important roles of the oxygenated products start from their interaction with G-protein-coupled receptors and involve cellular homeostasis, proliferation and differentiation, as well as the occurrence of other paths in pathophysiological processes.

The prototype substrate for these enzymes is arachidonic acid in animals, whereas linoleic and linolenic acids are used in plants. LOX and COX enzymes effect the first conversion to fatty acid peroxides, but COX enzymes proceed to the formation of endoperoxide products.

Interestingly, the steps of oxygenation taken by the enzymes are comparable to what happens during the chemical process of lipid peroxidation. However, in the case of enzymes, the control of oxygenation in terms of regio- and stereoselectivities leads to specific isomers with mechanisms that are still under examination (Schneider et al., 2007). This can explain the differences in activities between the enzymatic and chemical products because, depending on the stereochemistry, the biological roles are quite different. This is well-represented by the class of F2-isoprostanes, having a prostaglandin-like structure (like $PGF_{2\alpha}$) with elevated toxicity, that is also linked to several diseases (Morrow & Roberts, 1997). When prostaglandins are formed by cyclooxygenase, they exclusively have the two substituent chains on the isoprostane ring in the *trans* disposition, whereas the nonenzymatic formation of isoprostanes gives racemic mixtures containing the more thermodynamically *cis* stereochemistry, as shown in Fig. 15.5. One can use these products, in fact, as markers of lipid peroxidation.

Several chemical agents can cause lipid peroxidation. The general category of ROS is involved, and among them either $H_2O_2$ or hydroxyl radical (•OH) can possess the starting conditions for this chemical pathway. In the case of •OH radicals, they can directly effect the H-atom abstraction depicted as the first step in Fig. 15.5. Since the formation of hydroxyl radicals is also connected to radiation effects, one can use lipid peroxidation as the measurement of these effects on membranes.

The formation of $H_2O_2$ can be another primer of lipid peroxidation, due to the reaction with iron salts, in particular Fe(II), named for the first discoverer in 1950, the chemist H.J.K. Fenton. In this process, known also as metal-mediated peroxidation, •OH are formed (Reaction 15.1) (Gutteridge, 1995); therefore, the metal toxicity to membranes, that is evoked in certain diseases (Stohs & Baggi, 1995), is measured.

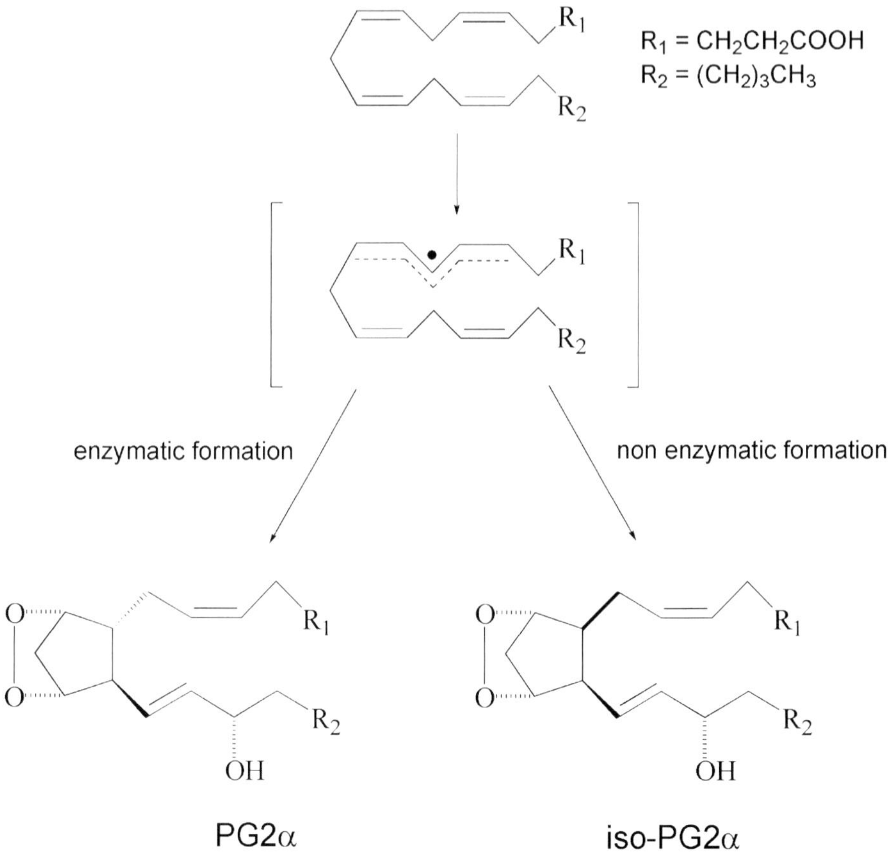


**Fig. 15.5.** Formation of isoprostanes with *trans* (left) and *cis* (right) stereochemistry.

$$H_2O_2 + Fe^{2+} \longrightarrow {}^{\bullet}OH + OH + Fe^{3+}$$

**Reaction 15.1.**

Also singlet oxygen produces lipid hydroperoxides by a mechanism known as ene-reaction, which is accelerated in the presence of sensitizers, such as chlorophyll, rose bengal, methylene blue, bilirubin, or porphyrin (photodynamic lipid peroxidation) (Girotti, 1990). This is the basic process that occurs in membrane phospholipids by illuminating erythrocytes in the presence of porphyrin or bilirubin, which leads to protein aggregation, inactivation of enzymes, and eventual hemolysis.

Figure 15.6 shows the general mechanism of lipid peroxidation as a radical chain reaction, starting with the abstraction of a hydrogen atom by an ROS and producing the bisallylic (or pentadienyl) radical $L^{\bullet}$. The next steps are the reaction of $L^{\bullet}$ with oxygen that forms peroxyl radicals $LOO^{\bullet}$ and the subsequent abstraction of a hydrogen atom from another lipid molecule (LH) that produces lipid hydroperoxide (LOOH) and another "fresh" $L^{\bullet}$ able to continue the chain (propagation steps).

The reaction of lipid radicals $L^{\bullet}$ with oxygen is close to a diffusion-controlled process but is also a reversible process, because the peroxyl radical can undergo a very rapid fragmentation ($10^6$ $s^{-1}$). Many of the antioxidant activities are measured by the ability of trapping this peroxyl radical intermediate. In the biological context, the proximity of the antioxidants to the peroxyl radical center is crucial for the effectiveness of the trapping. Detailed studies of the products of peroxidation were initiated in the 1970s (Porter et al., 1995; Yin & Porter, 2005), revealing complex mixtures of oxidized fatty acids. The first identified products were the hydroperoxides derived from the corresponding peroxyl radicals (Fig. 15.6). The distribution of hydroperoxides that are formed depends on the efficiency and concentration of the hydrogen atom donor present. For example, when the oxidation of linoleic acid occurs in the presence of α-tocopherol (α-Toc, <10 mM), *trans,cis* conjugated hydroperoxides are the major products. Instead, in the absence of a hydrogen donor, the fragmentation of the intermediate hydroperoxyl radicals gives conjugated dienes with the most stable *trans,trans* geometry (Tallman et al., 2004). The chain reactions have termination steps, which in this case consist of a radical-radical combination with other radical centers generated in the same environment. However, peroxyl lipids can continue their radical degradation cascade so that the hydrocarbon chain is fragmented with the formation of low molecular weight products, as truncated phospholipids and different types of oxygenated compounds. The aldehydes, such as malondialdehyde (MDA), 4-hydroxynonenale (HNE), and other related unsaturated aldehydes, were found as the products of cleavage of hydroperoxides. MDA attracted a great deal of attention in lipid peroxidation for many years that motivated the use of the thiobarbituric acid (TBA) to assay the peroxidation in vitro (Pryor & Stanley, 1975). Also HNE was individuated for its role in this degradation process (Esterbauer et al., 1991; Schneider et al., 2008), and was found to be particularly

$$X^{\bullet} + LH \longrightarrow X + L^{\bullet}$$

$$L^{\bullet} + O_2 \rightleftharpoons LOO^{\bullet}$$

$$LOO^{\bullet} + LH \longrightarrow LOOH + L^{\bullet}$$

**Fig. 15.6.** Mechanistic steps of lipid peroxidation.

toxic to mitochondria (Kristal et al., 1996). These structures containing a double bond, an aldehyde function, and a hydroxyl group are chemically very reactive, and they can easily form adducts with many functional groups, such as thiol and amino groups, widely present in the biological environment, for example, in proteins and the nucleotidic components of DNA. The adducts have a mutagenic potential and, in general, very strong toxicity effects (Crabb et al., 2002; Keller et al., 1997). These compounds can induce the production of antibodies, and it is currently spreading the use of HNE or MDA antibodies that are able to visualize their adducts directly in a tissue, helping in the assessment of the importance of these oxidative reactions in diseases and aging. For example, the modification of proteins with 4-HNE was detected in human peripheral blood lymphocytes by using two-dimensional gel electrophoresis followed by Western blotting with an antibody recognizing 4-HNE protein adducts (Poggioli et al., 2004). Analogously, such biomarkers are used to detect the occurrence of neurodegenerations (Kruman et al., 1997).

## *Products of Oxidative Transformation from Low-density Lipoproteins (LDL) and Membrane Phospholipids*

After the mechanistic demonstration of the free radical oxidation of phospholipids, a fruitful era started with a continuous flow of works devoted to chemistry, biochemistry, and medicine (Spiteller, 2007). As already mentioned, one can approach the simulation of such transformations by using models of fatty acid aggregates in aqueous media, such as micelles and liposomes, as well as complexes of lipids with proteins (Sabatini et al., 2006). Linoleic acid is frequently used as a model fatty acid in the studies of autoxidation, but arachidonic acid also is used, since both are the most abundant PUFA found in humans. The characteristic oxidative stability of PUFA in organized systems may be correlated with the specific physical properties of PUFA. Their tight conformation may result in the selective attack of free radicals and/or oxygen at the bisallylic position in PUFA. Consequently, naturally, some differences exist in the distribution of positional isomers of lipid hydroperoxides between the oxidation in aqueous micellar solutions of PUFA and the autoxidation of neat substrate in the air.

Perhaps, the most known process in this field is the oxidation of LDL. In experimental and clinical studies of atherosclerosis, LDL undergoes modifications that result in marked changes in its physicochemical properties, and these changes make the particle a much more effective inducer of pathological events. The phospholipid part of LDL, that accounts for up to ca. 20–25% of the whole particle (by weight), is the primary target of oxidation in an LDL particle. For this reason, the peroxidation process is seen as a potential cause in the early stages of atherogenesis (Berliner & Watson, 2005; Witzum, 1993). The in vitro oxidation of LDL caused the isolation of several oxidized phospholipids, and with the development of HPLC methods coupled with ion-spray mass spectrometry identifications of these primary products in the early stages of LDL oxidation occurred (Milne & Porter, 1995).

A major transformation is occurring on the fatty acid at the *sn*-2 position of the glycerophospholipid structure: it is truncated and transformed into an aldehyde derivative. For example, the prevalent major oxidized glycerophosphocholine lipids were recognized by electrospray ionization mass spectrometry and corroborated by chemical synthesis to be 1-palmitoyl-2-(9-oxononanoyl)glycerophosphocholine and 1-octadecanoyl-2-(7-hydroxy-hepta-5-enoyl)glycerophosphocholine. In this way, the substituents in the *sn*-2 position are transformed into γ-oxygenated-α,β-unsaturated aldehyde or carboxyl group functions (Harrison et al., 2000).

Interestingly, *sn*-2 truncated phospholipids are also a common feature of natural lipids, such as platelet-activating factor (PAF) (which contains an acetyl group in the *sn*-2 position).

The effect of oxidized PC structures on the membrane lipid organization is to disrupt the bilayer, with a tendency of moving toward the lipid–water interface (Megli et al., 2005). Biological assays showed that they are bioactive compounds, and they are really involved in the biological events associated with atherosclerosis. In fact, the uptake of oxidized LDL by the cells of the vascular wall plays a key role in atherogenesis. The modified particles either inhibit or induce (programmed) cell death, depending on the extent of lipoprotein oxidation and the dose. These effects can be initiated by minimally modified LDL (mmLDL) in which only the lipids are oxidized. The contribution of the individual lipids to the toxic effect of mmLDL on vascular cells is, however, far from clear.

The scenario regarding the modifications of unsaturated lipids would not be complete without mentioning the oxidation products of cholesterol esters from linoleic and arachidonic acids. These esters are incorporated into very low density lipoprotein that are then transformed into LDL. When this LDL is transferred to endothelial cells, the toxic products are liberated and induce cell damage. The damage is combined with structural changes that influence neighboring cells and cause an influx of $Ca^{+2}$ ions, with the activation of phospholipase first, that is responsible for the free fatty acid liberation from membranes, and secondly the activation of lipoxygenase enzymes, that produce lipid peroxides. When the level of free PUFA obtained from the phospholipase activity exceeds certain limits, lipoxygenase self-destructs, liberating iron ions. These ions react with lipid peroxides, and this is a production of peroxyl radicals via nonenzymatic reactions, which are able to attack any biological compounds and induce severe damage (Spiteller, 2005).

What are the membrane phospholipids most sensitive to oxidative damage? This question is the subject of several investigations that use model liposomes as well as living organisms. In rats, the ischemia-reperfusion injury to cardiac myocytes involved membrane damage with the most pronounced effects on cardiolipin, a lipid which is mostly present in mitochondria, with its oxidation products being involved in apoptosis and signaling (Houtkooper & Vaz, 2008; Paradies et al., 1999). One of the most indicative experimental protocols for investigating the damage of membrane lipids uses irradiation conditions. By employing oxidative lipidomics to qualitatively and quantitatively characterize phospholipid peroxidation in the small intestine of mice exposed to total body irradiation (TBI) of 10 and 15 Gy, two anionic phospholipids—cardiolipin in mitochondria and phosphatidylserine outside mitochondria—were established as the membrane components most involved in the oxidation. Phosphatidylcholine and phosphatidylethanolamine did not reveal any oxidative stress responses despite the presence of highly oxidizable docosahexaenoic fatty acid residues in their structures (Tyurina et al., 2008). Therefore, the sensitivity of the different lipid molecules can vary depending on the biological context and location.

From the available scientific data, lipid oxidation in vivo emerges to target membrane phospholipid components, considering the PUFA usually are located in the *sn*-2 position of the glycerol backbone (Fruhwirth et al., 2007).

## Health Effects of Radical-based Processes on Membrane Lipids

The connection between free radical processes and health effects has become more and more evident in these last decades, due to the amelioration of analytical techniques for lipid identification in biological samples. The ultimate goal to elucidate the lipidome of living organisms, including humans, is now much closer, but contacts and collaborations among different disciplines and expertise need to be improved to allow a straightforward application of chemical and biochemical knowledge to biology and medicine.

The term "oxidative stress" groups the radical processes that influence health and are connected to the overproduction of ROS and their damage potential to biomolecules. As described in this chapter, the comprehensive term "radical stress" is more representative of the lipid modifications that do not always imply an oxidative pathway. However, oxidative stress to lipids with the generation of lipid peroxides and other low molecular weight components is very popular nowadays, being evoked in the onset and the progression of diseases, as well as in aging.

More recently, the meaning of the word "stress" started to change: more than just an indication of biological damage. In fact, adaptation paths linked to cellular responses suggest that free radicals can act as inducers, and living organisms have always coped with free radical production or oxidative stress that occurs at the level of many biological activities, including exercise (Alessio et al., 1988; Crawford & Davies, 1994). Moreover, in response to stress, enzymatic and molecular systems are activated in distinct environments with specific radical-trapping activities that often act in synergy; their stimulation and adequate levels in each condition must be considered. The effectiveness of such systems is also associated with strategies for a more general control of radical production, thus, having an impact on therapeutic intervention as well as on prevention.

The effects of antioxidants and, in general, of radical trapping agents are well-documented and motivate a great deal of research and application to physiopathological conditions, including aging (Cutler & Rodriguez, 2003). In particular, thiols attract interest as trapping agents, due to their rapid reactivity with carbon-centered radicals, such as shown in Reaction 15.2 (Ferreri et al., 2005). This is the so-called "repair reaction."

$$X^{\bullet} + RSH \longrightarrow XH + RS^{\bullet}$$

**Reaction 15.2.**

Typical levels of intracellular nonprotein thiol (principally, glutathione, GSH) are in the order of 5 mM, although values of around 10 mM are reported (Smith et al., 1996). The total level of SH groups may approach or exceed that of GSH after taking into account the cysteine residues in metallothioneins and other abundant proteins. In considering the reactivity of thiols in the biological environment in repair reactions, some years ago the scavenging effect produced thiyl radicals ($RS^{\bullet}$) as counterparts that can display a damaging potential toward a series of compounds in the biological environment (Pogocki & Schoeneich, 2001). As mentioned in the section on lipid isomerization, thiyl radicals are indeed harmful for the natural *cis* geometry by catalyzing the formation of *trans* lipids. This information at the molecular level started only recently to be extrapolated to living systems in biology and medicine, and it will contribute to examining the scenario related to the thiol balance and integrity of lipid structures in health and diseases.

Many of the known effects due to the geometrical isomers, but still interpreted as being derived from dietary issues, can now be extended to the possibility that such isomers are generated by radical stress. In the evaluation of the changes of membrane lipidome during metabolic conditions, the inclusion of the geometrical features of lipids is actually needed.

## Trans *and Oxidized Lipids in Health*

Other chapters are dedicated to the importance of *trans* fatty acids in diseases, starting from the point of view of the dietary intake. Therefore, we are giving some examples of *trans* fatty acids generated under the conditions of radical stress that can influence the formation of *trans* isomers in vivo.

The former studies were made under "*trans*-free" conditions by using animals with a diet completely free of any *trans* lipid contribution (Zambonin et al., 2006). Membrane lipids of different tissues isolated from rats were analyzed, proving for the first time the spontaneous occurrence of endogenous *trans* fatty acids: *trans* C18:1 and *trans* C18:2 isomers were present in low amounts in the liver, heart, and kidney, whereas a higher content of these configurational isomers occurs in erythrocytes and adipose tissue. *Trans* isomers of arachidonic acid were present in high amounts in the liver, heart, kidney, and erythrocytes. Actually, the total content of *trans* fatty acids increases following the order of kidney < heart < adipose tissue < liver < erythrocytes, reaching the 0.93% of the total fatty acid content. Indeed, erythrocytes are the natural "deposit" of arachidonic acid as phospholipid residues. In the same study, an increase of *trans* lipids was also correlated to stress conditions by subjecting rats to an acute dose of $CCl_4$ (1200 mg/kg). A recent report gives further support to the *trans* fatty acid in vivo formation during aging (Zambonin et al., 2008).

On the basis of *trans*-free models, other physiopathological conditions are seen in association with the formation of *trans* isomers. In smokers, it is well-known that the production of radical species increases; therefore, it is reasonable to check for the *trans* lipid isomers. In the plasma of smokers, the average concentration of mono-*trans* arachidonic acid isomers (as free acids) was found to be 20.2 ng/mL (66.4 nM); particularly the mono-8-*trans* isomer, that was identified separately, reached 2.75 ± 0.39 ng/mL. The average levels of plasma F2-isoprostanes, that are a group of free-radical derived markers of arachidonic peroxidation in vivo, as previously mentioned, are between 0.1 and 0.9 nM; therefore, the levels of *trans* isomers are significantly higher. (Zghibeh et al., 2004).

*Trans* isomers were detected in dermatological diseases known to be associated with radical stress and the consumption of antioxidant defenses, such as atopic eczema/dermatitis in children. *Trans* lipid isomers were found in both the erythrocyte and T-lymphocyte membranes of these subjects, reaching a total content of 2.7 and 4.9% of the fatty acid composition, respectively (Ferreri et al., 2005a). Interestingly, *trans* isomers were found also in control subjects with a dietary contribution similar to the studied group, but the statistical significance of the subjects compared with the controls had a particular meaning, and it was high ($P < 0.001$).

Another case of *trans* isomer detection was recently reported in the case of the offspring of long-lived individuals (Puca et al., 2008a). Erythrocyte membranes were considered in evaluating the percentage content of all fatty acid families, including the *trans* isomers of oleic acid and the mono-*trans* isomers of arachidonic acid. This comprehensive analysis determined the basal differences in membrane composition, which also involve the natural fatty acid residues. A different content of some natural fatty acids was significant compared to controls, especially with the increased content of palmitoleic acid (9*cis*-C16:1), which cannot come from the diet, and the reduced content of C18:2n-6 and C20:4n-6. This fact recalls the concept of reduced lipid peroxidation and increased membrane integrity for favoring the life span; that is formulated as the membrane pacemaker theory of aging (Hulbert, 2003). Moreover, it showed the increased content of *trans* C18:1n-9, and total *trans* fatty acids, thus suggesting a threshold value of a *trans* content for playing the role of endogenous inducers of defense systems. These results also suggest that strategies to increase favorable factors for slowing aging should carefully evaluate the contribution of fatty acid families from diet or from a target supplementation (Puca et al., 2008b).

As far as the involvement of oxidized lipids in health is concerned, it started from the identification of fatty acid markers in atherosclerotic vascular disease, as previously described. The formation of lipid peroxides, similar to that in cardiovascular diseases, is found in inflammatory and neurodegenerative diseases, indicating a close relationship between the inducers of all these events (Spiteller, 2006).

Especially note that the formation of oxidized lipids in membranes influences the channels across the bilayer and, consequently, the flux of $Ca^{+2}$ ions. This activates phospholipase enzymes (PL), that are able to cleave to phospholipid structures, and among them $PLA_2$ is considered with great interest because it causes the hydrolysis of fatty acid residues at the *sn*-2 position (Farooqui et al., 2005; Sun et al., 2004). However, also, the presence of oxidized or truncated fatty acid residues in the *sn*-2 position of phospholipids is per se a signal for PL activation. The products are lysophospholipids that are recognized for having very important signalling activities, and attracted interest from various research teams in the last few years (Meyer et al., 2007) also for their pharmacological applications to diseases (Murph et al., 2006).

Membrane lipidomics and mediator lipidomics are expected to give an important contribution to the understanding of the molecular basis of human metabolic conditions.

## Some Hints for Preventive and Repair Strategies of Radical Stress

Clearly, radical stress can intervene in the modification of unsaturated lipids. PUFA consumption is detected in several diseases, including aging, and a crucial role is assigned to the balance between the two families of omega-6 and omega-3 PUFA, which has an epidemiological meaning, such as in the case of skin and allergy diseases (Logan, 2004). This motivated the application to health care of preventive and repair strategies targeting two directions: (i) normalizing the PUFA content and (ii) enhancing the protection against free radicals. In the latter case, antioxidant vitamin supplementation is the subject of numerous trials and studies still in progress. Actually, the antioxidant effect is interpreted in two opposite ways, taking into account the antioxidant and pro-oxidant activities. The case of vitamin E is a very seminal example of this behavior (Bowry & Stocker, 1993).

The supplementation with natural oils containing the PUFA families is also a double-faced subject, and literature data show excellent results in some cases but not always, leading to a contradictory scenario (Grundt & Nilsen, 2008). Interestingly, the well- known oxidizability of PUFA substrates is not considered during supplementation to patients with an unknown condition of oxidative stress.

Therefore, from the scenario described so far, the PUFA supplementation should not be done indiscriminately, but according to real needs and under protection from the radical degradation during the biodistribution.

Together with the lipid modifications described so far, another aspect to consider is the lipid reorganization at the level of fatty acid families and their balance in the membrane, occurring during the free radical events. In fact, during metabolism, the damage is processed: oxidized membrane phospholipids are removed, whereas for *trans* isomers no specific enzymes exist; therefore, they can remain at the membrane level and follow the same catabolism as the other lipids. The balance among the different types and families of fatty acids (MUFA vs SFA; PUFA omega-6 vs omega-3) is altered, and the intervention to restore membrane conditions and to eliminate radical stress cannot rely only on endogenous defenses because the diet must provide essential lipids and antioxidants.

Lipidomics intervenes at this moment to provide information at the molecular level and to offer a practical application to health. Given the levels of fatty acid families that are characteristic of each tissue and to ensure the proper membrane properties and functions (Lauritzen et al., 2001), membrane lipidomics allows for the follow-up of the individual fatty acid status concerning essential fatty acids (omega-6 and omega-3) and the effects of radical stress, and the individuation of the imbalance or loss of components. In this way, personalized intervention can be designed with the goal of restoring the natural membrane fatty acid balance, thus helping to preserve the composition and functionality of this important cell compartment.

## Acknowledgments

The scientific mentoring of Dr. Chryssostomos Chatgilialoglu is gratefully acknowledged. The author wishes to acknowledge the support and sponsorship concerted by COST Action CM0603 on "Free Radicals in Chemical Biology (CHEMBIORADICAL)".

### References

Alessio, H.-M.; A.H. Goldfarb. Lipid peroxidation and scavenger enzymes during exercise: adaptive response to training. *J. Appl. Physiol.* **1988**, *64*, 1333–1336.

Berdeaux, O.; J.M. Chardigny; J.L. Sébédio; T. Mairot; D. Poullain; J.M. Vatèle; J.P. Noël. Effects of a trans isomer of arachidonic acid on rat platelet aggregation and eicosanoid production. *J. Lipid Res.* **1996**, *37*, 2244–2250.

Berdeaux, O.; J.P. Blond; L. Bretillon; J.M. Chardigny; T. Mairot; J.M. Vatèle; D. Poullain; J.L. Sébédio. In vitro desaturation or elongation of monotrans isomers of linoleic scid by rat liver microsomes. *Mol. Cell. Biochem.* **1998**, *185*, 17–25.

Berliner, J.A.; A.D. Watson. A role for oxidized phospholipids in atherosclerosis, *N. Eng. J. Med.*, **2005**, *353*, 8–11.

Bjorkbom, A.; B. Ranstedt; J.P. Slotte. Phosphatidylcholine and sphingomyelin containing an elaidoyl fatty acid can form cholesterol-rich lateral domain in bilayer membranes. *BBABiomem-*

*branes* **2007**, *1768*, 1839–1847.

Bowry, V.W.; R. Stocker. Tocopherol-mediated peroxidation. The prooxidant effect of vitamin E on the radical-initiated oxidation of human low-density lipoprotein. *J. Am. Chem. Soc* **1993**, *115*, 6029–6044.

Breistøl, K.; J. Balzarini; M.M. Sandvold; F. Myhren; M. Martinsen; E. De Clerq; Ø. Fodstad. Antitumor activity of P-4055(elaidic acid-cytarabine) compared to cytarabine in metastatic and s.c. human tumor xenograft models. *Cancer Res.* **1999**, *59*, 2944–2949.

Brock, T.J.; J. Browse; J.L. Watts. Fatty acid desaturation and the regulation of adiposity in Caenorhabditis elegans. *Genetics*, **2007**, *176*, 865–875.

Broun, P.; J. Sankling; E. Whittle; C. Somerville. Catalytic plasticity of fatty acid modification enzymes underlying chemical diversity of plant lipids. *Science* **1998**, *282*, 1315–1317.

Cevc, G. *Phospholipids Handbook,* Marcel Dekker: New York, 1993.

Chatgilialoglu, C.; C. Ferreri; Trans lipids: the free radical path. *Acc. Chem. Res.* **2005**, *38*, 441–448.

Chatgilialoglu, C.; C. Ferreri. Cis-trans isomerization : from biology to supramolecular chemistry. *Fatty Acids and Phospholipids*; C. Dugave, Ed.; Wiley-VCH: Wienheim, 2006, pp. 92–112.

Chatgilialoglu, C.; C. Ferreri; M. Ballestri; Q.G. Mulazzani; L. Landi. Cis-trans-isomerization of monounsaturated fatty acid residues in phospholipids by thiyl radicals. *J. Am. Chem. Soc.* **2000**, *122*, 4593–4601.

Chatgilialoglu, C.; A. Samadi; M. Guerra; H. Fischer. The kinetics of Z/E isomerization of methyl oleate catalyzed by photogenerated thiyl radicals. *Chem. Phys. Chem.* 2005, *6*, 286–291.

Crabb, J.W.; J. O'Neil; M. Miyagi; K. West; H.F. Hoff. Hydroxynonenal inactivates cathepsin B by forming Michael adducts with active site residues. *Protein Sci.* **2002**, *11*, 831–840.

Crawford, D.R.; K.J.A. Davies. Adaptive response and oxidative stress. *Environ. Health Perspectives*, **1994**, *102*, 25–28.

Dianzani, M.U. 4-Hydroxynonenale and cell signaling, *Free Radical Res.* **1998**, *28*, 553–560.

Diefenbach, R.; H. Keweloh. Synthesis of trans unsaturated fatty acids in Pseudomonas putida P8 by direct isomerization of the double bond of lipids *Arch. Microbiol.* **1994**, *162*, 120–125.

Escribà, P.V. Membrane lipid therapy: a new approach in molecular medicine. *Trends Mol. Med.* **2006**, *12*, 34–43.

Esterbauer, H.; R.G. Schauer; H. Zollner. Chemistry and biochemistry of 4-hydroxynonenal, malondialdehyde and related aldehydes. *Free Radical Biol. Med.* **1991**, *11*, 81–128.

Evans, M.E.; J.M. Brown; M.K. McIntosh. Isomer-specific effects of conjugated linoleic acid (CLA) on adiposity and lipid metabolism. *J. Nutr. Biochem.* **2002**, *13*, 508–516.

Farooqui, A.A.; L.A. Horrocks. Signalling and interplay mediated by phospholipases $A_2$, C, and D in LA-N-1 cell nuclei. *Reprod. Nutr. Dev.* **2005**, *45*, 613–631.

Ferreri, C.; F. Angelini; C. Chatgilialoglu; S. Dellonte; V. Moschese; P. Rossi;L. Chini. Trans fatty acids and atopic eczema/dermatitis syndrome: the relationship with a free radical cis-trans isomerization of membrane lipids. *Lipids* **2005a**, *40*, 661–667.

Ferreri, C.; S. Kratzsch; L. Landi; O. Brede. Thiyl radicals in biosystems: effects on lipid structures and metabolism. *Cell. Mol. Life Sci.* **2005b**, *62*, 834–847.

Ferreri, C.; M.R. Faraone Mennella; C. Formisano; L. Landi; C. Chatgilialoglu. Arachidonate geometrical isomers generated by thiyl radicals: the relationship with trans lipids detected in biological samples. *Free Radical Biol. Med.* **2002**, *33*, 1516–1526.

Ferreri, C.; S. Pierotti; A. Barbieri; L. Zambonin; L. Landi; S. Rasi; P.L. Luisi; F. Barigelletti; C. Chatgilialoglu. Comparison of phosphatidylcholine vesicle properties related to geometrical isomerism. *Photochem. Photobiol.* **2006a**, *82,* 274–280.

Ferreri, C.; S. Pierotti; C. Chatgilialoglu; A. Barbieri; F. Barigelletti. Probing the influence of cis-trans isomers on model lipid membrane fluidity using cis-parinaric acid and stop-flow technique. *Chem. Commun.* **2006b**, 529–531.

Ferreri, C.; A. Samadi; F. Sassatelli; L. Landi; C. Chatgilialoglu. Regioselective cis–trans isomerization of arachidonic double bonds by thiyl radicals: the influence of phospholipid supramolecular organization. *J. Am. Chem. Soc.* **2004**, *126*, 1063–1072.

Fox, B.G; K.S. Lyle; C.E. Rogge. Reactions of the diiron enzyme stearoyl-acyl carrier protein desaturase. *Acc. Chem. Res.* **2004**, *37*, 421–429.

Fruhwirth, G.O.; A. Loidl; A. Hermetter. Oxidized phospholipids: from molecular properties to disease. *Biochim. Biophys. Acta* **2007**, *1772*, 718–736.

Fukuda, N.; N. Igari; T. Hidaka; M. Sugano. A comparison of the metabolism of cis,cis, cis,trans/trans,cis. and trans,trans-9,12-octadecadienoic acid in rat liver. *Nutr. Res.* **1993**, *13*, 779–786.

Funk, C.D. Prostaglandins and leukotrienes: advances in eicosanoid biology. *Science* **2001**, *294*, 1871–1875.

Girotti, A.W. Photodynamic lipid peroxidation in biological systems. *Photochem. Photobiol.* **1990**, *51*, 497–509.

Grundt, H.; D.W.T. Nilsen.. n-3 Fatty acids and cardiovascular disease. *Haematologica* **2008**, *93*, 807–812.

Gutteridge, J.M.C. Lipid peroxidation and antioxidants as biomarkers of tissue damage. *Clin. Chem.* **1995**, *41*, 1819–1828.

Halliwell, B.; J.M.C. Gutteridge; *Free Radicals in Biology and Medicine,* 4th ed.; Oxford University Press: Oxford, 2007.

Harrison, K.A.; S.S. Davies; G.K. Marathe; T. Mcintyre; S. Prescott; K.M.Reddy; J.R. Falck; R.C. Murphy. Analysis of oxidized glycerophosphocholine lipids using electrospray ionization mass spectrometry and microderivatization techniques. *J. Mass Spectrom.* **2000**, *35*, 224–236.

Heipieper, H.J.; R. Diefenbach; H. Keweloh. Conversion of cis unsaturated fatty acids to trans, a possible mechanism for the protection of phenol-degrading Pseudomonas putida P8 from substrate toxicity. *Appl. Environ. Microbiol.* **1992,** *58*, 1847–1852.

Heipieper, H.J.; F. Meinhardt; A. Segura. The cis-trans isomerase of unsaturated fatty acids in Pseudomonas and Vibrio: biochemistry, molecular biology and physiological function of a unique stress adaptive response. *FEMS Microbiol. Lett.* **2003,** *229*, 1–7.

Houtkooper, R.H.; F.M. Vaz. Cardiolipin, the heart of mitochondrial metabolism. *Cell. Mol. Life Sci.* **2008**, DOI 10.1007/s00018-008-8030-5.

Hu, F.B.; M.J. Stampfer; J.E. Manson; E. Rimm; G.A. Colditz; B.A. Rosner; C.H. Hennekens; W.C. Willett. Dietary fat intake and the risk of coronary artery disease in women. *N. Engl. J. Med.* **1997,** *337*, 1491–1499.

Hulbert, A.J. On the importance of fatty acid composition of membranes for aging. *J. Exp. Biol.* **2003**, *206*, 303–311.

Isken, S.; P. Santos; J.A.M. de Bont. Effects of solvent adaptation on the antibiotic resistance of Pseudomonas putida S12. *Appl. Microbiol. Biotechnol.*, **1997**, 642–647.

Kagan, V.E.; P.J. Quinn. Toward oxidative lipidomics of cell signaling, *Antioxid. Redox Signaling* **2004**, *6*, 199–202.

Keller, J.N.; R.J. Mark; A.J. Bruce; E. Blanc; J.D. Rothstein; K. Uchida;G. Waeg; M.P. Mattson. 4-Hydroxynonenal, an aldehydic product of membrane lipid peroxidation, impairs glutamate transport and mitochondrial function in synaptosomes. *Neuroscience* 1997, *80*, 685–696.

Kondoh, Y.; T. Kawada; R. Urade. Activation of caspase 3 in HepG2 cells by elaidic acid (t18:1), *BBA, Mol. Cell Biol. Lipids* **2007**, *1771*, 500–505.

Kristal, B.S.; B.K. Park; B.P. Yu.. 4-Hydroxyhexenal is a potent inducer of the mitochondrial permeability transition. *J. Biol. Chem.* **1996**, *271*, 6033–6038.

Kruman, I.; A.J. Bruce-Keller; D. Bredesen; G. Waeg; M.P. Mattson. Evidence that 4-hydroxynonenal mediates oxidative stress-induced neuronal apoptosis. *J. Neurosci.* 1997, *17*, 5089–5100.

Kummerow, F.A.; M.M. Mahfouz; Q. Zhou. Trans fatty acids in partially hydrogenated soybean oil inhibit prostacyclin release by endothelial cells in presence of high level of linoleic acid. *Prostaglandins Other Lipid Mediat.* **2007**, *84*, 138–153.

Kummerow, F.A.; Q. Zhou; M.M. Mahfouz. Effects of trans fatty acids on calcium influx into human arterial endothelial cells. *Am. J. Clin. Nutr.* **1999**, *70*, 832–838.

Kummerow, F.A.; Q. Zhou; M.M. Mahfouz; M.R. Smiricky; C.M. Grieshop; D.J. Schaeffer. Trans fatty acids in hydrogenated fat inhibited the synthesis of polyunsaturated fatty acids in the phospholipid of arterial cells. *Life Sci.* **2004**, *74*, 2707–3205.

Larquè, E.; P.-A. Garcia-Ruiz; F. Perez-Llamas; S. Zamora; A. Gil. Dietary trans fatty acids alter the composition of microsomes and mitochondria and the activities of microsome Δ6-fatty acid desaturase and glucose-6-phosphatase in livers of pregnant rats. *J. Nutr.* **2003**, *133*, 2526–2531.

Larquè, E.; S. Zamora; A. Gil. A. Dietary trans fatty acids in early life: a review. *Early Human Develop.* **2001**, *65*, S31–S41.

Lauritzen, L.; H.S. Hansen; M.H. Jørgensen; K.F. Michaelsen. The essentiality of long chain *n*-3 fatty acids in relation to development and function of the brain and retina. *Progr. Lipid Res.* **2001,** *40,* 1–94.

Logan, A.C. Omega-3, omega-6 and psoriasis: a different view. *Int. J. Dermatol.* **2004**, *44*, 527–528.

Marathe, G.K.; K. Harrison; R.C. Murphy; S.M. Prescott; G.A. Zimmerman; T.M. McIntyre. Bioactive phospholipids oxidation products. *Free Radical Biol. Med.* **2000**, *28*, 1762–1770.

Megli, F.M.; L. Russo; K. Sabatini. Oxidized phospholipids induce phase separation in lipid vesicles. *FEBS Lett.* **2005**, *579*, 4577–4584.

Metz, J.G.; et al. Polyketide synthase produce polyunsaturated fatty acids in both prokaryotes and eukaryotes. *Science* **2001**, *293*, 290–293.

Meyer, Z.U.; D. Heringdorf; K.H. Jacobs. Lysophospholipid receptors: signalling, pharmacology and regulation by lysophospholipid metabolism. *Biochim. Biophys. Acta* 2007, *1768*, 923–940.

Milne, G.L.; N.A. Porter. Separation and identification of phospholipid peroxidation products. *Lipids* **2001**, *36*, 1265–1275.

Morrow, J.D.; L.J. Roberts. The isoprostanes: unique bioactive products of lipid peroxidation. *Progr. Lipid Res.* **1997,** *36*, 1–21

Murakami, Y.; M. Tsuyama; Y. Kobayashi; H. Kodama; K. Iba.. Trienoic fatty acids and plant tolerance of high temperature. *Science* **2000**, *287*, 476–479.

Murph, M.; T. Tanaka; S. Liu; G.B. Mills. Of spiders and crabs: the emergence of lysophospholipids and their metabolic pathways as targets for therapy in cancer. *Clin. Cancer Res.* **2006**, *12*, 6598–6602.

Neumann, G.;N. Kabelitz; H.J. Heipieper. The regulation of the cis-trans isomerase of unsaturated fatty acids in Pseudomonas putida: correlation between cti activity and $K^+$-uptake systems. *Eur. J. Lipid Sci. Technol.* **2003**, *105*, 585–589.

Niki, E.; Y. Yoshida; Y. Saito; N. Nogichi. Lipid peroxidation: mechanisms, inhibition, and biological effects. *Biochem. Biophys. Res. Commun.* **2005**, *338*, 66–676.

Niu, S.-L.; D.C. Mitchell; B.J. Litman. Trans fatty acid derived phospholipids show increased membrane cholesterol and reduced receptor activation as compared to their cis analogs. *Biochemistry* **2005**, *44*, 4458–4465.

Okuyama, H.; N. Okajima; S. Sasaki; S. Higashi; N. Murata. The cis/trans isomerization of the double bond of a fatty acid as a strategy for adaptation to changes in ambient temperature in the psychrophilic bacterium, Vibrio sp strain ABE-1. *Biochim. Biophys. Acta* **1991**, *1084*, 13–20.

Paradies, G.; G. Petrosillo; M. Pistolese; N. Di Venosa; D. Serena; F.M.Ruggiero. Lipid peroxidation and alterations to oxidative metabolism in mitochondria isolated from rat heart subjected to ischemia and reperfusion. *Free Radical Biol. Med.* **1999**, *27*, 42–50.

Poggioli, S.; J. Mary; H. Bakala; B. Friguet. Evidence of Preferential Protein Targets for Age-Related Modifications in Peripheral Blood Lymphocytes. *Ann. N.Y. Acad. Sci.* **2004**, *1019*, 211–214.

Pogocki, D.; C. Schoeneich. Thiyl radicals abstract hydrogen atoms from carbohydrates: reactivity and selectivity. *Free Radical Biol. Med.* **2001**, *31*, 98–101.

Porter, N.A.; S.E. Caldwell; K.A. Mills. Mechanisms of free radical oxidation of unsaturated lipids. *Lipids* **1995**, *30*, 277–290.

Pryor, W.A.; J.P. Stanley. Suggested mechanism for the production of malonaldehyde during the autoxidation of polyunsaturated fatty acids. Nonenzymic production of prostaglandin endoperoxides during autoxidation. *J. Org. Chem.* **1975**, *40, 3615*–3617.

Puca, A.A.; C. Chatgilialoglu; C. Ferreri. Lipid Metabolism and Diet :Possible Mechanism of Slow Aging. *Int. J. Biochem. Cell Biol.* **2008**, *40*, 324–333.

Puca, A.A.; V. Novelli; C. Viviani; P. Andrew; F. Somalvico; N.A. Cirillo;C. Chatgilialoglu; C. Ferreri. Lipid profile of erythrocyte membranes as possible biomarker of longevity. *Rejuven. Res.* **2008a**, *11*, 63–72.

Roach, C.; S.E. Feller; J.A. Ward; S. Raza Shaikh; M. Zerouga; W. Stillwell. Comparison of cis and trans fatty acid containing phosphatidylcholines on membrane properties. *Biochemistry* **2004**, *43*, 6344–6351.

Roberts, T.L.; D.A. Wood; R.A. Riemersma; P.J. Gallagher; F.C. Lampe. Trans isomers of oleic and linoleic acids in adipose tissues and sudden cardiac death. *Lancet* **1995**, *345*, 278–282.

Roy, U.; O. Loreau; M. Balazy. Cytochrome P450/NADPH-dependent formation of trans epoxides from trans-arachidonic acids. *Bioorg. Med. Chem. Lett.* **2004**, *14*, 1019–1022.

Sabatini, K.; J.P. Mattila; F.M. Megli; P.K. Kinnunen. Characterization of two oxidatively modified phospholipids in mixed monolayers with DPPC. *Biophys. J.* **2006**, *90*, 4488–4499.

Sakamoto, T.; N. Murata. Regulation of the desaturation of fatty acids and its role in tolerance to cold and salt stress. *Curr. Opin. Microbiol.* **2002**, *5*, 206–210.

Schneider, C.; N.A. Porter; A.R. Brash. Routes to 4-hydroxynonenal: fundamental issues in the mechanisms of lipid peroxidation. *J. Biol. Chem.* **2008**, *283*, 15539–15543.

Schneider, C.; D.A. Pratt; N.A. Porter; A.R. Brash. Control of oxygenation in lipoxygenase and cyclooxygenase catalysis. *Chem. Biol.* **2007**, *14*, 473–488.

Schwarz, W. Trans unsaturated fatty acids in European nutrition. *Eur. J. Lipid Sci. Technol.* **2000**, *102*, 633–635.

Sébédio, J.L.; W.W. Christie. *Trans Fatty Acids in Human Nutrition;* The Oily Press: Dundee, 1998.

Serhan, C.N. Mediator lipidomics. *Prostaglandins Other Lipid Mediat.* **2005**, *77*, 4–14.

Sinensky, M. Homeoviscous adaptation: a homeostatic process that regulates the viscosity of membrane lipids in Escherichia coli. *Proc. Natl. Acad. Sci. USA* **1974**, *71*, 522–525.

Smith, C.V.; D.P. Jones; T.M. Guentner; L.H. Lash; B.H. Lanterburg. Contemporary issues in toxicology. Compartmentation of glutathione: implications for the study of toxicity and disease. *Toxicol. Appl. Pharmacol.* **1996**, *140*, 1–12.

Spiteller, G. Is atherosclerosis a multifactorial disease or is it induced by a sequence of lipid peroxidation reactions? *Ann. N. Y. Acad. Sci.* **2005**, *1043*, 355–366.

Spiteller, G. The important role of lipid peroxidation processes in aging and age dependent diseases. *Mol. Biotechnol.* **2007**, *37*, 5–12.

Spiteller, G. Peroxyl radicals: Inductors of neurodegenerative and other inflammatory diseases. Their origin and how they transform cholesterol, phospholipids, plasmalogens, polyunsaturated fatty acids, sugars and proteins into deleterious products. *Free Radical Biol. Med.* **2006**, *41*, 362–387.

Stachowska, E.; B. Dogowska; M. Olszewska; I. Gutowska; D. Chlubek. Isomers of trans fatty acids modify the activity of platelets 12-P lipoxygenase and cyclooxygenase/thromboxane synthase. *Nutrition* **2004**, *20*, 570–571.

Stender, S.; J. Dyerberg; G. Holmer; L. Ovesen; B. Sandström. The influence of trans fatty acids on health: a report from the Danish Nutrition Council. *Clin Sci.* **1995**, *88*, 375–392.

Stohs, S.J.; D. Baggi. Oxidative mechanisms in the toxicity of metal ions, *Free Radical Biol. Med.* **1995**, *18*, 321–336.

Sun, G.Y.; J. Xu; M.D. Jensen; A. Simonyi. Phospholipase $A_2$ in the central nervous system: implications for neurodegenerative diseases. *J. Lipid Res.* **2004**, *45*, 205–213.

Svensson, M.; A.-K. Mossberg; J. Pettersson; S. Linse; C. Svanborg. Lipids as cofactors in protein folding: Stereo-specific lipid-protein interactions are required to form HAMLET (human α-lactalbumin made lethal to tumor cells). *Protein Sci.* **2003**, *12*, 2805–2814.

Tallman, K.A.; B. Roschek, Jr.; N.A. Porter. Factors influencing the autoxidation of fatty acids: effect of olefin geometry of the nonconjugated diene. *J. Am. Chem. Soc.* **2004**, *126*, 9240–9247.

Tyurina, Y.Y.; V.A. Tyurin; M.W. Epperly; J.S. Greenberger; V.E. Kagan. Oxidative lipidomics of γ-irradiation-induced intestinal injury. *Free Radical Biol. Med.* **2008**, *44*, 299–314.

Vance, D.E.; J.E. Vance. *Biochemistry of Lipids, Lipoproteins and Membranes*, 4th ed.; Elsevier:Amsterdam, 2002.

van de Vijver, L.P.L.; et al. Association between trans fatty acid intake and cardiovascular risk factors in Europe: the TRANSFAIR study. *Eur. J. Clin. Nutr.* **2000**, *54*, 126–135.

Wakeldm, M.J..; T.R. Pettit; A.D. Postle. Lipidomic analysis of signaling pathways, *Methods Enzymol.* **2007**, *432*, 233–246.

Wältermann, M.; A. Steinbüchel. Neutral lipid-bodies in prokaryotes: recent insights into structure. Formation, and relationship to eukaryotic lipid depots. *J. Bacteriol.* **2005**, *187*, 3607–3619.

Watson, A.D. Lipidomics: a global approach to lipid analysis in biological systems. *J. Lipid Res.* **2006**, *47*, 2101–2111.

Wenk, M.R. The emerging field of lipidomics. *Nat. Rev. Drug Discov.* **2005**, *4*, 594–610.

Wilson, J.F. Long-suffering lipids gain respect. *The Scientist* **2003**, *17*, 34–36.

Witztum, J.L. Role of oxidized low density lipoprotein in atherogenesis. *Br. Heart J.* **1993**, *69*, S12–S18.

Yin, H.; N.A. Porter. New insights regarding the autoxidation of polyunsaturated fatty acids. *Antiox. Redox Signal.* **2005**, *7*, 170–184.

Zambonin, L.; C. Ferreri; L. Cabrini; C. Prata; C. Chatgilialoglu; L. Landi. Occurrence of trans fatty acids in rats fed a trans-free diet: a free radical-mediated formation? *Free Radical Biol. Med.* **2006**, *40*, 1549–1556.

Zambonin, L.; C. Prata; L. Cabrini; T. Maraldi; D. Fiorentini;; F. Vieceli Dalla Sega; G. Hakim; L. Landi. Effect of radical stress and ageing on the occurrence of *trans* fatty acids in rats fed a *trans*-free diet. *Free Radical Biol. Med.* **2008**, *44*, 594–601.

Zapolska-Downar, D.; A. Kosmider; M. Naruszewicz. Trans fatty acids induce apoptosis in human endothelial cells. *J. Physiol. Pharmacol.* **2005**, *56*, 611–625.

Zghibeh, C.M.; V. Raj Gopal; C.D. Poff; J.R. Falck; M. Balazy. Determination of *trans*-arachidonic acid isomers in human blood plasma. *Anal. Biochem.* **2004**, *332*,137–144.

# 16

# Ruminal Metabolism of Fatty Acids: Modulation of Polyunsaturated, Conjugated, and *trans* Fatty Acids in Meat and Milk

**Michel Doreau and Frédéric Glasser**
*INRA, UR 1213 Herbivore Research Unit, Site de Theix, F-63122 Saint-Genès Champanelle, France*

## Introduction

Milk and dairy products are major sources of lipids for humans in Western countries: in Europe and the United States, they represent 14–40% of total lipid intake and 27–57% of saturated fatty acid (FA) intake, as a consequence of their high concentration in saturated FA (Hulshof et al., 1999; Weinberg et al., 2004). Animals that produce milk for human consumption are mainly ruminants: cows, ewes, goats, and camels; only a very minor part of milk is produced by nonruminants, such as mare milk in central Asia. Ruminants also contribute to lipid intake through meat, but to a lower level. FAs from ruminant products are known to be rich in saturated FA (and particularly the short- and medium-chain ones in milk) and poor in polyunsaturated FA (PUFA), such as linoleic acid (18:2 n-6) and alpha-linolenic acid (ALA, 18:3 n-3). Increasing the content of PUFA and decreasing the saturated FA in ruminant products are challenges to improve the global health value of these products, which are an important part of the human diet now and in the future; however, obviously, dairy products and ruminant meat will never significantly contribute to meet human requirements in omega-3 FA. Less obviously, ruminant products are the only food to contain conjugated linoleic acids (CLAs), with the exception of pork from pigs fed synthetic CLA. Ruminant products also contain significant amounts of various nonconjugated *trans* FAs, especially monounsaturated isomers; they also are the only natural source of *trans* FA in the human diet, and represent 28–79% of *trans* FA intake in Europe (Hulshof et al., 1999). Now increasing data exist showing that these natural *trans* isomers would not have the deleterious effects of the *trans* isomers from industrial origin (margarines and other partially hydrogenated fats). For example, the well-known nurse's health epidemiologic study (Willett et al., 1993) showed that the relative risk was lower with animal than with vegetal *trans* sources: the latter lower HDL cholesterol as suggested by a study on healthy subjects (Chardigny et al., 2008).

Milk composition is very variable, mainly depending on dietary factors, and very few differences exist in FA composition between milk and dairy products. Other chapters of this book deal with milk FA composition. This chapter is devoted to the understanding of digestive processes that determine this composition, and the transfer of FAs from the gastrointestinal tract to mammary gland and muscle. Attention is drawn to PUFA and *trans* monounsaturated FAs; CLA variations in the rumen are less studied because 95% of milk CLA on average is of post-ruminal origin and is synthesized by the tissues from *trans* monounsaturated FA produced in the rumen (Glasser et al., 2008a).

## Rumen: Site of FA Metabolism in Ruminants

In humans as in monogastric animal species (pig, birds, rodents), FAs are absorbed in the small intestine without major alteration in the stomach, so that the composition of pork and poultry meat FA is close to the composition of dietary FAs. On the contrary, in ruminant species such as cattle, sheep, and goat, FAs are extensively metabolized in the rumen before their absorption in the small intestine, so that the FA composition of milk and meat from ruminants completely differs from that of their diet.

The rumen, together with its appendix the reticulum, is a large reservoir located after the esophagus, and corresponds to the first digestive compartment in ruminants. It contains feeds in fermentation. For a 700-kg cow, rumen contents may reach 100 kg. The digestive organs that follow the rumen are the omasum, the abomasum (which is the functional equivalent to a monogastric stomach), then the small intestine, and then the large intestine. In the rumen, a numerous and diversified microbial population is living as symbiotic organisms: bacteria, protozoa, archaea, and fungi. Owing to their enzymatic equipment, bacteria are responsible for carbohydrate fermentation into volatile FAs (mainly acetic, propionic, and butyric acids), which are the main energy substrates for ruminants. Although metabolically active, protozoa play a less important role. Ruminants can thus convert grass into animal products because rumen bacteria can convert cellulose into volatile FAs used as an energy substrate by animal metabolism. Detailed information of the ruminant gastrointestinal tract physiology is found in Church (1993).

FAs of ruminant feedstuffs are present as triglycerides, which are storage lipids; phospholipids, which are located in cell membranes; and glycolipids, specific of forage lipids. Forages and other standard ruminant feedstuffs such as cereals contain less than 4% of lipids. The main FA of grass or grass silage is ALA, which represents almost 50% of total FAs (Table 16.1); the main FA of cereals is linoleic acid that represents approximately 50% of total FAs. In addition, one can feed ruminants oleaginous seeds, rich in lipids (Table 16.1), and fish oil or fish products, with lipids rich in 20- and 22-carbon omega-3 FAs, mainly eicosapentaenoic acid (EPA, 20:5 n-3) and docosahexaenoic acid (DHA, 22:6 n-3). Technological treatments of lipid sources can also result in industrial feeds that are given to ruminants as powder supplements. Calcium salts of FAs are generally made from palm oil, but are sometimes based on

**Table 16.1. Mean Fatty Acid Composition (g/100 g Total FA) of Some Forages and Lipid Supplements Used in Ruminant Diets**

| | <C16 | C16:0 | C18:0 | C18:1 | C18:2 | C18:3 |
|---|---|---|---|---|---|---|
| Pasture | 1.6 | 18.2 | 1.9 | 2.7 | 14.2 | 48.9 |
| Grass silage | 1.7 | 20.6 | 2.6 | 3.9 | 16.6 | 48.2 |
| Grass hay | 2.6 | 23.5 | 3.4 | 6.8 | 18 | 37.8 |
| Alfalfa hay | 1.5 | 27.1 | 4.5 | 4.6 | 21.1 | 21.3 |
| Corn silage | 0.9 | 15.2 | 2.7 | 20.5 | 43.7 | 5.6 |
| Palm oil | 1.7 | 46.5 | 4.4 | 36.1 | 8.7 | 0.2 |
| Tallow | 3.5 | 25.4 | 17.2 | 39.9 | 4.4 | 0.4 |
| Rapeseed | 0.2 | 4.8 | 2.1 | 60.5 | 20.8 | 9.2 |
| Corn | 0.0 | 13.6 | 2.7 | 28.4 | 50.8 | 1.1 |
| Sunflower | 0.1 | 5.1 | 4.3 | 21.6 | 66.8 | 0.3 |
| Soybean | 0.1 | 11.3 | 4.1 | 22.4 | 53.5 | 7.2 |
| Linseed | 0.1 | 3.6 | 3.4 | 18.8 | 16.3 | 54.4 |

vegetable oils. Treating oils and oilseeds with formaldehyde can protect them from rumen degradation (see below). Crystallized or prilled fats are made of saturated or monounsaturated FAs, arising from native or hydrogenated sources.

Rumen is the site of many changes in FA flow and composition, due to several mechanisms that are summarized in Fig. 16.1. Rumen microbes modify dietary lipids through a series of enzymes. The first step of lipid metabolism in the rumen is lipolysis, which converts esterified FAs into free FAs. Among bacterial species, *Anaerovibrio lipolytica* is the main species responsible for this process, through a lipase. Lipolysis is very extensive, so that with standard feedstuffs few esterified FAs escape the rumen. After lipolysis, once the hydroxyl radical is free, FA can be isomerized and hydrogenated by microbial isomerases and hydrogenases. Some FAs are taken up by the microbes, which can also synthesize their own FAs.

Two main pathways of isomerization and hydrogenation are described for ALA and linoleic acid (*c*9*c*12-18:2) (Harfoot & Hazlewood, 1997). ALA is first isomerized to several *trans*-18:3 isomers (partly unknown), which are then hydrogenated to *t*11*c*15-18:2, then to *t*11-18:1, which can in turn be hydrogenated to 18:0. Linoleic acid is first isomerized to *c*9*t*11-18:2, which is then hydrogenated to *t*11-18:1, which can then be further hydrogenated to 18:0. Isomerases are active even after hydrogenation occurs. In certain conditions (high PUFA content of the diet, low rumen pH, modification of bacterial populations), an alternative pathway through *t*10*c*12-18:2 and *t*10-18:1 can prevail. These processes involve several enzymes that are

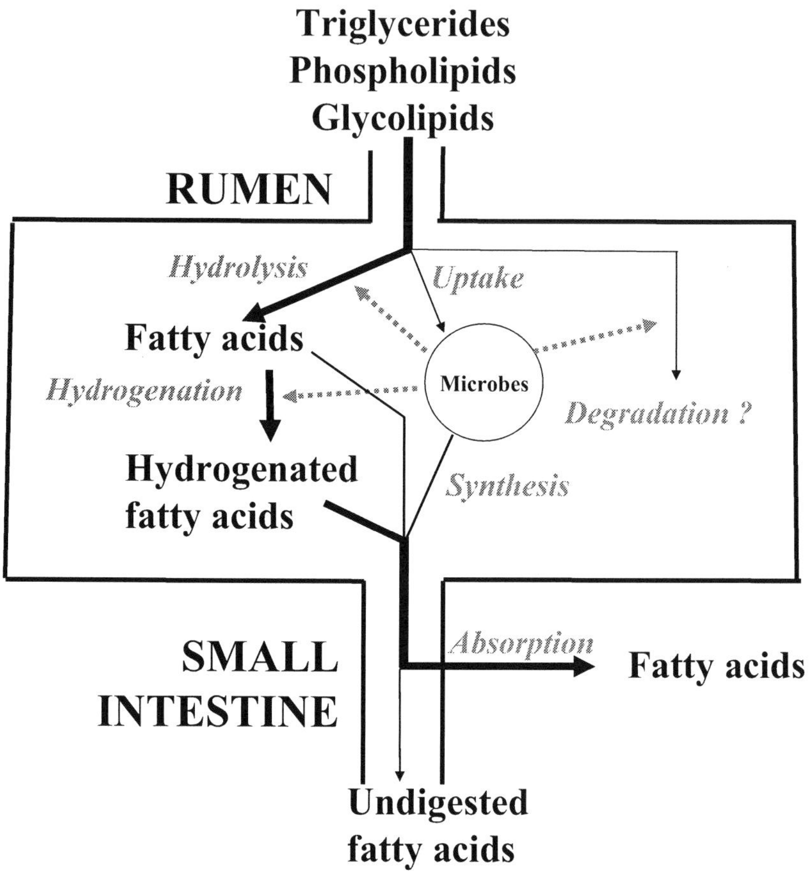


**Fig. 16.1.** Diagram of the main processes of FA digestion in ruminants.

present in different classes of bacteria. The main mechanisms are described by Harfoot and Hazlewood (1997), who summarized the hydrogenation capacities of various strains and split them into two groups named A and B, according to the hydrogenation and isomerization pathways they can perform. Group A comprises *Butyrivibrio fibrisolvens* and is necessary for the first steps of biohydrogenation. Group B, which mainly includes *Fusocillus* sp., could be the only group to hydrogenate *t*11-18:1 to produce stearic acid. Biohydrogenation is inhibited when ruminal protozoa decrease (Boeckaert et al., 2007), but protozoa probably do not act directly, but through the bacteria they have ingested (Jenkins et al., 2008). In fact, the actual mechanisms are much more complex (review by Jenkins & Bridges, 2007), imply numerous other 18:1, 18:2, and 18:3 isomers (that are present in the duodenal contents) (Fig. 16.2), and all biochemical pathways are not known. A well-known fact is that rumen digesta and bacteria contain a wide variety of *cis* and *trans* 18:1 isomers and several CLA isomers (Keeney, 1970). For example, Loor et al. (2005) found on chromatograms of duodenal contents, considered as the result of ruminal metabolism, seven nonconjugated 18:2 isomers, 9 peaks of CLAs, and 16 peaks of 18:1 *cis* and *trans* FAs. More than 100 peaks of FAs are generally found on chromatograms of duodenal contents. By using labeled oleic (*c*9-18:1) and elaidic acids (*t*9-18:1), Mosley et al. (2002) and Proell et al. (2002) showed that these FAs may be converted in a large number of other 18:1 isomers. This suggests that isomerases are very active on several FAs.

The C18 FAs reaching the duodenum are composed on an average of 70% of 18:0, 9% of *cis*-18:1, 11% of *trans*-18:1, 7% 18:2 (25% of which is *c*9*c*12-18:2), and 2% of 18:3 (Glasser et al., 2008b). Diets containing fish oil divide the percentage of 18:0 by a factor of 2, to the benefit of *trans*-18:1. Of course, dietary modifications alter the FA proportions around these means. When rumen microbial populations are disturbed (e.g., high-concentrate diets inducing a low rumen pH, high amounts of dietary PUFA), the last biohydrogenation step (*trans*-18:1 to 18:0) is generally the most affected one, leading to increases in *trans*-18:1 flow at the duodenum, at the expense of 18:0. The profile of *trans*-18:1 can also be modified, with a shift from *t*11-18:1 (the main isomer in standard conditions) to *t*10-18:1. Other intermediates (various 18:2 and 18:3 isomers) also increase following lipid supplementation.

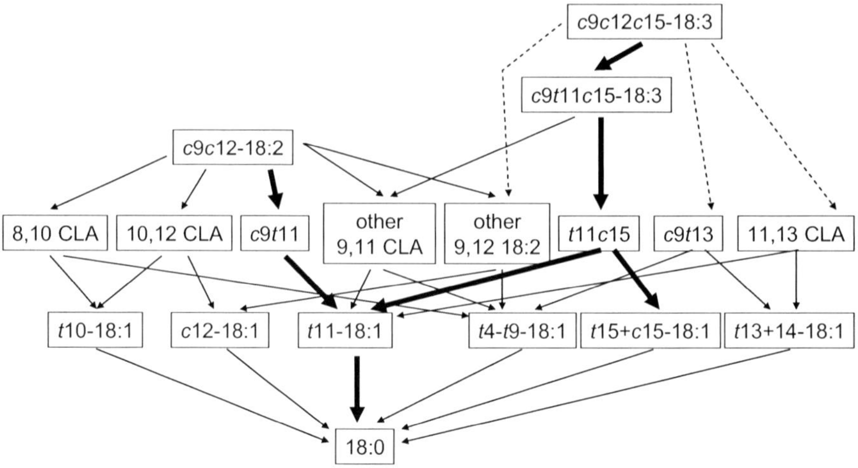


**Fig. 16.2.** Main putative biohydrogenation pathways of linoleic and linolenic acids. When *cis* or *trans* configurations are not mentioned, it means that the various *cis-cis*, *cis-trans*, and *trans*-trans configurations are included. Thick arrows represent the major pathways (Harfoot & Hazlewood, 1997); thin arrows represent other putative pathways, as suggested by increases in the corresponding isomers during in vitro incubations of pure linoleic and linolenic acids (Jouany et al., 2007); dotted arrows represent possibly indirect BH pathways (possibly including other intermediates). Not all FA are mentioned, and the numerous interconversions among 18:1 isomers (Mosley et al., 2002; Proell et al., 2002) are not represented on the figure. Figure from Chilliard et al. (2007), © Wiley-VCH Verlag GmbH & Co, reproduced with permission.

Bacterial proteins are synthesized from carbon chains and ammonia arising from feedstuff protein degradation by microbial enzymes. In the same way, bacteria can synthesize their own FAs, mainly from volatile FAs. Bacterial lipids are rich in even-chain FAs, but also contain very specific FAs as 15- and 17-carbon straight and branched-chain FAs (Vlaeminck et al., 2006). Theoretically, FAs are neither absorbed nor catabolized in the rumen. In fact, the flow of FAs leaving the rumen is often lower than FAs intake, especially with diets rich in lipids (Doreau & Ferlay, 1994; Schmidely et al., 2008); in vitro experiments suggest that some anaerobic mechanisms could be involved.

Besides the hydrogenation of a high proportion of the dietary FAs, rumen metabolism thus produces a complex mix of unsaturated FAs isomers, with many *trans* isomers, that later are found in ruminant products and sometimes also influence the animal's metabolism.

## Post-ruminal Absorption of FAs

When FAs resulting from ruminal metabolism reach the duodenum, they are generally adsorbed onto small feed particles and bacteria. Mechanisms of intestinal absorption are close to the general features in monogastric species, except that lipids enter the small intestine as free FAs. The absence of monoglycerides in the ruminant duodenum is compensated for by the presence of lysolecithins in bile, produced by phospholipases from bacterial phospholipids. FAs are desorbed and solubilized by bile salts and lysolecithins, then transferred to a micellar phase that enables absorption in the jejunum. One can only measure FA absorption in a reliable manner between the duodenum and ileum or feces by using animals fitted with duodenal and sometimes ileal cannulae. A literature survey revealed intestinal digestibility ranging between 55% and 92% (Doreau & Ferlay, 1994). Variability is not explained by the level of FA intake or the FA composition of the diet. Apparent digestibility coefficients determined from meta-analysis are 60%, 71%, 79%, and 78% for 12-, 14-, 16-, and 18-carbon FAs, respectively (unpublished data, means of respectively, 48, 69, 95, and 45 data). Less data exist for 20- and 22-carbon FAs; apparent digestibility is on average 70% for both C20 and C22 FAs (means of, respectively, 35 and 22 published data). Among 18-carbon FAs, absorption coefficients are lower for 18:0, 18:2, and 18:3 (74%, 72%, and 70%, respectively) than for 18:1 *cis* and *trans* (78% and 82%) (Glasser et al., 2008b).

The epithelial cells of the intestine are the site of FA esterification into triglycerides and phospholipids, transported into the lymph as chylomicrons and VLDL, and further into the blood where these lipoproteins are found together with LDL and HDL. Chylomicrons, LDL, and VLDL contain approximately 85%, 10–15%, and 60% of triglycerides, respectively (Demeyer & Doreau, 1999). Lipoproteins transport FA mainly to the mammary gland in dairy animals and mainly to adipose and muscle tissue in growing and fattening animals.

During the passage into the mammary gland or muscle, triglycerides are largely or completely hydrolyzed by a lipoprotein lipase located on the tissue membrane.

Additional details on mechanisms and on the role of adipose tissue for lipid storage are found in Chilliard (1993) and Demeyer & Doreau (1999).

## FA Transfer to Udder and Muscle and Their Effect on Tissue Metabolism

Meat and milk FAs come from two main sources: they can be taken up by the tissues from plasma or synthesized de novo by the tissues (mammary gland, adipose tissue, and muscle). FA uptake concerns both long-chain FAs from lipid mobilization (mainly during restricted feeding or during the first weeks of lactation in dairy cows) and long-chain FAs from dietary origin. In meat, the main synthesized FA is palmitic acid (16:0), followed by 14:0, whereas in milk, FAs from 4 to 16 carbon units are synthesized. No further modification of preformed FAs within these tissues occurs, except for desaturation of medium- and long-chain FAs by a delta-9 desaturase. This enzyme converts 14:0, 16:0, and 18:0 into *c*9-14:1, *c*9-16:1, and *c*9-18:1, adding a *cis* double bond on the carbon #9 of the FA chain. This enzyme also converts *t*11-18:1 (vaccenic acid) into *c*9*t*11-18:2, which is the main isomer of CLA in milk and meat, sometimes named rumenic acid. This enables partial compensation for the high saturation activity of rumen microbes, and decreases the melting point of body and milk fat, ensuring their fluidity at body temperature. The main desaturation site is within the tissue itself (adipocyte or mammary epithelial cell), but some desaturation activity is also present in the enterocyte during intestinal absorption.

The composition of FAs in animal products thus depends on the balance between these various processes (uptake, synthesis, and desaturation). Rumen digestion processes are major determinants of these processes: they directly determine the composition of the FAs at the duodenum that are available for absorption and then tissue uptake; some FA isomers from partial ruminal biohydrogenation are inhibitors of de novo synthesis, especially the *t*10*c*12-CLA (Baumgard et al., 2002), and also inhibitors of FA desaturation.

Since the apparent digestibilities of the FAs are similar, the composition of the FAs absorbed is close to the composition of the FAs at the duodenum. Moreover, we recently showed that the composition of milk C18 FAs is very similar to the composition of duodenal C18 FAs (Glasser et al., 2008a), once mammary desaturation is taken into account (i.e., when the substrates and products of desaturation are totaled). The various C18 FAs from dietary origin are apparently taken up by the mammary gland in amounts proportional to their composition at the duodenum. This is true for average FA composition at the duodenum, but some compensation could however exist: when some FAs are at a very high concentration at the duodenum (e.g., owing to protection from ruminal metabolism); their transfer efficiency to milk C18 FAs may be slightly lower than that of the other FAs.

Mammary desaturation activity was proportional to the amount of substrate FAs taken up by the mammary gland, and the amount of delta-9 desaturated

FA secreted in milk increases linearly with the uptake of its saturated precursors. However, it greatly differs between FAs, with a mean of 54% of 18:0 being apparently desaturated, compared to 21 – 22% for *t*11- and *t*13-18:1, respectively. This results in a tight relationship between the contents of the substrates and the products of delta-9 desaturase in meat and milk. The mammary desaturation of 18:0 contributes a mean of 80% to milk *c*9-18:1 content, and *t*11-18:1 desaturation almost 95% to milk *c*9*t*11-CLA (Glasser et al., 2008a). The amount of these FAs in animal products thus directly depends on the production of their precursors, resulting from rumen metabolism.

During the last decade, a great research effort was placed on the metabolic effects of some products of partial rumen biohydrogenation of PUFA. The main products studied were the CLAs, particularly *c*9*t*11- and *t*10*c*12-CLA, in part because they were the most easily chemically synthesized CLAs. The isomer *t*10*c*12-CLA proved to have a role in decreasing mammary de novo synthesis of FAs and also mammary desaturation (Baumgard et al., 2002). However, the duodenal flows of this isomer measured in vivo are very low (less than 0.50 g/day in most studies) compared to the amounts used in duodenal infusions to demonstrate its effect on milk fat synthesis and desaturation (3 to 50 g/day). Thus, decreases in milk-fat yield observed with diets promoting CLA production in the rumen cannot be attributed to *t*10*c*12-18:2 alone. Recently, other 18:2 isomers, such as *t*10*c*12-, *c*10*t*12-, *t*9*t*11-, or *t*9*c*11-CLA, were identified or suspected as being inhibitors of milk-fat synthesis (Roy et al., 2006; Saebo et al., 2005; Shingfield & Griinari, 2007). The *t*10-18:1 isomer was suspected to be an inhibitor of de novo synthesis, but this hypothesis was recently ruled out (Lock et al., 2007). The very high number of 18:2 and 18:3 isomers produced by rumen microbes lengthens the candidate list.

The response of milk FA composition to changes in diet composition is rapid (a few days) but may be transient in some cases (Roy et al., 2006), due to the progressive adaptation of the rumen flora to dietary changes. Long-term effects of lipid supplements on rumen metabolism and their effect on milk FA composition are not well-known up to date.

The data on meat FAs are scarcer, and no published data exist on the relationships between FAs at the duodenum (resulting from rumen digestion) and meat FAs composition. Nevertheless, indirect relationships are found. For example, the lower ruminal hydrogenation with diets low in forages results in a higher level of PUFA in muscle (Nuernberg et al., 2005). The relationship between ruminal metabolism and muscle FAs is less strong than with milk. Indeed, meat FA composition is the result of the dietary history of the animal, and not only of the last few weeks before slaughtering. Contrary to milk, meat FAs require a few weeks to be significantly altered, but their plasticity is also high (Scott et al., 1971). For example, the ALA content of muscle depends on the duration of grazing before slaughter because grass is rich in ALA (Noci et al., 2005). Apart from the diet, meat FA composition also varies according to the animal breeds, muscle site, sex (including castration), and age of the animal (De Smet et al., 2004; Wood et al., 2004). FA composition of muscle greatly differs between the main lipid classes, namely phospholipids and triglycerides; the phospholipids are richer in PUFA. In cattle, linoleic acid is specifically incorporated in muscle phospholipids, whereas in sheep, adipose tissue too incorporates linoleic acid in phospholipids (Wood et al., 2008). Thus, a major determinant of meat FA composition is the triglycerides:phospholipids ratio, that reflects the fat:lean ratio of the sample (Eichhorn et al., 1985). Fatter meat is thus richer in triglycerides and in saturated FA.

Diets based on grass or grass silage, a source of ALA, lead to higher meat content in ALA and other omega-3 FAs (such as EPA and DHA, synthesized by elongation from ALA) compared to animals fed on grain, which have a higher content of 18:2 (and also 20:4 n-6, from linoleic acid elongation) (Warren et al., 2008; Wood et al., 2004). The n-6:n-3 ratio in meat is thus more favorable with grass- or grass silage-fed animals. The response of the content in CLA and other *trans* FA to dietary modifications is variable between studies: it is sometimes higher with grain-based diets compared to grass-based diets (Aurousseau et al., 2004; Warren et al., 2008), and sometimes is reversed (Scollan et al., 2005). These differences likely originate from rumen FA metabolism, depending on the FA intake and other rumen parameters (pH, bacterial populations, etcetera). Increasing the animals' intakes of PUFA through oilseed supplementation also increases the respective PUFA content in the meat (e.g., linoleic acid with sunflower supplements, ALA with linseed supplements), but also numerous *trans* 18:1 and 18:2 isomers resulting from their partial biohydrogenation (Noci et al., 2007). The ALA content of meat obtained with linseed-supplemented diets is similar to that obtained with grass-based diets, but the levels of *trans*-18:1 and *trans*-18:2 are higher with linseed-supplemented diets (Noci et al., 2007). Besides the health effects, the FA composition influences the technological and gustatory qualities of the meat (firmness, flavor, sensitivity to oxidation, etcetera) (Wood et al., 2004).

## How to Increase PUFA Flows

Among PUFA, especially interesting, from a human health perspective, is increasing the content of omega-3 FA in milk and meat. Alpha-linolenic acid, EPA, and DHA are present in small amounts in the milk and the meat of ruminants. Despite the need for increasing the n-3:n-6 ratio in the human diet, an increase in omega-6 such as linoleic acid is also of interest, especially when it replaces saturated FAs. However, the nutritional interest for increasing omega-3 in ruminant products can be counterbalanced by negative effects on sensorial qualities, especially when animals are fed fish oil, but also high amounts of 18-carbon PUFA, as is shown for beef (Scollan et al., 2005). In this latter case, lipids are very sensitive to peroxidation, unless additional antioxidants such as vitamin E are given to animals (Scislowski et al., 2005). Because the FAs available for tissue metabolism are those resulting from rumen digestion, increasing the PUFA content of the animal product means increasing the PUFA content of duodenal FAs. This is performed in two ways: by increasing the intake of PUFA in the ruminant diets and by increasing the proportion of dietary PUFA that escape rumen biohydrogenation. In this section we first describe the results of ruminal metabolism with standard diets, and then the different nutritional ways to increase the escape of PUFA from the rumen.

The proportion of PUFA that escapes biohydrogenation is measured by the ratio of the duodenal flow of a FA to the intake of the same FA, measured using animals fitted with cannulae at the proximal duodenum, with the use of undigestible tracers of the digestive contents (see review by Fievez et al., 2007). The duodenal flow is considered the result of ruminal metabolism, since no FA absorption occurs in the omasum and the abomasum, situated between the rumen and the duodenum. The ruminal biohydrogenation of PUFA, estimated by the proportion of these FAs that disappear between the mouth and the duodenum, is on an average of 87% and 86% for linoleic acid and ALA, respectively (Glasser et al., 2008b). Few data deal with the biohydrogenation of 20- and 22-carbon FAs. Fish oil is the main source of EPA and DHA in ruminant diets. Algae are less used, but are also rich in EPA and DHA. From 23 published data, the mean biohydrogenation of EPA and DHA was at 80% on average for both of these FAs.

With most diets, the dietary concentration in PUFA has only a low influence on their ruminal biohydrogenation, so that the amount of PUFA absorbable in the small intestine is linearly related to PUFA intake. Standard feedstuffs for ruminants (forages, concentrates) do not differ to a large extent in the availability of their lipids. However, a high supply of oleaginous seeds results in a moderate decrease in ruminal biohydrogenation. Indeed, the presence of oil within the cell walls in a seed acts as a partial physical protection against biohydrogenation. This was shown, for example, for soybeans, but it may be very limited for linseeds, depending on the nature of the seed hull. Another natural protection can occur with red clover. This forage naturally contains an enzyme, polyphenol oxidase, which reduces both proteolysis and lipolysis in the rumen (Lee et al., 2007). The consequences on biohydrogenation measured in vivo remain to be assessed. Except diets containing feedstuffs "protected" against ruminal biohydrogenation, the only diets resulting in low ruminal biohydrogenation (less than 60% and 80% for linoleic and ALA, respectively) are diets containing more than 70% concentrates (and thus less than 30% roughages as grasses, silages, and hays) on a dry matter basis (Doreau et al., 1997). These diets are very scarce in dairy cow feeding, and more often are used in feedlot conditions, especially for beef fattening. The cause of this low biohydrogenation is a low pH in the rumen, which is a consequence of diets rich in concentrates. The value of ruminal pH, which is generally between 6 and 7 with most diets, can be lower than 5.5 with concentrate-based diets. The consequence of low pH is a decrease in the activity of microbial enzymes, lipases, and especially isomerases and hydrogenases, and was assessed by in vitro trials (Troegeler-Meynadier et al., 2006a; Van Nevel & Demeyer, 1996b).

For several decades, various means to protect dietary PUFA against ruminal biohydrogenation were investigated. A recent meta-analysis (Jenkins & Bridges,

2007) summarized the main conclusions. Until now, the only technique that was shown to increase significantly the amount of PUFA leaving the rumen was the encapsulation of lipids in a matrix of proteins treated with formaldehyde, which protects lipids from microbial attack. This chemical linkage between formaldehyde and proteins is disrupted in the abomasum due to the low pH, so that both amino acids and FAs can be absorbed in the small intestine. This technique, which was first used in the 1970s, is not easy to control because differences in processing result in variations in the level of protection. This protection may be incomplete in the rumen; this is reinforced by the effect of mastication, which contributes to a partial breakdown of the protein shell, leading to the release of free lipids in the rumen fluid. On the contrary, protection may be too strong so that the abomasal disrupting is incomplete, leading to a decrease in FA intestinal absorption. However, an extreme diet containing 20% of encapsulated linseed oil resulted in a proportion of 20% of ALA in milk FAs (McDonald & Scott, 1977). With a more reasonable supply of 5% of encapsulated linseed oil, milk FAs contained 6.4% of ALA (Goodridge et al., 2001). For linoleic acid, values as high as 35% of total milk FAs were reported with protected safflower oil (McDonald & Scott, 1977), but supplements that are used in practical conditions result in ca. 10–15% of linoleic acid in milk FAs (compared to 4–5% on average with unprotected supplements). Although efficient, this technique is seldom used in cow feeding due to its cost when the improvement of FA quality was not a major issue. Nowadays, it is never or very seldom used due to the bad image of chemical treatments of feedstuffs, especially by formaldehyde, and possible residues in the products. In some countries, this technique is even forbidden.

Other techniques of lipid protection, such as calcium salts, do not prevent the hydrogenation of PUFA, because salts are dissociated in the rumen at low pH (less than 6) that often occurs some hours after feeding (Ferlay et al., 1993). Although calcium salts do not disturb microbial metabolism in the rumen, they are all the more hydrogenated than FA are unsaturated and than ruminal pH is low, both factors increasing calcium salt dissociation (Sukhija & Palmquist, 1990; Van Nevel & Demeyer, 1996a). FA amides were experimented with for several years. The chemical protection allowed a slight increase in linoleic acid with soybean oil amides (Jenkins et al., 1996), but overall suffers from inconsistent results on PUFA protection (Jenkins & Bridges, 2007) and from the same drawback as encapsulation (i.e., the bad image of such feeding practices for the consumer). Another kind of physical treatment leads to crystallized or prilled fats, but the process is not adapted to fats rich in PUFA. Some recent attempts did aim toward the use of plant secondary metabolites that could inhibit specific steps of the hydrogenation process. For example, cinnamaldehyde was shown in vitro to reduce biohydrogenation of linoleic acid and ALA, with adverse effects on carbohydrate fermentation (Lourenço et al., 2008). Additional research is needed to find plant extracts that reduce biohydrogenation while maintaining a normal fermentative activity. Likely, the use of natural compounds as additives in animal feeding will be more easily acceptable by the consumer than the chemical treatment of feedstuffs.

## Modulation of *trans* and Conjugated FAs

According to present knowledge on the effect of *trans* monounsaturated FAs and CLAs on human health, increasing CLA content in ruminant products and limiting *t*9- and *t*10-18:1 might be desirable. Promoting *t*11-18:1 is questionable. A close relationship exists between *t*11-18:1 in duodenal contents and both *t*11-18:1 and *c*9*t*11-CLA in milk fat (Glasser et al., 2008a) and probably also in meat, due to the post-ruminal synthesis of the latter from the former. For this reason, to naturally increase *c*9*t*11-CLA while decreasing *t*11-18:1 in ruminant products is not possible. The effect of other FAs on human health is not known. Some of them, such as *t*11*c*15-18:2, can be present in high amounts in duodenal contents (as much as 4.7% of total FAs; Loor et al., 2005), which results in significant amounts in milk or meat, but nothing is known about the possible effects of this FA on human health.

CLAs are present in very small amounts in duodenal contents (less than 0.5% of total FAs). This low concentration is due to their rapid biohydrogenation to 18:1 isomers. Rumenic acid (*c*9*t*11-18:2) always represents less than half of total CLA and only 2–3% of total 18:2. The isomer *t*10*c*12-18:2 (whose beneficial action for human health was described) is either not detected or present in minute amounts (not more than 0.2% of milk FAs). *Trans* 18:1 FAs are present in higher amounts. At the duodenum, the proportion of total *trans* isomers among 18:1 isomers is generally higher than the proportion of *cis* isomers, and is comprised of between 64 and 72% on average, depending on the animal's diet (Table 16.2). Oleic acid (*c*9-18:1) represents on average 20% of the total 18:1 at the duodenum. Dietary polyunsaturated 20- and 22-carbon FAs, such as EPA and DHA, are extensively biohydrogenated and result in a large number of unsaturated C20 and C22 FAs and small amounts of saturated acids. In addition, these FAs inhibit the hydrogenation process of 18-carbon FAs (AbuGhazaleh & Jenkins, 2004; Chow et al., 2004).

The nature and level of the intake of dietary FAs determine the amount and composition of intermediates of biohydrogenation. Diets rich in ALA, such as fresh grass, grass silage, and diets containing linseeds, favor the production of *t*11*c*15-18-2 or *t*11*t*13-18:2, whereas diets rich in linoleic acid (e.g., from sunflower seeds or soybeans) favor the production of different 8,10- and 9,11-CLAs (Fig. 16.2). Results from in vivo experiments (Doreau et al., 2007; Loor et al., 2005) were confirmed by in vitro incubations of pure FA, either ALA or linoleic acid (Jouany et al., 2007). However, when PUFA intake is high, *t*10-18:1 can be considerably enhanced at the expense of *t*11-18:1, even when linseeds are given (Table 16.3).

Besides the nature of dietary FAs, other characteristics of the diet influence the composition of the intermediates of biohydrogenation. A high proportion of concentrates, together with a linoleic acid supply, results in a shift of *t*11-18:1 to *t*10-18-1 in the rumen (Loor et al., 2004). Rumen production of *trans*-18:1 can be increased by oilseed extrusion, and decreased by thermal treatments (Troegeler-Meynadier et al., 2006b). Various other dietary factors, such as the proportion of concentrate in the diet, the nature of the forage, and the feeding schedule influence

**Table 16.2.** Proportions of 18:1 Isomers at Duodenum (in g/100 g Duodenal 18:1).

| Isomer | Unsupplemented diets | Lipid-supplemented diets | Minimum | Maximum |
|---|---|---|---|---|
| *c*9 | 19.6 ± 10.8 | 21.2 ± 17.6 | 4.8 | 58.7 |
| *c*11 | 4.8 ± 3.1 | 6.1 ± 3.7 | 1.9 | 16.2 |
| *c*12 | 1.5 ± 0.6 | 1.8 ± 0.9 | 0.4 | 3.4 |
| *c*13 | 0.5 ± 0.1 | 0.4 ± 0.1 | 0.3 | 0.7 |
| *c*15 | 3.7 ± 3.3 | 3.2 ± 2.3 | 0.8 | 11.8 |
| *t*4 | 0.8 ± 0.3 | 0.5 ± 0.1 | 0.3 | 1.4 |
| *t*5 | 0.7 ± 0.5 | 0.7 ± 0.6 | 0.2 | 1.9 |
| *t*6+7+8 | 2.5 ± 0.9 | 2.3 ± 1.7 | 0.3 | 4.4 |
| *t*9 | 1.8 ± 0.5 | 2.1 ± 1.4 | 0.1 | 4.6 |
| *t*10 | 5.0 ± 3.2 | 16.2 ± 18.4 | 0.9 | 53.3 |
| *t*11 | 30.8 ± 12.3 | 20.4 ± 16.7 | 2.3 | 60.2 |
| *t*12 | 3.9 ± 1.1 | 2.9 ± 1.7 | 0.5 | 6.1 |
| *t*13+14 | 11.1 ± 3.4 | 10.5 ± 4.9 | 5.3 | 18.1 |
| *t*15 | 4.9 ± 2.5 | 4.5 ± 2.3 | 0.3 | 9.4 |
| *t*16 | 6.0 ± 2.6 | 3.1 ± 2.1 | 1 | 10.7 |
| Sum of *trans* | 63.9 ± 16.1 | 71.7 ± 17.4 | 25.2 | 90.5 |

From Glasser et al. (2008b), © The Animal Consortium, reproduced with permission.

**Table 16.3.** Effect of Increasing Linseed Incorporation in the Diet (0, 2, 4, and 6% of Supplemental FA in Dry Matter Intake) on Selected FA Concentration (g/100 g of Total FA) in Rumen Fluid.

| | 0 | 2 | 4 | 6 |
|---|---|---|---|---|
| C18:0 | 41.28 | 41.16 | 39.79 | 37.60 |
| *t*6,7,8 C18:1 | 0.50[a] | 0.72[b] | 0.98[c] | 1.00[c] |
| *t*9 C18:1 | 0.31[a] | 0.43[b] | 0.54[c] | 0.52[c] |
| *t*10 C18:1 | 0.81 | 1.14 | 2.31 | 4.61 |
| *t*11 C18:1 | 4.78 | 6.85 | 9.34 | 7.57 |
| *t*13+*t*14 C18:1 | 1.64[a] | 3.36[b] | 4.80[c] | 5.26[c] |
| *t*15+*c*15 C18:1 | 0.11[a] | 0.47[ab] | 0.81[c] | 1.22[d] |
| C18:2 n-6 | 6.69[a] | 4.6[b] | 3.08[c] | 2.80[c] |
| *c*9*t*11 C18:2 | 0.65 | 0.75 | 0.60 | 0.63 |
| *t*11*c*15 C18:2 | 0.44[a] | 2.34[b] | 4.11[c] | 6.09[d] |
| *t*11*t*13 C18:2 | 0.09[a] | 0.31[b] | 0.33[b] | 0.29[b] |
| C18:3 n-3 | 2.19 | 3.80 | 3.03 | 3.05 |

(Dangin et al., 2008)

the outcome of rumen FA metabolism through their effect on diet FA composition but also through their effect on global rumen parameters (pH, rumen outflow rate, bacterial populations), which, in turn, influence rumen FA metabolism and the composition of FAs at the duodenum. All of these changes at the ruminal level result in the possibility of the modulation of *trans* FA composition in milk (see the recent review by Chilliard et al., 2007; Shingfield et al., 2008) as in meat.

## Conclusion

Rumen FA metabolism plays an important role in modulating the FA composition of ruminant milk and meat. Most techniques that protect PUFA from ruminal hydrogenation by microbes, to increase the absorbed amounts of ALA and linoleic acid, are not used for consumer acceptability issues. Pasture- or grass silage-based diets, or linseed supplementation, can enhance the digestive flows of ALA, but to a limited extent. On the contrary, the intermediates of the biohydrogenation process, such as *trans*-18:1 and 18:2 isomers, widely change with dietary and rumen conditions. These numerous isomers are often specific to ruminant products. In most cases, their effects on human health remain unknown. In the future, if recommendations are available concerning their content in the human diet, it will be possible to propose specific feeding practices for ruminants to produce milk and meat that can contribute to meeting these recommendations.

### References

AbuGhazaleh, A.A.; T.C. Jenkins. Docosahexaenoic acid promotes vaccenic acid accumulation in mixed ruminal cultures when incubated with linoleic acid. *J. Dairy Sci.* **2004**, *87*, 1047–1050.

Aurousseau, B.; D. Bauchart; E. Calichon; D. Micol; A. Priolo. Effect of grass or concentrate feeding systems and rate of growth on triglyceride and phospholipid and their fatty acids in the *M. Longissimus thoracis* of lambs. *Meat Sci* **2004**, *66*, 531–541.

Baumgard, L.H.; B.A. Corl; D.A. Dwyer; D.E. Bauman. Effects of conjugated linoleic acids (CLA) on tissue response to homeostatic signals and plasma variables associated with lipid metabolism in lactating dairy cows. *J. Anim. Sci.* **2002**, *80*, 1285–1293.

Boeckaert, C.; V. Fievez; D. Van Hecke; W. Verstraete; N. Boon. Changes in rumen biohydrogenation intermediates and ciliate protozoa diversity after algae supplementation to dairy cattle. *Eur. J. Lipid Sci. Technol.* **2007**, *109*, 767–777.

Chardigny, J.M.; F. Destaillats; C. Malpuech-Brugere; J. Moulin; D.E. Bauman; A.L. Lock; D.M. Barbano; R.P. Mensink; J.B. Bezelgues; P. Chaumont; et al. Do *trans* fatty acids from industrially produced sources and from natural sources have the same effect on cardiovascular disease risk factors in healthy subjects? Results of the *trans* fatty acids collaboration (TRANSFACT) study. *Am. J. Clin. Nutr.* **2008**, *87*, 558–566.

Chilliard, Y. Dietary fat and adipose tissue metabolism in ruminants, pigs, and rodents: A review. *J. Dairy Sci.* **1993**, *76*, 3897–3931.

Chilliard, Y., F. Glasser; A. Ferlay; L. Bernard; J. Rouel; M. Doreau. Diet, rumen biohydrogenation, and nutritional quality of cow and goat milk fat. *Eur. J. Lipid Sci. Technol.* **2007**, *109*,

828-855.

Chow, T.T.; V. Fievez; A.P. Moloney; K. Raes; D. Demeyer; S. De Smet. Effect of fish oil on in vitro rumen lipolysis, apparent biohydrogenation of linoleic and linolenic acid and accumulation of biohydrogenation intermediates. *Anim. Feed Sci. Technol.* **2004**, *117*, 1–12.

Church, D.C. *The Ruminant Animal: Digestive Physiology and Nutrition*; Prentice Hall: Englewood Cliffs, NJ, 1993.

Dangin, M.; F. Glasser; C. Martin; A. Ferlay; Y. Chilliard; M. Doreau. *BSAS Annual Conference*; BSAS, Ed.; BSAS: Scarborough, UK, 2008; pp. 28.

De Smet, S.; K. Raes; Demeyer, D. Meat fatty acid composition as affected by fatness and genetic factors: A review. *Anim. Res.* **2004**, *53*, 81–98.

Demeyer, D.; M. Doreau. Targets and products for altering ruminant meat and milk lipids. *Proc. Nut. Soc.* **1999**, *58*, 593–607.

Doreau, M.; D.I. Demeyer; C.J. Van Nevel. Transformations and effects of unsaturated fatty acids in the rumen. Consequences on milk fat secretion. *Milk Composition, Production and Biotechnology.*; R.A.S. Welch, D.J.W. Burns, S.R. Davis, A.I. Popay, C.G. Prosser, Eds.; CAB International: Oxford, UK, 1997; pp. 73–92.

Doreau, M.; A. Ferlay. Digestion and utilisation of fatty acids by ruminants. *Anim. Feed Sci. Technol.* **1994**, *45*, 379–396.

Doreau, M.; D. Rearte; J. Portelli; J.L. Peyraud. Fatty acid ruminal metabolism and digestibility in cows fed perennial ryegrass. *Eur. J. Lipid Sci. Technol.* **2007**, *109*, 790–798.

Eichhorn, J.M.; C.M. Bailey; G.J. Blomquist. Fatty-acid composition of muscle and adipose-tissue from crossbred bulls and steers. *J. Anim. Sci.* **1985**, *61*, 892–904.

Ferlay, A.; J. Chabrot; Y. Elmeddah; M. Doreau. Ruminal lipid balance and intestinal digestion by dairy cows fed calcium salts of rapeseed oil fatty acids or rapeseed oil. *J. Anim. Sci.* **1993**, *71*, 2237–2245.

Fievez, V.; B. Vlaeminck; T. Jenkins; F. Enjalbert; M. Doreau. Assessing rumen biohydrogenation and its manipulation in vivo, in vitro and in situ. *Eur. J. Lipid Sci. Technol.* **2007**, *109*, 740–756.

Glasser, F.; A. Ferlay; M. Doreau; P. Schmidely; D. Sauvant; Y. Chilliard. Long-chain fatty acid metabolism in dairy cows: A meta-analysis of milk fatty acid yield in relation to duodenal flows and de novo synthesis. *J. Dairy Sci.* **2008a**, *91*, 2771–2795.

Glasser, F.; P. Schmidely; D. Sauvant; M. Doreau. Digestion of fatty acids in ruminants: A meta-analysis of flows and variation factors. 2. C18 fatty acids. *Animal* **2008b**, *2*, 691–704.

Goodridge, J.; J.R. Ingalls; G.H. Crow. Transfer of omega-3 linolenic acid and linoleic acid to milk fat from flaxseed or linola protected with formaldehyde. *Can. J. Anim. Sci.* **2001**, *81*, 525–532.

Harfoot, C.G.; G.P. Hazlewood. Lipid metabolism in the rumen. *The Rumen Microbial Ecosystem*; P.N. Hobson, C.S. Stewart, Eds.; Blackie Academic & Professional: London, **1997**; pp. 382–426.

Hulshof, K.F.A.M.; M.A. van Erp-Baart; M. Anttolainen;W. Becker; S.M. Church; C. Couet; E. Hermann-Kunz; H. Kesteloot; T. Leth; I. Martins; et al. Intake of fatty acids in western europe with emphasis on *trans* fatty acids: The transfair study. *Eur. J. Clin. Nutr.* **1999**, *53*, 143–157.

Jenkins, T.C.; H.G. Bateman; S.M. Block. Butylsoyamide increases unsaturation of fatty acids in plasma and milk of lactating dairy cows. *J. Dairy Sci.* **1996**, *79*, 585.

Jenkins, T.C.; W.C. Bridges, Jr. Protection of fatty acids against ruminal biohydrogenation in cattle. *Eur. J. Lipid Sci. Technol.* **2007**, *109*, 778–789.

Jenkins, T.C.; R.J. Wallace; P.J. Moate; E.E. Mosley. Recent advances in biohydrogenation of unsaturated fatty acids within the rumen microbial ecosystem. *J. Anim Sci.* **2008**, *86*, 397–412.

Jouany, J.P.; B. Lassalas; M. Doreau; F. Glasser. Dynamic features of the rumen metabolism of linoleic acid, linolenic acid, and linseed oil measured *in vitro*. *Lipids* **2007**, *42*, 351–360.

Keeney, M. Lipid metabolism in the rumen. *Physiology of Digestion and Metabolism in the Ruminant*; A.T. Philipson, Ed.; Oriel Press: Newcastle upon Tyne, UK, **1970**; pp. 489–503.

Lee, M.R.F.; L.J. Parfitt; N.D. Scollan; F.R. Minchin. Lipolysis in red clover with different polyphenol oxidase activities in the presence and absence of rumen fluid. *J. Sci. Food Agric.* **2007**, *87*, 1308–1314.

Lock, A.L.; C. Tyburczy; D.A. Dwyer; K.J. Harvatine; F. Destaillats; Z. Mouloungui; L. Candy; D.E. Bauman. *Trans*-10 octadecenoic acid does not reduce milk fat synthesis in dairy cows. *J. Nutr.* **2007**, *137*, 71–76.

Loor, J.J.; K. Ueda; A. Ferlay; Y. Chilliard; M. Doreau. Biohydrogenation, duodenal flow, and intestinal digestibility of *trans* fatty acids and conjugated linoleic acids in response to dietary forage: concentrate ratio and linseed oil in dairy cows. *J. Dairy Sci.* **2004**, *87*, 2472–2485.

Loor, J.J.; K. Ueda; A. Ferlay; Y. Chilliard; M. Doreau. Intestinal flow and digestibility of *trans* fatty acids and conjugated linoleic acids (CLA) in dairy cows fed a high-concentrate diet supplemented with fish oil, linseed oil, or sunflower oil. *Anim. Feed Sci. Technol.* **2005**, *119*, 203–225.

Lourenço, M.; P.W. Cardozo; S. Calsamiglia; V. Fievez. Effects of saponins, quercetin, eugenol, and cinnamaldehyde on fatty acid biohydrogenation of forage polyunsaturated fatty acids in dual-flow continuous culture fermenters. *J. Anim Sci.* **2008**, doi:10.2527/jas.2007-0708.

McDonald, I.W.; T.W. Scott. Foods of ruminant origin with elevated content of polyunsaturated fatty acids. *World Rev. Nutr. Diet* **1977**, *26*, 144–207.

Mosley, E.E.; G.L. Powell; M.B. Riley; T.C. Jenkins. Microbial biohydrogenation of oleic acid to *trans* isomers in vitro. *J. Lipid Res.* **2002**, *43*, 290–296.

Noci, F.; P. French; F.J. Monahan; A.P. Moloney. The fatty acid composition of muscle fat and subcutaneous adipose tissue of grazing heifers supplemented with plant oil-enriched concentrates. *J. Anim. Sci.* **2007**, *85*, 1062–1073.

Noci, F.; F.J. Monahan; P. French; A.P. Moloney. The fatty acid composition of muscle fat and subcutaneous adipose tissue of pasture-fed beef heifers: Influence of the duration of grazing. *J. Anim. Sci.* **2005**, *83*, 1167–1178.

Nuernberg, K.; D. Dannenberger; G. Nuernberg; K. Ender; J. Voigt; N.D. Scollan; J.D. Wood; G.R. Nute; R.I. Richardson. Effect of a grass-based and a concentrate feeding system on meat quality characteristics and fatty acid composition of longissimus muscle in different cattle breeds. *Livest. Prod. Sci.* **2005**, *94*, 137–147.

Proell, J.M.; E.E. Mosley; G.L. Powell; T.C. Jenkins. Isomerization of stable isotopically labeled elaidic acid to cis and *trans* monoenes by ruminal microbes. *J. Lipid Res.* **2002**, *43*, 2072–2076.

Roy, A.; A. Ferlay; K.J. Shingfield; Y. Chilliard. Examination of the persistency of milk fatty acid composition responses to plant oils in cows given different basal diets, with particular emphasis on *trans*-c18:1 fatty acids and isomers of conjugated linoleic acid. *Anim. Sci.* **2006**, *82*, 479–492.

Saebo, A.; P.C. Saebo; J.M. Griinari; K.J. Shingfield. Effect of abomasal infusions of geometric isomers of 10,12 conjugated linoleic acid on milk fat synthesis in dairy cows. *Lipids* **2005**, *40*, 823–832.

Schmidely, P.; F. Glasser; M. Doreau; D. Sauvant. Digestion of fatty acids in ruminants: A meta-analysis of flows and variation factors. 1. Total fatty acids. *Animal* **2008**, *2*, 677–690.

Scislowski, V.; D. Bauchart; D. Gruffat; P.M. Laplaud; D. Durand. Effects of dietary n-6 or n-3 polyunsaturated fatty acids protected or not against ruminal hydrogenation on plasma lipids and their susceptibility to peroxidation in fattening steers. *J. Anim. Sci.* **2005**, *83*, 2162–2174.

Scollan, N.D.; I. Richardson; S. De Smet; A.P. Moloney; M. Doreau; D. Bauchart; K. Nürnberg. Enhancing the content of beneficial fatty acids in beef and consequences for meat quality. *Indicators of Milk and Beef Quality*; J.F. Hoquette, S. Gigli, Eds.; Wageningen Academic Publishers: Wageningen, The Netherlands, **2005**; pp. 151–162.

Scott, T.W.; L.J. Cook; S.C. Mills. Protection of dietary polyunsaturated fatty acids against microbial hydrogenation in ruminants. *J. Am. Oil Chem. Soc.* **1971**, *48*, 358–364.

Shingfield, K.J.; Y. Chilliard; V. Toivonen; P. Kairenius; D.I. Givens. Bioactive components of milk *trans* fatty acids and bioactive lipids in ruminant milk. *Bioactive Components of Milk*; Z. Bösze, Ed.; Springer: New York, NY, **2008**; Vol. 606; pp. 3–65.

Shingfield, K.J.; J.M. Griinari. Role of biohydrogenation intermediates in milk fat depression. *Eur. J. Lipid Sci. Tech.* **2007**, *109*, 799–816.

Sukhija, P.S.; D.L. Palmquist. Dissociation of calcium soaps of long-chain fatty acids in rumen fluid. *J. Dairy Sci.* **1990**, *73*, 1784–1787.

Troegeler-Meynadier, A.; L. Bret-Bennis; F. Enjalbert. Rates and efficiencies of reactions of ruminal biohydrogenation of linoleic acid according to pH and polyunsaturated fatty acids concentrations. *Reprod. Nutr. Dev.* **2006a**, *46*, 713–724.

Troegeler-Meynadier, A.; M.C. Nicot; F. Enjalbert. Effects of heating process of soybeans on ruminal production of conjugated linoleic acids and *trans*-octadecenoic acids in situ. *Rev. Méd. Vét.* **2006b**, *157*, 509–514.

Van Nevel, C. J.; D.I. Demeyer. Effect of pH on biohydrogenation of polyunsaturated fatty acids and their Ca-salts by rumen microorganisms in vitro. *Arch. Anim. Nutr.* **1996a**, *49*, 151–157.

Van Nevel, C.J.; D.I. Demeyer. Influence of pH on lipolysis and biohydrogenation of soybean oil by rumen contents in vitro. *Reprod. Nutr. Dev.* **1996b**, *36*, 53–63.

Vlaeminck, B.; V. Fievez; D. Demeyer; R.J. Dewhurst. Effect of forage:concentrate ratio on fatty acid composition of rumen bacteria isolated from ruminal and duodenal digesta. *J. Dairy Sci.* **2006**, *89*, 2668–2678.

Warren, H.E.; N.D. Scollan; M. Enser; S.I. Hughes; R.I. Richardson; J.D. Wood. Effects of breed and a concentrate or grass silage diet on beef quality in cattle of 3 ages. I: Animal performance, carcass quality and muscle fatty acid composition. *Meat Sci* **2008**, *78*, 256–269.

Weinberg, L.G.; L.A. Berner; J.E. Groves. Nutrient contributions of dairy foods in the United States, continuing survey of food intakes by individuals, 1994–1996, 1998. *J. Am. Diet Assoc.*

**2004**, *104*, 895–902.

Willett, W.C.; M.J. Stampfer; J.E. Manson; G. A. Colditz; F.E. Speizer; B.A. Rosner; L.A. Sampson; C.H. Hennekens. Intake of *trans* fatty acids and risk of coronary heart disease among women. *Lancet* **1993**, *341*, 581–585.

Wood, J.D.; M. Enser; A.V. Fisher; G.R. Nute; P.R. Sheard; R.I. Richardson; S.I. Hughes; F.M. Whittington. Fat deposition, fatty acid composition and meat quality: A review. *Meat Sci.* **2008**, *78*, 343–358.

Wood, J.D.; R.I. Richardson; G.R. Nute; A.V. Fisher; M.M. Campo; E. Kasapidou; P.R. Sheard; M. Enser. Effects of fatty acids on meat quality: A review. *Meat Sci.* **2004**, *66*, 21–32.

# 17

# Fatty Acid Metabolism and Peroxisome Proliferator-activated Receptors

**Zivar Yousefipour and Mohammad Newaz**
*Center for Cardiovascular Diseases, Texas Southern University, Houston, Texas*

## Introduction

Fatty acids are aliphatic monocarboxylic acids, derived from an animal or vegetable fat, oil, or wax. Natural fatty acids commonly have a chain of 4 to 28 carbons (usually unbranched and even-numbered), which may be saturated (no double bonds) or unsaturated (one or more double bonds between the carbon atoms). The size of fatty acids determines whether they are either short-chain fatty acids that are absorbed directly into the blood via intestinal capillaries or long-chain fatty acids that are absorbed into the fatty walls of the intestine villi and subsequently reassembled again into triglycerides. Fatty acids can exist in the blood as free fatty acids (FFAs), chylomicrons (triglycerides coated with cholesterol and protein), very low density lipoproteins (VLDLs), low-density lipoproteins (LDLs), and high-density lipoproteins (HDLs).

Dietary fatty acids have multiple functions in the human body. They are an important energy source as well as an essential part of the phospholipid bilayer of membranes. They also function as precursors to several signaling molecules, such as the eicosanoids, by targeting nuclear receptors, such as the peroxisome proliferator-activated receptors (PPARs). Research done in the past few decades provides convincing evidence that changes in dietary fatty acid composition can profoundly influence health and disease. As is well-established, replacing dietary saturated fatty acids with n-6 mono- and polyunsaturated fatty acids leads to a decrease in the plasma concentration of LDL, a well-known risk factor for atherosclerosis (Nicolosi et al., 2004; Yamashita et al., 2005). Similarly, an increased consumption of n-3 fatty acids, especially eicosapentaenoic acid and docosahexaenoic acid present in fish oil, is associated with decreased plasma-triglyceride concentrations (Harris & Bulchandani, 2006), prevention of cardiac arrhythmias (Leaf, 2007), and improvement in visual acuity in preterm infants (Cheatham et al., 2006). Extensive earlier research shows that elevated plasma levels of cholesterol-rich LDLs are associated with an increased risk for coronary heart disease, while elevated levels of HDLs exert a protective influence (Abdel-Maksoud et al., 2008; Miller et al., 2008). Accordingly, raising HDL levels and especially lowering LDL levels have become the conventions for the nutritional and pharmacological prevention and treatment of coronary heart disease. Studies also indicate that the common causes of heart failure are associated with derangements in myocardial fuel utilization. Emerging evidence suggests that metabolic abnormalities may contribute to the development and progression of myocardial disease and that the quality of dietary lipids may be an important modulator in terms of the risks associated with metabolic syndrome (Berglund et al., 2007; Muzio et al., 2007).

A balance between lipid intake and lipid consumption is required for fatty acid homeostasis. This process involves several tissues specializing in fatty acid storage, such as white adipose tissue, or fatty acid catabolism, such as skeletal muscle, heart, and liver. Excessive amounts of dietary lipids associated with a lack of physical exercise create a profound disturbance in this balance, leading to metabolic diseases. PPARs, because of their unique functional ability as the transcriptional regulators, play a critical role in modulating physiological as well as pathological responses which depend on fatty acid metabolism. Different mechanisms may be involved that modulate the effects of dietary fatty acids on parameters influencing health and diseases. Historically, the main focus has been on changes in plasma-membrane fluidity as a result of changes in phospholipid composition, whereas the discovery of nuclear receptors like PPARs has gradually shifted the emphasis to the regulation of gene expression. Therefore, one must understand the integral role of PPARs in fatty acid metabolism.

Nuclear receptors play a major role in the regulation of lipid and lipoprotein metabolism, and are considered major drug targets for correcting abnormal lipids in the circulation (Chawla et al., 2001). These ligand-activated transcription factors alter gene transcription by direct binding to specific DNA-response elements in target genes (Aranda & Pascual, 2001). Nuclear receptors also modulate transcription by interfering with specific intracellular signaling pathways, thus impairing transcriptional activation by other transcription factors. As the primary regulators of lipid metabolism at the cellular level, the PPAR isotypes help to maintain metabolic homeostasis when the energy or lipid composition of the diet changes. PPARs regulate cardiac fuel metabolism at the gene-expression level (Madrazo & Kelly, 2008), and the unique distribution of the three members gives them an important role as transducers of developmental, physiological, and dietary modulators that influence fatty acid metabolism. This chapter elaborates on the PPARs and their significance in fatty acid metabolism.

## Fatty Acid Metabolism and Peroxisomes

### *Peroxisomes and Peroxisome Proliferators*

Peroxisomes are subcellular organelles encompassed by a single membrane with a crucial role both in cellular metabolism through the oxidation of fatty acids, bile salts, and cholesterol and in the conversion of hydrogen peroxide to a nontoxic compound. These organelles are metabolically complex because of their diverse enzyme contents. At present, nearly 100 different enzymes are identified in mammalian peroxisomes.

Some of these enzymatic activities are restricted to peroxisomes, whereas others have their counterparts in other organelles. The enzymatic reaction in peroxisomes is vitally important for the cells because it also includes the detoxification of reactive species. Disturbances in the peroxisomal system, as demonstrated by numerous inborn errors of peroxisomal metabolism leading to an accumulation or a shortage of certain metabolites, point to the importance of peroxisomal metabolism (Gootjes et al., 2004).

Peroxisome proliferation is a pleiotropic cellular response to diverse groups of chemicals, including herbicides and insecticides as well as certain patho-/physiological conditions, which result in drastic changes in cellular morphology and enzymatic activity. Fibric acid, a peroxisomal activator and its derivatives (e.g., clofibrate, fenofibrate, bezafibrate, ciprofibrate, and beclofibrate), reduces plasma triglycerides and, to a lesser extent, cholesterol levels in hyperlipidemic patients (Najib, 2002; Spieker et al., 2000). Fibrates also result in peroxisome proliferation in rats and mice which is most notable in the liver (Cornwell et al., 2004). Other compounds that can induce peroxisome proliferation include a range of xenobiotic compounds, such as phthalate and adipate ester plasticizers, herbicides, leukotriene antagonists, acetylsalicylic acid, and thio-substituted fatty acids (Cajaraville & Ortiz-Zarragoitia, 2007; Turunen et al., 1999; Venkata et al., 2006). Natural factors, such as high-fat diets, also cause peroxisome proliferation (Kjaer et al., 2008). Diets enriched in partially hydrogenated fish oils, which are poorly oxidized via the mitochondrial β-oxidation pathway, also have a profound effect on peroxisome proliferation (Miranda et al., 1997; Sülzle et al., 2004). Studies report that conditions with fatty acid overloads, such as increased dietary-fat intake in times of starvation (Lambert et al., 2006; Madsen & Berge, 1999) and uncontrolled diabetes mellitus (Asayama et al., 1999), can also induce peroxisome proliferation. These observations suggest that the peroxisome- proliferation response also occurs under certain patho/physiological conditions. One other factor that may play a role in the degree of responsiveness to peroxisome proliferators is the hormonal status of the animal. Male rats show a greater response to peroxisome proliferators than females (Amacher et al., 1997; Yamoto et al., 1996). Reportedly, dehydroepiandrosterone, an adrenal androgen, is also capable of producing a peroxisome-proliferative response in rodents (Depreter et al., 2002). Hormonal imbalances such as hyperthyroidism (Webb et al., 1996) and treatment with synthetic glucocorticoids, such as dexamethasone, were also reported to induce or enhance the enzymatic capacity of peroxisomes (Lawrence et al., 2001; Rao & Subbarao, 1997). Additionally, reports exist of the induction of the peroxisomal enzyme by certain vitamin derivatives, such as retinoic acid (Peehl & Feldman, 2004; Wang et al., 2007) or vitamin E (Kawada et al., 2004; Orfila et al., 2002; Sohlenius et al., 1996).

## *Peroxisome Proliferation and Nuclear Receptor*

Nuclear receptors are a group of proteins with a significant role in the regulation of lipoprotein metabolism. They are considered major drug targets for correcting abnormal plasma lipids (Chawla et al., 2001). Nuclear receptors are ligand activated transcription factors that directly bind to specific DNA-response elements in target genes, alter gene transcription (Aranda & Pascual, 2001), and modulate transcription by interfering with specific intracellular signaling pathways. A comparison of different nuclear receptors revealed that they share a common modular structure including a relatively well-conserved central DNA-binding domain and a C-terminal ligand-binding domain (LBD) (Aranda & Pascual, 2001). Several nuclear receptors, including the estrogen receptors (ERs), the oxysterol receptors (Liver X Receptor [LXRs]), the bile-acid receptors (Farnesoid X Receptor [FXRs]), and the fatty acid receptors (PPARs), are involved in the regulation of plasma lipoprotein metabolism. In this chapter, the emphasis is given to the role of PPARs in peroxisome proliferation and fatty acid metabolism.

A superfamily of nuclear receptors encompasses a related but diverse set of transcription factors that one can classify under four major subgroups according to their dimerization and DNA-binding properties (revised in Schoonjans et al., 1996): (i) The classic steroid receptors are classified as Class I. These receptors are localized in the cytoplasm, and are associated with heat-shock proteins that translocate to the nucleus upon the binding of their cognate ligand. They bind as homodimers to DNA half-sites arranged as inverted repeats. The well-known members of this class include the glucocorticoid receptor (GR), androgen receptor, progesterone receptor (PR), mineralocorticoid receptor, and ER. (ii) Those nuclear receptors that heterodimerize with the 9-*cis* retinoic-acid receptor (Retinoid X Receptor [RXR]) and bind to direct repeats separated by a variable number of bases or spacer nucleotides make up the Class II receptors. (iii) Nuclear localization of this class of receptors is independent of ligand activation. Members of this class include the thyroid receptor (TR), the RXR, the vitamin-D receptor (VDR), and the PPAR. Receptors such as the RXR, hepatocyte nuclear factor-4 (HNF-4), and chicken ovary upstream promoter (COUP)/a human orphan receptor which bind to direct DNA repeats as homodimers are classified as Class III. (iv) Receptors of Class IV, including Rev-erb-α (EAR-1), Rev-erb-β (RVR), NGF1-β, FTZ-F1-α, -β, SF-1, ELP and RZR-α, and ROR-α bind as monomers to a single hexameric core-recognition motif flanked by some additional sequences upstream of this motif. For the members of Class II receptors like PPARs, the binding of ligands to the receptor leads to the recruitment of co-activators and the dissociation of co-repressors, resulting in chromatin remodeling followed by the initiation of DNA transcription. The main function of these receptors is to act as lipid sensors by altering the rate of the transcription of specific genes in response to changes in lipid concentration (Chawla et al., 2001). These lipids include oxysterols, bile acids, and fat-soluble vitamins. Other receptors that mediate the effects of dietary fatty acids on gene expression include the sterol regulatory element-binding protein 1 and the nuclear factor κB (Sampath & Ntambi, 2005).

## Peroxisome Proliferator-activated Receptors (PPARs)

PPARs are ligand-activated transcription factors that belong to the nuclear-receptor superfamily. The first nuclear receptor to which peroxisome proliferators bind was discovered in 1990 by Issemann and Green (1990) which later was designated as PPAR-α. To date, three different types of PPARs—α, β (also referred to as NUC I, FAAR, or PPAR-δ), and γ—are identified. Primarily, scientists were able to clone the three isoforms in *Xenopus* (a genus of carnivorous frogs native to Africa), and shortly after they cloned an α–, δ-, and γ-type in man and mouse as well. Two slice variants exist of the mPPAR-γ isoforms, γ1 and γ2, differing only in their N-terminal 30 amino acids (Auwerx, 1999; Auwerx et al., 2003; Chawla et al., 2001; Desvergne & Wahli, 1999; Francis et al., 2003; Lee & Evans, 2002; Michalik & Wahli, 1999; Picard & Auwerx, 2002; Rosen & Spiegelman, 2001; Rosen et al., 2000; Sporn et al., 2001; Willson et al., 2001). These two isoforms are derived from the same gene by alternative promoter usage and splicing. Each PPAR-γ has a distinct expression pattern (Fajas et al., 1997, 1998). A differential splicing of the noncoding first exon was reported for mPPAR-α (Chew et al., 2003; Fajas et al., 1997; Fredenrich & Grimaldi, 2005) and also for retinoid and thyroid hormone receptors (Malartre et al., 2004). The relative selectivity of the PPARs' response to a given peroxisome proliferator is also an important factor: for instance, the WY-14643 mainly activates mPPAR-α; LY-171883 (a leukotriene inhibitor) activates mPPAR-γ; and linoleic acid activates mPPAR-δ. PPARs are widely present in human tissues and are capable of transactivating liver peroxisome acyl-CoA oxidase and apolipoprotein AII genes, but so far no clear demonstration about their role exists. Human PPAR-γ was activated by antidiabetic thiazolidinediones (Kiaei, 2008), this effect being incriminated in the lipogenic activity of these drugs.

## Expression of a PPAR and Its Tissue Distribution

The presence of multiple receptors in the same subfamily suggests different physiological functions for each isoform. Therefore, one must understand their tissue specificity and relative abundance. Most of the study of PPAR-tissue distribution was limited to the analysis of its mRNA distributions. According to reports, mPPAR-α is predominantly expressed in liver, heart, kidney, and brown adipose tissue with a lesser expression in other tissues, including small intestine, skeletal muscle, thymus, and testis (Kersten & Wahli, 2000). A high transcript of the δ-form (or NUC I and FAAR) was reported in various tissues including brain and fat, but a very low transcript in liver compared to other isoforms. In the mouse, mPPAR-α is present in the embryo only in the liver and adipose tissue, while in the adult it is also expressed in the heart and kidney and to a lesser extent in some other tissues (Braissant et al., 1996). The mPPAR-γ is abundant in adrenal glands; the mPPAR-γ2 is especially abundant in adipocytes and in brown adipose tissue (Fajas et al., 1997; Guan & Breyer, 2001); and the mPPAR-δ is highly expressed in the heart, adrenal glands, and intestine (Fredenrich & Grimaldi, 2005). The human PPAR-α (NUC-1) is well-expressed in the heart, lung, and kidney but weakly in the liver (Auboeuf et al., 1997; Braissant et al., 1996; Gonzalez, 1997; Palmer et al., 1998). Kliewer et al. (1994) proposed that the expression of mPPAR isotypes in the same tissue may present antagonistic properties that can result in a cellular effect based on their relative expression level. Of the two PPAR-γ isoforms, PPAR-γ1 exhibits a distribution pattern reminiscent of PPAR-α, whereas PPAR-γ2 is predominantly expressed in adipose tissue (Fajas et al., 1997; Guan & Breyer, 2001). Interestingly, the various PPAR types also display different developmental expression patterns in some species. For example, the analysis of a whole-mouse embryo RNA during mouse embryogenesis indicated an early expression of mPPAR-δ preceding the onset of mPPAR-α and mPPAR-γ expression, while no differential expression patterns are revealed for *Xenopus* (reviewed in Michalik et al., 2002). In adult *Xenopus*, xPPAR-α and xPPAR-β are ubiquitously expressed, while xPPAR-γ exhibits a tissue distribution pattern relatively similar to mPPAR-α, with the exception of the liver. Both xPPAR-α and xPPAR-β are detected during oogenesis, where xPPAR-γ is absent (reviewed in Michalik et al., 2002).

## Activators/Ligands of PPARs

The activation of PPARs and the subsequent gene expression prevent the accumulation of fatty acids and peroxisome proliferators. Among the possible ligands of PPARs might be the following compounds and their metabolically generated derivatives. CoA or carnitine esters were studied as factors mediating proxisome proliferator (PP) induction (Goll et al., 1999; Yu et al., 2001); they may be considered as specific ligands of PPARs. PPAR activation induces β-oxidation pathways, and in the absence of a cellular concerted response to fatty acid accumulation, β-oxidation products would increase. Apparently, the enhanced disposition of β-oxidation products appears to be associated with the enhanced oxidation of fatty acids in cells exposed to peroxisome proliferators. The β-oxidation products might also play a crucial role as the inductors of their enhanced cellular utilizations through PPAR activation. These potential inductors/ligands include (in the free or esterified forms) intramitochondrially generated acetyl-CoA (may stimulate ketone body genesis) (Meertens et al., 1998), hydroxyacetyl-CoA (may stimulate glycolylated sialic acid formation), and succinyl-CoA (Westin et al., 2005) (may stimulate gluconeogenesis from fatty acids) (reviewed in Kersten, 2002), as well as intraperoxisomally generated medium-chain acyl-CoA (Goetzman et al., 2005) and acetyl-CoA (Wanders et al., 2000) (may stimulate phospholipid synthesis). The stimulation of key gluconeogenesis enzymes through peroxisome proliferators (reviewed in Chevalier et al., 2000) causes provisional responses related to these ligands, which, in addition, are encoded by a peroxisome proliferator response element (PPRE)-containing gene. For instance, the ketone body genesis enzyme 3-Hydroxy-3-methylglutaryl CoA (HMG-CoA) synthase is encoded by a PPRE-containing gene (Hegardt, 1998).

Exogenous substances such as hypolipidemic fibrate drugs, phthalate ester plasticizers, and herbicides are known inducers of peroxisome proliferation, and do activate PPARs (Lampen et al., 2003; Lovekamp-Swan & Davis, 2003; Nakajima et al., 2002; Vu-Dac et al., 1998; Zhang et al., 2004). No concrete evidence suggests that these substances function as ligands for PPARs although fatty acids were proposed as the endogenous direct activators of PPARs. A high-fat diet and physiological conditions with a fatty acid overload characteristic can stimulate peroxisomal β-oxidation and peroxisome proliferation, and ample evidence shows that a range of fatty acids can activate different PPARs (Bragt & Popeijus, 2008; Gani, 2008). With the exception of short-chain fatty acids (<C10), very long-chain monounsaturated fatty acids, and dodecanedioic acid, all other fatty acids can activate PPARs to a variable extent in transient transfection systems. No evidence indicates the importance of number or position of unsaturated bonds in the increased activation potential of PPARs with the exception of xPPAR-α, which is better activated by polyunsaturated fatty acids (Dreyer & Ellinger-Ziegelbauer, 1996). Substituted fatty acids, which are not substrates for β-oxidation and are hence metabolized more slowly, are more potent PPAR activators than natural fatty acids. Therefore, the degree of PPAR activation may be inversely correlated to the degree of fatty acid β-degradation. Some studies clearly demonstrate that exogenous fatty acids activate PPARs, but they do not pinpoint whether the endogenous active form consists of the acid form or rather the thioester form. Enzyme acyl-CoA synthetase (ACS) converts some of the FFAs into active acyl-CoA thioesters based on the metabolic requirements of the cell, and these derivatives can either be stored complexed with an acyl-CoA-binding protein as an intracellular acyl-CoA ester pool or metabolized in various intracellular enzymatic pathways. Hence, their direct involvement in intracellular lipid metabolism (in contrast to FFAs), together with the finding that xenobiotic peroxisome proliferators also form acyl-CoA esters (Hunt et al., 2002; Knights & Drogemuller, 2000) are arguments for a putative role of acyl-CoAs as PPAR activators and/or ligands. These arguments are reinforced by the finding that acyl-CoA derivatives act as the direct ligands of the prokaryotic transcription factor FadR, which regulates the expression of prokaryotic genes involved in fatty acid transport and β-oxidation (Caviglia et al., 2004; Raman et al., 1997). However, comparing the efficiency of the activation of free acids with their corresponding acyl-CoA derivatives using transient expression assays indicates that the immediate inducer is rather the free-acid form. Consistent with the hypothesis that fatty acids or their metabolites may be the natural PPAR ligands, as demonstrated, the arachidonic acid-derived prostaglandin J metabolites are natural PPAR-γ ligands (Stoll, 2002; Yamakawa-Karakida et al., 2002). Since antidiabetic thiazolidinediones activate and also selectively bind with high affinity to the PPAR-γ subtype (Kameda et al., 2000; Zingarelli & Cook, 2005), they are considered as synthetic PPAR-γ ligands. Reports reveal that both thiazolidinediones (Boyd, 2007) and prostaglandins enhance adipocyte differentiation through the activation of PPAR-γ (Aubert et al., 2000).

Also several xenobiotic analogs of natural compounds exist which have a low-affinity binding for PPARs. PPARs' interaction with environmental nutriments or metabolites is through ligand-binding sites similar to the substrate-binding sites of intermediary metabolism enzymes, a situation that could hamper experimental evidence of ligand–receptor interactions. Among these metabolites are unsaturated fatty acids (i.e., linoleic, arachidonic and prostaglandins, but neither cholesterol,

25-OH-cholesterol, nor dehydroepiandrosterone) (Bull et al., 2003; Das, 2006; Wang et al., 2006). However, dehydroepiandrosterone-3-β-sulfate is required to activate PPAR-α and trigger gene activation (Ripp et al., 2002). Relatively efficient binding to *Xenopus* PPARs is obtained on 5,8,11,14-eicosatetraynic acid (Dreyer & Ellinger-Ziegelbauer, 1996), but the alkine arachidonic-acid homolog (inhibitor of lipoxygenase and cyclooxygenase) is 100-fold more potent than WY-14643. Therefore, PPAR activation requires the involvement of specific ligand-mediated mechanisms.

## PPAR-mediated Gene Expression that Involved Lipid Metabolism

### Gene Up-regulation

Studies by Osumi et al. in 1991 indicated that the 5' upstream region of the AOX gene from rat-liver peroxisomes contains a sequence that is able to bind to liver nuclear extracts from rats treated with peroxisome proliferators. Later on, Tugwood et al. (1992) and then Dreyer et a1. (1993) identified a PPRE binding to a PPAR. This PPRE is a direct repeat of the DRI pattern (TGACCT X TGTCCT). The DRI pattern (one spacing base between the two consensus motifs) is specific for the PPAR response as well as for RXR. To the contrary, other receptor-response elements contain either direct repeats from DRO to DRS, palindromic, or inverted palindromic sequences (Hsu et al. 1998). From the different works, several genes appear to be controlled by a common activation mechanism. These genes contain either an exact direct repeat of the "TGACCT" pattern of the DRI type or a closely related pattern. Each of these PPREs is capable of triggering the transcription of a gene reporter in a transfection assay when activated by the PPAR. All of the PPRE-containing genes encode proteins that are involved in lipid metabolic or energy-producing pathways (i.e., fat storing, fatty acid trafficking, fatty acid ω-hydroxylase, β-oxidation, ketogenesis, gluconeogenesis, or fatty acid synthesis). One may speculate that other strongly activated enzymes such as peroxisome, carnitine octanoyltransferase, or PMP 70 would contain PPREs in their genes.

### Down-regulated Genes

As is well-known, the treatment of hepatic cells or rats with peroxisome proliferators causes several enzymes to undergo a strong decrease of their specific mRNA level. Among these enzymes are: (i) transthyretin (Luci et al., 2006; Motojima et al., 1997); (ii) BIP/GAP78 protein (Barter & Rye, 2008); (iii) rat-liver apolipoproteins AI, AII, and AIV (Fu et al., 2004; Raspé et al., 1999); (iv) rat-liver lipase (Raspé et al., 1999), rat-liver lecithin-cholesterol acyltransferase (Bays & Stein, 2003); and (v) the FAS complex (Li et al., 2005). In the case of liver-spot 14 protein, available information indicates that the gene contains a PPRE-like sequence at least through –2 kb (Motojima et al., 1994), suggesting that the down-regulation of the encoding gene utilizes a negative control of elements that are activated in genes up-regulated by peroxisome proliferators (Kahn, 1997). Heterodimerization of the PPAR and an ARP-I (Clavey et al., 1999; Dana et al., 2001; Gervois et al., 2000) might be responsible for the down-regulation of the apo A-I gene expression. The PPAR is also involved in the down-regulation of the apolipoprotein CIII gene (Clavey et al., 1999; Dana et al., 2001; Gervois et al., 2000).

***Interaction of PPARs with Other Transcriptional Factors Involved in Lipid Metabolism***

In addition to being important *trans*-factors in the regulation of numerous genes, the PPARs also display a positive or negative interaction with other nuclear proteins. In most of these cases, a PPAR binds to a PPRE as a heterodimer with an RXR. Each of these receptor subunits binds to one of the consensus motifs "TGACCT" or a closely related motif (Palmer et al., 1995). On the other hand, antagonisms between a PPAR (in the heterodimer complex form) and: (i) either a COUP-TFI (chicken ovary upstream promoter, transcriptional factor) (Brandenbourg & Hu, 2005) or a COUP-TFII (Eubank et al., 2001) or (ii) either an ARP1 (a human orphan receptor which regulates apo A-I gene expression) or an Hepatic Nuclear Factor (HNF)-4 (a rat orphan receptor) (Patel et al., 2000) were pointed out. PPARs can form a heterodimer or interact with the thyroid hormone receptor (TRb) (Gurnell & Chatterjee, 2004) Jun (Khandoudi et al., 2002) and the ubiquitous transcription factor SPI (Sassa et al., 2004), with LXRa (Guan et al., 2003) or with ARF6 (Tontonoz et al., 1994).

## PPAR and Fatty Acid Metabolism

### *Fatty Acid Transport and Triglyceride Synthesis*

The cellular uptake of long-chain fatty acids is facilitated by fatty acid translocases (FATs), such as the fatty acid transporter protein (FATP) (Stahl et al., 2001) or the FAT itself (Bonen et al., 2000). Earlier studies indicate that the expression of both FATs in rat liver is enhanced by fibrate or fatty acid treatment (Stremmel et al., 2001). FFAs are transported across the plasma membrane through membrane transporters where they are esterified by the ACS-dependent to acyl-CoA derivatives. These changes prevent the efflux of FFAs from the cell. This process makes the uptake unidirectional, and activates the FFAs for utilization in both catabolic (β-oxidation) and/or anabolic pathways (conversion into more complex cellular lipids). Fibrates exert their hypolipidemic action not only via the enhanced catabolism of triglyceride-rich lipoproteins through their effects on LPL and apo C-III gene expression, but also by a concomitant increase in the hepatic uptake of the released FFAs (Martin et al., 1997). Fibrates and fatty acids induce the ACS gene expression and activity in a variety of tissues and cells (Jeong et al., 2004) mediated by a PPRE located in the C-ACS promoter. Furthermore, this induction results in the generation of acyl-CoA esters which are predominantly used for β-oxidation. The increased peroxisomal β-oxidation pathway after treatment with peroxisome proliferators is associated with a moderate induction of the mitochondrial β-oxidation pathway, decreasing the availability of acyl-CoA esters for triglyceride synthesis. A reduction in acetyl-CoA carboxylase (ACC) (Jeukendrup, 2002) and FAS (Li & Tian, 2004) activity will inhibit de novo fatty acid synthesis, thereby further diminishing the intracellular levels of FFAs available for triglyceride synthesis. In addition to increasing β-oxidation and decreasing triglyceride synthesis (Wagner et al., 2005), peroxisome proliferators also decrease apo B and VLDL production (Goldstein et al., 2006). As a consequence, a reduced secretion of VLDL particles together with an enhanced catabolism of triglyceride-rich particles seemingly accounts for the hypolipidemic effect of fibrates.

## *PPARs and β-Oxidation*

Since the discovery of PPARs, scientists have searched for clues to the role of PPARs in modulating the peroxisome-proliferator responsiveness to certain target genes. Many genes encoding the various enzymes of the peroxisomal β-oxidation pathway were among the first ones to be investigated since this pathway is responsible for the metabolism of long-chain fatty acids, and involves sequentially the enzymes acyl-CoA oxidase (ACO), enoyl-CoA hydratase 3-hydroxyacyl-CoA dehydrogenase (multifunctional enzyme), and 3-ketoacyl-CoA thiolase. Reportedly, peroxisome proliferators stimulate the activities of these enzymes through changes in the transcription rates of their genes (Kassam et al., 2000). The analysis of the ACO gene promoter has led to the identification of two PPREs conferring transcriptional activation by PPARs (Lambe et al., 1999). A PPRE resembling the ACO-PPREs was also identified in the regulatory sequences of the multifunctional enzyme (Kassam et al., 2001). Peroxisome proliferators stimulate the transcription of ketoacyl-CoA, but no functional PPRE was identified in its gene. The mutagenesis of the PPAR-α gene by homologous recombination has shed some light on the importance of the PPAR-α in the regulation of enzymes involved in β-oxidation. The mutant animals show resistance to the induction of the enzymes of the peroxisomal β-oxidation pathway by peroxisome proliferators (Kersten, 2002). Reports indicate that the treatment of rats with peroxisome proliferators also enhances ketogenesis (Cullingford et al., 2002) and mitochondrial β-oxidation (Yu et al., 2003). PPARs control the induction of the HMG-CoA synthase, a key mitochondrial enzyme in ketogenesis, via a PPRE located in the proximal promoter region of its gene (Iida et al., 2002). The PPAR binds to a pleiotropic element, called nuclear receptor regulatory element l (NRRE-1), in the regulatory sequences of the mitochondrial medium-chain acyl-CoA dehydrogenase (MCAD) gene, and thus mediates its transcriptional induction (Maehara et al., 2003). MCAD is one of the four different chain-length-specific mitochondrial enzymes catalyzing the initial reaction in mitochondrial β-oxidation.

Peroxisome proliferators also activate several cytosolic proteins including palmitoyl-CoA hydrolase (Hunt et al., 2000), malic enzyme (Shin et al., 1999), and the fatty acid binding proteins (FABP): aP2 (Fujimura et al., 2006), acyl-CoA-binding protein (ACBP) (Sandberg et al., 2005), and L-FABP (Nagasawa et al., 2006). The identification of functional PPRE-like sequences in these genes explains the regulatory effect of PPARs on these proteins. Considering the large number of genes carrying PPREs in their regulatory sequences, likely, the PPARs are crucial in intracellular, extracellular, and peroxisomal lipid metabolism.

## *PPARs and Triglyceride Metabolism*

LPL, a key enzyme in lipoprotein metabolism, hydrolyzes the triglyceride moiety of chylomicrons and VLDL particles. The oxidation of FFAs generates the adenosine triphosphate (ATP) in muscles, which is stored in adipose tissue, or is secreted in milk by the mammary gland. The LPL therefore occupies a pivotal position in both lipoprotein and energy metabolism. The importance of this enzyme in lipoprotein metabolism is illustrated by the severe hypertriglyceridemia and chylomicronemia in patients with familial LPL deficiency (Hooper et al., 2008). In contrast to LPL, apo C-III, which is synthesized in the liver and small intestine, appears to antagonize plasma-triglyceride metabolism. Reports exist of a positive correlation between apo C-III levels and plasma-triglyceride concentrations (Desroches et al., 2008). Apo C-III inhibits triglyceride hydrolysis by the LPL and hepatic lipase in vitro, and impairs the uptake of triglyceride-rich lipoproteins by the liver. The evidence for the casual involvement of apo C-III in hypertriglyceridemia came from transgenic animal studies, showing a correlation between plasma-triglyceride levels and plasma apo C-III concentrations and liver apo C-III gene expression (Park et al., 2008). An impaired clearance of triglyceride-rich lipoproteins due to interference with the apo E-mediated uptake of these particles is the primary abnormality in these animals. Reportedly, an increase in LPL activity is the reason for the hypotriglyceridemic action of fibrates (Srivastava et al., 2006). Studies of cultured hepatocyte and preadipocyte cells indicate that fibrates and fatty acids induce LPL gene expression via a PPRE, to which a PPAR binds (Schoonjans et al., 1996). In addition, fibrates reduce the expression of the rat apo C-Ill gene through a transcriptional mechanism (Anderson et al., 1999), which may involve competition by a PPAR for the binding of the strong hepatic transcription factor HNF-4 to the apo C-Ill promoter as well as a direct repression of an HNF-4 expression by fibrates (Marrapodi & Chiang, 2000). Furthermore, fenofibrate diminishes the expression and secretion apo C-III in primary human hepatocytes and the human hepatoma cell line Hep G2 (Staels et al., 1995). Turnover studies in humans demonstrate that fibrates reduce the apo C-III synthetic rates. The reduction in circulating apo C-III levels in response to fibrates should enhance both the LPL-mediated lipoprotein lipolysis and the clearance of VLDL particles. Consequently, this dual action of fibrates on the expression of the LPL and apoC-III provides a potential mechanism by which these drugs reduce plasma triglycerides and their subsequent beneficial effect on postprandial hypertriglyceridemia.

## *PPARs and Lipoprotein Metabolism*

Peroxisome proliferation in rodents is associated with a variety of changes affecting lipid metabolic pathways. Among metabolic steps stimulated in these circumstances, several were already shown to be catalyzed by proteins encoded by PPRE-containing genes. The discovery of PPARs and their role in the control of peroxisomal β-oxidation enzyme encoding genes were breakthroughs in understanding the regulation of lipid metabolism. Furthermore, the activating effect of fatty acids and related molecules put forward the lipids as gene modulators and the fatty acids as self-enzyme regulators.

HDL has two major protein constituents, apo A-I and apo A-II, and changes in the HDL level play an important role in the reverse cholesterol transport (Fielding & Fielding, 1995). This pathway has a protective role against coronary artery disease: therefore, possibly the reason for protection against atherosclerosis development that may be related to specific particles within HDL containing apo A-I and not apo A-II. Studies reported that, compared to Lp A-I, the ratio of LpA-I:A-II displays a decreased capacity to stimulate cholesterol efflux (Kontush & Chapman, 2006). Studies using transgenic animals also showed that an overexpression of human apo A-I confers resistance to early atherogenesis (Vergnes et al., 2000), whereas a simultaneous overexpression of human apo A-I and apo A-II is less protective (Hedrick et al., 2001). An overexpression of mouse apo A-II in transgenic mice which exhibit increased atherosclerotic lesion development (Rotllan et al., 2005) further confirms the protective role of apo A-I in these situations. All these studies indicate a less protective role of apo A-II relative to apo A-I against the development of coronary heart disease. Furthermore, in vivo studies indicated that fibrates and fish oils down-regulate the gene expression of liver apo A-I and apo A-II genes in rodents (Dallongeville et al., 2001; Gervois et al., 2000). On the other hand, an increased level of HDL and its major constituents' apo A-I and apo A-II to a variable extent was reported in human subjects treated with fibrates (Despres et al., 2004). Fibrates primarily increase the ratio of Lp A-I:A-II, whereas often a small decrease is observed in Lp A-I levels. Fibrates and FFAs exert an overall negative effect on the minimal apo A-I promoter (nt –41 to +91), which is independent of PPAR (Hennuyer et al., 1999). In humans, this negative effect of fibrates and FFAs on apo A-I transcription is counteracted by an interaction of a PPAR with a functional PPRE, localized in the A site of the human but not the rat apo A-I promoter, indicating that a PPAR positively regulates the human apo A-I gene. The apo A-I A site also binds other nuclear receptors such as ARP-1 and RXR (Ge et al., 1994). As a result of these two opposite mechanisms, the human apo A-I gene exhibits a complex regulation in response to fibrates, whereas the rodent apo A-I transcription is repressed. In humans, the final effects of fibrates on the apo A-I gene expression are the result of the interplay of these opposite mechanisms of apo A-I regulation.

## Conclusion

Fatty acids are important energy sources and mediators of biological processes in response to endogenous and exogenous stimuli. The fine tuning of fatty acids' metabolic pathway is the hallmark of healthy organisms. Lipid homeostasis depends on factors that participate directly in the transcriptional control of genes encoding proteins involved in key metabolic steps. PPAR, the prototype nuclear receptor, regulates the expression of several genes involved in fatty acid metabolism, including FAT, uptake by the cells, intracellular binding and activation, as well as catabolism or storage. A PPAR-$\alpha$-mediated change in the expression of genes involved in fatty acid metabolism lies at the basis of the phenomenon of peroxisome proliferation, a pleiotropic cellular response, mainly limited to the liver and kidney. The different isoforms of the PPAR are important messengers in the translation of nutritional, pharmacological, and metabolic stimuli into changes in the expression of genes, more specifically those genes involved in lipid metabolism. PPAR agonists have positive effects on glucose homeostasis and lipid metabolism, and can provide protection against cardiovascular events in obese–diabetic patients. The activation of PPAR-$\alpha$ increases lipolysis and the clearance of remnant particles, due to changes in LPL and apo C-III levels; stimulates cellular fatty acid uptake and their conversion to acyl-CoA derivatives by the induction of FAT, FATP, and ACS activity; induces fatty-acid $\beta$-oxidation pathways; reduces fatty acid and triglyceride synthesis; and finally decreases VLDL production. Both the enhanced catabolism of triglyceride-rich particles and the reduced secretion of VLDL particles are mechanisms that contribute to the hypolipidemic effect of fibrates. PPAR-$\gamma$ is a postprandial lipid- storing–glucose-utilizing regulator that increases both the storage capacity as well as the fatty acid flux in adipocytes. Saturated and unsaturated fatty acids are natural ligands of PPARs that cause the induction of proteins involved in lipid catabolism and cholesterol efflux. Because of PPARs' diverse roles in fatty acid metabolism, one must understand the mechanism of the PPAR-mediated regulation of fatty acid metabolism.

## References

Abdel-Maksoud, M.; V. Sazonov; S.W. Gutkin; J.E. Hokanson. Effects of modifying triglycerides and triglyceride-rich lipoproteins on cardiovascular outcomes. *J. Cardiovasc. Pharmacol.* **2008,** *51(4),* 331–351.

Amacher, D.E.; R. Beck; S.J. Schomaker; C.V. Kenny. Hepatic microsomal enzyme induction, beta-oxidation, and cell proliferation following administration of clofibrate, gemfibrozil, or bezafibrate in the CD rat. *Toxicol. Appl. Pharmacol.* **1997,** *142(1),* 143–150.

Andersson, Y.; Z. Majd; A.M. Lefebvre; G. Martin; A.V. Sechkin; V. Kosykh; J.C. Fruchart; J. Najib; B. Staels. Developmental and pharmacological regulation of apolipoprotein C-II gene expression. Comparison with apo C-I and apo C-III gene regulation. *Arterioscler. Thromb. Vasc. Biol.* **1999,** *19(1),* 115–121.

Aranda, A.; A. Pascual. Nuclear hormone receptors and gene expression. *Physiol. Rev.* **2001**, *81(3),* 1269–1304.

Asayama, K.; R. Sandhir; F.G. Sheikh; H. Hayashibe; T. Nakane; I. Singh. Mol Increased peroxisomal fatty acid beta-oxidation and enhanced expression of peroxisome proliferator-activated receptor-alpha in diabetic rat liver. *Cell Biochem.* **1999,** *194(1–2),* 227–234.

Aubert, J.; P. Saint-Marc; N. Belmonte; C. Dani; R. Négrel; G. Ailhaud. Prostacyclin IP receptor up-regulates the early expression of C/EBPbeta and C/EBPdelta in preadipose cells. *Mol. Cell. Endocrinol.* **2000,** *160(1–2),* 149–156.

Auboeuf, D.; J. Rieusset; L. Fajas; P. Vallier; V. Frering; J.P. Riou; B. Staels; J. Auwerx; M. Laville; H. Vidal. Tissue distribution and quantification of the expression of mRNAs of peroxisome proliferator-activated receptors and liver X receptor-alpha in humans: no alteration in adipose tissue of obese and NIDDM patients. *Diabetes* **1997,** *46(8),* 1319–1327.

Auwerx, J. PPARgamma, the ultimate thrifty gene. *Diabetologia* **1999,** *42,* 1033–1049.

Auwerx, J.; T.A. Cock; C. Knouff. PPAR-gamma: a thrifty transcription factor. *Nucl. Recept. Signal* **2003,** *1,* e006.

Barter, P.J.; K.A. Rye. Is there a role for fibrates in the management of dyslipidemia in the metabolic syndrome? *Arterioscler. Thromb. Vasc. Biol.* **2008,** *28(1),* 39–46.

Bays, H.; E.A. Stein. Pharmacotherapy for dyslipidaemia—current therapies and future agents. *Expert Opin. Pharmacother.* **2003,** *4(11),* 1901–1938.

Berglund, L.; M. Lefevre; H.N. Ginsberg; P.M. Kris-Etherton; P.J. Elmer; P.W. Stewart; A. Ershow; T.A. Pearson; B.H. Dennis; P.S. Roheim; et al. Comparison of monounsaturated fat with carbohydrates as a replacement for saturated fat in subjects with a high metabolic risk profile: studies in the fasting and postprandial states. *Am. J. Clin. Nutr.* **2007,** 86(6), 1611–1620.

Bonen, A.; J.J. Luiken; Y. Arumugam; J.F. Glatz; N.N. Tandon. Acute regulation of fatty acid uptake involves the cellular redistribution of fatty acid translocase. *J. Biol. Chem.* **2000,** *275,* 14501–14508.

Boyd, A.S. Thiazolidinediones in dermatology. *Int. J. Dermatol.* **2007,** *46(6),* 557–563.

Bragt, M.C.; H.E. Popeijus. Peroxisome proliferator-activated receptors and the metabolic syndrome. *Physiol. Behav.* **2008,** *94(2),* 187–197.

Braissant, O.; F. Foufelle; C. Scotto; M. Dauça; W. Wahli. Differential expression of peroxisome proliferator-activated receptors (PPARs): tissue distribution of PPAR-alpha, -beta, and -gamma in the adult rat. *Endocrinology* **1996,** *137(1),* 354–366.

Brandebourg, T.D.; C.Y. Hu. Regulation of differentiating pig preadipocytes by retinoic acid. *J. Anim. Sci.* **2005,** *83(1),* 98–107.

Bull, A.W.; K.R. Steffensen; J. Leers; J.J. Rafter. Activation of PPAR gamma in colon tumor cell lines by oxidized metabolites of linoleic acid, endogenous ligands for PPAR gamma. *Carcinogenesis* **2003,** *24(11),* 1717–1722.

Cajaraville, M.P.; M.Ortiz-Zarragoitia. Specificity of the peroxisome proliferation response in mussels exposed to environmental pollutants. *Aquat. Toxicol.* **2006,** *78 (Suppl. 1),* S117–123. Erratum in: *Aquat. Toxicol.* **2007,** *81(2),* 232.

Caviglia, J.M.; L.O. Li; S. Wang; C.C. DiRusso; R.A. Coleman; T.M. Lewin. Rat long chain acyl-CoA synthetase 5, but not 1, 2, 3, or 4, complements Escherichia coli fadD. *J. Biol. Chem.* **2004,** *279(12),* 11163–11169.

Chawla, J.; J. Repa; R.M. Evans; D.J. Mangelsdorf. Nuclear receptors and lipid physiology: opening the X-files. *Science* **2001**, *294(5548),* 1866–1870.

Cheatham, C.L.; J. Colombo; S.E. Carlson. N-3 fatty acids and congnitive and visual acuity development: methodologic and conceptual considerations. *Am. J. Clin. Nutr.* **2006**, *83,* 1458S–1466S.

Chevalier, S.; N. Macdonald; R.A. Roberts. PPAR alpha-mediated responses in the rodent liver: a holistic biochemical view. *Curr. Protein Pept. Sci.* **2000,** *1(4),* 325–338.

Chew, C.H; M.R. Samian; N. Najimudin; T.S. Tengku-Muhammad. Molecular characterisation of six alternatively spliced variants and a novel promoter in human peroxisome proliferator-activated receptor *alpha. Biochem. Biophys.Res. Commun.* **2003,** *305(2),* 235–243.

Clavey, V.; C. Copin; M.C. Mariotte; E. Baugé; G. Chinetti; J. Fruchart; J.C. Fruchart; J. Dallongeville; B. Staels. Cell culture conditions determine apolipoprotein CIII secretion and regulation by fibrates in human hepatoma HepG2 cells. *Cell Physiol. Biochem.* **1999,** *9(3),* 139–149.

Cornwell, P.D.; A.T. De Souza; R.G. Ulrich. Profiling of hepatic gene expression in rats treated with fibric acid analogs. *Mutat. Res.* **2004,** *549(1-2),* 131–145.

Cullingford, T.E.; C.T. Dolphin; H. Sato. The peroxisome proliferator-activated receptor alpha-selective activator ciprofibrate upregulates expression of genes encoding fatty acid oxidation and ketogenesis enzymes in rat brain. *Neuropharmacology* **2002,** *42(5),* 724–730.

Dallongeville, J.; E. Baugé; A. Tailleux; J.M. Peters; F.J. Gonzalez; J.C. Fruchart; B. Staels. Peroxisome proliferator-activated receptor alpha is not rate-limiting for the lipoprotein-lowering action of fish oil. *J. Biol. Chem.* **2001,** *276(7),* 4634–4639.

Dana, S.L.; P.A. Hoener; J.M. Bilakovics; D.L. Crombie; K.M. Ogilvie; R.F. Kauffman; R. Mukherjee; J.R. Paterniti, Jr. Peroxisome proliferator-activated receptor subtype-specific regulation of hepatic and peripheral gene expression in the Zucker diabetic fatty rat. *Metabolism* **2001,** *50(8),* 963–971.

Das, U.N. Biological significance of essential fatty acids. *J. Assoc. Physicians India* **2006,** *54,* 309–319.

Depreter, M.; J. Vandesompele; M. Espeel; F. Speleman; F. Roels. Modulation of the peroxisomal gene expression pattern by dehydroepiandrosterone and vitamin D: therapeutic implications. *J. Endocrinol.* **2002,** *175(3),* 779–792.

Després, J.P.; I. Lemieux; S.J. Robins. Role of fibric acid derivatives in the management of risk factors for coronary heart disease. *Drugs* **2004,** *64(19),* 2177–2198.

Desroches, S.; I.L. Ruel; Y. Deshaies; M.E. Paradis; W.R. Archer; P. Couture; N. Bergeron; B. Lamarche. Kinetics of plasma apolipoprotein C-III as a determinant of diet-induced changes in plasma triglyceride levels. *Eur. J. Clin. Nutr.* **2008,** *62(1),* 10–7.

Desvergne, B.; W. Wahli. Peroxisome proliferator-activated receptors: nuclear control of metabolism. *Endocrine Rev.* **1999,** *20(5),* 649–688.

Dreyer, C.; H. Ellinger-Ziegelbauer. Retinoic acid receptors and nuclear orphan receptors in the development of Xenopus laevis. *Int. J. Dev. Biol.* 1996, *40(1),* 255–262.

Dreyer, C.; H. Keller; A. Mahfoudi; V. Laudet; G. Krey; W. Wahli. Positive regulation of the peroxisomal beta-oxidation pathway by fatty acids through activation of peroxisome proliferator-activated receptors (PPAR). *Biol. Cell* **1993**, *77(1),* 67–76.

Eubank, D.W.; E. Duplus; S.C. Williams; C. Forest; E.G. Beale. Peroxisome proliferator-activated receptor gamma and chicken ovalbumin upstream promoter transcription factor II negatively regulate the phosphoenolpyruvate carboxykinase promoter via a common element. *J. Biol. Chem.* **2001,** *276(32),* 30561–30569.

Fajas, L.; D. Auboeuf; E. Raspé; K. Schoonjans; A.M. Lefebvre; R. Saladin; J. Najib; M. Laville; J.C. Fruchart; S. Deeb; A. Vidal-Puig; J. Flier; M.R. Briggs; B. Staels; H. Vidal; J. Auwerx. The organization, promoter analysis, and expression of the human PPARgamma gene. *J. Biol. Chem.* **1997,** *272(30),* 18779–87.

Fajas, L.; J.C. Fruchart; J. Auwerx. PPARgamma3 mRNA: a distinct PPARgamma mRNA subtype transcribed from an independent promoter. *FEBS Lett.* **1998,** *438(1-2)*, 55–60.

Fielding, C.J.; P.E. Fielding. Molecular physiology of reverse cholesterol transport. *J. Lipid Res.* **1995,** *36,* 211–228.

Francis, G.A.; E. Fayard; F. Picard; J. Auwerx. Nuclear receptors and the control of metabolism. *Annu. Rev. Physiol.* **2003,** *65,* 261–311.

Fredenrich, A.; P.A. Grimaldi. PPAR *delta*: an uncompletely known nuclear receptor. *Diabetes & Metabolism.* **2005,** *31(1),* 23–27.

Fu, T.; D. Mukhopadhyay; N.O. Davidson; J. Borensztajn. The peroxisome proliferator-activated receptor alpha (PPARalpha) agonist ciprofibrate inhibits apolipoprotein B mRNA editing in low density lipoprotein receptor-deficient mice: effects on plasma lipoproteins and the development of atherosclerotic lesions. *J. Biol. Chem.* **2004,** *279(27),* 28662–28669.

Fujimura, T.; C. Kimura; T. Oe; Y. Takata; H. Sakuma; I. Aramori; S. Mutoh. A selective peroxisome proliferator-activated receptor gamma modulator with distinct fat cell regulation properties. *J. Pharmacol. Exp. Ther.* **2006,** *318(2),* 863–871.

Gani, OA. Are fish oil omega-3 long-chain fatty acids and their derivatives peroxisome proliferator-activated receptor agonists? *Cardiovasc. Diabetol.* **2008,** *7,* 6.

Ge, R.; M. Rhee; S. Malik; S.K. Karathanasis. Transcriptional repression of apolipoprotein AI gene expression by orphan receptor ARP-1. *J. Biol. Chem.* **1994,** *269(18),* 13185–13192.

Gervois, P.; I.P. Torra; J.C. Fruchart; B. Staels. Regulation of lipid and lipoprotein metabolism by PPAR activators. *Clin. Chem. Lab. Med.* **2000,** *38(1),* 3–11.

Goetzman, E.S.; L. Tian; P.A. Wood. Differential induction of genes in liver and brown adipose tissue regulated by peroxisome proliferator-activated receptor-alpha during fasting and cold exposure in acyl-CoA dehydrogenase-deficient mice. *Mol. Genet. Metab.* **2005,** *84(1),* 39–47.

Goldstein, B.J.; J. Rosenstock; D. Anzalone; C. Tou; K.P. Ohman. Effect of tesaglitazar, a dual PPAR alpha/gamma agonist, on glucose and lipid abnormalities in patients with type 2 diabetes: a 12-week dose-ranging trial. *Curr. Med. Res. Opin.* **2006,** *22(12),* 2575–2590.

Goll, V.; E. Alexandre; C. Viollon-Abadie; L. Nicod; D. Jaeck; L. Richert. Comparison of the effects of various peroxisome proliferators on peroxisomal enzyme activities, DNA synthesis, and apoptosis in rat and human hepatocyte cultures. *Toxicol. Appl. Pharmacol.* **1999,** *160(1),* 21–32.

Gonzalez, FJ. The role of peroxisome proliferator activated receptor alpha in peroxisome proliferation, physiological homeostasis, and chemical carcinogenesis. *Adv. Exp. Med. Biol.* **1997,** *422,* 109–125.

Gootjes, J.; F. Schmohl; P.A. Mooijer; C. Dekker; H. Mandel; M. Topcu; M. Huemer; M. Von Schütz; T. Marquardt; J.A. Smeitink; H.R. Waterham; R.J. Wanders. Identification of the molecular defect in patients with peroxisomal mosaicism using a novel method involving culturing of cells at 40 degrees C: implications for other inborn errors of metabolism. *Hum. Mutat.* **2004,** *24(2),* 130–139.

Guan, Y.F.; M.D. Breyer. Peroxisome proliferators-activated receptors (PPARs): Novel therapeutic targets in renal disease. *Kidney Int.* **2001,** *60,* 14–30.

Guan, J.Z.; N. Tamasawa; H. Murakami; J. Matsui; K. Yamato; T. Suda. Clofibrate, a peroxisome-proliferator, enhances reverse cholesterol transport through cytochrome P450 activation and oxysterol generation. *Tohoku J. Exp. Med.* **2003,** *201(4),* 251–259.

Gurnell, M.; V.K. Chatterjee. Nuclear receptors in disease: thyroid receptor beta, peroxisome-proliferator-activated receptor gamma and orphan receptors. *Essays Biochem.* **2004,** *40,* 169–189.

Harris, W.S.; D. Bulchandani. Why do omega-3 fatty acids lower serum triglycerides? *Curr. Opin. Lipidol.* **2006**, *17*, 387–393.

Hedrick, C.C.; L.W. Castellani; H. Wong; A.J. Lusis. In vivo interactions of apoA-II, apoA-I, and hepatic lipase contributing to HDL structure and antiatherogenic functions. *J. Lipid Res.* ***2001,*** *42(4),* 563–570.

Hegardt, F.G. Transcriptional regulation of mitochondrial HMG-CoA synthase in the control of ketogenesis. *Biochimie* **1998,** *80(10),* 803–806.

Hennuyer, N.; P. Poulain; L. Madsen; R.K. Berge; L.M. Houdebine; D. Branellec; J.C. Fruchart; C. Fiévet; N. Duverger; B. Staels. Beneficial effects of fibrates on apolipoprotein A-I metabolism occur independently of any peroxisome proliferative response. *Circulation* **1999,** *99(18),* 2445–2451.

Hooper, A.J.; G.M. Crawford; J.M. Brisbane; K. Robertson; G.F. Watts; F.M. van Bockxmeer; J.R. Burnett. Familial lipoprotein lipase deficiency caused by known (G188E) and novel (W394X) LPL gene mutations. *Ann. Clin. Biochem.* **2008,** *45(Pt 1),* 102–105.

Hsu, M.H.; C.N. Palmer; W. Song; K.J. Griffin; E.F. Johnson. A carboxyl-terminal extension of the zinc finger domain contributes to the specificity and polarity of peroxisome proliferator-activated receptor DNA binding. *J. Biol. Chem.* **1998,** *273(43),* 27988–27997.

Hunt, M.C.; P.J. Lindquist; J.M. Peters; F.J. Gonzalez; U. Diczfalusy; S.E. Alexson. Involvement of the peroxisome proliferator-activated receptor alpha in regulating long-chain acyl-CoA thioesterases. *J. Lipid Res.* **2000,** *41(5),* 814–823.

Hunt, M.C.; K. Solaas; B.F. Kase; S.E. Alexson. Characterization of an acyl-coA thioesterase that functions as a major regulator of peroxisomal lipid metabolism. *J. Biol. Chem.* **2002,** *277(2),* 1128–1138.

Iida, K.T.; Y. Kawakami; H. Suzuki; H. Sone; H. Shimano; H. Toyoshima; Y. Okuda; N. Yamada. PPAR gamma ligands, troglitazone and pioglitazone, up-regulate expression of HMG-CoA synthase and HMG-CoA reductase gene in THP-1 macrophages. *FEBS Lett.* **2002,** *520(1-3),* 177–181.

Issemann, I.; S. Green. Activation of a member of the steroid hormone receptor superfamily by peroxisome proliferators. *Nature* **1990,** *347,* 645–650.

Jeong, S.; M. Kim; M. Han; H. Lee; J. Ahn; M. Kim; Y.H. Song; C. Shin; K.H. Nam; T.W. Kim; G.T. Oh; M. Yoon. Fenofibrate prevents obesity and hypertriglyceridemia in low-density lipoprotein receptor-null mice. *Metabolism* **2004,** *53(5),* 607–613.

Jeukendrup, A.E. Regulation of fat metabolism in skeletal muscle. *Ann. N.Y. Acad. Sci.* **2002,** *967,* 217–235.

Kahn, A. Transcriptional regulation by glucose in the liver. *Biochimie* **1997,** *79(2-3),* 113–118.

Kameda, N.; S. Okuya; Y. Oka. Rosiglitazone (BRL-49653). *Nippon Rinsho* **2000,** *58(2),* 401–404.

Kassam, A.; J.P. Capone; R.A. Rachubinski. The short heterodimer partner receptor differentially modulates peroxisome proliferator-activated receptor alpha-mediated transcription from the peroxisome proliferator-response elements of the genes encoding the peroxisomal beta-oxidation enzymes acyl-CoA oxidase and hydratase-dehydrogenase. *Mol. Cell. Endocrinol.* **2001,** *176(1–2),*

49–56.

Kassam, A., C.J. Winrow; F. Fernandez-Rachubinski; J.P. Capone; R.A. Rachubinski. The peroxisome proliferator response element of the gene encoding the peroxisomal beta-oxidation enzyme enoyl-CoA hydratase/3-hydroxyacyl-CoA dehydrogenase is a target for constitutive androstane receptor beta/9-cis-retinoic acid receptor-mediated transactivation. *J. Biol. Chem.* **2000,** *275(6),* 4345–4350.

Kawada, Y.; M. Khan; A.K. Sharma; D.B. Ratnayake; K. Dobashi; K. Asayama, H.W. Moser; M.A. Contreras; I. Singh. Inhibition of peroxisomal functions due to oxidative imbalance induced by mistargeting of catalase to cytoplasm is restored by vitamin E treatment in skin fibroblasts from Zellweger syndrome-like patients. *Mol. Genet. Metab.* **2004,** *83(4),* 297–305.

Kersten, S. Peroxisome proliferator activated receptors and obesity. *Eur. J. Pharmacol.* **2002,** *440(2–3),* 223–234.

Kersten, S.; W. Wahli. *New Approches to Drug Development;* P. Jolles, Ed.; Birkhauser Verlag: Switzerland, 2000.

Khandoudi, N.; P. Delerive; I. Berrebi-Bertrand; R.E. Buckingham; B. Staels; A. Bril. Rosiglitazone, a peroxisome proliferator-activated receptor-gamma, inhibits the Jun NH(2)-terminal kinase/activating protein 1 pathway and protects the heart from ischemia/reperfusion injury. *Diabetes* **2002,** *51(5),* 1507–1514.

Kiaei, M. Peroxisome Proliferator-Activated Receptor-gamma in Amyotrophic Lateral Sclerosis and Huntington's Disease. *PPAR Res.* **2008,** *2008,* 418765.

Kjaer, M.A.; A. Vegusdal; T. Gjøen; A.C. Rustan; M. Todorcević; B. Ruyter. Effect of rapeseed oil and dietary n-3 fatty acids on triacylglycerol synthesis and secretion in Atlantic salmon hepatocytes. *Biochim. Biophys. Acta* **2008,** *1781(3),* 112–22.

Kliewer, S.A.; B.M. Forman; B. Blumberg; E.S. Ong; U. Borgmeyer; D.J. Mangel-dorf; K. Umesono; R.M. Evans. Differential expression and activation of family of peroxisome proliferators-activated receptors. *Proc. Natl. Acad. Sci. U.S.A.* **1994,** *91,* 7355–7359.

Knights, K.M.; C.J. Drogemuller. Xenobiotic-CoA ligases: kinetic and molecular characterization. *Curr. Drug Metab.* **2000,** *1(1),* 49–66.

Kontush, A.; M.J. Chapman. Functionally defective high-density lipoprotein: a new therapeutic target at the crossroads of dyslipidemia, inflammation, and atherosclerosis. *Pharmacol. Rev.* **2006,** *58(3),* 342–374.

Lambe, K.G.; N.J. Woodyatt; N. Macdonald; S. Chevalier; R.A. Roberts. Species differences in sequence and activity of the peroxisome proliferator response element (PPRE) within the acyl CoA oxidase gene promoter. *Toxicol. Lett.* **1999,** *110(1-2),* 119–127.

Lambert, G.; A.L. Jarnoux; T. Pineau; O. Pape; M. Chetiveaux; C. Laboisse; M. Krempf; P. Costet. Fasting induces hyperlipidemia in mice overexpressing proprotein convertase subtilisin kexin type 9: lack of modulation of very-low-density lipoprotein hepatic output by the low-density lipoprotein receptor. *Endocrinology* **2006,** *147(10),* 4985–4995.

Lampen, A.; S. Zimnik; H. Nau. Teratogenic phthalate esters and metabolites activate the nuclear receptors PPARs and induce differentiation of F9 cells. *Toxicol. Appl. Pharmacol.* **2003,** *188(1),* 14–23.

Lawrence, J.W.; G.K. Wollenberg; J.D. Frank; J.G. DeLuca. Dexamethasone selectively inhibits

WY14,643-induced cell proliferation and not peroxisome proliferation in mice. *Toxicol. Appl. Pharmacol.* **2001,** *170(2),* 113–123.

Leaf, A. Omega-3 fatty acids and prevention of arrhythmias. *Curr. Opin. Lipidol.* **2007**, *18*, 31–34.

Lee C.H.; R.M. Evans. Peroxisome proliferator-activated receptor-gamma in macrophage lipid homeostasis. *Trends Endocrinol. Metab.* **2002,** *13,* 331–335.

Li, X.; P.A. Hansen, L. Xi; R.A. Chandraratna; C.F. Burant. Distinct mechanisms of glucose lowering by specific agonists for peroxisomal proliferator activated receptor gamma and retinoic acid X receptors. *J. Biol. Chem.* **2005,** *280(46),* 38317–38327.

Li B.H.; W.X. Tian. Inhibitory effects of flavonoids on animal fatty acid synthase. *J. Biochem.* **2004,** *135(1),* 85–91.

Lovekamp-Swan, T.; B.J. Davis. Mechanisms of phthalate ester toxicity in the female reproductive system. *Environ. Health Perspect.* **2003,** *111(2),* 139–145.

Luci, S.; H. Kluge; F. Hirche; K. Eder. Clofibrate increases hepatic triiodothyronine (T3)- and thyroxine (T4)-glucuronosyltransferase activities and lowers plasma T3 and T4 concentrations in pigs. *Drug Metab. Dispos.* **2006,** *34(11),* 18871892.

Madrazo, J.A.; D.P. Kelly. The PPAR trio: regulators of myocardial energy metabolism in health and disease. *J. Mol. Cell Cardiol.* **2008**, *44(6)*, 968–975.

Madsen, L.; R.K. Berge. 3-Thia fatty acid treatment, in contrast to eicosapentaenoic acid and starvation, induces gene expression of carnitine palmitoyltransferase-II in rat liver. *Lipids* **1999,** *34(5),* 447–456.

Maehara, K.; T. Hida; Y. Abe; A. Koga; K. Ota; E. Kutoh. Functional interference between estrogen-related receptor alpha and peroxisome proliferator-activated receptor alpha/9-cis-retinoic acid receptor alpha heterodimer complex in the nuclear receptor response element-1 of the medium chain acyl-coenzyme A dehydrogenase gene. *J. Mol. Endocrinol.* **2003,** *31(1),* 47–60.

Malartre, M.; S. Short; C. Sharpe. Alternative splicing generates multiple SMRT transcripts encoding conserved repressor domains linked to variable transcription factor interaction domains. *Nucleic Acids Res.* **2004,** *32(15),* 4676–4686.

Marrapodi, M.; J.Y. Chiang. Peroxisome. Proliferator-activated receptor alpha (PPARalpha) and agonist inhibit cholesterol 7alpha-hydroxylase gene (CYP7A1) transcription. *J. Lipid Res.* **2000,** *41(4),* 514–520.

Martin, G.; K. Schoonjans; A.M. Lefebvre; B. Staels; J. Auwerx. Coordinate regulation of the expression of the fatty acid transport protein and acyl-CoA synthetase genes by PPARalpha and PPARgamma activators. *J. Biol. Chem.* **1997,** *272(45),* 28210-28217.

Meertens, L.M.; K.S. Miyata; J.D. Cechetto; R.A. Rachubinski; J.P. Capone. A mitochondrial ketogenic enzyme regulates its gene expression by association with the nuclear hormone receptor *PPARalpha. EMBO J.* **1998,** *17(23),* 6972–6978.

Michalik, L.; B. Desvergne; C. Dreyer; M. Gavillet; R.N. Laurini; W. Wahli. PPAR expression and function during vertebrate development. *Int. J. Dev. Biol.* **2002,** *46(1),* 105–114.

Michalik, L.; W. Wahli. Peroxisome proliferator-activated receptors: three isotypes for a multitude of functions. *Curr. Opin. Biotechnol.* **1999,** *10,* 564–570.

Miller, M.; H.N. Ginsberg; E.J. Schaefer. Relative atherogenicity and predictive value of non-high-density lipoprotein cholesterol for coronary heart disease. *Am. J. Cardiol.* **2008,** *101(7),* 1003–1008.

Miranda, S.; V. Vollrath; A.M. Wielandt; G. Loyola; M. Bronfman; J. Chianale. Overexpression of mdr2 gene by peroxisome proliferators in the mouse liver. *J. Hepatol.* 1997, *26(6),* 1331–1339.

Motojima, K.; M. Isaka; Y. Takino; S. Goto. Transient induction of fatty acid synthase in rat liver after removal of a peroxisome proliferator. *FEBS Lett.* **1994,** *356,* 122–124.

Motojima, K.; J.M. Peters; F.J. Gonzalez. PPAR alpha mediates peroxisome proliferator-induced transcriptional repression of nonperoxisomal gene expression in mouse. *Biochem. Biophys. Res. Commun.* **1997,** *230(1),* 155–158.

Muzio, F.; L. Mondazzi; W.S. Harris; D. Sommariva; A. Branchi. Effects of moderate variations in the macronutrient content of the diet on cardiovascular disease risk factors in obese patients with the metabolic syndrome. *Am. J. Clin. Nutr.* **2007,** *86(4),* 946–951.

Nagasawa, T.; Y. Inada; S. Nakano; T. Tamura; T. Takahashi; K. Maruyama; Y. Yamazaki; J. Kuroda; N. Shibata. Effects of bezafibrate, PPAR pan-agonist, and GW501516, PPARdelta agonist, on development of steatohepatitis in mice fed a methionine- and choline-deficient diet. *Eur. J. Pharmacol.* **2006,** *536(1–2),* 182–191.

Najib, J. Fenofibrate in the treatment of dyslipidemia: a review of the data as they relate to the new suprabioavailable tablet formulation. *Clin. Ther.* **2002,** *24(12),* 2022–2050.

Nakajima, T.; G. Ichihara; M. Kamijima; S. Itohara; T. Aoyama. Functional activation of peroxisome proliferator-activated receptor alpha (PPARalpha) by environmental chemicals in relation to their toxicities. *Nagoya J. Med. Sci.* **2002,** *65(3–4),* 85–94.

Nicolosi R.J.; B. Woolfrey; T.A. Wilson; P. Scollin; G. Handelman; R. Fisher. Decreased aortic early atherosclerosis and associated risk factors in hypercholesterolemic hamsters fed a high- or mid-oleic acid oil compared to a high-linoleic acid oil. *J. Nutr. Biochem.* **2004,** *15(9),* 540–547.

Orfila, L.; S. Mendoza; J. Rodríguez; F. Arvelo. Participation of dexamethasone and E and C vitamins in the modulation of the hepatotoxic effect induced by fomesafen and 2,4-D amino herbicides, in rats. *Acta Cient Venez* **2002,** *53(1),* 60–65.

Osumi, T.; J.K. Wen; T. Hashimoto. Two cis-acting regulatory sequences in the peroxisome proliferators-responsive enhancer region of rat acyl-CoA oxidase gene. *Biochem. Biophys. Res. Commun.* **1991,** *175,* 866–871.

Palmer, C.N.; M.H. Hsu; H.J. Griffin; E.F. Johnson. Novel sequence determinants in peroxisome proliferator signaling. *J. Biol. Chem.* **1995,** *(27),* 16114–16121.

Palmer, C.N.A.; M.H. Hsu; K.J. Griffin; J.L. Raucy; E.F. Johnson. Peroxisome proliferator activated receptor-*alpha* expression in human liver. *Mol. Pharmacol.* **1998,** *53(1),* 14–22.

Park, S.H.; M.S.Choi; T. Park. Changes in the hepatic gene expression profile in a rat model of chronic ethanol treatment. *Food Chem. Toxicol.* **2008,** *46(4),* 1378–1388.

Patel, D.D.; B.L. Knight; A.K. Soutar; G.F. Gibbons; D.P. Wade. The effect of peroxisome-proliferator-activated receptor-alpha on the activity of the cholesterol 7 alpha-hydroxylase gene. *Biochem. J.* **2000,** *351 Pt 3,* 747–753.

Peehl, D.M.; D. Feldman. Interaction of nuclear receptor ligands with the Vitamin D signaling pathway in prostate cancer. *J. Steroid Biochem. Mol. Biol.* **2004,** *92(4),* 307–315.

Picard, F.; J. Auwerx. PPAR(gamma) and glucose homeostasis. *Annu. Rev. Nutr.* **2002,** *22,*

167–197.

Raman, N.; P.N. Black; C.C. DiRusso. Characterization of the fatty acid-responsive transcription factor FadR. Biochemical and genetic analyses of the native conformation and functional domains. *J. Biol. Chem.* **1997,** *272(49),* 30645–30650.

Rao, M.S.; V. Subbarao. Effect of dexamethasone on ciprofibrate-induced cell proliferation and peroxisome proliferation. *Fundam. Appl. Toxicol.* **1997,** *35(1),* 78–83.

Raspé, E.; L. Madsen; A.M. Lefebvre; I. Leitersdorf; L. Gelman; J. Peinado-Onsurbe; J. Dallongeville; J.C. Fruchart; R. Berge; B. Staels. Modulation of rat liver apolipoprotein gene expression and serum lipid levels by tetradecylthioacetic acid (TTA) via PPAR activation. *J. Lipid Res.* **1999,** *40,* 2099–2110.

Ripp, S.L.; J.L. Fitzpatrick; J.M. Peters; R.A. Prough. Induction of CYP3A expression by dehydroepiandrosterone: involvement of the pregnane X receptor. *Drug Metab. Dispos.* **2002,** *30(5),* 570–575.

Rosen, E.D.; B.M. Spiegelman. PPARgamma: a nuclear regulator of metabolism, differentiation, and cell growth. *J. Biol. Chem.* **2001,** *276,* 37731–37734.

Rosen, E.D.; C.J. Walkey; P. Puigserver; B.M. Spiegelman. Transcriptional regulation of adipogenesis. *Genes Dev.* **2000,** *14,* 1293–1307.

Rotllan, N.; V. Ribas; L. Calpe-Berdiel; J.M. Martín-Campos; F. Blanco-Vaca; J.C. Escolà-Gil. Overexpression of human apolipoprotein A-II in transgenic mice does not impair macrophage-specific reverse cholesterol transport in vivo. *Arterioscler. Thromb. Vasc. Biol.* **2005,** *25(9),* e128–132.

Sampath, H.; J.M. Ntambi. Polyunsaturated fatty acid regulation of genes of lipid metabolism. *Annu. Rev. Nutr.* **2005,** *25,* 317–340.

Sandberg, M.B.; M. Bloksgaard; D. Duran-Sandoval; C. Duval; B. Staels; S. Mandrup. The gene encoding acyl-CoA-binding protein is subject to metabolic regulation by both sterol regulatory element-binding protein and peroxisome proliferator-activated receptor alpha in hepatocytes. *J. Biol. Chem.* **2005,** *280(7),* 5258–5266.

Sassa, Y.; Y. Hata; L.P. Aiello; Y. Taniguchi; K. Kohno; T. Ishibashi. Bifunctional properties of peroxisome proliferator-activated receptor gamma1 in KDR gene regulation mediated via interaction with both Sp1 and Sp3. *Diabetes* **2004,** *53(5),* 1222–1229.

Schoonjans, K.; J. Peinado-Onsurbe; A.M. Lefebvre; R.A. Heyman; M. Briggs; S. Deeb; B. Staels; J. Auwerx. PPARalpha and PPARgamma activators direct a distinct tissue-specific transcriptional response via a PPRE in the lipoprotein lipase gene. *EMBO J.* **1996,** *15(19),* 5336–5348.

Shin, M.; M. Ohnishi; S. Iguchi; K. Sano; C. Umezawa. Peroxisome-proliferator regulates key enzymes of the tryptophan-NAD+ pathway. *Toxicol. Appl. Pharmacol.* **1999,** *158(1),* 71–80.

Sohlenius, A.K.; M. Reinfeldt; K. Bäckström; A. Bergstrand; J.W. DePierre. Hepatic peroxisome proliferation in vitamin A-deficient mice without a simultaneous increase in peroxisomal acyl-CoA oxidase activity. *Biochem. Pharmacol.* **1996,** *51(6),* 821–827.

Spieker, L.E.; G. Noll; M. Hannak; T.F. Lüscher. Efficacy and tolerability of fluvastatin and bezafibrate in patients with hyperlipidemia and persistently high triglyceride levels. *J. Cardiovasc. Pharmacol.* **2000,** *35(3),* 361–365.

Sporn, M.B.; N. Suh; D.J. Mangelsdorf. Prospects for prevention and treatment of cancer with selective PPARgamma modulators (SPARMs). *Trends Mol. Med.* **2001,** *7,* 395–400.

Srivastava, R.A.; R. Jahagirdar; S. Azhar; S. Sharma; C.L. Bisgaier. Peroxisome proliferator-activated receptor-alpha selective ligand reduces adiposity, improves insulin sensitivity and inhibits atherosclerosis in LDL receptor-deficient mice. *Mol. Cell. Biochem.* **2006,** *285(1-2),* 35–50.

Staels, B.; N. Vu-Dac; V. Kosykh; R. Saladin; J.C. Fruchart; J. Dallongeville; J. Auwerx. Fibrates downregulate apolipoprotein C-III expression independent of induction of peroxisomal acyl coenzyme A oxidase. A potential mechanism for the hypolipidemic action of fibrates. *J. Clin. Invest.* **1995,** *95,* 705–712.

Stahl, A.; R.E. Gimeno; L.A. Tartaglia; H.F. Lodish. Fatty acid transport proteins: a current view of a growing family. *Trends Endocrinol. Metab.* **2001,** *12,* 266–273.

Stoll, BA. N-3 fatty acids and lipid peroxidation in breast cancer inhibition. *Br. J. Nutr.* **2002,** *87(3),* 193–198.

Stremmel, W.; L. Pohl; A. Ring; T. Herrmann. A new concept of cellular uptake and intracellular trafficking of long-chain fatty acids. *Lipids* **2001,** *36(9),* 981–989.

Sülzle, A.; F. Hirche; K. Eder. Thermally oxidized dietary fat upregulates the expression of target genes of PPAR alpha in rat liver. *J. Nutr.* **2004,** *134(6),* 1375–1383.

Tontonoz, P.; R.A. Graves; A.I. Budavari; H. Erdjument-Bromage; M. Lui; E. Hu; P. Tempst; B.M. Spiegelman. Adipocyte-specific transcription factor ARF6 is a heterodimeric complex of two nuclear hormone receptors, PPAR gamma and RXR alpha. *Nucleic Acids Res.* **1994,** *22(25),* 5628–5634.

Tugwood, J.T.; I. Issemann; R.G. Anderson; K. Bundell; W. McPheat; S. Green. The mouse peroxisome proliferator receptor recognizes a response element in the 5' flanking sequence of the rat acyl CoA oxidase gene. *EMBO J.* **1992,** *11,* 433–439.

Turunen, M.; P. Sindelar; G. Dallner. Induction of endogenous coenzyme Q biosynthesis by administration of peroxisomal inducers. *Biofactors* **1999,** *9(2–4),* 131–139.

Venkata, N.G.; J.A. Robinson; P.J. Cabot; B. Davis; G.R. Monteith; S.J. Roberts-Thomson. Mono(2-ethylhexyl)phthalate and mono-n-butyl phthalate activation of peroxisome proliferator activated-receptors alpha and gamma in breast. *Toxicol. Lett.* **2006,** *163(3),* 224–234.

Vergnes, L.; N. Baroukh; M.A. Ostos; G. Castro; N. Duverger; M.N. Nanjee; J. Najib; J.C. Fruchart; N.E. Miller; M.M. Zakin; A. Ochoa. Expression of human apolipoprotein A-I/C-III/A-IV gene cluster in mice induces hyperlipidemia but reduces atherogenesis. *Arterioscler. Thromb. Vasc. Biol.* **2000,** *20(10),* 2267–2274.

Vu-Dac, N.; S. Chopin-Delannoy; P. Gervois; E. Bonnelye; G. Martin; J.C. Fruchart; V. Laudet; B. Staels. The nuclear receptors peroxisome proliferator-activated receptor alpha and Rev-erbalpha mediate the species-specific regulation of apolipoprotein A-I expression by fibrates. *J. Biol. Chem.* **1998,** *273(40),* 25713–25720.

Wagner, J.A.; P.J. Larson; S. Weiss; J.L. Miller; T.W. Doebber; M.S. Wu; D.E. Moller; K.M. Gottesdiener. Individual and combined effects of peroxisome proliferator-activated receptor and γ-agonists, fenofibrate and rosiglitazone, on biomarkers of lipid and glucose metabolism in healthy nondiabetic volunteers. *J. Clin. Pharmacol.* **2005,** *45(5),* 504–513.

Wanders, R.J.; E.G. van Grunsven; G.A. Jansen. Lipid metabolism in peroxisomes: enzymology, functions and dysfunctions of the fatty acid alpha- and beta-oxidation systems in humans.

*Biochem. Soc. Trans.* **2000,** *28(2),* 141–149.

Wang, Z.J.; C.L. Liang; G.M. Li; C.Y. Yu; M. Yin. Neuroprotective effects of arachidonic acid against oxidative stress on rat hippocampal slices. *Chem. Biol. Interact.* **2006,** *163(3),* 207–217.

Wang, L.; Y. Tang; D.C. Rubin; M.S. Levin. Chronically administered retinoic acid has trophic effects in the rat small intestine and promotes adaptation in a resection model of short bowel syndrome. *Am. J. Physiol. Gastrointest. Liver Physiol.* **2007,** *292(6),* G1559–1569.

Webb, S.J.; G.H. Xiao; T.E. Geoghegan; R.A. Prough. Regulation of CYP4A expression in rat by dehydroepiandrosterone and thyroid hormone. *Mol. Pharmacol.* **1996,** *49(2),* 276–287.

Westin, M.A.; M.C. Hunt; S.E. Alexson. The identification of a succinyl-CoA thioesterase suggests a novel pathway for succinate production in peroxisomes. *J. Biol. Chem.* **2005,** *280(46),* 38125–38132.

Willson, T.M.; M.H. Lambert; S.A. Kliewer. Peroxisome proliferator-activated receptor gamma and metabolic disease. *Ann. Rev. Biochem.* **2001,** *70,* 341–367.

Yamakawa-Karakida, N.; K. Sugita; T. Inukai; K. Goi; M. Nakamura; K. Uno; H. Sato; K. Kagami; N. Barker; S. Nakazawa. Ligand activation of peroxisome proliferator-activated receptor gamma induces apoptosis of leukemia cells by down-regulating the c-myc gene expression via blockade of the Tcf-4 activity. *Cell Death Differ.* **2002,** *9(5),* 513–526.

Yamashita, T.,; E. Oda; T. Sano; T. Yamashita; Y. Ijiru; J.C. Giddings;J. Yamamoto. Varying the ratio of dietary n-6/n-3 polyunsaturated fatty acid alters the tendency to thrombosis and progress of atherosclerosis in apoE-/- LDLR-/- double knockout mouse. *Thromb. Res.* **2005,** *116(5),* 393–401.

Yamoto, T.; Y. Ohashi; T. Furukawa; M. Teranishi; S. Manabe; T. Makita. Change of the sex-dependent response to clofibrate in F344 rat liver during postnatal development. *Toxicol. Lett.* **1996,** *85(2),* 77–83.

Yu, X.X.; J. Odle; J.K. Drackley. Differential induction of peroxisomal beta-oxidation enzymes by clofibric acid and aspirin in piglet tissues. *Am. J. Physiol. Regul. Integr. Comp. Physiol.* **2001,** *281(5),* R1553–1561.

Yu, S.; S. Rao; J.K. Reddy. Peroxisome proliferator-activated receptors, fatty acid oxidation, steatohepatitis and hepatocarcinogenesis. *Curr. Mol. Med.* **2003,** *3(6),* 561–572.

Zhang, F.; B. Lavan; F.M. Gregoire. Peroxisome proliferator-activated receptors as attractive anti-obesity targets. *Drug News Perspect.* **2004,** *17(10),* 661–669.

Zingarelli, B.; J.A. Cook. Peroxisome proliferator-activated receptor-gamma is a new therapeutic target in sepsis and inflammation. *Shock* **2005,** *23(5),* 393–399.

PART 3

# Fatty Acids and Health Promotion

# 18

# Fatty Acids in Membrane Lipids: Role in Disease Causation and Prevention

**Breanne Anderson and David W.L. Ma**

*Dept. of Human Health and Nutritional Sciences, Animal Science/Nutrition Building, Room 342, College of Biological Science, University of Guelph, Guelph, Ontario, Canada N1G 2W1.*

## Introduction

Dietary lipids contribute significantly to human health and chronic diseases. A greater understanding of the fundamental basis by which dietary lipids contribute to human health and pathology may lead to the development of effective strategies for the prevention, management, or treatment of major chronic diseases. In recent years, focus has increased on the role of specific dietary fatty acids and their role in health promotion and disease progression. Given this significant and growing body of knowledge, it is no longer possible to consider dietary fat a single entity but rather a composition of distinct fatty acids with specific structural and functional properties that combine to modulate human health and disease. Therefore, this review focuses on the specific effects of major classes of fatty acids on chronic diseases, including cancer, cardiovascular disease (CVD), and insulin resistance (IR). Potential mechanisms of action are also highlighted, including the effects on membrane rafts (MRs), inflammation, and transcription factors. This review focuses predominantly on studies published from the year 2000 onward.

## Fatty Acids

Four main types of fatty acids are present in the diet: saturated, monounsaturated, polyunsaturated, and *trans* fats. Saturated fatty acids (SFAs) are hydrocarbon chains with no double bonds. Monounsaturated fatty acids (MUFAs) have one double bond, whereas polyunsaturated fatty acids (PUFAs) consist of a hydrocarbon chain with two or more double bonds. PUFAs are classified as either n-6 or n-3, referring to the location of the first double bond from the methyl carbon. In addition to the International Union of Pure and Applied Chemistry (IUPAC) convention of the "n" designation, the classical naming system using omega-6 and omega-3 terminology is still commonly used. The double bond present in both PUFAs and MUFAs is in the *cis* configuration, while *trans* fatty acids (TFAs) refer to MUFAs and PUFAs which contain double bonds in the *trans* configuration. TFAs are present naturally in the diet, but the majority is consumed through TFAs produced by the food industry in a process known as hydrogenation.

## n-3 PUFA

Alpha-linolenic acid (ALA; 18:3n-3), the parent fatty acid of the n-3 PUFA family, is found in some leafy vegetables, nuts, seeds, and vegetable oils. ALA is considered an essential fatty acid which mammals can not synthesize; it must be consumed through the diet. In mammals, limited conversion of ALA occurs to eicosapentaenoic acid (EPA; 20:5n-3) and docosahexaenoic acid (DHA; 22:6n-3) through a series of elongation and desaturation steps. Alternatively, mammals can directly consume EPA and DHA in the diet from marine sources such as salmon, tuna, mackerel, and other fatty fish.

Intakes of ALA, EPA, and DHA vary considerably across different populations. For example, the estimated daily intake of n-3 PUFA in Japan is 2.4–2.9 g per person as EPA + DHA (Yamada et al., 2000), whereas the typical North American consumes 0.1–0.2 g of EPA + DHA and approximately 1.4 g of ALA per day (Kris-Etherton et al., 2003).

## n-6 PUFA and Conjugated Linoleic Acid

Linoleic acid (LA; 18:2n-6), the parent fatty acid of the n-6 PUFA family, is found in vegetable oils, seeds, and nuts. LA is also an essential fatty acid that can be further metabolized to arachidonic acid (AA; 20:4n-6). One can also directly consume AA in the diet from animal fat. Relative to n-3 PUFA, n-6 PUFA-intake levels are much higher. The ratio of n-6 to n-3 PUFA intake is estimated to be upward of 20:1 in a modern Western diet, a figure that has changed dramatically from centuries ago when our Paleolithic ancestors ate a diet of roughly 1:1–2 n-6:n-3 PUFA (DeFilippis & Sperling, 2006; Simopoulos, 2002).

Conjugated linoleic acid (CLA) is a collective term for isomers of LA containing conjugated double bonds. The predominant isomers studied in the literature are *cis*9, *trans*11-CLA (*c*9,*t*11) and *trans*10, *cis*12-CLA (*t*10,*c*12). Commercially produced supplements contain an equal mixture of *c*9,*t*11 and *t*10*c*12-CLA, while dairy products and ruminant animal fat are the predominant sources of *c*9,*t*11 CLA (Ma et al., 1999). The latter isomer is the main isomer in the human diet, accounting for more than 90% of total CLA intake (Tricon et al., 2005), which is estimated to be less than 500 mg/day in the U.S. population (Ritzenthaler et al., 2001) and less than 100 mg/day in Canada (Ens et al., 2001).

## MUFAs

Common MUFAs—including palmitoleic acid (16:1n-7), *cis*-vaccenic acid (18:1n-7), and oleic acid (OA) (18:1n-9)—are found in foods such as avocado, nuts, and oils.

Olive oil is a key component of the Mediterranean diet, widely regarded as being cardioprotective (Perez-Martinez et al., 2007). OA constitutes approximately 75% of olive oil, and thus has received considerable attention for its role in modifying blood-lipid profiles. People have also studied it for its potential insulin-sensitizing and anti-oncogenic effects.

### *SFAs and TFAs*

SFAs are found in high-fat milk products; fatty meats; eggs; lard; and coconut, palm, and palm-kernel oils. High intakes of SFA raise low-density lipoprotein (LDL) cholesterol, and may increase the risk of developing IR (Roche, 2005). TFAs, such as *trans*-vaccenic acid (18:1*t*-11), are found naturally in a few foods such as dairy products, beef, and lamb. Typically, TFAs are consumed as man-made hydrogenated fats, used by food companies to increase the stability and shelf life of their products. In addition to raising LDL-cholesterol, high-density lipoprotein (HDL) cholesterol is decreased by TFA, leading to an increased risk of developing CVD and potentially numerous other diseases (Ascherio, 2006).

Worldwide consumption of TFA varies, with the lowest intakes typically found in Korea and Japan (0.6 g/person/day and 0.1–0.3 g/person/day, respectively) (Craig-Schmidt, 2006). The contribution of TFA to total daily-energy intake is approximately 2.6% or 5.3 g/day for Americans, in comparison to that of SFAs, which is estimated to be about 12.5% or 25 g/day (Allison et al., 1999). For Canadians, the estimated mean daily intake of TFA is 6.4% of energy or 7 g/day and 25.7% of energy or 27.9 g/day of SFA (Statistics Canada, 2003). With the advent of regulations requiring TFA labelling on food products in Canada and the United States in December 2005 and January 2006, respectively, a decline in TFA intake is expected due to increased consumer awareness and product reformulation (Craig-Schmidt, 2006).

## Role of Fatty Acids in Cancer, Insulin Resistance, and Cardiovascular Disease

Geographical differences in the incidence rates of certain diseases prompted research into potential causes for these observations. For instance, breast cancer rates are up to five times higher in developed countries than in those reported from Asian regions, which have the lowest incidences of this cancer (Greenlee et al., 2000). As well, CVD rates in Inuit populations tend to be markedly lower than in other regions, despite their very high intake of fat (Dyerberg et al., 1978). Interestingly, when immigrants leave a low-incidence region of a particular disease and move to a region with high-incidence rates, they do not immediately assume the host country's rate. After two to three generations, however, the risk of their descendants approaches that of their adopted country, indicating that environmental factors contribute to health and disease (Kelsey & Bernstein, 1996; Kuller, 1995; Lopez-Otin & Diamandis, 1998; Ziegler et al., 1993). Epidemiologic and experimental studies suggest a role for specific dietary fatty acids in the etiology of diseases including cancer, IR and, CVD, which are discussed in the following sections.

## Cancer

Cancer is among the main causes of mortality worldwide, and is the second leading cause of death in Canada and the United States (Canadian Cancer Society/National Cancer Institute of Canada, 2008; Jemal et al., 2006). The most common sites of tumor development for North Americans include the lung, colon, breast, and prostate (Canadian Cancer Society/National Cancer Institute of Canada, 2008; Jemal et al., 2006); by all estimates, approximately 30% of cancer risk is associated with diet (Colditz et al., 2002). Dietary lipids, in particular, have been studied extensively for their tumor-promoting and tumor-protective effects. Many retrospective case-control investigations in humans have linked increased fat intake with increased cancer risk (Kushi & Giovannucci, 2002). However, due to recall bias and confounding variables, definitive conclusions are not possible (Dennis et al., 2004). Results from the European Prospective Investigation into Cancer and Nutrition (EPIC) did not support a strong association between fat intake and cancer development in adults (Gonzalez, 2006). Thus, one can make no clear associations currently between dietary-fat consumption and cancer in humans. In contrast, results from animal studies support a relationship between dietary fatty acids and cancer. Independent of caloric supply, studies suggest a fatty acid specific effect (Bartsch et al., 1999; Kolonel et al., 1999; Rose, 1997; Wynder et al., 1997), which is discussed in the context of breast cancer as follows.

### *n-3 PUFA and Breast Cancer*

Several case-control studies demonstrated significant inverse associations between breast cancer risk and dietary intake of n-3 PUFA. Bagga et al. (2002) showed a decreased risk of breast cancer development with an increase in both EPA and DHA consumption, while others showed that an increased intake of ALA alone or in combination with DHA has a similar protective effect (Bagga et al., 2002; Klein et al., 2000; Maillard et al., 2002). Case-control studies assessing erythrocyte n-3 PUFA levels show an inverse association with breast cancer risk, regardless of geographical location (Kuriki et al., 2007; Shannon et al., 2007). Contrary to these findings, however, a study of 23,693 postmenopausal women from Denmark concluded that increased fish consumption was associated with a higher breast cancer rate, but only in estrogen receptor (ER)+ breast cancers (Stripp et al., 2003).

Animal studies have generally pointed to a protective effect of n-3 PUFA in mammary tumorigenesis (Cave, Jr., 1997; Chajes & Bougnoux, 2003; Hubbard et al., 1998; Stoll, 1998). Further, some rodent studies suggested that the timing of exposure to n-3 PUFA might affect mammary-gland development and response to a cancer challenge. Feeding an n-3:n-6 PUFA ratio of 1:2 (versus 1:17) to prepubertal rats conferred protection to carcinogen-induced mammary tumorigenesis but only in a low-fat diet context (16% versus 39% total energy from fat) (Hilakivi-Clarke et al.,

2005; Olivo & Hilakivi-Clarke, 2005). In contrast, increasing n-3:n-6 PUFA ratios in the presence of a constant overall PUFA:SFA diet did not suppress the incidence or reduce the latency of rat mammary-tumor development in a separate study (Sasaki et al., 1998). Others showed that feeding rats ALA-rich flaxseed from conception to weaning decreases the number of terminal-end buds and increases differentiation to lobulo-alveolar structures (Tou & Thompson, 1999; Ward et al., 2000). These developmental markers are typically associated with a reduced risk of mammary-tumor development.

Cell-culture studies have supported a protective role for n-3 PUFA in breast cancer, providing new mechanistic insight into the etiology of breast cancer. Studies showed that n-3 PUFA exerted anti-proliferative effects (Barascu et al., 2006; Chamras et al., 2002), which may be mediated through decreased fatty acid synthase (FAS) activity (Menendez et al., 2004), a possible oncogene that is up-regulated in breast cancers (Hunt et al., 2007). Menendez et al. (2006) studied BT-474 and SkBr-3 breast cancer cells, which naturally amplify the HER-2 oncogene, and found that ALA suppressed the HER-2 coded p185 HER-2/neu oncogene expression. Further, DHA was found to down-regulate HER-2 action.

### *n-6 PUFA, CLA, and Breast Cancer*

The relationship between n-6 PUFA and breast cancer risk is inconclusive. Human studies correlated high n-6 PUFA intake with an increased breast cancer risk (Stoll, 1998), whereas other analyses found no association (Shannon et al., 2007; Thiebaut et al., 2005), and others still found negative associations (Rissanen et al., 2003). In addition, several studies identified positive associations between breast cancer risk and low n-3:n-6 PUFA ratios (Maillard et al., 2002; Simonsen et al., 1998a), causing difficulty in determining the nature in which the low n-3 PUFA or high n-6 PUFA intake contributes to the relationship. In a study examining the association between n-3:n-6 PUFA ratios and breast cancer, Goodstine et al. (2003) concluded that neither overall fat intake or specific fatty acid intake was related to breast cancer risk. Subgroup analyses, however, suggested that a higher n-3:n-6 PUFA ratio may reduce the risk of breast cancer in premenopausal but not postmenopausal women.

Positive associations between n-6 PUFA and breast cancer risk were identified in animal and cell-culture studies supporting a potential tumor-promoting effect of this group of fatty acids (Cave, Jr., 1997; Fay & Freedman, 1997; Hilakivi-Clarke et al., 1997; Luijten et al., 2007; Rose, 1997). Escrich et al. (2004) demonstrated that high corn-oil diets, rich in n-6 PUFA, promoted the development of 7,12-dimethylbenz(alpha)anthracene (DMBA) induced mammary tumors in rats. Interestingly, Chamras and colleagues (2002) found that AA inhibited MCF-7 cell growth in vitro by 30%, whereas LA had no effect and, further, was found to increase HER-2 oncogene expression (Menendez et al., 2006). Although the results from animal and cell-culture models generally show a negative effect of n-6 PUFA on breast cancer risk, a need remains for further research to substantiate these effects in humans and an understanding of the mechanisms of action.

In contrast, CLA is effective at inhibiting angiogenesis in mice in a dose-dependent manner (Masso-Welch et al., 2002), and reduces the risk of N-methyl-N-nitrosourea (MNU)-induced mammary carcinogenesis in adult rats (Ip et al., 1995). Recently, however, CLA demonstrated a stimulatory effect on mammary tumorigenesis in transgenic mice overexpressing erbB2, which is overexpressed in 20–30% of human breast cancer cases (Ip et al., 2007). The *t*10,*c*12-CLA isomer accelerated mammary-tumor development by ≈100 days, and increased metastasis by 42% compared with the control group. Conversely, cell-culture studies generally support an anti-cancer role for CLA, and exert growth-inhibitory efforts on human breast cancer cells (O'Shea et al., 2000). CLA augments the anti-cancer effects of Docetaxel, a common drug used in breast cancer therapy, in vitro (Fite et al., 2007). In humans, associations between CLA intake and breast cancer risk are less clear. McCann et al. (2004) found no association between total CLA consumption and the overall risk of pre- or postmenopausal breast cancer, although compared with premenopausal women in the lowest quartile of *c*9,*t*11-CLA intake, those in the highest quartile had a marginally significant reduction in the risk of having an ER-negative tumor (Aro et al., 2000).

### *MUFA and Breast Cancer*

A potential tumor-protective role for OA was observed in southern European populations where olive oil consumption was high (Lipworth et al., 1997; Martin-Moreno et al., 1994; Simonsen et al., 1998b). In a recent case-control analysis of the erythrocyte-membrane composition of postmenopausal women, the percentage of total MUFA in red blood cells (RBCs) was lower in cases, suggesting a tumor-protective effect of this group of fatty acids (Shannon et al., 2007). However, epidemiologic studies involving OA and breast cancer have been inconclusive. A recent review reported inconsistent results ranging from neutral to tumor-growth-promoting effects of OA (Escrich et al., 2007). These study results may depend on whether OA or olive oil is used; the latter contains minor bioactive compounds including phenols, flavonoids and lignans, which can further confound experimental results (Hashim et al., 2005; Kitts, 1994). Therefore, no clear conclusions regarding the role of OA in breast cancer can be made at this time.

### *SFA, TFA, and Breast Cancer*

Limited and controversial evidence exists regarding the potential tumor-promoting effect of SFAs and TFAs on breast cancer risk. In a study of breast cancer and RBC composition in Japan, no association was found between dietary intake of SFA and breast cancer risk; however, erythrocyte levels of SFA were especially higher in women who developed breast cancer (Kuriki et al., 2007). These results corroborate the findings of Shannon et al. (2007) who, in addition to establishing a positive relationship between erythrocyte SFA and breast cancer risk, found a significant direct association between palmitic acid and breast cancer. Conversely, in a recent prospective cohort study, no association between SFA intake and breast cancer risk was observed (Lof et al., 2007). But in rats fed SFA, MNU-induced mammary carcinogenesis resulted in a greater number of adenocarcinomas and a higher cell proliferation relative to controls (Wei et al., 2007).

Several case-control studies have assessed dietary-TFA intake in humans and breast cancer risk. Conflicting outcomes resulted from trials assessing breast cancer risk and consumption of *trans* vaccenic acid versus *trans* elaidic acid (18:1*t*-9). In postmenopausal women, *trans* elaidic acid intake was associated with increased breast cancer risk (Kohlmeier et al., 1997). In contrast, a study of premenopausal women concluded that no association existed between 18:1*t*9 intake and breast cancer risk (Saadatian-Elahi et al., 2002). Rissanen et al. (2003) found a positive association between increased *trans* vaccenic acid intake and breast cancer risk, whereas, Aro et al. (2000) reported that increased *trans* vaccenic acid consumption was associated with decreased breast cancer risk. Results from a large prospective cohort study ($n$ = 88,795) indicated no association existed between TFA intake and postmenopausal breast cancer incidence (Holmes, 1999). The relationship between intakes of SFA and TFA and breast cancer risk has yet to be established and more research in this area is warranted.

## *Insulin Resistance*

IR is a key component of type 2 diabetes (T2D), which exists when insulin levels are elevated relative to blood-glucose levels (Shanik et al., 2008). IR is also a key component of other health issues such as obesity and metabolic syndrome. Dietary modifications, including reduced energy intake, are beneficial in mitigating the progression of the disease, and research on how specific nutrients, including fat, might affect IR is well underway. A brief review of the literature involving IR and the fatty acid groups follows.

### *n-3 PUFA and Insulin Resistance*

Results from studies suggest an inverse association between n-3 PUFA and IR. Several human studies demonstrated anti-diabetic effects of n-3 PUFA, including decreased body-fat mass, increased metabolic rate, and increased thermogenic response to food (Couet et al., 1997; Jones & Schoeller, 1988). Browning et al. (2007) reported that after 12 weeks of n-3 PUFA supplementation in overweight women, a significant reduction in inflammatory markers was observed, although whether the effect of n-3 PUFA on insulin is mediated through inflammatory mechanisms was unclear. In contrast, Kusunoki et al. (2007) did not identify any correlation between dietary intakes of EPA and DHA and IR, as measured by homeostasis model assessment resistance index (HOMA-R).

Animal studies involving n-3 PUFA and IR tend to be more consistent and support an anti-diabetic effect. Numerous rodent studies demonstrated that EPA improves IR in several models of obesity and diabetes (Mori et al., 1997, 1999;

Nobukata et al., 2000), and elevated systemic concentrations of insulin-sensitizing adiponectin were found in mice fed high-fat diets enriched in EPA and DHA (Flachs et al., 2006). Ghafoorunissa et al. (2005) demonstrated that substituting one-third of dietary LA with ALA improved insulin sensitivity and decreased blood-lipid levels in sucrose-induced IR rats. Using the ob/ob mouse model of leptin resistance, ALA demonstrated significantly improved insulin sensitivity (Mustad et al., 2006), as measured by a plasma-glucose response to a standard meal and an insulin challenge. In general, findings from fish-oil studies suggest a beneficial effect of long-chain PUFAs; however, at present too few studies are available on ALA in this area of research to define its role.

### *n-6 PUFA, CLA, and Insulin Resistance*

Research surrounding n-6 PUFA, CLA, and IR is inconsistent. Epidemiological studies suggested that a low dietary intake of LA is associated with IR (Vessby et al., 1994, 2002); however, this association might not apply to populations with preexisting, compromised insulin sensitivity. A review of nutrition in prediabetics recommended, among other lifestyle modifications, a shift from n-6 PUFA to n-3 PUFA as a cost-effective tool in overcoming the burden of T2D (Bhoraskar, 2005). More specifically, in a study on Indian Asian males at increased risk for coronary heart disease (CHD), subjects were assigned to either a moderate or high n-6:n-3 PUFA diet for 6 weeks (Minihane et al., 2005). The high n-6:n-3 diet showed a trend toward decreased insulin sensitivity and significantly increased fasting insulin levels. Interestingly, supplementing with 4 g/day of fish oil for 6 weeks as a follow-up seemed to ameliorate the unfavorable effects of an elevated n-6 intake (Brady et al., 2004). In contrast, a randomized controlled crossover study in normolipidemic and type 2 diabetics demonstrated that an n-6 PUFA-rich diet improved insulin sensitivity, as measured by a euglycemic clamp, when substituted for an SFA-rich diet after only 5 weeks (Summers et al., 2002). Further, a significant reduction in visceral fat was noted after the n-6 PUFA diet, as compared to the SFA diet. Reasonably, we can conclude that, to date, too few published studies exist, and a lack of consistency therein, to draw any firm conclusions about n-6 PUFA and IR.

Several animal studies suggest that CLA can improve insulin sensitivity and can favorably modify body composition (Moloney et al., 2007; Moon et al., 2008; Park et al., 1997; Shimomura et al., 1990), whereas other investigations found either neutral or positive associations between pro-diabetic outcomes and CLA (Poirier et al., 2006; Roche et al., 2002). Human trials involving CLA in particular were extensive, due to the promising body composition and plasma-lipid alterations observed in animal studies. A consistent reproduction of the results from animal investigations, however, has yet to occur. Tricon et al. (2005) reviewed the literature on CLA with respect to human-body composition, and found little consistency in the results. Of the 17 studies summarized, 8 found no effect of supplementation on body weight, fat mass, or body mass index (BMI), markers known to be associated with decreased insulin sensitivity. The remaining 9 found moderate improvements in body composition, but to varying degrees. Thrush et al. (2007) found that 4 g/day of CLA supplementation resulted in a significant decrease in insulin sensitivity in overweight, nondiabetic subjects, whereas another supplementation study in healthy volunteers showed no effect on risk markers of fasting insulin or glucose concentrations (Raff et al., 2008). Conversely, a commercial CLA-isomer mixture impaired insulin sensitivity in type 2 diabetics (Moloney et al., 2004), and the *t*10*c*12 isomer, specifically, impaired insulin sensitivity in abdominally obese men at only 1% of total-energy intake (Riserus et al., 2002a).

From these summaries and recent literature reviews (Salas-Salvado et al., 2006; Silveira et al., 2007), we can conclude that no clear associations between CLA and IR currently exist, although possibly the *t*10*c*12 isomer is the most potent fatty acid at impairing insulin sensitivity (Riserus, 2006). More research is needed to elucidate the individual effects of the CLA isomers and to clarify inconsistencies between animal and human trials.

***MUFA and Insulin Resistance***

Studies suggest that MUFA contribute to favorable disease-related outcomes, mediated through changes in IR. Vessby et al. (2001) compared insulin sensitivity and secretion in 162 healthy subjects fed an isoenergetic diet high in either MUFA or SFA. At total-fat intakes below 37% of energy, insulin sensitivity was 12.5% lower on the SFA diet and 8.8% higher on the MUFA diet. No change in insulin secretion was observed for either group. Similarly, an increase in insulin sensitivity was observed, as determined by glucose-suppression testing and Oral Glucose Tolerance Tests (OGTTs), in both healthy and IR subjects when a MUFA-rich diet was consumed versus an SFA-rich one (Paniagua et al., 2007; Perez-Jimenez et al., 2001). Piers et al. (2002) assessed whole-body fat-oxidation rates in men following the consumption of a high-fat isocaloric breakfast rich in either MUFA or SFA. In the 5 hours following the MUFA breakfast meal, postprandial oxidation rates were increased for fats and decreased for carbohydrates, compared to the SFA breakfast. In addition, the thermic effect of the MUFA breakfast was elevated for those with a waist circumference of 99 cm or more, but not for leaner individuals. This difference was not detected in the SFA breakfast group. In a separate study, the effect of feeding an isoenergetic MUFA- or SFA-rich diet for 4 weeks in overweight or obese men was assessed (Piers et al., 2003). Body weight and fat mass were decreased following the MUFA-rich diet as compared to these values following the SFA-rich diet. No differences in energy or fat intake, energy expenditure, or self-reported physical activity were detected between groups. While the results seem promising, notably, they apply to overweight and obese subjects, and evidence shows that the benefits of MUFA may not extend to lean individuals. Lovejoy et al. (2002) showed that insulin sensitivity and secretion in lean subjects were not affected by MUFA, SFA, and TFA diets. Further, a recent study on fasting blood serum from nonobese type 2 diabetics suggested that MUFA positively correlated with HOMA-R, an index of IR (Kusunoki et al., 2007).

Although the majority of human trials demonstrate a trend toward improved insulin sensitivity with MUFA-rich diets, notably, many studies use diets very high in SFA or TFA for comparison. Since these fatty acids are implicated in a range of detrimental health-related outcomes, the difficulty lies in elucidating this quandary: whether MUFAs apparent insulin-sensitizing effects are the result of merely decreased SFA and/or TFA consumption or if a MUFA-specific beneficial effect exists.

### *SFA, TFA, and Insulin Resistance*

The general consensus from dietary studies in humans and animals is that SFAs and TFAs have unfavorable effects on insulin sensitivity and body composition. Rodent studies reported elevated levels of fasting plasma insulin when fed TFA- and SFA-enriched diets (Ibrahim et al., 2005), or a decreased metabolic rate and increased weight gain and body-fat content with a high-SFA diet (Takeuchi et al., 1995). In human studies assessing insulin sensitivity, SFA-rich diets tend to produce less favorable outcomes when compared to MUFA- or PUFA-rich diets, as previously reviewed in the n-6 PUFA and MUFA sections. Further, while this effect was most often demonstrated in short-term studies, its persistence lasted over long-term periods (Heine et al., 1989). Similarly, a study was recently conducted to assess the long-term effects of feeding TFA-enriched diets on insulin sensitivity and body composition. In a study of 42 monkeys with a 6-year follow-up, TFA- versus MUFA-fed monkeys gained significant weight, with increased intra-abdominal fat deposition, even in the absence of caloric excess (Kavanagh et al., 2007). Significant postprandial hyperinsulinemia was also observed in the TFA-fed group. In a randomized crossover study of 14 healthy women consuming either a MUFA- or TFA-rich diet, no effect was observed on glucose or insulin metabolism for either group (Louheranta et al., 1999); however, the 4-week per diet study duration might not have been long enough to observe any significant metabolic changes. As recently reviewed (Riserus, 2006), human intervention studies produced mixed results, posing a challenge to assert any conclusions regarding TFA intake and IR. In terms of SFA, however, a recent review of dietary intervention trials suggested that the removal of this fatty acid, as verified by changes in plasma fatty acid composition, can have a direct effect on insulin sensitivity (Roche, 2005). This was supported in a recent analysis that found SFAs to be positively correlated with HOMA-R (Kusunoki et al., 2007).

## *Cardiovascular Disease*

CVD is the leading cause of death in developed nations. In the United States alone, CVD is responsible for approximately 40% of all deaths, resulting in health-care costs exceeding $430 billion annually (Albert, 2007). As a result, much research has been focused on the potential causes and contributing factors of this disease. Now, plasma lipids and lipoproteins are well-established biomarkers of CVD risk, along with fasting blood glucose and insulin, inflammatory markers, lipoprotein(a), blood pressure, and clotting factors (Psota et al., 2006). Clinical trials and epidemiological studies consistently support a relationship between total and LDL-cholesterol levels and CHD (Sacks & Katan, 2002). Dietary fatty acids have, in turn, received considerable attention due to their significant effects on cholesterol levels, as well as HDLcholesterol and triglycerides (TGs), which are potential independent-lipid risk factors (Psota et al., 2006).

### *n-3 PUFA and Cardiovascular Disease*

The inverse relationship between n-3 PUFA consumption and CVD risk is well-established, and in 2002, the American Heart Association (AHA) released a statement endorsing the use of n-3 PUFA in both the primary and secondary prevention of CVD (Kris-Etherton et al., 2002). Epidemiological and dietary intervention trials support a cardioprotective role of n-3 PUFAs and their beneficial anti-arrhythmic, anti-inflammatory, and anti-thrombotic effects. A recent randomized crossover intervention trial supplemented two groups of women with n-3 PUFA: one a reference group and a second group with a known raised inflammatory status (Browning et al., 2007). TGs were reduced in all n-3-supplemented subjects, and the inflammatory markers C-reactive protein (CRP) and interleukin-6 (IL-6) were significantly lower after 12 weeks in the raised inflammatory status group when the women were receiving n-3 PUFA. This corroborates findings from the Nurses' Health Study which, in addition to CRP and IL-6, found an inverse relationship between E-selectin, a soluble intercellular cell-adhesion molecule 1 and a soluble vascular cell- adhesion molecule 1, and n-3 PUFA (Lopez-Garcia et al., 2004). A recent review of 97 placebo-controlled randomized trials of different lipid-lowering interventions concluded that the most favorable effects of treatment were observed with statins and n-3 PUFA (Psota et al., 2006). This is impressive, as fish oil was shown to have similar efficacy as a widely prescribed pharmacological agent. Further, levels of n-3 PUFA required to reduce TGs were achievable from the diet, thus providing compelling evidence for effective dietary CVD therapy (Brady et al., 2004; Lovegrove et al., 2004; Minihane et al., 2000; Roche & Gibney, 2000). A similar conclusion was drawn regarding the effectiveness of n-3 PUFA as an agent for the secondary prevention of cardiovascular events following a review of four recent secondary prevention trials (DeFilippis & Sperling, 2006). All four trials reduced secondary cardiac events when 1.0—1.8 g/day of fish-oil capsules, 1 serving of fish per day, ALA supplementation of ≈2.9 g/day, or a Mediterranean diet including ALA-rich rapeseed-oil spreads was consumed.

### *n-6 PUFA, CLA, and Cardiovascular Disease*

In addition to n-3 PUFA, n-6 PUFA also reduce CVD risk based on favorable changes in total cholesterol and LDL-cholesterol. Many studies assessing the outcome of an n-6 intake do so by replacing SFA in the diet. A summary of four randomized clinical trials that replaced dietary SFA with LA, mainly as soybean oil, found that coronary-event rates, including stroke, myocardial infarction and sudden death, were significantly reduced in three of the four trials (Sacks & Katan, 2002). This is most likely attributable to the decrease in LDL observed with SFA replacement by PUFA. ALA increased in the n-6 PUFA/soybean-oil groups as well, however, causing difficulty in determining if the reduced coronary-event rates are the result of LA, ALA, or other components present in soybean oil. Another soybean-oil study determined that palm-oil users were significantly more likely to suffer a myocardial infarction than LA-rich soybean-oil users (Odds Ratio [OR] = 1.33) (Kabagambe et al., 2005). Although, again, clear conclusions regarding LA are difficult to make, given oils contain multiple, potentially confounding, constituents. Laaksonen et al. (2005) recently assessed the association of dietary LA and total PUFA intake with cardiovascular mortality in middle-aged men. Men with LA and total PUFA intake in the upper third were less likely to die of CVD than men in the lower third. This association was similar for serum-esterified LA and PUFA levels, and persisted after adjustment for age and energy intake. Interestingly, the cardioprotective effects were stronger for LA, specifically, than for total PUFA.

The effects of CLA on cardiovascular health are inconsistent and less clear than the well-established inverse relationship between n-3 and n-6 PUFA and CVD. CLA supplementation in humans decreased HDL levels (Blankson et al., 2000; Mougios et al., 2001), an effect that tends to be more apparent in obese subjects, raising safety concerns. Conversely, several supplementation studies showed no effect of CLA on plasma total cholesterol, LDL, HDL, or TG concentrations (Benito et al., 2001; Petridou et al., 2003; Smedman & Vessby, 2001). The aforementioned supplementation studies used a mixture of *c*9,*t*11 and *t*10,*c*12 CLA isomers, and more research on the effects of the individual isomers on a CVD risk is warranted. When obese men with signs of metabolic syndrome received 3.4 g of *t*10,*c*12 CLA for 3 months, CRP was markedly increased (+110%) compared to the olive-oil placebo (Riserus et al., 2002b), suggesting a potentially detrimental effect of this isomer on cardiovascular health and inflammation. Unclear, however, is whether these results reflect a detrimental effect of CLA or a cardioprotective effect of olive oil, known to be a rich source of OA and antioxidants. When apolipoprotein E knockout mice received *t*10,*c*12 CLA, it had a profound pro-atherogenic effect, while mice receiving the *c*9,*t*11 isomer had impeded development of atherosclerosis (Silveira et al., 2007). This indicates mechanistic differences between CLA isomers, but warrants more work to elucidate the effects of individual CLA isomers on CVD outcomes.

### *MUFA and Cardiovascular Disease*

Since the observation that residents of Mediterranean countries enjoy superior cardiovascular health, research has focused on dietary elements consumed in abundance in these regions, including MUFA, and their effects on CVD outcomes. A comparison of the CVD-risk profile of an average American diet (AAD) versus an AHA low-fat diet and three different high-MUFA diets revealed a reduction in total and LDLcholesterol by 10% and 14%, respectively, in the high-MUFA diets, which was comparable to the AHA-diet reductions (Kris-Etherton et al., 1999). TG concentrations were 13% lower in high-MUFA fed subjects versus AAD, whereas the AHA diet raised TG levels by 11% (versus AAD). Overall, high-MUFA diets decreased CVD risk by approximately 21%, while the AHA diet decreased the risk by only 12%, demonstrating more favorable effects on the CVD profiles of MUFA-rich diets. LDL-cholesterol levels were also reduced from baseline in a separate study, when 162 healthy volunteers were fed isoenergetic diets rich in MUFA (Vessby et al., 2001).

Another dietary study reported decreased circulating markers of endothelial activation in MUFA-fed subjects compared to low-fat, high-carbohydrate or high-fat, high-SFA diet-fed individuals (Perez-Martinez et al., 2007), suggesting an anti-atherogenic effect of this group of fatty acids. In a 16-week supplementation study, 26 healthy university students received 33 g of SFA/100 g of total fat substituted with MUFA, and a reduction in platelet aggregation and postprandial factor VIIc response resulted (Smith et al., 2003). Factor VIIc, a coagulation factor thought to be associated with ischemic heart disease (Mennen et al., 1997), was also lower, as well as LDL and TGs in subjects consuming a MUFA-rich diet in a separate crossover study (Iman-Farinelli et al., 2005).

Research surrounding MUFA and CVD is not without inconsistencies. Fuentes et al. (2001) reported an improved flow-mediated dilatation (FMD) in hypercholesterolemic patients receiving a MUFA-rich diet, whereas no differences in FMD were observed in a similar dietary comparison by de Roos et al. (2001). In a recent review, Brown et al. (2007) detail the inconsistencies between epidemiological data and experimental evidence. Human epidemiological studies suggest a potential protective effect of a Mediterranean diet against atherosclerosis; however, animal experiments directly measuring the extent of atherosclerosis following dietary intervention do not demonstrate atheroprotective effects of MUFA. Brown et al. (2007) highlight the need to determine which specific aspects of the Mediterranean diet are indeed heart-healthy.

### *SFA, TFA, and Cardiovascular Disease*

The detrimental effects of SFA and TFA intake on cardiovascular health are well-documented. Mensink and Katan (1990) determined that a diet enriched with elaidic acid increased total and LDL-cholesterol concentrations, and decreased HDL as compared to an OA-enriched diet. Similarly, a crossover study of 14 healthy women consuming a TFA-rich diet for 4 weeks demonstrated an increase in TGs and the total/HDL-cholesterol ratio, as compared to the MUFA-rich diet phase (Louheranta et al., 1999). Tanasescu et al. (2004) estimated, based on results from the Nurses' Health Study, that the replacement of 5% of energy from SFA with MUFA is associated with a 37% decreased risk of CVD. SFA intake is also positively associated with factor VII levels (Lefevre et al., 2004), indicating their potential involvement in blood coagulation, and thus, their potentially adverse role in the etiology of CVD.

Several studies compared the effects of SFA versus TFA intake, often reporting a more deleterious effect of TFA on cardiovascular health-related outcomes. A review of numerous trials demonstrating a dose-dependent relationship between TFA intake and the LDL:HDL ratio concluded that the magnitude of this effect is about twice greater for TFA versus SFA, when OA was replaced in the diet (Ascherio, 2006). In addition, a recent analysis of TFA consumption from cooking oils in 7158 Iranian homes reported that the replacement of TFA with SFA would prevent 31% of CHD events (Mozaffarian et al., 2007). Further, if TFAs were replaced by *cis*-unsaturated fats, one could prevent 39% of CHD events.

As is well-documented, in addition to raising total and LDLcholesterol, TFAs also lower HDLcholesterol. Not surprisingly, a meta-analysis of investigations comparing the effects of various butters and margarines on blood lipids indicated that hard, high-*trans* margarines yielded poorer lipid profiles than soft, low-*trans* margarines (Zock & Katan, 1997). Despite these and other findings by numerous studies indicating an elevated risk of CHD in people consuming TFA (Ascherio, 2006), many epidemiologic studies suggest that typical levels of TFA intake from ruminant fat are not related to an increased CHD risk (Mensink & Katan, 1990). Clearly, more research is required to resolve these inconsistencies and to determine if differences exist between CHD risk and the type of TFA consumed.

## Potential Mechanisms of Action

Several mechanisms of action are currently studied to understand the role of fatty acids in human health and disease, including effects on inflammation and transcription factors. While much progress has been made in these areas of research, new investigations on the effects of fatty acids on membrane rafts (MRs) are rapidly expanding our basic knowledge. Our current understanding of the effects of fatty acids on MRs is reviewed as follows.

### *Membrane Rafts*

MRs are classically known as lipid rafts, lipid microdomains, detergent-resistant membranes (DRMs), and Triton-X insoluble membranes. MRs are distinct plasma-membrane regions ≈100 nm–200 nm in diameter (Pike, 2003), with reduced fluidity due to their enrichment in cholesterol, glycosphingolipids, and phospholipids (Brown & London, 2000; Hancock, 2006; Parton et al., 2006). The phospholipid fatty acid side chains tend to have a higher degree of saturation than those in the surrounding membrane, which facilitates close packing with the saturated acyl chains of sphingolipids and contributes to phase separation (Pike, 2003).

Caveolae, viewed as a subset of lipid rafts, are ≈100-nm diameter flask-shaped invaginations of the plasma membrane, rich in cholesterol, glycosphingolipids, and the cholesterol-binding protein caveolin (Murata et al., 1995; Parton et al., 2006). Caveolin is thought to contribute to the structural stability of membrane invaginations (Fra et al., 1995; Le et al., 2002); however, increasingly, this protein is being implicated in numerous signalling pathways as our understanding of caveolae and its constituents expands. Three major isoforms of caveolin have been identified.

Caveolin-1 and -2 are expressed in epithelial, endothelial and immune cells, and in adipocytes, while caveolin-3 is only found in cardiac and muscle tissues (Parton et al., 2006).

MRs are thought to play an important role in signal transduction as well as ion-channel function, trafficking, protein sorting, and apoptosis (Brown & London, 1998, 2000; Pike, 2003; Simons & Ehehalt, 2002; Simons & Toomre, 2000). Many acylated proteins, including Src family kinases and heterotrimeric G-proteins (Melkonian et al., 1999; Moffett et al., 2000; Young et al., 2003), are targeted to lipid rafts, and from this family of proteins alone, one can easily speculate how lipid rafts could play an important role in health promotion and disease progression.

A few potential mechanisms exist by which MRs regulate cell signalling. In one proposed model, lipid rafts act as signalling platforms that serve to co-localize the various elements involved in the signalling pathway, including receptors, coupling factors, effector enzymes, and substrates (Pike, 2003). In theory, the proximity of the signalling constituents would facilitate rapid and efficient signal transduction.

Another proposed mechanism involves the initial segregation of signalling components in different rafts. Upon stimulation of the cell with a hormone or growth factor, the rafts assemble into larger structures, promoting the interaction of cell-signalling constituents and signal transduction (Hancock, 2006). Similarly, a participant in a given signalling pathway that would normally be localized in the nonraft portion of the membrane may be recruited into the raft, co-localizing the various components involved and leading to the activation of that pathway. In this scenario, rafts are providing regulation through compartmentalization and physically separating proteins that would otherwise interact (Pike, 2003).

MRs are involved in endocytic events (Le et al., 2002), thus implicating them in signal termination. They may limit cell signalling by internalizing specific components, thereby preventing the endocytized constituent from participating in a particular pathway (Pike, 2003).

The above-proposed models in which MRs are implicated in cell signalling provide plausible and intriguing mechanisms that require further elucidation to determine the specific nature and extent of their involvement.

### *Membrane-raft Modification by Fatty Acids*

MR-function is influenced by changes in membrane-lipid composition. The tightly packed structure rich in cholesterol and phospholipids facilitates the targeting of many proteins involved in cellular processes, as mentioned in the previous section. Thus, structural alteration of MRs can potentially influence numerous signalling pathways, with a wide range of possible cellular outcomes, and ultimately affect health promotion and/or disease progression. In fact, a structural alteration of MRs by multiple classes of fatty acids, particularly PUFAs, has been documented.

### *Membrane-raft Modification by PUFA*

Compositional analyses of extracted lipids from MRs demonstrate that alterations in dietary PUFA supply can modify specific cellular responses. In Jurkat T-cells, the displacement of LAT and the Src family kinases Lck and Fyn was observed following treatment with PUFA, and a subsequent decrease in signal transduction (Stulnig et al., 1998, 2001; Zeyda et al., 2002). Similarly, stimulation-induced protein kinase C (PKC) translocation into T-cell MRs was suppressed by n-3 PUFA (Fan et al., 2004), and still a separate investigation revealed the inhibition of Fyn localization by AA, EPA, and DHA treatment in COS-1 cells (Webb et al., 2000). These in vitro outcomes demonstrate that T-cell structure and function were altered due to the incorporation of PUFA into MRs, which were further corroborated by in vivo data. Several studies demonstrated that dietary n-3 PUFA can alter mouse lipid-raft composition (Fan et al., 2003, 2004; Switzer et al., 2004), which has functional consequences such as a decreased PKCθ translocation into T-cell MRs (Fan et al., 2004; Switzer et al., 2004). In vivo experimental evidence demonstrates that T-cell apoptosis is also mediated by raft structure and indirectly influenced by n-3 PUFA (Switzer et al., 2004).

Apart from T-cells, n-3 PUFA enrichment of MRs was demonstrated in mammary, colon, and epithelial cells, affecting various signalling pathways depending on the cell type involved (Ma et al., 2004; Schley et al., 2007). N-3 PUFA incorporation into MRs displaces cholesterol from MRs, an effect which enhanced apoptosis in epithelial prostate, mammary, and cancer cells via Akt inactivation, as previously reviewed (Li et al., 2006). Briefly, Akt/protein kinase B is a cell-survival regulator that, when activated, inactivates pro-apoptotic proteins and concurrently up-regulates anti-apoptotic genes. Previous studies suggested the involvement of lipid rafts in Akt inactivation (Panka et al., 2001; Shimamura et al., 2003), a process which was subsequently identified to be mediated through raft-cholesterol depletion (Li et al., 2006).

### *Membrane-raft Modification by MUFA*

Very little work has been done assessing the impact of MUFA status on lipid rafts. One investigation compared the degree of phase separation in monolayers and bilayers resulting from the addition of OA versus DHA (Shaikh et al., 2002). Specifically, interactions of sphingomyelin (SM), cholesterol, OA-containing phospholipid (POPE), and DHA-containing phospholipid (PDPE) were assessed. Close proximity of cholesterol to POPE was observed, even in the presence of SM, indicating a lack of phase separation. In contrast, PDPE elicited lateral phase separation similarly reported in previous studies (Dumaual et al., 2000; Litman & Mitchell, 1996), thus corroborating the hypothesis that PUFA may play an important role in lipid-raft stability. Similar results were found with palmitoylated OA phosphatidylethanolamine (PE) and palmitoylated DHA PE in the presence or absence of cholesterol (Shaikh et al., 2004). Cholesterol was observed to elicit a two fold greater increase in order in the OA PE than the DHA PE, and phase separation was greater for DHA PE. Furthermore, the amount of fatty acid associated with raft-rich detergent-resistant membranes was almost twice as great for OA than for DHA in detergent experiments conducted on cardiomyocytes (Shaikh et al., 2004). While little research is available on the effects of MUFA on lipid rafts, the studies conducted suggest OA associates closely with cholesterol and SM, and does not contribute to lateral phase separation.

***Membrane-raft Modification by TFA***

Recent research demonstrated the ability of TFA to alter adipocyte plasma-membrane phospholipid fatty acid composition and adipocyte plasma-membrane fluidity (Ibrahim et al., 2005; Saravanan et al., 2005). Only one study investigated the effects of TFA on lipid-raft association. Bjorkbom et al. (2007) assessed the bilayer-membrane properties of elaidic acid in SM and phosphatidylcholine (PC), and evaluated their interactions with cholesterol. Both elaidic acid–SM and elaidic acid–PC were incorporated into sterol and SFA-rich lateral-membrane domains. In fact, elaidic acid–SM and –PC also formed sterol-rich domains without any SFA present.

Overall, MR structure is modified by fatty acid incorporation into phospholipid-membrane bilayers. PUFA incorporation, in particular, leads to lateral-phase separation and alterations in the downstream cellular process that may have important health implications with respect to immune response and progression of various chronic diseases. While research on PUFA modification of membranes is well underway, more work is required to characterize the nature and extent of MUFA and TFA involvement with MRs.

## Conclusion

Significant advances have been made in understanding the effects of specific groups of fatty acids. Nevertheless, a lack of fundamental knowledge remains of the mechanisms of action by which specific fatty acids contribute to health and disease. This is necessary to provide a direct linkage between a given fatty acid and an outcome measure. State-of-the-art research is continuing to incrementally shed new light on the role of fatty acids. In particular, the effect of fatty acids on MRs has markedly changed our appreciation of how fatty acids influence membrane structure, signalling, regulation, and ultimately cellular function. Clearly, dietary fatty acid composition modulates health and chronic-disease risk, and therein is a potential solution to the prevention, treatment, and management of chronic diseases, thus improving the quality of life.

### References

Albert, M.A. Inflammatory biomarkers, race/ethnicity and cardiovascular disease. *Nutr. Rev.* **2007,** *65,* S234–S238.

Allison, D.B.; S.K. Egan; L.M. Barraj; C. Caughman; M. Infante; J.T. Heimbach. Estimated intakes of trans fatty and other fatty acids in the US population. *J. Am. Diet. Assoc.* **1999,** *99,* 166–174.

Aro, A.; S. Mannisto; I. Salminen; M.L. Ovaskainen; V. Kataja; M. Uusitupa. Inverse association between dietary and serum conjugated linoleic acid and risk of breast cancer in postmenopausal women. *Nutr. Cancer* **2000,** *38,* 151–157.

Ascherio, A. Trans fatty acids and blood lipids. *Atheroscler. Suppl.* **2006,** *7,* 25 27.

Bagga, D.; K.H. Anders; H.J. Wang; J.A. Glaspy. Long-chain n-3-to-n-6 polyunsaturated fatty acid ratios in breast adipose tissue from women with and without breast cancer. *Nutr. Cancer* **2002,** *42,* 180–185.

Barascu, A.; P. Besson; F.O. Le; P. Bougnoux; M.L. Jourdan. CDK1-cyclin B1 mediates the inhibition of proliferation induced by omega-3 fatty acids in MDA-MB-231 breast cancer cells. *Int. J. Biochem. Cell Biol.* **2006,** *38,* 196–208.

Bartsch, H.; J. Nair; R.W. Owen. Dietary polyunsaturated fatty acids and cancers of the breast and colorectum: emerging evidence for their role as risk modifiers. *Carcinogenesis* **1999,** *20,* 2209–2218.

Benito, P.; G.J. Nelson; D.S. Kelley; G. Bartolini; P.C. Schmidt; V. Simon. The effect of conjugated linoleic acid on plasma lipoproteins and tissue fatty acid composition in humans. *Lipids* **2001,** *36,* 229–236.

Bhoraskar, A. Nutrition in prediabetes. *J. Indian Med. Assoc.* **2005,** *103,* 596, 598–599.

Bjorkbom, A.; B. Ramstedt; J.P. Slotte. Phosphatidylcholine and sphingomyelin containing an elaidoyl fatty acid can form cholesterol-rich lateral domains in bilayer membranes. *Biochim. Biophys. Acta* **2007,** *1768,* 1839–1847.

Blankson, H.; J.A. Stakkestad; H. Fagertun; E. Thom; J. Wadstein; O. Gudmundsen. Conjugated linoleic acid reduces body fat mass in overweight and obese humans. *J. Nutr.* **2000,** *130,* 2943–2948.

Brady, L.M.; S.S. Lovegrove; S.V. Lesauvage; B.A. Gower; A.M. Minihane; C.M. Williams; J.A. Lovegrove. Increased n-6 polyunsaturated fatty acids do not attenuate the effects of long-chain n-3 polyunsaturated fatty acids on insulin sensitivity or triacylglycerol reduction in Indian Asians. *Am. J. Clin. Nutr.* **2004,** *79,* 983–991.

Brown, D.A.; E. London. Structure and origin of ordered lipid domains in biological membranes. *J. Membr. Biol.* **1998,** *164,* 103–114.

Brown, D.A.; E. London. Structure and function of sphingolipid- and cholesterol-rich membrane rafts. *J. Biol. Chem.* **2000,** *275,* 17221–17224.

Brown, J.M.; G.S. Shelness; L.L. Rudel. Monounsaturated fatty acids and atherosclerosis: opposing views from epidemiology and experimental animal models. *Curr. Atheroscler. Rep.* **2007,** *9,* 494–500.

Browning, L.M.; J.D. Krebs; C.S. Moore; G.D. Mishra; M.A. O'Connell; S.A. Jebb. The impact of long chain n-3 polyunsaturated fatty acid supplementation on inflammation, insulin sensitivity and CVD risk in a group of overweight women with an inflammatory phenotype. *Diabetes Obes. Metab.* **2007,** *9,* 70–80.

Canadian Cancer Society/National Cancer Institute of Canada. *Canadian Cancer Statistics 2008;* Toronto, Canada, 2008. Ref Type: Generic

Cave, W.T., Jr. Omega-3 polyunsaturated fatty acids in rodent models of breast cancer. *Breast Cancer Res. Treat.* **1997,** *46,* 239–246.

Chajes, V.; P. Bougnoux. Omega-6/omega-3 polyunsaturated fatty acid ratio and cancer. *World Rev. Nutr. Diet.* **2003,** *92,* 133–151.

Chamras, H.; A. Ardashian; D. Heber; J.A. Glaspy. Fatty acid modulation of MCF-7 human breast cancer cell proliferation, apoptosis and differentiation. *J. Nutr. Biochem.* **2002,** *13,* 711–716.

Colditz, G.A.; M. Samplin-Salgado; C.T. Ryan; H. Dart; L. Fisher; A. Tokuda; B. Rockhill. Harvard report on cancer prevention, volume 5: fulfilling the potential for cancer prevention: policy approaches. *Cancer Causes Control* **2002,** *13,* 199–212.

Couet, C.; J. Delarue; P. Ritz; J.M. Antoine; F. Lamisse. Effect of dietary fish oil on body fat mass and basal fat oxidation in healthy adults. *Int. J. Obes. Relat. Metab. Disord.* **1997,** *21,* 637–643.

Craig-Schmidt, M.C. World-wide consumption of trans fatty acids. *Atheroscler. Suppl.* **2006,** *7,* 1–4.

de Roos, N.M.; M.L. Bots; E. Siebelink; E. Schouten; M.B. Katan. Flow-mediated vasodilation is not impaired when HDL-cholesterol is lowered by substituting carbohydrates for monounsaturated fat. *Br. J. Nutr.* **2001,** *86,* 181–188.

DeFilippis, A.P.; L.S. Sperling. Understanding omega-3's. *Am. Heart J. 151* **2006,** 564–570.

Dennis, L.K.; L.G. Snetselaar; B.J. Smith; R.E. Stewart; M.E. Robbins. Problems with the assessment of dietary fat in prostate cancer studies. *Am. J. Epidemiol.* **2004,** *160,* 436–444.

Dumaual, A.C.; L.J. Jenski; W. Stillwell. Liquid crystalline/gel state phase separation in docosahexaenoic acid-containing bilayers and monolayers. *Biochim. Biophys. Acta* **2000,** *1463,* 395–406.

Dyerberg, J.; H.O. Bang; E. Stoffersen; S. Moncada; J.R. Vane. Eicosapentaenoic acid and prevention of thrombosis and atherosclerosis? *Lancet* **1978,** *2,* 117–119.

Ens J.G.; D.W. Ma; K.S. Cole; C.J. Field; M.T. Clandinin. An assessment of *c*9,*t*11 linoleic acid intake in a small group of young Canadians. *Nutr.Res.* **2001,** *21,* 955–960.

Escrich, E.; R. Moral; G. Garcia; I. Costa; J.A. Sanchez; M. Solanas. Identification of novel differentially expressed genes by the effect of a high-fat n-6 diet in experimental breast cancer. *Mol. Carcinog.* **2004,** *40,* 73–78.

Escrich, E.; R. Moral; L. Grau; I. Costa; M. Solanas. Molecular mechanisms of the effects of olive oil and other dietary lipids on cancer. *Mol. Nutr. Food Res.* **2007,** *51,* 1279–1292.

Fan, Y.Y.; L.H. Ly; R. Barhoumi; D.N. McMurray; R.S. Chapkin. Dietary docosahexaenoic acid suppresses T cell protein kinase C theta lipid raft recruitment and IL-2 production. *J. Immunol.* **2004,** *173,* 6151–6160.

Fan, Y.Y.; D.N. McMurray; L.H. Ly; R.S. Chapkin. Dietary (n-3) polyunsaturated fatty acids remodel mouse T-cell lipid rafts. *J. Nutr.* **2003,** *133,* 1913–1920.

Fay, M.P.; L.S. Freedman. Meta-analyses of dietary fats and mammary neoplasms in rodent experiments. *Breast Cancer Res.Treat.* **1997,** *46,* 215–223.

Fite, A.; M. Goua; K.W. Wahle; A.C. Schofield; A.W. Hutcheon; S.D. Heys. Potentiation of the anti-tumour effect of docetaxel by conjugated linoleic acids (CLAs) in breast cancer cells in vitro. *Prostaglandins, Leukotrienes Essent. Fatty Acids* **2007.** *77,* 87–96.

Flachs, P.; V. Mohamed-Ali; O. Horakova; M. Rossmeisl; M.J. Hosseinzadeh-Attar; M. Hensler; J. Ruzickova; J. Kopecky. Polyunsaturated fatty acids of marine origin induce adiponectin in mice fed a high-fat diet. *Diabetologia* **2006,** *49,* 394–397.

Fra, A.M.; E. Williamson; K. Simons; R.G. Parton. De novo formation of caveolae in lymphocytes by expression of VIP21-caveolin. *Proc. Natl. Acad. Sci. U.S.A.* **1995,** *92,* 8655 8659.

Fuentes, F.; J. Lopez-Miranda; E. Sanchez; F. Sanchez; J. Paez; E. Paz-Rojas; C. Marin; P. Gomez; J. Jimenez-Pereperez; J.M. Ordovas; F. Perez-Jimenez. Mediterranean and low-fat diets improve endothelial function in hypercholesterolemic men. *Ann. Intern. Med.* **2001,** *134,* 1115–1119.

Ghafoorunissa; A. Ibrahim; S. Natarajan. Substituting dietary linoleic acid with alpha-linolenic acid improves insulin sensitivity in sucrose fed rats. *Biochim. Biophys. Acta* **2005,** *1733,* 67–75.

Gonzalez, C.A. The European Prospective Investigation into Cancer and Nutrition (EPIC). *Public Health Nutr.* **2006,** *9,* 124–126.

Goodstine, S.L.; T. Zheng; T.R. Holford; B.A. Ward; D. Carter; P.H. Owens; S.T. Mayne. Dietary (n-3)/(n-6) fatty acid ratio: possible relationship to premenopausal but not postmenopausal breast cancer risk in U.S. women. *J. Nutr.* **2003,** *133,* 1409–1414.

Greenlee, R.T.; T. Murray; S. Bolden; P.A. Wingo. Cancer statistics, 2000. *CA Cancer J. Clin.* **2000,** *50,* 7–33.

Hancock, J.F. Lipid rafts: contentious only from simplistic standpoints. *Nat. Rev. Mol. Cell Biol.* **2006,** *7,* 456–462.

Hashim, Y.Z.; M. Eng; C.I. Gill; H. McGlynn; I.R. Rowland. Components of olive oil and chemoprevention of colorectal cancer. *Nutr. Rev.* **2005,** *63,* 374–386.

Heine, R.J.; C. Mulder; C. Popp-Snijders; M.J. van der; V. van d. Linoleic-acid-enriched diet: long-term effects on serum lipoprotein and apolipoprotein concentrations and insulin sensitivity in noninsulin-dependent diabetic patients. *Am. J. Clin. Nutr.* **1989,** *49,* 448–456.

Hilakivi-Clarke, L.; R. Clarke; I. Onojafe; M. Raygada; E. Cho; M. Lippman. A maternal diet high in n-6 polyunsaturated fats alters mammary gland development, puberty onset, and breast cancer risk among female rat offspring. *Proc. Natl. Acad. Sci. U.S.A.* **1997,** *94,* 9372–9377.

Hilakivi-Clarke, L.; S.E. Olivo; A. Shajahan; G. Khan; Y. Zhu; A. Zwart; E. Cho; R. Clarke. Mechanisms mediating the effects of prepubertal (n-3) polyunsaturated fatty acid diet on breast cancer risk in rats. *J. Nutr.* **2005,** *135,* 2946S–2952S.

Holmes M.D.; D.J. Hunter; G.A. Colditz; M.J. Stampfer; S.E. Hankinson; F.E. Speizer; B. Rosner; W.C. Willett. Association of dietary intake of fat and fatty acids with risk of breast cancer. *JAMA* **1999,** *281,* 914–920.

Hubbard, N.E.; D. Lim; K.L. Erickson. Alteration of murine mammary tumorigenesis by dietary enrichment with n-3 fatty acids in fish oil. *Cancer Lett.* **1998,** *124,* 1–7.

Hunt, D.A.; H.M. Lane; M.E. Zygmont; P.A. Dervan; R.A. Hennigar. MRNA stability and overexpression of fatty acid synthase in human breast cancer cell lines. *Anticancer Res.* **2007,** *27,* 27–34.

Ibrahim, A.; S. Natrajan; R. Ghafoorunissa. Dietary trans-fatty acids alter adipocyte plasma membrane fatty acid composition and insulin sensitivity in rats. *Metabolism* **2005,** *54,* 240–246.

Ip, M.M.; S.O. McGee; P.A. Masso-Welch; C. Ip; X. Meng; L. Ou; S.F. Shoemaker. The t10,c12 isomer of conjugated linoleic acid stimulates mammary tumorigenesis in transgenic mice over-expressing erbB2 in the mammary epithelium. *Carcinogenesis* **2007,** *28,* 1269–1276.

Ip, C.; J.A. Scimeca; H. Thompson. Effect of timing and duration of dietary conjugated linoleic acid on mammary cancer prevention. *Nutr. Cancer* **1995,** *24,* 241–247.

Jemal, A.; R. Siegel; E. Ward; T. Murray; J. Xu; C. Smigal; M.J. Thun. Cancer statistics, 2006. *CA Cancer J. Clin.* **2006,** *56,* 106–130.

Jones, P.J.; D.A. Schoeller. Polyunsaturated:saturated ratio of diet fat influences energy substrate utilization in the human. Metabolism **1988,** *37,* 145–151.

Kabagambe, E.K.; A. Baylin; A. Ascherio; H. Campos. The type of oil used for cooking is associated with the risk of nonfatal acute myocardial infarction in costa rica. *J. Nutr.* **2005,** *135,* 2674–2679.

Kavanagh, K.; K.L. Jones; J. Sawyer; K. Kelley; J.J. Carr; J.D. Wagner; L.L. Rudel. Trans fat diet induces abdominal obesity and changes in insulin sensitivity in monkeys. *Obesity(SilverSpring)* **2007,** *15,* 1675–1684.

Kelsey, J.L.; L. Bernstein. Epidemiology and prevention of breast cancer. *Annu. Rev. Public Health* **1996,** *17,* 47–67.

Kitts, D.D. Bioactive substances in food: identification and potential uses. *Can. J. Physiol. Pharmacol.* **1994,** *72,* 423–434.

Klein, V.; V. Chajes; E. Germain; G. Schulgen; M. Pinault; D. Malvy; T. Lefrancq; A. Fignon; F.O. Le; C. Lhuillery; P. Bougnoux. Low alpha-linolenic acid content of adipose breast tissue is associated with an increased risk of breast cancer. *Eur. J. Cancer* **2000,** *36,* 335–340.

Kohlmeier L.; N. Simonsen; V. van; J.J. Strain; J.M. Martin-Moreno; B. Margolin; J.K. Huttunen; N.J. Fernandez-Crehuet; B.C. Martin; M. Thamm; A.F. Kardinaal; F.J. Kok. Adipose tissue trans fatty acids and breast cancer in the European Community Multicenter Study on Antioxidants, Myocardial Infarction, and Breast Cancer. *Cancer Epidemiol.Biomarkers Prev.* **1997,** *6,* 705–710.

Kolonel, L.N.; A.M. Nomura; R.V. Cooney. Dietary fat and prostate cancer: current status. *J. Natl. Cancer Inst.* **1999,** *91,* 414–428.

Kris-Etherton, P.M.; W.S. Harris; L.J. Appel. Fish consumption, fish oil, omega-3 fatty acids, and cardiovascular disease. *Arterioscler. Thromb. Vasc. Biol.* **2003,** *23,* e20–e30.

Kris-Etherton, P.M.; W.S. Harris; L.J. Appel. Fish consumption, fish oil, omega-3 fatty acids, and cardiovascular disease. *Circulation* **2002,** *106,* 2747–2757.

Kris-Etherton, P.M.; T.A. Pearson; Y. Wan; R.L. Hargrove; K. Moriarty; V. Fishell; T.D. Etherton. High-monounsaturated fatty acid diets lower both plasma cholesterol and triacylglycerol concentrations. *Am. J. Clin. Nutr.* **1999,** *70,* 1009–1015.

Kuller, L.H. The etiology of breast cancer—from epidemiology to prevention. *Public Health Rev.* **1995,** *23,* 157–213.

Kuriki, K.; K. Hirose; K. Wakai; K. Matsuo; H. Ito; T. Suzuki; A. Hiraki; T. Saito; H. Iwata; M. Tatematsu; K. Tajima. Breast cancer risk and erythrocyte compositions of n-3 highly unsaturated fatty acids in Japanese. *Int. J. Cancer* **2007,** *121,* 377–385.

Kushi, L.; E. Giovannucci. Dietary fat and cancer. *Am. J. Med.* **2002,** *113(Suppl. 9B),* 63S–70S.

Kusunoki, M. K. Tsutsumi; M. Nakayama; T. Kurokawa; T. Nakamura; H. Ogawa; Y. Fukuzawa; M. Morishita; T. Koide; T. Miyata. Relationship between serum concentrations of saturated fatty acids and unsaturated fatty acids and the homeostasis model insulin resistance index in Japanese patients with type 2 diabetes mellitus. *J. Med. Invest.* **2007,** *54,* 243–247.

Laaksonen, D.E.; K. Nyyssonen; L. Niskanen; T.H. Rissanen; J.T. Salonen. Prediction of cardiovascular mortality in middle-aged men by dietary and serum linoleic and polyunsaturated fatty acids. *Arch. Intern. Med.* **2005,** *165,* 193–199.

Le, P.U.; G. Guay; Y. Altschuler; I.R. Nabi. Caveolin-1 is a negative regulator of caveolae-mediated endocytosis to the endoplasmic reticulum. *J. Biol. Chem.* **2002,** *277,* 3371–3379.

Lefevre, M.; P.M. Kris-Etherton; G. Zhao; R.P. Tracy. Dietary fatty acids, hemostasis, and cardiovascular disease risk. *J. Am. Diet. Assoc.* **2004,** *104,* 410–419.

Li, Y.C.; M.J. Park; S.K. Ye; C.W. Kim; Y.N. Kim. Elevated levels of cholesterol-rich lipid rafts in cancer cells are correlated with apoptosis sensitivity induced by cholesterol-depleting agents. *Am. J. Pathol.* **2006,** *168,* 1107–1118.

Lipworth, L.; M.E. Martinez; J. Angell; C.C. Hsieh; D. Trichopoulos. Olive oil and human cancer: an assessment of the evidence. *Prev. Med.* **1997,** *26,* 181–190.

Litman, B.J.; D.C. Mitchell. A role for phospholipid polyunsaturation in modulating membrane protein function. *Lipids* **1996,** *31(Suppl.),* S193–S197.

lman-Farinelli, M.A.; K. Gomes; E.J. Favaloro; P. Petocz. A diet rich in high-oleic-acid sunflower oil favorably alters low-density lipoprotein cholesterol, triglycerides, and factor VII coagulant activity. *J. Am. Diet. Assoc.* **2005,** *105,* 1071–1079.

Lof, M.; S. Sandin; P. Lagiou; L. Hilakivi-Clarke; D. Trichopoulos; H.O. Adami; E. Weiderpass. Dietary fat and breast cancer risk in the Swedish women's lifestyle and health cohort. *Br. J. Cancer* **2007,** *97,* 1570–1576.

Lopez-Garcia, E.; M.B. Schulze; J.E. Manson; J.B. Meigs; C.M. Albert; N. Rifai; W.C. Willett; F.B. Hu. Consumption of (n-3) fatty acids is related to plasma biomarkers of inflammation and endothelial activation in women. *J. Nutr.* **2004,** *134,* 1806–1811.

Lopez-Otin, C.; E.P. Diamandis. Breast and prostate cancer: an analysis of common epidemiological, genetic, and biochemical features. *Endocr. Rev.* **1998,** *19,* 365–396.

Louheranta, A.M.; A.K. Turpeinen; H.M. Vidgren; U.S. Schwab; M.I. Uusitupa. A high-trans fatty acid diet and insulin sensitivity in young healthy women. *Metabolism* **1999,** *48,* 870–875.

Lovegrove, J.A.; S.S. Lovegrove; S.V. Lesauvage; L.M. Brady; N. Saini; A.M. Minihane; C.M. Williams. Moderate fish-oil supplementation reverses low-platelet, long-chain n-3 polyunsaturated fatty acid status and reduces plasma triacylglycerol concentrations in British Indo-Asians. *Am. J. Clin. Nutr.* **2004,** *79,* 974–982.

Lovejoy, J.C.; S.R. Smith; C.M. Champagne; M.M. Most; M. Lefevre; J.P. DeLany; Y.M. Denkins; J.C. Rood; J. Veldhuis; G.A. Bray. Effects of diets enriched in saturated (palmitic), monounsaturated (oleic), or trans (elaidic) fatty acids on insulin sensitivity and substrate oxidation in healthy adults. *Diabetes Care* **2002,** *25,* 1283–1288.

Luijten, M.; A. Verhoef; J.A. Dormans; R.B. Beems; H.W. Cremers; N.J. Nagelkerke; H. Adlercreutz; J.L. Penalvo; A.H. Piersma. Modulation of mammary tumor development in Tg.NK (MMTV/c-neu) mice by dietary fatty acids and life stage-specific exposure to phytoestrogens. *Reprod. Toxicol.* **2007,** *23,* 407–413.

Ma, D.W.; J. Seo; L.A. Davidson; E.S. Callaway; Y.Y. Fan; J.R. Lupton; R.S. Chapkin. n-3 PUFA alter caveolae lipid composition and resident protein localization in mouse colon. *FASEB J.* **2004,** *18,* 1040–1042.

Ma, D.W.; A.A. Wierzbicki; C.J. Field; M.T. Clandinin. Conjugated linoleic acid in canadian dairy and beef products. *J. Agric. Food Chem.* **1999,** *47,* 1956–1960.

Maillard, V.; P. Bougnoux; P. Ferrari; M.L. Jourdan; M. Pinault; F. Lavillonniere; G. Body; F.O. Le; V. Chajes. N-3 and N-6 fatty acids in breast adipose tissue and relative risk of breast cancer in a case-control study in Tours, France. *Int. J. Cancer* **2002,** *98,* 78–83.

Martin-Moreno, J.M.; W.C. Willett; L. Gorgojo; J.R. Banegas; F. Rodriguez-Artalejo; J.C. Fernandez-Rodriguez; P. Maisonneuve; P. Boyle. Dietary fat, olive oil intake and breast cancer risk. *Int. J. Cancer* **1994,** *58,* 774–780.

Masso-Welch, P.A.; D. Zangani; C. Ip; M.M. Vaughan; S. Shoemaker; R.A. Ramirez; M.M. Ip. Inhibition of angiogenesis by the cancer chemopreventive agent conjugated linoleic acid. *Cancer Res.* **2002,** *62,* 4383–4389.

McCann, S.E.; C. Ip; M.M. Ip; M.K. McGuire; P. Muti; S.B. Edge; M. Trevisan; J.L. Freudenheim. Dietary intake of conjugated linoleic acids and risk of premenopausal and postmenopausal breast cancer, Western New York Exposures and Breast Cancer Study (WEB Study). *Cancer Epidemiol. Biomarkers Prev.* **2004,** *13,* 1480–1484.

Melkonian, K.A.; A.G. Ostermeyer; J.Z. Chen; M.G. Roth; D.A. Brown. Role of lipid modifications in targeting proteins to detergent-resistant membrane rafts. Many raft proteins are acylated, while few are prenylated. *J. Biol. Chem.* **1999,** *274,* 3910–3917.

Menendez, J.A.; I. Mehmi; V.A. Verma; P.K. Teng; R. Lupu. Pharmacological inhibition of fatty acid synthase (FAS): a novel therapeutic approach for breast cancer chemoprevention through its ability to suppress Her-2/neu (erbB-2) oncogene-induced malignant transformation. *Mol. Carcinog.* **2004,** *41,* 164–178.

Menendez, J.A.; A. Vazquez-Martin; S. Ropero; R. Colomer; R. Lupu. HER2 (erbB-2)-targeted effects of the omega-3 polyunsaturated fatty acid, alpha-linolenic acid (ALA; 18:3n-3), in breast cancer cells: the "fat features" of the "Mediterranean diet" as an "anti-HER2 cocktail." *Clin. Transl. Oncol.* **2006,** *8* 812–820.

Mennen, L.I.; J.C. Witteman; J.H. den Breeijen; E.G. Schouten; P.T. de Jong; A. Hofman; D.E. Grobbee. The association of dietary fat and fiber with coagulation factor VII in the elderly: the Rotterdam Study. *Am. J. Clin. Nutr.* **1997,** *65,* 732–736.

Mensink, R.P.; M.B. Katan. Effect of dietary trans fatty acids on high-density and low-density lipoprotein cholesterol levels in healthy subjects. *N. Engl. J. Med.* **1990,** *323,* 439–445.

Minihane, A.M.; L.M. Brady; S.S. Lovegrove; S.V. Lesauvage; C.M. Williams; J.A. Lovegrove. Lack of effect of dietary n-6:n-3 PUFA ratio on plasma lipids and markers of insulin responses in Indian Asians living in the UK. *Eur. J. Nutr.* **2005,** *44,* 26–32.

Minihane, A.M.; S. Khan; E.C. Leigh-Firbank; P. Talmud; J.W. Wright; M.C. Murphy; B.A. Griffin; C.M. Williams. ApoE polymorphism and fish oil supplementation in subjects with an atherogenic lipoprotein phenotype. *Arterioscler. Thromb. Vasc. Biol.* **2000,** *20* 1990–1997.

Moffett, S.; D.A. Brown; M.E. Linder. Lipid-dependent targeting of G proteins into rafts. *J. Biol. Chem.* **2000,** *275,* 2191–2198.

Moloney, F.; S. Toomey; E. Noone; A. Nugent; B. Allan; C.E. Loscher; H.M. Roche. Antidiabetic effects of cis-9, trans-11-conjugated linoleic acid may be mediated via anti-inflammatory effects in white adipose tissue. *Diabetes* **2007,** *56,* 574–582.

Moloney, F.; T.P. Yeow; A. Mullen; J.J. Nolan; H.M. Roche. Conjugated linoleic acid supplementation, insulin sensitivity, and lipoprotein metabolism in patients with type 2 diabetes mellitus. *Am. J. Clin. Nutr.* **2004,** *80,* 887–895.

Moon, H.S.; H.G. Lee; J.H. Seo; C.S. Chung; T.G. Kim; Y.J. Choi; C.S. Cho. Antiobesity effect of PEGylated conjugated linoleic acid on high-fat diet-induced obese C57BL/6J (ob/ob) mice: attenuation of insulin resistance and enhancement of antioxidant defenses. *J. Nutr. Biochem.* **2008.**

Mori, Y.; Y. Murakawa; S. Katoh; S. Hata; J. Yokoyama; N. Tajima; Y. Ikeda; H. Nobukata; T. Ishikawa; Y. Shibutani. Influence of highly purified eicosapentaenoic acid ethyl ester on insulin resistance in the Otsuka Long-Evans Tokushima Fatty rat, a model of spontaneous non-insulin-dependent diabetes mellitus. *Metabolism* **1997,** *46,* 1458–1464.

Mori, Y.; Y. Murakawa; J. Yokoyama; N. Tajima; Y. Ikeda; H. Nobukata; T. Ishikawa; Y. Shibutani. Effect of highly purified eicosapentaenoic acid ethyl ester on insulin resistance and hypertension in Dahl salt-sensitive rats. *Metabolism* **1999,** *48,* 1089–1095.

Mougios, V.; A. Matsakas; A. Petridou; S. Ring; A. Sagredos; A. Melissopoulou; N. Tsigilis; M. Nikolaidis. Effect of supplementation with conjugated linoleic acid on human serum lipids and body fat. *J. Nutr. Biochem.* **2001,** *12,* 585–594.

Mozaffarian, D.; M. Abdollahi; H. Campos; A. Houshiarrad; W.C. Willett. Consumption of trans fats and estimated effects on coronary heart disease in Iran. *Eur. J. Clin. Nutr.* **2007,** *61,* 1004–1010.

Murata, M.; J. Peranen; R. Schreiner; F. Wieland; T.V. Kurzchalia; K. Simons. VIP21/caveolin is a cholesterol-binding protein. *Proc. Natl. Acad. Sci. U.S.A.* **1995,** *92* 10339–10343.

Mustad, V.A.; S. Demichele; Y.S. Huang; A. Mika; N. Lubbers; N. Berthiaume; J. Polakowski; B. Zinker. Differential effects of n-3 polyunsaturated fatty acids on metabolic control and vascular reactivity in the type 2 diabetic ob/ob mouse. *Metabolism* **2006,** *55,* 1365–1374.

Nobukata, H.; T. Ishikawa; M. Obata; Y. Shibutani. Long-term administration of highly purified eicosapentaenoic acid ethyl ester prevents diabetes and abnormalities of blood coagulation in male WBN/Kob rats. *Metabolism* **2000,** *49,* 912–919.

O'Shea, M.; R. Devery; F. Lawless; J. Murphy; C. Stanton. Milk fat conjugated linoleic acid (CLA) inhibits growth of human mammary MCF-7 cancer cells. *Anticancer Res.* **2000,** *20,* 3591–3601.

Olivo, S.E.; L. Hilakivi-Clarke. Opposing effects of prepubertal low- and high-fat n-3 polyunsaturated fatty acid diets on rat mammary tumorigenesis. *Carcinogenesis* **2005,** *26,* 1563–1572.

Paniagua, J.A.; S.A. Gallego de la; I. Romero; A. Vidal-Puig; J.M. Latre; E. Sanchez; P. Perez-Martinez; J. Lopez-Miranda; F. Perez-Jimenez. Monounsaturated fat-rich diet prevents central body fat distribution and decreases postprandial adiponectin expression induced by a carbohydrate-rich diet in insulin-resistant subjects. *Diabetes Care* **2007,** *30,* 1717–1723.

Panka, D.J.; T. Mano; T. Suhara; K. Walsh; J.W. Mier. Phosphatidylinositol 3-kinase/Akt activity regulates c-FLIP expression in tumor cells. *J. Biol. Chem.* **2001,** *276,* 6893–6896.

Park, Y.; K.J. Albright; W. Liu; J.M. Storkson; M.E. Cook; M.W. Pariza. Effect of conjugated linoleic acid on body composition in mice. *Lipids* **1997,** *32,* 853–858.

Parton, R.G.; M. Hanzal-Bayer; J.F. Hancock. Biogenesis of caveolae: a structural model for caveolin-induced domain formation. *J. Cell Sci.* **2006,** *119,* 787–796.

Perez-Jimenez, F.; J. Lopez-Miranda; M.D. Pinillos; P. Gomez; E. Paz-Rojas; P. Montilla; C. Marin; M.J. Velasco; A. Blanco-Molina; J.A. Jimenez Pereperez; J.M. Ordovas. A Mediterranean and a high-carbohydrate diet improve glucose metabolism in healthy young persons. *Diabetologia* **2001,** *44,* 2038–2043.

Perez-Martinez, P.; J. Lopez-Miranda; L. Blanco-Colio; C. Bellido; Y. Jimenez; J.A. Moreno; J. gado-Lista; J. Egido; F. Perez-Jimenez. The chronic intake of a Mediterranean diet enriched in virgin olive oil, decreases nuclear transcription factor kappaB activation in peripheral blood mononuclear cells from healthy men. *Atherosclerosis* **2007,** *194,* e141–e146.

Petridou, A.; V. Mougios; A. Sagredos. Supplementation with CLA: isomer incorporation into serum lipids and effect on body fat of women. *Lipids* **2003,** *38,* 805–811.

Piers, L.S.; K.Z. Walker; R.M. Stoney; M.J. Soares; K. O'Dea. Substitution of saturated with monounsaturated fat in a 4-week diet affects body weight and composition of overweight and obese men. *Br. J. Nutr.* **2003,** *90,* 717–727.

Piers, L.S.; K.Z. Walker; R.M. Stoney; M.J. Soares; K. O'Dea. The influence of the type of dietary fat on postprandial fat oxidation rates: monounsaturated (olive oil) vs saturated fat (cream). *Int. J. Obes. Relat. Metab. Disord.* **2002,** *26,* 814–821.

Pike, L.J. Lipid rafts: bringing order to chaos. *J. Lipid Res.* **2003,** *44,* 655–667.

Poirier, H.; J.S. Shapiro; R.J. Kim; M.A. Lazar. Nutritional supplementation with trans-10, cis-12-conjugated linoleic acid induces inflammation of white adipose tissue. *Diabetes* **2006,** *55,* 1634–1641.

Psota, T.L.; S.K. Gebauer; P. Kris-Etherton. Dietary omega-3 fatty acid intake and cardiovascular risk. *Am. J. Cardiol.* **2006,** *98,* 3i–18i.

Raff, M.; T. Tholstrup; S. Basu; P. Nonboe; M.T. Sorensen; E.M. Straarup. A diet rich in conjugated linoleic acid and butter increases lipid peroxidation but does not affect atherosclerotic, inflammatory, or diabetic risk markers in healthy young men. *J. Nutr.* **2008,** *138,* 509–514.

Riserus, U. Trans fatty acids and insulin resistance. *Atheroscler. Suppl.* **2006,** *7,* 37–39.

Riserus, U.; P. Arner; K. Brismar; B. Vessby. Treatment with dietary trans10cis12 conjugated linoleic acid causes isomer-specific insulin resistance in obese men with the metabolic syndrome. *Diabetes Care* **2002a,** *25,* 1516–1521.

Riserus, U.; S. Basu; S. Jovinge; G.N. Fredrikson; J. Arnlov; B. Vessby. Supplementation with conjugated linoleic acid causes isomer-dependent oxidative stress and elevated C-reactive protein: a potential link to fatty acid-induced insulin resistance. *Circulation* **2002b,** *106,* 1925–1929.

Rissanen, H.; P. Knekt; R. Jarvinen; I. Salminen; T. Hakulinen. Serum fatty acids and breast cancer incidence. *Nutr. Cancer* **2003,** *45,* 168–175.

Ritzenthaler, K.L.; M.K. McGuire; R. Falen; T.D. Shultz; N. Dasgupta; M.A. McGuire. Estimation of conjugated linoleic acid intake by written dietary assessment methodologies underestimates actual intake evaluated by food duplicate methodology. *J. Nutr.* **2001,** *131,* 1548–1554.

Roche, H.M. Fatty acids and the metabolic syndrome. *Proc. Nutr. Soc.* **2005,** *64,* 23–29.

Roche, H.M.; M.J. Gibney. Effect of long-chain n-3 polyunsaturated fatty acids on fasting and postprandial triacylglycerol metabolism. *Am. J. Clin. Nutr.* **2000,** *71,* 232S–237S.

Roche, H.M.; E. Noone; C. Sewter; B.S. Mc; D. Savage; M.J. Gibney; S. O'Rahilly; A.J. Vidal-Puig. Isomer-dependent metabolic effects of conjugated linoleic acid: insights from molecular markers sterol regulatory element-binding protein 1c and LXRalpha. *Diabetes* **2002,** *51,* 2037–2044.

Rose, D. Effects of dietary fatty acids on breast and prostate cancers: evidence from in vitro experiments and animal studies. *Am. J. Clin. Nutr.* **1997,** *66,* 1513S–1522S.

Sacks, F.M.; M. Katan. Randomized clinical trials on the effects of dietary fat and carbohydrate on plasma lipoproteins and cardiovascular disease. *Am. J. Med.* **2002,** *113(Suppl. 9B),* 13S–24S.

Saadatian-Elahi, M.; P. Toniolo; P. Ferrari; J. Goudable; A. Akhmedkhanov; A. Zeleniuch-Jacquotte; E. Riboli. Serum fatty acids and risk of breast cancer in a nested case-control study of the New York University Women's Health Study. *Cancer Epidemiol.Biomarkers Prev.* **2002,** *11,* 1353–1360.

Salas-Salvado, J.; F. Marquez-Sandoval; M. Bullo. Conjugated linoleic acid intake in humans: a systematic review focusing on its effect on body composition, glucose, and lipid metabolism. *Crit. Rev. Food Sci. Nutr.* **2006,** *46,* 479–488.

Saravanan, N.; A. Haseeb; N.Z. Ehtesham; Ghafoorunissa.Differential effects of dietary saturated and trans-fatty acids on expression of genes associated with insulin sensitivity in rat adipose tissue. *Eur. J. Endocrinol.* **2005,** *153,* 159-165.

Sasaki, T.; Y. Kobayashi; J. Shimizu; M. Wada; S. In'nami; Y. Kanke; T. Takita. Effects of dietary n-3-to-n-6 polyunsaturated fatty acid ratio on mammary carcinogenesis in rats. *Nutr. Cancer* **1998,** *30,* 137–143.

Schley, P.D.; D.N. Brindley; C.J. Field. (n-3) PUFA alter raft lipid composition and decrease epidermal growth factor receptor levels in lipid rafts of human breast cancer cells. *J. Nutr.* **2007,** *137,* 548–553.

Shaikh, S.R.; M.R. Brzustowicz; N. Gustafson; W. Stillwell; S.R. Wassall. Monounsaturated PE does not phase-separate from the lipid raft molecules sphingomyelin and cholesterol: role for polyunsaturation? *Biochemistry* **2002,** *41,* 10593–10602.

Shaikh, S.R.; A.C. Dumaual; A. Castillo; D. LoCascio; R.A. Siddiqui; W. Stillwell; S.R. Wassall. Oleic and docosahexaenoic acid differentially phase separate from lipid raft molecules: a comparative NMR, DSC, AFM, and detergent extraction study. *Biophys. J.* **2004,** *87,* 1752–1766.

Shanik, M.H.; Y. Xu; J. Skrha; R. Dankner; Y. Zick; J. Roth. Insulin resistance and hyperinsulinemia: is hyperinsulinemia the cart or the horse? *Diabetes Care* **2008,** *31(Suppl. 2)* S262–S268.

Shannon, J.; I.B. King; R. Moshofsky; J.W. Lampe; D.L. Gao; R.M. Ray; D.B. Thomas. Erythrocyte fatty acids and breast cancer risk: a case-control study in Shanghai, China. *Am. J. Clin. Nutr.* **2007,** *85,* 1090–1097.

Shimamura, H.; Y. Terada; T. Okado; H. Tanaka; S. Inoshita; S. Sasaki. The PI3-kinase-Akt pathway promotes mesangial cell survival and inhibits apoptosis in vitro via NF-kappa B and Bad. *J. Am. Soc. Nephrol.* **2003,** *14,* 1427–1434.

Shimomura, Y.; T. Tamura; M. Suzuki. Less body fat accumulation in rats fed a safflower oil diet than in rats fed a beef tallow diet. *J. Nutr.* **1990,** *120,* 1291–1296.

Silveira, M.B.; R. Carraro; S. Monereo; J. Tebar. Conjugated linoleic acid (CLA) and obesity. *Public Health Nutr.* **2007,** *10,* 1181–1186.

Simons, K.; R. Ehehalt. Cholesterol, lipid rafts, and disease. *J. Clin. Invest.* **2002,** *110,* 597–603.

Simons, K.; D. Toomre. Lipid rafts and signal transduction. *Nat. Rev. Mol. Cell Biol.* **2000,** *1,*

31–39.

Simonsen, N.; V.P. van't; J.J. Strain; J.M. Martin-Moreno; J.K. Huttunen; J.F. Navajas; B.C. Martin; M. Thamm; A.F. Kardinaal; F.J. Kok; L. Kohlmeier. Adipose tissue omega-3 and omega-6 fatty acid content and breast cancer in the EURAMIC study. European Community Multicenter Study on Antioxidants, Myocardial Infarction, and Breast Cancer. *Am. J. Epidemiol.* **1998a,** *147,* 342–352.

Simonsen, N.R.; N.J. Fernandez-Crehuet; J.M. Martin-Moreno; J.J. Strain; J.K. Huttunen; B.C. Martin; M. Thamm; A.F. Kardinaal; V.P. van't; F.J. Kok; L. Kohlmeier. Tissue stores of individual monounsaturated fatty acids and breast cancer: the EURAMIC study. European Community Multicenter Study on Antioxidants, Myocardial Infarction, and Breast Cancer. *Am. J. Clin. Nutr.* **1998b,** *68,* 134–141.

Simopoulos, A.P. Omega-3 fatty acids in inflammation and autoimmune diseases. *J. Am. Coll. Nutr.* **2002,** *21,* 495–505.

Smedman, A.; B. Vessby. Conjugated linoleic acid supplementation in humans—metabolic effects. *Lipids* **2001,** *36,* 773–781.

Smith, R.D.; C.N. Kelly; B.A. Fielding; D. Hauton; K.D. Silva; M.C. Nydahl; G.J. Miller; C.M. Williams. Long-term monounsaturated fatty acid diets reduce platelet aggregation in healthy young subjects. *Br. J. Nutr.* **2003,** *90,* 597–606.

Statistics Canada. *Food Statistics 2002*; Catalogue no. 21-020-XIE 2 (1&2). 2003.
Ref Type: Generic

Stoll, B.A. Breast cancer and the western diet: role of fatty acids and antioxidant vitamins. *Eur. J. Cancer* **1998,** *34,* 1852–1856.

Stripp, C.; K. Overvad; J. Christensen; B.L. Thomsen; A. Olsen; S. Moller; A. Tjonneland. Fish intake is positively associated with breast cancer incidence rate. *J. Nutr.* **2003,** *133,* 3664–3669.

Stulnig, T.M.; M. Berger; T. Sigmund; D. Raederstorff; H. Stockinger; W. Waldhausl. Polyunsaturated fatty acids inhibit T cell signal transduction by modification of detergent-insoluble membrane domains. *J. Cell Biol.* **1998,** *143,* 637–644.

Stulnig, T.M.; J. Huber; N. Leitinger; E.M. Imre; P. Angelisova; P. Nowotny; W. Waldhausl. Polyunsaturated eicosapentaenoic acid displaces proteins from membrane rafts by altering raft lipid composition. *J. Biol. Chem.* **2001,** *276,* 37335–37340.

Summers, L.K.; B.A. Fielding; H.A. Bradshaw; V. Ilic; C. Beysen; M.L. Clark; N.R. Moore; K.N. Frayn. Substituting dietary saturated fat with polyunsaturated fat changes abdominal fat distribution and improves insulin sensitivity. *Diabetologia* **2002,** *45,* 369–377.

Switzer, K.C.; Y.Y. Fan; N. Wang; D.N. McMurray; R.S. Chapkin. Dietary n-3 polyunsaturated fatty acids promote activation-induced cell death in Th1-polarized murine CD4+ T-cells. *J. Lipid Res.* **2004,** *45,* 1482–1492.

Takeuchi, H.; T. Matsuo; K. Tokuyama; Y. Shimomura; M. Suzuki. Diet-induced thermogenesis is lower in rats fed a lard diet than in those fed a high oleic acid safflower oil diet, a safflower oil diet or a linseed oil diet. *J. Nutr.* **1995,** *125,* 920–925.

Tanasescu, M.; E. Cho; J.E. Manson; F.B. Hu. Dietary fat and cholesterol and the risk of cardiovascular disease among women with type 2 diabetes. *Am. J. Clin. Nutr.* **2004,** *79,* 999–1005.

Thiebaut, A.C.; V. Chajes; F. Clavel-Chapelon; M. Gerber.[Unsaturated fatty acids intake and breast cancer risk: epidemiological data review]. *Bull. Cancer* **2005,** *92,* 658–669.

Thrush, A.B.; A. Chabowski; G.J. Heigenhauser; B.W. McBride; M. Or-Rashid; D.J. Dyck. Conjugated linoleic acid increases skeletal muscle ceramide content and decreases insulin sensitivity in overweight, non-diabetic humans. *Appl. Physiol. Nutr. Metab.* **2007,** *32,* 372–382.

Tou, J.C.; L.U. Thompson. Exposure to flaxseed or its lignan component during different developmental stages influences rat mammary gland structures. *Carcinogenesis* **1999,** *20,* 1831–1835.

Tricon, S.; G.C. Burdge; C.M. Williams; P.C. Calder; P. Yaqoob. The effects of conjugated linoleic acid on human health-related outcomes. *Proc. Nutr. Soc.* **2005,** *64,* 171–182.

Vessby, B.; I.B. Gustafsson; S. Tengblad; M. Boberg; A. Andersson. Desaturation and elongation of Fatty acids and insulin action. *Ann. N.Y. Acad. Sci.* **2002,** *967* 183–195.

Vessby, B.; S. Tengblad; H. Lithell. Insulin sensitivity is related to the fatty acid composition of serum lipids and skeletal muscle phospholipids in 70-year-old men. *Diabetologia* **1994,** *37,* 1044–1050.

Vessby, B.; M. Unsitupa; K. Hermansen; G. Riccardi; A.A. Rivellese; L.C. Tapsell; C. Nalsen; L. Berglund; A. Louheranta; B.M. Rasmussen; et al. Substituting dietary saturated for monounsaturated fat impairs insulin sensitivity in healthy men and women: The KANWU Study. *Diabetologia* **2001,** *44,* 312–319.

Ward, W.E.; F.O. Jiang; L.U. Thompson. Exposure to flaxseed or purified lignan during lactation influences rat mammary gland structures. *Nutr. Cancer* **2000,** *37,* 187–192.

Webb, Y.; L. Hermida-Matsumoto; M.D. Resh. Inhibition of protein palmitoylation, raft localization, and T cell signaling by 2-bromopalmitate and polyunsaturated fatty acids. *J. Biol. Chem.* **2000,** *275,* 261–270.

Wei, N.; M.T. Mi; B. Wang; J.D. Zhu; D.P. Zhu; J.L. Yuan. [Effects of different dietary fatty acid on expression of nuclear receptor genes in breast cancer of rats]. *Zhonghua Yu Fang Yi.Xue.Za Zhi.* **2007,** *41,* 271–276.

Wynder, E.L.; L.A. Cohen; J.E. Muscat; B. Winters; J.T. Dwyer; G. Blackburn. Breast cancer: weighing the evidence for a promoting role of dietary fat. *J. Natl. Cancer Inst.* **1997,** *89,* 766–775.

Yamada, T.; J.P. Strong; T. Ishii; T. Ueno; M. Koyama; H. Wagayama; A. Shimizu; T. Sakai; G.T. Malcom; M.A. Guzman. Atherosclerosis and omega-3 fatty acids in the populations of a fishing village and a farming village in Japan. *Atherosclerosis* **2000,** *153,* 469–481.

Young, R.M.; D. Holowka; B. Baird. A lipid raft environment enhances Lyn kinase activity by protecting the active site tyrosine from dephosphorylation. *J. Biol. Chem.* **2003,** *278,* 20746–20752.

Zeyda, M.; G. Staffler; V. Horejsi; W. Waldhausl; T.M. Stulnig. LAT displacement from lipid rafts as a molecular mechanism for the inhibition of T cell signaling by polyunsaturated fatty acids. *J. Biol. Chem.* **2002,** *277,* 28418–28423.

Ziegler, R.G.; R.N. Hoover; M.C. Pike; A. Hildesheim; A.M. Nomura; D.W. West; A.H. Wu-Williams; L.N. Kolonel; P.L. Horn-Ross; J.F. Rosenthal; M.B. Hyer. Migration patterns and breast cancer risk in Asian-American women. *J. Natl. Cancer Inst.* **1993,** *85,* 1819–1827.

Zock, P.L.; M.B. Katan. Butter, margarine and serum lipoproteins. *Atherosclerosis* **1997,** *131,* 7–16.

# 19

# Linoleic Acids and Cancer Cell Functions

**Donato F. Romagnolo[1], Andreas J. Papoutsis[1], Stephanie C. Degner, and Ornella Selmin[2]**

*Departments of Nutritional Sciences and Veterinary Science and Microbiology, The University of Arizona, Tucson, Arizona*

## Introduction

Dietary fats are important risk factors in the etiology of several diseases including some types of cancer. In general, the intake of total fat, types, and source of fat appear to influence the cancer process. The ratio of n-6 to n-3 may influence the risk of cancer, with n-6 polyunsaturated fatty acids having a stronger promoting effect compared to saturated fats and n-3 fatty acids (Terry et al., 2003). However, some epidemiological studies have failed to find an association between the intake of fats and the risk for some types of cancer including prostate (Leitzmann et al., 2004) and breast cancer (Cho et al., 2003; Holmes et al., 1999; Prentice et al., 2006).

The objective of this chapter is to provide an overview of the mechanisms through which linoleic acids (LAs) and metabolic products such as conjugated linoleic acid (CLA) and arachidonic acid (AA) may influence cancer-cell functions. Particular emphasis is given to cellular and molecular processes that play a role in cell proliferation, apoptosis, and the production of inflammatory factors in cancer cells. We also discuss the results of studies that investigated the effects of LA and CLA on the cancer process in preclinical animal models and human populations.

### *Chemistry of LA and CLA*

LA is an essential unsaturated fatty acid containing 2 double bonds and 18 carbon atoms with the stereochemistry of the double bonds in the *cis* formation. By starting from the carboxyl-end of LA, the *cis* double bonds are at carbons 9 and 12, to which the name is attributed: *cis*9,*cis*12-octadecadienoic acid, often abbreviated as *c*9,*c*12-18:2. Alternatively, the n- or ω-system is used, and the double bonds are numbered by starting from the methyl-end. In the latter system, the first double bond of LA is 6 carbons distant from the methyl group, and is represented as n-6 or ω-6. Therefore, by utilizing this nomenclature, one can identify LA as 18:2ω6 or 18:2n-6.

LA, along with α-linolenic acid (ALA), is an essential fatty acid. Mammalian cells are unable to introduce double bonds on the methyl side of the n-9 double bond. Therefore, LA must be provided in the diet. In humans, clinical symptoms of ω-6 fatty acid deficiency include decreased growth in infants and children, increased epidermal water loss (dermatitis), impaired healing, and alterations of reproductive functions (Chapkin, 1992). In general, the typical American diet more than meets the requirements (1–2% of daily caloric intake) for LA, so deficiency of LA is extremely rare. In addition to providing energy, LA is a structural component of the cell membrane, acts as a carrier of fat-soluble vitamins and antioxidants, and serves as a precursor for the synthesis of eicosanoids.

Modifications of LA include desaturation and elongation to AA (20:4ω6), from which eicosanoids are derived. This process occurs mostly in the liver. The first step in the pathway that leads to the conversion of LA (18:2ω6) to γ-linolenic acid (GLA, 18:3ω6) is the addition of a third double bond via Δ-6-desaturase, followed by enzymatic elongation via elongase to dihomo-γ-linolenic acid (DGLA) (20:3ω6), and finally to AA via Δ-5-desaturase. Further elongation and desaturation generate 22:4ω6 and 22:5ω6. The physiological functions of the latter fatty acids are not clear although their synthesis increases during ALA deficiency. The metabolic product AA can enter the cycloxygenase (COX) pathway to produce prostaglandins (PGs) and thromboxanes (TXAs), the lipoxygenase (LOX) pathway to produce leukotrienes, or the cytochrome P450 pathway to generate epoxyeicosatrienoic acids (Fig. 19.1). These eicosanoids are signaling molecules that may function as autocrine and/or paracrine mediators. PGs and TXAs produced via the COX pathway are involved in blood coagulation, inflammation, and in cardiovascular and renal function. The leukotrienes formed via the LOX pathway are involved in the tissue response to inflammatory stimuli. The epoxyeicosatrienoic acids modulate vascular resistance and blood pressure (Stipanuk, 2006).

A series of positional and geometric isomers of *c*9,*c*12-octadecadienoic acid are collectively known as CLAs. Starting from the carboxyl-end of the molecule, these octadecadienoic acids contain conjugated double bonds with no methylene group separating them at positions 7,9; 8,10; 9,11; 10,12; 11,13; and 12,14. Geometrically, these isomers can occur in the *cis,cis; trans,trans; cis,trans;* or *trans,cis* configurations (Sehat et. al., 1998). Although 24 isomers of CLAs were characterized, the major isomer found in natural products is *c*9,*t*11-octadecadienoic acid (Christie et al., 1997), which accounts for about 70–85% of CLA intake in the human diet.

## Dietary Sources of LA and CLA

LA is present in various amounts in almost all vegetable fats. It is found in the highest amounts in safflower oil (77%), sunflower oil (60–68%), corn oil (57%), soybean oil (53%), cottonseed oil (52%), sesame oil (44%), peanut oil (31%), rice-bran oil (31%), rapeseed/canola oil (22%), palm oil (10–15%), olive oil (7%), and coconut oil (2%) (Akoh, 2006; Akoh & Min, 2008; Chow, 2008; Gunstone, 1996). LA is also present in less commercially popular oils from poppyseed (76%), acacia seed (40–55%), hemp (60%), prickly pear (70%), and mapleseed (40–70%) (Chow, 2008). Although the

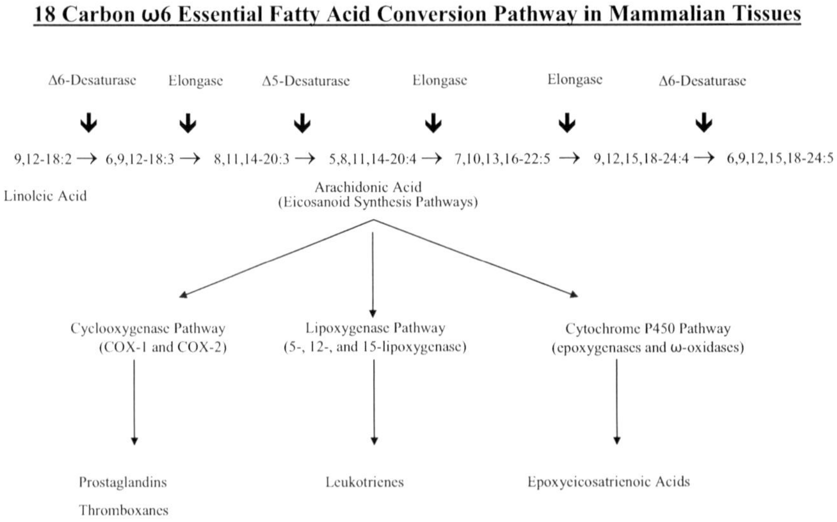


**Fig. 19.1.** Schematic representation of 18-carbon ω6 fatty acid conversion in mammalian tissues.

major sources of LA are vegetable oils, it is present at much lower levels in animal fats and fish oils. The content of LA found in fruits and vegetables is influenced by plant species, geographic location, soil type, climate, moisture, temperature, seed maturity, agricultural practice, cultivar, and measurement techniques.

The *c*9,*t*11 CLA isomer is most abundant in meats and dairy products preferentially produced during the bacterial isomerization of LA in the fermentative environment of the rumen (Chin et al., 1992). This reaction is catalyzed by the anaerobic bacterium *Butyrivibrio fibrisolvens,* which possesses LA isomerase (linoleate Δ*c*12, Δ *t*11-isomerase) activity. However, rumen bacteria are not the only producers of CLA since it is found in nonruminant meats such as pork, chicken, and turkey. Also contributing to the content of CLA in foods is the cooking and grilling process where the application of high temperatures increases CLA concentrations (Ha et al., 1989).

The main source of CLA in the Western diet is from dairy products with CLA concentrations ranging from 0.55 to 24 mg/g of fat; cheese contains the highest levels of CLA (Fritsche & Steinhart, 1998). Variations in the content of CLA in milk and dairy products are due to the content of fat in the milk (about 10 mg/g of milk fat) (Jiang et al., 1996) and nutrition (Shantha & Decker, 1993). Milk from grazing cows had a higher content of CLA than cows on grain diets and housed indoors. The supplementation with either rapeseed or soybean concentrates increased milk CLA (Dhiman et al., 2000). Seasonal variations in CLA content in milk were observed, with the highest levels detected between May and September. Individual cow variations due to the number of lactations were also reported; milk CLA content ranged from 1.6 to 16.0 mg/g of fat (Stanton et al., 1997). CLA is found also in beef muscle at concentrations ranging from 1.2 to 9.9 mg/g of fat (Shantha et al., 1994). It is also present in lesser amounts in nonruminant meats from turkey (2.5 mg/g of fat) (Ha et al., 1989), chicken (0.9 mg/g of fat), and pork (0.6 mg/g of fat); and in egg yolk (0.6 mg/g of fat) (MacDonald, 2000). Some seafood and vegetable oils contain small amounts of CLA. Commercial preparations of CLA usually have the *c*9,*t*11- and *c*10,*t*12-CLA isomers in equal proportions (Dijkstra et al., 2008; Wahle et al., 2004).

## Mechanisms of Action of LAs

Realizing that many studies and excellent reviews have been published during the last two decades on the effects of fatty acids on health promotion, and in particular on the effects of LA and CLA on the cancer process, we knew our citation of the available scientific literature could not be exhaustive due to space constraints. The association between the intake of LA and the incidence of various types of cancer was the subject of many reviews (Kelley et al., 2007). Compared to ALA and eicosapentaenoic acid (EPA), which exerted strong cancer-chemopreventative activities (Sauer et al., 2000), LA promoted rodent-tumor growth (Schoenberg & Krokan, 1995). Earlier studies corroborated these results in reporting that diets rich in LA were tumor-promoting in rodents (Cohen, 1997; Rose et al., 1993) and humans (Lanson et al., 1990). Conversely, studies reported that GLA and CLA exerted protective effects against the development of several types of tumors. A study that compared the effects of LA and CLA on the growth of several tumor-cell lines concluded that LA exerted different effects, ranging from inhibitory, neutral, or even promoting growth. In contrast, CLA inhibited cell growth in all tumor-cell lines tested (Maggiora et al., 2004). The mechanisms responsible for the differential effects of LA and CLA on the cancer process are still under investigation. In this chapter, potential candidate mechanisms are reviewed, and include the effects of LA on the regulation of eicosanoid synthesis, cell proliferation, the regulation of the signal transduction pathway, the transcription activity of nuclear receptors, and the expression of proinflammatory genes. Because the mechanisms of carcinogenesis may vary between men and women and among cancers, one must be cautious when interpreting the data from studies that investigated the effects of LA and CLA on the cancer process (Laakasonen et al., 2004). For example, whereas many studies reported the anti-proliferative and anticarcinogenic effects of CLA, a recent report indicated that a selected isomer of CLA (*t*10,*c*12) stimulated mammary-tumor progression in Her2/ErbB2 mice through the activation of both proliferative and survival pathways (Meng et al., 2008). On the other hand, combinatorial strategies that used conjugated double bonds and an (n-3) highly unsaturated fatty acid (EPA, C20:5) produced stronger protective effects through apoptosis and lipid peroxidation than EPA or CLA alone (Tsuzuki et al., 2004). Moreover, the etiology of tumors with specific genetic aberrations mediates the effects of CLA. In a cohort study of ≈120,000 Dutch subjects, the intake of LA, which was the most abundant fatty acid in the diet, was associated with an increase in the risk of colon cancer with only a KRAS (v-Ki-ras2 Kirsten rat sarcoma viral oncogenic homolog) and no additional APC (adenomatous polyposis coli) mutation or lack of MLH1 (mutL homolog 1). Conversely, LA intake was not associated with the risk of colon tumors without these combined gene defects, or tumors harboring aberrations in either MLH1 or APC (Weijenberg et al., 2007). Therefore, one should consider many factors—including processing, interactions of LA and CLA acids with other dietary factors, and genetic background—when extrapolating experimental data to develop dietary recommendations.

## *Effects of LA on Synthesis of Eicosanoids and Hydroxyeicosatetraenoic Acids*

The metabolism of LA by the enzyme Δ-6-desaturase generates GLA, which is elongated to DGLA. Through the action of acyl transferases, DGLA is incorporated into the cell membrane or converted to AA by the enzyme Δ-5-desaturase. In turn, AA is either metabolized to PG through the action of COX-2, or metabolized by LOX to hydroxyeicosatetraenoic acids (5- and 12-HETE), which inhibit apoptosis, stimulate angiogenesis, and induce the secretion of proteolytic enzymes that assist tumor cells in the invasion process (Liu et al., 1996). The formation of AA from DGLA is under the negative regulation of AA and specific nutritional factors including sesamin found in sesame seeds (Hrelia et al., 1996) and the fish oil EPA (Barham et al., 2000). In contrast to LA (n-6), fatty acids of the n-3 family inhibit the activity of the enzyme Δ-6-desaturase, and reduce the production of 5- and 12-HETE (Rose & Connolly, 1999). Through these opposite actions, LA and n-3 fatty acids may either promote or prevent tumor growth. Dietary fats that are predominantly rich in LA compared to fish oils may increase the susceptibility to cancer development. The metabolism of LA to PG may increase the risk of cancer through the PG-dependent stimulation of COX-2 expression. Studies by Wang et al. (2005) documented that $PGE_2$ enhanced the cell proliferation of colorectal cells through the activation of the Ras-MAPK pathway. Similarly, the generation of HETE metabolites through the LOX pathway stimulated the proliferation of cancer cells mediated by the activation of MEL/ERK1-2 and the PI3K/Akt pathways (Ding et al., 2003). The knowledge that the metabolism of AA by COX-2 generates tumor-promoting eicosanoids stimulated the interest to develop selective inhibitors of COX-2. Unfortunately, therapeutic intervention with COX-2 inhibitors was linked to an increased risk of myocardial infarction. Therefore, dietary strategies are important to reduce the intake of tumor-prone fatty acids including LA.

## *Effects of LA on Cell Proliferation*

Several studies report that, at micromolar concentrations, fatty acids are toxic to cancer cells both in vivo and in vitro (Hawkins et al., 1998). The toxicity of fatty acids appeared to be inversely related to the chain length and degree of saturation

(Andrade et al., 2005). Whereas the mechanisms responsible for this toxicity are largely unknown, recent investigations compared the effects of saturated and unsaturated fatty acids on cell viability. In S91 murine melanoma cells, the treatment with LA and AA was the most effective in inducing the loss of membrane integrity and DNA fragmentation compared to EPA (C20:5). The toxic effect of LA was attributed to lipid accumulation in the cytosol, mitochondrial depolarization, and changes in the expression of c-MYC and p53 (Cury-Boaventura et al., 2004). In rat C6 glioma cells, the treatment with LA-enhanced lipid peroxidation, induced the loss of membrane integrity, and promoted giant DNA fragmentation (Higuchi & Yoshimoto, 2004). Whereas short-term treatment with LA induced apoptosis, long-term continuous treatment with LA induced quiescence and dormancy with possible induction of cancer stem and/or progenitor phenotype (Kuniyasu, 2008).

## *Effects of GLA on Cancer Cells*

GLA is the precursor of DGLA, which is accumulated in the plasma membrane. The metabolism of DGLA by COX-2 generates eicosanoids of the series-1 ($PGE_1$) and thromboxane-1 ($TXA_1$). Both $PGE_1$ and $TXA_1$ exert anti-inflammatory properties. In addition, the generation of 15-hydroxyeicosatrienoic acid (HETrE) inhibits the enzyme 5-LOX, which participates in the generation of leukotriene $B_4$ (Ziboh et al., 2000). Several studies document that GLA inhibits the proliferation of various types of cancer cells (Menendez et al., 2004; Watkins et al., 2005). Several mechanisms were advocated for the anti-cancer effects of GLA, including the induction of apoptosis (Menendez et al., 2004) and the down-regulation of estrogen receptors in breast-cancer cells. In combination with tamoxifen, GLA improved the efficacy of tamoxifen therapy in breast-cancer patients (Kenny et al., 2000).

## *Effects of CLA on Cancer-cell Functions*

In general, most studies investigated the effects of two common dietary CLA isomers, *c*9,*t*11-CLA and *t*10,*c*12-CLA, although the *c*9,*t*11-CLA isomer is the most abundant in dairy and meat products. CLAs exhibit isomer-specific biological effects (Ou et al., 2008). For example, the *t*9, *c*11-CLA inhibited the COX-2 pathway, whereas the *t*10, *c*12-CLA inhibited the LOX pathway (Kelley et al., 2007). However, the molecular mechanisms responsible for these differential effects are still unclear (Murphy et al., 2007). For example, diets containing 0.1% of *c*9,*t*11-CLA or *t*10,*c*12-CLA were equally effective in inhibiting colon-cancer cell metastasis in vivo. However, only *c*9,*t*11-CLA, but not *t*10,*c*12-CLA, inhibited colon-cancer cell migration (Soel et al., 2007). The type of cell tumor and the degree of malignancy may influence the effects of CLA isomers. Compared to nonmalignant mammary epithelial MCF-10A cells, the treatment of breast-cancer MCF-7 cells with CLA stimulated the expression of 4-hydroxy-2-nonenal (4-HNE), a product of lipid peroxidation. The expression of 4-HNE was augmented in MCF-7 cells by the co-treatment with hydrogen peroxide (200 μM). The expression of 4-HNE increased the expression of the tumor-suppressor gene p21 (Barrera et al., 2002), which is also activated by the redox-sensitive factor p53. Consistent with these findings, CLA alone or in combination with hydrogen peroxide induced (in MCF-7, but not in MCF-10A cells) the nuclear localization of phosphorylated p53Ser15, reduced BrdU incorporation, and phosphorylated histone-3. Thus, CLA may increase in breast cancer, but not in normal mammary epithelial cells, the susceptibility to oxidative stress (Albright et al., 2005). This biological difference between normal and breast-cancer cells may be useful to improve targeted anti-proliferative therapies based on CLA alone or in combination with other agents.

The inhibition of cell proliferation by the CLA isomer *t*9,*t*11-CLA was also observed in human colon-cancer cells (Bocca et al., 2007). The treatment of Caco-2 cells with CLA reduced the expression levels of Raf-1 and the phosphorylation of ERK1/2. These changes were accompanied by a reduction in the expression of the downstream transcription factor c-myc. Investigations with Caco-2 cells (Beppu et al., 2006) documented that the treatment with CLA reduced the levels of Bcl-2 without changing the expression of Bax, suggesting that CLA may increase the susceptibility of cancer cells to lipid peroxidation and induce apoptosis. The anti-proliferative effects of CLA were further documented in human osteosarcoma (MG-63) cells in which the treatment with a mixture of *t,t* isomers of CLA induced apoptosis. This effect was characterized by morphological changes and DNA fragmentation: increased Bax expression, reduced Bcl-2 expression, release of cytochrome-c from mitochondria to the cytosol, and activation of caspase-3 (Kim et al., 2008). Moreover, the same study documented that the incorporation of *t,t*-CLA into the membrane phospholipids reduced the content of AA. Therefore, CLA may exert anti-proliferative effects by limiting the pool of AA available for the synthesis of eicosanoids and hydroxyeicosatetraenoic acids, which are associated with the stimulation of cell growth. The proapoptotic effects of CLA were further documented in estrogen-receptor negative MDA-MB-231 cells. The occurrence of apoptosis in these cells was accompanied by a reduction in ERK1/2 and anti-apoptotic Bcl-$x_L$, upregulation of the pro-apoptotic protein Bak, translocation of cytochrome-c from mitochondria to the cytosol, and cleavage of procaspase-9 and -3 (Miglietta et al., 2006). Apoptosis induced by the *t*10,*c*12-CLA isomer appeared to be mediated by an atypical endoplasmic-reticulum (ER) response characterized by the dilation of the ER lumen. This change was accompanied by the induction of the pro-apoptotic C/EBP-homologous protein and the cleavage of caspase-12 (Ou et al., 2008). One of the mechanisms through which the *t*10,*c*12-CLA isomer may induce apoptosis is the induction of a stress response at the level of ER, thus preventing normal post-translational protein modifications such as disulfide-bond formation and glycosylation.

Investigations with metastatic mouse mammary-tumor cells indicated that CLA reduced the invasiveness and expression levels of matrix metalloproteinase (MMP)-2. Moreover, the activity of MMP-9 was decreased by CLA, whereas the mRNA and protein levels of the tissue inhibitors of metalloproteinase-1 (TIMP-1) and TIMP-2, which are inhibitors of MMP, were increased by CLA. Therefore, CLA may exert protective effects through the repression of MMP activity (Hubbard et al., 2007)

One mechanism through which CLA may influence cancer-cell functions is the inhibition of receptor-mediated signal-transduction pathways. The overexpression of members of the ErB family of receptor tyrosine kinases was implicated in the etiology of various types of cancers. In colon-cancer HT-29 cells, the *t*10,*c*12-CLA isomer inhibited the expression of ErB3, a member of the ErB family of receptor tyrosine kinases that regulate the activity of downstream pathways including the mitogen-activated protein (MAP) kinase and phosphoinositide-3-kinase (PI3K) (Cho et al., 2005). The same study revealed that *t*10,*c*12-CLA, but not *c*9,*t*11-CLA, repressed the phosphorylation of Akt, a downstream target of PI3K. These results suggest that the modulation of the ErB/PI3K/Akt axis may be limited to selected isomers including *t*10,*c*12-CLA. Experiments performed in hepatoma 7288CTC cells documented that the isomer *t*10,*c*12-CLA, but not *c*9,*t*11-CLA, decreased cAMP content and ERK1/2 phosphorylation (Sauer et al., 2004). Studies that investigated the anti-proliferative effects of CLA in breast-cancer and colon-cancer cells reported that CLA inhibited cell proliferation through the activation of p53 and p21 and the arrest in the G0/G1 phase of the cell cycle (Kemp et al., 2003). Investigations with colon-cancer cells suggested that CLA inhibited the growth of colon-cancer cells with either wild-type or mutated p53 through the cdk inhibitor p21 (Lim et al., 2005).

Several transcription factors that may be targeted, directly or indirectly, by CLA include the activator protein-1 (AP-1) and the aryl hydrocarbon receptor (AhR). In vitro studies with breast-cancer MCF-7 cells illustrated that the co-treatment with CLA reduced the binding of AP-1 to the COX-2 promoter, thus reducing COX-2 transcription. In addition, CLA counteracted the TPA-dependent induction of COX-2 protein, the phosphorylation of c-Jun, and the activation of SAPK/JNK (Degner et al., 2006). Similarly, CLA reduced in MCF-7 cells the binding of the AhR to the COX-2 promoter, thus reducing the activation of the COX-2 transcription by the AhR ligand TCDD (2,3,7,8-tetrachlorodibenzo-*p*-dioxin) (Degner et al., 2007). Overall, these studies point to the COX-2 gene as a suitable target for prophylactic strategies based on CLA. By antagonizing the stimulatory effects of AP-1 and AhR on the transcriptional activation of COX-2, CLA may lower the cellular levels of COX-2, thus reducing the metabolism of LA to PG, a process that requires the participation of COX-2. A parallel mechanism through which selected CLA isomers (*t*10,*c*12-CLA) may exert anti-cancer effects is the reduction of 5-hydroxyeicosatetraenoic acid (5-HETE) production by competing with the LOX substrate, AA (Kim et al., 2006).

CLA may exert anti-cancer properties through the modulation of the peroxisome proliferator-activated receptor (PPAR), which includes three members, PPARα, PPARβ/δ, and PPARγ. Through direct or indirect PPARγ activation, the treatment of human glioblastoma cells (ADF) with CLA (25 μM) or a PPARγ agonist (GW347845X) inhibited cell proliferation and invasiveness, while inducing apoptosis

(Cimini et al., 2005). The effects of CLA were reverted by a co-treatment with the PPARγ antagonist GW259662. The potential role of PPAR in the CLA-dependent effects on cancer growth was further documented by studies with male F344 rats given subcutaneous injections with the colon-carcinogen azoxymethane (AOM). The accumulation of CLA in liver tissue through the administration of seed oil from bitter melon (*Momordica Charantia*), which is rich in CLA, was associated with an increased expression of PPARγ and a reduced incidence and a multiplicity of colonic adenocarcinoma (Kohno et al., 2004). Other studies with HT29 and Caco-2 colon-cancer cells attributed the preventative effects of CLA (*c*9,*t*11-CLA) to the repression of PPARδ expression, an inhibition of AP-1 activity, and a reduced expression of c-jun and cyclin D1. These changes were associated with CLA-induced cell differentiation and a reduced expression of β-catenin (Lampen et al., 2005).

Studies that compared the effects of LA and CLA on the growth of several tumor- cell lines documented that CLA was more effective than LA in inhibiting cell proliferation and that this effect was dependent on the type and degree of the malignancy of the cell line tested (Maggiora et al., 2004). The growth-promoting effects of LA were more noticeable with less-differentiated prostate-cancer (PC3 and SG65) cell lines. In contrast, the more malignant mammary-tumor cell line MDA-MB-231 was the least affected by CLA, whereas CLA strongly inhibited the growth of bladder- (639V) and prostate- (LNCaP, PC3) cancer cell lines. The anti-proliferative effects of CLA were associated with the presence or increased expression of PPARγ and PPARβ/δ proteins. In general, the effects of CLA were seen at concentrations (≈5 μM) that approached physiological levels, suggesting that one may achieve the health benefits of CLA through diet.

The preventative properties of CLA against chemical carcinogenesis were first reported by Pariza and Hargraves (1985), who documented that applications of CLA inhibited, in a skin mouse model, 7,12-dimethylbenz(a)anthracene (DMBA)-induced epidermal papillomas, and decreased tumor incidence. Studies with Sprague-Dawley rats also informed us that the isomer *c*9, *t*11-CLA mediated the anti-carcinogenic effects of vaccenic acid (18:1) against mammary tumors induced by methylnitrosourea. The protective effects of vaccenic acid depended on its metabolism to *c*9, *t*11-CLA by the enzyme Δ9-desaturase since the inhibition of Δ9-desaturase activity with cyclopropenoic acids supplied by sterculic oil attenuated the preventative effects of vaccenic acid (Lock et al., 2004).

The age of CLA intake is an important factor in breast-cancer prevention. In a rat mammary-tumor model, the supplementation with 1% of CLA from 55 days to 6 months of age exerted the best protective effects (54% inhibition) against DMBA-induced mammary carcinogenesis compared with supplementation from weaning to 50 days of age (49% inhibition) or from weaning to 6 months of age (35% inhibition) (Thompson et al., 1997). Diets supplemented with 1% of a CLA diet during early post-weaning to the pubertal period (from 21 to 42 days of age) reduced tumorigenesis induced by a single dose of methylnitrosourea given at 56 days of age (Ip et al., 1995).

Taken together, these results suggest that CLA may exert a protective effect during mammary-gland development.

Additional evidence of the anti-carcinogenic properties of CLA came from in vivo studies involving a mouse model in which a synthetic mixture of CLA decreased (by 50%) benzo(a)pyrene-induced forestomach tumors (Ha et al., 1990). Similarly, CLA reduced the number of 2-amino-3-methylimidazo[4.5-*f*]quinoline (IQ)-induced colonic foci in rats (Liew et al., 1995). A more recent study reported that the supplementation of CLA (1% of the diet) led to a reduction in the development of colon tumors and peritoneal metastasis (Park et al., 2004).

## Effects of LA and CLA in Epidemiological Studies

Epidemiological studies investigated the links between the dietary intake of fats and the incidence of various types of cancer. The intake of LA assessed in case-control studies through the validation of food-frequency questionnaires was inversely related to the incidence of renal-cell carcinoma in a population of 1534 Italian subjects (Bidoli et al., 2008), and the risk of hepatocellular carcinoma (Polesel et al., 2007). An assessment through dietary food records of fatty acid consumption in a population-based cohort of ≈2000 middle-aged Finnish men reported that diets rich in LA tended to be inversely correlated with the incidence of prostate cancer (Laaksonen et al., 2004). However, the same study concluded that the effects of diets containing higher levels of LA on the incidence of prostate cancer could be due to other nutrients associated with vegetable fats. Other studies that examined a population of nearly 48,000 U.S. men concluded that the intake of LA was unrelated to the risk of prostate cancer (Leitzmann et al., 2004). Prospective studies using a cohort of approximately 60,000 Swedish women reported that high intakes of high-fat dairy foods and CLA may reduce the risk of colorectal cancer (Larsson et al., 2005).

The most promising evidence for the use of CLA as a preventative agent in humans arises from studies that linked CLA consumption with the incidence of breast cancer. In a study of 4697 initially cancer-free Finnish women, ages 15 years or over, a significant inverse relationship was found between milk intake and the incidence of breast cancer over a 25-year follow-up period (Knekt et al., 1996). The women subjects that consumed more than 620 mL of milk each day had half the risk of breast cancer compared with those that consumed less than 370 mL of milk each day. In contrast, other studies involving 213 French women with invasive breast carcinoma and 84 control patients with benign breast disease reported that CLA content in breast adipose tissue was not associated with the risk of breast cancer (Chajes et al., 2002). In this case-control study, adipose-tissue samples analyzed by gas chromatography identified *c*9,*t*11-CLA as the major isomer, and found no significant difference in mean CLA levels in patients with breast cancer (0.44% of total fatty acids) compared to patients with benign-breast pathologies (0.43% of total fatty acids). However, a potential confounding factor for the latter study was whether or not adipose-tissue CLA levels served as an accurate biomarker of previous CLA dietary intake when food questionnaires were not done.

A cohort study in The Netherlands found a higher intake of CLA to be associated with a slight increase in the risk of breast cancer in 941 postmenopausal women who had developed breast cancer with a 6.3-year follow-up (Voorrips et al., 2002). In this study, patients' dietary intake was derived from a 150-item food-frequency questionnaire which was linked with the TRANSFAIR Study, a market-basket study in 14 European countries. The dietary intake of total CLA and *c*9,*t*11-CLA among 1122 women with breast cancer and 2036 control cases was not linked to breast-cancer risk in either premenopausal or postmenopausal women. However, among the premenopausal women, a small reduced risk of ER-negative tumors was found between the highest quartile compared with the lowest quartile of *c*9,*t*11 CLA intake (McCann et al., 2004).

A few studies evaluated the effects of CLA intake on the incidence of gastrointestinal cancers. The Swedish Mammography Cohort Study examined the association between the consumption of CLA and the incidence of colorectal cancers. During a follow-up period of ≈15 years, 798 cases of colorectal cancer were diagnosed out of 60,708 women of 40 to 76 years of age who participated in the study. A 35% reduction in the risk of distal colon cancer was observed in women that consumed ≥3 servings of cheese each day compared to women who consumed <1 serving each day (Larsson et al., 2005). However, the inverse association between high-fat dairy food consumption and the risk of colorectal cancer was attributed to other components of high-fat dairy products, such as sphingomyelin, that are known to reduce the risk of colorectal cancer (Dillehay et al., 1994; Lemonnier et al., 2003). Although several studies support the protective effects of fatty acids in dairy products, milk, and/or cheese against colorectal cancer (Nkondjock et al., 2003; Theodoratou et al., 2007), other reviews of epidemiological evidence found no clear association (Norat & Riboli, 2003).

## CLA and Human Clinical Studies

To our knowledge, no human clinical studies have examined the effects of dietary CLA intake or supplementation on tumor incidence. Although human clinical trials investigated the effects of CLA supplementation on inflammation and obesity, which are conditions interrelated to various types of cancer, comparisons across various human clinical trials are difficult due to the differences in CLA-isomer preparations as well as the duration of the studies (Gaullier et al., 2002).

A recent meta-analysis summarized 18 human clinical trials that investigated whether or not CLA supplementation influenced body composition (Whigham et al., 2007). Overall, results from this analysis suggested that CLA supplementation at 3.2 g/day produced a modest, but significant, fat-mass reduction in humans. Interestingly, mixed CLA-isomer supplementation altered energy expenditure and fat oxidation during sleep in overweight subjects, as measured using whole-room indirect calorimetry and stable isotope-labeled oleate and palmitate (Close et al., 2007).

Adverse side effects from CLA supplementation include fatty livers and lipodystrophy, although these effects seem to be limited mostly to mouse models

(Pariza, 2004). In a 12-month clinical trial conducted with obese subjects, no adverse side effects regarding liver function, serum lipids, serum glucose, serum insulin, and blood counts were noted in individuals who were given 6 g/day of a commercially available CLA supplement compared to the placebo control group (Whigham et al., 2004). The CLA supplementation was well-tolerated in healthy, overweight humans over a period of 24 months (Gauiller et al., 2005).

An important safety concern is whether or not CLA induces oxidative stress, and unfavorably alters lipid profiles. CLA supplementation (4.2 g/day) for three months significantly increased both 8-iso-$PGF_{2\alpha}$ and 15-keto-dihydro-$PGF_{2\alpha}$— markers of lipid peroxidation in the urine of healthy subjects compared to the control group (Basu et al., 2000). Additional concern stems from a study in which a CLA supplement containing primarily *t*10,*c*12-CLA resulted in elevated urinary isoprostane, increased C-reactive protein, reduced HDL, and increased very low density lipoprotein (VLDL) (Riserus et al., 2002). In the same study, the extent of these adverse side effects was much lower in subjects who took a CLA supplement containing equal amounts of *t*10,*c*12-CLA and *c*9,*t*11-CLA. In healthy young men, a supplementation with 115 g/day of CLA-rich fat increased plasma 8-iso-$PGF_{2\alpha}$ concentrations compared to the control without altering fasting glucose and insulin concentrations, or any other markers of cardiovascular disease and inflammation (Raff et al., 2008).

Although the majority of animal studies seem to indicate that CLA may have anti-diabetic properties, the supplementation with *t*10,*c*12-CLA for men with metabolic syndrome increased insulin resistance (Riserus et al., 2002). In patients with type-2 diabetes, CLA supplementation had adverse effects on insulin and glucose metabolism (Moloney et al., 2004). Other studies reported no adverse effect or improvement of insulin sensitivity with CLA supplementation (Eyjolfson et al., 2004; Whigham et al., 2007). In patients with type-2 diabetes, an improvement in serum insulin was noted following CLA supplementation (6 g/day) for 2 weeks (Belury et al., 2003).

In healthy young adults, CLA supplementation reduced the levels of circulating inflammatory cytokines tumor necrosis factor alpha (TNFα) and interleukin beta (ILβ), while increasing the levels of the anti-inflammatory cytokine IL-10 (Song et al., 2005). In the latter study, plasma glucose, lipids, and the lymphocyte profile were not changed significantly by CLA. After a 12-month clinical trial with healthy obese subjects, CLA supplementation resulted in slightly elevated leukocyte concentrations (Larsen et al., 2005). In healthy males receiving CLA supplements containing a 50:50 mixture of *c*9, *t*11-CLA and *t*10,*c*12-CLA, more subjects produced elevated levels of protective antibodies in response to the hepatitis B vaccine than control subjects (Albers et al., 2003). In summary, human clinical trials investigating CLA supplementation indicate that the type of CLA-isomer preparation, the duration of supplementation, and the disease state of the patient influence whether or not CLA supplementation exerts beneficial or adverse effects. Therefore, any CLA supplementation strategy designed regarding cancer prevention or treatment should consider the potential beneficial effects as well as adverse effects.

## References

Akoh, C. *Handbook of Functional Lipids;* Taylor and Francis Group: Boca Raton, FL, 2006; pp. 489–512.

Akoh, C.; D. Min. *Food Lipids: Chemistry, Nutrition, and Biotechnology;* Taylor and Francis Group: Boca Raton, FL, 2008; pp. 683–703.

Albers, R.; R.P. van der Wielen; E.J. Brink; H.F. Hendriks; V.N. Dorovska-Taran; I.C. Mohede. Effects of *cis*-9, *trans*-11 and *trans*-10, *cis*-12 conjugated linoleic acid (CLA) isomers on immune function in healthy men. *Eur. J. Clin. Nutr.* **2003,** *57,* 595ñ603.

Albright, C.D.; E. Klem; A.A. Shah; P. Gallagher. Breast cancer cell-targeted oxidative stress: enhancement of cancer cell uptake of conjugated linoleic acid, activation of p53, and inhibition of proliferation. *Exp. Mol. Pathol.* **2005,** *79(2),* 118–125.

Andrade, L.N.; T.M. de Lima; R. Curi; A.M. Castrucci. Toxicity of fatty acids on murine and human melanoma cell lines. *Toxicol. In Vitro* **2005,** *19(4),* 553–560.

Angelucci, A.; S. Garofalo; S. Speca; A. Bovadilla; G.L. Gravina; P. Muzi; C. Vicentini; M. Bologna. Arachidonic acid modulates the crosstalk between prostate carcinoma and bone stromal cells. *Endocr. Relat. Cancer* **2008,** *15(1),* 91–100.

Barham, J.B.; M.B. Edens; A.N. Fonteh; M.M. Johnson; L. Easter; F.H. Chilton. Addition of eicosapentaenoic acid to gamma-linolenic acid-supplemented diets prevents serum arachidonic acid accumulation in humans. *J. Nutr.* **2000,** *130(8),* 1925–1931.

Barrera, G.; S. Pizzimenti; S. Laurora; E. Moroni; B. Giglioni; M.U. Dianzani.

4-Hydroxynonenal affects pRb/E2F pathway in HL-60 human leukemic cells. *Biochem. Biophys. Res. Commun.* **2002,** *295(2),* 267–275.

Basu, S.; A. Smedman; B. Vessby. Conjugated linoleic acid induces lipid peroxidation in humans. *FEBS Lett.* **2000,** *468(1),* 33–36.

Belury, M.A.; A. Mahon; S. Banni. The conjugated linoleic acid (CLA) isomer, t10c12-CLA, is inversely associated with changes in body weight and serum leptin in subjects with type 2 diabetes mellitus. *J. Nutr.* **2003,** *133(1),* 257S–260S.

Beppu, F.; M. Hosokawa; L. Tanaka; H. Kohno; T. Tanaka; K. Miyashita. Potent inhibitory effect of trans9, trans11 isomer of conjugated linoleic acid on the growth of human colon cancer cells. *J. Nutr. Biochem.* **2006,** *17(12),* 830–836.

Bidoli, E.; R. Talamini; A. Zucchetto; J. Polesel; C. Bosetti; E. Negri; D. Maruzzi; M. Montella; S. Franceschi; C. La Vecchia. Macronutrients, fatty acids, cholesterol and renal cell cancer risk. *Int. J. Cancer* **2008,** *122(11),* 2586–2589.

Bocca, C.; F.L. Bozzo; A. Gabriel; A. Miglietta. Conjugated linoleic acid inhibits Caco-2 cell growth via ERK-MAPK signaling pathway. *J. Nutr. Biochem.* **2007,** *18(5),* 332–340.

Chajes, V.; F. Lavilloniere; P. Ferrari; M.L. Jourdan; M. Pinualt; V. Maillard; J.L. Sebedio; P. Bougnoux. Conjugated linoleic acid content in breast adipose tissue is not associated with the relative risk of breast cancer in a population of French patients. *Cancer Epidemiol. Biomarkers Prev.* **2002**, *11,* 672–673.

Chapkin, R.S. Reappraisal of the essential fatty acids. *Fatty Acids in Foods and Their Health Implications;* Dekker: New York, NY**,** 1992; pp. 429–436.

Chin, S.F.; W. Liu; J.M. Storkson; Y.L. Ha; M.W. Pariza. Dietary sources of conjugated dienoic isomers of linolcic acid, a newly recognized class of anticarcinogens. *J. Food Comp. Anal.* **1992,** *5,* 185–197.

Cho, H.J.; W.K. Kim; J.I. Jung; E.I. Kim; S.S. Lim; D.Y. Kwon; J.H. Park. *Trans*-10,*cis*-12, not *cis*-9,*trans*-11, conjugated linoleic acid decreases ErbB3 expression in HT-29 human colon cancer cells. G1-S progression in HT-29 human colon cancer cells. *J. Nutr.* **2006,** *World J. Gastroenterol.* *11,* 5142–5150.

Cho, H.J.; E.J. Kim; S.S. Lim; M.K. Kim; M.K. Sung; J.S. Kim; J.H. Park. *Trans*-10,*cis*-12, not *cis*-9,*trans*-11, conjugated linoleic acid inhibits G1-S progression in HT-29 human colon cancer cells. *J. Nutr.* **2006,** *136(4),* 893–898.

Cho, E.; D. Spiegelman; D.J. Hunter; W.Y. Chen; M.J. Stampfer; G.A. Colditz; W.C. Willett. Premenopausal fat intake and risk of breast cancer. *J. Natl. Cancer Inst.* **2003,** *95(14),* 1079–1085.

Chow, C.K. *Fatty Acids in Foods and their Health Implications,* 3rd ed.; Taylor and Francis Group: Boca Raton, FL, **2008; pp.** 263–302.

Christie, W.W.; G. Dobson; F.D. Gunstone. Isomers in commercial samples of conjugated linoleic acid. *Lipids* **1997**, *32,* 1231.

Cimini, A.; L. Cristiano; S. Colafarina; E. Benedetti; S. Di Loreto; C. Festuccia; F. Amicarelli; R.A. Canuto; M.P. CerÃ. PPARgamma-dependent effects of conjugated linoleic acid on the human glioblastoma cell line (ADF). *Int. J. Cancer* **2005,** *117(6),* 923–933.

Close, R.N.; D.A. Schoeller; A.C. Watras; E.H. Nora. Conjugated linoleic acid supplementation alters the 6-mo change in fat oxidation during sleep. *Am. J. Clin. Nutr.* **2007,** *86(3),* 797–804.

Cohen, L.A. Breast cancer risk in rats fed a diet high in n-6 polyunsaturated fatty acids during pregnancy. *J. Natl. Cancer Inst.* **1997,** *89(9),* 662–663.

Cury-Boaventura, M.F.; C. Pompéia; R. Curi. Comparative toxicity of oleic acid and linoleic acid on Jurkat cells. *Clin. Nutr.* **2004,** *23(4),* 721–732.

Degner, S.C.; M.Q. Kemp; G.T. Bowden; D.F. Romagnolo. Conjugated linoleic acid attenuates cyclooxygenase-2 transcriptional activity via an anti-AP-1 mechanism in MCF-7 breast cancer cells. *J. Nutr.* **2006,** *136(2),* 421–427.

Degner, S.C.; M.Q. Kemp; J.K. Hockings; D.F. Romagnolo. Cyclooxygenase-2 promoter activation by the aromatic hydrocarbon receptor in breast cancer mcf-7 cells: repressive effects of conjugated linoleic acid. *Nutr. Cancer* **2007,** *59(2),* 248–257.

Dhiman, T.R.; L. Satter; M. Pariza; M. Galli; K. Albright; M. Tolosa. Conjugated linoleic acid (CLA) content of milk from cows offered diets rich in linoleic and linolenic acids. *J. Dairy Sci.* **2000,** *83,* 1016–1027.

Dijkstra, A.J.; R.J. Hamilton; W. Hamm. *Trans Fatty Acids;* Blackwell Publishing: Oxford, UK, 2008; pp. 54–101.

Dillehay, D.L.; S.K. Webb; E.M. Schmelz; A.H. Merrill, Jr. Dietary sphingomyelin inhibits 1,2-dimethylhydrazine-induced colon cancer in CF1 mice. *J. Nutr.* **1994**, *124,* 615–620.

Ding, X.Z.; W.G. Tong; T.E. Adrian. Multiple signal pathways are involved in the mitogenic effect of 5(S)-HETE in human pancreatic cancer. *Oncology* **2003,** *65(4),* 285–294.

Eyjolfson, V.; L.L. Spriet; D.J. Dyck. Conjugated linoleic acid improves insulin sensitivity in young, sedentary humans. *Med. Sci. Sports Exerc***. 2004,** *36,* 814–820.

Field, C.J.; P.D. Schley. Evidence for potential mechanisms for the effect of conjugated linoleic acid on tumor metabolism and immune function: lessons from n-3 fatty acids. *Am. J. Clin. Nutr.* **2004,** *79(Suppl. 6),* 1190S–1198S. (Review.).

Fite, A.; M. Goua; K.W. Wahle; A.C. Schofield; A.W. Hutcheon; S.D. Heys. Potentiation of the anti-tumour effect of docetaxel by conjugated linoleic acids (CLAs) in breast cancer cells in vitro. *Prostaglandins, Leukotrienes Essent. Fatty Acids* **2007,** *77(2),* 87–96.

Fritsche, J.; H. Steinhart. Analysis, occurrence, and physiological properties of *trans* fatty acids (TFA) with particular emphasis on conjugated linoleic acid isomers (CLA)—a review. *Fett-Lipid* **1998**, *100,* 190–210.

Gaullier, J.M.; G. Berven; H. Blankson; O. Gudmundsen. Clinical trial results support a preference for using CLA preparations enriched with two isomers rather than four isomers in human studies. *Lipids* **2002,** *37,* 1019–1025.

Gaullier, J.M.; J. Halse; K. Høye; K. Kristiansen; H. Fagertun; H. Vik; O. Gudmundsen. Supplementation with conjugated linoleic acid for 24 months is well tolerated by and reduces body fat mass in healthy, overweight humans. *J. Nutr.* **2005,** *135(4),* 778–784.

Gebauer, S.K.; T.L. Psota; P.M. Kris-Etherton. The diversity of health effects of individual *trans* fatty acid isomers. *Lipids* **2007,** *42(9),* 787–799. (Review)

Gunstone, F. *Fatty Acid and Lipid Chemistry;* Blackie Academic and Professional: Glasgow, UK, 1996; pp. 61–86.

Ha, Y.L.; N.K. Grimm; M.W. Pariza. Newly recognized anticarcinogenic fatty acids: identification and quantification in natural and processed cheeses. *J. Agric. Food Chem.* **1989**, *37,* 75–81.

Ha, Y.L.; J.M. Storkson; M.W. Pariza. Inhibition of benzo[a]pyrene-induced mouse forestomach neoplasia by conjugated dienoic derivatives of linoleic acid. *Cancer Res.* **1990**, *50,* 1097–1101.

Hawkins, R.A.; K. Sangster; M.J. Arends. Apoptotic death of pancreatic cancer cells induced by polyunsaturated fatty acids varies with double bond number and involves an oxidative mechanism. *J. Pathol.* **1998**, *185(1),* 61–70.

Higuchi, Y.; T. Yoshimoto. Promoting effects of polyunsaturated fatty acids on chromosomal giant DNA fragmentation associated with cell death induced by glutathione depletion. *Free Radical Res.* **2004,** *38(6),* 649–658.

Holmes, M.D.; D.J. Hunter; G.A. Colditz; M.J. Stampfer; S.E. Hankinson; F.E. Speizer; B. Rosner; W.C. Willett. Association of dietary intake of fat and fatty acids with risk of breast cancer. *JAMA* **1999,** *281(10),* 914–920.

Hrelia, S.; A. Bordoni; P. Biagi; C.A. Rossi; L. Bernardi; D.F. Horrobin; A. Pession. gamma-Linolenic acid supplementation can affect cancer cell proliferation via modification of fatty acid composition. *Biochem. Biophys. Res. Commun.* **1996,** *225(2),* 441–447.

Hubbard, N.E.; D. Lim; K.L. Erickson. Conjugated linoleic acid alters matrix metalloproteinases of metastatic mouse mammary tumor cells. *J. Nutr.* **2007,** *137(6),* 1423–1429.

Ip, C.; J.A. Scimeca; H. Thompson. Effect of timing and duration of dietary conjugated linoleic acid on mammary cancer prevention. *Nutr. Cancer* **1995**, *24,* 241–247.

Jiang, J.; L. Bjoerck; R. Fonden; M. Emanuelson. Occurrence of conjugated *cis*-9,*trans*-11-octadecadienoic acid in bovine milk: effects of feed and dietary regimen. *J. Dairy Sci.* **1996**, *79,* 438–445.

Kelley, N.S.; N.E. Hubbard; K.L. Erickson. Conjugated linoleic acid isomers and cancer. *J. Nutr.* **2007,** *137(12),* 2599–2607. (Review)

Kemp, M.Q.; B.D. Jeffy; D.F. Romagnolo. Conjugated linoleic acid inhibits cell proliferation through a p53-dependent mechanism: effects on the expression of G1-restriction points in breast and colon cancer cells. *J. Nutr.* **2003,** *133(11),* 3670–3677.

Kenny, F.S.; S.E. Pinder; I.O. Ellis; J.M. Gee; R.I. Nicholson; R.P. Bryce; J.F. Robertson. Gamma linolenic acid with tamoxifen as primary therapy in breast cancer. *Int. J. Cancer* **2000,** *85(5),* 643–648.

Kim, Y.S.; R.M. Cerbo; C.K. Hah; K.N. Bahn; J.O. Kim; Y.L. Ha. Growth inhibition of osteosarcoma cell MG-63 by a mixture of *trans,trans* conjugated linoleic acid isomers: possible mechanistic actions. *J. Food Sci.* **2008,** *73(1),* T7–15.

Kim, J.H.; N.E. Hubbard; V. Ziboh; K.L. Erickson. Attenuation of breast tumor cell growth by conjugated linoleic acid via inhibition of 5-lipoxygenase activating protein. *Biochim. Biophys. Acta* **2005a,** *1736(3),* 244–250.

Kim, J.H.; N.E. Hubbard; V. Ziboh; K.L. Erickson. Conjugated linoleic acid reduction of murine mammary tumor cell growth through 5-hydroxyeicosatetraenoic acid. *Biochim. Biophys. Acta* **2005b,** *1687(1-3),* 103–109.

Kim, E.J.; H.K. Shin; J.S. Cho; S.K. Lee; M.H. Won; J.W. Kim; J.H. Park. *trans*-10,*cis*-12 conjugated linoleic acid inhibits the G1-S cell cycle progression in DU145 human prostate carcinoma cells. *J. Med. Food* **2006,** *9(3),* 293–299.

Knekt, P.; R. Jarvinen; R. Seppanen; E. Pukkala; A Aromaa. Intake of dairy products and the risk of breast cancer. *Br. J. Cancer* **1996**, *73,* 687–691.

Kohno, H.; Y. Yasui; R. Suzuki; M. Hosokawa; K. Miyashita; T. Tanaka. Dietary seed oil rich in conjugated linolenic acid from bitter melon inhibits azoxymethane-induced rat colon carcinogenesis through elevation of colonic PPARγ expression and alteration of lipid composition. *Int. J. Cancer* **2004,** *110(6),* 896–901.

Kuhnt, K.; A. Wagner; J. Kraft; S. Basu; G. Jahreis. Dietary supplementation with 11trans- and 12trans-18:1 and oxidative stress in humans. *Am. J. Clin. Nutr.* **2006,** *84(5),* 981–988.

Kuniyasu, H. The roles of dietary PPARγ ligands for metastasis in colorectal cancer. *PPAR Res.* **2008,** 1–7 [doi:10.1155/2008/529720].

Laaksonen, D.E.; J.A. Laukkanen; L. Niskanen; K. Nyyssönen; T.H. Rissanen; S. Voutilainen; E. Pukkala; A. Hakkarainen; J.T. Salonen. Serum linoleic and total polyunsaturated fatty acids in relation to prostate and other cancers: a population-based cohort study. *Int. J. Cancer* **2004,** *111(3),* 444–450.

Lampen, A.; M. Leifheit; J. Voss; H. Nau. Molecular and cellular effects of *cis*-9, *trans*-11-conjugated linoleic acid in enterocytes: effects on proliferation, differentiation, and gene expression. *Biochim. Biophys. Acta* **2005,** *1735(1),* 30–40.

Lanson, M.; P. Bougnoux; P. Besson; J. Lansac; B. Hubert; C. Couet; O. Le Floch. *Br. J. Cancer* **1990,** *61(5),* 776–778. N-6 polyunsaturated fatty acids in human breast carcinoma phosphatidylethanolamine and early relapse.

Larsen, T.M.; S. Toubro; O. Gudmundsen; A. Astrup. Conjugated linoleic acid supplementation for 1 y does not prevent weight or body fat regain. *Am. J. Clin. Nutr.* **2006,** *83,* 606–612.

Larsson, S.C.; L. Bergkvist; A. Wolk. High-fat dairy food and conjugated linoleic acid intakes in relation to colorectal cancer incidence in the Swedish Mammography Cohort. *Am. J. Clin. Nutr.* **2005,** *82,* 894–900.

Leitzmann, M.F.; M.J. Stampfer; D.S. Michaud; K. Augustsson; G.C. Colditz; W.C. Willett; E.L. Giovannucci. Dietary intake of n-3 and n-6 fatty acids and the risk of prostate cancer. *Am. J. Clin. Nutr.* **2004,** *80(1),* 204–216.

Lemonnier, L.A.; D.L. Dillehay; M.J. Vespremi; J. Abrams; E. Brody; E.M. Schmelz. Sphingomyelin in the suppression of colon tumors: prevention versus intervention. *Arch. Biochem. Biophys.* **2003**, *419,* 129–138.

Liew, C.; H.A.J. Schut; S.F. Chin; M.W. Pariza; R.H. Dashwood. Protection of conjugated linoleic acids against 2-amio-3-methylimidazo[4,5-*f*]quinoline-induced colon carcinogenesis in the F344 rat: a study of inhibitory mechanisms. *Carcinogenesis* **1995**, *16,* 3037–3043.

Lim, D.Y.; A.L. Tyner; J.B. Park; J.Y. Lee; Y.H. Choi; J.H. Park. Inhibition of colon cancer cell proliferation by the dietary compound conjugated linoleic acid is mediated by the CDK inhibitor p21CIP1/WAF1. *J. Cell. Physiol.* **2005,** *205(1),* 107–113.

Liu, X.H.; J.M. Connolly; D.P. Rose. Eicosanoids as mediators of linoleic acid-stimulated invasion and type IVcollagenase production by a metastatic human breast cancer cell line. *Clin. Exp. Metastasis* **1996,** *14(2),* 145–152.

Lock, A.L.; B.A. Corl; D.M. Barbano; D.E. Bauman; C. Ip. The anticarcinogenic effect of *trans*-11 18:1 is dependent on its conversion to *cis*-9, *trans*-11 CLA by delta9-desaturase in rats. *J. Nutr.* **2004,** *134(10),* 2698–2704.

MacDonald, H.B. Conjugated linoleic acid and disease prevention: a review of current knowledge. *J. Am. Coll. Nutr.* **2000**, *19,* 111–118S.

Maggiora, M.; M. Bologna; M.P. CerÃ; L. Possati; A. Angelucci; A. Cimini; A. Miglietta; F. Bozzo; C. Margiotta; G. Muzio; R.A. Canuto. An overview of the effect of linoleic and conjugated-linoleic acids on the growth of several human tumor cell lines. *Int. J. Cancer* **2004,** *112(6),* 909–919.

McCann, S.E.; C. Ip; M.M. Ip; M.K. McGuire; P. Muti; S.B. Edge; M. Trevisan; J.L. Freudenheim. Dietary intake of conjugated linoleic acids and risk of premenopausal and postmenopausal breast cancer, Western New York Exposures and Breast Cancer Study (WEB Study). *Cancer Epidemiol. Biomarkers Prev.* **2004**, *13,* 1480–1484.

Menendez, J.A.; R. Colomer; R. Lupu. Omega-6 polyunsaturated fatty acid gamma-linolenic acid (18:3n-6) is a selective estrogen-response modulator in human breast cancer cells: gamma-linolenic acid antagonizes estrogen receptor-dependent transcriptional activity, transcriptionally represses estrogen receptor expression and synergistically enhances tamoxifen and ICI 182,780 (Faslodex) efficacy in human breast cancer cells. *Int. J. Cancer* **2004,** *109(6),* 949–954.

Meng, X.; S.F. Shoemaker; S.O. McGee; M.M. Ip. t10,c12-Conjugated linoleic acid stimulates mammary tumor progression in Her2/ErbB2 mice through activation of both proliferative and survival pathways. *Carcinogenesis* **2008,** *29(5),*1013–1021.

Miglietta, A.; F. Bozzo; C. Bocca; L. Gabriel; A. Trombetta; S. Belotti; R.A. Canuto. Conjugated linoleic acid induces apoptosis in MDA-MB-231 breast cancer cells through ERK/MAPK signalling and mitochondrial pathway. *Cancer Lett.* **2006,** *234(2),* 149–157.

Moloney, F.; T.P. Yeow; A. Mullen; J.J. Nolan; H.M. Roche. Conjugated linoleic acid supplementation, insulin sensitivity, and lipoprotein metabolism in patients with type 2 diabetes mellitus. *Am. J. Clin. Nutr.* **2004,** *80(4),*887–895.

Murphy, E.F.; G.J. Hooiveld; M. Muller; R.A. Calogero; K.D. Cashman. Conjugated linoleic acid alters global gene expression in human intestinal-like Caco-2 cells in an isomer-specific manner. *J. Nutr.* **2007,** *137(11),* 2359–2365.

Nkondjock, A.; B. Shastenstein; P. Maisonneuve; P. Ghadirian. Specific fatty acids and human colorectal cancer: an overview. *Cancer Detect. Prev.* **2003**, *27,* 55–66.

Norat, T.; E. Riboli. Dairy products and colorectal cancer. A review of possible mechanisms and epidemiological evidence. *Eur. J. Clin. Nutr.* **2003**, *57,* 1–17.

Ou, L.; Y. Wu; C. Ip; X. Meng; Y.C. Hsu; M.M. Ip. Apoptosis induced by t10,c12-conjugated linoleic acid is mediated by an atypical endoplasmic reticulum stress response. *J. Lipid Res.* **2008,** *49(5),* 985–994.

Pariza, M.W. Perspective on the safety and effectiveness of conjugated linoleic acid. *Am. J. Clin. Nutr.* **2004,** *79(Suppl. 6),* 1132S–1136S.

Pariza, M.W.; W.A. Hargraves. A beef-derived mutagenesis modulator inhibits initiation of mouse epidermal tumors by 7,12-dimethylbenz[a]anthracene. *Carcinogenesis* **1985**, *6,* 591–593.

Park, H.S.; H.Y. Cho; Y.L. Ha; J.H. Park. Dietary conjugated linoleic acid increases the mRNA ratio of Bax/Bcl-2 in the colonic mucosa of rats. *J. Nutr. Biochem.* **2004**, *15,* 229–235.

Polesel, J.; R. Talamini; M. Montella; L.D. Maso; M. Crovatto; M. Parpinel; F. Izzo; L.G. Tommasi; D. Serraino; C. La Vecchia; S. Franceschi. Nutrients intake and the risk of hepatocellular carcinoma in Italy. *Eur. J. Cancer* **2007,** *43(16),* 2381–2387.

Prentic, R.L.; B. Caan; R.T. Chlebowski; R. Patterson; L.H. Kuller; J.K. Ockene; K.L. Margolis; M.C. Limacher; J.E. Manson; L.M. Parker; et al. Low-fat dietary pattern and risk of invasive breast cancer: the Women's Health Initiative Randomized Controlled Dietary Modification Trial. *JAMA* **2006,** *295(6),* 629–642.

Raff, M.; T. Tholstrup; S. Basu; P. Nonboe; M.T. Sørensen; E.M. Straarup. A diet rich in conjugated linoleic acid and butter increases lipid peroxidation but does not affect atherosclerotic, inflammatory, or diabetic risk markers in healthy young men. *J. Nutr.* **2008,** *138(3),* 509–514.

Risérus, U.; S. Basu; S. Jovinge; G.N. Fredrikson; J. Arnlöv; B. Vessby. Supplementation with conjugated linoleic acid causes isomer-dependent oxidative stress and elevated C-reactive protein: a potential link to fatty acid-induced insulin resistance. *Circulation* **2002,** *106(15),* 1925–1929.

Riserus, U.; B. Vessby; J. Arnlov; S. Basu. Effects of *cis*-9,*trans*-11 conjugated linoleic acid supplementation on insulin sensitivity, lipid peroxidation, and proinflammatory markers in obese men. *Am. J. Clin. Nutr.* **2004,** *80,* 279–283.

Rose, D.P.; J.M. Connolly. Omega-3 fatty acids as cancer chemopreventive agents. *Pharmacol. Ther.* **1999,** *83(3),* 217–244.

Rose, D.P.; M.A. Hatala; J.M. Connolly; J. Rayburn. Effect of diets containing different levels of linoleic acid on human breast cancer growth and lung metastasis in nude mice. *Cancer Res.* **1993,** *53(19),* 4686–4690.

Sauer, L.A.; D.E. Blask; R.T. Dauchy. Dietary factors and growth and metabolism in experimental tumors. *J. Nutr. Biochem.* **2007,** *18(10),* 637–649. (Review.)

Sauer, L.A.; R.T. Dauchy; D.E. Blask. Mechanism for the antitumor and anticachectic effects of n-3 fatty acids. *Cancer Res.* **2000**, *60,* 5289–5295.

Sauer, L.A.; R.T. Dauchy; D.E. Blask; J.A. Krause; L.K. Davidson; E.M. Dauchy; K.J. Welham; K. Coupland. Conjugated linoleic acid isomers and *trans* fatty acids inhibit fatty acid transport in hepatoma 7288CTC and inguinal fat pads in Buffalo rats. *J. Nutr.* **2004,** *134,* 1989–1997.

Schønberg, S.; H.E. Krokan. The inhibitory effect of conjugated dienoic derivatives (CLA) of linoleic acid on the growth of human tumor cell lines is in part due to increased lipid peroxidation. *Anticancer Res.* **1995,** *15(4),* 1241–1246.

Sehat, N.; M.P. Yurawecz; J.A. Roach; M.M. Mossoba; J.K. Kramer; Y. Ku. Silver-ion high performance liquid chromatographic separation and identification of conjugated linoleic acid isomers. *Lipids* **1998**, *33,* 217–221.

Shantha, N.C.; A.D. Crum; E.A. Decker. Evaluation of conjugated linoleic acid concentrations in cooked beef. *J. Agric. Food Chem.* **1994**, *42,* 1757–1760.

Shantha, N.C.; E.A. Decker. Conjugated linoleic acid concentrations in processed cheese containing hydrogen donors, iron and dairy based additives. *Food Chem.* **1993**, *47,* 257–261.

Soel, S.M.; O.S. Choi; M.H. Bang; J.H. Yoon Park; W.K. Kim. Influence of conjugated linoleic acid isomers on the metastasis of colon cancer cells in vitro and in vivo. *J. Nutr. Biochem.* **2007,** *18(10),* 650–657.

Song, H.J.; I. Grant; D. Rotondo; I. Mohede; N. Sattar; S.D. Heys; K.W. Wahle. Effect of CLA supplementation on immune function in young healthy volunteers. *Eur. J. Clin. Nutr.* **2005,** *59(4),* 508–517.

Stanton, C.; F. Lawless; G. Kjellmer; D. Harrington; R. Devery; J.F. Connolly; J. Murphy. Dietary influences on Bovine milk *cis*-9,*trans*-11-conjugated linoleic acid content. *J. Food Sci.* **1997**, *62,* 1083–1086.

Stipanuk, M.H. *Biochemical, Physiological, & Molecular Aspects of Human Nutrition;* 2nd ed.; Saunders Elsevier: St. Louis, MO, 2006; pp. 518–540.

Terry, P.D.; T.E. Rohan; A. Wolk. Intake of fish and marine fatty acids and the risks of cancers of the breast and prostate and of other hormone-related cancers: a review of the epidemiologic evidence. *Am. J. Clin. Nutr.* **2003,** *77,* 532–543.

Theodoratou, E.; G. McNeill; R. Cetnarskyj; S.M. Farrington; A. Tenesa; R. Barnetson; M. Porteous; M. Dunlop; H. Campbell. Dietary fatty acids and colorectal cancer: a case-control study. *Am. J. Epidemiol.* **2007**, *166,* 181–195.

Thompson, H.; Z.J. Zhu; S. Banni; K. Darcy; T. Loftus; C. Ip. Morphological and biochemical status of the mammary gland as influenced by conjugated linoleic acid: implication for a reduction in mammary cancer risk. *Cancer Res.* **1997,** *57,* 5067–5072.

Tsuzuki, T.; M. Igarashi; T. Miyazawa. Conjugated eicosapentaenoic acid (EPA) inhibits transplanted tumor growth via membrane lipid peroxidation in nude mice. *J. Nutr.* **2004,** *134(5),* 1162–1166.

Voorrips, L.E.; H.A. Brants; A.F. Kardinaal; G.J. Hiddink; P.A. van den Brandt; R.A. Goldbohm. Intake of conjugated linoleic acid, fat, and other fatty acids in relation to postmenopausal breast cancer: the Netherlands Cohort Study on Diet and Cancer. *Am. J. Clin. Nutr.* **2002**, *76,* 873–882.

Wahle, K.W.; S.D. Heys; D. Rotondo. Conjugated linoleic acids: are they beneficial or detrimental to health? *Prog. Lipid Res.* **2004,** *43(6),* 553–587. (Review).

Wang, D.; F.G. Buchanan; H. Wang; S.K. Dey; R.N. DuBois. Prostaglandin E2 enhances intestinal adenoma growth via activation of the Ras-mitogen-activated protein kinase cascade. *Cancer Res.* **2005,** *65(5),* 1822–1829.

Wang, J.; E.M. John; P.L Horn-Ross; S.A. Ingles. Dietary fat, cooking fat, and breast cancer risk in a multiethnic population. *Nutr. Cancer* **2008,** *60(4),* 492–504.

Watkins, G.; T.A. Martin; R. Bryce; R.E. Mansel; W.G. Jiang. Gamma-Linolenic acid regulates the expression and secretion of SPARC in human cancer cells. *Prostaglandins Leukotrienes Essent. Fatty Acids* **2005,** *72(4),* 273–278.

Weijenberg, M.P.; M. Lüchtenborg; A.F. de Goeij; M. Brink; G.N. van Muijen; A.P. de Bruïne; R.A. Goldbohm; P.A. van den Brandt. Dietary fat and risk of colon and rectal cancer with aberrant MLH1 expression, APC or KRAS genes. *Cancer Causes Control* **2007,** *18(8),* 865–879.

Whigham, L.D.; M. O'Shea; I.C. Mohede; H.P. Walaski; R.L. Atkinson. Safety profile of conjugated linoleic acid in a 12-month trial in obese humans. *Food Chem. Toxicol.* **2004,** *42(10),* 1701–1709.

Whigham, L.D.; A.C. Watras; D.A. Schoeller. Efficacy of conjugated linoleic acid for reducing fat mass: a meta-analysis in humans. *Am. J. Clin. Nutr.* **2007,** *85(5),* 1203–1211.

Ziboh, V.A.; C.C. Miller; Y. Cho. Metabolism of polyunsaturated fatty acids by skin epidermal enzymes: generation of antiinflammatory and antiproliferative metabolites. *Am. J. Clin. Nutr.* **2000,** *71(Suppl. 1),* 361S–366S.

# 20

# Effects of Dietary Fatty Acids on Human Microbes: Role in Health

**Edward R. Farnworth[1], Delphine Sène[1,2], and Claude P. Champagne[1]**
[1]*Food Research and Development Centre, Agriculture and Agri-Food Canada; 3600 Casavant West, St. Hyacinthe, QC, J2S 8E3 Canada;* [2]*Graduate student, Laval University, Quebec City, QC, G1K 7P4, Canada*

## Introduction

Food that is consumed passes down through the gastrointestinal tract (GIT), where it is digested and absorbed. Any undigested food is voided from the body. Many researchers have held this simplified view of nutrition and digestion for a long time.

But in fact, fully one-third of fecal matter is composed of bacteria (Goldin, 2003). Thus, microbiologists and some nutritionists increasingly understand that the GIT is inhabited by a large number, and a large variety, of microorganisms (bacteria) that play an important role in the host's digestion, immune function, disease resistance, health, and well-being. To live, grow, reproduce, and carry out metabolic functions, these bacteria digest and consume food as it passes down the GIT. Like their host, the endogenous bacteria have nutrient requirements. However, when one looks at the lipid requirements of bacteria, in general, they are often not well-defined. This may be due to the fact that the methodologies to define the lipid requirements of bacteria are difficult, in part, because of the very small quantities of lipid found in the bacterial cell, and because of the ability of the bacteria to produce lipids de novo.

This chapter describes three aspects of the interrelations between fatty acids (FA), the GIT flora, and human health: (i) what is known about the lipid requirements of bacteria and, in particular, the role that dietary FAs play on the GIT microbiota, (ii) how GIT bacteria modify lipids critical in FA metabolism, and (iii) clinical trials that show how changes in the dietary fat content impact the gut microbiota and how this, in turn, influences the health and well-being of the host.

## The Human Intestinal Microflora

### *Composition*

The human GIT system contains over 400 bacterial species and is therefore quite complex (Bauer et al., 2006; Goldin, 2003). A picture of what are believed to be the main species is provided in Table 20.1. Obviously, the genera evolve as a function of the location along the GIT, and the microbiota gradually shift from facultative anaerobic organisms to strict anaerobes.

**Table 20.1. Major Bacterial Groups in the Human Gastrointestinal Tract of Adults (Bourlioux, 1994; Goldin, 2003)**

| Region | Genera or group | Estimated population (number per mL of content) |
|---|---|---|
| Mouth and pharynx | *Streptococcus* | |
| | *Staphylococcus* | |
| | *Veillonella* | |
| Stomach | Total | $10^2$ |
| | *Streptococcus* | $10^1 - 10^2$ |
| | *Lactobacillus* | $10^1 - 10^2$ |
| Duodenum - jejunum | Total (dominant = facultative) | $10^4 - 10^6$ |
| | *Streptococcus / Enterococcus* | $10^2 - 10^4$ |
| | *Lactobacillus* | $10^2 - 10^4$ |
| | *Veillonella* | $10^2 - 10^4$ |
| Ileum— Cecum | Total (dominant = anaerobic) | $10^8$ |
| | *Bacteroides* | $10^4 - 10^8$ |
| | *Lactobacillus* | |
| | *Clostridium* | |
| | *Streptococcus / Enterococcus* | |
| | *Enterobacteriacae Bifidobacterium* | |
| Colon—Feces | Total (anaerobic >99%) | Almost $10^{12}$ |
| | *Bacteroides* | $10^{10} - 10^{11}$ |
| | *Peptococcus* | $10^{10} - 10^{11}$ |
| | *Eubacterium* | $10^{10} - 10^{11}$ |
| | *Bifidobacterium* | $10^9 - 10^{11}$ |
| | *Clostridium* | $10^{10}$ |
| | *Streptococcus / Enterococcus* | $10^9 - 10^{10}$ |
| | *Lactobacillus* | $10^6 - 10^8$ |
| | *Enterobacteriacae* | $10^7$ |

Unfortunately, this picture might, in fact, be imprecise. Indeed, comparison between microscopic plate counts and hybridization techniques indicates that a significant fraction of the microbiota can escape cultivation using traditional selective media techniques (Konstantinov et al., 2002). Genomic analyses are very useful in filling this knowledge gap, but they nevertheless have limits. Indeed, comparative genomics require well-studied, defined isolates and genetic sequences, which are unavailable because many microbes are not yet isolated.

The microbiota evolve with age. Only 48 hours after birth, the GIT contains a population of between $10^9$ and $10^{10}$ CFU/gram (Bourlioux, 1994). The effect of diet on the microbiota composition is more easily observed during these early years because diet is initially milk-based and a major change occurs at weaning. Newborns, particularly breastfed children, have a bacterial population mainly composed of bifidobacteria, presumably because of the high content of oligosaccharides and other selective ingredients (e.g., lysozyme) in human milk. This flora evolves (Bauer et al., 2006), and between the ages of 2 and 4 it starts to resemble an adult microbiota. As the diet shifts to include cereals, fruits, vegetables, and meats, the *Bacteroides* and *Eubacterium* genera become the main occupants (Table 20.1). Much later in life, the fecal microbiota of the elderly show increased *Lactobacillus, Clostridium,* and *Enterobacter* populations with a concomitant decrease in *Bifidobacterium* (Goldin, 2003).

In addition to the location within the GIT and the age, numerous other parameters influence the GIT ecology: antibiotics, host genotype, GIT disorders, disease states, surgery, radiation treatment, and diet. The goal of this chapter is to focus on the latter.

## Effect of Diet

Bacteria have very variable growth needs, and foods show a wide range of pH and chemical or nutrient composition. Therefore, one assumes that diet would strongly influence bacterial populations in the GIT, as is observed with food-spoilage floras. Dietary studies indicate that food matrices modify some bacterial populations but that wide-ranging and long-term shifts in the composition of the microbiota do not occur. Thus, one study comparing a Western-style diet and a Japanese traditional diet showed that the subjects on the Japanese diet had higher counts in some enterococci, lactobacilli, bifidobacteria, and eubacteria species while having lower counts in *Bacteroides* and *Clostridium* (Rasic, 2003). However, another study reported that shifting from an omnivorous to a vegetarian diet did not induce changes in the predominant organisms in the fecal flora (Goldin, 2003). The Japanese diet had less fat, but to what extent this affected results remains to be ascertained. These data suggest that other factors combine with diet to influence the GIT microbiota.

Many foods, such as canned or heated products, contain very low bacterial populations as they enter the GIT. Furthermore, foods contain aerobic organisms that are not subsequently found in the feces. Therefore, foods are not the sole source of microorganisms that will eventually inhabit the GIT. Indeed, ingested food is constantly inoculated by cells adhered to the intestinal walls or to the mucus. This constant inoculation system partially explains the microbiota stability. Consequently, the importance of the ability of bacteria to adhere to GIT walls seems critical in modulating the GIT microbiota (Bourlioux, 1994). This justifies the studies carried out on the effect of FAs on the adhesion of probiotic bacteria to GIT components, which is detailed later.

Do FAs in the form of triglycerides affect bacterial growth? The presence of milk fat in yogurt may affect the growth of the starter cultures, but this is often in combination with processing steps (Lanciotti et al., 2004). The limited effect of triglycerides on the growth of lactic acid bacteria (LAB) is linked to the fact that these cultures generally do not have high lipolytic activities (Cagno et al., 2006; Hickey et al., 2007). However, in the GIT, FAs are released by pancreatic lipases, and numerous studies show that free FAs can be stimulatory or highly inhibitory to bacterial growth as a function of the type and concentration of the FA (Partanen et al., 2001). The effect of such free FAs on probiotic bacteria is further addressed later. Nevertheless, fat hydrolysis has the potential of strongly influencing the mortality or the growth of GIT microbiota. FAs released by the digestion of neutral fats in milk can damage bacteria by disrupting their cell membranes and thus exert antiviral, antibacterial, and antiprotozoal activity (Bauer et al., 2006). A few studies on the effects of FAs on microbiota of single-stomach species were reviewed by Bauer et al. (2006) and show the effects of fat on the microbiota. In humans, however, most of the FAs are absorbed in the intestine (Goldin, 2003). Therefore, the effect of the FAs on the GIT microbiota might principally occur on populations in the small intestine and not be as significant in the colon.

## FAs and the Growth of Some GIT Bacteria

Most of the organic matter of the bacterial cell consists of macromolecules that belong to four classes: nucleic acids, proteins, polysaccharides, and complex lipids. Lipids are a class of cell constituents that include triglycerides, phospholipids, steroids, isoprenoids, and poly-β-hydroxybutyrate. They have different functions such as energy reserve material (poly-β-hydroxybutyrate), membrane constituents (phospholipids and glycolipids), or components of the lipopolysaccharide wall layer, the last two being their main functions. Unlike the three other classes of macromolecules, complex lipids are more variable and heterogeneous in composition; their precursors include FAs, polyalcohols, simple sugars, amines, and amino acids (Stanier et al., 1986).

### *FA Biosynthesis*

Different FAs in bacteria contain different numbers of carbon atoms (most of them containing an even number of carbon atoms), are straight-chained or branched, and they may or may not contain double bonds, -OH groups, and cyclopropane rings. Although polyunsaturated FAs (PUFAs) are common constituents of the lipids of eukaryotes, they are less frequent among prokaryotes (Stanier et al, 1986).

The study of the membrane lipids of *Escherichia coli* and *Salmonella typhimurium* has contributed greatly to our understanding of the synthesis and functions of bacterial membrane lipids in general. In addition to all the other advantages of studying these organisms, their lipid composition is among the simplest found in biology (Cronan & Rock, 1987).

The enzymes of lipid biosynthesis are distributed between the cytosol and the inner membrane (Cronan & Rock, 1987). FAs are synthesized separately and esterified to form complex lipids. One can discuss the reactions of their synthesis in terms of initiation reaction, elongation reaction, and product diversification. The precursors for FA biosynthesis are derived from the acetyl coenzyme A (CoA) pool, and a protein known as "acyl carrier protein" (ACP) plays a vital role by acting as an acetyl group carrier. ACP is a small protein (MW 10,000) that is functionally and chemically analogous to CoA. In the initiation reaction, the formation of long-chain FAs starts with the transfer of an acetyl group from CoA to ACP by the action of acetyl transacylase. This is the only step in which an acetate unit is directly used in FA biosynthesis (Cronan & Rock, 1987; Stanier et al., 1986). The acetyl–ACP complex that is formed serves as an acceptor to which successive $C_2$ units are transferred during the elongation reaction; the $C_2$ donor is malonyl-ACP. The product of $C_2$ transfer carries a terminal acetyl group, which in subsequent reactions is sequentially reduced, dehydrated, and reduced again, yielding an unsaturated acyl–ACP complex with two additional carbon atoms. Repetitions of this set of reactions progressively lengthen the FA chain until the length that is characteristic of the particular bacterium (usually $C_{14}$ to $C_{18}$) is reached (Stanier et al., 1986). During product diversification reactions, a specific dehydrase enzyme catalyzes a key reaction at the point at which the biosynthesis of unsaturated FAs diverges from that of saturated FAs (Cronan & Rock, 1987).

## Beneficial Effects of FAs on Probiotic Bacteria

Very few studies were made on the role of FAs in the nutrition of microorganisms. In his review, Nieman (1954) reports the growth-stimulating effect of FAs in three ways.

First, FAs are required as essential growth factors for bacteria (Das, 2002). In this case, the FA acts as an indispensable growth factor with the medium containing all other known growth factors for the microorganism. This essential function of FAs was demonstrated with several *Lactobacteriaceae* as well as several other organisms (Nieman, 1954). As an example, Partanen et al. (2001) showed that strains of *Lactobacillus delbrueckii* needed an external source of unsaturated FAs like oleic acid ($C_{18:1}$) as essential growth factors. It is now well-known that oleic acid is incorporated into the membranes of LAB grown in medium supplemented with Tween 80 (polyoxyethylene-sorbitan-mon-oleate), a water-soluble derivative of oleic acid. The addition of Tween 80 to the growth medium enhances the growth of many LAB, and Tween 80 is therefore added in the growth medium of lactobacilli [e.g., the standard De Man Rogosa Sharpe (MRS) medium (de Man et al., 1960)]. In the previously mentioned study (Partanen et al., 2001), only one of the six strains studied could grow in modified MRS medium lacking any FA supplement. Johnsson et al. (1995) compared the cellular FA profile of 10 strains of lactobacilli grown on MRS medium with and without Tween 80. They observed that the main cellular FAs detected in the strains examined were myristic (C14:0), palmitic (C16:0), hexadecenoic (C16:1), stearic (C18:0), oleic, *cis*-vaccenic, dihydrosterculic (C19:0; *cis*-9,10-methyleneoctadecanoic), and lactobacillic (C19:0; *cis*-11,12-methyleneoctadecanoic) acids. Strains cultivated without Tween 80 lacked oleic and dihydrosterculic acids among the cellular FAs, which indicates that oleic acid was not synthesized by these strains. Prior to these studies, authors also reported the requirements for FAs by certain rumen bacteria belonging to *Borellia* and *Bacteroides* species (Wegner & Foster, 1960).

Secondly, without being essential, FA can simply increase bacterial growth rates. This is not unusual, since bacteria act in the same fashion in the presence of amino acids, vitamins, and nucleotides.

Thirdly, FA can act as a biotin substitute. Apparently, when biotin is totally absent from the medium, various unsaturated FAs can take over its function. This biotin-like activity was demonstrated by oleic, elaidic vaccenic, linoleic, and linolenic acids on bacterial strains such as *Lactobacillus casei* and *Lactobacillus arabinosus* (Nieman, 1954).

## *Detrimental Effect of FAs on the Microbiota*

Lipids can also inhibit bacterial growth. Their bactericidal activity depends on their nature (e.g., chain length, saturation, stereochemistry of the double bond, their concentration) and on the bacterial strain involved.

In a comparative study of the effect of ten human milk FAs on bacterial growth, the four bifidobacteria strains studied were more inhibited than the gram-negative *E. coli* and *S. typhimurium*. During a general observation, the growth of bifidobacteria decreased with the increase of FA concentration (Powell & May, 1981). Although this suggests that gram-positive bacteria could be more sensitive to FAs than gram-negative bacteria, FA-sensitive gram-negative bacteria were recently described, and a diversity of responses is observed among species and strains.

Researchers reported that certain strains of *Lactococcus lactis* can use large amounts of oleic acid during their growth, while other strains of lactococci and lactobacilli are inhibited by this FA. Those authors showed that mixed starters used for the production of sour creams, *Streptococcus thermophilus* and *Lactobacillus delbrueckii* ssp. *bulgaricus*, are inhibited by capric acid. This FA also inhibits the proteolytic activity of certain strains of *Lc. lactis* or *Lb. bulgaricus*. The inhibition effect of FA on the growth of streptococci, lactobacilli, and *Leuconostoc* was also reported (Desmazaud, 1983). *Salmonella typhimurium* is unaffected by 10 ppm of a mixture of FA, but growth is hindered by values above 100 ppm (Kulshrestha & Marth, 1975). On the other hand, Sprong et al. (2001) showed bactericidal effects of milk FAs on the following pathogen bacteria (among which we can find gram-positive and gram-negative bacteria): *Campylobacter jejuni*, *S. enteritidis*, *E. coli* O:157:H7, *Clostridium perfringens,* and *Listeria monocytogenes*. Results showed that, within concentrations used, short-chain FAs and saturated $C_{18}$ were not bactericidal. Predominantly medium-chain and unsaturated $C_{18}$ FAs were bactericidal, whereas $C_{10:0}$ and $C_{12:0}$ were toxic to all of the test pathogens. Since the FA concentrations tested were in the range of those found in human intestinal juice (since digestion cleaves FAs from triglycerides), their result suggests that $C_{10:0}$ and $C_{12:0}$ liberated during digestion of milk fat may affect gastrointestinal infections. Indeed, providing a mixture of triglycerides and a lipase active in the gastric environment significantly reduced the lactobacilli and *E. coli* flora in the gastric and duodenum environment by a factor of 10 in canulated pigs (Dierick et al., 2002). These data suggest that the rapid release of FA in the GIT can indeed modify the microbiota and help prevent bacterial infections of the GIT of farm animals. This approach could be very useful in animal production practices to reduce the use of antibiotics, but could also find applications in human medicine.

The nature of the FA has an important impact on its antibacterial properties. Saturated and unsaturated FAs have different antimicrobial properties, and, in general, the bactericidal activity increases with chain length and unsaturation. However, saturated FAs can also act as growth inhibitors, the bacteriostatic properties being optimal at chain lengths around 12 carbons (Nieman, 1954).

The importance of the unsaturation of FAs with respect to growth-promoting ability for bacteria is evidenced by the fact that the stimulating effect decreases with an increase in the number of double bonds (Nieman, 1954). In vitro studies showed that PUFAs at very low concentrations ($10^{-5}$ mol) have a very strong bactericidal effect on a total colonic flora and on *Bacteroides fragilis* in pure culture. On the other hand, EPA (eicosapentanoic acid, an ester of PUFA of marine origin), in the form of the ethyl-ester (7 g/L), inhibits the growth of *Bacteroides thetaiotaomicron*, a dominant species of the normal flora of healthy humans, while *E. coli* are resistant to concentrations up to 100 g/L of that same FA (Juste, 2005).

Stereochemical structure of unsaturated FAs, moreover, influences the growth stimulation of microorganisms. Compounds with *cis*-configuration seem to be more active than the corresponding *trans*-isomers (Endo et al., 2006; Nieman, 1954). A study on the role of position, configuration, and number of double bonds in the FA on the growth of five *Lactobacillus* strains showed that conjugated linoleic and stearic acids having *trans* double bonds were able to promote the growth of the lactobacili at all concentrations. However, their results also suggested that only linoleic and α-linolenic acids with *cis* double bonds could promote growth at low concentrations, but not at high concentrations (Endo et al., 2006). The authors also obtained results showing a stimulating effect of *trans*-rich free FA, regardless of the different positions of double bonds and carbon chain length. This last result is of interest since *trans* FAs are associated with coronary heart disease: their excessive intake is unfavorable for human health.

Fernandez-Lopez et al. (2005) described a high-throughput assay that allowed them to identify unsaturated FAs (oleic and linoleic acids) as inhibitors of bacterial conjugation in *E. coli* strains. Since conjugation is largely responsible for multiple antibiotic resistances in human pathogens, these results suggest that conjugation inhibitors may provide a means to control the spread of antibiotic resistance.

## Dietary Fat and Health

A review of the scientific literature reveals that surprisingly very few clinical studies are reported describing the effects of dietary fat or FAs on the intestinal microbiota and the resulting impact on the host's health (Bauer et al., 2006). The relatively abundant literature on the effect of FAs on bacteria suggests many potential effects on health via the GIT. However, it is difficult to attempt to correlate in vitro data with in vivo studies. One reason is that the GIT is a very rich and dynamic system where digestion, hydrolysis, and absorption reactions happen at the same time. The microorganisms are in contact with the ingested and partially digested food as well as a mixture of digestive agents (enzymes, biles salts, etcetera). In vivo studies with humans can be invasive, but more of them are necessary to confirm the results obtained in vitro and their applications.

Generally, under normal physiological conditions in humans, digestion and absorption of dietary lipids are very efficient. Lipid reaching the colon (5–8 g/day) comes from the diet, from endogenous sources (e.g., sloughed cells), and from intestinal bacteria. Thus, various lipids, including FAs, may be available to intestinal bacteria. By all estimates, although the concentration of free FAs in milk is approximately 1 µg $mL^{-1}$, the action of lipases could increase this to over 400 µg $mL^{-1}$ (Kankaanpää et al., 2001). Lipid that is not absorbed in the proximal small intestine is utilized or absorbed in the colon; fecal material generally is low in fat (Carey & Hernell, 1992; Juste, 2005).

As detailed already, the free FAs that are liberated during the digestive process interact with the resident bacteria in two major ways: (i) stimulatory, bacteriostatic, and antibacterial properties (Boyaval et al., 1995; Kankaanpää et al., 2001) and (ii) incorporation into the bacterial membranes, thereby changing cell membrane characteristics and function (Jenkins & Courtney, 2003).

In either case, this interaction between dietary fat may alter the makeup of the population of bacteria and/or their metabolic activity (see Fig. 20.1).

## *Dietary Fat and Cancer*

The area of research that has received the most attention is the role that dietary fat plays on the development of colon cancer, and how the intestinal microbiota may be contributing to this effect (Goldin, 1986; Hambly et al., 1977).

Early epidemiological studies comparing data from different countries (including from Europe, America, Asia, Oceania, and Africa) reported that total fat, meat, and animal protein intake were positively correlated with both colon and rectum cancer in both men and women (Armstrong & Doll, 1975; Drasar & Irving, 1973). At the same time, researchers were showing that the diet affected the makeup of the population of intestinal bacteria (Reddy et al., 1975). Several studies were soon published that attempted to show some characteristic of the gut bacterial population that could be linked to the onset of colon cancer. Reasonably, the activity of some bacterial enzymes such as β-glucuronidase, azoreductase, and nitroreductase could result in the production of mutagens and carcinogens in the gut, and that cancer could be the long-term consequence. However, these enzymes are mainly linked to the bioconversions of carbohydrate or nitrogenous compounds and not of FA. Therefore, an effect of FAs on these three enzyme levels could only be indirect. Goldin & Gorbach (1976) did show that, in rats, changing from a grain-based diet to a meat-based (cooked and juices discarded) diet did cause 1.5- to 2.5-fold increases in the activities of these target enzymes. However, few studies were reported in humans where the effects of dietary fat, per se, on fecal enzyme activity were measured. Cummings et al. (1978) reported no effect on the β-glucuronidase activity in six subjects when they consumed a diet with either a low (62 g/day) or a high (152 g/day) animal fat content. They found no changes in the bacterial makeup (seven different bacteria) of fecal samples obtained during the feeding periods of the two fat levels. Sugawara et al. (1992) reported a similar lack of effect on the microbiota population (13 bacterial groups) and enzyme activity (β-glucuronidase, β-glucosidase, nitroreductase) in Japanese subjects fed a high-fat, low dietary fiber diet. Supplementing a low-fat or a high-fat diet (30% versus 50% energy from fat) with fish oil or corn oil (4.4 g/day n-3 fatty acids versus 4.4 n-6 FAs/day) also had no effect on fecal enzyme activity (Bartram et al., 1996).

A second hypothesis was suggested that links dietary fat, the gut microbiota, and colon cancer (Hill et al., 1971; McGarr et al., 2005). Bile acids are excreted into the intestinal lumen to carry out the digestion and absorption of dietary cholesterol, fat-soluble vitamins, and lipids. Normally, about 95% of the bile acids then return to the liver via the enterohepatic circulation system. Bile acids that are not recycled pass down into the colon where they are metabolized into secondary bile acids such as deoxycholic acid and lithocholic acid by bacteria in the genus *Clostridium* (Doerner et al., 1997). Secondary bile acids were shown to be carcinogenic (Hamada et al., 1994; Zusman et al., 1992). These observations were made: populations with a high incidence of colon cancer had increased concentrations of certain possible cancer-causing metabolites such as sterols and bile acids (Reddy & Wynder, 1973); subjects with colon cancer had high levels of certain fecal constituents (Reddy & Wynder, 1977); and increasing dietary fat increases some bile acids in fecal material (Cummings et al., 1978; Reddy et al., 1975) These led to the conclusion that the production of secondary bile salts in the colon may explain the relationship between dietary fat consumption and colon cancer. However, supplementing a high- or low-fat diet with corn oil or fish oil had no effect on fecal bile acid concentrations (Bartram et al., 1996).

Notably, the initial international comparisons of cancer incidence and diet patterns may have included confounding variables such as the intake of red meat and animal protein and the possibility of other lifestyle factors such as smoking and exercise that affected the interpretation of results linking dietary fat and colon cancer. This has led some to question if, in fact, the consumption of dietary fat is as important a factor in cancer statistics as originally proposed (Wakai et al., 2006; Willet, 1990, 1998, 2001). However, the intake of a Western-type diet (high in fat, cholesterol, red meat, processed foods; low in fruits, vegetables, poultry, and fish), dietary fat in general and particular FAs, continues to be quoted as a possible causal factor in the etiology of colon cancer, and its recurrence after diagnosis (Meyerhardt et al., 2007; Oba et al., 2006; Sharma & O'Keefe, 2007; You et al., 2002).

## *Diet, Intestinal Microbiota, and Obesity*

Obesity is a multifactorial condition that results in the storage of excessive amounts of fat. The microbiota of obese people are different than lean people, and changes in the intestinal microbiota were reported when obese people lost weight (Ley et al., 2006). Bäckhed et al. (2007) showed that germ-free mice raised on a low-fat diet, inoculated with the cecal microbiota of conventionally raised mice, and then fed a Western diet (41% of the calories from fat) had significantly increased weight gains and fat-pad weights and decreased locomotor activity compared to germ-free animals fed the same diet. This group also showed that the gut microbiota of conventional mice induce the deposition of dietary FAs in adipocytes by suppressing the fasting-induced adipose factor (Bäckhed et al., 2004).

The gut microbiota appear to be able to influence how dietary energy is extracted during digestion, and also how this energy is utilized or stored by the host. The exact mechanism that links dietary fat, the gut microbiota, and obesity is not yet established.

## *PUFAs and Probiotic Bacteria*

Free FAs such as PUFAs are found in the intestinal lumen at concentrations which affect the growth, metabolism, and function of probiotic bacteria, and this in turn could influence the ability of these bacteria to exert their beneficial effects on the host.

The generation of free FAs in the gut during the digestive process may affect the growth and function of beneficial bacteria (probiotics) added to the diet. The PUFAs γ-linolenic acid (18:3 n-6) and arachidonic acid (20:4 n-6) suppressed the growth of three probiotic bacteria (*Lactobacillus* GG, *Lb. casei* Shirota, and *Lb. bulgaricus*). Although growth was suppressed, the viability of the bacteria was not affected, suggesting that PUFAs are not lethal to these bacteria, but may only alter their metabolism (Kankaapää et al., 2001).

The intestinal mucus is mainly composed of protein and carbohydrate components. Sugars in the food matrix do affect bacterial adhesion (Bourlioux, 1994) and consequently modulate the microbiota in the mucus. FAs also affect adhesion. The presence of PUFAs modifies the hydrophobic and hydrophilic properties of probiotic bacteria, which could influence their adhesion to the GIT wall. Strains of *Lactobacillus* sp. can uptake free FAs present in their growth media to include them in their membranes (Jenkins et al., 2003; Kankaanpää et al., 2004). Low levels of α-linolenic acid significantly increased adherence to Caco-2 cells in vitro of *L. casei* Shirota, while high levels ($\geq$10 μg/mL) of n-3 and n-6 long-chain PUFAs inhibited the adhesion of each of the three probiotic bacteria to intestinal mucus in vitro (Kankaapää et al., 2001). These two observations may partly explain the differences in the adhesion and retention of different probiotic bacteria in the gut. With respect to bacterial populations, as such, no one knows whether FAs modify adhesion sufficiently to influence microbiota populations in humans. Data, however, exist in other species.

In fish (arctic charr), adding 7% linoleic acid to the diet increased the frequency of LAB in the intestinal system (Ringo et al., 1998).

Conjugated linoleic acids (CLAs) were reported to have potential beneficial effects on human metabolism and health (Li & Watkins, 2006; Tricon et al., 2005). CLAs are synthesized in the rumen of cows by *Butyrovibrio* as well as *Megasphaera,* and a fraction of these rumen CLAs are incorporated into milk fat (Sieber et al., 2004). *Butyrovibrio* was also isolated from the humans' GIT which raises the potential of CLA synthesis by the human microbiota. Many lactobacilli and streptococci also have the ability to convert linoleic acid into CLAs (Sieber et al., 2004). This raises the possibility of influencing the synthesis of CLA for human benefits in two ways. The first is through the use of CLA-producing lactic starter cultures for cheese and fermented milk manufacture. In this case, the milk products would contain the CLAs. This approach has its challenges: cultures need to be induced for CLA production during the starter manufacturing process, availability of free linoleic acid is limiting, and the presence of lactose in the milk reduces this enzymatic activity (Lin, 2000). This explains why blue cheese and Emmenthal are good candidates for this bioconversion in dairy foods. The second approach is the use of probiotic cultures in functional foods or dietary supplements. In this instance, the CLAs are produced in the GIT. Bifidobacteria and propionibacteria show potential for this application (Sieber et al., 2004).

Evidence shows that the human colonic microbiota modify FAs and carry out bioconversions as they pass down the GIT. Some bacteria found in the GIT are capable of hydrogenation and hydration (or hydroxylation) of free FAs (Howard & Henderson, 1999; Thomas, 1972), thus altering their properties and function (see Fig. 20.1). For example, bacterial production of 10-hydroxysteric acid from oleic acid is implicated in nonpancreatic origin steatorrhea in humans (Kim & Spritz, 1968). Thus, links between FA bioconversions and GIT microbiota are of interest.

## *Short-chain FAs (SCFAs)*

The rationale for initial research on probiotics was the interest in SCFAs, which were considered to be linked to "fermentation" in preference to phenolic compounds that were linked to "putrefaction" (Tannock, 1999). The SCFAs are not delivered by foods, but rather by fermentation of carbohydrates by some probiotic bacteria. Increasing evidence shows that the consumption of probiotic bacteria increases SCFA levels (Alander et al., 1999; Bourlioux et al., 2003). Acetic acid is produced by the bifidobacteria, while propionic acid is synthesized by *Propionibacterium.*

The SCFAs have numerous effects on human physiology (Table 20.2). Since the FAs released by triglyceride hydrolysis are mostly absorbed in the small intestine, likely few SCFA generated by diet will reach the colon. Therefore, the SCFAs found in the colon are the result of bacterial activity. Since the SCFAs in the colon are mainly generated through carbohydrate fermentation, consumption of prebiotics is a method of increasing SCFA levels in the colon. Therefore, when examining the effect of FA on health and the links with the microbiota, consider the metabolism of SCFAs.

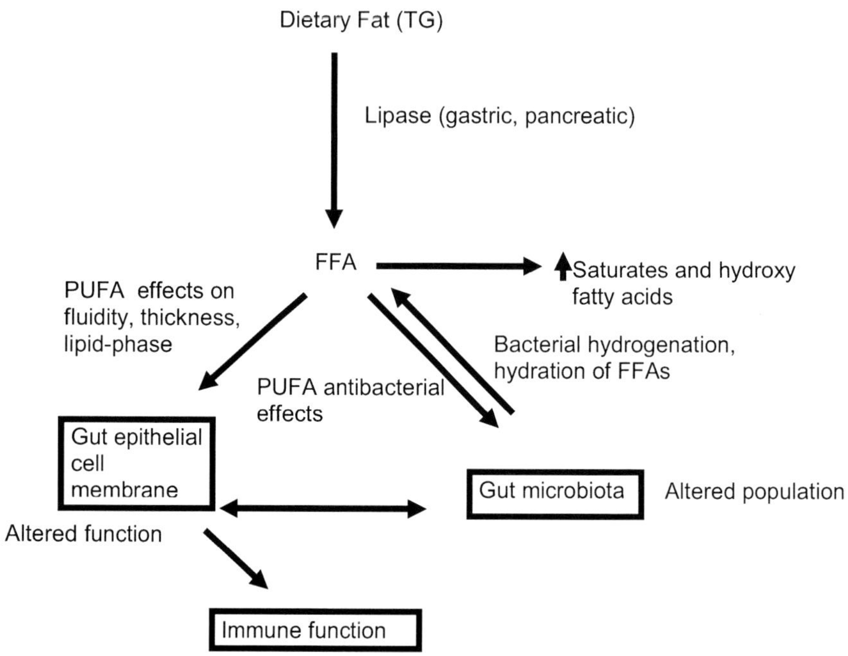


**Fig. 20.1.** Interactions of dietary fatty acids with the intestinal microbiota and gut epithelial cells.

**Table 20.2. Some Potential Benefits of Short-Chain Fatty Acids (SCFA) Produced by Probiotic Bacteria in the GIT**

| SCFA | Effect | Reference |
|---|---|---|
| Acetic, butyric | Antimutagenicity (Ames test) | Shah, 2000 |
| Acetic | Antimicrobial activity | Shah, 2000 |
| Butyric | Growth regulator epithelial cells of the colon | Puupponen-Pimia et al., 2004 |
| Propionic | Liver; cholesterol metabolism | Puupponen-Pimia et al., 2004 |
| Butyric | Affects cytokine and IL-10 production | Watzl et al., 2005 |
| Butyric | Affects lymphocyte proliferation in GALT | Watzl et al., 2005 |
| Acetic | Muscles, energy | Puupponen-Pimia et al., 2004 |

Modification of cell-wall properties can also result in changes in the virulent factors of pathogenic bacteria. Results show that strains of *S. typhimurium* develop an acid resistance when exposed to SCFAs like acetate and propionate (Kwon & Ricke, 1998). Anaerobiosis significantly enhanced this acid resistance, and the authors found that the resistance of *S. typhimurium* to other stress conditions, including reactive oxygen and high osmolarity, was also increased by exposure to the mixture of SCFAs in concentrations similar to those in the large intestines of animals. On the other hand, the growth of *Helicopbacter pylori* (responsible for gastric and duodenal ulcers and gastritis) was completely inactivated in a lipase-hydrolyzed cow milk, while counts of *E. coli* and *S. typhi* slightly decreased (Orozco et al., 2007), and this was linked to free soluble FAs like butyric, hexanoic, octanoic, and decanoic acids.

### *Bacterial Overgrowth and Fat Absorption*

The small intestine generally does not have populations of bacteria above $10^8$ per gram (Table 20.1). When gastric acid production is decreased, bacterial overgrowth in the small intestine can occur. This affects carbohydrate, protein, vitamin $B_{12}$, and fat metabolism. The most common clinical manifestation of this bacterial overgrowth is the malabsorption of fats or fat-soluble vitamins (Goldin, 2003). Therefore, the microbiota affect fat metabolism/digestion, as an indirect consequence of impaired gastric physiology.

### *Other Effects*

Researchers show in animals the indirect effects of FAs on the intestinal microbiota. Dänicke et al. (1999) showed changes in the digesta viscosity, intestinal transit time, and digestion occurring in the small intestine in chickens that might impact the gut bacterial population. No studies are reported to show similar effects in humans.

## Conclusion

Many interactions occur between FAs, the GIT microbiota, and health. When considering future perspectives, the potential of probiotic bacteria to interact with FAs needs to be explored. Fat components in foods can be modified by selected lactic cultures for targeted health effects, such as were shown for CLAs. Bioconversions of FAs by selected probiotic bacteria could also be enhanced.

Feta, parmesan, and blue cheeses are manufactured to enable lipolysis and to contain significant amounts of free FAs. However, whether these products do affect the GIT microbiota and whether potential FA bioconversions, which could be carried out during production and storage of the cheeses, would benefit health are yet to be determined.

FAs as bioactive ingredients for health have limited applications in foods because of flavor problems. Encapsulation offers the potential of preventing the off-flavors linked to FA. This was applied to n-3 oils of fish or plant origin. And with targeted release in the GIT possible by selecting the encapsulation matrix, generating FA effects in the colon in addition to the small intestine is possible, thereby expanding the bioactivity of these molecules.

## References


Alander, M.; I. de Smet; L. Nollet; W. Verstraete; A.von Wright; T. Mattila-Sandholm. The effect of probiotic strains on the microbiota of the simulator of the human intestinal microbial ecosystem (SHIME). *Int. J. Food Microbiol.* **1999,** *46*, 71–79.

Armstrong, B.; R. Doll. Environmental factors and cancer incidence and mortality in different countries with special reference to dietary practices. *Int. J. Cancer* **1975,** *15*, 617–631.

Bäckhed, F.; H. Ding; T. Wang; L.V. Hooper; G.Y. Koh; A. Nagy; C.F. Semenkovich; J.I. Gordon. The gut microbiota as an environmental factor that regulates fat storage. *Proc. Natl. Acad. Sci. USA* **2004,** *101*, 15718–15723.

Bäckhed, F.; J.K. Manchester; C.F. Semenkovich; J.I. Gordon. Mechanisms underlying the resistance to diet-induced obesity in germ-free mice. *Proc. Natl. Acad. Sci. USA* **2007,** *104*, 979–984.

Bartram, H-P.; A. Gostner; E. Kelber; G. Dusel; A. Weimer; W. Scheppach; H. Kasper. Effects of fish oil on fecal bacterial enzymes and steroid excretion in healthy volunteers: implications for colon cancer prevention. *Nutr. Cancer* **1996,** *25*, 71–78.

Bauer, E.; B.A. Williams; H. Smidt; R. Mosenthin; M.W.A. Verstegen. Influence of dietary components on development of the microbiota in single-stomached species. *Nutr. Res. Rev.* **2006,** *19*, 63–78.

Bourlioux, P. Écologie microbienne du tractus digestif humain. *Bactéries Lactiques;* H. de Roissard, F.M. Luquet, Eds.; Lorica: Uriage, 1994; Vol. 2, pp. 369–381.

Bourlioux, P.; B. Koletzko; F. Guarner; V. Braesco. The intestine and its microflora are partners for the protection of the host: report on the danone symposium "the intelligent intestine." *Am. J. Clin. Nutr.* **2003,** *78*, 675–683.

Boyaval, P.; C. Corre; C. Dupuis; E. Roussel. Effects of free fatty acids on propionic acid bacteria. *Lait* **1995,** *75*, 17–29.

Cagno, R. di; M. Quinto; A. Corsetti; F. Minervini; M. Gobbetti. Assessing the proteolytic and lipolytic activities of single strains of mesophilic lactobacilli as adjunct cultures using a Caciotta cheese model system. *Int. Dairy J.* **2006,** *16*, 119–130.

Carey, M.C.; O. Hernell. Digestion and absorption of fat. *Semin. Gastrointest. Dis.* **1992,** *3*, 189–208.

Cronan, J.E., Jr.; C.O. Rock. Biosynthesis of membrane lipids. *Escherichia coli and Salmonella tiphymurium, Cellular and Molecular Biology;* F.C. Neidhardt, J.L. Ingraham, K.B. Low, B. Magasanik, M. Schaechter, H.E. Umbarger, Eds.;American Society for Microbiology: Washington, DC, 1987; Vol. 1, 475–497.

Cummings, J.H.; H.S. Wiggins; D.J.A. Jenkins; H. Houston; T. Jivraj; B.S. Drasar; M.J. Hill. Influence of diets high and low in animal fat on bowel habit, gastrointestinal transit time, fecal microflora, bile acid, and fat excretion. *J. Clin. Invest.* **1978,** *61*, 953–963.

Dänicke, S.; W. Vahjen; O. Simon; H. Jeroch. Effects of dietary fat type and xylanase supplementation to rye-based broiler diets on selected bacterial groups adhering to the intestinal epithelium, on transit time of feed, and on nutrient digestibility. *Poult. Sci.* **1999,** *78*, 1292–1299.

Das, U.N. Essential fatty acids as possible enhancers of the beneficial actions of probiotics. *Nutrition* **2002,** *18*, 786–789.

DeMan, J.E.; M. Rogosa; M.E. Sharpe. A medium for the cultivation of lactobacilli. *J. App. Bacteriol.* **1960,** *23*, 130–135.

Desmazaud, M. L'état des connaissances en matière de nutrition des bactéries lactiques. *Lait* **1983,** *63*, 267–316.

Dierick, N.A.; J.A. Decuypere; K. Molly; E.V. Beek; E. Vanderbeke. The combined use triacylglycerols (TAGs) containing medium chain fatty acids (MCFAs) and exogenous lipolytic enzymes as an alternative to nutritional antibiotics in piglet nutrition. II. In vivo release of MCFAs in gastric cannulated and slaughtered piglets by endogenous and exogenous lipases; effects on the luminal gut flora growth performance. *Livestock Prod. Sci.* **2002,** *76*, 1–16.

Doerner, K.; F. Takamine; C.P. LaVoie; D.H. Mallonee; P.B. Hylemon. Assessment of fecal bacteria with bile acid 7α-dehydroxylating activity for the presence of bai-like genes. *Appl. Environ. Microbiol.* **1997,** *63*, 1185–1188.

Drasar, B.S.; D. Irving. Environmental factors and cancer of the colon and breast. *Br. J. Nutr.* **1973,** *17*, 167–172.

Endo Y.; S. Kamisada; K. Fujimoto; T. Saito. Trans fatty acids promote the growth of some Lactobacillus strains. *J. Gen. Appl. Microbiol.* **2006,** *52,* 29–35.

Fernandez-Lopez R.; C. Machòn; C.M. Longshaw; S. Martin; S. Molin; E.L. Zechner; M. Espinosa; E. Lankaand; F. De la Cruz. Unsaturated fatty acids are inhibitors of bacterial conjugation. *Microbiology,* **2005,** *151*, 3517–3526.

Goldin, B.R. Microflora of the intestine. *Encyclopedia of Food Science and Nutrition,* 2nd ed.; B. Caballero, L.C. Trugo, P.M. Finglas, Eds.; Academic Press: Amsterdam, 2003; pp. 3904–3911.

Goldin, B.R. The metabolism of the intestinal microflora and its relationship to dietary fat, colon and breast cancer. *Dietary Fat and Cancer;* C. Ip, D.F. Birt, A.E. Rogers, C. Mettlin, Eds.; Alan R. Liss Inc.: New York, 1986; pp. 655–685.

Goldin, B.R.; S.L. Gorbach. The relationship between diet and rat fecal bacterial enzymes implicated in colon cancer. *J. Natl. Cancer Inst.* **1976,** *57*, 371–375.

Hamada, K.; A. Umemoto; A. Kajikawa; M.J. Seraj; Y. Monden. In vitro formation of DNA adducts with bile acids. *Carcinogenesis* **1994,** *15*, 1911–1915.

Hambly, R.J.; C.J. Rumney; J.M.E. Fletcher; P.J. Rijken; I.R. Rowland. Effects of high- and low-risk diets on gut microflora-associated biomarkers of colon cancer in human flora-associated rats. *Nutr. Cancer,* **1977,** *27*, 250–255.

Hickey, D.K.; K.N. Kilcawley; T.P. Beresford; E.M. Sheehan; M.G. Wilkinson. Starter strain related effects on the biochemical and sensory properties of cheddar cheese. *J. Dairy Res.* **2007,** *74*, 9–17.

Hill, M.J.; B.S. Drasar; V. Aries; J.S. Crowther; G. Hawksworth; R.E.O. Williams. Bacteria and the aetiology of cancer of large bowel. *Lancet* **1971,** *Jan 16*, 95–100.

Howard, F.A.; C. Henderson. Hydrogenation of polyunsaturated fatty acids by human colonic bacteria. *Lett. Appl. Microbiol.* **1999,** *29*, 193–196.

Jenkins, J.K.; P.D. Courtney. Lactobacillus growth and membrane composition in the presence of linoleic or conjugated linoleic acid. *Can. J. Microbiol.* **2003,** *49*, 51–57.

Johnsson, T.; P. Nikkilä; L. Toivonen; H. Rosenqvist; S. Laasko. Cellular fatty acid profiles of *Lactobacillus* and *Lactococcus* strains in relation to the oleic content of the cultivation medium. *Appl. Environ. Microbiol.* **1995,** *62*, 4497–4499.

Juste, C. Dietary fatty acids, intestinal microbiota and cancer. *Bull. Cancer* **2005,** *92*, 708–721.

Kankaanpaa, P.; B. Yang; H. Kallio; E. Isolauri; S. Salminen. Effects of polyunsatured fatty acids in growth medium on lipid composition and on physicochemical surface properties of lactobacilli. *Appl. Environ. Microbiol.* **2004,** *70*, 129–136.

Kankaanpää, P.E.; S.J. Salminem; E. Isolauri; Y.K. Lee. The influence of polyunsaturated fatty acids on probiotic growth and adhesion. *FEMS Microbiol. Lett.* **2001,** *194*, 149–153.

Kim, Y.S; N. Spritz. Hydroxy acid excretion in steatorrhea of panceatic and nonpancreatic origin. *N. Engl. J. Med.* **1968,** *279*, 1424–1426.

Konstantinov. S.R.; N. Fitzsimons; E. Vaughan; A.D.L. Akkermans. From composition to functionality of the intestinal microbial communities. *Probiotics: Where Are We Going?* G.W. Tannock, Ed.; Caister: Norfolk, UK., 2002; pp. 59–84.

Kulshrestha, D.C.; E.H. Marth. Inhibition of *Streptococcus lactis* and *Salmonella typhimurium* by mixtures of some volatile and non-volatile compounds associated with milk. *J. Milk Food Technol.* **1975,** *38*, 138–141.

Kwon, Y.M.; S.C. Ricke. Induction of acid resistance of *Salmonella typhimurium* by exposure to short-chain fatty acids. *Appl. Environ. Microbiol.* **1998,** *64*, 3458–3463.

Lanciotti, R.; L. Vannini; P. Pittia; M.E. Guerzoni. Suitability of high-dynamic-pressure-treated milk for the production of yoghurt. *Food Microbiol.* **2004,** *21*, 753–760.

Ley, R.E.; P.J. Turnbaugh; S. Klein; J I. Gordon. Human gut microbes associated with obesity. *Nature* **2006,** *444*, 1022–1023.

Li, Y.; B.A. Watkins. CLA in human nutrition and health: human studies. *Handbook of Functional Lipids;* C.C. Akoh, Ed.; Taylor & Francis Group: Boca Raton, 2006; pp. 363–388.

Lin, T.Y. Conjugated linoleic acid concentration as affected by lactic cultures and additives. *Food Chem.* **2000,** *69*, pp. 27–31.

McGarr, S.E.; J.M. Ridlon; P.B. Hylemon. Diet, anaerobic bacterial metabolism, and colon cancer. *J. Clin. Gastroenterol.* **2005,** *39*, 98–109.

Meyerhardt, J.A.; D. Niedzwiecki; D. Hollis; L.B. Saltz; F.B. Hu; R.J. Mayer; H. Nelson; R. Whittom; A. Hantel; J. Thoma.; C.S. Fuchs. Association of dietary patterns with cancer recurrence and survival in patients with stage III colon cancer. *JAMA.* **2007,** *298*, 754–764.

Nieman, C. Influence of trace amounts of fatty acids on the growth of microorganisms. *Bacteriological Rev.* **1954,** *18*, 147–163.

Oba, S.; N. Shimizu; C. Nagata; H. Shimizu; M. Kametani; N. Takeyama; T. Ohnuma; S. Matsushita. The relationship between the consumption of meat, fat, and coffee and the risk of colon cancer: a prospective study in Japan. *Cancer Lett.* **2006,** *244*, 260–267.

Orozco, A.; T. Ogura; T. Hirosawa; R. Garduño; I. Kubo. In hydrolyzed cow's milk *Helicobacter pylori* becomes nonculturable and the growth of *Salmonella typhi* and *Escherichia coli* is inhibited. *J. Food Sci.* **2007,** *72*, M306–309.

Partanen, L.; N. Marttinen; T. Alatossawa. Fats and fatty acids as growth factors for *Lactobacillus delbrueckii. System. Appl. Microbiol.* **2001,** *24*, 500–506.

Powell, H.J.; J.T. May. Effect of various lipids found in human milk on the growth of infant bifidobacteria. *J. Gen. Appl. Microbiol.* **1981,** *27*, 185–193.

Puupponen-Pimia, R.; A.M. Aura; S. Karppinen; K.M. Oksman-Caldentey. Interactions between plant bioactive food ingredients and intestinal flora. Effects on human health. *Biosci. Microflora* **2004,** *23*, 67–80.

Rasic, J.L. Probiotics. *Encyclopedia of Food Science and Nutrition*; 2nd ed.; B. Caballero, L.C. Trugo, P.M. Finglas, Eds.; Academic Press: Amsterdam, 2003; pp. 3911–3915.

Reddy, B.S.; E.L. Wynder. Large-bowel carcinogenesis: fecal constituents of populations with diverse incidence rates of colon cancer. *J. Natl. Cancer Inst.* **1973,** *50*, 1437–1442.

Reddy, B.S.; E.L. Wynder. Metabolic epidemiology of colon cancer: fecal bile acids and neutral sterols in colon cancer patients and patients with adenomatous polyps. *Cancer* **1977,** *39*, 2533–2539.

Reddy, R.S.; J.H. Weisburger; E.L. Wynder. Effects of high risk and low risk diets for colon carcinogenesis on fecal microflora and steroids in man. *J. Nutr.* **1975,** *105*, 878–884.

Ringo, E.; H.R. Bendiksen; S.J. Gausen; A. Sundsfjord; R.E. Olsen. The effect of dietary fatty acids on lactic acid bacteria associated with the epithelial mucosa and from faecalia of Arctic charr, *Salvelinus alpinus* (L.). *J. Appl. Microbiol.* **1998,** *85*, 855–864.

Shah, N. Some beneficial effects of probiotic bacteria. *Biosci. Microflora*, **2000,** *19*, 99–106.

Sharma, S.; S.J. O'Keefe. Environmental influences on the high mortality from colorectal cancer in African Americans. *Postgrad. Med. J.* **2007,** *83*, 583–589.

Sieber, R.; M. Collomb; A. Aeschlimann; P. Jelen; H. Eyer. Impact of microbial cultures on conjugated linoleic acid in dairy products: A review. *Internat. Dairy J.* **2004,** *14*, 1–15.

Sprong, C.R.; M.F.E. Hulstein; R. Van Der Meer. Bactericidal activities of milk lipids. *Antimicrob. Agents Chemother;* **2001,** *45*, 1298–1301.

Stanier, R.Y.; J.L. Ingraham; M.L. Wheelis; P.R. Painter. *The Microbial World;* 5thed.; Prentice-Hall: Englewood Cliffs, New Jersey, 1986; pp. 120–124.

Sugawara, M.; K. Suzuki; K. Endo; Y. Tashiro; K. Nakamura; K. Suzuki; T. Fujisawa; N. Shiragami; T. Mitsuoka. Effect of dietary fat and fiber on fecal flora, bacterial metabolites, and fecal properties in Japanese volunteers. *J. Nutr. Sci. Vitaminol.* **1992,** *38*, 317–328.

Tannock, G.E. A fresh look at the intestinal microflora. *Probiotics: A Critical Review*; Horizon Scientific Press: Wymondham, UK, 1999; pp. 5–14.

Thomas, P.J. Identification of some enteric bacteria which convert oleic acid to hydroxystearic acid in vitro. *Gastroenterol.* **1972,** *62,* 430–435.

Tricon. S.; G.C. Burdge; C.M. Williams; P.C. Calder; P. Yaqoob. The effects of conjugated linoleic acid on human health-related outcomes. *Proc. Nutr. Soc.* **2005,** *64*, 171–182.

Wakai, K.; K. Hirose; K. Matsuo; H. Ito; K. Kuriki,; T. Suzuki; T. Kato; T. Hirai; Y. Kanemitsu; K. Tajima. Dietary risk factors for colon and rectal cancers: a comparative case-control study. *J. Epidemiol.* **2006,** *16*, 125–135.

Watzl, B.; S. Girrbach; M. Roller. Inulin, oligofructose and immunomodulation. *Br. J. Nutr.* **2005,** *93*, *Suppl. 1*, S49–S55.

Wegner, G.H.; E.M. Foster. Fatty acid requirements of some rumen bacteria. *J. Dairy Sci.* **1960,** *43*, 566–568.

Willett, W.C. Diet and cancer: one view at the start of the millennium. *Cancer Epidemiol. Biomarkers Prev.* **2001,** *10*, 3–8.

Willett, W.C. Dietary fat intake and cancer risk: a controversial and instructive story. *Semin. Cancer Biol.* **1998,** *8*, 245–253.

Willett, W.C.; M.J. Stampfer; G.A. Colditz; B.A. Rosner; F.E. Speizer. Relation of meat, fat, and fiber intake to the risk of colon cancer in a prospective study among women. *N. Engl. J. Med.* **1990,** *323*, 1664-1672.

You, W.C.; F. Jin; S. Devesa; G. Gridley; A. Schatzkin; G. Yang; P. Rosenberg; Y.B. Xiang; Y.R. Hu; Q. Li. Rapid increase in colorectal cancer rates in urban Shanghai, 1972–97, in relation to dietary changes. *J. Cancer Epidemiol. Prev.* **2002,** *7*, 143–146.

Zusman, I.; M. Chevion; N. Kitrosski. Effects of N'methyl-N'-nitrosoguanidine and deoxycholic acid on the content of free radicals in rat serum. *Exp. Toxicol Pathol.* **1992,** *44*, 187–189.

# 21

# Fatty Acids and Lipids in Neurobiology: A Brief Overview

**John R. Moffett[1], John A. Ives[2] and Aryan M. A. Namboodiri[1]**

[1]*Department of Anatomy, Physiology & Genetics, Uniformed Services University of the Health Sciences, 4301 Jones Bridge Road, Bethesda, MD 20814;* [2]*Samueli Institute, 1737 King Street, Alexandria, VA 22314*

## Overview

Lipid metabolism in the central nervous system (CNS) is more complex than in any other organ system. In tissues such as liver, lipid metabolism is primarily directed toward either membrane lipid (phosphoglyceride) and sterol synthesis for cellular structure and physiology, or triglyceride synthesis for energy-storage purposes. In contrast, lipid synthesis and utilization in the brain are far more complex, involving many molecular mechanisms unique to the nervous system. The unique structural and functional roles that lipids perform in the CNS include the facilitation of nerve conduction, providing continuous *de novo* vesicular membrane for synaptic neurotransmission, and the regulation of nervous-system-specific intracellular- and intercellular-signaling pathways. Complex and robust lipid- synthesis mechanisms are required to maintain nervous-system functions, and disorders of the lipid synthetic and degradatory pathways lead to many CNS pathologies. Essential long-chain polyunsaturated fatty acids (PUFAs) are important for brain function, and therefore the dietary content of these lipids has relevance for brain development and activity. We briefly review the basic neurobiology of fatty acids and lipids in the brain, and the connections between the fatty acid content of the diet, and the nervous-system function and dysfunction.

## Introduction

The brain is second only to adipose tissue in terms of lipid content, and as such, the brain has an enormous capacity for lipid synthesis and metabolism. However, unlike adipose tissue, which primarily produces storage fats (triglycerides), the brain must synthesize and metabolize a vast array of different lipid molecules with elaborate structures and varied functions. To synthesize many of these brain lipids, humans require certain fatty acids in their diet. These so-called essential fatty acids come in two forms known as omega-6 and omega-3 essential fatty acids, and the lipid products derived from each of these types are critical for human health. But the sources of omega 3 essential fatty acids are very limited, occurring predominantly in fish and mollusks. Omega-6 fatty acids are found predominantly in vegetable oils, whose widespread introduction to the human diet is relatively recent. This has some interesting evolutionary implications in terms of what is known about early hominid habits and diet. Specifically, fossil evidence indicates that humans exploited the aquatic food chain, both marine and freshwater, during the period of geographic expansion and rapid brain evolution, suggesting that the transition to modern humans occurred at the land/water interface (Crawford et al., 1999; Eaton et al., 1997; Eaton & Konner, 1985). Supposedly, Neolithic diets were rich in fish and shellfish, with omega-6 to omega-3 fatty acid ratios approaching 1:1. In contrast, modern Western diets often have an imbalance of 15:1 or greater for omega-6 versus omega-3 fatty acids. Accordingly, with the advent of agriculture, the increased use of vegetable oils in the human diet, and a reduction in seafood intake, an imbalance occurred with respect to the two types of essential fatty acids that are required for human health.

In all cells of the body, complex lipid synthesis is required to maintain plasma-membrane and internal-membrane structure and function. Cell membranes are composed of complex lipid molecules arranged in the classic bilayer configuration, with polar head groups facing the aqueous environments on either side of the membrane and fatty acid chains forming the central portion of the bilayer. In general, cellular membranes perform four primary roles: a hydrophobic barrier to solute diffusion, a critical operating environment for proteins and supramolecular complexes, a source of stored metabolic energy, and a reservoir of numerous lipid substrates for critical cellular-signaling pathways. In certain metabolically active tissues, including the immune system and the brain, lipid synthesis employs diverse lipogenic pathways to produce highly specialized lipids. Brain lipid metabolism, in particular, is extremely complex and poorly understood, and many aspects of brain lipid synthesis are distinct from those in other tissues of the body (D'Adamo, Jr., et al., 1968; Gross et al., 2005). The total number of enzymes involved in lipid synthesis, trafficking, and breakdown in the nervous system is uncertain, but in yeast cells that express a much simpler lipidome, the number of enzymes involved in lipid metabolism involves at least 493 enzymes and carriers, or approximately 9% of the expressed proteins in these cells (Natter et al., 2005). This highlights the extreme complexity of lipid metabolism in eukaryotic cells. The question facing modern biologists studying this complex field of lipid metabolism is how to analyze and understand such complexity.

## Lipidomics

In the post-genomic era, mass spectrometric techniques were combined with bioinformatics, or the use of computers to analyze complex data sets, to revolutionize the study of proteins, ushering in the era of proteomics. The "proteome" is the sum total of the proteins expressed in all the cells of the body, and the field of proteomics is dedicated to the elucidation of the entire proteome in the human body. The field of biology that concentrates on the study of fatty acids, and lipids is presently undergoing a similar revolution (Adibhatla et al., 2006). The term "lipidomics," borrowing from the terms "proteomics" and "genomics," was coined to describe this emerging field of biology (Han & Gross, 2005). Mass spectroscopy techniques, especially electrospray ionization mass spectrometry, enabled the characterization of large numbers of lipids differing in fatty acid composition from relatively crude extracts of biological samples. For example, over 100 cardiolipin molecular species were identified and quantified during embryonic development using so-called shotgun lipidomic methods (Cheng et al., 2008). Other studies showed specific changes in lipids at the earliest clinically recognizable stage of Alzheimer's disease (Han et al., 2002). In a more recent study, a lipidomic analysis of the retina in a rat model of Smith-Lemli-Opitz syndrome showed alterations in the docosahexaenoic acid (DHA) content of phospholipid molecular species (Ford et al., 2008). The power of mass spectrometry is only beginning to be realized in the field of lipidomics, and major new discoveries regarding the roles of specific lipids in neurobiology and pathogenesis of various nervous system disorders are likely to be forthcoming in the near future.

## Major Lipid Classes in the Brain

A comprehensive classification system was recently proposed for lipids (Fahy et al., 2005). Fatty acid groups form the major building blocks of complex lipids, and also, in the case of eicosanoid fatty acids such as the prostaglandins, act as signaling molecules in all types of cells. A unique aspect of lipid synthesis in the nervous system is the requirement for specialized lipids necessary to make the myelin sheaths that surround neuronal axons. Myelin in the CNS is produced by glial cells called oligodendrocytes. Myelin sheaths are composed of thin concentric wrappings of oligodendrocyte cytoplasm and phospholipid membrane bilayer, with thicker layers of myelin-associated lipids and proteins. The synthesis of myelin lipids is a metabolically demanding task that is shared by oligodendrocytes and neurons, with neurons supplying many of the building blocks for complex lipid synthesis. In general, one can divide lipids into fatty acids and complex lipids. Fatty acids act as the basic building blocks for complex lipids, such as the phospholipids that are the predominant lipids making up cell membranes. In the case of phospholipids like phosphatidylethanolamine, two fatty acids and a phosphate group are coupled to a molecule of glycerol. Despite the large number and complexity of the lipids in the nervous system, they fall into a relatively small number of major groups.

### *Fatty Acids*

Fatty acids have relatively simple molecules composed of long chains of carbon atoms (typically 16 to 22 carbons). Complex lipids that make up cell membranes are composed of various fatty acids coupled to a common backbone molecule such as glycerol. In many complex lipids, fatty acids are coupled to the glycerol backbone by ester linkages (esterification).

### Glycerophospholipids

Membrane phospholipids, such as phosphatidylcholine, phosphatidylserine, and phosphatidylethanolamine, are major components of cellular and vesicular membranes. Glycerophospholipids have two fatty acids coupled to glycerol via ester bonds. A plasmalogen is a modified type of membrane phospholipid (e.g., an ethanolamine plasmalogen is a variation of phosphatidylethanolamine). Plasmalogens have an ether linkage instead of an ester linkage to the glycerol backbone.

### Sphingolipids

Sphingolipids are formed from sphingosine, a long-chain amino alcohol, instead of glycerol. Both the amino group and the alcohol group can be substituted to produce various sphingolipids. The attachment of an acyl group to the amino position of sphingosine produces a family of complex lipids called ceramides. Sphingolipids also can be phosphorylated or glycosylated.

### Sterol Lipids

Sterol lipids, such as cholesterol, are important constituents of plasma membranes and myelin, and neuroactive steroids, such as dehydroepiandrosterone and allopregnanolone, are derived from cholesterol.

### Triacylglycerols

Triacylglycerols are another common type of complex lipid, which have three fatty acids esterified to the three hydroxyl groups of glycerol. Triacylglycerols act as energy-storage molecules, and are the primary lipids stored in adipose tissue. They have high levels of saturated fatty acids esterified to glycerol, and low levels of PUFAs. The brain contains very low levels of triacylglycerides, and instead contains complex lipids rich in PUFAs. Unsaturated fatty acids tend to increase the fluidity of the lipid membranes into which they are incorporated, whereas saturated fatty acids and cholesterol tend to decrease membrane fluidity.

## Fatty Acid Synthesis

Fatty acids are relatively simple molecules consisting of chains of carbon atoms (alkyl chains) with a carboxylic acid group (COOH) at the beginning of the chain and a methyl group at the terminus. Fatty acids are typically categorized as saturated, monounsaturated, and polyunsaturated, based on the number of double bonds present in the carbon chain. Monounsaturated fatty acids contain only a single carbon-carbon double bond in the alkyl chain, whereas PUFAs contain two or more double bonds. Fatty acids form the hydrophobic portions of many important complex lipids, such as glycerophospholipids, but to synthesize these more complex lipids, long-chain fatty acids must first be generated from smaller 2-carbon units. The primary building blocks for fatty acid synthesis come from acetyl coenzyme A (acetyl-CoA) derived from the citric acid produced in mitochondria. For any carbon-containing molecule, such as the two-carbon molecule acetate, to participate in fatty acid synthesis, it must first be "activated," meaning that it must be coupled to CoA to enter a lipogenic metabolic pathway. Free acetate molecules are not used for fatty acid synthesis unless coupled to CoA, and enzymes that couple acetate to CoA, known as acetate-CoA ligases, or acetyl-CoA synthetases (Ace-CS), are found in all living organisms.

Acetyl-CoA is produced primarily via pyruvate oxidation within mitochondria when glucose is available. However, fatty acid synthesis occurs in various cytoplasmic compartments of cells, rather than in mitochondria. The acetyl-CoA produced in the citric-acid cycle can not cross the mitochondrial membrane, and therefore mitochondria manufacture and export citrate, which can then be converted back to acetyl-CoA in the cytoplasm of cells by the enzyme ATP citrate lyase. Acetyl-CoA is then carboxylated in the cytoplasm to form malonyl-CoA, which then goes on to provide the substrate for the elongation of fatty acid chains by the action of fatty acid synthase (FAS) (see Fig. 21.1). FAS is a complex, multifunctional enzyme that performs sequential biosynthetic reactions to form the product palmitate (palmitic acid), a 16-carbon saturated fatty acid. Fatty acid elongases act to add additional two-carbon units to palmitate to produce longer chain fatty acids. Fatty acid elongase enzymes can act on both dietary and FAS-synthesized fatty acids (Jakobsson et al., 2006). Fatty acyl-CoA desaturase enzymes in the endoplasmic reticulum act to produce unsaturated fatty acids, but these enzymes can not introduce sites of unsaturation beyond the ninth carbon (C9), and therefore they cannot synthesize either linoleic acid or linolenic acid. As such, these two PUFAs are considered essential, meaning that they, or their longer chain analogs, must be acquired from the diet (see below).

## Essential Fatty Acids

Although we have long recognized dietary fat as an important source of energy for mammals, it wasn't until the late 1920s that researchers demonstrated the dietary requirement for particular fatty acids. These came to be known as essential fatty acids, but their importance in the diet remained controversial. It was not until the advent of intravenous feeding that the importance of essential fatty acids became widely accepted. This was due, in part, to the fact that clinical signs of essential-fatty acid deficiency are generally observed only in patients on total parenteral nutrition who received mixtures devoid of essential fatty acids, or in patients with malabsorption syndromes. Important signs of essential-fatty acid deficiency include dermatitis and changes in visual and neural functions. Over the past 40 years, an increasing number of physiological functions, such as immunomodulation, has been attributed to the essential fatty acids and their metabolites, and this area of research is expanding rapidly (Dangour & Uauy, 2006; Uauy & Dangour, 2006; Yehuda et al., 2005).

The cells of the body can synthesize most of the fatty acids necessary for complex lipid synthesis. However, the so-called omega-3 and omega-6 fatty acids can not be synthesized from simpler molecules in mammals. Omega-3 fatty acids are a subtype of the so-called long-chain PUFAs. PUFAs contain two or more carbon-carbon double bonds, and form one of the three main classes of fatty acids. The two other groups

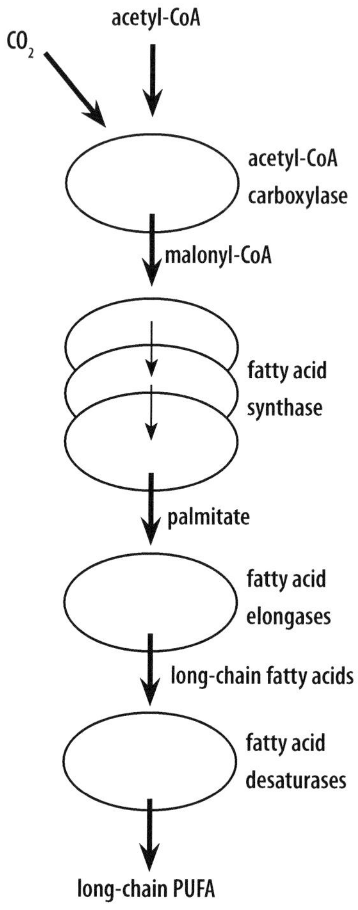


**Fig. 21.1.** Simplified diagram of the basic steps in eukaryotic fatty acid synthesis. Acetyl-CoA is carboxylated in the cytoplasm of cells by the action of the enzyme acetyl-CoA carboxylase to form malonyl-CoA. Malonyl-CoA and additional acetyl-CoA are substrates for the multifunctional enzyme fatty acid synthase (FAS). The final product released from the FAS complex is the 16-carbon saturated fatty acid palmitate. Palmitate is acted upon by fatty acid elongase enzymes to create longer chain fatty acids. Fatty acid desaturase enzymes introduce double bonds to fatty acids, generating long-chain monounsaturated fatty acids, and long-chain polyunsaturated fatty acids (long-chain PUFA). Because human desaturase enzymes can not introduce double bonds beyond the $9^{th}$ carbon in fatty acids, the long-chain PUFA with double bonds near the end of the fatty acids (omega-3 and omega-6) can not be synthesized, and must be acquired in the diet.

of fatty acids include saturated (no double bonds) and monounsaturated (a single double bond in the carbon chain). The PUFAs are subdivided into the omega-3 series (n-3, where the first double bond is 3 carbons from the terminal methyl carbon) and the omega-6 series (n-6, where the first double bond is 6 carbons from the terminal methyl carbon). The omega-3 PUFAs are derived from alpha-linolenic acid, whereas the omega-6 PUFAs are synthesized from linoleic acid; both are 18-carbon atom-containing fatty acids. Linoleic acid and alpha-linolenic acid are considered essential unsaturated fatty acids because mammals can not synthesize them from precursors, and therefore they must be present in the diet (Ruxton et al., 2004).

Fatty acids are further classified by a numbering system that indicates the number of carbon atoms in the carbon chain and the number of double bonds present in the chain. Therefore, a 16- carbon saturated fatty acid (e.g., palmitate) is given the number 16:0 to indicate 16 carbon atoms in the chain, with no carbon-carbon double bonds. A PUFA with 20 carbon atoms and 4 double bonds [e.g., arachidonic acid (AA)] is therefore designated 20:4. Because AA is an omega-6 fatty acid, its full designation is 20:4n-6, indicating 20 carbon atoms and 4 double bonds, with the first double bond being 6 carbon atoms from the methyl terminus of the fatty acid chain.

A series of biosynthetic reactions can convert the omega-6 PUFA linoleic acid into other omega-6 fatty acids (see Fig. 21.2). These include the 18-carbon gamma-linolenic acid, two 20-carbon fatty acids, AA, and dihomogammalinolenic acid. AA is a critical cellular- signaling agent, and figures prominently in the section on neuroinflammation. The omega-3 PUFA alpha-linolenic acid can likewise be converted to longer chain omega-3 fatty acids, such as the 20-carbon eicosapentaenoic acid (EPA) and 22-carbon docosahexaenoic acid (DHA). These long-chain PUFA (LC-PUFA) are important for brain function, as is discussed below. Even though linoleic acid and alpha-linolenic acid can be converted into their longer length metabolites in the body, the rate of conversion in humans is very slow, resulting in an estimated 2 to 10% of alpha-linolenic acid being converted to DHA or EPA in the liver, with very little conversion occurring in the brain itself. Liver can thus convert some alpha-linolenic acid in the diet into DHA and EPA, which can then supply the nervous system with these essential fatty acids (Rapoport et al., 2007). Because the conversion rates in liver are low, and almost undetectable in the brain, the longer chain omega-3 PUFA species EPA and DHA are also important dietary constituents. Dietary supplementation with DHA- and EPA-rich food sources such as fish oils can significantly increase the levels of both of these omega-3 PUFAs in the tissues of the body, including the brain. Omega-6 fatty acids compete with omega-3 fatty acids for access to elongase and desaturase enzymes (see below), and therefore, if the diet is rich in omega-6, but poor in omega-3 fatty acids, then the synthesis of critical omega-3 PUFA is hampered.

Elongase and desaturase enzymes in the liver act to produce a variety of longer chain fatty acids including AA, EPA, DPA, and DHA, which are known collectively as LC-PUFA. Among these LC-PUFAs, AA (20:4n-6) and DHA (22:6n-3) are the

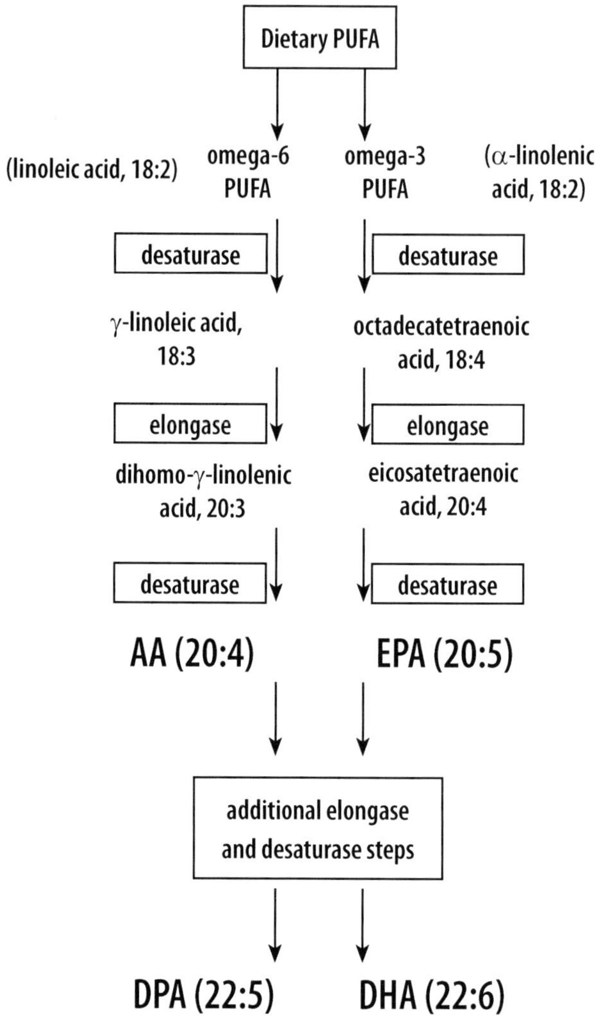


**Fig. 21.2.** Long-chain polyunsaturated fatty acid (LCPUFA) synthesis starting from the essential fatty acids linoleic acid (omega-6) and alpha-linolenic acid (omega-3). The numbering system indicates the number of carbon atoms in the fatty acid chain, and the number of double carbon-carbon bonds in the chain, respectively. Elongase enzymes add additional 2-carbon units to the fatty acid chains, whereas desaturase enzymes increase the number of double bonds. Western diets are rich in essential omega-6 fatty acids (7–8% dietary intake), and relatively poor in essential omega-3 fatty acids (0.3–0.4% dietary intake). The LCPUFAs derived from essential fatty acids are necessary for the synthesis of eicosanoids. Abbreviations: AA = arachidonic acid, EPA = eicosapentaenoic acid, DPA = docosapentaenoic acid, DHA = docosahexaenoic acid.

predominant essential-fatty acid derivatives in the brain, and both are important for brain function and response to injury. They must be synthesized in the liver from shorter chain analogs, or they must be present in the diet.

Although researchers are beginning to understand the roles of LC-PUFA in the brain, much remains to be discovered. What is clear is their importance in the diet. This is underscored by the observation that the LC-PUFA composition of complex membrane lipids in the brain is differential across regions. For example, the frontal cortex of the brain has a high proportion of the omega-3 LC-PUFA DHA compared with other brain regions, and DHA levels there are more sensitive to the dietary deprivation of omega-3 fatty acids (Carrie et al., 2000).

## Sources of Brain Lipids in Development: Local Synthesis versus Circulation Derived

Myelination of nerve-cell axons by oligodendrocytes occurs predominantly after birth in mammals (reviewed in Moffett et al., 2007). Cholesterol is an important constituent of the myelin sheath surrounding axons, and cholesterol accumulates in the brain during the period of rapid myelination that takes place after birth. The cholesterol accumulation in myelin during this period occurs primarily by local synthesis, and neither diet nor production by other organs such as the liver plays a significant role (Jurevics & Morell, 1995). Also, studies indicate that during brain growth and myelination, the major saturated and monounsaturated fatty acids in complex brain lipids are exclusively produced locally by *de novo* biosynthesis (Edmond et al. 1998). However, the situation is different in the case of the important PUFA, including AA and DHA. Evidence indicates that the liver converts the essential dietary PUFAs alpha-linolenic and linoleic acids into AA and DHA, and makes them available to the brain via the circulation, because the ability of the brain to synthesize them from linoleic or alpha-linolenic acid is minimal (Rapoport et al., 2007).

## Phospholipid Synthesis

Phospholipids are the most abundant complex lipids making up cell membranes. Phosphatidic acid is the precursor molecule for the synthesis of complex lipids, such as glycerophospholipids, that form the major constituents of cell membranes. The basic steps in glycerolipid and glycerophospholipid synthesis are shown in Fig. 21.3. Fatty acids must first be activated to participate in complex lipid synthesis, just as the precursors of fatty acids, such as acetate, must be activated by coupling to CoA. Acyl CoA synthases perform this function by coupling fatty acids to CoA to form as many species of acyl-CoA as there are types of fatty acids. These acyl CoA molecules are then combined with glycerol 3-phosphate to form lyso-phosphatidic acid by the action of the enzyme glycerol 3-phosphate acyltransferase. The enzyme 1-acylglycerol-3-phosphate acyltransferase then acts on the lyso-phosphatidic acid to form phosphatidic acid, the basic building block of more complex glycerolipids. Phosphatidic acid phosphatase then converts phosphatidic acid to diacylglycerol, which can be further converted to

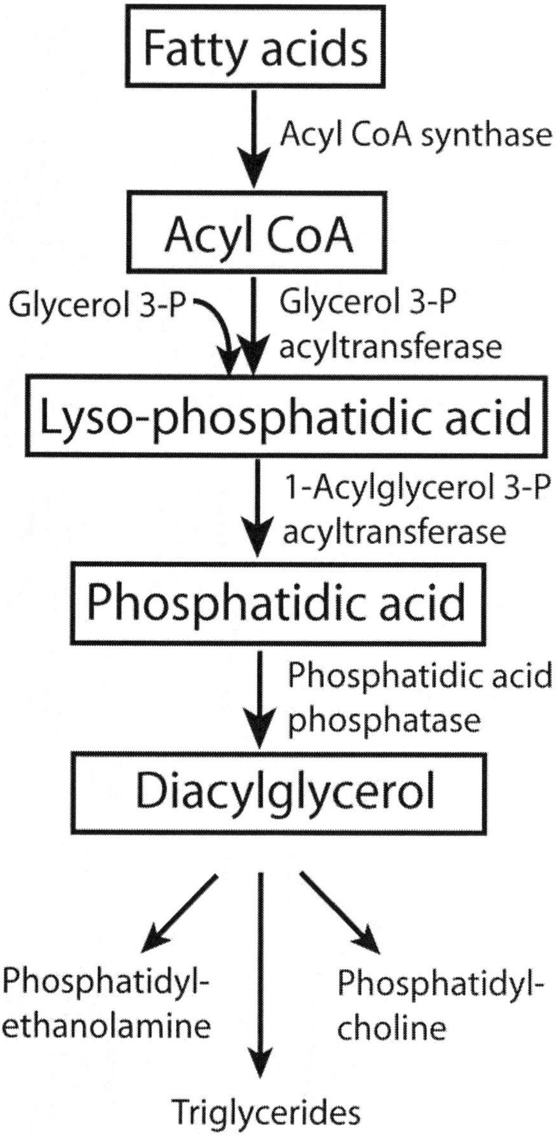


**Fig. 21.3.** Simplified diagram of the basic steps in glycerophospholipid synthesis. Fatty acids of all types are activated by the enzyme acyl-CoA synthase to produce various acyl-CoA molecules. The acyl-CoA molecules go through several additional enzymatic steps to produce phosphatidic acid, and then diacylglycerol. Diacylglycerol can then go on to participate in the synthesis of triglycerides and glycerophospholipids, such as phosphatidylethanolamine and phosphatidylcholine. Abbreviation: glycerol 3-P = glycerol 3-phosphate.

triglycerides or to membrane phospholipids such as phosphatidylethanolamine and phosphatidylcholine by the actions of a number of enzymes.

## Brain Lipids

Many complex lipids are so-called glycerolipids, meaning that fatty acids and other compounds, including phosphate, are coupled to a glycerol backbone. Glycerol is a three-carbon molecule with three alcohol groups, one on each carbon atom (Fig. 21.4). Therefore, glycerol has three chemical attachment sites through the alcohol groups designated *sn*-1, *sn*-2, and *sn*-3. When other molecules such as fatty acids are attached to an alcohol group of glycerol, the chemical bond is known as an ester bond, and hence, adding fatty acids to glycerol is a process known as esterification. Glycerolipids with a single fatty acid chain attached to glycerol are called monoacylglycerols; those with two fatty-acyl chains are known as diacylglycerols; and those with three fatty-acyl groups esterified to glycerol are the triacylglycerols. The "*sn*" designation for the three alcohol attachment sites stands for "stereospecific numbering system," and the three sites on glycerol are not equivalent regarding the fatty acids and other compounds that are typically bound to them in complex lipids. For example, triacylglycerols are nutritional/storage lipids that have three fatty acids esterified to glycerol, and the triacylglycerols in human milk have the fatty acid palmitate coupled to the *sn*-2 position 60% of the time, as opposed to the 33% expected at this position for random distribution among the three binding sites (Lopez-Lopez et al., 2002). As another example, glycerophospholipids have two fatty acid groups coupled to the *sn*-1 and *sn*-2 positions of glycerol and a phosphate group or modified phosphate group coupled to the *sn*-3 position. Often, saturated fatty acids are coupled to the *sn*-1 position, whereas unsaturated fatty acids are coupled to the *sn*-2 position. Many of the enzymes that synthesize and degrade membrane lipids are selective regarding the three different attachment sites in glycerolipids.

Phosphoglycerides (glycerophospholipids) comprise one of the major constituents making up cellular membranes. These amphipathic molecules have two fatty acid chains coupled to a glycerol backbone, and a phosphate group is attached to the third carbon (*sn*-3) of the glycerol backbone in phosphoglycerides. Membrane phospholipids include two major classes:(i) standard membrane phosphoglycerides, such as phosphatidylcholine, phosphatidylserine, and phosphatidylethanolamine and (ii) a unique class called plasmalogens (Farooqui & Horrocks, 2001; Gross et al., 2005). The brain has particularly high levels of plasmalogen phospholipids (up to 20% of brain phosphoglycerides), which differ from standard membrane phospholipids in that they have a different type of chemical linkage to one of the fatty acid groups. Rather than having the standard ester linkage, they have an enol-ether linkage between the glycerol backbone and the first alky group (*sn*-1 position). Plasmalogens are thought to confer different electrical and biophysical characteristics to neural membranes.

Sphingolipids are a very important class of complex lipids in the nervous system. Discovered in the 1800s in neural tissues, these complex lipids were named sphingolipids after the Sphinx, due to their unusual characteristics (van Echten-

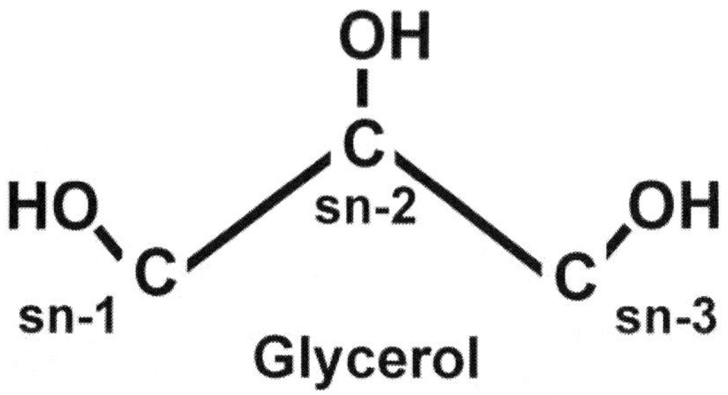


**Fig. 21.4.** Glycerol forms the backbone for all glycerolipids. This 3-carbon molecule has three alcohol (OH = hydroxyl groups), one on each carbon atom. These provide three attachment sites for fatty acids or other functional groups such as phosphate. The three attachment sites are designated *sn*-1, *sn*-2, and *sn*-3, and the enzymes that attach and remove fatty acids and other groups are often selective as to which of the three sites they act on. (Note: hydrogen atoms on carbons not shown).

Deckert & Herget, 2006). Unlike glycerolipids, which are based on a glycerol backbone, sphingolipids do not contain glycerol. Rather, sphingolipids are based on sphingosine, a long-chain (18-carbon) amino alcohol. Sphingosine has an alcohol group at carbon 1, an amine group at carbon 2, and another alcohol group at carbon 3; like glycerol, three chemical attachment sites exist for fatty acids or functional groups. Ceramide is an important sphingolipid that is composed of sphingosine coupled to a fatty acid by an amide bond. The fatty acid composition of various sphingolipids is different than that of glycerolipids, and typically includes very long chain saturated and monounsaturated alkyl chains. Ceramide is synthesized starting from palmitoyl-CoA and serine to form 3-ketosphinganine, which is then converted to sphinganine, and then dihydroceramide. The enzyme dihydroceramide desaturase adds a carbon-carbon double bond to dihydroceramide to form ceramide, which is the basic building block for all sphingolipids. Phosphosphingolipids, such as sphingomyelin (ceramide with esterification of the alcohol with phosphocholine); glycosphingolipids, such as galactocerebrosides (ceramide with glycosylation of an alcohol group with the sugar galactose); and sulfated forms (sulfated on position 3 of galactose) called sulfatides are all important constituents of cell membranes and myelin (Marcus et al., 2000). The galactose-containing sphingolipids galactocerebroside and sulfatide are key constituents of the myelin sheath of axons, as well as components in cell membranes. Because they contain the sugar galactose, they are typically present in the external face of the plasma membranes of brain cells, with the hydrophilic galactose moiety facing the extracellular space. Galactolipids most likely interact with the extracellular matrix to provide structural support; galactolipid-deficient mice have reduced myelin and less compact myelin (Coetzee et al., 1999), suggesting that galactolipids are important structural elements of normal myelin.

## Cell Signaling and Neuroinflammation

Complex lipids, such as glycerophospholipids and sphingolipids, are the predominant constituents of all cellular membranes, but because of their highly diverse fatty acid content, complex lipids also serve as a reservoir for specific fatty acid molecules that act as cellular-signaling agents and second messengers. Specialized enzymes that are activated in response to a number of signals act to break membrane lipid molecules apart, releasing one of the fatty acid chains. The freed fatty acids derived from glycerophospholipid and sphingolipid breakdown are converted by another series of enzymes into metabolites that act as second messengers in all cells of the body.

The complex membrane lipids of brain cells are exceptionally rich in PUFAs, particularly DHA and AA, and these two essential fatty acids are critically important for brain development, function, and responses to injury. When cells are stressed or damaged, one initial reaction is the stimulation of enzymes that break down a small proportion of the complex lipid molecules making up the cell membrane, releasing some of the fatty acids of which they are composed. Additional enzymes act upon these fatty acids released from cell-membrane lipids and convert them into cellular-signaling agents, many of which act as inflammation modulators. Both omega-6 and omega-3 PUFAs act as biosynthetic precursors for important cell-signaling molecules including the prostaglandins, thromboxanes, leukotrienes, and resolvins, which are known collectively as eicosanoids. Because these critical cellular-signaling agents are derived from omega-6 and omega-3 PUFAs, the lack of these essential fatty acids in the diet can lead to various pathologies. The brain has the highest levels of AA and DHA of any organs in the body, and therefore these two PUFAs are especially critical precursors for the synthesis of eicosanoid signaling agents in the nervous system.

When the brain is injured, resident immune cells known as microglia are some of the first responders to the damage. Resting microglia are rapidly transformed into reactive microglia which become mobile and move to the site of the injury to begin the processes of clearing debris and pathogens and recruiting immune cells from the peripheral circulation to enter the damaged brain tissue. The first immune cells to arrive from the blood are polymorphonucleocytes, which bind to endothelial cells near the injury and move across the capillaries into the brain (Farooqui et al., 2007a). Macrophages, which are the primary phagocytic cells of the immune system, arrive after polymorphonucleocytes. Together, reactive microglia, polymorphonucleocytes, and macrophages clear the cellular debris left behind from destroyed brain cells, and begin the process of healing the remaining living tissue.

During the initial process of reacting to brain damage, microglia and other cells release signaling molecules, including cytokines that act to initiate the inflammatory response. Cytokines and other pro-inflammatory signaling agents stimulate a group of lipid-degrading enzymes known as phospholipase A2 enzymes ($PLA_2$). $PLA_2$ enzymes act to break down membrane lipids, releasing the PUFAs AA and DHA, which have generally opposing effects on inflammation (Farooqui et al., 2007a). AA (20:4n-6) is distributed rather evenly in membrane lipids throughout the brain, but

DHA is highly enriched in neurons and their synapses. The frontal cortex of the brain is particularly rich in DHA (Carrie et al., 2000). AA and DHA are often esterified at the *sn*-2 position of brain membrane glycerophospholipids, from where the actions of selective $PLA_2$ enzymes can release them. After release, the bulk of the free AA or DHA enters the acyl-CoA pool and is reincorporated into an unesterified *sn*-2 position of a lysophospholipid via the actions of an acyl-CoA synthetase and acyltransferase (Rapoport et al., 2007). Enzymes involved in fatty acid synthesis, including acyl-CoA synthetases, are up-regulated in the CNS even in response to inflammation occurring outside the brain (Benani et al., 2003). Some proportion of the AA and DHA that are freed from membrane lipids by the action of $PLA_2$ enzymes is then acted upon by other enzymes that turn them into eicosanoid-signaling agents.

Prostaglandins and leukotrienes are members of the eicosanoid family of fatty acid-derived cellular-signaling agents that play important roles in the regulation of cell physiology and inflammation. Prostaglandins are generated from PUFA by the action of enzymes known as cyclooxygenases (COX), whereas leukotrienes are synthesized from PUFA by the action of enzymes called lipoxygenases (LOase). The prostaglandins and leukotrienes are produced from dihomo-gamma-linolenic acid and AA (omega-6 PUFA), as well as from EPA (omega-3 PUFA). The long-chain omega-6 fatty acid AA (20:4n-6) is the precursor of a group of eicosanoids that include series-2 prostaglandins and series-4 leukotrienes, which tend to be pro-inflammatory. The omega-3 fatty acid, EPA (20:5n-3), is the precursor to a group of eicosanoids that includes series-3 prostaglandins and series-5 leukotrienes, which tend to be more anti-inflammatory (see Fig. 21.5). Injury or stress will induce the synthesis of AA-derived pro-inflammatory series-2 prostaglandins and series-4 leukotrienes. EPA-derived anti-inflammatory series-3 prostaglandins are also formed during injury or stress, but their synthesis is delayed relative to the production of pro-inflammatory eicosanoids. These anti-inflammatory series-3 prostaglandins work to attenuate the effects of the excessive levels of series-2 prostaglandins. Thus, adequate production of the series-3 prostaglandins tends to have anti-inflammatory effects in the body, and may protect against diseases with an inflammatory component, such as heart disease and stroke as well as arthritis, lupus, and asthma.

EPA (omega-3) decreases the production of the pro-inflammatory cytokines, interleukin 1β (IL-1β) and tumor necrosis factor α (TNF-α), which are involved in the expression of the adhesion molecules necessary for leukocyte adhesion and movement from the circulatory system into tissues (Simopoulos, 2008). EPA has other anti-inflammatory effects through its elongation product, DPA (22:5n-3), which is then metabolized to DHA (22:6n-3)—the precursor for the metabolite called 10,17*S*-docosatriene (Marcheselli et al., 2003), which is part of a family of compounds called resolvins (Serhan et al., 2004). Resolvins counteract the pro-inflammatory actions of infiltrating leukocytes by blocking IL-1 β-induced nuclear factor-κB activation and cyclooxygenase-2 expression, and are found in the brain in response to an ischemic insult (Hong et al., 2003). The exact mechanism responsible

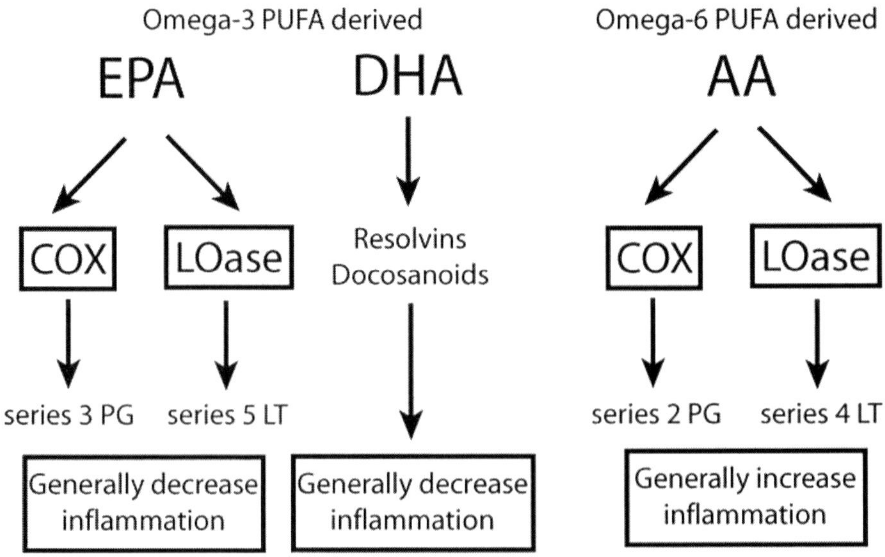


**Fig. 21.5.** Highly simplified depiction of eicosanoid synthesis from omega-3 and omega-6 PUFAs. Phospholipase A2 enzymes cleave PUFA from the *sn*-2 position of membrane glycerophospholipids, and these are then available for conversion to eicosanoids. Omega-3- and omega-6-derived eicosanoids often have opposing effects on inflammatory reactions. Abbreviations: AA = arachidonic acid, EPA = eicosapentaenoic acid, DHA = docosahexaenoic acid, COX = cyclooxygenase enzymes, LOase = lipoxygenase enzymes, LT = leukotrienes, PG = prostaglandins.

for the suppression of cytokine production by omega-3 LC-PUFA is uncertain. Because the omega-3 and omega-6 fatty acids compete for common enzymes in the fatty acid-eicosanoid metabolic pathways, including desaturase enzymes, $PLA_2$, cyclooxygenases, and lipoxygenases, possibly, the suppression of omega-6-derived eicosanoid production by omega-3 fatty acids may be involved.

In addition to the eicosanoid cellular-signaling systems that function by converting PUFAs into cellular-signaling agents, other membrane lipids are also targeted by specific enzymes that convert them into second messengers. For example, phosphatidylinositol bisphosphate ($PIP_2$) is a di-phosphorylated form of the membrane lipid phosphatidylinositol. $PIP_2$ is formed from the membrane lipid phosphatidylinositol by the action of phosphoinositide kinases present in cell membranes. The membrane-bound enzyme phospholipase C (PLC) cleaves $PIP_2$ into inositol triphosphate ($IP_3$) and diacylglycerol (DAG), two important cellular-signaling molecules. The DAG generated remains associated with the cell membrane and engages a signal cascade by activating protein kinase C (PKC) which, in turn, activates other cytosolic proteins by way of phosphorylation. Many cellular functions are regulated by PKC-dependent protein phosphorylation. $IP_3$ acts as a second messenger by entering the cytoplasm and activating $IP_3$ receptors to mobilize calcium from intracellular stores, such as smooth endoplasmic reticulum and mitochondria, raising cytosolic calcium levels, and activating a number of other protein systems.

Finally, sphingolipid degradation products also act as cellular-signaling agents (Ledeen & Wu, 2008; Merrill, Jr. et al., 1997). For example, the enzyme sphingomyelinase acts to degrade sphingolipids, leading to the production of ceramide, sphingosine, and sphingosine phosphate, which act as signaling agents in the cytoplasm and nucleus of cells.

## Fatty Acids and Lipids in CNS Diseases

Essential fatty acids are intimately involved in the regulation of pro- and anti-inflammatory responses. As such, a lack of or an imbalance in essential-fatty acid intake is associated with disorders involving acute or chronic inflammation. Deficiencies in omega-3 fatty acids, or an imbalance in the ratio of omega-6 to omega-3 fatty acids, are implicated in various disorders affecting the CNS, including Alzheimer's disease (Farooqui et al., 2007b), Parkinson's disease (Chen et al., 2003), stroke, schizophrenia, and mood disorders, among others (Adibhatla & Hatcher, 2008).

The exact mechanism for the role of fatty acid in disease is unclear, but various animal and human studies suggest several possible biological mechanisms. A positive association exists between the intake of omega-3 PUFA and the reduction of cardiovascular risk and adverse outcomes (Breteler, 2000). One mechanism linking fatty acids and cognitive function or dementia may be atherosclerosis and thrombotic events (Kalmijn, 2000). All of these may be a function of inflammation, and that may, in part, explain the role that omega-3 fatty acids play in dementia (Blok et al., 1996).

Amyotrophic lateral sclerosis (ALS) is an adult-onset neurodegenerative disease of uncertain origin. Diet affects the likelihood of developing ALS. High omega-3 PUFA intake is associated with a significantly reduced risk for developing ALS (Veldink et al., 2007). This effect was enhanced by a high intake of vitamin E, which acted synergistically with omega-3 PUFA to reduce the chances for developing ALS later in life. The level of intake of other compounds including flavonols, lycopene, vitamin C, vitamin $B_2$, glutamate, calcium, or phytoestrogens was not associated with the risk of developing ALS. Such findings are consistent with the possibility that a pro-inflammatory imbalance in omega-6 and omega-3 PUFAs could have some role in the development of ALS.

Studies with animal models support the importance of omega-3 fatty acids in learning and memory (Hashimoto et al., 2006). These findings were extended to Alzheimer's disease models, demonstrating evidence of protection against cognitive decline. Dietary DHA improved memory, increased synapse density, and decreased amyloid beta toxicity (Calon et al., 2004) and beta amyloid load (Lim et al., 2005) in the mouse models of Alzheimer's disease. This protection is positively correlated with increased synaptosomal plasma-membrane fluidity in the cerebral cortex, and this membrane fluidity plays an important role in the protection against memory loss provided by DHA. One characteristic of Alzheimer's disease is a reduction in the level of neuroactive steroids, with significantly lower amounts of pregnenolone and dehydroepiandrosterone (Adibhatla & Hatcher, 2008). These neuroactive steroids act on gamma-amino butyric acid (GABA) and glutamate receptors, and they have neuroprotective properties. Whether the reduced neuroactive steroid levels are etiologically involved in Alzheimer's disease, or are a secondary consequence of the disease is unknown.

Alterations in GABA and glutamate neurotransmission in the brain are thought to be involved in both schizophrenia and bipolar disorders. Because neuroactive steroids such as pregnenolone and dehydroepiandrosterone act to modulate glutamate and GABA receptors, possibly, these psychiatric disorders are associated with a disruption of steroid synthesis in the brain. Reportedly, schizophrenia patients have reduced levels of AA and DHA, and this deficiency may have some role in the pathogenesis of these disorders. Furthermore, dietary supplementation with the essential fatty acid EPA showed beneficial effects on schizophrenia and bipolar disorder (Adibhatla & Hatcher, 2008).

Proper brain functioning requires a balance between excitatory and inhibitory neural activities, and these are mediated by different types of nerve cells. Excitatory neurons release transmitters such as the amino acid glutamate, whereas inhibitory neurons release neurotransmitters such as GABA. Proper brain function requires that the release of the excitatory neurotransmitter glutamate be counterbalanced by the release of GABA from inhibitory neurons. GABA prevents glutamate from over-activating neurons, which can lead to seizures. When brain damage results in the loss of inhibitory neurons in part of the brain, the results can be excessive excitation of neurons and seizures.

Epilepsy is a CNS disorder that is associated with seizures of varying severity and duration, which are often caused by ineffective inhibitory neural activity. Anti-epileptic drugs work by a number of mechanisms, including either enhancing the inhibitory actions of GABA or blocking the excitatory actions of glutamate. However, a dietary approach was found that is also effective in reducing seizures in patients with epilepsy. This approach is known as the ketogenic diet because it is meant to increase the level of so-called ketone bodies in the blood through altering the dietary intake of fats. It is now well-established that the ketogenic diet is an effective nonpharmacological approach to the symptomatic treatment for epilepsy (Bough et al., 2002; Bough & Eagles, 1999). Dietary fats are increased dramatically, and carbohydrates are nearly eliminated. The result is a drastic shift in blood metabolites away from free glucose to increased levels of ketone bodies, including hydroxybutyrate, aceoacetate, and acetone. These can enter the brain and are used as energy sources in the place of glucose. Shifting the brain's primary energy source from glucose to ketone bodies has a powerful effect on reducing seizure frequency in epilepsy patients. Although the effectiveness of the ketogenic diet was established as long as 80 years ago, the biochemical mechanisms involved are still unknown. Research is currently underway to understand the physiological basis of the efficacy of ketogenic diets in the control of epileptic seizures.

## Membrane Formation and Synaptic Membrane Turnover

Nerve cells communicate using neurotransmitters that are packaged and released from synaptic vesicles. Neural synapses are the structures by which nerve cells communicate through neurotransmitter release from presynaptic endings and receptor activation on postsynaptic membranes. To release neurotransmitters, synapses must constantly synthesize new membrane to produce synaptic vesicles, which store and release neurotransmitters into the synaptic cleft. The brain must synthesize new membrane lipids or recycle lipids from synaptic vesicles that were already released. This means that neural synapses are sites of rapid lipid turnover due to synaptic membrane synthesis and recycling.

Omega-3 fatty acids increase phosphatidylcholine levels and synaptic protein levels in the brain, whereas omega-6 PUFAs do not (Cansev & Wurtman, 2007). Specifically, in gerbils given DHA or EPA, glycerophospholipid levels were increased throughout the brain, including the cortex, striatum, hippocampus, brainstem, and cerebellum. In addition, the levels of synaptic-associated proteins were also increased, probably indicating a more rapid turnover of synaptic vesicle membranes. Giving gerbils the omega-6 PUFA AA had no effect on synaptic protein or membrane lipid levels, demonstrating that omega-3 fatty acids have a more profound effect on brain lipid composition and protein expression than omega-6 fatty acids. When rats are given diets poor in alpha-linolenic acid through two generations, the offspring have poorer learning performance and altered synaptic vesicle morphology in the hippocampus, possibly by reducing the rate of synaptic vesicle synthesis and turnover (Yoshida et al., 1997). In addition, chronic omega-3 PUFA dietary deficiency alters the density of dopamine-containing synaptic vesicles in the frontal cortex of rats (Zimmer et al., 2000).

To release neurotransmitters from synaptic vesicles, the vesicles must fuse with the internal face of the synaptic membrane and then create a pore through which transmitter molecules can enter the synaptic cleft. $PLA_2$ enzymes are involved in the synaptic vesicle fusion process by their ability to produce free PUFAs from membrane phospholipids, and these, in turn, may regulate the action of proteins known as syntaxins, which are involved in the vesicle fusion process (Darios et al., 2007).

## Myelin Synthesis in the CNS

One of the primary functions of the nervous system is to transmit nerve impulses rapidly over significant distances between neural centers. Myelin is a major lipid component of the nervous system which is critical for the proper conduction of nerve impulses, as well as for the survival of neuronal axons. Oligodendrocytes are glial cells of the CNS that produce the myelin sheaths that surround neuronal axons (Sherman

& Brophy, 2005). Oligodendrocytes are metabolically active cells, and require large inputs of basic substrates to synthesize and maintain the myelin sheaths surrounding fast-conducting nerve-cell axons. Myelin lipid synthesis and axonal myelination by oligodendrocytes require considerable substrate input from neuronal axons themselves. Neuronally derived substrates that become incorporated into myelin include serine, choline, acetate, palmitate, phosphate, and ethanolamine (Ledeen, 1984). One unique aspect of myelin lipid synthesis in the CNS is the involvement of the highly concentrated brain metabolite *N*-acetylaspartate (NAA) (reviewed in Moffett et al., 2006, 2007). In addition to the compounds listed above, NAA also provides a critical substrate for central myelin lipid synthesis. NAA is synthesized in neurons (Goldstein, 1969; Moffett et al., 1991; Moffett & Namboodiri, 1995) from aspartate and acetyl-CoA, and is transferred to oligodendrocytes where the NAA-degrading enzyme aspartoacylase (ASPA) is localized (Klugmann et al., 2003; Madhavarao et al., 2004). NAA is catabolized in oligodendrocytes into free acetate and aspartate, and the NAA-derived acetate is used to synthesize some portion of the lipids that comprise myelin (Burri et al., 1991; Chakraborty et al., 2001; D'Adamo et al., 1968; Madhavarao et al., 2005; Wang et al., 2007). This lipogenic pathway is thought to be specific to the nervous system.

## Unique Aspects of CNS Lipid Synthesis

D'Adamo and colleagues first demonstrated the incorporation of the acetate moiety of NAA into fatty acids in the brain during myelination, and showed that incorporation from NAA was three times greater than from free acetate ( D'Adamo, Jr. et al., 1968; D'Adamo, Jr. & Yatsu, 1966). They noted the growing body of evidence indicating that fatty acid and lipid syntheses in the CNS were different from those in other tissues. Evidence has since accumulated showing that brain lipid synthesis differs mechanistically from lipid synthesis in many peripheral tissues. Lipid synthesis requires a continuous supply of acetyl CoA, as does the synthesis of NAA. However, the generation of acetyl CoA is a complex and poorly understood aspect of lipid synthesis (Nikolau et al., 2000). Further, the various sources of acetate other than that which is directly generated from the citric-acid cycle as acetyl-CoA remain uncertain. In many peripheral tissues, cells are thought to produce most or all of the acetyl-CoA required for fatty acid synthesis by the action of the cytoplasmic enzyme ATP citrate lyase (EC 2.3.3.8) (Goldberg & Brunengraber, 1980; Jones & Ashton, 1976). The major source of carbon units for lipid synthesis through this critical lipogenic pathway is glucose, by way of pyruvate produced in the glycolytic pathway (Bauer et al., 2005). The pyruvate produced from glucose enters the citric acid cycle in mitochondria as acetyl Co-A, which is then converted to citrate that is exported to the cytoplasm to be reconverted to acetyl Co-A. In this ATP citrate lyase-dependent lipogenic pathway, free-acetate molecules are not involved at any step, and this is one reason why the role of free acetate in brain lipid synthesis is neglected. In the cytosol of most cell types, ATP citrate lyase catalyzes the reaction of citrate and CoA to produce oxaloacetate and acetyl-CoA, and the acetyl-CoA synthesized can then be used for the synthesis of cellular lipids.

However, when highly available sources of free acetate for lipid synthesis exist, certain cell types make direct use of this acetate for lipogenesis. Studies of fatty acid synthesis in intestinal colonocytes highlight the distinct mechanisms of lipid synthesis from free acetate. Intestinal colonocytes are rapidly dividing cells that synthesize the bulk of their own cholesterol and fatty acids from substrates such as acetate and butyrate derived from bacterial metabolism in the gut. When colonocytes are incubated with [$^{14}$C]-labeled substrates including glucose, glutamine, propionate, hydroxybutyrate, butyrate, and acetate, acetate provides more carbon to lipids than the other substrates (Zambell et al., 2003). This indicates that citric-acid cycle-generated acetyl-CoA was not significantly involved in *de novo* lipid synthesis in these cells. Further, hydroxycitrate, an inhibitor of the ATP citrate lyase enzyme, did not inhibit acetate incorporation into lipids, suggesting that the ATP citrate lyase reaction was not critical for lipid synthesis in colonocytes. Therefore, unlike liver cells, intestinal colonocytes do not use citric-acid cycle-derived acetyl-CoA as the primary carbon source for lipid synthesis. Like intestinal colonocytes, oligodendrocytes in the brain may also make use of a similar alternate pathway of acetyl-CoA production involving free acetate. In support of this, an ATP citrate lyase-independent pathway of acetate incorporation into sterols has been reported in calf-brain oligodendrocytes in culture (Pleasure et al., 1979).

The concentration of NAA in the brain is exceptionally high, ranging between 8 and 12 mM (Moffett et al., 2007). This provides ample levels of free acetate for fatty acid synthesis as long as the enzymes required to degrade NAA, and then synthesize acetyl-CoA from free acetate and CoA, are expressed in the CNS. Oligodendrocytes are known to strongly express the NAA-degrading enzyme aspartoacylase (Baslow et al., 1999; Klugmann et al., 2003; Madhavarao et al., 2004), but little is known about the expression of acetyl-CoA synthase enzymes in the brain. The acetyl-CoA synthase-1 expression is developmentally regulated, with increased expression in the brain and spinal cord during embryogenesis (Loikkanen et al., 2002). This correlates well with studies showing that the expression of ASPA in the brain is also developmentally regulated, with the highest expression occurring during the peak period of postnatal myelination in the CNS (Kirmani et al., 2003). At least two forms of acetyl-CoA synthase enzymes (also called acetate-CoA ligases) are known to be expressed in the brain, acetyl-CoA synthetase-1 (ACS1; EC 6.2.1.1), which appears to be a nucleocytoplasmic enzyme, and ACS2, a mitochondrial enzyme. ACS1 is the most likely candidate for a lipogenic enzyme in the brain capable of converting the acetate derived from NAA into acetyl-CoA, and then fatty acids.

Radiolabeled carbon infusion and feeding experiments show a much more rapid turnover of the acetate carbon in NAA than the aspartate moiety (Karelson et al., 2003), suggesting that the acetate from NAA is highly active in brain metabolism, particularly lipid synthesis associated with CNS myelination. ATP citrate lyase is strongly expressed in the developing brain, and ATP citrate lyase-deficient mice die early in development, highlighting the essential role of this reaction in lipid synthesis in many cell types and the fact that ACS1 can not compensate for the loss of the ATP citrate lyase pathway (Beigneux et al., 2004). Likely, the brain uses both of these acetyl-CoA synthesizing pathways together to meet the strong demand for lipid synthesis in the CNS during postnatal myelination. The ASPA–ACS1 pathway in this view is a parallel pathway for acetyl-CoA production and lipogenesis (Fig. 21.6).

This emerging view of parallel lipogenic pathways for myelin lipid synthesis in the CNS involving both citrate and NAA as substrates is a departure from the traditional view. In this role, NAA is seen as an adjunct mitochondrial export from neuronal mitochondria (in addition to citrate). The NAA is then transferred to the cytoplasm of oligodendrocytes for myelin lipid synthesis. The purpose of this arrangement is unknown, but could be due to a lack of transport mechanisms for

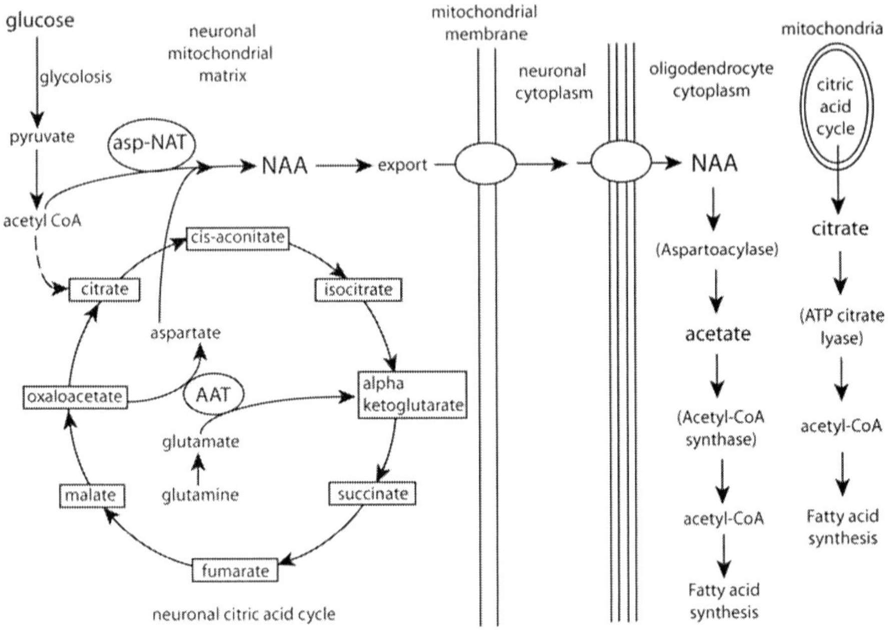


**Fig. 21.6.** Dual substrate sources for myelin-lipid synthesis in oligodendrocytes. Neuronal mitochondria synthesize and export NAA, which is then transported from the cytoplasm of neurons to the cytoplasm of oligodendrocytes. In oligodendrocytes, the NAA is broken down into aspartate and free acetate by the enzyme aspartoacylase, and the acetate is then converted to acetyl-CoA, probably by the action of acetyl-CoA synthase. Oligodendrocyte mitochondria export citrate, which acts as a primary source of substrate for acetyl-CoA synthesis in the cytoplasm of oligodendrocytes. The NAA pathway of fatty acid synthesis in oligodendrocytes is a secondary, but essential, source of acetyl-CoA during postnatal CNS myelination. Abbreviations: asp-NAT = aspartate *N*-acetyltransferase (NAA synthetic enzyme), AAT = aspartate aminotransferase (enzyme in neuronal mitochondria), NAA = *N*-acetylaspartate.

citrate from neurons to oligodendrocytes. In this hypothesis, NAA is produced, in part, to be transported specifically to oligodendrocytes to provide additional substrate for fatty acid synthesis. As such, NAA synthesized in neuronal mitochondria and citrate synthesized in oligodendrocyte mitochondria both participate in CNS myelin lipid synthesis. This bipartite system for delivering substrates to lipogenic pathways in oligodendrocytes may be necessary for the demanding task of postnatal CNS myelination. Both neurons and oligodendrocytes provide the basic substrates for myelin lipid synthesis, and the interaction is necessary for the survival of both types of cell.

# Conclusion

Essential PUFAs are critical for normal brain function and for the brain's response to injury or disease. Modern Western diets are notoriously low in essential omega-3 fatty acids due to the increasing use of vegetable and animal oils and fats and the reduced intake of fish and shellfish. This resulted in an imbalance in the essential omega-3 to omega-6 fatty acid ratios in the tissues of the populations of many developed countries. Omega-3 and omega-6 fatty acids are the precursors for the synthesis of critical eicosanoid cellular-signaling agents, but these two types of fatty acid are converted into cellular-signaling agents with generally opposing effects on inflammatory responses. Omega-3 PUFAs are converted into eicosanoids with predominantly anti-inflammatory properties, whereas omega-6 PUFAs are converted into eicosanoids with pro-inflammatory properties. This shift in dietary intake may be responsible for many pathological conditions that are associated with chronic inflammation. Increasing the dietary intake of omega-3 PUFAs has many beneficial effects on health, and may prove to be useful in treating CNS disorders ranging from Alzheimer's disease to schizophrenia.

## References

Adibhatla, R.M.; J.F. Hatcher. Altered lipid metabolism in brain injury and disorders. *Subcell. Biochem.* **2008,**48, nihpa41041.

Adibhatla, R.M.; J.F. Hatcher; R.J. Dempsey. Lipids and lipidomics in brain injury and diseases. *AAPS. J.* **2006,** *8,* E314–E321.

Baslow, M.H.; R.F. Suckow; V. Sapirstein;B.L. Hungund. Expression of aspartoacylase activity in cultured rat macroglial cells is limited to oligodendrocytes. *J. Mol. Neurosci.* **1999,** *13,* 47–53.

Bauer, D.E.; G. Hatzivassiliou; F. Zhao; C. Andreadis;C.B. Thompson. ATP citrate lyase is an important component of cell growth and transformation. *Oncogene* **2005,** *24,* 6314–6322.

Beigneux, A.P.; C. Kosinski; B. Gavino; J.D. Horton; W.C. Skarnes; S.G. Young. ATP-citrate lyase deficiency in the mouse. *J. Biol. Chem.* **2004,** 279, 9557–9564.

Benani, A.; C. Vol; T. Heurtaux; C. Asensio; M. Dauca; F. Lapicque; P. Netter; A. Minn. Up-regulation of fatty acid metabolizing-enzymes mRNA in rat spinal cord during persistent peripheral local inflammation. *Eur. J. Neurosci.* **2003,** *18,* 1904–1914.

Blok, W.L.; M.B. Katan; J.W. van der Meer. Modulation of inflammation and cytokine production by dietary (n-3) fatty acids. *J. Nutr.* **1996,** *126,* 1515–1533.

Bough, K.J.; D.A. Eagles. A ketogenic diet increases the resistance to pentylenetetrazole-induced seizures in the rat. *Epilepsia* **1999,** *40,* 138–143.

Bough, K.J.; K. Gudi; F.T. Han; A.H. Rathod; D.A. Eagles. An anticonvulsant profile of the ketogenic diet in the rat. *Epilepsy Res.* **2002,** *50,* 313–325.

Breteler, M.M. Vascular involvement in cognitive decline and dementia. Epidemiologic evidence from the Rotterdam Study and the Rotterdam Scan Study. *Ann. N.Y. Acad. Sci.* **2000,** *903,* 457–465.

Burri, R.; C. Steffen; N. Herschkowitz; N. N-acetyl-L-aspartate is a major source of acetyl groups for lipid synthesis during rat brain development. *Dev. Neurosci.* **1991,** *13,* 403–412.

Calon, F.; G.P. Lim; F. Yang; T. Morihara; B. Teter; O. Ubeda; P. Rostaing; A. Triller; N. Salem, Jr.; K.H. Ashe; S.A. Frautschy;G.M. Cole. Docosahexaenoic acid protects from dendritic pathology in an Alzheimer's disease mouse model. *Neuron* **2004,** *43,* 633–645.

Cansev, M.; R.J. Wurtman. Chronic administration of docosahexaenoic acid or eicosapentaenoic acid, but not arachidonic acid, alone or in combination with uridine, increases brain phosphatide and synaptic protein levels in gerbils. *Neurosci.* **2007,** *148,* 421–431.

Carrie, I.; M. Clement; J.D. de; H. Frances;J.M. Bourre. Specific phospholipid fatty acid composition of brain regions in mice. Effects of n-3 polyunsaturated fatty acid deficiency and phospholipid supplementation. *J. Lipid Res.* **2000,** *41,* 465–472.

Chakraborty, G.; P. Mekala; D. Yahya; G. Wu;R.W. Ledeen. Intraneuronal N-acetylaspartate supplies acetyl groups for myelin lipid synthesis: evidence for myelin-associated aspartoacylase. *J. Neurochem.* **2001,** *78,* 736–745.

Chen, H.; S.M. Zhang; M.A. Hernan; W.C. Willett; A. Ascherio. Dietary intakes of fat and risk of Parkinson's disease. *Am. J. Epidemiol.* **2003,** *157,* 1007–1014.

Cheng, H.; D.J. Mancuso; X. Jiang; S. Guan; J. Yang; K. Yang; G. Sun; R.W. Gross;X. Han. Shotgun lipidomics reveals the temporally dependent, highly diversified cardiolipin profile in the mammalian brain: temporally coordinated postnatal diversification of cardiolipin molecular species with neuronal remodeling. *Biochemistry* **2008.**

Coetzee, T.; K. Suzuki; K.A. Nave; B. Popko. Myelination in the absence of galactolipids and proteolipid proteins. *Mol. Cell Neurosci.* **1999,** *14,* 41–51.

Crawford, M.A.; M. Bloom; C.L. Broadhurst; W.F. Schmidt; S.C. Cunnane; C. Galli;K. Gehbremeskel; F. Linseisen; J. Lloyd-Smith;J. Parkington. Evidence for the unique function of docosahexaenoic acid during the evolution of the modern hominid brain. *Lipids* **1999,** *34,* (Suppl.) S39–S47.

D'Adamo, A.F.; L.I. Gidez; F.M. Yatsu. Acetyl transport mechanisms. Involvement of N-acetyl aspartic acid in *de novo* fatty acid biosynthesis in the developing rat brain. *Exp. Brain Res.* **1968,** *5,* 267–273.

D'Adamo, A.F., Jr.; L.I. Gidez; F.M. Yatsu. Acetyl transport mechanisms. Involvement of N-acetyl aspartic acid in *de novo* fatty acid biosynthesis in the developing rat brain. *Exp. Brain Res.* **1968,** *5,* 267–273.

D'Adamo, A.F., Jr.; F.M. Yatsu. Acetate metabolism in the nervous system. N-acetyl-L-aspartic acid and the biosynthesis of brain lipids. *J. Neurochem.* **1966,** *13,* 961–965.

Dangour, A.D.; R. Uauy. Nutrition challenges for the twenty-first century. *Br. J. Nutr.* **2006,** *96* (Suppl. 1), S2–S7.

Darios, F.; E. Connell; B. Davletov. Phospholipases and fatty acid signalling in exocytosis. *J. Physiol.* **2007,** *585,* 699–704.

Eaton, S.B.; S.B. Eaton, III; M.J. Konner. Paleolithic nutrition revisited: a twelve-year retrospective on its nature and implications. *Eur. J. Clin. Nutr.* **1997,** *51,* 207–216.

Eaton, S.B.; M. Konner. Paleolithic nutrition. A consideration of its nature and current implications. *N. Engl. J. Med.* **1985,** *312,* 283–289.

Edmond, J.; T.A. Higa; R.A. Korsak; E.A. Bergner; W.N. Lee. Fatty acid transport and utilization for the developing brain. *J. Neurochem.* **1998,** *70,* 1227–1234.

Fahy, E.; S. Subramaniam; H.A. Brown; C.K. Glass;A.H. Merrill, Jr.: R.C. Murphy; C.R. Raetz; D.W. Russell; Y. Seyama; W. Shaw; T. Shimizu; F. Spener; M.G. van; M.S. VanNieuwenhze; S.H. White; J.L. Witztum; E.A. Dennis. A comprehensive classification system for lipids. *J. Lipid Res.* **2005,** *46,* 839–861.

Farooqui, A.A.; L.A. Horrocks. Plasmalogens: workhorse lipids of membranes in normal and injured neurons and glia. *Neuroscientist* **2001,** *7,* 232–245.

Farooqui, A.A.; L.A. Horrocks; T. Farooqui. Modulation of inflammation in brain: a matter of fat. *J. Neurochem.* **2007a,** *101,* 577–599.

Farooqui, A.A.; W.Y. Ong; L.A. Horrocks; P. Chen; T. Farooqui. Comparison of biochemical effects of statins and fish oil in brain: the battle of the titans. *Brain Res. Rev.* **2007b,** *56,* 443–471.

Ford, D.A.; J.K. Monda; R.S. Brush; R.E. Anderson; M.J. Richards; S.J. Fliesler. Lipidomic analysis of the retina in a rat model of Smith-Lemli-Opitz syndrome: alterations in docosahexaenoic acid content of phospholipid molecular species. *J. Neurochem.* **2008,** *105,* 1032–1047.

Goldberg, R.P.; H. Brunengraber. Contributions of cytosolic and mitochondrial acetyl-CoA syntheses to the activation of lipogenic acetate in rat liver. *Adv. Exp. Med. Biol.* **1980,** *132,* 413–418.

Goldstein, F.B. The enzymatic synthesis of N-acetyl-L-aspartic acid by subcellular preparations of rat brain. *J. Biol. Chem.* **1969,** *244,* 4257–4260.

Gross, R.W.; C.M. Jenkins; J. Yang; D.J. Mancuso;X. Han. Functional lipidomics: the roles of specialized lipids and lipid-protein interactions in modulating neuronal function. *Prostaglandins Other Lipid Mediat.* **2005,** *77,* 52–64.

Han, X.; R.W. Gross. Shotgun lipidomics: multidimensional MS analysis of cellular lipidomes. *Expert. Rev. Proteomics.* **2005,** *2,* 253–264.

Han, X.; M. Holtzman; D.W. McKeel, Jr.; J. Kelley; J.C. Morris. Substantial sulfatide deficiency and ceramide elevation in very early Alzheimer's disease: potential role in disease pathogenesis. *J. Neurochem.* **2002,** *82,* 809–818.

Hashimoto, M.; S. Hossain; T. Shimada; O. Shido. Docosahexaenoic acid-induced protective effect against impaired learning in amyloid beta-infused rats is associated with increased synaptosomal membrane fluidity. *Clin. Exp. Pharmacol. Physiol.* **2006,** *33,* 934–939.

Hong, S.; K. Gronert; P.R. Devchand; R.L. Moussignac; C.N. Serhan. Novel docosatrienes and 17S-resolvins generated from docosahexaenoic acid in murine brain, human blood, and glial cells. Autacoids in anti-inflammation. *J. Biol. Chem.* **2003,** *278,* 14677–14687.

Jakobsson, A.; R. Westerberg; A. Jacobsson. Fatty acid elongases in mammals: their regulation and roles in metabolism. *Prog. Lipid Res.* **2006,** *45,* 237–249.

Jones, C.T.; I.K. Ashton. Lipid biosynthesis in liver slices of the foetal guinea pig. *Biochem. J.* **1976,** *154,* 149–158.

Jurevics, H.; P. Morell. Cholesterol for synthesis of myelin is made locally, not imported into brain. *J. Neurochem.* **1995,** *64,* 895–901.

Kalmijn, S. Fatty acid intake and the risk of dementia and cognitive decline: a review of clinical and epidemiological studies. *J. Nutr. Health Aging* **2000,** *4,* 202–207.

Karelson, G.; A. Ziegler; B. Kunnecke; J. Seelig. Feeding versus infusion: a novel approach to study the NAA metabolism in rat brain. *NMR Biomed.* **2003,** *16,* 413–423.

Kirmani, B.F.; D.M. Jacobowitz; M.A. Namboodiri. Developmental increase of aspartoacylase in oligodendrocytes parallels CNS myelination. *Brain Res. Dev. Brain Res.* **2003,** *140,* 105–115.

Klugmann, M.; C.W. Symes; B.K. Klaussner;C.B. Leichtlein; T. Serikawa; D. Young;M.J. During. Identification and distribution of aspartoacylase in the postnatal rat brain. *Neuroreport* **2003,** *14,* 1837–1840.

Ledeen, R.W. Lipid-metabolizing enzymes of myelin and their relation to the axon. *J. Lipid Res.* **1984,** *25,* 1548–1554.

Ledeen, R.W.;G. Wu. Thematic Review Series: Sphingolipids. Nuclear sphingolipids: metabolism and signaling. *J. Lipid Res.* **2008,** *49,* 1176–1186.

Lim, G.P.; F. Calon; T. Morihara; F. Yang; B. Teter; O. Ubeda; N. Salem, Jr.; S.A. Frautschy;G.M. Cole. A diet enriched with the omega-3 fatty acid docosahexaenoic acid reduces amyloid burden in an aged Alzheimer mouse model. *J. Neurosci.* **2005,** *25,* 3032–3040.

Loikkanen, I.; S. Haghighi; S. Vainio; A. Pajunen. Expression of cytosolic acetyl-CoA synthetase gene is developmentally regulated. *Mech. Dev.* **2002,** *115,* 139–141.

Lopez-Lopez, A.; M.C. Lopez-Sabater; C. Campoy-Folgoso; M. Rivero-Urgell; A.I. Castellote-Bargallo. Fatty acid and sn-2 fatty acid composition in human milk from Granada (Spain) and in infant formulas. *Eur. J. Clin. Nutr.* **2002,** *56,* 1242–1254.

Madhavarao, C.N.; P. Arun; J.R. Moffett; S. Szucs; S. Surendran; R. Matalon; J. Garbern; D. Hristova; A. Johnson; W. Jiang;M.A. Namboodiri. Defective N-acetylaspartate catabolism reduces brain acetate levels and myelin lipid synthesis in Canavan's disease. *Proc. Natl. Acad. Sci. U.S.A.* **2005,** *102,* 5221–5226.

Madhavarao, C.N.; J.R. Moffett; R.A. Moore; R.E. Viola; M.A. Namboodiri; D.M. Jacobowitz. Immunohistochemical localization of aspartoacylase in the rat central nervous system. *J. Comp. Neurol.* **2004,** *472,* 318–329.

Marcheselli, V.L.; S. Hong; W.J. Lukiw; X.H. Tian; K. Gronert; A. Musto; M. Hardy;J.M. Gimenez; N. Chiang; C.N. Serhan;N.G. Bazan. Novel docosanoids inhibit brain ischemia-reperfusion-mediated leukocyte infiltration and pro-inflammatory gene expression. *J. Biol. Chem.* **2003,** *278,* 43807–43817.

Marcus, J.; J.L. Dupree; B. Popko. Effects of galactolipid elimination on oligodendrocyte development and myelination. *Glia* **2000,** *30,* 319–328.

Merrill, A.H., Jr.; E.M. Schmelz; D.L. Dillehay;S. Spiegel; J.A. Shayman; J.J. Schroeder; R.T. Riley; K.A. Voss; E. Wang.Sphingolipids—the enigmatic lipid class: biochemistry, physiology, and pathophysiology. *Toxicol. Appl. Pharmacol.* **1997,** *142,* 208–225.

Moffett, J.R.; M.A. Namboodiri. Differential distribution of N-acetylaspartylglutamate and N-acetylaspartate immunoreactivities in rat forebrain. *J. Neurocytol.* **1995,** *24,* 409–433.

Moffett, J.R.; M.A. Namboodiri; C.B. Cangro;J.H. Neale. Immunohistochemical localization of N-acetylaspartate in rat brain. *Neuroreport* **1991,** *2,* 131–134.

Moffett, J.R.; B. Ross; P. Arun; C.N. Madhavarao;A.M. Namboodiri. N-Acetylaspartate in the CNS: From neurodiagnostics to neurobiology. *Prog. Neurobiol.* **2007,** *81,* 89–131.

Moffett, J.R.; S.B. Tieman; D.R. Weinberger; J.T. Coyle; M.A. Namboodiri. *N-Acetylaspartate: A Unique Neuronal Molecule in the Central Nervous System;* Springer Science + Business Media: New York, NY, 2006.

Natter, K.; P. Leitner; A. Faschinger; H. Wolinski;S. McCraith; S. Fields; S.D. Kohlwein. The spatial organization of lipid synthesis in the yeast Saccharomyces cerevisiae derived from large scale green fluorescent protein tagging and high resolution microscopy. *Mol. Cell Proteomics.* **2005,** *4,* 662–672.

Nikolau, B.J.; D.J. Oliver; P.S. Schnable; E.S. Wurtele. Molecular biology of acetyl-CoA metabolism. *Biochem. Soc. Trans.* **2000,** *28,* 591–593.

Pleasure, D.; C. Lichtman; S. Eastman; M. Lieb;O. Abramsky; D. Silberberg. Acetoacetate and D-(-)-beta-hydroxybutyrate as precursors for sterol synthesis by calf oligodendrocytes in suspension culture: extramitochondrial pathway for acetoacetate metabolism. *J. Neurochem.* **1979,** *32,* 1447–1450.

Rapoport, S.I.; J.S. Rao; M. Igarashi. Brain metabolism of nutritionally essential polyunsaturated fatty acids depends on both the diet and the liver. *Prostaglandins Leukotrienes Essent. Fatty Acids* **2007,** *77,* 251–261.

Ruxton, C.H.; S.C. Reed; M.J. Simpson;K.J. Millington. The health benefits of omega-3 polyunsaturated fatty acids: a review of the evidence. *J. Hum. Nutr. Diet.* **2004,** *17,* 449–459.

Serhan, C.N.; M. Arita; S. Hong; K. Gotlinger. Resolvins, docosatrienes, and neuroprotectins, novel omega-3-derived mediators, and their endogenous aspirin-triggered epimers. *Lipids* **2004,** *39,* 1125–1132.

Sherman, D.L.; P.J. Brophy. Mechanisms of axon ensheathment and myelin growth. *Nat. Rev. Neurosci.* **2005,** *6,* 683–690.

Simopoulos, A.P. The omega-6/omega-3 fatty acid ratio, genetic variation, and cardiovascular disease. *Asia Pac. J. Clin. Nutr.* **2008,** *17* (Suppl. 1), 131–134.

Uauy, R.; A.D. Dangour. Nutrition in brain development and aging: role of essential fatty acids. *Nutr. Rev.* **2006,** *64,* S24–S33.

van Echten-Deckert, G.; T. Herget. Sphingolipid metabolism in neural cells. *Biochim. Biophys. Acta* **2006,** *1758,* 1978–1994.

Veldink, J.H.; S. Kalmijn; G.J. Groeneveld; W. Wunderink; A. Koster; J.H. de Vries; L.J. van der; J.H. Wokke; L.H. van den Berg. Intake of polyunsaturated fatty acids and vitamin E reduces the risk of developing amyotrophic lateral sclerosis. *J. Neurol. Neurosurg. Psychiatry* **2007,** *78,* 367–371.

Wang, J.; R. Matalon; G. Bhatia; G. Wu; H. Li;T. Liu; Z.H. Lu; R.W. Ledeen. Bimodal occurrence of aspartoacylase in myelin and cytosol of brain. *J. Neurochem.* **2007 .**

Yehuda, S.; S. Rabinovitz; D.I. Mostofsky. Essential fatty acids and the brain: from infancy to aging. *Neurobiol. Aging* **2005,** *26* (Suppl. 1), 98–102.

Yoshida, S.; A. Yasuda; H. Kawazato; K. Sakai;T. Shimada; M. Takeshita; S. Yuasa; T. Kobayashi; S. Watanabe; H. Okuyama. Synaptic vesicle ultrastructural changes in the rat hippocampus induced by a combination of alpha-linolenate deficiency and a learning task. *J. Neurochem.* **1997,** *68,* 1261–1268.

Zambell, K.L.; M.D. Fitch; S.E. Fleming. Acetate and butyrate are the major substrates for *de novo* lipogenesis in rat colonic epithelial cells. *J. Nutr.* **2003,** *133,* 3509–3515.

Zimmer, L.; S. Delpal; D. Guilloteau; J. Aioun;G. Durand; S. Chalon. Chronic n-3 polyunsaturated fatty acid deficiency alters dopamine vesicle density in the rat frontal cortex. *Neurosci. Lett.* **2000,** *284,* 25–28.

—•● 22 ●•—

# Fatty Acids in Immunomodulation: Role in Disease Prevention and Causation

**John W.C. Sijben[1], Günter Boehm[2,3], and Philip C. Calder[4]**

*[1]Danone Research—Centre for Specialised Nutrition, Bosrandweg 20, P.O. Box 7005, 6700 CA Wageningen, The Netherlands; [2]Danone Research—Centre for Specialised Nutrition, Bahnstr. 14–30, 61381 Friedrichsdorf, Germany; [3]Sophia's Children Hospital, Erasmus University, Rotterdam 3015 GE, The Netherlands; [4]Institute of Human Nutrition, School of Medicine, University of Southampton, IDS Building, MP887 Southampton General Hospital, Tremona Road, Southampton SO16 6YD, United Kingdom*

## Introduction

Over the course of the twentieth century, the dietary intake of fats in Western diets substantially changed. For example, in the United States the share of calories derived from fat increased from 32% during 1909–1913 to 43% in 1984 (Raper & Marston, 1986). This gain in fat intake was almost entirely due to an increase in fat from vegetable sources. Fat from vegetable oil more than tripled, from 21–70 g per capita per day in this period, an increase of the relative proportion of fat intake from 17–42%. Because vegetable oils, compared with animal fats, are very rich in polyunsaturated fatty acids (PUFAs), particularly of the n-6 type, the contribution of the major n-6 PUFA, linoleic acid (LA; 18:2n-6), increased from 2–7% of the total energy intake between the early twentieth century and 1984 in the United States (Raper & Marston, 1986). LA is now estimated to contribute up to 9% of the total energy intake in the United States (Hibbeln et al., 2006). LA, rather than $\alpha$-linolenic acid (ALA; 18:3n-3), an n-3 PUFA, is the predominant essential fatty acid (EFA) in the Western diet, resulting in a dietary n-6 to n-3 EFA ratio of 5–30 in present-day Western societies (Burdge & Calder, 2005). The apparent trend of the changing EFA intake is observed already at the first stages of life. For example, the proportion of LA in milk from women in the United States increased from 6–7% to 15–16% of total fatty acids (FAs) between the 1940s and the 1990s (see Ailhaud et al., 2006 for references). As the percentage of ALA remained essentially the same over this period, the LA to linolenic acid (LNA) ratio increased at the same rate as the LA level.

The dietary intakes of the longer chain, more unsaturated PUFAs are very much lower than those of the EFAs (British Nutrition Foundation, 1992, 1999). However, these longer chain, more unsaturated PUFAs appear to be readily incorporated into the membranes in a variety of cells and tissues, and they serve as precursors of bioactive molecules. Thus, likely, an important functional significance is related to the differences in the intake of these FAs. Some plant oils contain γ-linolenic acid (GLA: 18:3n-6), dihomo-γ-linolenic acid (DGLA; 20:3n-6), and stearidonic acid (STA; 18:4n-3), but typical intakes of these FAs from the diet are likely to be <10 mg/day. Arachidonic acid (AA; 20:4n-6) is found in meat and eggs, and intakes are estimated to be 50–500 mg/day. Eicosapentaenoic acid (EPA; 20:5n-3), docosapentaenoic acid (DPA; 22:5n-3), and docosahexaenoic acid (DHA; 22:6n-3) are mainly found in fish and other seafood, with oily fish being a rich source providing 1.5–3.5 grams of n-3 long-chain PUFA [PUFA with C >18, long-chain (LC)PUFA] per portion (British Nutrition Foundation, 1999). Little information is available on longitudinal trends in the consumption of LC-PUFA. In 1985 in the United States, the consumption of both EPA and DHA was similar to that during 1935–1939 (i.e., 124 versus 118 mg/day, respectively) (Raper et al., 1992). The significant decline in the use of fatty fish in this period was compensated by an increased supply from other foods that contain low amounts of these FAs, such as poultry. Due to a marked increase in the use of vegetable oils, the proportion of n-3 LC-PUFA as a percentage of total fat or of total PUFA declined from 0.09% to 0.07% and from 0.8% to 0.4%, respectively, over this period. The current AA to DHA ratio of breast milk from women in Western countries is between approximately 1.6 and 3.2 (Yuhas et al., 2006), whereas the ratio in breast milk from women in non-Western countries is closer to 1.0 (Jensen, 1999; Yuhas et al., 2006) which is close to the estimated value for early *homo sapiens* (Muskiet et al., 2006). In children the daily ingestion of cod-liver oil, a source of n-3 LC-PUFA, was very common until the mid-twentieth century, but this decreased dramatically once vitamins A and D were artificially synthesized. Thus, the alterations in the food chain over the past century are likely to have led to significant alterations in absolute and relative n-6 and n-3 EFA and LC-PUFA intakes throughout life.

The increased dietary n-6 to n-3 PUFA ratio—due to alterations in the food chain and the increased consumption of vegetable oils over the past century—was raised as a public-health concern (Simopoulos, 1999). In a recent workshop by the UK Food Standards Agency, the concept of n-6 to n-3 PUFA ratio as a useful dietary marker was discussed (Stanley et al., 2007). The conclusion was that absolute levels of specific n-6 PUFA and n-3 PUFA are preferred dietary markers because they are of greater relevance for physiological outcomes related to the risk of chronic disease. Hence, this information warrants a more detailed description of the potential effects of changed food trends in the twentieth century on immune function.

Human immune cells contain roughly equal proportions of saturated fatty acids, monounsaturated fatty acids, and PUFAs (Kew et al., 2004). Within the PUFA fraction, n-6 PUFAs are five to six times more abundant than n-3 PUFAs (Kew et al., 2004). In immune cells, LC-PUFAs exceed EFAs, accounting for 20–25% of total FAs, mainly as AA ( Kew et al., 2004; Miles et al., 2004; Rees et al., 2006; Thies et al., 2001; Yaqoob et al., 2000). Since the intake of LC-PUFA is less than 1% of total FAs in most individuals, these FAs are accumulated in immune cells, which may indicate a major functional importance. Indeed, the functionally most important PUFAs are LC-PUFAs because they can serve as precursors for the synthesis of bioactive lipid mediators, including prostaglandins (PGs), leukotrienes (LTs), lipoxins, and resolvins (Lewis et al., 1990; Serhan et al., 2004; Tilley et al., 2001; Vachier et al., 2002).

The FA composition of immune cells is susceptible to changes in the dietary intake of certain FAs. Changed habitually, PUFA intake can affect immune-cell FA compositions in a variety of ways. Firstly, an increased intake of LA may increase n-6 PUFA in peripheral blood mononuclear cells (PBMCs) (Damsgaard et al., 2008). Secondly, the conversion of ALA to EPA is reduced at high absolute intakes of LA (Goyens et al., 2006), which may result in a reduced incorporation of EPA into immune cells at times of a high dietary intake of LA. Thirdly, an increased intake of GLA results in an increased content of DGLA in human immune cells (Miles et al., 2004; Yaqoob et al., 2000) . Fourthly, an increased intake of ALA or STA increases the EPA content of human immune cells (Kew et al., 2003; Miles et al., 2004). Fifthly, the absolute and relative proportions of AA, EPA, and DHA in human immune cells are affected by the consumption of AA (Thies et al., 2001) or of n-3 LC-PUFAs (Rees et al., 2006; Yaqoob et al., 2000). The incorporation of n-3 LC-PUFA occurs in a dose-dependent manner (Healy et al., 2000; Rees et al., 2006), and is partly at the expense of AA, although proportions of other n-6 PUFAs, such as DGLA, are also decreased when n-3 LC-PUFAs are incorporated (Rees et al., 2006). Finally, increased intakes of *trans* FAs, including *trans*-18:1 isomers and conjugated LA isomers, result in an increased appearance of *trans* FAs that are normally found in very low amounts in human immune cells (Burdge et al., 2004; Kelley et al., 2001; Kuhnt et al., 2007). Again this incorporation of *trans* FAs into human immune cells occurs in a dose-dependent manner (Burdge et al., 2004).

Through this variety of mechanisms, the relative presence of n-6 LC-PUFAs—DGLA and AA—and of n-3 LC-PUFAs—EPA and DHA—can be changed; this can modify the functional activities of the cells involved and the immune response as a whole (Calder, 1996, 1998, 2001a, 2002, 2006b, 2007; Hwang, 2000; Sijben & Calder, 2007; Stulnig & Zeyda, 2004; Yaqoob, 2004). In brief, the dominance of AA, relative to n-3 LC-PUFA, in immune-cell phospholipids could, via its eicosanoid precursor function, potentiate inflammatory processes, and therefore could predispose to or exacerbate inflammatory diseases (Lewis et al., 1990; Tilley et al., 2001). This was proposed as a potential etiological factor for numerous disorders that are characterized by exaggerated inflammation and excessive formation of inflammatory eicosanoids and cytokines, such as allergies, asthma, chronic obstructive pulmonary disease (COPD), and inflammatory bowel diseases (IBDs). The suspicion of a possible causal role of dietary PUFA intake in these disorders has particularly risen because their increased prevalence in the past decades (Bach, 2002) coincides with the increased intake of n-6 PUFA described above. On the other hand, an increased intake of n-3 PUFA may dampen excessive inflammation (Calder, 2006b) and therewith exert suppressive effects on the pathogenesis of inflammatory diseases. In the current chapter, we aim to review the current evidence and plausibility of the role of dietary FAs as an environmental contributor to inflammatory disorders, in both early life and during adult life and aging.

## General Concept of Immunomodulation with Dietary Fatty Acids

The key link between FAs, inflammation, and immunity is that eicosanoids, which are among the most important mediators and regulators of inflammation and immune responses, are generated from the 20-carbon PUFAs—DGLA, AA, and EPA. Because inflammatory cells typically contain a high proportion of the n-6 PUFA AA and low proportions of other 20-carbon PUFAs (Calder, 2001a), AA is usually the major substrate for eicosanoid synthesis. Eicosanoids, which include prostaglandins (PGs), thromboxanes, leukotrienes (LTs), and other oxidized derivatives, are generated from AA by the action of cyclooxygenase and lipoxygenase enzymes as summarized in Fig. 22.1. These mediators are involved in modulating the intensity and duration of inflammatory responses (see Lewis et al., 1990 and Tilley et al., 2001 for reviews),

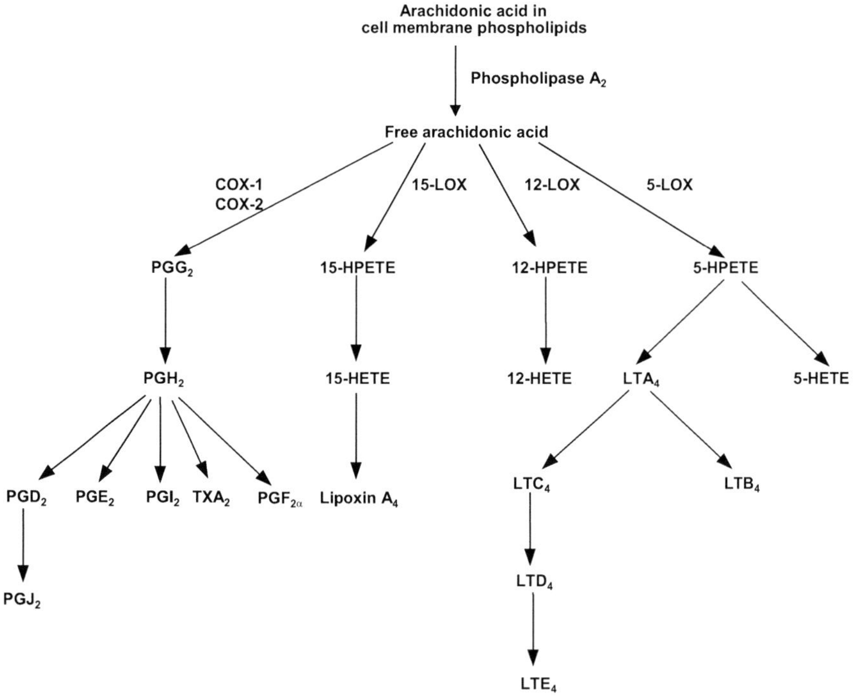


**Fig. 22.1.** Outline of the pathway of eicosanoid synthesis from arachidonic acid. COX, cyclooxygenase; HETE, hyroxyeicosatetraenoic acid; HPETE, hydroperoxyeicosatetraenoic acid; LOX, lipoxygenase; LT, leukotriene; PG, prostaglandin; TX, thromboxane (Calder, 2006a).

have cell- and stimulus-specific sources, and frequently have opposing effects (Calder, 2006b). Thus, the overall physiological (or pathophysiological) outcome will depend on the cells present, the nature of the stimulus, the timing of eicosanoid generation, the concentrations of different eicosanoids generated, and the sensitivity of target cells and tissues to the eicosanoids generated. In general, pro-inflammatory roles are ascribed to $PGE_2$ and 4-series LTs derived from AA. For example, $PGE_2$ induces fever, pain, vasodilation, and vascular permeability, while $LTB_4$ is chemotactic for leukocytes, and induces the release of reactive oxygen species by neutrophils and of inflammatory cytokines [tumor necrosis factor (TNF)-α, interleukin (IL)-1β, IL-6] by macrophages (Lewis et al., 1990; Tilley et al., 2001). With regard to cell-mediated immunity, $PGE_2$ inhibits T-cell proliferation and the production of T-helper 1-type cytokines [IL-2, interferon (IFN)-γ] by T cells and promotes immunoglobulin-E (IgE) production by B cells. In contrast, $LTB_4$ promotes the production of IL-2 and IFN-γ by T cells, and enhances natural killer (NK) cell activity.

Animal-feeding studies show a strong positive relationship between the amount of AA in immune cells and the ability of those cells to produce eicosanoids such as $PGE_2$ (Peterson et al., 1998); this was confirmed in humans (Rees et al., 2006). In turn, one can increase the amount of AA in inflammatory cells by including it in the diet of rats (Peterson et al., 1998) or by increasing the amount of it in the diet of humans (Thies et al., 2001c). The amount of AA in inflammatory cells may also be influenced by the dietary intake of its precursor, LA, although the range of LA intake over which this relationship occurs has not been defined for humans. The role of AA as a precursor for the synthesis of eicosanoids indicates the potential for dietary n-6 PUFA (LA or AA) to influence inflammatory and immune processes. The influence of increased dietary AA on immune outcomes was investigated in two studies in healthy humans. In one study, healthy young males supplemented their diets with 1.5 grams of AA per day for 7 weeks. This resulted in a marked increase in the production of $PGE_2$ and $LTB_4$ by bacterial lipopolysaccharide (LPS)-stimulated mononuclear cells (Kelley et al., 1998). However, the production of TNF-α, IL-1β, and IL-6 by the latter was not significantly altered (Kelley et al., 1998). Likewise, no effect was made on T-cell proliferation in response to mitogens (Kelley et al., 1997), on NK-cell activity (Kelley et al., 1997), or on IL-2 production by mitogen-stimulated T cells (Kelley et al., 1997). Thus, an increased AA intake may result in changes indicative of selectively increased inflammation or inflammatory responses in humans. In another study, elderly subjects supplemented their diets with 0.7 grams of AA per day for 12 weeks (Thies et al., 2001a,b,c). This had no effect on the LPS-stimulated production of TNF-α, IL-1β, or IL-6 by mononuclear cells (Thies et al., 2001a), mitogen-stimulated T-cell proliferation (Thies et al., 2001c), the production of IL-2 and IFN-γ by T cells in response to mitogen (Thies et al., 2001c), or NK-cell activity (Thies et al., 2001b). Taken together, these studies suggest: (i) a modestly increased intake of AA by healthy subjects results in the incorporation of AA into cells involved in inflammatory responses (Thies et al., 2001c), but (ii) this does not affect the production of inflammatory cytokines, T-cell responses, or NK-cell activity (Thies et al., 2001a,b,c), although the production of inflammatory eicosanoids is increased (Kelley et al., 1998).

The increased consumption of the n-3 LC-PUFAs EPA and DHA (found in fish oil) results in increased proportions of those FAs in inflammatory-cell phospholipids (Caughey et al., 1996; Endres et al., 1989; Gibney & Hunter, 1993; Healy et al., 2000; Lee et al., 1985; Sperling et al., 1993; Yaqoob et al., 2000). The incorporation of EPA and DHA into human inflammatory cells occurs in a dose-response fashion (Healy et al., 2000; Rees et al., 2006), partly at the expense of AA. Since less substrate is available for the synthesis of eicosanoids from AA, fish-oil supplementation of the human diet resulted in a decreased production of AA-derived eicosanoids by inflammatory cells (see Calder, 2006b for references). Although these studies used fish oil to provide both EPA and DHA, Kelley et al. (1999) demonstrated that 6 grams of DHA per day resulted in a decreased production of $PGE_2$ (by 60%) and $LTB_4$ (by 75%) by LPS-stimulated mononuclear cells.

EPA is also able to act as a substrate for both cyclooxygenase and lipoxygenase enzymes, giving rise to eicosanoids with a slightly different structure than those formed from AA (Calder, 2006b). These enzymes are not specific for a single substrate, and therefore the relative presence of different possible substrates is a determinant for the production of either n-6 or n-3 PUFA-derived eicosanoids. Thus, fish-oil supplementation of the human diet resulted in an increased production of 5-series LTs and 5-hydroxyeicosapentaenoic acid by inflammatory cells (see Calder, 2006b for references). The functional significance of this is that the mediators formed from EPA are frequently less potent than those formed from AA (Bagga et al., 2003; Goldman et al., 1983; Lee et al., 1984), although this is not always the case (Dooper et al., 2002; Miles et al., 2002, 2003). The reduction in the generation of AA-derived mediators which accompany fish-oil consumption led to the idea that fish oil is anti-inflammatory and immunomodulatory.

In addition to n-3 LC-PUFAs modulating the generation of eicosanoids from AA and to EPA acting as a substrate for the generation of alternative eicosanoids, recent studies identified a novel group of mediators, termed "E- and D-series resolvins," formed from EPA and DHA (Fig. 22.2), respectively, that appear to exert potent anti-inflammatory and immunomodulatory actions (see Serhan et al., 2004, 2005 for reviews). This is an exciting new area since the discovery of resolvins and related molecules indicates an entirely novel mechanism by which n-3 LC-PUFAs are anti-inflammatory. Furthermore, the implications of this discovery to a variety of inflammatory conditions may be of great importance since the potency of resolvins is high, at least in the experimental systems in which they were examined.

Through the changed profiles of the production of eicosanoids and other mediators, n-3 LC-PUFAs are expected to influence inflammatory processes and immune responses (Calder, 2003a, 2006b; Sijben & Calder, 2007). Cell-culture and animal experiments indicate that this is the case, although these have often involved

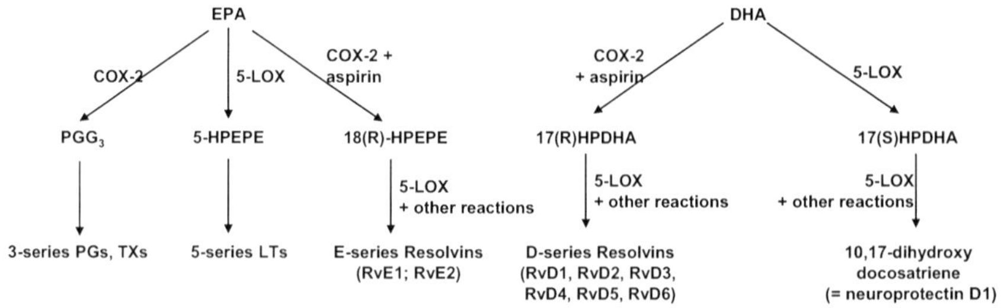


**Fig. 22.2.** Outline of the pathway of synthesis of resolvins and related mediators from EPA and DHA. COX, cyclooxygenase; HPDHA, hydroperoxydocosahexaenoic acid; HPEPE, hydrodoperoxy-eicosapentaenoic acid; LOX, lipoxygenase; LT, leukotriene; PG, prostaglandin; Rv, resolvin; TX, thromboxane (Calder, 2006b).

high levels of exposure to the FAs under study and other experimental conditions that are not transferable to the human setting. Data from cell culture and animal models reporting inflammatory and immune outcomes were reviewed in detail elsewhere (Calder, 2001a, 2002, 2003a, 2006b), and are not further discussed here. More specified and detailed descriptions of the general concept of the modulation of inflammation and immunity by altering PUFA supply are provided elsewhere for some of the areas addressed in this chapter: that is, immune development and maturation (Calder et al., 2006b); immunomodulation and exaggerated inflammation (Calder, 2005, 2007); allergies, atopy, and asthma (Calder, 2003b, 2006b; Prescott & Calder, 2004; Sala-Vila et al., 2008); IBDs (Calder, 2006b, 2008a); and rheumatoid arthritis (RA) (Calder, 2006b, 2008b; Calder & Zurier, 2001).

## Current Evidence of the Role of Dietary Fatty Acids in Immune Development, Disease Causation, and Prevention

### *LC-PUFA Requirements for the Developing Immune System*

A clear physiological requirement for LC-PUFA is apparent during fetal growth, particularly in membrane-rich tissues. Both the cardiovascular and central nervous systems (CNSs) are among the most rapidly growing membrane-rich tissues before birth. Both have a very high and specific requirement for LC-PUFA: AA is the predominant FA in blood vessels, and DHA is the predominant FA in the brain (Crawford et al., 1997). The LC-PUFA levels in these tissues are much greater than those of EFA, pointing to a preferential incorporation of LC-PUFA rather than EFA. A similar process might very well be the case in the developing immune system, since in immune cells LC-PUFAs usually greatly exceed EFAs, accounting for 20–25% of total FAs (Kew et al., 2004; Miles et al., 2004; Rees et al., 2006; Thies et al., 2001c; Yaqoob et al., 2000). Only a few data regarding the FA composition of immune cells in neonates are available. One study analyzed the FA profiles of the lymphocyte phospholipids of a preterm infant of 42 days of age (Field et al., 2000). These data suggest that LC-PUFAs, particularly AA, are the most predominant FAs in these cells and that their proportions are higher with the availability of a dietary source. In view of the role of LC-PUFAs in immune regulation, immunological immaturity of neonates and the critical development, and the maturation steps of the immune system in the neonatal period, conceivably anadequate availability of LC-PUFAs for the immune system is critical (Field et al., 2001) and coincides with relatively high requirements for other rapidly developing tissues. An adequate maternal supply of LC-PUFAs is therefore essential to meet the requirements of the fetus and the breast-fed infant. One further aspect is the limited capacity to convert LC-PUFAs from 18-carbon PUFA (Burdge, 2006; Plourde & Cunnane, 2007), indicating the likely necessity for a sufficient dietary supply of LC-PUFAs to meet the physiological requirements. Human- intervention studies on PUFAs and immune function in early life mainly focused on the effects of n-3 LC-PUFAs during pregnancy and lactation, the mixtures of AA and DHA in infancy, and again n-3 LC-PUFAs in late infancy and childhood. In the respective stages of life, these are the dietary PUFAs that are generally considered most critical for immune development and function.

### *Prenatal Dietary PUFAs: Role in Immune Maturation and Allergy Prevention*

Studies using food-frequency questionnaires reported intakes of 0.05 grams of EPA per day and 0.085 grams of DHA per day among lactating women and 0.08 grams of EPA per day and 0.14 grams of DHA per day among pregnant women in the Netherlands (Otto et al., 2001a,b). Similar intakes (0.08 grams of EPA per day and 0.16 grams of DHA per day) were found for pregnant Canadian women (Innis & Elias, 2003). The International Society for the Study of Fatty Acids and Lipids (ISSFAL) recommended an adequate intake of ≥0.3 grams of DHA per day for pregnant women (Simopoulos et al., 1999). In a more recent consensus statement that was jointly developed by several societies including ISSFAL, numerous international experts indicated that "no evidence was identified that demonstrates a need for changing the dietary fatty acids composition of pregnant and lactating women, with regard to intake of saturated, *trans*-isomeric, monounsaturated, and polyunsaturated fatty acids relative to the recommended intakes for the general population, except for the intake of n-3 LC-PUFA" (Koletzko et al., 2007). The required dietary intake of DHA, for deposition of adequate amounts in brain and other tissues during fetal and early postnatal life, was estimated to be at least 0.2 grams per day. Both recommendations are primarily based on estimated DHA requirements for accretion in the CNS. The study among pregnant Canadian women by Innis and Elias indicates that 60% had an intake of <0.15 grams of DHA per day, and only 16% consumed >0.3 grams of DHA per day. Hence, the picture emerges that pregnant and lactating women in Western societies, in very large numbers, are unlikely to meet the dietary requirement of DHA for the developing fetal CNS. Thus, in view of the important role of n-3 LC-PUFA for balanced immune development and function, the available n-3 LC-PUFA supply to immune cells might also be suboptimal in many fetal and also in many neonatal lives.

Several retrospective and prospective studies, suggesting that high fish consumption during pregnancy is associated with a lower risk of allergic diseases in offspring (Calvani et al., 2006; Miyake et al., 2007; Romieu et al., 2007; Salam et al., 2005; Sausenthaler et al., 2007; Willers et al., 2007), support the view that an adequate prenatal n-3 LC-PUFA supply enhances the maturation of the fetus' immune system. This might be particularly important for the prevention of exaggerated immune responses during the sensitization phase, which is an important determinant of the risk of allergy onset and perhaps also autoimmune disorders later in life.

Several intervention studies investigated the effect of n-3 LC-PUFA supplements on maternal and infant immune functions. A recent European multicenter trial on the effects of a fish-oil supplement providing 0.5 grams of DHA per day and 0.15 grams of EPA per day confirmed firstly that an enhanced maternal dietary intake of DHA increased fetal supply, as indicated by higher DHA concentrations in cord blood (Krauss-Etschmann et al., 2007). EPA was not evaluated in the cord blood because of the high number of values below the detection limit. Secondly, the study investigated whether this supplement, from 22 weeks of pregnancy until delivery, altered fetal Th1/Th2-related parameters and inflammatory cytokines (Krauss-Etschmann et al., 2008). The mRNA transcripts for IFN-γ, CX chemokine receptor 3, IL-4, IL-13, chemoattractant receptor homologous-molecule expressed on Th2 cells, chemokine receptor 4, TNF-α, IL-1, and TGF-β were quantified in 197 maternal and 195 cord blood samples. Fish-oil supplementation was associated with increased TGF-β mRNA in both maternal and cord blood; decreased IL-1β, TNF-α, and IFN-γ mRNA in mothers only; and decreased IL-4, IL-13, and CCR4 mRNA in cord blood only (Krauss-Etschmann et al., 2008). Cord-blood IL-13 and chemokine receptor 4 mRNA levels correlated inversely with cord-plasma DHA levels, while maternal peripheral blood IL-1β mRNA was correlated inversely with maternal plasma DHA at delivery. In a subcohort, the frequencies of chemokine receptor $4^{+}$T cells and NK cells in cord blood were significantly lower in the n-3 LC-PUFA group. An Australian placebo-controlled study in pregnant women whose babies would be at an increased risk of allergic disease studied the effects of a very high intake of n-3 LC-PUFAs, 1.1 grams of EPA per day and 2.2 grams of DHA per day, from week 20 of pregnancy on cord-blood cytokine levels, cytokine and eicosanoid production in response to stimulation, and later disease outcome (Dunstan et al., 2003a,b). Cord plasma from the fish-oil group was less likely to exhibit a detectable level of IL-13, and plasma IL-13 levels were significantly lower in the fish-oil group (Dunstan et al., 2003b). Cord-blood mononuclear IL-13, IL-10, IL-5, and IFN-γ production following ex vivo stimulation by various allergens were lower in the fish-oil group, although only significantly for the IL-10 production in response to the house-dust mite and cat-hair extract (Dunstan et al., 2003a). The $LTB_4$ production by cord-blood-derived neutrophils was significantly lower in neonates whose mothers had received fish oil, and was inversely correlated with erythrocyte membrane n-3 LC-PUFA levels (Prescott et al., 2007). Also a trend was detected toward a lower production of

5 hydroxyeicosatetraenoic acid (5-HETE), another major lipoxygenase product of AA metabolism, in this group. $LTB_5$ was below detectable levels in many samples, but nevertheless a trend for increased levels in the fish-oil group was found, and the levels were positively correlated with membrane n-3 LC-PUFA levels (Prescott et al., 2007). Neonates with lower $LTB_4$ production also had a lower production of IL-6 and IL-10 by LPS-stimulated neonatal mononuclear cells, and a trend was discovered for lower IFN-$\gamma$ and IL-13 production in the fish-oil group following polyclonal stimulation. At 1 year of age, infants of mothers in the fish-oil group were less likely to be sensitized to a range of allergens, determined by skin-prick testing, particularly to egg, and were less likely to have severe atopic dermatitis (Dunstan et al., 2003a). In a workshop report on early nutrition and immunity, Calder and co-authors (2006) reviewed these studies of increased fish-oil intake during pregnancy, and concluded that "these data do not indicate a selective effect on either Th1 or Th2 responses. Rather, it is possible the "dominant" immune responses (i.e. Th2 responses in neonates and Th1 responses in adults) might be primarily targeted." In the absence of a clear mechanistic explanation, perhaps the increased TGF-$\beta$ mRNA levels in both cord and maternal peripheral blood point toward an induction of certain types of adaptive regulatory T (Treg) cells (Calder et al., 2006). The data on modified neonatal immune response in the Australian study were not available at that time. In children with established allergic disease, local $LTB_4$ production in airways is a measure of disease activity and airway inflammation (Montuschi et al., 2005). Although animal data suggest that $LTB_4$ is required for allergic Th2 responses (Terawaki et al., 2005), the predictive value of the early down-regulation of $LTB_4$ in human newborns is unclear. Hence, these observations are supportive of a possible causal relationship: the prevalence of severe atopic dermatitis and positive skin-prick tests to egg at one year was found less in the children from the group with lower $LTB_4$ responses. In a recent study from Denmark, the effect of maternal supplementation of fish oil—providing 2.7 grams of EPA + DHA per day, from 30 weeks of gestation until delivery—on asthma occurrences at a 16-year follow-up was investigated (Olsen et al., 2008). The study was conducted in a population-based sample of 533 women with normal pregnancies who were randomly assigned 2:1:1 to receive fish-oil, olive-oil, or no-oil capsules. Compared with the olive-oil placebo, the hazard rate of asthma was reduced by 63%, and the hazard rate of allergic asthma was reduced by 87%. However, no differences were found between the fish-oil and no-oil control. According to the investigators, the most likely explanation for this result is an increased intake of fish oil in the no-oil placebo groups due to several factors, including participants' knowledge of the original study hypothesis that fish oil would reduce the risk of preterm delivery and low birth weight, and the awareness of other potential benefits and a wide availability of the studied fish-oil preparation.

Collectively, these studies provide evidence that increased n-3 LC-PUFA intake during pregnancy modulates immune function in mother and neonate. Limited data suggest that this may reduce the susceptibility to the onset of allergic diseases, but more data from well-designed studies with long-term follow-up examining clinical outcomes are required for firm conclusions.

### *Neonatal Dietary PUFA: Role in Allergy Prevention*

In neonatal nutrition, two major issues in the field of FAs and immune function were the subjects of scientific debate: the increased intake of LA and the importance of LC-PUFAs. The increased proportion of LA in human milk (e.g., 6–7% to 15–16% of FA between the 1940s and the 1990s in U.S. samples) (see Ailhaud et al., 2006 for references) coincided with an increased prevalence of atopic disease, and a causal relationship was suggested (Black & Sharpe, 1997; Hodge et al., 1994; Kankaanpaa et al., 1999). The essence of this hypothesis is that the increased consumption of LA over the last decades resulted in an enhanced capacity to synthesize AA and that, through the action of $PGE_2$ on T and B cells, a situation favoring skewing toward IgE production by B cells occurred (Prescott & Calder, 2004). Twelve prospective and cross-section studies explored human-milk PUFA in relation to allergy development in children (see review by Sala-Vila et al., 2008 for references). The results of these studies are highly inconsistent: of the 12 studies comparing breast-milk samples consumed by infants who went on to develop atopy compared with matched controls, higher concentrations of LA, DGLA, ALA, and DHA were reported in 2, 1, 1, and 2 studies, respectively. On the other hand, of these 12 studies, lower concentrations of LA, DGLA, ALA, EPA, and DHA consumed by infants who went on to develop atopy were reported in 1, 2, 1, 2, and 1 study, respectively. Hence, most studies reported no significant differences in these FA levels, and no studies found different concentrations of GLA and AA in breast milk consumed by atopic children compared to controls. Thus, no evidence is found for the proposed increase of LA and AA levels in the breast milk of mothers of atopic children. Neither is any other consistent result from these studies shown to support a possible contribution of breast-milk PUFA composition to atopic disease onset. Moreover, currently, no data were extracted from controlled intervention studies available in the area of atopic disease and/or allergy prevention with different levels of LA intake during infancy to provide stronger evidence.

Another hypothesis possibly linking dietary n-6 FA as a causal factor to the atopic-disease process is the suspected insufficient Δ6-desaturase activity in atopic individuals (Calder, 2006a; Calder & Miles, 2000). This enzyme is responsible for the conversion of LA to GLA and of ALA to STA. According to this hypothesis, the provision of dietary FAs that do not require Δ6-desaturase for desaturation, such as GLA, STA, or LC-PUFA, might be effective in preventing atopic disease by overcoming the inadequate synthesis of these FAs from their precursors. Two primary prevention studies of dietary GLA enrichment in neonates were based on this principle (Kitz et al., 2006; van Gool et al., 2003). In the first, double-blind, randomized placebo-controlled study in the Netherlands, formula-fed infants with a maternal history of atopic disease received a borage-oil supplement, proving 0.1 gram of GLA per day for the first 6 months of life (van Gool et al., 2003). Although at 1 year, total serum IgE, atopic dermatitis prevalence, parent-reported itching, medication use, and positive food-allergen tests were not affected by GLA enrichment, the severity of atopic dermatitis tends to be lower in the GLA group, and the increase of GLA status from 0 to 3 months was inversely correlated with the severity of atopic dermatitis. In the second prospective controlled study, newborns at increased atopic risk received GLA-enriched breast milk or formula for the first 5 months of life (Kitz et al., 2006). This study found no effect of GLA enrichment on the development of atopic dermatitis at 12 months, but IgE levels were lower in GLA-supplemented atopic subjects. We are not aware of any studies on atopy and/or allergy prevention in newborns with dietary STA, EPA, or DHA enrichment. The Childhood Allergy Prevention Study (Mihrshahi et al., 2001) started dietary supplementation with n-3 LC-PUFA at 6 months; this is addressed later in this chapter.

Thus, currently no substantial evidence was gleaned from human studies to support the view that high neonatal LA intake is a risk factor for atopic disease and allergies. No controlled intervention studies are available in this field to generate more conclusive evidence. Some, but inconsistent, data suggest a possible protective role of neonatal dietary GLA enrichment, and we identify an obvious data gap in a possible protective effect of an n-3 LC-PUFA enrichment against allergies.

## *Neonatal Dietary LC-PUFA: Role in Immune Development*

Breast milk contains a number of immunologically active components that are absent in all or many infant formulas (e.g., lactoferrin, antibodies, cytokines, hormones, oligosaccharides, and LC-PUFAs) (Field, 2005). Based on the overall body of evidence in developed countries, the conclusion is that breast-feeding, compared with formula-feeding, is associated with a reduction in the risk of acute otitis media, nonspecific gastroenteritis, severe lower-respiratory-tract infections, atopic dermatitis, asthma (in young children), type 1 diabetes, and several other diseases with a less clear immunological origin (Ip et al., 2007). The presence of LC-PUFAs in breast milk (Brenna et al., 2007; Jensen, 1999) and their only recent large-scale introduction into infant-milk formulas (starting in the early 1990s in Europe and in the early 2000s in the United States) posed the possibility of dietary LC-PUFAs' role in the developing immune system that might have contributed to the observed different disease patterns of breast- and formula-fed infants. This point is particularly relevant since the accretion of DHA, but not AA, in the brain of breast-fed infants is higher than in formula-fed infants. This indicates that particularly the conversion of DHA from LNA is insufficient to fully meet the infant's physiological requirements (Farquharson et al., 1992; Makrides et al., 1994).

Two intervention studies investigated the role of LC-PUFAs on immune development by a comparison of formula feeding with and without added LC-PUFAs from single-cell oils in a randomized-controlled setting (Field et al., 2000, 2008a,b). Both studies included a nonrandomized breast-fed control group. In the first study, preterm infants received formula that contained no or 0.5% AA + 0.35% DHA, expressed as the percentage of total FAs, from 8 until 42 days of postnatal life (Field et al., 2000). The content of DHA in peripheral blood lymphocytes was insignificantly different between groups and that of AA significantly higher in the LC-PUFA group. Phenotyping of lymphocytes indicated that infants in the breast-milk and LC-PUFA groups had a lower ratio of CD4 to CD3 cells compared with those receiving the control formula, a greater increase in CD20+ cells (B cells), and a higher number of CD14+ cells (monocytes). Compared with the control formula, CD4+ cells from the LC-PUFA and breast-milk groups expressed more CD45R0 (antigen mature) and less CD45RA (antigen naïve). Ex vivo IL-10 production by mononuclear cells upon stimulation with phytohaemagglutinin (PHA) was lower in the control-formula group, but not in the LC-PUFA-formula group, compared with the breast-milk reference group, and sIL2-R production was lower in the LC-PUFA-formula group than in the control-formula group. In a similar designed study, term infants were fed formula without or with LC-PUFA (0.2% of DHA and 0.34% of AA of total FAs) from 2 to 6 weeks after birth (Field et al., 2008a,b). Compared with those fed control formula, infants fed LC-PUFA-containing formula had higher levels of total CD3, CD3+CD44+, CD8+CD28+, and CD4+CD28+ cells and lower levels of CD20+ cells. For most markers, the values in the LC-PUFA group were closest to those in the breast-milk group. Other phenotypes were not different between infant-formula groups. Lymphocyte proliferation following phytohaemagglutinin (PHA) stimulation was higher in the breast-milk group than in the LC-PUFA group, and TNF-α production was higher in the control-formula group than in the LC-PUFA-formula and breast-milk groups. The production of other cytokines was similar between formulas (Field et al., 2008a). Ex vivo cytokine responses, lymphocyte proliferation, and phenotypes (after incubation with potential food allergens following this intervention) were reported separately (Field et al., 2008b). Lymphocyte proliferation did not differ between formula groups. At 6 weeks, infants fed the LC-PUFA formula produced 3.2-fold more TNF-α after incubation with soy protein and 3.3-fold more IFN-γ after incubation with β-lactoglobulin than infants fed control formula or breast milk. Compared with the breast-fed infants, only the infants fed the control formula produced more IL-6 after incubation with β-lactoglobulin. The implications of these results are not yet clear because clinical implications were not assessed. These studies illustrate immunomodulatory effects by dietary LC-PUFAs in neonates, and some, but not all, data suggest that the addition of LC-PUFAs to infant formula results in lymphocyte-membrane compositions, populations, and function that are more similar to the breast-fed reference. However, current knowledge of the ontology of neonatal immune development is insufficient for clear conclusions regarding the meaning of the observed effects on immune markers.

The effect of high n-3 LC-PUFA intake during infancy on immune function was studied by breast-milk enrichment via fish-oil supplementation, providing 1.5 grams per day of n-3 LC-PUFA, during the first 4 months of lactation (Lauritzen et al.,

2005). After 4 months, the milk of the mothers in the fish-oil group contained more EPA and DHA than the milk of the control mothers: 0.30% versus 0.13% and 1.34% versus 0.41% of total FAs, respectively (Lauritzen et al., 2004). The n-6 LC-PUFA levels were the same in the milk from both groups. At 2.5 years, plasma IgE levels and cytokine production in LPS-stimulated whole-blood cultures were measured. Plasma IgE and LPS-induced IL-10 production were not different between treatments, and LPS-induced IL-4 and IL-12 production did not reach detection levels in most children. LPS-induced IFN-γ production was four-fold higher in the fish-oil group compared with the control group, and the fish-oil group had a higher ratio of the production of IFN-γ to IL-10 (Lauritzen et al., 2005). Both IFN-γ production and the IFN-γ to IL-10 ratio at 2.5 years were positively correlated with the EPA to AA ratio in red blood cells (RBCs) at 4 months. The clinical significance of the observed immunomodulation and possible improved immune maturation is not yet clear. One prospective open-label observation study compared one LC-PUFA-containing formula with a heterogeneous group of formulas with lower LC-PUFA levels or no LC-PUFA on the prevalence of common illnesses at 1, 3, 5, 7, 9, and 12 months (Pastor et al., 2006). The incidence of bonchiolitis/bronchitis was lower at 5, 7, and 9 months in the infants who received the formula with higher LC-PUFA levels, but not at 1, 3, and 12 months. The incidence of other respiratory illnesses, pharyngitis, otitis, and conjunctivitis was similar between groups, with the exception of lower incidences of rhinitis at 1 month and of upper-respiratory-tract infections at 1 and 12 months in the higher LC-PUFA group (Pastor et al., 2006). Clearly, since the study was not blinded and randomized, one should interpret the results with caution due to potential confounding factors.

In conclusion, the available evidence suggests that the role of dietary LC-PUFAs in neonatal immune function is potentially beneficial, benchmarked against the breast milk as the "golden standard," but the potential benefits on clinical outcomes, such as incidence and prevalence of infectious diseases, remain to be investigated in well-designed studies. Although the effects in both studies by Field and co-workers (2000, 2005), are promising, the interventions were rather short, and one should advisably study these effects in interventions of at least 6 months. In a recent consensus recommendation regarding dietary LC-PUFAs for neonates, an international group of experts recommended that infant formulas should contain between 0.2 and 0.5% of total FAs as DHA, at least the same level of AA, and a level of EPA that does not exceed the level of DHA (Koletzko et al., 2008). This recommendation is primarily based on the required levels to achieve benefits on functional neurodevelopmental endpoints. The upper recommended level is determined by the lack of published systematic evaluations of higher levels. In their recommendation for future LC-PUFA research, a further evaluation of the effects on immune outcomes, such as allergies and inflammatory disorders, is advised. In addition, they advise studying the effects according to interindividual differences, such as genetic variation in FA desaturase activities or gender. Indeed, a recent study in two large cohorts of children indicated that the IQ-increasing effect of breast-feeding, often attributed to LC-PUFAs, depended on the genetic control of FA pathways (Caspi et al., 2007), suggesting that the physiological requirements and health effects of dietary LC-PUFAs in neonates depend on the genotype. Therefore, particularly interesting would be studying the immunological relevance of a dietary LC-PUFA supply in children in combination with their genetic variation in FA metabolism because this might improve the sensitivity of such an intervention study.

### *Dietary LC-PUFA During Childhood: Effects on Immune Maturation and Infectious-disease Prevention*

Historically, many children were given cod-liver oil each day as a source of vitamins A and D, with the usual dose being a teaspoonful (approximately 5 mL). At that time, vitamin A was known as an "anti-infective" vitamin, and several studies in the United States and WesternEurope between 1920 and 1940, involving over 4000 children, were conducted to investigate the efficacy of cod-liver oil as an "anti-infective" prophylactic therapy and an "anti-infective" therapy for specific diseases (see Semba, 1999 for references). Several, but not all, of these historical studies on cod-liver oil showed reductions in the incidence of respiratory infections and therapeutic effects in acute measles, typhoid fever, and tuberculosis. Although the use of cod-liver oil has markedly declined, this supplement is still available in many countries and is recommended for infants in Norwegian national dietary guidelines. More recently the notion—that the presence of n-3 LC-PUFAs in this traditional supplement may have immunomodulatory effects as well—placed the questions regarding the potential health benefits of cod-liver oil in a somewhat broader perspective. In two recent studies among children in New York, a daily teaspoonful of cod-liver oil—providing daily 0.46–0.5 grams of EPA; 0.5–0.55 grams of DHA; vitamins A, D and E, in combination with a multi-vitamin supplement—reduced the number of upper-respiratory-tract infections (Linday et al., 2004), and also reduced the antibiotic use for otitis media (Linday et al., 2002). The investigators of these studies hypothesized that the supplement reduced the complications from viral illnesses by reducing the inflammation of the respiratory and sinonasal mucosa that is produced by the viruses (Linday et al., 2004).

A randomized-controlled study in Denmark investigated the effects of a daily teaspoonful of fish oil—providing an average of 0.57 grams per day of EPA and 0.38 grams per day of DHA— for 3 months on a number of immune markers in infants of 12 months of age (Damsgaard et al., 2007). The intervention had no effect on plasma C-reactive protein (CRP), IgE, and soluble IL-2R concentrations. The fish-oil supplement increased *Lactobacillus paracasei*-induced IFN-$\gamma$ production, and tended to reduce LPS + PHA-induced IL-10 production in whole-blood cultures. The RBC EPA content was inversely correlated with LPS + PHA-induced IL-10 production. Fish oil did not affect TNF-$\alpha$ production, LPS + PHA-induced IFN-$\gamma$ production, *L. paracasei*-induced IL-10 production, or the ratio between IFN-$\gamma$ and IL-10, but the

*L. paracasei*-induced IFN-γ to IL-10 ratio was two times higher in the fish-oil group compared to the controls (Damsgaard et al., 2007). A rise in IFN-γ and the IFN-γ to IL-10 ratio suggests a more Th-1 cell-dominant responsiveness, which at this age might be indicative of a more mature immune function. A double-blind controlled Israeli study investigated the effects of 12 weeks of 0.18 grams of EPA + 0.12 grams of DHA per day on cytokine production in children between 8 and 12 years of age (Vaisman et al., 2005). Plasma IL-6 and TNF-α were not different between the fish-oil and control groups, but IL-6, TNF-α, IL-1β, IL-10, and IL-1RA productions by blood mononuclear cells were all higher in the fish-oil group both in nonstimulated and LPS-stimulated cultures. This finding is different from similar studies in adults, usually using higher intake levels (Sijben & Calder, 2007), and unclear is whether this is due to different responsiveness in children, the relatively low-intake level, or other factors related to the design and biochemical analyses. Finally, in a recently published, randomized, double-blind, placebo-controlled Canadian study, children of the ages of 5–7 years with a daily DHA intake below 0.078 grams per day received a dietary supplement providing 0.020–0.30 grams of AA and 0.014–0.021 grams of DHA per day or a placebo (Mazurak et al., 2008). After 7 months, immune-cell populations were phenotyped, and mononuclear cells were stimulated with a series of antigens and antigen expression on macrophages, T and B cells, and cytokine production measured. No differences existed between groups regarding the proportions of CD4+, CD8+, B cell, CD14+, and CD54+ cells and IL-4, IL-6, IFN-γ, and TNF-α production after stimulation. However, in the AA + DHA group, fewer CD8+ cells expressed CD25 and CD80 after exposure to different mitogens, CD54+ cell numbers were higher, and CD14+ cell numbers were lower after stimulation with ibuprofen and β-lactoglobulin, and IL-2 and IL10 productions were greater in pokeweed mitogen-stimulated mononuclear cells. These results suggest that even a relatively small increase in LC-PUFA intake may have immunomodulatory effects, although the clinical significance of these changes is unclear.

The effects of tuna oil, a fish oil with a relatively high DHA to EPA ratio, on the clinical outcome were investigated in a series of studies in Thai primary-school children (Thienprasert et al., 2006, 2007). In a randomized, double-blind, placebo-controlled study, children of the ages of 6–12 years were allocated to receive either placebo, 0.1, 0.3, 0.6, or 1 gram of DHA on every school day for 4 months (Thienprasert et al., 2006). Incidence of illness was assessed, and severity was measured by days with symptoms or absent days from school. The investigators reported that the duration of the illness was inversely correlated with the dose of DHA; the reductions were 9, 10, 23, and 31% from the lowest to the highest dose, respectively; and T-cell count was increased in the tuna-oil groups compared with the placebo (Thienprasert et al., 2006). In a second study the highest dose from the first study, proving 1 gram of DHA + 0.2 grams of EPA on every school day for 6 months, the episodes and severity of the illness were less than in the soybean-oil placebo group. Plasma IL-6 at 6 months was lower in the tuna-oil group than in the control, and TGF-β2 increased less during the study in the tuna-oil group compared with the control group (Thienprasert et al., 2007).

Except for the study by Mazurak and co-workers (2008), studies on the immunomodulatory effects of PUFA in children from 6 months and older used n-3 LC-PUFAs without a concomitant supply of AA. Indeed, studies in older infants suggest: (i) that the dietary supply of DHA is required to maintain DHA status during breast-feeding and (ii) that the AA status in RBCs is maintained at a much higher level regardless of the presence of a source of supplemental AA (Damsgaard et al., 2007; Hoffman et al., 2003, 2004; Makrides et al., 2002). Hence, these data indicate that, after 6 months particularly, a dietary source of n-3 LC-PUFA is critical to maintain LC-PUFA status at breast-feeding levels. Recent studies indicate that the mean intake of DHA among toddlers (Minns et al., 2008) and children ages 4 to 8 years (Madden et al., 2008) in North America is very low, at 22 mg per day and 44 mg per day, respectively. Collectively, these data suggest that adequate dietary n-3 LC-PUFA is probably the most limiting factor and most critical to meet the requirements of balanced immune development and function during childhood.

### *Role of Dietary PUFA during Childhood in the Prevention of Atopy, Asthma, and Allergies*

In addition to a possible role of n-3 LC-PUFA in infectious-disease prevention, several studies suggested a protected effect of fish consumption during childhood for the onset of childhood asthma and allergic diseases (Chatzi et al., 2007; Hodge et al., 1996; Nafstad et al., 2003) and of adult asthma (Laerum et al., 2007). In contrast, others report a higher prevalence among children with higher fish intake (Takemura et al., 2002) or no association of fish intake with allergic disorders (Dunder et al., 2001; Farchi et al., 2003; Hijazi et al., 2000 ).

A primary prevention study that links an increased consumption of n-3 LC-PUFA to a clinical outcome is the Childhood Asthma Prevention Study. In this study, infants at risk of developing asthma received fish oil, providing 0.15 grams of EPA + DHA per day or placebo from 6 months of age and older. No effect was noted of fish oil on the sensitization to inhaled or ingested allergens, determined by skin-prick testing at 18 months of age, but a decreased prevalence was noted of wheeze ever and wheeze >1 week and a trend for decreased visits to the doctor for wheeze in the fish-oil group (Mihrshahi et al., 2003). No effect of fish oil was observed on other wheeze indicators, diagnosed asthma, medication use, and dermatitis. Higher plasma levels of total n-3 PUFA at 18 months were associated with reduced wheeze, visits to the doctor because of wheeze, coughing during sleep, and bronchodilator use (Mihrshahi et al., 2004). No effect of fish oil was indicated on total serum IgE at 18 or 36 months of age (Mihrshahi et al., 2004; Peat et al., 2004). At 36 months of age the intervention resulted in a decreased prevalence of a cough and an atopic cough, but no effect occurred on the prevalence of asthma, wheeze, atopic dermatitis, or sensitization to ingested or inhaled allergens (Peat et al., 2004). At 5 years of age, no effect of fish oil was detected on the prevalence of asthma, wheezing, atopy, and eczema (Marks et al., 2006). Further analysis at this age indicated that plasma FAs at 18 months, 3 years, and 5 years were not associated with any respiratory or allergic outcome at 5 years of age (Almqvist et al., 2007).

Three studies on childhood asthma treatment with fish oil containing dietary supplements were performed (Hodge et al., 1998; Nagakura et al., 2000; Schubert et al., in press), with mixed results. An extensive overview of studies on disease treatment is beyond the scope of this chapter, and is found elsewhere (Schachter et al., 2004; Thien et al., 2004). Briefly, one study providing 0.72 grams of EPA + 0.48 grams of DHA per day for 6 months found no effect on the clinical severity of asthma (Hodge et al., 1998). The next study reported decreased asthma-symptom scores and bronchial hyper responsiveness to an acetylcholine challenge after 40 weeks of daily EPA (11–27 mg/kg) + DHA (7–11.5 mg/kg) (Nagakura et al., 2000). The most recent study, which is not included in the reviews, found that nitric oxide exhalation after allergen stimulation decreased and lung function, tested in response to methacholine, improved after 5 weeks of a supplement proving LA, ALA, STA, GLA, EPA, and DHA (Schubert et al., in press).

Several studies on the use of GLA to treat atopic disease were conducted and reviewed in detail elsewhere (Calder & Miles, 2000; Hoare et al., 2000; van Gool et al., 2004). Briefly, some of these studies, particularly the smaller studies, report benefits, but other studies do not (see Calder & Miles, 2000; Hoare et al., 2000; van Gool et al., 2004 for references). One study found a dose-dependent clinical improvement with evening-primrose oil (Wright & Burton, 1982), a source of GLA, but a more recent extensive study was unable to confirm the clinical benefits of a high-GLA intake, provided as borage oil (Takwale et al., 2003).

In conclusion, epidemiological studies provide some, but inconsistent, support of the protective effects of n-3 PUFA consumption against the onset of allergies. A modest short-term effect exists of dietary n-3 LC-PUFAs in primary prevention, but the long-term benefit is disappointing.

## *Type I Diabetes: Possible Protective Role of n-3 LC-PUFA*

Type 1 diabetes mellitus is an autoimmune disease that is characterized by the destruction of insulin-producing beta-cells in the pancreatic islets. Inflammatory cytokines were implicated in the inflammatory processes leading to the destruction of Islets of Langerhans in type 1 diabetes (Mandrup-Poulsen et al., 1989). Studies suggested that increased perinatal consumption of cod-liver oil may have a protective role in the etiology of the autoimmune process that leads to clinical disease. In a Norwegian pilot case-control study, a strong association between the maternal use of cod-liver oil during pregnancy and a lower risk of type 1 diabetes in the offspring was found, and an insignificant trend that cod-liver oil use during the first year of life reduced that risk was reported (Stene et al., 2000). In a larger case-control study from the same investigators, the use of cod-liver oil in the first year of life was associated with a lower risk of childhood type 1 diabetes even after an adjustment for confounders such as the duration of breast-feeding and maternal education (Stene & Joner, 2003).

However, the effects of maternal cod-liver oil from the pilot study were not repeated, and no effects of the use of other vitamin D supplements by the mothers or infants were found. Hence, these results suggest that EPA and DHA—present in cod-liver oil at approximately 0.4 grams of EPA + 0.6 grams of DHA per daily dose—account for the possible protective effect against type 1 diabetes. More recently, data from the Diabetes Autoimmunity Study in the Young (DAISY) provided further evidence of the role of dietary FAs (Norris et al., 2007). In this cohort, consisting of 1770 children with an increased risk of type 1 diabetes, defined as either the possession of a high diabetes risk HLA genotype or having a sibling or parent with type 1 diabetes, the total n-3 PUFA intake from 1 year and older was inversely associated with the risk of type 1 diabetes. This association was strengthened when the definition of the outcome was limited to those positive for two or more autoantibodies. With the latter definition, a trend of the protective effects of n-3 LC-PUFAs also appeared. The total RBC content of n-3 PUFA was also inversely correlated with the risk of islet autoimmunity. Thus, these studies suggest that the ingestion of n-3 PUFA during infancy and childhood may reduce the risk of type 1 diabetes onset.

### *Role of Dietary PUFA in the Onset of Inflammatory Bowel Diseases*

Ulcerative colitis (UC) and Crohn's Disease (CD) are chronic inflammatory diseases of the alimentary tract. In UC, the mucosa of the colon is mainly affected, while in CD any part of the alimentary tract from the mouth to the anus can be affected, although it is usually the ileum and colon. In both diseases, the intestinal mucosa contains elevated levels of inflammatory eicosanoids such as $LTB_4$ (Sharon & Stenson, 1984) and cytokines. Particularly, the activation of IL-2 and IFN-γ-producing Th1 cells in the lamina propria of a CD-affected gut plays a pivotal role in pathogenesis (Hommes & van Deventer, 2000). Several studies indicate that the incidence of IBD has greatly increased in the past decades (Loftus, 2004). Pediatric IBD increased similarly. For instance, in Scotland the incidence of pediatric IBD increased from 1 to 3.1 per 100.000 between the early 1970s to the early 1990s (Armitage et al., 2001). A prospective study in the United Kingdom indicated: (i) that UC was more common in second- generation migrants from South Asia, a region with low IBD incidence, than in the first generation and (ii) that the rates in the second-generation migrants were comparable to those in Europe (Carr & Mayberry, 1999). These examples suggest that, in addition to genetic predisposition, environmental factors, such as high LA and low n-3 LC-PUFA intake, may contribute to the onset of IBD (Innis & Jacobson, 2007). One epidemiological study from Japan—reporting that an increased incidence of CD between 1966 and 1985 correlated with an increased n-6 PUFA intake and an increased dietary n-6 to n-3 ratio—supports this view (Shoda et al., 1996). A case-control trial that found an inverse relation of fish consumption as well as an n-3 LC-PUFA intake and the risk of pediatric CD further supports the role of dietary lipids in CD onset (Amre et al., 2007). Tissue levels of n-3 LC-PUFAs are likely to have decreased as a result of such change in the dietary pattern. This is illustrated by several fish-oil supplementation studies in active IBD, resulting in an increased n-3 LC-PUFA incorporation into gut mucosal tissue and a modification of inflammatory-mediator profiles such as eicosanoids (see Calder, 2006b for references). Fish-oil supplements providing 2.7 grams of EPA + DHA per day markedly increased the n-3 LC-PUFA levels in the PBMCs of patients with CD, and decreased the production of $PGE_2$ and IFN-$\gamma$ by circulating monocytes and macrophages (Trebble et al., 2004). Hence, these observations provide one potential mechanistic basis to explain a possible link between dietary lipids and an IBD occurrence.

Currently, no primary IBD-prevention studies with dietary lipid intervention are available, but several studies investigated the role of an increased n-3 LC-PUFA intake for "secondary prevention," (i.e., a relapse in CD or UC patients in remission). In two studies by Belluzzi et al. (1996, 1997), patients with CD in remission were randomly assigned to receive placebo or 2.7 grams of enteric-coated n-3 LC-PUFA per day for one year. The proportion of patients who relapsed over 12 months was significantly lower in the fish-oil group, and, likewise, the number of patients who remained in remission at 1 year was higher in the fish-oil group. One relatively small study in pediatric CD reported a similar advantageous effect on a relapse in the group receiving 0.6 grams of enteric-coated EPA + DHA per day in addition to an amino-salicylic-acid treatment (Romano et al., 2005). In contrast, no effect on the relapse of 4.3 grams of EPA + DHA per day for one year was observed by Lorenz-Meyer and co-workers (1996). A Cochrane-pooled analysis on omega-3 FAs for the maintenance of remission in CD included these four studies, and reported a borderline significance for an overall favorable effect of fish oil (Turner et al., 2007b). Statistical significance was reached in a subanalysis including only the three studies using enteric-coated n-3 LC-PUFA capsules. However, more recent results of two large randomized controlled trials (RCTs) on enteric-coated omega-3 FFAs for the maintenance of the remission of CD failed to demonstrate clear benefits of n-3 LC-PUFAs on a one-year risk of a relapse (Feagan et al., 2008). Both studies randomized approximately 380 patients in remission to receive either a placebo or daily 2.6 to 3.4 grams of free EPA + DHA. Primary endpoint was a clinical relapse. In both studies, the proportion of patients in remission was higher during most of the one year study period, but no significant differences were noted on a relapse at one year.

A Cochrane review from 2007 evaluated the efficacy of fish oil for the maintenance of a remission in UC (Turner et al., 2007a). Three studies (Hawthorne et al., 1992; Loeschke et al., 1996; Mantzaris et al., 1996) using between 5 and 6 grams of EPA + DHA per day for one to two years were included in the analysis. For the pooled analysis, 138 patients were enrolled and showed a similar relapse rate in the fish-oil-treated patients and controls (Turner et al., 2007a). One study that used a combination of GLA, EPA, and DHA found no reduction of a relapse of UC either (Middleton et al., 2002). In addition, several RCTs of fish oil in active IBD studied disease severity, induction of remission, and other outcomes such as gut histology and the use of corticosteroids; however, these are beyond the scope of this chapter and are reviewed elsewhere (Calder, 2006b, 2008a; De Ley et al., 2007).

Thus, besides the presence of parallel trends of changed dietary lipid intakes and an increased prevalence of IBD, some evidence suggests an etiological role of dietary lipids. Despite a possible role in disease onset and a clear mechanistic basis of a disease-modifying role of n-3 LC-PUFAs, the overall evidence base of the favorable effects of n-3 LC-PUFAs in the prevention of a relapse of disease is moderate for CD and absent for UC.

## *Role of Dietary PUFA in the Onset of COPD*

In the United States, the age-adjusted death rates for COPD increased by 163% between 1965 and 1998; worldwide it was the fifth leading cause of death in 2000 (Pauwels & Rabe, 2004), and is projected to move to third place by 2020 (Murray & Lopez, 1997). COPD is actually a group of diseases characterized by the pathological limitation of airflow in the airway, including obstructive bronchitis and emphysema. It is most often caused by tobacco smoking, but can also be caused by other airborne irritants such as coal dust, and occasionally by genetic abnormalities, such as $\alpha_1$–antitrypsin deficiency (Barnes, 2008). COPD is characterized by chronic inflammation in the small airways and lung parenchyma accompanied by an infiltration of neutrophils and macrophages. This inflammation mediates excess mucous production, fibrosis, and proteolysis via neutrophil recruitment. The most important neutrophil chemotactic factors implicated in COPD are IL-8, TNF-$\alpha$, and $LTB_4$ (see review by Barnes, 2008 for references). The principal clinical symptom is reduced airflow on expiration due to airway obstruction, which is usually measured as forced expiratory volume in 1 second (FEV1).

Several studies investigated the relationship between fish and/or FA intake and respiratory symptoms or clinically manifested COPD. Shahar et al. (1994) showed a strong beneficial association between fish intake and the prevalence of COPD in former and current smokers. In the Honolulu Heart Program, smokers with a high fish consumption had a higher FEV1 than smokers with a low fish intake (Sharp et al., 1994). These results suggest that fish consumption may limit the damage of smoking on the lung, which can eventually progress to clinically manifest as COPD. Higher FEV1 in subjects with high fish intake were also shown in the National Health and Nutrition Examination Survey (NHANES), but in this study the magnitude of the effect was slightly higher after the exclusion of smokers (Schwartz & Weiss, 1994). On the other hand, no relationship between the fish intake and the FEV1 decline after a 5-year follow-up was found in a population- based study in the United Kingdom (Butland et al., 2000). One population-based cohort study that investigated the specific effects of n-3 FAs showed that the intake of fish, EPA, and DHA was inversely associated with 25-year COPD mortality (Tabak et al., 1998). In contrast, no association was observed for baseline fish consumption and a 20-year COPD mortality (Walda et al., 2002). More recently, two cross-sectional studies investigated the effects of FA status (Kompauer et al., 2008) and FA intake (McKeever et al., 2008) on lung function. DHA concentration in serum phospholipids was positively associated with FEV1, and in men an inverse correlation between FEV1 and DGLA status was observed (Kompauer et al., 2008). Similarly, inverse correlations between the dietary intake of several n-6 FAs and FEV1 were found, but in this study the DHA intake in the highest quintile was associated with the lowest FEV1 (McKeever et al., 2008). A high n-6 LC-PUFA intake was associated with an increased risk of COPD, and small insignificant inverse correlations were found between a high n-3 LC-PUFA intake and the risk of COPD in this Dutch cohort with a relatively low fish consumption (McKeever et al., 2008). One controlled intervention study in COPD patients, which provided 0.6 grams of EPA + DHA per day for 2 years, found a lower number of acute exacerbations in the n-3 PUFA group during the observation period that reached a borderline significance (Matsuyama et al., 2005).

Together, these studies provide some, but inconsistent, evidence that n-3 LC-PUFA consumption levels above population averages may improve lung function and reduce the risk of COPD. High n-6 LC-PUFA intake may be a risk factor for impaired lung function and COPD onset. The reasons for inconsistent findings can be manifold including differences in the types of studies and habitual FA intakes. One factor that might particularly add to the interindividual variance of interaction between an EPA + DHA intake and a COPD onset is the presence of TNF-α-308 polymorphism (Schols, 2003). Polymorphism in this gene was associated with the presence of COPD and the extent of emphysematous changes in these patients (Sakao et al., 2001, 2002), while the effect of dietary fish oil on TNF-α production by monocytes depends on this polymorphism (Grimble et al., 2002).

## *Role of Dietary PUFA in the Onset of Rheumatoid Arthritis*

Rheumatoid arthritis (RA) is a chronic inflammatory disease characterized by joint inflammation that manifests as swelling, pain, functional impairment, morning stiffness, osteoporosis, and muscle wasting. Joint lesions are characterized by the infiltration of activated macrophages, T lymphocytes, and plasma cells into the synovium (the tissue lining the joints) and by the proliferation of synovial cells called synoviocytes. Synovial biopsies from patients with RA contain high levels of TNF-α, IL-1β, IL-6, IL-8, and granulocyte/macrophage-colony stimulating factor (GM-CSF), and synovial cells cultured ex vivo produce TNF-α, IL-1β, IL-6, IL-8, and GM-CSF for extended periods of time without additional stimulus (Feldmann & Maini, 1999). Cyclooxygenase-2 expression is increased in the synovium of RA patients and in the joint tissues in rat models of arthritis (Sano et al., 1992). $PGE_2$, $LTB_4$, 5-hydroxyeicosatetraenoic acid, and also platelet-activating factor are found in the synovial fluid of patients with active RA (Sperling, 1995). The efficacy of nonsteroidal anti-inflammatory drugs (NSAIDS) in RA indicates the importance of pro-inflammatory cyclooxygenase-pathway products in the pathophysiology of the disease. Thus, these data provide a mechanistic basis for the possible benefits of an n-3 LC-PUFA consumption for the prevention or treatment of RA. At least 20 placebo-controlled studies of fish oil in RA were reported (see review by Calder, 2008b for references). The dose of n-3 LC-PUFA used in these trials was between 1.6 and 7.1

grams per day and averaged about 3.5 grams per day. Almost all of these trials showed some benefits of fish oils, including reduced duration of morning stiffness, reduced number of tender or swollen joints, reduced joint pain, reduced time to fatigue, increased grip strength, and decreased use of NSAIDS. However, relatively few studies investigated the role of dietary FAs as a potential etiological factor in RA.

Based on the observation that the prevalence of RA is low among Inuit (Kromann & Green, 1980), David Horrobin suggested that their high EPA intake might have a major role in RA prevention (1987). This suggestion is supported by further observations that, despite a higher prevalence of a genotype associated with an increased susceptibility to RA in Japan, the prevalence of RA is about 0.4%, compared with about 1% in Australia and the United States (Cleland & James, 2002). The possible inverse association between the prevalence of RA and n-3 LC-PUFA intake may be further supported by the results of a case-control study among 324 women with the disease and 1243 controls (Shapiro et al., 1996). Results indicated that higher fish consumption in five years before the onset of symptoms was associated with a reduced risk of RA, and the association was stronger in seropositive RA cases. The protective effect was found for the category of "broiled or baked fish," which was reported to most probably include salmon, mackerel, brook trout, bluefish, and herring. No effect of the number of servings of tuna was found. Moderately positive effects were confirmed by an earlier finding of a Greek case-control study that reported a weak protective effect of fish consumption (Linos et al., 1991). However, a second study by the same investigators found no effect of fish consumption on the risk of RA (Linos et al., 1999). In a Danish prospective cohort, a high intake of fat fish was associated with a reduced risk of RA. In contrast, a high intake of medium-fat fish (3–7 grams of fat per 100 grams of fish) was associated with an increased risk of RA, while no association was found with dietary LC-PUFA (Pedersen et al., 2005). Finally, in the Nurses' Health Study prospective cohort, no association was observed between fish consumption and the risk of RA (Benito-Garcia et al., 2007).

Thus, despite the strong evidence of the clinical benefits of a high n-3 LC-PUFA intake in RA, remarkably little high- quality information regarding a possible role of these nutrients in disease etiology exists. The available, apparently inconsistent, case-control and prospective cohort studies provide little insight into the true long-term n-3 LC-PUFA-intake levels. Too low and/or narrow intake ranges within the studied populations limit the predictive value of these studies for potential effects within a wider range of n-3 LC-PUFA intake. Given the strong potential of fish oils in RA treatment and their possible role in RA onset, a clear need exists for a well-powered systematic evaluation of a wide range of individual n-3 LC-PUFA-intake levels and a long-term risk of RA.

## *Emerging Link between Dietary n-3 LC-PUFA and Neuroinflammatory Conditions*

In the previous sections, we described the role of dietary lipids in clear "immunological" conditions and diseases (i.e., perinatal immune development, autoimmune diseases, allergic diseases, chronic inflammatory diseases, and infectious diseases). In these conditions, the general view is that immune-cell function is the principal disturbed phenomenon that ultimately results in clinical-disease symptoms. Hence, based on the general concept of immune modulation by dietary FAs outlined earlier in this chapter, an obvious rationale explains why dietary lipids can be a factor in the process of disease initiation and manifestation. Another class of disorders where dietary lipids were implicated to play a potentially etiological role is some neurological conditions (see Freeman et al., 2006 for references). Examples of such conditions are: several common and overlapping childhood neurodevelopmental disorders including attention-deficit/hyperactivity disorder, dyslexia, dyspraxia, and autistic-spectrum disorders; psychiatric disorders like major depression, bipolar disorder, and schizophrenia; and neurodegenerative disorders like Alzheimer's disease (AD) and Parkinson's disease (PD). In recent years, researchers have widely appreciated that, in addition to the diseases classically associated with inflammation, uncontrolled inflammation influences the pathogenesis of several other prevalent diseases including depression (Dantzer et al., 2008), AD, and PD (Rogers et al., 2007). At the same time, the newly discovered EPA- and DHA-derived mediators termed "resolvins" and "protectins," that appear to play a role in the resolution of inflammation (Serhan et al., 2008) and are neuroprotective (Mukherjee et al., 2007), open a new area that links immunomodulation with dietary lipids to neural function.

For example, in an experimental model of stroke, DHA and a neuroprotectin D1 (NPD1) infusion in the brain decreased inflammatory markers, including leukocyte infiltration (Marcheselli et al., 2003). As NPD1 had a more pronounced effect than DHA, the effects of DHA on the markers of neuroinflammation may be due to DHA metabolism to NPD1. NPD1 was identified in human neural tissue, and levels of DHA as well as NPD1 are decreased in postmortem brain samples from patients with AD (Lukiw et al., 2005). Although a lower consumption of DHA was linked to an increased risk of AD (Morris et al., 2003), still unclear is whether the observed decreased NPD1 (and DHA) in AD brains is the result or cause of the AD process. Furthermore, TNF-$\alpha$ is possibly involved in the neuroinflammation and pathogenesis of AD (Tarkowski et al., 2003a,b), while, in a case-report, the perispinal administration of a TNF-$\alpha$ antagonist improved the symptoms in AD patients (Tobinick & Gross, 2008). Based on these observations, one can surmise that possible concepts might be that DHA-derived, neuroprotective docosanoid-signaling counteracts proinflammatory, cytokine-triggered, cell-damaging events.

To this point, the mechanism underlying some of the observed effects of an increased n-3 LC-PUFA intake on clinical outcomes in some neurological conditions is substantially unclear. For instance, pure EPA showed benefits in several clinical trials for psychiatric disorders like depression, while studies using either pure DHA, or more DHA than EPA, for such disorders were negative (Stahl et al., 2008). Such observations appear to be paradoxical because DHA, but not EPA, is a critical, structural component of neuronal membranes. Although numerous mechanisms, including the moderation of inflammation, were proposed as possible modes of action (Richardson,

2008; Stahl et al., 2008), the mechanisms underlying the apparent differences between EPA and DHA in treatment effects remain a matter of speculation.

Thus, future research in the area of dietary EPA and DHA, their lipid mediators, and neuroinflammation may contribute to a better understanding of the complex relationships between immune regulation, dietary lipids, and treatment effects seen in psychiatric and neurodegenerative disorders and their possible roles in the etiology and pathogenesis thereof. A better understanding of this area may also provide more insights into potential dietary prevention strategies for neurological disorders like depression and AD, regardless of their degree of classification as inflammatory conditions.

## Conclusion

Alterations in the food chain over the past century are likely to have led to significant changes in absolute and relative n-6 and n-3 EFA and LC-PUFA intakes throughout life. The FA composition of immune cells is susceptible to such changes. Through a variety of mechanisms, the relative presence of LC-PUFAs can modify the functional activities of immune cells and the immune response as a whole. The dominance of AA, relative to n-3 LC-PUFAs, could, via its eicosanoid-precursor function, potentiate inflammatory processes, and so could predispose someone to, or exacerbate, inflammatory diseases. This was proposed as a potential etiological factor for numerous disorders that are characterized by exaggerated inflammation. The suspicion has particularly arisen because their increased prevalence in the past decades coincides with an increased intake of n-6 PUFA. On the other hand, an increased intake of n-3 PUFA may dampen excessive inflammation, and thereby exert suppressive effects on the pathogenesis of inflammatory diseases.

Human intervention studies provide clear support for the general concept that concentrations of dietary lipid-derived mediators, such as eicosanoids, are susceptible to changed dietary lipids, particularly of high-intake levels of n-3 LC-PUFAs. The concept of dietary immunomodulation is further supported by numerous human intervention studies showing changes in cytokine profiles and other immune markers, which might be mediated by shifts in produced eicosanoids, or other eicosanoid-independent pathways. Hence, these observations provide a robust basis for the hypothesis that structural changes in FA intake may cause changes in immune reactivity, and that such changes, on a population basis, contribute to a great or lesser occurrence of some diseases, particularly those characterized by uncontrolled inflammatory responses.

Studies of an increased prenatal n-3 LC-PUFA supply via maternal supplementation of fish oil indicate that higher EPA and DHA supplies modulate neonatal immune function in a manner that may favorably affect susceptibility to the onset of allergic diseases. Increased neonatal LA and AA intakes most likely are risk factors for an atopic-disease onset, but the current body of evidence provides no support for this, although controlled intervention studies are lacking. Some inconsistent data suggest that neonatal dietary GLA may protect against the onset of allergic diseases.

Intervention studies investigated the effects of DHA + AA in infant milk formula on a range of immune markers, relative to breast-milk reference groups. The outcomes are not entirely consistent, but the values of some, but not all, markers are closest to the breast-milk groups in those infants receiving formula with LC-PUFAs. Future research should elucidate whether these observations reflect a role of LC-PUFAs in the maturation of the immune system and the longevity of effects seen. In older infants and children, most research focused on the effects of fish-oil preparations for the prevention of allergic diseases and, to a lesser extent, infections. Some data suggest that a higher consumption of these FAs reduces a short-term risk of allergic symptoms and infections. On the other hand, the evidence for long-term benefits of such interventions is scarce, and data from prospective studies on fish consumption and the risk of allergies and asthma are conflicting, so no conclusive evidence exists that either low fish intake or high LA intake has contributed to the rise of atopy, allergies, and asthma. A too-low consumption of EPA + DHA was implicated as a risk factor for autoimmune diseases. Several prospective and case-control studies suggest that a higher intake of these FAs reduces the prevalence of type I diabetes and RA, although this is not consistent throughout studies. Moreover, no primary-prevention studies in either disease were conducted. Likewise, ecological and case-control reports suggest that a higher n-3 LC-PUFA and a lower n-6 intake reduce the risk of an IBD and a COPD onset, but no data from intervention studies are available to verify this. The evidence base of the favorable effects of n-3 LC-PUFAs in the prevention of a relapse in IBD is moderate for CD and absent for UC. In addition to these "classical" inflammatory diseases, evidence is emerging that uncontrolled inflammation is possibly involved in the pathogenesis of some neurological disorders like depression and AD. Possibly, part of the observed preventive effects of n-3 LC-PUFAs in these disorders is mediated by newly discovered n-3 LC-PUFA-derived docosanoids that counteract neuroinflammation.

Together, substantial support of a possible involvement of dietary lipids in the onset of diseases is characterized by excessive inflammation. Overall, the type of information is highly heterogeneous and relatively inconsistent, and too-little high-quality data are available to draw conclusions regarding possible causal relations. In general, low EPA and DHA consumption is reported more often as a risk factor of disease onset than a high-LA intake. Large-scale, well-powered primary- prevention intervention studies with long-term follow-up in the areas discussed in this chapter are required to generate conclusive evidence. Such an approach should also prevent false-negative and false-positive outcomes due to insufficient statistical power and too narrowly studied intake ranges.

## References

Ailhaud, G.; F. Massiera; P. Weill; P. Legrand; J.M. Alessandri; P. Guesnet. Temporal changes in dietary fats: role of n-6 polyunsaturated fatty acids in excessive adipose tissue development and relationship to obesity. *Prog. Lipid Res.* **2006,** *45(3),* 203–236.

Almqvist, C.; F. Garden; W. Xuan; S. Mihrshahi; S.R. Leeder; W. Oddy; K. Webb; G.B. Marks. Omega-3 and omega-6 fatty acid exposure from early life does not affect atopy and asthma at age 5 years. *J. Allergy Clin. Immunol.* **2007,** *119(6),* 1438–1444.

Amre, D.K.; S. D'Souza; K. Morgan; G. Seidman; P. Lambrette; G. Grimard; D. Israel; D. Mack; P. Ghadirian; C. Deslandres; et al. Imbalances in dietary consumption of fatty acids, vegetables, and fruits are associated with risk for Crohn's disease in children. *Am. J. Gastroenterol.* **2007,** *102(9),* 2016–2025.

Armitage, E.; H.E. Drummond; D.C. Wilson; S. Ghosh . Increasing incidence of both juvenile-onset Crohn's disease and ulcerative colitis in Scotland. *Eur. J. Gastroenterol. Hepatol.* **2001,** *13(12),* 1439–1447.

Bach, J.F. The effect of infections on susceptibility to autoimmune and allergic diseases. *N. Engl. J. Med.* **2002,** *347(12),* 911–920.

Bagga, D.; L. Wang; R. Farias-Eisner; J.A. Glaspy; S.T. Reddy. Differential effects of prostaglandin derived from omega-6 and omega-3 polyunsaturated fatty acids on COX-2 expression and IL-6 secretion. *Proc. Natl. Acad. Sci. U.S.A.* **2003,** *100(4),* 1751–1756.

Barnes, P.J. Immunology of asthma and chronic obstructive pulmonary disease. *Nat. Rev. Immunol.* **2008,** *8(3),* 183–192.

Belluzzi, A.; C. Brignola; M. Campieri; A. Pera; S. Boschi; M. Miglioli. Effect of an enteric-coated fish-oil preparation on relapses in Crohn's disease. *N. Engl. J. Med.* **1996,** *334(24),* 1557–1560.

Belluzzi, A.; M. Campieri; C. Belloli; S. Boschi; M. Cottone; F. Rizzello. A new enteric coated [reparation of omega-3 fatty acids for preventing post-surgical recurrence in Crohn's disease. *Gastroenterology* **1997,** *112(4),* A930.

Benito-Garcia, E.; D. Feskanich; F.B. Hu; L.A. Mandl; E. W. Karlson. Protein, iron, and meat consumption and risk for rheumatoid arthritis: a prospective cohort study. *Arthritis Res. Ther.* **2007**, *9(1),* R16.

Black, P.N.; S. Sharpe. Dietary fat and asthma: is there a connection? *Eur. Respir. J.* **1997,** *10(1),* 6–12.

Brenna, J.T.; B. Varamini; R.G. Jensen; D.A. Diersen-Schade; J.A. Boettcher; L. M. Arterburn. Docosahexaenoic and arachidonic acid concentrations in human breast milk worldwide. *Am. J. Clin. Nutr.* **2007,** *85(6),* 1457–1464.

British Nutrition Foundation. Report of the Task Force on Unsaturated Fatty Acids. Nutritional and Physiological Significance; Chapman & Hall: London, 1992.

British Nutrition Foundation. Briefing Paper: n-3 Fatty Acids and Health; British Nutrition Foundation: London.

Burdge, G.C. Metabolism of alpha-linolenic acid in humans. *Prostaglandins, Leukotrienes Essent. Fatty Acids* **2006,** *75(3),* 161–168.

Burdge, G.C.; P.C. Calder. Conversion of alpha-linolenic acid to longer-chain polyunsaturated fatty acids in human adults. *Reprod. Nutr. Dev.* **2005,** *45(5),* 581–597.

Burdge, G.C.; B. Lupoli; J.J. Russell; S. Tricon; S. Kew; T. Banerjee; K.J. Shingfield; D.E. Beever; R.F. Grimble; C. M. Williams; et al. Incorporation of cis-9,trans-11 or trans-10,cis-12 conjugated linoleic acid into plasma and cellular lipids in healthy men. *J. Lipid Res.* **2004,** *45(4),* 736–741.

Butland, B.K.; A.M. Fehily; P.C. Elwood. Diet, lung function, and lung function decline in a cohort of 2512 middle aged men. *Thorax* **2000,** *55(2),* 102–108.

Calder, P.C. Sir David Cuthbertson Medal Lecture. Immunomodulatory and anti-inflammatory effects of n-3 polyunsaturated fatty acids. *Proc. Nutr. Soc.* **1996,** *55(2),* 737–774.

Calder, P.C. Dietary fatty acids and lymphocyte functions. *Proc. Nutr. Soc.* **1998,** *57(4),* 487–502.

Calder, P.C. N-3 polyunsaturated fatty acids, inflammation and immunity: pouring oil on troubled waters or another fishy tale? *Nutr. Res.* **2001a,** *21(1–2),* 309–341.

Calder, P.C. Polyunsaturated fatty acids, inflammation, and immunity. *Lipids* **2001b,** *36(9),* 1007–1024.

Calder, P.C. N-3 polyunsaturated fatty acids and inflammation: from molecular biology to the clinic. *Lipids* **2003a,** *38(4),* 343–352.

Calder, P.C. Polyunsaturated fatty acids and cytokine profiles: a clue to the changing prevalence of atopy? *Clin. Exp. Allergy* **2003b,** *33(4),* 412–415.

Calder, P.C. Polyunsaturated fatty acids and inflammation. *Biochem. Soc. Trans.* **2005,** *33(Pt. 2),* 423–427.

Calder, P.C. Abnormal fatty acid profiles occur in atopic dermatitis but what do they mean? *Clin. Exp. Allergy* **2006a,** *36(2),* 138–141.

Calder, P.C. n-3 Polyunsaturated fatty acids, inflammation, and inflammatory diseases. *Am. J. Clin. Nutr.* **2006b,** *83(6),* S1505–1519.

Calder, P.C. Immunomodulation by omega-3 fatty acids. *Prostaglandins, Leukotrienes Essent. Fatty Acids* **2007,** *77(5–6),* 327–335.

Calder, P.C. Polyunsaturated fatty acids, inflammatory processes and inflammatory bowel diseases. *Mol. Nutr. Food Res.* **2008a,** *152*, 885–897.

Calder, P.C. Polyunsaturated fatty acids, inflammatory processes and rheumatoid arthritis. *Proc. Nutr. Soc.* **2008b,** *67*, 409–418.

Calder, P.C.; S. Krauss-Etschmann; E.C. de Jong; C. Dupont; J.S. Frick; H. Frokiaer; J. Heinrich; H. Garn; S. Koletzko; G. Lack; et al. Early nutrition and immunity— progress and perspectives. *Br. J. Nutr.* **2006,** *96(4),* 774–790.

Calder, P.C.; E.A. Miles. Fatty acids and atopic disease. *Pediatr. Allergy Immunol.* **2000,** *11(Suppl. 13),* 29–36.

Calder, P.C.; P. Yaqoob; F. Thies; F.A. Wallace; E.A. Miles. Fatty acids and lymphocyte functions. *Br. J. Nutr.* **2002,** *87(Suppl. 1),* S31–48.

Calder, P.C.; R.B. Zurier. Polyunsaturated fatty acids and rheumatoid arthritis. *Curr. Opin. Clin. Nutr. Metab. Care* **2001,** *4(2),* 115–121.

Calvani, M.; C. Alessandri; S.M. Sopo; V. Panetta; G. Pingitore; S. Tripodi; D. Zappala; A.M. Zicari. Consumption of fish, butter and margarine during pregnancy and development of allergic sensitizations in the offspring: role of maternal atopy. *Pediatr. Allergy Immunol.* **2006,** *17(2),* 94–102.

Carr, I.; J.F. Mayberry. The effects of migration on ulcerative colitis: a three-year prospective study among Europeans and first- and second-generation South Asians in Leicester (1991–1994). *Am. J. Gastroenterol.* **1999,** *94(10),* 2918–2922.

Caspi, A.; B. Williams; J. Kim-Cohen; I.W. Craig; B.J. Milne; R. Poulton; L.C. Schalkwyk; A. Taylor; H. Werts; T.E. Moffitt. Moderation of breastfeeding effects on the IQ by genetic variation in fatty acid metabolism. *Proc. Natl. Acad. Sci. U.S.A.* **2007,** *104(47),* 18860–18865.

Caughey, G.E.; E. Mantzioris; R.A. Gibson; L.G. Cleland; M.J. James. The effect on human tumor necrosis factor alpha and interleukin 1 beta production of diets enriched in n-3 fatty acids from vegetable oil or fish oil. *Am. J. Clin. Nutr.* **1996,** *63(1),* 116–122.

Chatzi, L.; M. Torrent; I. Romieu; R. Garcia-Esteban; C. Ferrer; J. Vioque; M. Kogevinas; J. Sunyer. Diet, wheeze, and atopy in school children in Menorca, Spain. *Pediatr. Allergy Immunol.* **2007,** *18(6),* 480–485.

Cleland, L.G.; M.J. James. The role of fats in the lifecycle stages. Adulthood—prevention: rheumatoid arthritis. *Med. J. Aust.* **2002,** *176(Suppl,)* S119–120.

Crawford, M.A.; K. Costeloe; K. Ghebremeskel; A. Phylactos; L. Skirvin; F. Stacey. Are deficits of arachidonic and docosahexaenoic acids responsible for the neural and vascular complications of preterm babies? *Am. J. Clin. Nutr.* **1997,** *66(Suppl. 4),* 1032S–1041S.

Damsgaard, C.T.; H. Frokiaer; L. Lauritzen. The effects of fish oil and high or low linoleic acid intake on fatty acid composition of human peripheral blood mononuclear cells. *Br. J. Nutr.* **2008,** *99(1),* 147–154.

Damsgaard, C.T.; L. Lauritzen; T.M. Kjaer; P.M. Holm; M.B. Fruekilde; K.F. Michaelsen; H. Frokiaer. Fish Oil Supplementation Modulates Immune Function in Healthy Infants. *J. Nutr.* **2007,** *137(4),* 1031–1036.

Dantzer, R.; J.C. O'Connor; G.G. Freund; R.W. Johnson; K.W. Kelley. From inflammation to sickness and depression: when the immune system subjugates the brain. *Nat. Rev. Neurosci.* **2008,** *9(1),* 46–56.

De Ley, M.; R. de Vos; D.W. Hommes; P. Stokkers. Fish oil for induction of remission in ulcerative colitis. *Cochrane Database Syst. Rev.* **2007,** 4, CD005986.

Dooper, M.M.; L. Wassink; L. M'Rabet; Y.M. Graus. The modulatory effects of prostaglandin-E on cytokine production by human peripheral blood mononuclear cells are independent of the prostaglandin subtype. *Immunology* **2002,** *107(1),* 152–159.

Dunder, T.; L. Kuikka; J. Turtinen; L. Rasanen; M. Uhari. Diet, serum fatty acids, and atopic diseases in childhood. *Allergy* **2001,** *56(5),* 425–428.

Dunstan, J.A.; T.A. Mori; A. Barden; L.J. Beilin; A.L. Taylor; P.G. Holt; S.L. Prescott. Fish oil supplementation in pregnancy modifies neonatal allergen-specific immune responses and clinical outcomes in infants at high risk of atopy: a randomized, controlled trial. J. *Allergy Clin. Immunol.* **2003a,** *112(6),* 1178–1184.

Dunstan, J.A.; T.A. Mori; A. Barden; L.J. Beilin; A.L. Taylor; P.G. Holt; S.L. Prescott. Maternal fish oil supplementation in pregnancy reduces interleukin-13 levels in cord blood of infants at high risk of atopy. *Clin. Exp. Allergy* **2003b,** *33(4),* 442–448.

Endres, S.; R. Ghorbani; V.E. Kelley; K. Georgilis; G. Lonnemann; J.W. van der Meer; J.G. Cannon; T.S. Rogers; M.S. Klempner; P.C. Weber; et al. The effect of dietary supplementation with n-3 polyunsaturated fatty acids on the synthesis of interleukin-1 and tumor necrosis factor by mononuclear cells. *N. Engl. J. Med.* **1989,** *320(5),* 265–271.

Farchi, S.; F. Forastiere; N. Agabiti; G. Corbo; R. Pistelli; C. Fortes; V. Dell'Orco; C.A. Perucci.

Dietary factors associated with wheezing and allergic rhinitis in children. *Eur. Respir. J.* **2003,** *22(5),* 772–780.

Farquharson, J.; F. Cockburn; W.A. Patrick; E.C. Jamieson; R.W. Logan. Infant cerebral cortex phospholipid fatty-acid composition and diet. *Lancet* **1992,** *340(8823),* 810–813.

Feagan, B.G.; W.J. Sandborn; U. Mittmann; S. Bar-Meir; G. D'Haens; M. Bradette; A. Cohen; C. Dallaire; T.P. Ponich; J.W. McDonald; et al. Omega-3 free fatty acids for the maintenance of remission in Crohn disease: the EPIC Randomized Controlled Trials. *Jama* **2008,** *299(14),* 1690–1697.

Feldmann, M.; R.N. Maini. The role of cytokines in the pathogenesis of rheumatoid arthritis. *Rheumatology (Oxford)* **1999,** *38(Suppl. 2),* 3–7.

Field, C.J. The immunological components of human milk and their effect on immune development in infants. *J. Nutr.* **2005,** *135(1),* 1–4.

Field, C.J.; M.T. Clandinin; J.E. Van Aerde.Polyunsaturated fatty acids and T-cell function: implications for the neonate. *Lipids* **2001,** *36(9),* 1025–1032.

Field, C.J.; C.A. Thomson; J.E. Van Aerde; A. Parrott; A. Euler; E. Lien; M.T. Clandinin. Lower proportion of CD45R0+ cells and deficient interleukin-10 production by formula-fed infants, compared with human-fed, is corrected with supplementation of long-chain polyunsaturated fatty acids. *J. Pediatr. Gastroenterol. Nutr.* **2000,** *31(3),* 291–299.

Field, C.J.; J.E. Van Aerde; L.E. Robinson; M.T. Clandinin. Effect of providing a formula supplemented with long-chain polyunsaturated fatty acids on immunity in full-term neonates. *Br. J. Nutr.* **2008a,** *99(1),* 91–99.

Field, C.J.; J.E. Van Aerde; L.E. Robinson; M.T. Clandinin. Feeding a formula supplemented with long chain polyunsaturated fatty acids modifies the 'ex vivo' cytokine responses to food proteins in infants at low risk for allergy. *Pediatr. Res.* **2008b.**

Freeman, M.P.; J.R. Hibbeln; K.L. Wisner; J.M. Davis; D. Mischoulon; M. Peet; P.E. Keck, Jr.; L.B. Marangell; A.J. Richardson; J. Lake; A.L. Stoll. Omega-3 fatty acids: evidence basis for treatment and future research in psychiatry. *J. Clin. Psychiatry* **2006,** *67(12),* 1954–1967.

Gibney, M.J.; B. Hunter. The effects of short- and long-term supplementation with fish oil on the incorporation of n-3 polyunsaturated fatty acids into cells of the immune system in healthy volunteers. *Eur. J. Clin. Nutr.* **1993,** *47(4),* 255–259.

Goldman, D.W.; W.C. Pickett; E.J. Goetzl. Human neutrophil chemotactic and degranulating activities of leukotriene B5 (LTB5) derived from eicosapentaenoic acid. *Biochem. Biophys. Res. Commun.* **1983,** *117(1),* 282–288.

Goyens, P.L.; M.E. Spilker; P.L. Zock; M.B. Katan; R.P. Mensink. Conversion of alpha-linolenic acid in humans is influenced by the absolute amounts of alpha-linolenic acid and linoleic acid in the diet and not by their ratio. *Am. J. Clin. Nutr.* **2006,** *84(1),* 44–53.

Grimble, R.F.; W.M. Howell; G. O'Reilly; S.J. Turner; O. Markovic; S. Hirrell; J.M. East; P.C. Calder. The ability of fish oil to suppress tumor necrosis factor alpha production by peripheral blood mononuclear cells in healthy men is associated with polymorphisms in genes that influence tumor necrosis factor alpha production. *Am. J. Clin. Nutr.* **2002,** *76(2),* 454–459.

Hawthorne, A.B.; T.K. Daneshmend; C.J. Hawkey; A. Belluzzi; S.J. Everitt; G.K. Holmes; C. Malkinson; M.Z. Shaheen; J.E. Willars. Treatment of ulcerative colitis with fish oil supplementation: a prospective 12 month randomised controlled trial. *Gut* **1992,** *33(7),* 922–928.

Healy, D.A.; F.A. Wallace; E.A. Miles; P.C. Calder; P. Newsholm. Effect of low-to-moderate amounts of dietary fish oil on neutrophil lipid composition and function. *Lipids* **2000,** *35(7),* 763–768.

Hibbeln, J.R.; L.R. Nieminen; T.L. Blasbalg; J.A. Riggs; W.E. Lands. Healthy intakes of n-3 and n-6 fatty acids: estimations considering worldwide diversity. *Am. J. Clin. Nutr.* **2006,** *83(Suppl. 6),* 1483S–1493S.

Hijazi, N.; B. Abalkhail; A. Seaton. Diet and childhood asthma in a society in transition: a study in urban and rural Saudi Arabia. *Thorax* **2000,** *55(9),* 775–779.

Hoare, C.; A. Li Wan Po; H. Williams. Systematic review of treatments for atopic eczema. *Health Technol. Assess.* **2000,** *4(37),* 1–191.

Hodge, L.; J.K. Peat; C. Salome. Increased consumption of polyunsaturated oils may be a cause of increased prevalence of childhood asthma. *Aust. N.Z. J. Med.* **1994,** *24(6),* 727.

Hodge, L.; C. Salome; J. Hughes; D. Liu-Brennan; J. Rimmer; M. Allman; D. Pang; C. Armour; A. Woolcock. Effect of dietary intake of omega-3 and omega-6 fatty acids on severity of asthma in children. *Eur. Respir. J.* **1998,** *11(2),* 361–365.

Hodge, L.; C.M. Salome; J.K. Peat; M.M. Haby; W. Xuan; A.J. Woolcock. Consumption of oily fish and childhood asthma risk. *Med. J. Aust.* **1996,** *164(3),* 137–140.

Hoffman, D.R.; E.E. Birch; Y.S. Castaneda; S.L. Fawcett; D. H. Wheaton; D.G. Birch; R. Uauy. Visual function in breast-fed term infants weaned to formula with or without long-chain polyunsaturates at 4 to 6 months: a randomized clinical trial. *J. Pediatr.* **2003,** *142(6),* 669677.

Hoffman, D.R.; R.C. Theuer; Y.S. Castaneda; D.H. Wheaton; R.G. Bosworth; A.R. O'Connor; S.E. Morale; L.E. Wiedemann; E.E. Birch. Maturation of visual acuity is accelerated in breast-fed term infants fed baby food containing dha-enriched egg yolk. *J. Nutr.* **2004,** *134(9),* 2307–2313.

Hommes, D.W.; S.J. van Deventer. Anti- and proinflammatory cytokines in the pathogenesis of tissue damage in Crohn's disease. *Curr. Opin. Clin. Nutr. Metab. Care* **2000,** *3(3),* 191–195.

Horrobin, D.F. Low prevalences of coronary heart disease (CHD), psoriasis, asthma and rheumatoid arthritis in Eskimos: are they caused by high dietary intake of eicosapentaenoic acid (EPA), a genetic variation of essential fatty acid (EFA) metabolism or a combination of both? *Med. Hypotheses* **1987,** *22(4),* 421–428.

Hwang, D. Fatty acids and immune responses—a new perspective in searching for clues to mechanism. *Annu. Rev. Nutr.* **20**, 431–456.

Innis, S.M.; S.L. Elias. Intakes of essential n-6 and n-3 polyunsaturated fatty acids among pregnant Canadian women. *Am. J. Clin. Nutr.* **2003,** *77(2),* 473–478.

Innis, S.M.; K. Jacobson. Dietary lipids in early development and intestinal inflammatory disease. *Nutr.Rev.* **2007,** *65,* 188–193.

Ip, S.; M. Chung; G. Raman; P. Chew; N. Magula; D. DeVine; T. Trikalinos; J. Lau. Breastfeeding and maternal and infant health outcomes in developed countries. *Evid Rep. Technol. Assess. (Full Rep)***2007,** *153,* 1–186.

Jensen, R.G. Lipids in human milk. *Lipids* 1999, *34(12),* 1243–1271.

Kankaanpaa, P.; Y. Sutas; S. Salminen; A. Lichtenstein; E. Isolauri. Dietary fatty acids and allergy. *Ann. Med.* **1999,** *31(4),* 282–287.

Kelley, D.S.; V.A. Simon; P.C. Taylor; I.L. Rudolph; P. Benito; G.J. Nelson; B.E. Mackey; K.L. Erickson. Dietary supplementation with conjugated linoleic acid increased its concentration in human peripheral blood mononuclear cells, but did not alter their function. *Lipids* **2001,** *36(7),* 669–674.

Kelley, D.S.; P.C. Taylor; G.J. Nelson; B.E. Mackey. Arachidonic acid supplementation enhances synthesis of eicosanoids without suppressing immune functions in young healthy men. *Lipids* **1998,** *33(2),* 125–130.

Kelley, D.S.; P.C. Taylor; G.J. Nelson; P.C. Schmidt; A. Ferretti; K.L. Erickson; R. Yu; R.K. Chandra; B.E. Mackey. Docosahexaenoic acid ingestion inhibits natural killer cell activity and production of inflammatory mediators in young healthy men. *Lipids* **1999,** *34(4),* 317–324.

Kelley, D.S.; P.C. Taylor; G.J. Nelson; P.C. Schmidt; B.E. Mackey; D. Kyle. Effects of dietary arachidonic acid on human immune response. *Lipids* **1997,** *32(4),* 449–456.

Kew, S.; T. Banerjee; A.M. Minihane; Y.E. Finnegan; R. Muggli; R. Albers; C.M. Williams; P.C. Calder. Lack of effect of foods enriched with plant- or marine-derived n-3 fatty acids on human immune function. *Am. J. Clin. Nutr.* **2003,** *77(5),* 1287–1295.

Kew, S.; M.D. Mesa; S. Tricon; R. Buckley; A.M. Minihane; P. Yaqoob. Effects of oils rich in eicosapentaenoic and docosahexaenoic acids on immune cell composition and function in healthy humans. *Am. J. Clin. Nutr.* **2004,** *79(4),* 674–681.

Kitz, R.; M.A. Rose; H. Schonborn; S. Zielen; H.J. Bohles. Impact of early dietary gamma-linolenic acid supplementation on atopic eczema in infancy. *Pediatr. Allergy Immunol.* **2006,** *17(2),* 112–117.

Koletzko, B.; I. Cetin; J.T. Brenna. Dietary fat intakes for pregnant and lactating women. *Br. J. Nutr.* **2007,** *98(5),* 873–877.

Koletzko, B.; E. Lien; C. Agostoni; H. Bohles; C. Campoy; I. Cetin; T. Decsi; J.W. Dudenhausen; C. Dupont; S. Forsyth; et al. The roles of long-chain polyunsaturated fatty acids in pregnancy, lactation and infancy: review of current knowledge and consensus recommendations. *J. Perinat. Med.* **2008,** *36(1),* 5–14.

Kompauer, I.; H. Demmelmair; B. Koletzko; G. Bolte; J. Linseisen; J. Heinrich. Association of fatty acids in serum phospholipids with lung function and bronchial hyperresponsiveness in adults. *Eur. J. Epidemiol.* **2008,** *23(3),* 175–190.

Krauss-Etschmann, S.; D. Hartl; P. Rzehak; J. Heinrich; R. Shadid; M. Del Carmen Ramirez-Tortosa; C. Campoy; S. Pardillo; D.J. Schendel; T. Decsi; et al. Decreased cord blood IL-4, IL-13, and CCR4 and increased TGF-beta levels after fish oil supplementation of pregnant women. *J. Allergy Clin. Immunol.* **2008,** *121(2),* 464–470 e6.

Krauss-Etschmann, S.; R. Shadid; C. Campoy; E. Hoster; H. Demmelmair; M. Jimenez; A. Gil; M. Rivero; B. Veszpremi; T. Decsi; B.V. Koletzko. Effects of fish-oil and folate supplementation of pregnant women on maternal and fetal plasma concentrations of docosahexaenoic acid and eicosapentaenoic acid: a European randomized multicenter trial. *Am. J. Clin. Nutr.* **2007,** *85(5),* 1392–400.

Kromann, N.; A. Green. Epidemiological studies in the Upernavik district, Greenland. Incidence of some chronic diseases 1950–1974. *Acta Med. Scand.* **1980,** *208(5),* 401–406.

Kuhnt, K.; J. Kraft; H. Vogelsang; K. Eder; J. Kratzsch; G. Jahreis. Dietary supplementation with trans-11- and trans-12-18 : 1 increases cis-9, trans-11-conjugated linoleic acid in human immune cells, but without effects on biomarkers of immune function and inflammation. *Br. J. Nutr.* **2007,** *97(6),* 1196–205.

Laerum, B.N.; T. Wentzel-Larsen; A. Gulsvik; E. Omenaas; T. Gislason; C. Janson; C. Svanes. Relationship of fish and cod oil intake with adult asthma. *Clin. Exp. Allergy* **2007,** *37(11),* 1616-1623.

Lauritzen, L.; C. Hoppe; E.M. Straarup; K.F. Michaelsen. Maternal fish oil supplementation in lactation and growth during the first 2.5 years of life. *Pediatr. Res.* **2005,** *58(2),* 235–242.

Lauritzen, L.; M.H. Jorgensen; T.B. Mikkelsen; M. Skovgaard; E.M. Straarup; S.F. Olsen; C.E. Hoy; K.F. Michaelsen. Maternal fish oil supplementation in lactation: effect on visual acuity and n-3 fatty acid content of infant erythrocytes. *Lipids* **2004,** *39(3),* 195–206.

Lauritzen, L.; T.M. Kjaer; M.B. Fruekilde; K.F. Michaelsen; H. Frokiaer. Fish oil supplementation of lactating mothers affects cytokine production in 2 1/2-year-old children. *Lipids* **2005,** *40(7),* 669–676.

Lee, T.H.; R.L. Hoover; J.D. Williams; R.I. Sperling; J. Ravalese, III; B.W. Spur; D.R. Robinson; E.J. Corey; R.A. Lewis; K.F. Austen. Effect of dietary enrichment with eicosapentaenoic and docosahexaenoic acids on in vitro neutrophil and monocyte leukotriene generation and neutrophil function. *N. Engl. J. Med.* **1985,** *312(19),* 1217–1224.

Lee, T.H.; J.M. Menica-Huerta; C. Shih; E.J. Corey; R.A. Lewis; K.F. Austen. Characterization and biologic properties of 5,12-dihydroxy derivatives of eicosapentaenoic acid, including leukotriene B5 and the double lipoxygenase product. *J. Biol. Chem.* **1984,** *259(4),* 2383–2389.

Lewis, R.A.; K.F. Austen; R.J. Soberman.Leukotrienes and other products of the 5-lipoxygenase pathway. Biochemistry and relation to pathobiology in human diseases. *N. Engl. J. Med.* **1990,** *323(10),* 645–655.

Linday, L.A.; J.N. Dolitsky; R.D. Shindledecker; C.E. Pippenger. Lemon-flavored cod liver oil and a multivitamin-mineral supplement for the secondary prevention of otitis media in young children: pilot research. *Ann. Otol. Rhinol. Laryngol.* **2002,** *111(7 Pt 1),* 642–652.

Linday, L.A.; R.D. Shindledecker; J. Tapia-Mendoza; J.N. Dolitsky. Effect of daily cod liver oil and a multivitamin-mineral supplement with selenium on upper respiratory tract pediatric visits by young, inner-city, Latino children: randomized pediatric sites. *Ann. Otol. Rhinol. Laryngol.* **2004,** *113(11),* 891–901.

Linos, A.; V.G. Kaklamani; E. Kaklamani; Y. Koumantaki; E. Giziaki; S. Papazoglou; C.S. Mantzoros. Dietary factors in relation to rheumatoid arthritis: a role for olive oil and cooked vegetables? *Am. J. Clin. Nutr.* **1999,** *70(6),* 1077–1082.

Linos, A.; E. Kaklamanis; A. Kontomerkos; Y. Koumantaki; S. Gazi; G. Vaiopoulos; G.C. Tsokos; P. Kaklamanis. The effect of olive oil and fish consumption on rheumatoid arthritis—a case control study. *Scand. J. Rheumatol.* **1991,** *20(6),* 419–426.

Loeschke, K.; B. Ueberschaer; A. Pietsch; E. Gruber; K. Ewe; B. Wiebecke; W. Heldwein; R. Lorenz. n-3 fatty acids only delay early relapse of ulcerative colitis in remission. *Dig. Dis. Sci.* **1996,** *41(10),* 2087-2094.

Loftus, E.V., Jr. Clinical epidemiology of inflammatory bowel disease: Incidence, prevalence, and environmental influences. *Gastroenterology* **2004**, *126(6)*, 1504–1517.

Lorenz-Meyer, H.; P. Bauer; C. Nicolay; B. Schulz; J. Purrmann; W.E. Fleig; C. Scheurlen; I. Koop; V. Pudel; L. Carr. Omega-3 fatty acids and low carbohydrate diet for maintenance of remission in Crohn's disease. A randomized controlled multicenter trial. Study Group Members (German Crohn's Disease Study Group). *Scand. J. Gastroenterol.* **1996,** *31(8),* 778–785.

Lukiw, W.J.; J.G. Cui; V.L. Marcheselli; M. Bodker; A. Botkjaer; K. Gotlinger; C.N. Serhan; N.G. Bazan. A role for docosahexaenoic acid-derived neuroprotectin D1 in neural cell survival and Alzheimer disease. *J. Clin. Invest.* **2005,** *115(10),* 2774–-2783.

Madden, S.M.; C.F. Garrioch; B.J. Holub. *Omega-3 Intakes in Canadian Children Aged 4 to 8 by Direct Analyses;* 8th Meeting of the International Society for the Study of Fatty Acids & Lipids, Kansas City; 2008.

Makrides, M.; J.S. Hawkes; M.A. Neumann; R.; A. Gibson. Nutritional effect of including egg yolk in the weaning diet of breast-fed and formula-fed infants: a randomized controlled trial. *Am. J. Clin. Nutr.* **2002,** *75(6),* 1084–1092.

Makrides, M.; M.A. Neumann; R.W. Byard; K. Simmer; R. A. Gibson. Fatty acid composition of brain, retina, and erythrocytes in breast- and formula-fed infants. *Am. J. Clin. Nutr.* **1994,** *60(2),* 189–194.

Mandrup-Poulsen, T.; S. Helqvist; J. Molvig; L.D. Wogensen; J. Nerup. Cytokines as immune effector molecules in autoimmune endocrine diseases with special reference to insulin-dependent diabetes mellitus. *Autoimmunity* **1989,** *4(3),* 191–218; discussion 219–-234.

Mantzaris, G.; E. Archavlis; C. Zografos; K. Petraki; C. Spiliades; G. Triantafyllou. A prospective, randomized, placebo controlled study of fish oil in ulcerative colitis. *Hell. J. Gastoenterol.* **1996,** *9,* 138–141.

Marcheselli, V.L.; S. Hong; W.J. Lukiw; X.H. Tian; K. Gronert; A. Musto; M. Hardy; J.M. Gimenez; N. Chiang; C.N. Serhan; N.G. Bazan. Novel docosanoids inhibit brain ischemia-reperfusion-mediated leukocyte infiltration and pro-inflammatory gene expression. *J. Biol. Chem.* **2003,** *278(44),* 43807–43817.

Marks, G.B.; S. Mihrshahi; A.S. Kemp; E.R. Tovey; K. Webb; C. Almqvist; R.D. Ampon; D. Crisafulli; E.G. Belousova; C.M. Mellis; et al. Prevention of asthma during the first 5 years of life: a randomized controlled trial. *J. Allergy Clin. Immunol.* **2006,** *118(1),* 53–61.

Matsuyama, W.; H. Mitsuyama; M. Watanabe; K. Oonakahara; I. Higashimoto; M. Osame; K. Arimura. Effects of omega-3 polyunsaturated fatty acids on inflammatory markers in COPD. *Chest* **2005**, *128(6),* 3817–3827.

Mazurak, V.C.; V. Lien; C.J. Field; S.D. Goruk; K. Pramuk; M.T. Clandinin. Long-chain polyunsaturated fat supplementation in children with low docosahexaenoic acid intakes alters immune phenotypes compared with placebo. *J. Pediatr. Gastroenterol. Nutr.* **2008,** *46(5),* 570–579.

McKeever, T.M.; S.A. Lewis; P.A. Cassano; M. Ocke; P. Burney; J. Britton; H.A. Smit. The relation between dietary intake of individual fatty acids, FEV1 and respiratory disease in Dutch adults. *Thorax* **2008,** *63(3),* 208–214.

Middleton, S.J.; S. Naylor; J. Woolner; J.O. Hunter. A double-blind, randomized, placebo-controlled trial of essential fatty acid supplementation in the maintenance of remission of ulcerative colitis. *Aliment. Pharmacol. Ther.* **2002,** *16(6),* 1131–1135.

Mihrshahi, S.; J.K. Peat; G.B. Marks; C.M. Mellis; E.R. Tovey; K. Webb; W.J. Britton; S.R. Leeder. Eighteen-month outcomes of house dust mite avoidance and dietary fatty acid modification in the Childhood Asthma Prevention Study (CAPS). *J. Allergy Clin. Immunol.* **2003,** *111(1),* 162–168.

Mihrshahi, S.; J.K. Peat; K. Webb; W. Oddy; G.B. Marks; C.M. Mellis. Effect of omega-3 fatty acid concentrations in plasma on symptoms of asthma at 18 months of age. *Pediatr. Allergy Immunol.* **2004,** *15(6),* 517–522.

Mihrshahi, S.; J.K. Peat; K. Webb; E.R. Tovey; G.B. Marks; C.M. Mellis; S.R. Leeder. The childhood asthma prevention study (CAPS): design and research protocol of a randomized trial for the primary prevention of asthma. *Control Clin. Trials* **2001,** *22(3),* 333–354.

Miles, E.A.; E. Allen; P.C. Calder. In vitro effects of eicosanoids derived from different 20-carbon fatty acids on production of monocyte-derived cytokines in human whole blood cultures. *Cytokine* **2002,** *20(5),* 215–223.

Miles, E.A.; L. Aston; P.C. Calder. In vitro effects of eicosanoids derived from different 20-carbon fatty acids on T helper type 1 and T helper type 2 cytokine production in human whole-blood cultures. *Clin. Exp. Allergy* **2003,** *33(5),* 624–632.

Miles, E.A.; T. Banerjee; P.C. Calder. The influence of different combinations of gamma-linolenic, stearidonic and eicosapentaenoic acids on the fatty acid composition of blood lipids and mononuclear cells in human volunteers. *Prostaglandins, Leukotrienes Essent. Fatty Acids* **2004,** *70(6),* 529–538.

Minns, L.M.; E.H. Kerling; M.R. Curtis; J.R. Goetz; D.K. Sullivan; S.E. Carlson. *Docosahexaenoic Acid Intake and Status of US Toddlers;* 8th Meeting of the International Society for the Study of Fatty Acids & Lipids, Kansas City; **2008**.

Miyake, Y.; S. Sasaki; K. Tanaka; Y. Ohya; S. Miyamoto; I. Matsunaga; T. Yoshida; Y. Hirota; H. Oda. Fish and fat intake and prevalence of allergic rhinitis in Japanese females: the Osaka Maternal and Child Health Study. *J. Am. Coll. Nutr.* **2007**, *26(3),* 279–287.

Montuschi, P.; S. Martello; M. Felli; C. Mondino; P.J. Barnes; M. Chiarotti. Liquid chromatography/mass spectrometry analysis of exhaled leukotriene B4 in asthmatic children. *Respir. Res.* **2005,** *6,* 119.

Morris, M.C.; D.A. Evans; J.L. Bienias; C.C. Tangney; D.A. Bennett; R.S. Wilson; N. Aggarwal; J. Schneider. Consumption of fish and n-3 fatty acids and risk of incident Alzheimer's disease. *Arch. Neurol.* **2003**, *60(7),* 940–946.

Mukherjee, P.K.; A. Chawla; M.S. Loayza; N.G. Bazan. Docosanoids are multifunctional regulators of neural cell integrity and fate: significance in aging and disease. *Prostaglandins, Leukotrienes Essent. Fatty Acids* **2007,** *77(5–6),* 233–238.

Murray, C.J. and A.D. Lopez. Alternatieve projects of mortality and disability by cause 1990-2020: Global Burden of Disease Study. *The Lancet* **1997,** *349(9064),* 1498–1504.

Muskiet, F.A.; S.A. van Goor; R.S. Kuipers; F.V. Velzing-Aarts; E.N. Smit; H. Bouwstra; D.A. Dijck-Brouwer; E.R. Boersma; M. Hadders-Algra. Long-chain polyunsaturated fatty acids in maternal and infant nutrition. *Prostaglandins, Leukotrienes Essent. Fatty Acids* **2006,** *75(3),* 135–144.

Nafstad, P.; W. Nystad; P. Magnus; J.J. Jaakkola. Asthma and allergic rhinitis at 4 years of age in relation to fish consumption in infancy. *J. Asthma* **2003,** *40(4),* 343–348.

Nagakura, T.; S. Matsuda; K. Shichijyo; H. Sugimoto; K. Hata. Dietary supplementation with fish oil rich in omega-3 polyunsaturated fatty acids in children with bronchial asthma. *Eur. Respir. J.* **2000,** *16(5),* 861–865.

Norris, J.M.; X. Yin; M.M. Lamb; K. Barriga; J. Seifert; M. Hoffman; H.D. Orton; A.E. Baron; M. Clare-Salzler; H.P. Chase; et al. Omega-3 polyunsaturated fatty acid intake and islet autoimmunity in children at increased risk for type 1 diabetes. *Jama* **2007,** *298(12),* 1420–1428.

Olsen, S.F.; M.L. Osterdal; J.D. Salvig; L.M. Mortensen; D. Rytter; N.J. Secher; T.B. Henriksen. Fish oil intake compared with olive oil intake in late pregnancy and asthma in the offspring: 16 y of registry-based follow-up from a randomized controlled trial. *Am. J. Clin. Nutr.* **2008,** *88(1),* 167–175.

Otto, S.J.; A.C. van Houwelingen; A. Badart-Smook; G. Hornstra. Changes in the maternal essential fatty acid profile during early pregnancy and the relation of the profile to diet. *Am. J. Clin. Nutr.* **2001a,** *73(2),* 302–307.

Otto, S.J.; A.C. van Houwelingen; A. Badart-Smook; G. Hornstra. Comparison of the peripartum and postpartum phospholipid polyunsaturated fatty acid profiles of lactating and nonlactating women. *Am. J. Clin. Nutr.* **2001b,** *73(6),* 1074–1079.

Pastor, N.; B. Soler; S.H. Mitmesser; P. Ferguson; C. Lifschitz. Infants fed docosahexaenoic acid- and arachidonic acid-supplemented formula have decreased incidence of bronchiolitis/bronchitis the first year of life. *Clin. ediatr. (Phila.)* **2006,** *45(9),* 850–855.

Pauwels, R.A.; K.F. Rabe. Burden and clinical features of chronic obstructive pulmonary disease (COPD). *Lancet* **2004,** *364(9434),* 613–620.

Peat, J.- K.; S. Mihrshahi; A.S. Kemp; G.B. Marks; E.R. Tovey; K. Webb; C.M. Mellis; S.R. Leeder. Three-year outcomes of dietary fatty acid modification and house dust mite reduction in the Childhood Asthma Prevention Study. *J. Allergy Clin. Immunol.* **2004,** *114(4),* 807–813.

Pedersen, M.; C. Stripp; M. Klarlund; S.F. Olsen; A.M. Tjonneland; M. Frisch. Diet and risk of rheumatoid arthritis in a prospective cohort. *J. Rheumatol.* **2005,** *32(7),* 1249–1252.

Peterson, L.D.; N.M. Jeffery; F. Thies; P. Sanderson; E.A. Newsholme; P.C. Calder. Eicosapentaenoic and docosahexaenoic acids alter rat spleen leukocyte fatty acid composition and prostaglandin E2 production but have different effects on lymphocyte functions and cell-mediated immunity. *Lipids* **1998,** *33(2),* 171–180.

Plourde, M.; S.C. Cunnane. Extremely limited synthesis of long chain polyunsaturates in adults: implications for their dietary essentiality and use as supplements. *Appl. Physiol. Nutr. Metab.* **2007,** *32(4),* 619–634.

Prescott, S.L.; A.E. Barden; T.A. Mori; J.A. Dunstan. Maternal fish oil supplementation in pregnancy modifies neonatal leukotriene production by cord-blood-derived neutrophils. *Clin. Sci. (Lond.)* **2007,** *113(10),* 409–416.

Prescott, S.L.; P.C. Calder. N-3 polyunsaturated fatty acids and allergic disease. *Curr. Opin. Clin. Nutr. Metab. Care* **2004,** *7(2),* 123–129.

Raper, N.R.; F.J. Cronin; J. Exler. Omega-3 fatty acid content of the US food supply. *J. Am. Coll. Nutr.* **1992,** *11(3),* 304–308.

Raper, N.R.; R.M. Marston. Levels and sources of fat in the U.S. food supply. *Prog. Clin. Biol. Res.* **1986,** *222,* 127–152.

Rees, D.; E.A. Miles; T. Banerjee; S.J. Wells; C.E. Roynette; K.W. Wahle; P.C. Calder. Dose-related effects of eicosapentaenoic acid on innate immune function in healthy humans: a comparison of young and older men. *Am. J. Clin. Nutr.* **2006,** *83(2),* 331–342.

Richardson, A.J. n-3 Fatty acids and mood: the devil is in the detail. *Br. J. Nutr.* **2008,** *99(2),* 221–223.

Rogers, J.; D. Mastroeni; B. Leonard; J. Joyce; A. Grover. Neuroinflammation in Alzheimer's disease and Parkinson's disease: are microglia pathogenic in either disorder? *Int. Rev. Neurobiol.* **2007,** *82,* 235–246.

Romano, C.; S. Cucchiara; A. Barabino; V. Annese; C. Sferlazzas. Usefulness of omega-3 fatty acid supplementation in addition to mesalazine in maintaining remission in pediatric Crohn's disease: a double-blind, randomized, placebo-controlled study. *World J. Gastroenterol.* **2005,** *11(45),* 7118–7121.

Romieu, I.; M. Torrent; R. Garcia-Esteban; C. Ferrer; N. Ribas-Fito; J.M. Anto; J. Sunyer. Maternal fish intake during pregnancy and atopy and asthma in infancy. *Clin. Exp. Allergy* **2007,** *37(4),* 518–525.

Sakao, S.; K. Tatsumi; H. Igari; Y. Shino; H. Shirasawa; T. Kuriyama. Association of tumor necrosis factor alpha gene promoter polymorphism with the presence of chronic obstructive pulmonary disease. *Am. J. Respir. Crit. Care Med.* **2001,** *163(2),* 420–422.

Sakao, S.; K. Tatsumi; H. Igari; R. Watanabe; Y. Shino; H. Shirasawa; T. Kuriyama. Association of tumor necrosis factor-alpha gene promoter polymorphism with low attenuation areas on high-resolution CT in patients with COPD. *Chest* **2002,** *122(2),* 416–420.

Salam, M.T.; Y.F. Li; B. Langholz; F.D. Gilliland. Maternal fish consumption during pregnancy and risk of early childhood asthma. *J. Asthma* **2005,** *42(6),* 513–518.

Sala-Vila, A.; E.-A. Miles; P.C. Calder. Fatty acid composition abnormalities in atopic disease: evidence explored and role in the disease process examined. *Clin. Exp. Allergy* 2008 (in press).

Sano, H.; T. Hla; J.A. Maier; L.J. Crofford; J.P. Case; T. Maciag; R.L. Wilder. In vivo cyclooxygenase expression in synovial tissues of patients with rheumatoid arthritis and osteoarthritis and rats with adjuvant and streptococcal cell wall arthritis. *J. Clin. Invest.* **1992,** *89(1),* 97–108.

Sausenthaler, S.; S. Koletzko; B. Schaaf; I. Lehmann; M. Borte; O. Herbarth; A. von Berg; H.E. Wichmann; J. Heinrich. Maternal diet during pregnancy in relation to eczema and allergic sensitization in the offspring at 2 y of age. *Am. J. Clin. Nutr.* **2007,** *85(2),* 530–537.

Schachter, H.M.; J. Reisman; K. Tran; B. Dales; K. Kourad; D. Barnes; M. Sampson; A. Morrison; I. Gaboury; J. Blackman. Health effects of omega-3 fatty acids on asthma. *Evid. Rep. Technol. Assessment No. 91 (Prepared by University of Ottawa Evidence-Based Practice Center under Contract No. 290-02-0021). AHRQ Publication No. 04-E013-2;* Agency for Health Care Research and Quality: Rockville, MD, March 2004.

Schols, A.M. Nutritional and metabolic modulation in chronic obstructive pulmonary disease management. *Eur. Respir. J. Suppl.* **2003,** *46,* 81s–86s.

Schubert, R.; R. Kitz; C. Beermann; M.A. Rose; A. Lieb; P.C. Sommerer; J. Moskowitz; H. Alberternst; H.J. Böhles; S. Zielen. Anti-inflammatory effect of n-3 polyunsaturated fatty acids in allergic asthma after low dose allergen challenge. *Clin. Exp. Allergy* (in press).

Schwartz, J.; S.T. Weiss. The relationship of dietary fish intake to level of pulmonary function in the first National Health and Nutrition Survey (NHANES I). *Eur. Respir. J.* **1994,** *7(10),*

1821 1824.

Semba, R.D. Vitamin A as "anti-infective" therapy, 1920–1940. *J. Nutr.* **1999,** *129(4),* 783–791.

Serhan, C.N. Novel eicosanoid and docosanoid mediators: resolvins, docosatrienes, and neuroprotectins. *Curr. Opin. Clin. Nutr. Metab. Care* **2005,** *8(2),* 115–121.

Serhan, C.N.; M. Arita; S. Hong; K. Gotlinger. Resolvins, docosatrienes, and neuroprotectins, novel omega-3-derived mediators, and their endogenous aspirin-triggered epimers. *Lipids* **2004,** *39(11),* 1125–1132.

Serhan, C.N.; N. Chiang; T.E. Van Dyke. Resolving inflammation: dual anti-inflammatory and pro-resolution lipid mediators. *Nat. Rev. Immunol.* **2008,** *8(5),* 349–361.

Shahar, E.; A.R. Folsom; S.L. Melnick; M.S. Tockman; G.W. Comstock; V. Gennaro; M.W. Higgins; P.D. Sorlie; W.J. Ko; M. Szklo. Dietary n-3 polyunsaturated fatty acids and smoking-related chronic obstructive pulmonary disease. Atherosclerosis Risk in Communities Study Investigators. *N. Engl. J. Med.* **1994,** *331(4),* 228–233.

Shapiro, J.A.; T.D. Koepsell; L.F. Voigt; C.E. Dugowson; M. Kestin; J.L. Nelson. Diet and rheumatoid arthritis in women: a possible protective effect of fish consumption. *Epidemiology* **1996,** *7(3),* 256–263.

Sharon, P.; W.F. Stenson; Enhanced synthesis of leukotriene B4 by colonic mucosa in inflammatory bowel disease. *Gastroenterology* **1984,** *86(3),* 453–460.

Sharp, D.S.; B.L. Rodriguez; E. Shahar; L.J. Hwang; C. M. Burchfiel. Fish consumption may limit the damage of smoking on the lung. *Am. J. Respir. Crit. Care Med.* **1994,** *150(4),* 983–987.

Shoda, R.; K. Matsueda; S. Yamato; N. Umeda. Epidemiologic analysis of Crohn's disease in Japan: increased dietary intake of n-6 polyunsaturated fatty acids and animal protein relates to the increased incidence of Crohn's disease in Japan. *Am. J. Clin. Nutr.* **1996,** *63(5),* 741–745.

Sijben, J.W.; P.C. Calder. Differential immunomodulation with long-chain n-3 PUFA in health and chronic disease. *Proc. Nutr. Soc.* **2007,** *66(2),* 237–259.

Simopoulos, A.P. Essential fatty acids in health and chronic disease. *Am. J. Clin. Nutr.* **1999,** *70(Suppl. 3),* 560S–569S.

Simopoulos, A.P.; A. Leaf; N. Salem, Jr. Workshop on the essentiality of and recommended dietary intakes for omega-6 and omega-3 fatty acids. *J. Am. Coll. Nutr.* **1999,** *18(5),* 487–489.

Sperling, R. I. Eicosanoids in rheumatoid arthritis. *Rheum. Dis. Clin. North Am.* **1995,** *21(3),* 741–758.

Sperling, R.I.; A.I. Benincaso; C.T. Knoell; J.K. Larkin; K.F. Austen; D.R. Robinson. Dietary omega-3 polyunsaturated fatty acids inhibit phosphoinositide formation and chemotaxis in neutrophils. *J. Clin. Invest.* **1993,** *91(2),* 651–660.

Stahl, L.A.; D.P. Begg; R.S. Weisinger; J. Sinclair. The role of omega-3 fatty acids in mood disorders. *Curr. Opin. Investig. Drugs* **2008,** *9(1),* 57–64.

Stanley, J.C.; R.L. Elsom; P.C. Calder; B.A. Griffin; W.S. Harris; S.A. Jebb; J.A. Lovegrove; C.S. Moore; R.A. Riemersma; T.A. Sanders. UK Food Standards Agency Workshop Report: the effects of the dietary n-6:n-3 fatty acid ratio on cardiovascular health. *Br. J. Nutr.* **2007,** *98(6),* 1305–1310.

Stene, L.C.; G. Joner. Use of cod liver oil during the first year of life is associated with lower risk of childhood-onset type 1 diabetes: a large, population-based, case-control study. *Am. J. Clin. Nutr.* **2003,** *78(6),* 1128–1134.

Stene, L.C.; J. Ulriksen; P. Magnus; G. Joner. Use of cod liver oil during pregnancy associated with lower risk of Type I diabetes in the offspring. *Diabetologia* **2000,** *43(9),* 1093–1098.

Stulnig, T.M.; M. Zeyda. Immunomodulation by polyunsaturated fatty acids: impact on T-cell signaling. *Lipids* **2004,** *39(12),* 1171–1175.

Tabak, C.; E.J. Feskens; D. Heederik; D. Kromhout; A. Menotti; H.W. Blackburn. Fruit and fish consumption: a possible explanation for population differences in COPD mortality (The Seven Countries Study). *Eur. J. Clin. Nutr.* **1998,** *52(11),* 819–825.

Takemura, Y.; Y. Sakurai; S. Honjo; A. Tokimatsu; M. Gibo; T. Hara; A. Kusakari; N. Kugai. The relationship between fish intake and the prevalence of asthma: the Tokorozawa childhood asthma and pollinosis study. *Prev. Med.* **2002,** *34(2),* 221–225.

Takwale, A.; E. Tan; S. Agarwal; G. Barclay; I. Ahmed; K. Hotchkiss; J.R. Thompson; T. Chapman; J. Berth-Jones. Efficacy and tolerability of borage oil in adults and children with atopic eczema: randomised, double blind, placebo controlled, parallel group trial. *Bmj* **2003,** *327(7428),* 1385.

Tarkowski, E.; N. Andreasen; A. Tarkowski; K. Blennow. Intrathecal inflammation precedes development of Alzheimer's disease. *J. Neurol. Neurosurg. Psychiatry* **2003a,** *74(9),* 1200–1205.

Tarkowski, E.; A.M. Liljeroth; L. Minthon; A. Tarkowski; A. Wallin; K. Blennow. Cerebral pattern of pro- and anti-inflammatory cytokines in dementias. *Brain Res. Bull.* **2003b,** *61(3),* 255–260.

Terawaki, K.; T. Yokomizo; T. Nagase; A. Toda; M. Taniguchi; K. Hashizume; T. Yagi; T. Shimizu. Absence of leukotriene B4 receptor 1 confers resistance to airway hyperresponsiveness and Th2-type immune responses. *J. Immunol.* **2005,** *175(7),* 4217–4225.

Thien, F.C.K.; R. Woods; S. De Luca; M.J. Abramson. Dietary marine fatty acids (fish oil) for asthma in adults and children. *Cochrane Database Syst. Rev.* **2004,** *2,* CD001283.

Thienprasert, A.; K. Pattanapanyasat; K. Sukapirom. Dose Effect of Docosahexaenoic Acid on Severity of Illness in Thai Schoolchildren: A Randomized Double Blind Placebo Controlled Intervention Trial; The 7th Congress of the International Society for the Study of Fatty Acids & Lipids: Cairns, Australia, 2006.

Thienprasert, A.; S. Samuhaseneetoo; K. Popplestone; A. West; E.A. Miles; P.C. Calder. Omega-3 Fatty Acids Supplementation Reduces Episodes and Severity of Illnesses in Schoolchildren: A Double Blind Randomized Placebo Controlled Trial; The 5th Euro Fed Lipid Congress: Gothenburg, Sweden, 2007.

Thies, F.; E.A. Miles; G. Nebe-von-Caron; J.R. Powell; T.L. Hurst; E.A. Newsholme; P.C. Calder. Influence of dietary supplementation with long-chain n-3 or n-6 polyunsaturated fatty acids on blood inflammatory cell populations and functions and on plasma soluble adhesion molecules in healthy adults. *Lipids* **2001a,** *36(11),* 1183–1193.

Thies, F.; G Nebe-von-Caron; J.R. Powell; P. Yaqoob; E.A. Newsholme; P.; C. Calder. Dietary supplementation with eicosapentaenoic acid, but not with other long-chain n-3 or n-6 polyunsaturated fatty acids, decreases natural killer cell activity in healthy subjects aged >55 y. *Am. J. Clin. Nutr.* **2001b,** *73(3),* 539–548.

Thies, F.; G. Nebe-von-Caron; J.R. Powell; P. Yaqoob; E.A. Newsholme; P.C. Calder. Dietary supplementation with gamma-linolenic acid or fish oil decreases T lymphocyte proliferation in healthy older humans. *J. Nutr.* **2001c,** *131(7),* 1918–1927.

Tilley, S.L.; T.M. Coffman; B.H. Koller. Mixed messages: modulation of inflammation and immune responses by prostaglandins and thromboxanes. *J. Clin. Invest.* **2001,** *108(1),* 15–23.

Tobinick, E.L.; H. Gross. Rapid cognitive improvement in Alzheimer's disease following perispinal etanercept administration. *J. Neuroinflammation.* **2008,** *5,* 2.

Trebble, T.M.; N.K. Arden; S.A. Wootton; P.C. Calder; M.A. Mullee; D.R. Fine; M.A. Stroud. Fish oil and antioxidants alter the composition and function of circulating mononuclear cells in Crohn's disease. *Am. J. Clin. Nutr.* **2004,** *80(5),* 1137–1144.

Turner, D.; A.H. Steinhart; A.M. Griffiths. Omega 3 fatty acids (fish oil) for maintenance of remission in ulcerative colitis. *Cochrane Database Syst. Rev.* **2007a,** *3,* CD006443.

Turner, D.; S.H. Zlotkin; P.S. Shah; A.M. Griffiths. Omega 3 fatty acids (fish oil) for maintenance of remission in Crohn's disease. *Cochrane Database Syst. Rev.* **2007b,** *2,* CD006320.

Vachier, I.; P. Chanez; C. Bonnans; P. Godard; J. Bousquet; C. Chavis. Endogenous anti-inflammatory mediators from arachidonate in human neutrophils. *Biochem. Biophys. Res. Commun.* **2002,** *290(1),* 219–224.

Vaisman, N.; Y. Zaruk; I. Shirazi; N. Kaysar; V. Barak. The effect of fish oil supplementation on cytokine production in children. *Eur. Cytokine Netw.* **2005,** *16(3),* 194–198.

van Gool, C.J.; C. Thijs; C.J. Henquet; A.C. van Houwelingen; P.C. Dagnelie; J. Schrander; P.P. Menheere; P.A. van den brandt. Gamma-linolenic acid supplementation for prophylaxis of atopic dermatitis—a randomized controlled trial in infants at high familial risk. *Am. J. Clin. Nutr.* **2003,** *77(4),* 943–951.

van Gool, C.J.; M.P. Zeegers; C. Thijs. Oral essential fatty acid supplementation in atopic dermatitis—a meta-analysis of placebo-controlled trials. *Br. J. Dermatol.* **2004,** *150(4),* 728–740.

Walda, I.C.; C. Tabak; H.A. Smit; L. Rasanen; F. Fidanza; A. Menotti; A. Nissinen; E.J. Feskens; D. Kromhout. Diet and 20-year chronic obstructive pulmonary disease mortality in middle-aged men from three European countries. *Eur. J. Clin. Nutr.* **2002,** *56(7),* 638–643.

Willers, S.M.; G. Devereux; L.C. Craig; G. McNeill; A.H. Wijga; W. Abou El-Magd; S.W. Turner; P.J. Helms; A. Seaton. Maternal food consumption during pregnancy and asthma, respiratory and atopic symptoms in 5-year-old children. *Thorax* **2007,** *62(9),* 773–779.

Wright, S.; J.L. Burton. Oral evening-primrose-seed oil improves atopic eczema. *Lancet* **1982,** *320(8308),* 1120–1122.

Yaqoob, P. Fatty acids and the immune system: from basic science to clinical applications. *Proc. Nutr. Soc.* **2004,** *63(1),* 89–104.

Yaqoob, P.; H.S. Pala; M. Cortina-Borja; E.A. Newsholme; P.C. Calder. Encapsulated fish oil enriched in alpha-tocopherol alters plasma phospholipid and mononuclear cell fatty acid compositions but not mononuclear cell functions. *Eur. J. Clin. Invest.* **2000,** *30(3),* 260–274.

Yuhas, R.; K. Pramuk; E.L. Lien. Human milk fatty acid composition from nine countries varies most in DHA. *Lipids* **2006,** *41(9),* 851–858.

# 23

# Modulation of Cytokine Action by Fatty Acids: Role in Health

**Renata Gorjão[1], Thaís Martins de Lima[2], Maria Fernanda[3], Cury Boaventura[3], and Rui Curi[4]**

[1]*Department of Physiology and Biophysics, Institute of Biomedical Sciences, University of São Paulo, Lineu Prestes, 1524, 05508-900, Butantã, São Paulo, Brazil;* [2]*Department of Physiology and Biophysics, Institute of Biomedical Sciences, University of São Paulo, Lineu Prestes, 1524, 05508-900, Butantã, São Paulo, Brazil;* [3]*Program of Post-Graduation Studies in Physical Education, Center of Biological Sciences and Health, Cruzeiro do Sul University, São, Paulo, Brazil;* [4]*Dr. Rui Curi, Department of Physiology and Biophysics, Institute of Biomedical, Sciences, University of São Paulo, Brazil*

## Introduction

Cytokines are a group of pharmacologically active and low molecular weight polypeptides that are humoral mediators in a highly complex and coordinated network regulating inflammatory and immune responses with the participation of different cytokine-associated signaling pathways (Navarro-Gonzáles & Mora-Fernández, 2008). These molecules cluster into several classes (i.e., interleukins, tumor necrosis factors, interferons, colony-stimulating factors, transforming growth factors, and chemokines). Cytokines are produced by a wide variety of cells in addition to leukocytes, playing an important role in many physiological responses (Balkwill & Burke, 1989). Any alteration in cytokine production or in the signaling pathways activated by them can serve as a tool for intervention in several diseases.

Interleukin (IL)-1β, tumor necrosis factor (TNF)-α, and IL-6 are often designated as pro-inflammatory cytokines. They are mainly produced by mononuclear phagocytic cells, including circulating monocytes and tissue macrophages (Fig. 23.1). These cytokines mediate the response of the host to inflammatory stimuli. They induce fever, activation of B and T lymphocytes and endothelial cells, synthesis of acute phase proteins by the liver, and many other effects that are all part of the acute-phase response (Dinarello, 1991). The term "acute phase response" refers to a set of local and systemic neurologic, endocrine, and metabolic changes through which the organism reacts to various stimuli, including infections and forms of sterile inflammation such as autoimmune disease, bleeding, injury, and heavy exercise (Blok et al., 1996).

The cytokines involved in these processes lead leukocytes to secrete other inflammatory mediators, including other cytokines such as the T lymphocyte products (IFN)-γ and IL-2 and lipid mediators such as prostaglandins, leukotrienes,

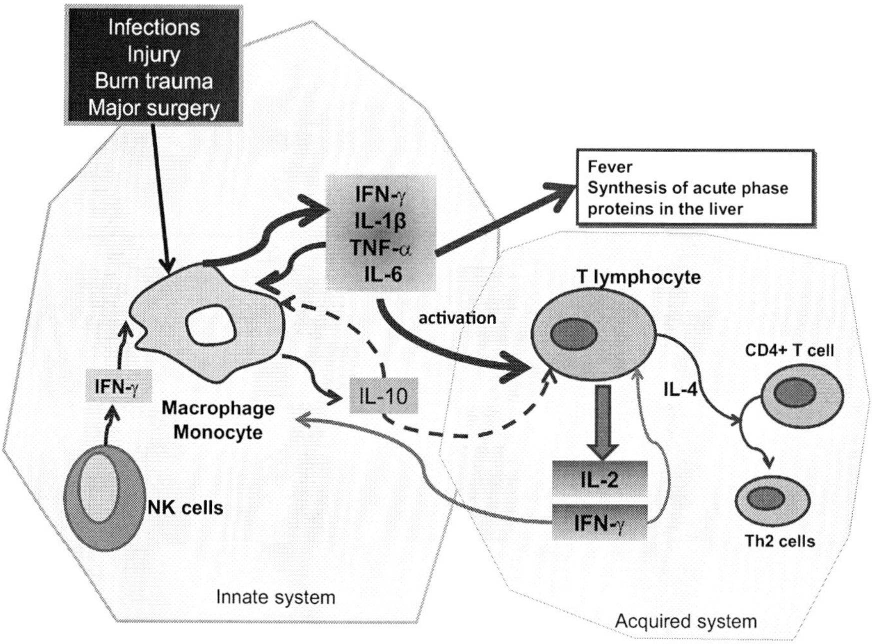


**Fig. 23.1.** Cytokine production by leukocytes. Interleukin-1β (IL-1β), tumor necrosis factor-α (TNF-α), and interleukin-6 (IL-6) are often designated as pro-inflammatory cytokines, and are mainly produced by circulating monocytes and tissue macrophages. They induce fever, activation of B and T lymphocytes and endothelial cells, synthesis of acute phase proteins by the liver, and many other effects that are all part of the acute-phase inflammatory response. T lymphocyte secretes mainly IL-2, IFN-γ, and IL-4 that activate other leukocytes. IL-10 is secreted by macrophages and is related to the inhibition of pro-inflammatory cytokine production and leukocyte activation. Filled arrows indicate protein activation, and hatched arrows indicate the inhibition of protein phosphorylation.

and platelet-activating factor. Elevated plasma concentrations of IL-6, TNF-α, or IL-1β are observed in patients with infections, endotoxemia, trauma, or burns, but also in acute bouts of autoimmune diseases such as rheumatoid arthritis and systemic lupus erythematosus, and in patients undergoing organ transplant rejection (Dinarello, 1992). IL-4 is also produced by T lymphocytes, and it stimulates B lymphocytes and T lymphocyte proliferation, and $CD4^+$ T cell differentiation into Th2 cells.

IL-10 is produced primarily by monocytes and to a lesser extent by lymphocytes. This cytokine has pleiotropic effects in immunoregulation and inflammation. IL-10 down-regulates the expression of Th1 cytokines, MHC class II antigens presentation, and costimulatory molecules in macrophages. It also enhances B cell survival, proliferation, and antibody production. This cytokine can block nuclear factor κB (NF-κB) activity, inhibiting synthesis of pro-inflammatory cytokines.

Modulation of cytokine production by fatty acids (FAs) is associated with alteration in leukocyte functions such as lymphocyte proliferation, neutrophil chemiotaxis, and macrophage recruitment. Omega-3 (ω-3) FAs are often associated with a decrease in pro-inflammatory cytokine production, whereas omega-6 (ω-6) FAs are related to pro-inflammatory cytokine stimulation. However, these effects depend on the concentration of the FA. In this chapter, the effect of FAs on cytokine production and on intracellular signaling pathways activated by cytokines is discussed.

# Effect of FAs on Cytokine Production

## *In vitro Studies*

### *Eicosapentaenoic Acid (EPA) and Docosahexaenoic Acid (DHA)*

#### Macrophages

EPA competes with arachidonic acid (AA) as a substrate of cyclooxygenase and lipoxygenase for the production of eicosanoids (Calder, 2003). However, several studies suggest that the effects of ω-3 polyunsaturated fatty acids (PUFAs) on pro-inflammatory cytokine production might occur downstream of altered eicosanoid synthesis or may occur independent of this activity.

Weldon et al. (2007) investigated the differential effects of pure EPA and DHA on cytokine expression and NF-κB activation in human THP-1 monocyte-derived macrophages. NF-κB plays a key role in regulating cytokine gene transcription, and it is located in the cytoplasm associated with the inhibitory protein IκB. Extracellular signals can activate IκB kinase (IKK). This enzyme phosphorylates the IκBα protein, which results in the dissociation of IκBα from NF-κB, and eventual degradation of IκBα by the proteosome. The activated NF-κB is then translocated into the nucleus where it binds to specific sequences of DNA called response elements (RE) and activates cytokine transcription. Pre-treatment with 100 μM EPA and DHA significantly decreased the LPS-stimulated THP-1 macrophage production of TNF-α, IL-1β, and IL-6, compared to control cells. Both FAs reduced TNF-α, IL-1β, and IL-6 mRNA expression. However, in all cases, the effect of DHA was significantly more potent than that of EPA. Furthermore, a low dose (25 μM) of DHA had a greater inhibitory effect than that of EPA on IL-1β and IL-6 production by macrophage following LPS stimulation. Both EPA and DHA down-regulated LPS-induced NF-κB/DNA binding in THP-1 macrophages. On the other hand, only DHA significantly decreased macrophage nuclear p65 expression and increased cytoplasmic IκB expression. These findings suggest that DHA may be more effective than EPA in alleviating LPS-induced pro-inflammatory cytokine production by macrophages, an effect that may be mediated by NF-κB.

A recent study by Skuladottir et al. (2007) showed that ω-3 PUFAs increased TNF-α secretion by resident peritoneal macrophages probably by a direct effect on the cells. The ω-3 PUFAs, however, did not affect IL-10 secretion by the cells but decreased the number of cells secreting IL-10, possibly by affecting cell recruitment, maturation, or proliferation. These results are indicative that FA can exert distinct effects on different cell lines.

### Lymphocytes

Verlengia et al. (2004a) reported that EPA and DHA promoted an inhibitory effect on IL-2, IL-10, and IFN-γ production by Jurkat cells (a leukemic lineage of human T lymphocytes). In a lineage of human B lymphocytes (Raji cells), EPA and DHA decreased IL-10, TNF-α, and IFN-γ production (Verlengia et al. 2004b). In these studies, the suppressive effect of EPA on cytokine production was always more pronounced as compared to DHA.

### Endothelial Cells

The interaction between lymphocytes, cytokines, and endothelial cells (EC) is a key step in the inflammation that leads to atherosclerosis. Khalfoun et al. (1997) examined the effects of PUFA on IL-6 production by human unstimulated EC or stimulated with TNF-α, IL-4, LPS, or allogeneic peripheral blood lymphocytes. The production of IL-6 by stimulated EC cells was potentiated by PUFA after 24 hours in culture in comparison to unstimulated EC. The addition of ω-3 PUFA into culture medium (100 μg/mL DHA or EPA) significantly reduced IL-6 production by either unstimulated or stimulated EC, whereas the ω-6 PUFA (AA), even at the high concentration, was ineffective. This inhibitory effect of PUFA was more pronounced by EPA than DHA and was dose-dependent.

### *Conjugated Linoleic Acid (CLA)*

CLA also modulates cytokine production by macrophages. RAW macrophages incubated with 50 and 100 μM *c*9,*t*11-CLA for 24 hours prior to LPS stimulation presented lower TNF-α production (reduction by 40% and 60%, respectively) (Yang & Cook, 2003).

In dendritic cells (DC), however, *c*9,*t*11-CLA presented different effects. Treatment of DC with 50 μM *c*9,*t*11-CLA for 48 hours suppressed LPS-induced IL-12 production, but enhanced IL-10R expression and IL-10 production at the transcriptional and protein levels. The *c*9,*t*11-CLA decreased NF-κB:DNA binding after LPS stimulation, which was concomitant with delayed translocation of the NF-κB p65 subunit into the nucleus and an increased content of IκB (Loscher et al., 2005).

In Jurkat cells, treatment with 50 μM of CLA for 48 hours caused a significant inhibitory effect on Jurkat proliferation but increased the expression of IL-2 and IFN-γ (Luongo et al., 2003).

### *α-Linolenic Acid, Linoleic and Oleic Acids*

α-Linolenic acid (ALA) and, to a certain extent, linoleic acid (LA), γ-linolenic acid (GLA), and di-γ-linolenic acid (DGLA) can suppress TNF-α and IL-2 production by stimulated human lymphocytes after a 24-hour treatment at 10–20 μg/mL. On the other hand, DGLA and AA enhanced, whereas EPA inhibited IL-4 synthesis by these cells. DGLA, AA, and EPA did not alter the secretion of IL-6 by stimulated human lymphocytes (Das, 1994).

Pereira et al. (2008) studied the release of TNF-α, IL-1β, CINC 2α/β, and VEGF-α by neutrophils treated with oleic acid (OA) and LA. Neutrophils were treated with OA or LA (5, 25, 50, 100, and 200 μM) for 4 and 18 hours. A dose-dependent increase of VEGF-α and IL-1β production by neutrophils treated with OA and LA was observed. OA was also able to stimulate the production of CINC-2α/β by incubated neutrophils. These FAs did not modify TNF-α production by neutrophils in the conditions used.

## *In vivo* Studies

### *Animal Studies*

Olive oil, an abundant fundamental constituent of the Mediterranean diet, is also able to modulate immune function. This oil contains various components that possess biological activities, including OA. Classically, monounsaturated FAs (MUFAs) are considered as neutral FAs and are often applied as a placebo in studies investigating the anti-inflammatory properties of other FAs. However, several studies show that MUFAs, such as OA, modulate lymphocyte function (Gorjão et al., 2007; Verlengia et al., 2003).

For 8 or 12 weeks, the administration of diets containing olive oil produced an increase of IL-2 production by lymphocytes in mice (Yaqoob & Calder, 1995). For 4 weeks, IL-4 production was increased in mice after the administration of a diet containing olive oil (Puertollano et al., 2004). In contrast, the production of IL-10, a cytokine with an anti-inflammatory function, was decreased after the administration of a diet containing olive oil (Yaqoob et al., 1994).

In mice fed a diet containing olive oil, the production of pro-inflammatory cytokines such as IL-1, IL-6, and TNF-α was modified by a *Listeria. monocytogenes* infection, especially at 24 hours after the challenge (Puertollano et al., 2007). Diets containing high amounts of olive oil may be related to the suppression of pro-inflammatory cytokine production, but this effect was not as severe as that produced by the administration of a fish oil-rich diet (i.e., a ω-3 FA-rich oil).

Tappia and Grimble (1996) observed that after 4 weeks macrophages from fish oil- and olive oil-fed animals showed an enhanced production of IL-6 when compared to animals fed corn oil. However, IL-1β production, after 8 weeks of dietary treatment, was greatest by macrophages from animals fed corn and olive oils. Peritoneal macrophages from rats fed a diet rich in fish oil presented lower TNF-α production (Somers & Erickson, 1994; Wallace et al., 2000) that seems to be associated with a decrease in NF-κB activation (Novak et al., 2003).

Peritoneal resident macrophages from mice fed a CLA- or a corn oil-supplemented diet for 6 weeks were obtained for measuring TNF-α and nitric oxide production after an in vitro exposure to IFN- γ and/or LPS. TNF-α production did not change. However, in the same study, the production of IL-2 was elevated and that of IL-4 was decreased in CLA-fed mice when splenocytes were stimulated with ConA for 44 hours (Yang & Cook., 2003).

Mice were fed for 6 weeks on a low-fat diet or on high-fat diets containing coconut (rich in the medium-chain saturated FAs capric, lauric, and myristic acids), safflower (rich in linoleic acid), or fish (rich in EPA and DHA) oils as the main fat sources. IL-2 production was higher by ConA-stimulated spleen lymphocytes after feeding the coconut fat-rich diet. IFN-γ production was decreased by safflower-oil or fish-oil feeding. IL-4 production was not significantly affected by the diets, although production was low by lymphocytes from fish oil-fed mice (Wallace et al., 2001).

Regarding the suppressive effect of ω-3 FA on T lymphocyte proliferation, Jolly et al. (1998) observed that EPA and DHA suppressed IL-2 receptor α (IL-2Rα) subunit mRNA levels, but they did not affect IL-2 mRNA expression in splenic lymphocytes from mice supplemented with these FAs. These results are indicative that the suppressed IL-2 secretion and impaired proliferative response observed in other studies (Aggarwal et al., 1994) were not due to a reduction in IL-2 mRNA levels. However, IL-2Rα gene transcription may play a role in blunting the T-lymphocyte proliferative response.

Fritsche et al. (2000) showed that ω-3 FAs from different sources have the same effect. They tested the effect of supplementation with different ω-3 FAs on murine cytokine production in vivo. Weanling female C3H mice were fed for 4 weeks with diets containing 20% by weight of different sources of ω-3 (one with purified EPA esters only, another with purified DHA esters only, one with equal amounts of purified DHA and EPA esters, and one with menhaden fish oil). The control diet contained purified olive oil ethyl esters. Mice were then challenged with live *L. monocytogenes* or sterile PBS, and in 24 hours after infection all ω-3 PUFA-fed mice had significantly lower circulating levels of IL-12 and IFN-γ than mice fed the control diet ($P < 0.01$). In addition, splenic cytokine mRNA levels for IL-12, TNF-α, and IL-1β were lower in infected mice fed ω-3 PUFA-containing diets than in mice fed the olive oil ethyl esters control diet (Fritsche et al., 2000).

### *Human Studies*

Most studies on FA supplementation in humans were performed with ω-3 FA. The dosage of ω-3 FAs used in different studies may be responsible for the conflicting results.

Low doses of fish oil supplementation (<2 g/day) did not affect the production of IL-6, TNF-α, IL-1β, and IL-10 by mononuclear cells (Trebble et al., 2003; Wallace et al., 2003). However, Trebble et al. (2003) found a dose- responsive increase of IFN-γ production by peripheral blood mononuclear cells from the baseline that reached significance ($P < 0.05$) at 2 g of EPA plus DHA per day. Gorjão et al. (2006), in a study performed with DHA-rich fish oil supplementation (that provided 1.62 and 0.78 g/day of DHA and EPA, respectively), also reported an increase of IFN-γ production by lymphocytes (a cytokine produced by the Th1-type cells). In both studies, lower doses of EPA and DHA were used as compared to those that showed inhibitory effects of fish oil on cytokine production by the Th1-type cells. Therefore, supplementary DHA intakes of ≤2 g/day may result in increased cytokine production by the Th1-type cells;

however, an inhibitory effect may occur from EPA and DHA at a higher daily intake or after a prolonged period of treatment even at low doses. This issue remains to be examined.

A high intake of EPA plus DHA decreased production of IFN-γ and IL-2 by lymphocytes. Gallai et al. (1995) also reported a decrease in PHA-induced IL-2 production as well as ConA-induced IFN-γ production by lymphocytes following supplementation with 5.2 g of EPA plus DHA per day.

Production of pro-inflammatory cytokines by macrophages and monocytes, such as TNF-α, IL-1β, and IL-6, was investigated. Blok et al. (1997) supplemented volunteers for one year with 0, 3, 6, or 9 g/day of fish oil providing 0, 1.1, 2.13, or 3.2 g of ω-3 FA per day, and evaluated circulating cytokine levels and the ex vivo LPS-stimulated production of cytokines by monocytes. In this study, endotoxin-stimulated whole-blood cytokine production was measured at 26 and 52 weeks immediately after the beginning and at 4, 8, and 26 weeks after a cessation of supplementation. In all groups, no change of IL-1β, IL-6, and TNF-α circulating levels was detected after a one-year supplementation at any given dose. No differences were observed in an ex vivo LPS-stimulated secretion of the cytokines between the placebo and supplemented groups, although IL-1β production was higher during supplementation and decreased afterwards.

The studies described above are indicative that cytokine production by lymphocyte is more affected by ω-3 FAs than monocytes.

**Factors that Influence Cytokine Production in Human Studies**

Some of the contradictory effects of fish oil supplementation on cytokine production may be due to genetic polymorphisms. Grimble et al. (2002) suggested that the sensitivity to the suppressive effects of ω-3 PUFA on TNF-α production by monocytes is linked to the inherent level of the production of the cytokine before supplementation and to the genetic variation associated with TNF-α 308 and lymphotoxin 252 SNPs. Paradoxically, fish oil appears to enhance TNF-α production in some subjects. These results, together with other studies about the effects of fish oil supplements on TNF-α production, indicate that the association of ω-3 PUFA intake and cytokine biology is complex. The different sensitivities of patients to the effect of fish oil—because of the genetic variation and other individual factors that influence the inherent level of cytokine production by the cells of the subject—may limit the effectiveness of moderate doses of fish oil as an anti-inflammatory agent. An analysis of genotype is required to establish the relationship between the effect of gene polymorphisms on TNF-α production, and a person's sensitivity to fish oil is to be fully understood. A better understanding of the precise nature of the genomic determinants of the ability of fish oil to act as an anti-inflammatory agent will enable supplementation to be used more effectively in suppressing inflammation.

Some of the inconsistent results from the studies performed with fish oil on cytokine production also may be due to a healthy versus an infected state, as the immune function of subjects is different in these two states, or if the level of vitamin E ingested is not the same. Vitamin E is an antioxidant agent that prevents lipid peroxidation. Several studies show information on the doses of vitamin E supplements. This is important information since some authors attribute several effects of ω-3 FA to the content of vitamin E. Therefore, the amount of vitamin E used in the studies cannot be elevated much. Trebble et al. (2003) showed that antioxidant co-supplementation (30 mg/day of vitamin E) increases the incorporation of ω-3 PUFA into phospholipid at supplemental intakes of <2.0 g/day, and augments the inhibitory effect of supplementary ω-3 PUFA intakes <1.0 g/day on PBMC function.

***Parenteral Lipid Emulsions and Cytokines***

Intravenous fat emulsions are an integral part of parenteral nutrition. The incorporation of lipids into nutritional therapy seems to optimize the provision of energy requirements and essential FAs, and may prevent many metabolic disturbances associated with the intravenous feeding of amino acids and glucose alone (Carpentier & Hacquebard, 2006; Wanten & Calder, 2007).

Intravenous lipid emulsions are made of a triglyceride-rich core surrounded by a monolayer of phospholipids with some free cholesterol. The first well-tolerated lipid emulsion was based on soybean oil or safflower oil, which is composed by triacylglycerol rich in ω-6 PUFA, mainly LA. More recently, lipid emulsions with different FA compositions that decrease the proportion of ω-6 PUFA and/or increase the medium-chain triacylglycerols (MCT), ω-3 PUFA, and/or monounsaturated fatty acids (MUFA) were introduced into the market. Actually, commercially available fat emulsions are also derived from: coconut oil/soybean oil (50:50), containing a large portion of MCT; olive oil/soybean oil (80:20), containing a large portion of ω-9 FA; fish oils, containing a large portion of ω-3 PUFA; and a fat emulsion, containing a mixture of these four lipid sources: soybean oil, MCT, olive oil, and fish oil (30:30:25:15) (Carpentier & Hacquebard, 2006; Wanten & Calder, 2007).

Parenteral fat emulsions have a significant impact on immune function (Carpentier & Hacquebard, 2006; Wanten & Calder, 2007). The increase of susceptibility to infection in patients on parenteral nutrition is associated with the immunosuppressor effects of fat emulsions (Battistella et al., 1997; Fischer et al., 1980; Freeman et al, 1990; Muller et al., 1986; Sosenko et al., 1993). Intravenous fat emulsions showed a varying immunomodulatory effect, depending on the FA composition.

One factor associated with the adverse effect of lipid emulsion on immunomodulation is the excess of PUFA that leads to the alteration of FA metabolism, causing lipid peroxidation and an imbalance of eicosanoid and cytokine production. The ω-6 and ω-3 PUFAs participate directly in the inflammatory and immune responses, serving as substrates for eicosanoid synthesis, consequently modulating cytokine production. High conversion of ω-6 PUFAs (mainly LA and AA) may lead to the overproduction of pro-inflammatory eicosanoids (2-series prostaglandins and 4-series leukotrienes) and cytokines. The ω-3 PUFAs generally lead to a decrease in the production of AA-derived mediators (Calder, 2003; Carpentier & Hacquebard, 2006; Wanten & Calder, 2007).

Studies with soybean oil-based emulsion (SOE) showed decreased IL-2 production and IL-2 receptor expression in lymphocytes (Granato et al., 2000; Moussa et al., 2000). In addition, lymphocyte proliferative responses to IL-2 in vitro are inhibited in the presence of SOE and MCT/SOE (Sedman et al., 1990,; 1991). On the other hand, some studies indicated neither an effect (Jarstrand et al., 1978; Nordenstrom et al., 1979) nor an increase (Helms et al., 1983; Ota et al., 1978) of lymphocyte proliferation by SOE. Olive oil-based emulsion (OOE) had little or no effect on IL-2 production by lymphocytes, and prevented the inhibition of the IL-2 receptor expression (Granato et al., 2000; Moussa et al., 2000), suggesting that OOE offers a neutral alternative to SOE with respect to their effects on the immune system. Recent study also observed no effect of an olive oil-based emulsion on various clinical or inflammatory markers over a 3-month period of determination in plasma (Reimund et al., 2005).

A recent work also observed that OOE has no effect on basal and LPS-induced expression of TNF-α, IL-1β, and IL-8 in the neutrophils. In contrast, SOE and SO/MCT decreased both IL-1β mRNA levels and protein expression evoked by LPS in peripheral blood mononuclear cells (Buenestado et al., 2006). Another study demonstrated that OOE was less effective than SOE and SOE/MCT in reducing basal TNF-α and IL-1β production by PBMC, whereas IL-6 and IL-8 were not affected. After monocyte activation by LPS/PHA, only the IL-1β expression was decreased by SOE (Reimund et al., 2004).

Wanten et al. (2002) observed that after ex vivo stimulation with *Candida albicans,* SOE/MCT, but not SOE, decreased IFN-γ and increased IL-10, IL-1β, and TNF-α production, suggesting an increased susceptibility to fungal infections. The same authors also observed no effect of lipids on TNF-α, IL-16, and IL-18 production by mononuclear cells in the absence of a stimulus and after stimulation with LPS and PHA (Wanten et al., 2002).

A previous study, however, reported that SOE amplified the plasma level of IL-6 in severely stressed patients but had no effect on moderately stressed patients (Furukawa et al., 2002). Krogh-Madsen et al. (2008) observed a pronounced systemic inflammatory response with an increase of TNF-α and IL-6 plasma levels during SOE after endotoxemia stimulation in humans. In contrast, Li et al. suggested that SOE infusion does not alter cytokine plasma concentration in adult and pediatric patients undergoing moderate gastrointestinal surgery (Li et al., 2007, 2008).

When compared with SOE, fish oil emulsion (FOE) suppressed the production of pro-inflammatory cytokine production after 2–4 days in septic patients. However, after 14 days, the effects of these two emulsions were not different. Both lipids also suppressed IL-10 production by macrophages (Mayer et al., 2003). The timing of nutritional interventions appears to be critical. A recent work demonstrates that fish oil emulsion markedly suppressed the monocyte release of TNF-α, IL-1, IL-6, and IL-8 in healthy volunteers and patients with sepsis (Mayer et al., 2003). McCann et al. (2000) also showed a decrease of TNF-α production by monocytes after FOE infusion and an increase with SOE infusion. Weiss et al. (2002) showed that FOE reduced TNF-α and IL-6 release by monocytes and preserved the expression of leukocyte antigen HLA-DR (Weiss et al., 2002). Another study demonstrated that FOE prevented the suppression of IL-2 and decreased IL-10 production and TGF-β release by splenocytes, a pro-inflammatory mediator that led to immunosuppression during sepsis (Lanza-Jacoby et al., 2001).

In patients with large-bowel surgery, the FO/SO-based emulsion (5:1) prevented the drop in IFN-γ release by lymphocytes observed in patients receiving soybean oil-based emulsion and increased plasma IL-2, TNF-α, and IL-2R levels compared to parenteral nutrition without fat (Schauder et al., 2002). Lin et al. (2006) demonstrated that FO/SO-based emulsion (1:1) administration promoted Th1 lymphocyte cytokine production as compared with soybean oil- based emulsion in rats with total gastrectomy (Lin et al., 2006).

Major progress was made in understanding the role of lipid emulsions on immune function and cytokine release. Studies on lipid emulsion are required to indentify adverse effects and to generate knowledge to develop adequate preparations for the targeted delivery of specific constituents to immune cells. In the near future, lipid emulsions will be prepared with an ideal combination of FAs for each patient's disease.

## Intracellular Signaling

### *Modulation of IL-2 Action by FAs*

IL-2 plays an essential role in lymphocyte proliferation (Wang et al., 2004). We recently showed that DHA, EPA, palmitic acid, and stearic acid decreased the stimulatory effect of IL-2 on human lymphocyte proliferation, increasing the percentage of cells in the G1 phase and decreasing the proportion of cells in the S and G2/M phases (Gorjão et al., 2007). DHA, EPA, palmitic acid, and stearic acid inhibited the signaling pathway activated by this cytokine after a short period of treatment (1 hour). The IL-2R consists of three subunits: α, β, and γ chains. The IL-2-induced heterodimerization of β and γ chains results in intermolecular transphosphorylation of their corresponding receptor-associated Janus kinase 1 (JAK1) and JAK3 (Kirken et al., 1995; Russell et al., 1994). Members of the STAT (signal transducer and activator of transcription) family of transcription factors, downstream effectors of the JAK, are also regulated by IL-2. The IL-2-induced tyrosine phosphorylation of STAT5 allows src homology 2 domain-mediated homodimerization or heterodimerization, with a resulting induction of nuclear migration and a sequence-specific DNA binding by the STATs (Darnell et al., 1994). PA, SA, DHA, and EPA decreased JAK1, JAK3, STAT5, ERK ½, and Akt phosphorylation induced by IL-2.

OA and LA increased lymphocyte proliferation, and this effect was related to a decrease in PKC-ζ phosphorylation. In conclusion, the inhibitory effect of PA, SA, DHA, and EPA on lymphocyte proliferation was attributed to a decrease in JAK/STAT, ERK, and Akt pathways activated by IL-2. Probably, OA and LA stimulated lymphocyte proliferation by increasing ERK1/2 phosphorylation through PKC-ζ activation. The inhibition of JAK1, JAK3, STAT5, ERK1/2, and Akt phosphorylation caused by DHA, SA, and PA is associated with an alteration of the CD25 expression at the cell surface. Therefore, these FAs inhibit lymphocyte proliferation by altering the protein phosphorylation state (Fig. 23.2).

### *Modulation of TNF-α Action by FAs*

Xue et al. (2006) investigated the effects of EPA and DHA on mitogen-activated protein kinases (MAPK) in the endothelium. They measured kinase activities in TNF-α-activated endothelial cells from human umbilical vein (HUVEC). EPA or DHA alone significantly reduced the TNF-α-induced activation of p38 and JNK kinases at a concentration of 20 μM, but EPA was a more potent inhibitor than DHA. In contrast,

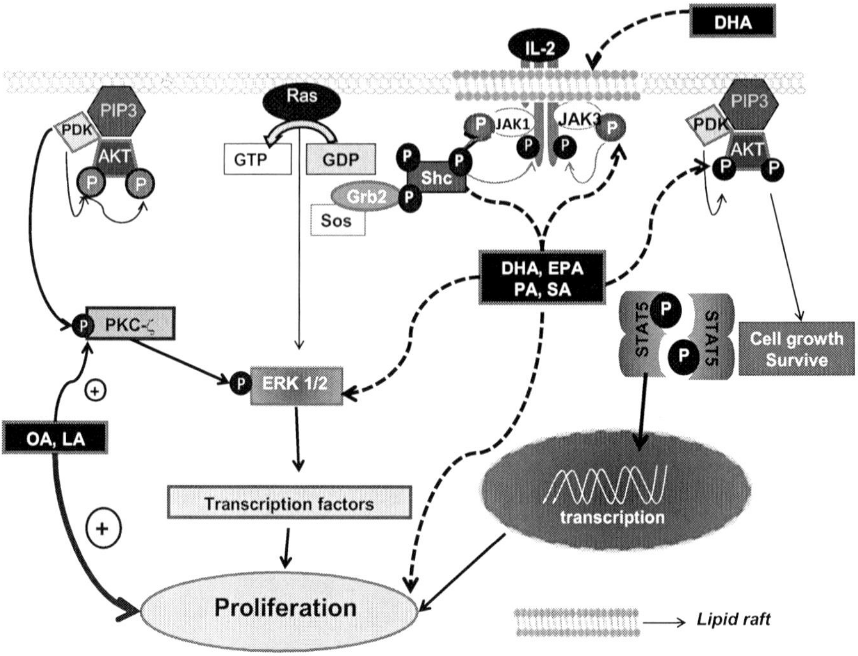


**Fig. 23.2**. Regulation of IL-2 signaling by fatty acids in human lymphocytes. The IL-2-induced heterodimerization of β and γ chains results in the activation of JAK1 and 3 that phosphorylate tyrosine residues in IL-2R, creating docking sites to STAT5 and Shc ligation. STAT5 is phosphorylated and acts as a transcription factor regulating the expression of several genes associated with proliferation. Shc leads to ERK1/2 and Akt activation that also induces cell proliferation. Palmitic (PA), stearic (SA), docosahexaenoic (DHA), and eicosapentaenoic (EPA) acids inhibited lymphocyte proliferation and decreased JAK1 and 3, STAT5, ERK ½, and Akt phosphorylation induced by IL-2. Oleic (OA) and linoleic (LA) acids stimulated lymphocyte proliferation through PKC-ζ activation that phosphorylates ERK1/2. Filled arrows indicate protein activation and hatched arrow indicates inhibition of protein phosphorylation.

both EPA and DHA significantly counteracted the TNF-α-mediated deactivation of ERK1/2 kinases. Meanwhile, both EPA and DHA significantly attenuated the TNF-α-induced expression of p38 and ERK1/2 mRNA. DHA, but not EPA, also reduced the TNF-α-induced JNK mRNA expression.

Chen et al. (2005) observed that DHA plays a central role in antagonizing cytokine-induced adhesion molecule expression by attenuating NF-κB signaling in the early steps of inflammation in human vascular endothelial cells. These cells contain the cognate receptors for TNF-α and IL-1β, and the activation of these receptors leads to the increased activity of NF-κB. Up-regulation of inflammatory cytokines, especially TNF-α (Limb et al., 1996, 1997, 1999), IL-1β (Kowluru & Odenbach, 2004), and VEGF (Aiello et al., 1995) along with their corresponding receptors, were well-documented in the eyes of diabetic patients and in diabetic animal models. These cytokines induce the expression of adhesion molecules (cultured human retinal endothelial cells) which is then mediated by NF-κB. Therefore, DHA can inhibit adhesion molecule expression through a decrease in NF-κB activity, blocking the action of pro-inflammatory cytokines.

The modulatory potential of CLA on cytokine-induced eicosanoid production from smooth muscle cells (SMCs), which contributes to the chronic inflammatory response associated with atherosclerosis, was investigated (Ringseis et al., 2006). *Cis*-9, *trans*-11 CLA and *trans*-10, *cis*-12 CLA were shown to reduce proportions of the eicosanoid precursor AA in SMC total lipids and to inhibit TNF-α-induced expression of inducible enzymes involved in eicosanoid formation (cPLA2, COX-2, mPGES) and, thus, the production of the prostaglandins PGE2 and PGI2. These effects were not exclusively related to the decrease in the content of the PG precursor AA. CLA treatment of SMC for 24 hours diminished NF-κB DNA-binding activity induced by TNF-α.

FA also alters TNF-α signaling in fibroblast-like synovial cells (FLS). Electrophoretic mobility shift assays (EMSA) revealed that TNF-α activates NF-κB in FLS, but this was inhibited by ALA at a concentration of 1 mM. TNF-α-induced IKK mediated the phosphorylation of GST-IκB; the pre-treatment with α-LA inhibited this pathway (Lee et al., 2008).

### *Modulation of IL-1β Action by FAs*

Hirafuji et al. (2002) showed that DHA increases NO production by VSMCs by potentiating iNOS expression induced by IL-1β. DHA significantly potentiated the IL-1β-induced phosphorylation of p44/42 MAPK but had no significant effect on p38 MAPK phosphorylation.

### *Toll-like Receptors Activation by FAs*

The nuclear transcription factor NF-κB is one of the most important transcription factors involved in cytokine production by leukocytes. NF-κB pathway plays an important role in the TLR4-mediated immunomodulatory effect including cytokine synthesis. Toll-like receptors (TLRs) are transmembrane receptors that play a critical role in the detection of microbial infection and in the induction of inflammatory and immune responses against conserved microbial structures, called pathogen-associated molecular patterns (Aderem & Ulevitch, 2000). Eleven members of the TLR family were identified so far, and they are ubiquitously expressed in human tissues (Zarember & Godowski, 2002). Genetic and biochemical evidence demonstrated that TLR4 confers responsiveness to lipopolysaccharide (LPS) derived from gram-negative bacteria (Qureshi et al., 1999; Rhee & Hwang, 2000). The FAs present in LPS lipid A are the sites for the interaction with TLR4. So, FA may modulate cytokine production through activation or inhibition of Toll-like receptors signaling.

Lee et al. (2001) demonstrated that saturated FAs induce NF-κB activation, expression of COX-2, and other inflammatory markers, such as cytokines, in a murine monocytic cell line (RAW264.7) through TLR4 activation (Lee et al., 2001). NF-κB inhibitors significantly suppressed the palmitate-induced TNF-α mRNA expression and secretion in these cells (Suganami et al., 2007). In addition, the inhibition of LPS-induced NF-κB activation and COX-2 expression by unsaturated FAs was also mediated through TLR4-derived signaling pathways (Lee et al., 2001). DHA suppressed NF-κB activation and COX-2 expression induced by the activation of TLR4 in RAW264.7. LPS-induction of COX-2 expression was decreased in blood peripheral monocytes by the consumption of food containing fish oil (Lee et al., 2003). In fact, ω-3 PUFAs are much more potent inhibitors of TLR4 and TLR2 activation as compared with ω-6 PUFAs or saturated FAs. This may explain why ω-3 PUFAs are considered the most effective anti-inflammatory FAs (Hashimoto et al., 2003).

FA can also modulate cytokine production by microglia cells (resident macrophage of the central nervous system). DHA is a major component of brain plasma membrane phospholipids (Salem et al., 2001), representing up to 30% of phosphatidylethanolamine (PE) and phosphatidylserine fatty acyl chains in synaptosomes and synapse vesicle membranes (Breckenridge et al., 1972). De Smedt-Peyrusse et al. (2008) studied molecular targets of DHA in microglia cells. The authors observed that DHA, when added exogenously, is specifically enriched in membrane phospholipids but not in lipid rafts of microglial cells. DHA incorporation in a membrane-impaired the surface presentation of LPS receptors CD-14 and TLR-4 but not their membrane subdomain localization. The innate immune recognition of LPS is based on the binding of LPS to CD14 (Wright et al., 1990) that is a glycosylphosphatidylinositol-linked protein and transduces the signal by associating with other partners, especially TLR4 (Chow et al., 1999; Lien et al., 2000; Poltorak et al., 1998). The activation of TLR4 by LPS initiates downstream signaling cascades leading to up-regulation of NF-κB and MAPK, and to expression of pro-inflammatory cytokines (Chow et al., 1999). LPS-induced NF-κB activation was inhibited by DHA, consequently the LPS-induced synthesis of IL-1β and TNF-α was strongly attenuated. This anti-inflammatory action of DHA in microglia cells occurred by targeting the LPS receptor surface location, therefore reducing LPS action on microglia. Pro-inflammatory cytokine release in the brain is the result of innate immune response that is mainly mediated by microglia cells (Aloisi, 2001). Although transient activation of these cells is beneficial for defense processes against pathogens, either chronic activation or overactivation can lead to neurodegeneration, which causes (or even exacerbates) neurodegenerative diseases such as Alzheimer's (Lehnardt et al., 2003; McGeer & McGeer, 2002).

### *Cytokine Receptor Displacement From Lipid Rafts by FAs*

Lipid rafts are specialized plasma-membrane microdomains that contain high concentrations of cholesterol and sphingolipids, and their polar lipids predominantly contain saturated fatty acyl residues (Schroeder et al., 1994). Cytoplasmic and transmembrane proteins are targeted toward lipid rafts mostly by acylation with saturated fatty acyl moieties (palmitoyl and myristoyl) that link these proteins to the cytoplasmic lipid leaflet of the microdomains (Li et al., 2005). Therefore, lipid rafts serve as signaling platforms to facilitate efficient and specific signal transduction in living cells. Lipid rafts are found in large quantities in the plasma membranes of leukocytes and several proteins involved in cell signaling and cytokine action such as Src-family protein tyrosine kinases, LAT (linker for activation of T-cells) and IL-2 receptors are concentrated in rafts because of post-translational palmitoylation, indicating the role of lipid rafts cell signalling (Kane et al., 2000).

PUFAs are incorporated into membrane phospholipids and, hence, modulate membrane structure and function. On the basis of the original fluid mosaic model of cellular membranes (Li et al., 2005), the incorporation of PUFAs highly alters their general biophysical properties such as microviscosity. However, PUFAs also affect the composition of lipid rafts. Fan et al. (2004) observed that dietary ω-3 PUFAs decreased lipid raft sphingolipid content and altered raft FA composition after 48 hours of treatment.

Li et al. (2005) showed that the IL-2 receptor (IL-2R) is located in these microdomains in Jurkat cells (a T cell lineage). When T-cells were treated with DHA for 48 hours, the ω-3 PUFAs (GLA, EPA, and DHA) were significantly enriched in raft fractions compared with those of control cells. DHA treatment resulted in a considerable increase of unsaturated fatty acyl chains in rafts from DHA-treated T-cells compared with control cells. Distinct saturated FAs, such as myristic and palmitic acids, were also increased in raft fractions of DHA-treated cells compared with control cells; however, stearic and oleic acids were markedly decreased. This alteration indicated that DHA-treated cells aim to maintain lipid composition in rafts by changing the saturated or monounsaturated fatty environment. In this study, the authors found that after the IL-2 stimulation of Jurkat T-cells, IL-2Rα, IL-2Rβ, and IL-2Rγ chain proteins were detected in the fractions of membrane lipid rafts. After DHA treatment, these proteins were removed from the lipid rafts. These partial IL-2R chains displacement from lipid rafts to soluble membrane fractions were very important for the DHA-induced suppression of the IL-2R signaling pathway.

## FAs, Cytokines, and Diseases

The first evidence of the importance of the dietary intake of ω-3 PUFAs for the immune function was derived from epidemiological studies indicating a low incidence of autoimmune and inflammatory disorders, such as psoriasis, asthma, and rheumatoid arthritis, as well as the complete absence of multiple sclerosis, in a population of Greenland Eskimos compared with gender- and age-matched groups living in Denmark (Kromann & Green, 1980). Most of these diseases are characterized by inappropriate activation of T cells, resulting in the destruction of host tissues. Since then, substantial progress in the understanding of the mechanisms of FA effects on autoimmune diseases has occurred. Several studies show that the protective effects of FA are related to the modulation of cytokine production.

### *Rheumatoid Arthritis*

Sundrarjun et al. (2004) observed that both a diet low in ω-6 FAs and supplemented with ω-3 FAs and a diet low in ω-6 FAs but with no supplementation decreased IL-6 and TNF-α plasma levels in rheumatoid arthritis patients. Circulating monocytes from rheumatoid arthritis patients supplemented with GLA also showed lower TNF-α production when compared to the control group (Watson et al., 1993).

### *Sepsis*

Chiu et al. (2008) supplemented rats with FO for 10 days before sepsis was induced. The control and experimental groups were fed a common semi-purified diet with soybean oil as the main fat source. In other groups, rats were fed an identical diet except that 20% of the soybean oil was replaced by the FO. The FO contained 34% of EPA, 27% of DHA, and 72% of total ω-3 FAs, whereas the concentration of mixed tocopherols was 2.4 mg/g according to the manufacturer. This model mimics the septic complications in patients with abdominal surgery for which preventive use of an FO-supplemented enteral diet is recommended. Sepsis was induced by cecal ligation and puncture (CLP). Total parenteral nutrition (TPN) was administered for 3 days after CLP because the authors found that the total number of Peyer's patches on the serosal side of the intestine was much greater on the third day than on any other day after CLP. Sepsis induced by CLP resulted in impaired intestinal absorption. This work demonstrated that the CD4 distribution and CD4/CD8 ratio in the group without FO supplementation were lower than those in the control group, whereas no differences were noted between the FO-supplemented groups and the control groups. These findings indicate that sepsis results in a lower CD4 percentage and that FO supplementation before and/or after CLP helps to maintain the systemic helper T-lymphocyte percentage and the CD4/CD8 ratio. The mRNA expressions of IL-2 and TNF-α in splenocytes were higher in the FO than in the control and soybean groups. The IL-10 mRNA expression in the FO group was higher than in the control and the soybean groups. These results are indicative that FO administration before and/or after CLP maintained blood T-lymphocyte subpopulations and modulated T-helper type 1 and 2 cytokine mRNA expressions in rats with polymicrobial sepsis.

### *Wound Healing*

Cutaneous wound healing is a highly coordinated process that restores skin integrity. This process involves the production of soluble mediators and extracellular matrix components produced by resident cells (keratinocytes, fibroblasts, endothelial cells, and nerve cells), and the infiltration of leukocytes. Tissue repair shows a specific signaling network involving different cells and can be modulated by FAs. McDaniel et al. (2008) studied the effects of marine-derived ω-3 EPA and DHA on pro-inflammatory cytokines in wound serum and the time to complete wound healing in healthy human skin. Volunteers were supplemented for 4 weeks with total daily intake of 1.6 g of EPA and 1.1 g of DHA, and eight small blisters on participants' forearms were generated. Pro-inflammatory cytokines IL-1β, IL-6, and TNF-α were quantified in blister fluid at 5 and 24 hours after generation. They found significantly higher IL-1β levels in 24-hour blister fluid in the supplemented group, and the time to complete wound closure was somewhat longer. These results suggest that EPA and DHA may increase pro-inflammatory cytokine production at the wound sites and thus, depending on the clinical context, may have noninvasive and therapeutic potential to affect cutaneous wound healing.

## Conclusion

FAs can alter cytokine production by different cell types, but these effects are dependent on the doses used and other factors such as antioxidant co-supplementation and genetic variation. Recent, studies show that FAs modulate cellular function through alteration in the intracellular proteins activated by cytokines, TLRs activation, and change in lipid raft organization. However, the precise mechanisms involved still remain to be completely elucidated and consist of a stimulating field of research.

### References

Aderem, A.; R.J. Ulevitch. Toll-like receptors in the induction of the innate immune response. *Nature.* **2000**, *406*, 782-787.

Aggarwal, S.; S. Lee; A. Mathur; S. Gollapudi; S. Gupta. 12-Deoxyphorbol-13-O-phenylacetate 20 acetate [an agonist of protein kinase C beta 1 (PKC beta 1)] induces DNA synthesis, interleukin-2 (IL-2) production, IL-2 receptor alpha-chain (CD25) and beta-chain (CD122) expression, and translocation of PKC beta isozyme in human peripheral blood lymphocytes: evidence for a role of PKC beta 1 in human T cell activation. *J Clin Immunol.* **1994**, *14*, 248-56.

Aiello, L.P.; J.M. Northrup; B.A. Keyt; H. Takagi; M.A. Iwamoto. Hypoxic regulation of vascular endothelial growth factor in retinal cells. *Arch Ophthalmol.* **1995**, 113, 1538-44.

Aloisi F. Immune function of microglia. *Glia.* **2001**, *36*, 165-79.

Balkwill, F.R.; F. Burke. The cytokine network. *Immunol Today.* **1989**, *10,* 299-304.

Battistella, F.D.; J.T. Widergren; J.T. Anderson; J.K. Siepler; J.C. Weber; K. MacColl. A prospective, randomized trial of intravenous fat emulsion administration in trauma victims requiring total parenteral nutrition. *J Trauma.* **1997**, *43*, 52-60.

Blok, W.L.; J.P. Deslypere; P.N. Demacker; J. van der Ven-Jongekrijg; M.P. Hectors; J.W. van der

Meer; M.B. Katan. Pro- and anti-inflammatory cytokines in healthy volunteers fed various doses of fish oil for 1 year. *Eur J Clin Invest.* **1997,** *27*, 1003-8.

Blok, W.L.; M.B. Katan; J.W. Van der Meer. Modulation of inflammation and cytokine production by dietary (n-3) fatty acids. *J Nutr.* **1996,** *126*, 1515-33.

Breckenridge, W.C.; G. Gombos; I.G. Morgan. The lipid composition of adult rat brain synaptosomal plasma membranes. *Biochim Biophys Acta.* **1972**, *266*, 695-707.

Buenestado, A.; J. Cortijo; M.J. Sanz; Y. Naim-Abu-Nabah; M. Martinez-Losa; M. Mata; A.C. Issekutz; E. Martí-Bonmatí; E.J. Morcillo. Olive oil-based lipid emulsion's neutral effects on neutrophil functions and leukocyte-endothelial cell interactions. *JPEN J Parenter Enteral Nutr.* **2006**, *30*, 286-96.

Calder, P.C. N-3 polyunsaturated fatty acids and inflammation: from molecular biology to the clinic. *Lipids.* **2003**, *38*, 343-52.

Calder, P.C. Lipids and the critically ill patient. *Nestle Nutr Workshop Ser Clin Perform Programme.* **2003**, *8*, 75-98.

Carpentier, Y.A.; M. Hacquebard. Intravenous lipid emulsions to deliver omega 3 fatty acids. *Prostaglandins Leukot Essent Fatty Acids.* **2006**, *75*, 145-8.

Chen, W.; W.J. Esselman; D.B. Jump; J.V. Busik. Anti-inflammatory effect of docosahexaenoic acid on cytokine-induced adhesion molecule expression in human retinal vascular endothelial cells. *Invest Ophthalmol Vis Sci.* **2005**, *46,* 4342-7.

Chiu, W.C.; S.S. Tsou; C.L. Yeh; Y.C. Hou; S.L. Yeh. Effects of omega-3 fatty acids on inflammatory mediators and splenocyte cytokine mRNA expressions in rats with polymicrobial sepsis. *Nutrition.* **2008**, *24*, 484-91.

Chow, J.C.; D.W. Young; D.T. Golenbock; W.J. Christ; F. Gusovsky. Toll-like receptor-4 mediates lipopolysaccharide-induced signal transduction. *J Biol Chem.* **1999**, *274*, 10689-92.

Darnell, J.E. Jr.; I.M. Kerr; G.R. Stark. Jak-STAT pathways and transcriptional activation in response to IFNs and other extracellular signaling proteins. *Science.* **1994,** *264*, 1415-21.

Das U.N. Beneficial effect of eicosapentaenoic and docosahexaenoic acids in the management of systemic lupus erythematosus and its relationship to the cytokine network. *Prostaglandins Leukot Essent Fatty Acids.* **1994**, *51*, 207-13.

De Smedt-Peyrusse, V.; F. Sargueil; A. Moranis; H. Harizi; S. Mongrand; S. Layé. Docosahexaenoic acid prevents lipopolysaccharide-induced cytokine production in microglial cells by inhibiting lipopolysaccharide receptor presentation but not its membrane subdomain localization. *J Neurochem.* **2008**, *105*, 296-307.

Dinarello, C.A. Inflammatory cytokines: interleukin-1 and tumor necrosis factor as effector molecules in autoimmune diseases. *Curr Opin Immunol.* **1991**, *3*, 941-8.

Dinarello, C.A. The role of interleukin-1 in host responses to infectious diseases. *Infect Agents Dis.* **1992**, *1*, 227-36.

Fan, Y.Y.; L.H. Ly; R. Barhoumi; D.N. McMurray; R.S. Chapkin. Dietary docosahexaenoic acid suppresses T cell protein kinase C theta lipid raft recruitment and IL-2 production. *J Immunol.* **2004,** *173*, 6151-60.

Fischer, G.W.; K.W. Hunter; S.R. Wilson; A.D. Mease. Diminished bacterial defences with intralipid. *Lancet.* **1980**, *2*, 819-20.

Freeman, J.; D.A. Goldmann; N.E. Smith; D.G. Sidebottom; M.F. Epstein; R. Platt. Association of intravenous lipid emulsion and coagulase-negative staphylococcal bacteremia in neonatal intensive care units. *N Engl J Med.* **1990**, *323*, 301-8.

Fritsche, K.L.; M. Anderson; C. Feng. Consumption of eicosapentaenoic acid and docosahexaenoic acid impair murine interleukin-12 and interferon-gamma production in vivo. *J Infect Dis.* **2000**, *182,* S54-61.

Furukawa, K.; H. Yamamori; K. Takagi; N. Hayashi; R. Suzuki; N. Nakajima; T. Tashiro. Influences of soybean oil emulsion on stress response and cell-mediated immune function in moderately or severely stressed patients. *Nutrition.* **2002**, *18*, 235-40.

Gallai, V.; P. Sarchielli ; A. Trequattrini ; M. Franceschini ; A. Floridi ; C. Firenze ; A. Alberti ; D. Di Benedetto; E. Stragliotto. Cytokine secretion and eicosanoid production in the peripheral blood mononuclear cells of MS patients undergoing dietary supplementation with n-3 polyunsaturated fatty acids. *J Neuroimmunol.* **1995**, *56*, 143-53.

Gorjão, R.; M.F. Cury-Boaventura; T.M. de Lima; R Curi. Regulation of human lymphocyte proliferation by fatty acids. *Cell Biochem Funct.* **2007**, *25*, 305-15.

Gorjão, R.; R. Verlengia; T.M. Lima; F.G. Soriano; M.F. Boaventura; C.C. Kanunfre; C.M. Peres; S.C. Sampaio; R. Otton; A. Folador; E.F. Martins; T.C. Curi; E.P. Portiolli; P. Newsholme; R. Curi. Effect of docosahexaenoic acid-rich fish oil supplementation on human leukocyte function. *Clin Nutr.* **2006**, *25*, 923-38.

Granato, D.; S. Blum; C. Rössle ; J. Le Boucher; A. Malnoë; G. Dutot. Effects of parenteral lipid emulsions with different fatty acid composition on immune cell functions in vitro. *JPEN J Parenter Enteral Nutr.* **2000**, *24,* 113-8.

Grimble, R.F.; W.M. Howell; G. O'Reilly; S.J. Turner; O. Markovic; S. Hirrell; J.M. East; P.C. Calder. The ability of fish oil to suppress tumor necrosis factor alpha production by peripheral blood mononuclear cells in healthy men is associated with polymorphisms in genes that influence tumor necrosis factor alpha production. *Am J Clin Nutr.* **2002**, *76*, 454-9.

Hashimoto, M. Y Asai; T. Ogawa. Trponemal phospholipids inhibit innate immune responses induced by pathogen-associated molecular patterns. *J. Biol. Chem.* **2003,** *278,* 44205-44213.

Helms, R.A.; H.G. Herrod; G.J. Burckart; M.L. Christensen. E-rosette formation, total T-cells, and lymphocyte transformation in infants receiving intravenous safflower oil emulsion. *JPEN J Parenter Enteral Nutr.* **1983,** *7*, 541-5.

Hirafuji, M.; T. Machida; M. Tsunoda; A. Miyamoto; M. Minami. Docosahexaenoic acid potentiates interleukin-1beta induction of nitric oxide synthase through mechanism involving p44/42 MAPK activation in rat vascular smooth muscle cells. *Br J Pharmacol.* **2002**, *136*, 613-9.

Jarstrand, C.; L. Berghem; G. Lahnborg. Human granulocyte and reticuloendothelial system function during intralipid infusion. *JPEN J Parenter Enteral Nutr.* **1978**, *2*, 663-70.

Jolly, C.A.; D.N. McMurray; R.S. Chapkin. Effect of dietary n-3 fatty acids on interleukin-2 and interleukin-2 receptor alpha expression in activated murine lymphocytes. Prostaglandins *Leukot Essent Fatty Acids.* **1998**, *58*, 289-93.

Kane, L.P.; J. Lin; A. Weiss. Signal transduction by the TCR for antigen. *Curr Opin Immunol.* **2000**, *12*, 242-9.

Khalfoun, B.; F. Thibault; H. Watier; P. Bardos; Y. Lebranchu. Docosahexaenoic and eicosapentaenoic acids inhibit in vitro human endothelial cell production of interleukin-6. *Adv Exp Med Biol.* **1997**, *400*B:589-97.

Kirken, R.A; H. Rui; M.G. Malabarba; O.M. Howard; M. Kawamura; J.J. O'Shea; W.L. Farrar. Activation of JAK3, but not JAK1, is critical for IL-2-induced proliferation and STAT5 recruitment by a COOH-terminal region of the IL-2 receptor beta-chain. *Cytokine.* **1995**, *7*, 689-700.

Kowluru, R.A.; S. Odenbach. Effect of long-term administration of alpha-lipoic acid on retinal capillary cell death and the development of retinopathy in diabetic rats. *Diabetes. 2004, 53*, 3233–8.

Krogh-Madsen, R.; P. Plomgaard; T. Akerstrom; K. Møller; O. Schmitz; B.K. Pedersen. Effect of short-term intralipid infusion on the immune response during low-dose endotoxemia in humans. *Am J Physiol Endocrinol Metab.* **2008**, *294*, E371-9.

Kromann, N; A. Green. Epidemiological studies in the Upernavik district, Greenland. Incidence of some chronic diseases 1950-1974. *Acta Med Scand.* **1980**, *208*, 401-6.

Lanza-Jacoby, S.; J.T. Flynn; S. Miller. Parenteral supplementation with a fish-oil emulsion prolongs survival and improves rat lymphocyte function during sepsis. *Nutrition.* **2001**, *17,* 112-6.

Lee, C.K.; E.Y. Lee; Y.G. Kim; S.H. Mun; H.B. Moon; B. Yoo. Alpha-lipoic acid inhibits TNF-alpha induced NF-kappa B activation through blocking of MEKK1-MKK4-IKK signaling cascades. *Int Immunopharmacol.* **2008**, *8*, 362-70.

Lee, J.Y.; A. Plakidas; W.H. Lee; A. Heikkinen; P. Chanmugam; G. Bray; D.H. Hwang. Differential modulation of toll-like receptors by fatty-acids: preferential inhibition by ω-3 polyunsaturated fatty acids. *J Lipid Res.* **2003**, *44*, 479-486.

Lee, J.Y.; K.H. Sohn; S.H. Rhee; D. Hwang. Saturated fatty acids, but not unsaturated fatty acids, induce the expression of cyclooxygenase-2 mediated through toll-like receptor 4. *J. Biol. Chem.* **2001**, *276*, 16683-16689.

Lehnardt, S.; L. Massillon; P. Follett; F.E. Jensen; R. Ratan; P.A. Rosenberg; J.J. Volpe; T. Vartanian. Activation of innate immunity in the CNS triggers neurodegeneration through a Toll-like receptor 4-dependent pathway. *Proc Natl Acad Sci U S A.* **2003**, *100,* 8514-9.

Li, Q.; M. Wang; L. Tan; C. Wang; J. Ma; N. Li; Y. Li; G. Xu; J. Li. Docosahexaenoic acid changes lipid composition and interleukin-2 receptor signaling in membrane rafts. *J Lipid Res.* **2005**, *46*, 1904-13.

Li, X.; J. Ying; S. Zeng; Y. Li; H. Yang; L. Shen; J. Han; J. Chen; H. Shen. A short-term long-chain triglycerides infusion has no influence on immune function of adult patients undergoing gastrointestinal surgery. *JPEN J Parenter Enteral Nutr.* **2007**, *31*, 167-72.

Li, X.; J. Ying; S. Zeng; Y. Li; H. Yang; L. Shen; J. Han; J. Chen; H. Shen. The effects of a short-term long-chain-triglyceride infusion on the postoperative immune function of pediatric patients receiving a gastrointestinal surgical procedure. *JPEN J Parenter Enteral Nutr.* **2008**, *32*, 72-7.

Lien, E.; T.K. Means; H. Heine; A. Yoshimura; N. Qureshi; B. Monks; R.W. Finberg; R.R. Ingalls; D.T. Golenbock. Toll-like receptor 4 imparts ligand-specific recognition of bacterial lipopolysaccharide. *J Clin Invest.* **2000**, *105*, 497-504.

Limb, G.A.; A.H. Chignell; W. Green; F. LeRoy; D.C. Dumonde. Distribution of TNF alpha and its reactive vascular adhesion molecules in fibrovascular membranes of proliferative diabetic retinopathy. *Br J Ophthalmol.* **1996**, *80*, 168-73.

Limb, G.A.; C.J. Cole; O. Earley; R.D. Hollifield; W. Russell; M.R. Stanford. Expression of hematopoietic cell markers by retinal pigment epithelial cells. *Curr Eye Res.* **1997**, *16*, 985-91.

Limb, G.A.; H. Soomro; S. Janikoun; R.D. Hollifield; J. Shilling. Evidence for control of tumour necrosis factor-alpha (TNF-alpha) activity by TNF receptors in patients with proliferative diabetic retinopathy. *Clin Exp Immunol.* **1999**, *115*, 409-14.

Lin, M.T.; S.L. Yeh; C.L. Yeh; Y.N. Lai; K.J. Chang; P.H. Lee; W.J. Chen; Parenteral N-3 fatty acids modulate inflammatory and immune response in rats undergoing total gastrectomy. *Shock.* **2006**, *25*, 56-60.

Loscher, C.E.; E. Draper; O. Leavy; D. Kelleher; K.H. Mills; H.M. Roche. Conjugated linoleic acid suppresses NF-kappa B activation and IL-12 production in dendritic cells through ERK-mediated IL-10 induction. *J Immunol.* **2005**, *175*, 4990-8.

Luongo, D.; P. Bergamo; M. Rossi. Effects of conjugated linoleic acid on growth and cytokine expression in Jurkat T cells. *Immunol Lett.* **2003**, *90*, 195-201.

Mayer, K.; S. Gokorsch; C. Fegbeutel; K. Hattar; S. Rosseau; D. Walmrath; W. Seeger; F. Grimminger. Parenteral nutrition with fish oil modulates cytokine response in patients with sepsis. *Am J Respir Crit Care Med.* **2003**, *167*, 1321-8.

McCann, M.E.; J.N. Moore; J.B. Carrick; M.H. Barton. Effect of intravenous infusion of omega-3 and omega-6 lipid emulsions on equine monocyte fatty acid composition and inflammatory mediator production in vitro. *Shock.* **2000**, *14*, 222-8.

McDaniel, J.C.; M. Belury; K. Ahijevych; W. Blakely. Omega-3 fatty acids effect on wound healing. *Wound Repair Regen.* **2008**, *16*, 337-45.

McGeer, P.L.; E.G. McGeer. Local neuroinflammation and the progression of Alzheimer's disease. *J Neurovirol.* **2002**, *8*, 529-38.

Miles, E.A.; T. Banerjee; M.M. Dooper; L. M'Rabet; Y.M. Graus; P.C. Calder. The influence of different combinations of gamma-linolenic acid, stearidonic acid and EPA on immune function in healthy young male subjects. *Br J Nutr.* **2004**, *91,* 893-903.

Mølvig, J.; F. Pociot; H. Worsaae; L.D. Wogensen; L. Baek; P. Christensen; T. Mandrup-Poulsen; K. Andersen; P. Madsen; J. Dyerberg. Dietary supplementation with omega-3-polyunsaturated fatty acids decreases mononuclear cell proliferation and interleukin-1 beta content but not monokine secretion in healthy and insulin-dependent diabetic individuals. *Scand J Immunol.* **1991**, *34*, 399-410.

Moussa, M.; J. Le Boucher; J. Garcia; J. Tkaczuk; J. Ragab; G. Dutot; E. Ohayon; J. Ghisolfi; J.P. Thouvenot. In vivo effects of olive oil-based lipid emulsion on lymphocyte activation in rats. *Clin Nutr.* **2000**, *19*, 49-54.

Müller, J.M.; H.W. Keller; U. Brenner. Fats and immunocompetence. *Beitr Infusionther Klin Ernahr.* **1986,** *13*, 128-41.

Navarro-González, J.F.; C. Mora-Fernández. The role of inflammatory cytokines in diabetic nephropathy. *J Am Soc Nephrol.* **2008,** *19*, 433-42.

Nordenström, J.; C. Jarstrand; A. Wiernik. Decreased chemotactic and random migration of leukocytes during Intralipid infusion. *Am J Clin Nutr.* **1979**, *32*, 2416-22.

Novak, T.E.; T.A. Babcock; D.H. Jho; W.S. Helton; N.J. Espat. NF-kappa B inhibition by omega -3 fatty acids modulates LPS-stimulated macrophage TNF-alpha transcription. *Am J Physiol*

*Lung Cell Mol Physiol.* **2003**, *284*, L84-9.

Ota, D.M.; E.M. Copeland 3rd; J.N. Corriere Jr; E.R. Richie; K. Jacobson; S.J. Dudrick. The effects of a 10% soybean oil emulsion on lymphocyte transformation. *JPEN J Parenter Enteral Nutr.* **1978**, *2*, 112-5.

Pereira, L.M.; E. Hatanaka; E.F. Martins; F. Oliveira; E.A. Liberti; S.H. Farsky; R. Curi; T.C. Pithon-Curi. Effect of oleic and linoleic acids on the inflammatory phase of wound healing in rats. *Cell Biochem Funct.* **2008**, *26*, 197-204.

Poltorak, A.; X. He; I. Smirnova; M.Y. Liu; C. Van Huffel; X. Du; D. Birdwell; E. Alejos; M. Silva; C. Galanos; M. Freudenberg; P. Ricciardi-Castagnoli; B. Layton; B. Beutler; Defective LPS signaling in C3H/HeJ and C57BL/10ScCr mice: mutations in Tlr4 gene. *Science.* **1998**, *282*, 2085-8.

Puertollano, M.A.; E. Puertollano; A. Ruiz-Bravo; M. Jiménez-Valera; M.A. De Pablo; G.A. De Cienfuegos. Changes in the immune functions and susceptibility to Listeria monocytogenes infection in mice fed dietary lipids. *Immunol Cell Biol.* **2004**, *82*, 370-6.

Puertollano, M.A.; E. Puertollano; G. Alvarez de Cienfuegos; M.A. de Pablo. Significance of olive oil in the host immune resistance to infection. *Br J Nutr.* **2007,** *98*, S54-8.

Qureshi, S.T.; L. Lariviere; G. Leveque; S. Clermont; K.J. Moore; P. Gros; D. Malo. Endotoxin-tolerant mice have mutations in Toll-like receptor e (Tlr4) *J. Exp. Med.* **1999**, *189*, 615-625.

Reimund, J.M.; G. Rahmi; G. Escalin; G. Pinna; G. Finck; C.D. Muller; B. Duclos; R. Baumann. Efficacy and safety of an olive oil-based intravenous fat emulsion in adult patients on home parenteral nutrition. *Aliment Pharmacol Ther.* **2005**, *21*, 445-54.

Reimund, J.M.; O. Scheer; C.D. Muller; G. Pinna; B. Duclos; R. Baumann. In vitro modulation of inflammatory cytokine production by three lipid emulsions with different fatty acid compositions. *Clin Nutr.* **2004**, *23*, 1324-32.

Rhee, S.H.; D. Hwang. Murine Toll-like receptor 4 confers lipolysaccharide responsiveness as determine by activation of NF kappa B and expression of the inducible cyclooxgenase. *J. Biol. Chem.* **2000**, *275*, 34035-34040.

Ringseis, R.; S. Gahler; C. Herter; K. Eder. Conjugated linoleic acids exert similar actions on prostanoid release from aortic and coronary artery smooth muscle cells. *Int J Vitam Nutr Res.* **2006**, *76*, 281-9.

Russell, S.M.; J.A. Johnston; M, Noguchi; M, Kawamura; C,M, Bacon; D,W, McVicar; B,A, Witthuhn; O. Silvennoinen. Interaction of IL-2R beta and gamma c chains with Jak1 and Jak3: implications for XSCID and XCID. *Science.* **1994**, *266,* 1042-5.

Salem, N. Jr.; B. Litman; H.Y. Kim; K. Gawrisch. Mechanisms of action of docosahexaenoic acid in the nervous system. *Lipids.* **2001**, *36*, 945-59.

Schauder, P.; U. Röhn; G. Schäfer; G. Korff; H.D. Schenk. Impact of fish oil enriched total parenteral nutrition on DNA synthesis, cytokine release and receptor expression by lymphocytes in the postoperative period. *Br J Nutr.* **2002**, *87*, S103-10.

Schroeder, R.; E. London; D. Brown. Interactions between saturated acyl chains confer detergent resistance on lipids and glycosylphosphatidylinositol (GPI)-anchored proteins: GPI-anchored proteins in liposomes and cells show similar behavior. *Proc Natl Acad Sci U S A.* **1994**, *91*, 12130-4.

Sedman, P.C.; C.W. Ramsden; T.G. Brennan; .PJ. Guillou. Pharmacological concentrations of lipid emulsions inhibit interleukin-2-dependent lymphocyte responses in vitro. *JPEN J Parenter Enteral Nutr.* **1990**, *14*, 12-7.

Sedman, P.C.; S.S. Somers; C.W. Ramsden; T.G. Brennan; P.J. Guillou. Effects of different lipid emulsions on lymphocyte function during total parenteral nutrition. *Br J Surg.* **1991**, *78*, 1396-9.

Skuladottir, I.H.; D.H. Petursdottir; I. Hardardottir. The effects of omega-3 polyunsaturated fatty acids on TNF-alpha and IL-10 secretion by murine peritoneal cells in vitro. *Lipids.* **2007**, *42*, 699-706.

Somers, S.D.; K.L. Erickson. Alteration of tumor necrosis factor-alpha production by macrophages from mice fed diets high in eicosapentaenoic and docosahexaenoic fatty acids. *Cell Immunol.* **1994**, *153*, 287-97.

Sosenko, I.R.; M. Rodriguez-Pierce; E. Bancalari. Effect of early initiation of intravenous lipid administration on the incidence and severity of chronic lung disease in premature infants. *J Pediatr.* **1993**, *123*, 975-82.

Suganami, T.; K. Tanimoto-Koyama; J. Nishida; M. Itoh; X. Yuan; S. Mizuarai; H. Kotani; S. Yamaoka; K. Miyake; S. Aoe; Y. Kamei; Y. Ogawa. Role of the Toll-like receptor 4/NF-kappaB pathway in saturated fatty acid-induced inflammatory changes in the interaction between adipocytes and macrophages. *Arterioscler Thromb Vasc Biol.* **2007**, *27*, 84-91.

Sundrarjun, T.; S. Komindr; N. Archararit; W. Dahlan; O. Puchaiwatananon; S. Angthararak; U. Udomsuppayakul; S. Chuncharunee. Effects of n-3 fatty acids on serum interleukin-6, tumour necrosis factor-alpha and soluble tumour necrosis factor receptor p55 in active rheumatoid arthritis. *J Int Med Res.* **2004**, *32*, 443-54.

Tappia, P.S.; R.F. Grimble. The relationship between altered membrane composition, eicosanoids and TNF-induced IL1 and IL6 production in macrophages of rats fed fats of different unsaturated fatty acid composition. *Mol Cell Biochem.* **1996**, *165*, 135-43.

Trebble, T.; N.K. Arden; M.A. Stroud; S.A. Wootton; G.C. Burdge; E.A. Miles; A.B. Ballinger; R.L. Thompson; P.C. Calder. Inhibition of tumour necrosis factor-alpha and interleukin 6 production by mononuclear cells following dietary fish-oil supplementation in healthy men and response to antioxidant co-supplementation. *Br J Nutr.* **2003,** *90*, 405-12.

Verlengia, R.; R. Gorjão; C.C. Kanunfre; S. Bordin; T.M. de Lima; P. Newsholme; R. Curi. Genes regulated by arachidonic and oleic acids in Raji cells. *Lipids.* **2003**, *38*, 1157-65.

Verlengia, R.; R. Gorjão; C.C. Kanunfre; S. Bordin; T.M. de Lima; E.F. Martins; R. Curi. Comparative effects of eicosapentaenoic acid and docosahexaenoic acid on proliferation, cytokine production, and pleiotropic gene expression in Jurkat cells. *J Nutr Biochem.* **2004a**, *15*, 657-65.

Verlengia, R.; R. Gorjão; C.C. Kanunfre; S. Bordin; T.M. de Lima; E.F. Martins; P. Newsholme; R. Curi. Effects of EPA and DHA on proliferation, cytokine production, and gene expression in Raji cells. *Lipids.* **2004b,** *39*, 857-64.

Wallace, F.A.; E.A. Miles; P.C. Calder. Activation state alters the effect of dietary fatty acids on pro-inflammatory mediator production by murine macrophages. *Cytokine.* **2000**, *12,* 1374-9.

Wallace, F.A.; E.A. Miles; C. Evans; T.E. Stock; P. Yaqoob; P.C. Calder. Dietary fatty acids influence the production of Th1- but not Th2-type cytokines. *J Leukoc Biol.* **2001**, *69*, 449-57.

Wallace, F.A.; E.A. Miles; P.C. Calder. Comparison of the effects of linseed oil and different doses of fish oil on mononuclear cell function in healthy human subjects. *Br J Nutr.* **2003**, *89*, 679-89.

Wang, H.; X. Xie; W.G. Lu; D.F. Ye; H.Z. Chen; X. Li; Q. Cheng. Ovarian carcinoma cells inhibit T cell proliferation: suppression of IL-2 receptor beta and gamma expression and their JAK-STAT signaling pathway. *Life Sci.* **2004**, *74,* 1739-49.

Wanten, G.J.; P.C. Calder. Immune modulation by parenteral lipid emulsions. *Am J Clin Nutr.* **2007**, *85*, 1171-84.

Wanten, G.J.; M.G. Netea; T.H. Naber; J.H. Curfs; L.E. Jacobs; T.J. Verver-Jansen. B.J. Kullberg. Parenteral administration of medium- but not long-chain lipid emulsions may increase the risk for infections by Candida albicans. *Infect Immun.* **2002**, *70*, 6471-4.

Watson, J.; M.L. Byars; P. McGil; A.W. Kelman. Cytokine and prostaglandin production by monocytes of volunteers and rheumatoid arthritis patients treated with dietary supplements of blackcurrant seed oil. *Br J Rheumatol.* **1993**, *32*, 1055-8.

Weiss, G.; F. Meyer; B. Matthies; M. Pross; W. Koenig; H. Lippert. Immunomodulation by perioperative administration of n-3 fatty acids. *Br J Nutr.* **2002**, *87*, S89-94.

Weldon, S.M.; A.C. Mullen; C.E. Loscher; L.A. Hurley; H.M. Roche. Docosahexaenoic acid induces an anti-inflammatory profile in lipopolysaccharide-stimulated human THP-1 macrophages more effectively than eicosapentaenoic acid. *J Nutr Biochem.* **2007**, *18,* 250-8.

Wright, S.D.; R.A. Ramos; P.S. Tobias; R.J. Ulevitch; J.C. Mathison. CD14, a receptor for complexes of lipopolysaccharide (LPS) and LPS binding protein. *Science.* **1990**, *249,* 1431-3.

Xue, H.; M. Wan; D. Song; Y. Li; J. Li. Eicosapentaenoic acid and docosahexaenoic acid modulate mitogen-activated protein kinase activity in endothelium. *Vascul Pharmacol.* **2006**, *44,* 434-9.

Yang, M.; M.E. Cook. Dietary conjugated linoleic acid decreased cachexia, macrophage tumor necrosis factor-alpha production, and modifies splenocyte cytokines production. *Exp Biol Med,* **2003**, *228*, 51-8.

Yaqoob, P.; P.C. Calder. The effects of dietary lipid manipulation on the production of murine T cell-derived cytokines. *Cytokine.* **1995**, *7*, 548-53.

Yaqoob, P.; E.A. Newsholme; P.C. Calder. The effect of dietary lipid manipulation on rat lymphocyte subsets and proliferation. *Immunology.* **1994**, *82*, 603-10.

Zarember, K.A.; P.J. Godowski. Tissue expression of human Toll-like receptors and differential regulation of Toll-like receptor mRNAsin leukocytes in response to microbes, their products, and cytokines. *J. Immunol.* **2002,** *168*, 554-561.

## PART 4

# Omega-3 Fatty Acids and Health

# 24

# From ADHD to Alzheimer's: Omega-3 Fatty Acids and Mental Health

**Natalie Sinn, Catherine Milte, and Peter R.C. Howe**
*Nutritional Physiology Research Centre/Sansom Institute, University of South Australia, Adelaide SA, Australia*

## Introduction

The World Health Organization (WHO) (2008) defines mental health as "a state of well-being in which every individual realizes his or her own potential, can cope with the normal stresses of life, can work productively and fruitfully, and is able to make a contribution to her or his community." About 450 million people worldwide do not enjoy this state of well-being, and it is estimated that one in four people will suffer from mental illness at some stage in their lifetime, causing enormous personal suffering, social and financial burdens, and associated physical illnesses (WHO, 2004). The identification of preventable risk factors and effective treatments therefore constitutes an international priority.

Nutrition has an important role in mental health because the brain relies on both macro- and micronutrients for effective functioning. In particular, suboptimal levels of omega-3 polyunsaturated fatty acids (n-3 PUFAs) are emerging as a potentially modifiable risk factor for mental illness. Since their discovery in the 1970s as key components of brain tissue (Crawford & Sinclair, 1971), long-chain (LC) n-3 PUFAs have been postulated to serve critical roles in brain development and function, and a lack of these essential fatty acids was implicated in a number of mental-health conditions across the lifespan: developmental disorders and mental retardation in childhood; depression, bipolar disorder, schizophrenia, and borderline personality disorder in adulthood; and cognitive decline, dementia, and Alzheimer's disease in late adulthood.

Although the etiology of these disorders is clearly multifactorial and subject to individual variation, the number of clinical trials addressing suboptimal PUFA levels as a possible underlying biological contributor to associated symptoms (and importantly, symptoms that often co-occur and overlap between these disorders) is steadily growing. This chapter provides an overview of n-3 PUFAs and their role in the brain, and then discusses the current state of evidence for their association with, and their role in alleviating symptoms of, psychopathology from childhood throughout adulthood.

# Omega-3 PUFA

## Overview

The omega-6 (n-6) and n-3 families of PUFAs have numerous biological roles in cellular structure and function. Alpha linolenic acid (ALA; 18:3n-3), parent n-3 PUFA, and linoleic acid (LA; 18:2n-6), parent n-6 PUFA, cannot be synthesized by humans: the diet must provide them. They are therefore termed "essential fatty acids" (EFAs). Humans can obtain ALA through their diet via various green leafy vegetables, nuts, and seeds. EFAs have 18 carbon atoms with double-carbon bonds. These chains undergo further processes of elongation and desaturation (an insertion of additional double bonds) to form highly unsaturated LC-PUFA. Our bodies can perform these conversions, although not always very efficiently. LC derivatives of ALA, eicosapentaenoic acid (EPA), and docosahexaenoic acid (DHA) are made by phytoplankton and transferred via the foodchain to marine organisms, particularly cold-water fish and marine animals. Therefore, humans can also obtain these elongated n-3 PUFAs directly via algal or fish sources.

Unlike saturated fats, which are relatively inactive and chiefly used for insulation and energy generation, PUFAs are chemically active lipids that are required for essential life processes. The naturally occurring double bonds in PUFAs form bends or "kinks" in fatty- acid molecules which render them more fluid and mobile, and therefore able to keep cell membranes supple (Lauritzen et al., 2001). Structurally, PUFAs form the major components of phospholipids, comprising cellular and intracellular membranes. They govern growth and vitality through oxidation (metabolism of food to produce energy required for cellular processes), chemical activities, and transportation. As well as being instrumental in constructing membranes and generating and moving electrical impulses, LC-PUFAs are required for the synthesis of eicosanoids, important signaling hormones with numerous complex functions. Those derived from n-3 LC-PUFAs are generally anti-inflammatory, anti-thrombotic and vasodilatory, counteracting the pro-inflammatory, vasoconstrictor actions of eicosanoids derived from n-6 LC-PUFAs (Simopoulos, 1991). The cardiovascular benefits of n-3 PUFAs are largely attributed to these eicosanoid properties, and they may also have important roles in brain function.

## Omega-3 PUFA and the Brain

Lipids constitute approximately 60% of the dry weight of the brain. DHA and arachidonic acid (AA) are the most highly concentrated PUFAs in neural phospholipids, which include subcellular membranes such as synaptosomes, synaptic vesicles, mitochondria, microsomes, and nerve- growth cones (Hamilton et al., 2000; Horrocks & Yeo, 1999; Salem et al., 2001; Youdim et al., 2000). Although the circulation contains at least 10 times more n-6 than n-3 PUFAs, DHA predominates in the retina, brain, and nervous system (Salem et al., 2001). Furthermore, DHA is particularly concentrated at neural synapses (Horrobin, 1999).

Importantly, DHA levels in neural membranes vary according to dietary oil intake (Hamilton et al., 2000; Tacconi et al., 1997; Yehuda et al., 1998; Youdim et al., 2000), and evidence shows that low-PUFA and high-cholesterol levels reduce phospholipid fluidity (Yehuda et al., 1998, 2002). Animal studies and human-infant autopsies also show that when insufficient n-3 PUFAs are available during early neural development, a decrease occurs in the DHA content of the brain. Furthermore, increased n-6 to n-3 PUFA ratios can also alter the fatty acid composition of neural membranes (Tiemeier et al., 2003). High–n-6 and low–n-3 intake can result in higher levels of the n-6 LC-PUFA, docosapentaenoic acid (DPA) (Hamilton et al., 2000; Lauritzen et al., 2001; Moriguchi et al., 2001; Wainwright et al., 1999; Youdim et al., 2000). Therefore, n-6 DPA can substitute for DHA in neural membranes when DHA supplies are low, and may impact negatively on various functions involving neurotransmission (Hibbeln & Salem, Jr., 1995), enzyme activity, retinal and brain development, and performance on learning tasks (Hamilton et al., 2000).

Various reviews outline the biological mechanisms for n-3 PUFAs in brain function (e.g., Assisi et al., 2006; Haag, 2003; Young & Conquer, 2005). In particular, and in line with a long-standing focus on the role of neurotransmitters such as dopamine (DA) and serotonin in mental illness, research has focused on the associations between PUFAs and central nervous system activity (Leaf & Kang, 2001). Evidence points to the role of eicosanoids in healthy brain functioning, and phospholipid membranes in neural cell signalling (Hamilton et al., 2000; Horrobin, 1998; Yehuda et al., 1998; Youdim et al., 2000). Levels of n-3 PUFAs were associated with monoaminergic neurotransmitter levels (Chalon, 2006; Chalon et al., 2001; Lauritzen et al., 2001; Youdim et al., 2000). In animal studies, an n-3 deficiency was also found to reduce the levels of phosphatidylserine (PS) in the brain, which is thought to play an important function in neural-signalling activities (Hamilton et al., 2000). In alcoholics, DHA deficiency predicted reduced 5-hydroxyindoleacetic acid (5-HIAA) concentrations in cerebrospinal fluid, an indicator of a low-serotonin turnover rate in the frontal cortex (Hibbeln et al., 1998).

How n-3 PUFAs influence neurotransmission is not precisely known. Studies indicate that they may affect receptor properties or the activation of signal transduction by receptors (Lauritzen et al., 2001). Electrical impulse conduction is dependent on the exchange of ions through the cell membrane, which relies on the fluidity and physiological structure of cell membranes. Furthermore, indications show that PUFAs are involved in the synthesis and activities of brain peptides (Yehuda et al., 1998), which are involved in modulating the activities of neurotransmitters (Froehlich, 1997). The n-3 PUFAs also influence the gene expression of a range of enzymes required for important neural functions including synaptic transduction, ion channel formation, energy metabolism, and the formulation of proteins vital for brain development and function (Assisi et al., 2006).

The regular delivery of oxygen and nutrients via the blood is also critical for optimal brain function, and psychopathology is associated with both reduced cerebral blood flow and the transportation of glucose, the brain's primary energy source, to brain regions as required. In this regard, n-3 PUFAs are associated with the production of nitric oxide (Mori et al., 2000), as well as anti-inflammatory and vasodilatory eicosanoids [notably prostacyclin ($PGI_2$)], and assist in endothelial-dependent vasodilation (Simopoulos, 1991). They have also been associated with substantially increased transport of glucose across the blood-brain barrier (da Silva et al., 2002; Pifferi et al., 2005). Therefore, primary influences of n-3 PUFA on brain function may also include improved cerebral blood flow and blood-brain barrier integrity (Sinn & Howe, 2008). This notion is supported by the high co-morbidity between cardiovascular disease (CVD) and psychopathology, indicative of a common underlying vascular pathology that lifestyle factors such as suboptimal levels of n-3 PUFAs may mediate (Hooijmans & Kiliaan, 2008).

## *Animal Studies*

Numerous animal studies have demonstrated a link between dietary n-3 PUFAs and cognitive performance (Gamoh et al., 1999; Kaplan & Greenwood, 1998; Lim & Suzuki, 2000). In a spatial memory test, the performance of rats given a soybean-oil diet (51% LA; 7% ALA) was superior to that of rats on a lard diet (high in saturated fat with 10% LA; 1% ALA) after controlling for other physiological variables (Kaplan & Greenwood, 1998). Kaplan and Greenwood (1998) reported further studies examining the effects of n-3 PUFAs on specific aspects of learning and memory that rely on different regions of the brain. Animals on a lard diet showed deficits in spatial memory, short- and long-term temporal memories, and in learning various maze problems. The authors concluded that the effects of PUFA deficiency may be generalized across different brain regions rather than being specific to certain areas of the brain.

Studies on animals with reduced maternally-derived DHA revealed impaired performance on various neurological tasks (Salem et al., 2001). Gamoh et al. (1999) tested the effects of DHA supplementation on the learning ability in rats fed fish-oil-deficient diets over three generations. The DHA-supplemented group showed significantly fewer reference-memory errors than the control group, although working-memory results were inconclusive. The supplemented group also had a significant increase in DHA and AA concentrations in the hippocampus and cerebral-cortex regions of the brain, which are both important for memory formation and, therefore, learning. Importantly, this indicated that DHA supplementation may be able to reverse chronic n-3 deficiencies and improve learning ability. DHA uptake into the brain also appeared to be selective because the increase that was found in the cerebral cortex and hippocampus was not found in the cerebellum and brain stem. This may indicate that DHA was taken up by brain regions where it was either most deficient and/or most needed for specific brain functions. DHA intake also improved maze-learning performance in both young and old mice compared to control groups (Lim & Suzuki, 2000), even though old mice performed less well and had lower brain DHA levels. The improvement of the maze-learning ability following

DHA supplementation was replicated in a later controlled trial, and the effects were measured over various time periods. Learning did not improve until two weeks after the DHA levels had increased in mice brains, indicating that DHA needs time to be incorporated into neural membranes before learning outcomes are influenced. A different study found reduced levels of DHA and AA in the hippocampus of older rats and associated impairments in long-term potentiation (LTP), an indicator of learning and memory. After supplementation with EPA and AA for 8 weeks, the levels of EPA and AA increased in the hippocampus, and this was associated with a reversal in the age-related impairment in LTP (Martin et al., 2002).

Animal studies have also found abnormalities in dopaminergic systems consistent with behavioral abnormalities associated with an n-3 deficiency. Dopaminergic projections to the frontal lobes influence motivational behavior, emotional functions, and cognitive functions such as a working memory (Chalon et al., 2001; Zimmer et al., 2002). Thus, the effects of an n-3 deficiency in animals on decreased learning ability, sensory, motor, or motivational processes may be attributable to alterations in monoaminergic neurotransmission. To investigate the hypothesis, brain monoamine levels in rats fed diets deficient in ALA were compared to a control group (Chalon et al., 2001). The main difference observed was a 40–60% decrease in DA levels in the frontal cortex. Overall, a chronic n-3 deficiency affected the mesocortical and mesolimbic systems, which is consistent with studies relating an n-3 deficiency to motivation, response to reward, and learning ability. More recent work also associated n-3 PUFA levels with the neurotransmitter serotonin (Chalon, 2006), low levels of which are thought to play a role in depressive disorders and aggression.

Lauritzen et al. (2001) reviewed controlled animal studies and concluded that evidence exists of a role for n-3 PUFAs in improving learning and behavior. A large body of research has investigated n-3 PUFAs and infant development, which is covered in a separate chapter of this book (see Smithers & Makrides). This chapter focuses on mental health problems in childhood through to older adulthood.

## PUFA and Mental Illness

PUFA deficiencies have been reported in people with a range of psychiatric problems (Assisi et al., 2006; Haag, 2003; Richardson, 2006; Young & Conquer, 2005), including developmental disorders such as attention deficit hyperactivity disorder (ADHD), depression, bipolar disorder, aggression, hostility and criminality, and dementia. A small but growing body of clinical research trials have been conducted with variable outcomes. These are reviewed here.

### *Attention Deficit Hyperactivity Disorder (ADHD)*

Increasing attention has been given to the role of EFAs in childhood developmental disorders such as autistic spectrum disorder (Bell et al., 2000, 2004); dyslexia (Baker, 1985; Richardson et al., 1997; Richardson & Puri, 2000; Stordy, 2000; Taylor et al., 2000; Taylor & Richardson, 2000); dyspraxia (Richardson & Montgomery, 2005); and ADHD (Richardson, 2006; Sinn & Bryan, 2007), all of which involve learning and behavioral difficulties. Given that brain development continues throughout childhood (Thatcher, 1991; Toga et al., 2006), PUFA supplementation may have a beneficial effect during developmental milestones, particularly in children with developmental disorders that might be related to problems with PUFA metabolism and/or deficiency.

Researchers have found lower levels of n-3 and n-6 PUFAs in the blood analyses of hyperactive children compared with matched controls (Arnold et al., 1989; Burgess et al., 2000; Chen et al., 2004; Colquhoun & Bunday, 1981; Mitchell et al., 1983, 1987; Stevens et al., 1995, 1996). Mitchell et al. (1987) found significantly lower plasma levels of dihomo-gamma-linolenic acid (DGLA), AA, and DHA in hyperactive children. EPA was also lower in hyperactive children than controls ($M$ = 17.9 and 20.7 μg/mL serum, respectively); however, significance levels and effect sizes were not reported. Stevens et al. (1995) found significantly lower levels of AA, EPA, and DHA in plasma and red blood cells (RBCs) in a group of ADHD children, but no differences in DGLA. In the latter study, average n-3 levels were lower in the ADHD group; however, mean n-6 concentrations did not differ between the groups, and therefore the ratio of total n-6 to n-3 fatty acids was significantly higher in the ADHD group. A study in Taiwan found significantly lower levels of LA, AA, and DHA in the RBCs of children with ADHD compared with controls. They also found lower EPA levels in the ADHD children, but the difference was not significant. No difference was noted in the total n-6 fatty acids between the groups, and the ADHD children had significantly lower total n-3 fatty acids in RBCs, resulting in higher n-6 to n-3 ratios (Chen et al., 2004). Interestingly, in this study, levels of n-3 PUFA in plasma were not significantly different between ADHD children and controls, indicating a possible problem with PUFA incorporation into cellular membranes. More recently, however, Stevens et al. (2003) reported significantly lower levels of n-6 fatty acids DGLA and AA as well as n-3 PUFA ALA, EPA, and DHA in the plasma of children with ADHD. All in all, given the importance of the PUFAs DHA, AA, EPA, and DGLA for brain function and the fact that suboptimal levels of these PUFA were identified in children with ADHD, growing numbers of clinical trials are investigating the effects of PUFA supplementation on ADHD-related symptoms.

Early-intervention trials showed little or no improvement in alleviating hyperactive symptoms of ADHD with evening primrose oil, which contains the n-6 PUFA gamma-linolenic acid (GLA) (Aman et al., 1987; Arnold et al., 1989). Following these studies and with an increasing awareness of the importance of n-3 PUFAs, seven randomized, double-blind, placebo-controlled PUFA supplementation trials have been completed with children displaying ADHD-related symptoms, with varying results.

In the first study, supplementation with 345 mg of DHA daily over four months in 6–12-year-old children diagnosed with ADHD did not significantly improve the objective or subjective measurements of symptoms, even though a significant increase occurred in the RBC levels of DHA in the DHA group (Voigt et al., 2001). In this study, a stimulant medication was ceased 24 hours before laboratory measurements. However, parents completed the subjective scales (Child Behaviour Checklist and Conners' Rating Scales) while the children were still receiving stimulant medication. This may have influenced the results by masking their symptoms and making it difficult to detect any improvements. Moreover, children who had experienced ineffective treatment with stimulant medication or had a previous diagnosis of mood, anxiety, thought, or bipolar disorder were excluded from the study. Presumably, the rationale for this was to select a group of children with "pure" ADHD symptoms. This may not be entirely practical due to the high co-morbidity prevalent in ADHD, and, as discussed below, the heterogeneity of ADHD and its overlap with other neurodevelopmental disorders need to be explored within a phospholipid framework (Richardson, 2003a).

Another study using both DHA and EPA (Hirayama et al., 2004) also found no significant treatment effects of fish oil-enriched bread (supplying 3600 mg of DHA and 700 g of EPA weekly) on symptoms of ADHD in a two-month placebo-controlled, double-blind trial with 40 children ages 6–12 years who were mostly drug-free (34/40). The placebo bread contained olive oil. Paradoxically, the control group had significant improvements on visual short-term memory and errors of commission, possibly due to practice effects. These improvements were not seen in the treatment group. Blood samples were not measured so it is not clear whether this sample had low n-3 PUFA levels at baseline. Given that the study was conducted in Japan, known to have a high fish consumption, it is likely that baseline levels were relatively high. It is also possible that two months may have been an insufficient time for effects to become observable, as it may take longer to elevate the fatty acid composition of neural membranes (Bourre et al., 1989; Moriguchi et al., 2001).

The other five interventions reported improvements in symptoms with a combination of n-6 and n-3 PUFAs, including both EPA and DHA. In a pilot study, 41 British children ages 8–12 years with ADHD-related symptoms and specific learning disabilities (dyslexia) were given a PUFA supplement or olive-oil placebo over 12 weeks (Richardson & Puri, 2002). The PUFA supplement in this study provided a daily dose of 186 mg of EPA, 480 mg of DHA, 864 mg of LA, and 42 mg of AA, as well as $\alpha$-tocopherol (vitamin E). These children all had above-average scores on parent ratings of ADHD symptoms and average general ability yet low reading achievement. Baseline measures on learning and behavior did not differ between the groups, but the PUFA group showed improvements on global ADHD indices and subscale ratings of cognitive problems/inattention, hyperactivity, restlessness/impulsivity, psychosomatic complaints, and anxiety/shyness on the Conners' Parent Rating Scale following 12 weeks of supplementation, with medium-effect sizes reported.

Similarly, another study investigated the effects of PUFA supplementation, providing a daily dose of 80 mg of EPA, 480 mg of DHA, 40 mg of AA, 96 g of GLA, and 24 mg of $\alpha$-tocopherol, or olive-oil placebo over four months in American children with ADHD-like symptoms, selected for thirst and skin problems indicative of a fatty acid deficiency (Stevens et al., 2003). Plasma proportions of DHA, EPA, and α-tocopherol increased in the intervention group following supplementation, and a significant drop occurred in n-6 to n-3 ratios, although the olive-oil group demonstrated a small increase in ALA. Significant treatment effects were found for only 2 of 16 outcome measures compared to placebo: parent ratings of conduct and teacher ratings of attention. Oppositional defiant-behavior scores significantly improved from clinical to nonclinical levels, and significant relationships were reported between changes in RBC PUFA and the magnitude of outcome measures. Increased levels of EPA and DHA were associated with decreases in teacher ratings of inattention and increased levels of EPA with parent ratings of reduced disruptive behavior. Methodological issues in this study included increased n-3 plasma levels in the placebo (olive oil) group and the small sample size ($n$ = 50 plus 17 dropouts).

Two larger double-blind, placebo-controlled trials have been conducted to investigate the effects of PUFA on ADHD symptoms. The first study (Richardson & Montgomery, 2005) included 117 children diagnosed with dyspraxia, or Developmental Coordination Disorder (DCD), and a third of the sample had scores ≥2 SD above the population mean on the DSM-IV ADHD subscale of the Conners' Teacher Rating Scales (CTRS). The children were functioning, on average, about a year behind their chronological age in reading and spelling. The active supplement provided a high ratio of EPA:DHA with a daily dose of 552 mg of EPA, 168 mg of DHA, 60 mg of DGLA, and 9.6 mg of α-tocopherol. Although no improvements were detected on the core DCD symptom of poor motor function, significant improvements were reported in reading, spelling, and behavior in the treatment group compared to placebo over three months, and significant treatment effects were observed for teacher ratings of oppositional behavior, cognitive problems/inattention, hyperactivity, anxiety/shyness, and global/DSM-IV ADHD indices. Following a one-way crossover to active treatment, the placebo group demonstrated similar improvements in mean scores, while the original treatment group's scores continued to improve.

The second intervention included 132 Australian children, all with ADHD symptoms >$90^{th}$ percentile and therefore in the clinical range for a possible diagnosis (Sinn & Bryan, 2007). Children received the same treatment as above (a daily dose of 552 mg of EPA, 168 mg of DHA, 60 mg of DGLA, and 9.6 mg of α-tocopherol) with or without a micronutrient supplement or a placebo for 15 weeks, and then all groups crossed over to active treatment for a further 15 weeks. Significant improvements were observed on parent ratings of inattention, hyperactivity, and impulsivity in both PUFA groups over 15 weeks, which were then mirrored in the placebo group after switching to active treatment for 15 weeks. Objective improvements were found in the children's ability to switch and control their attention, and on vocabulary scores, and these mediated parent-reported improvements in hyperactivity, impulsivity, and inattention (Sinn et al., 2008). This study also found that the fatty acid-deficiency symptoms used as a selection criterion by Stevens et al. (2003) improved in both the treatment and placebo groups over 15 weeks, and concluded that these symptoms are more likely to be an indicator of n-6 rather than n-3 deficiency (Sinn, 2007).

A more recent study was conducted in Sweden with a similar supplement and study design as the previous two large trials but including 75 children ages 8–18 years with ADHD (Johnson et al., 2008). They found the response to supplementation similar to the previous two trials; however, when dividing the sample into subgroups according to co-morbid symptoms, they found that responders were more likely to have the inattentive subtype of ADHD and associated neurodevelopmental disorders (i.e., autistic symptoms and learning difficulties).

Therefore, evidence shows that children with ADHD-related symptoms may respond to PUFA supplementation and that those with the attention subtype and/or learning difficulties may be more likely to respond. Interestingly, studies using a combination of n-3 and n-6 fatty acids have been more effective than those with DHA or GLA (DGLA precursor) alone. However, the relative importance of EPA, DHA, and GLA remains to be determined due to methodological issues in other studies including small-sample size, length of supplementation, and selection criteria. Our group is currently investigating this in a three-way crossover study over 12 months comparing EPA-rich with DHA-rich oils versus a sunflower-oil placebo. This study is also measuring the RBC levels of PUFAs to help determine likely responders.

Functions of PUFA in neural membranes and synapses complement existing models of neurotransmitter actions in ADHD (Richardson & Puri, 2000). Symptoms of ADHD are particularly related to known symptoms of dopaminergic malfunction, such as problems with attention, motivation, and reactivity to stimuli and rewards. This is related to animal studies that linked n-3 deficiency to impaired dopaminergic systems, particularly in the frontal cortex of the brain (Zimmer et al., 2002). Further indications that are difficult to explain with a neurotransmitter model alone include the higher prevalence of ADHD and other neurological disorders such as schizophrenia, dyslexia, and dyspraxia in males. This is consistent with observations that males are more susceptible to EFA deficiencies (Richardson et al., 2000). Symptoms consistent with PUFA deficiency have also been observed in patients with schizophrenia (Horrobin, 1998), dyslexia (Baker, 1985), and autism and Asperger's syndrome (Bell et al., 2000). These indications provide further support for the hypothesis that the overlap between neurologically based disorders may be explained by phospholipid abnormalities (Horrobin, 1998; Richardson, 2003b). Considering the widespread prevalence of suboptimal n-3 levels, possibly maternal and dietary n-3 deficiencies result in behavioral disorders when combined with abnormalities in EFA metabolism. Furthermore, research suggests that genetic abnormalities in phospholipid metabolism may be exacerbated by environmental influences such as diet, stress, or pollution to create neurological deficits (Ward, 2000).

## *Other Developmental Disorders*

PUFAs have also been also implicated in other developmental disorders including dyslexia (Baker, 1985; Richardson et al., 2000; Stordy, 2000; Taylor et al., 2000;

Taylor & Richardson, 2000). Some evidence suggests that autism may involve functional deficiencies or imbalances in n-3 PUFAs. Studies on the profiles of PUFAs in children with autism that found defects of PUFAs and phospholipids, the major constituents of cell membranes, have had conflicting results. Vancassel et al. (2001) examined phospholipid fatty acids in the plasma of a population of children with autism compared to intellectually disabled controls. They reported a 23% reduction of DHA levels in the children with autism compared with controls. Reduced RBC levels of n-3 PUFAs and increased levels of saturated fatty acids (SFAs) were also reported in individuals with autism (Bell et al., 2000, 2004). Additionally, evidence shows that n-3 PUFAs can assist in inflammatory bowel disorders (Belluzi, 2002), which are often found in children with autism, and may play a role in the disorders' etiology (Horvath & Perman, 2002).

Few studies have investigated the effects of n-3 PUFA supplementation in autism. A case report noted improvements in the symptoms of a boy with autism following EPA supplementation that was increased from 1 g daily to 3 g daily over 4 weeks, with improvements continuing after an eight-month follow-up (Johnson & Hollander, 2003). An uncontrolled open-label study completed by 18 out of 20 children reported significant within-group improvements after three months of combined n-3, n-6, and n-9 PUFA supplementation (1 g/day) (Patrick & Salik, 2006). Only one randomized controlled trial (RCT) involving n-3 PUFA supplementation in autism has been published (Amminger et al., 2007). This six-week pilot RCT in 13 children with autism reported a trend for improvements in hyperactivity and stereotypy in the group receiving the n-3 PUFAs. Menhaden fish oil was used with daily doses of 840 mg of EPA and 700 mg of DHA.

A three-month crossover RCT was conducted in Durham by Dr. Madeleine Portwood, and is yet to be published. The daily doses of PUFAs used were 558 mg of EPA and 174 mg of DHA. Results regarding outcome measures were inconclusive and postulated to be due to a failure to reach a ceiling effect of the PUFAs over three months. After a one-way crossover, however, improvements were observed after six months of active n-3 PUFA supplementation. Therefore, further studies examining active versus placebo treatment over six months are warranted. Taken together, these studies highlight the importance of the length of supplementation relative to the dosage for any improvements to be observed. Considering the complexity of autism, n-3 PUFAs may also be best investigated as an adjunctive therapy.

## *Mental Retardation*

To date, fatty acid researchers have not focused specifically on the heterogeneous group of disorders that characterize mental retardation. Many people with mental retardation are likely to display co-morbid symptoms including hyperactivity, impulsivity, aggression, anxiety, and DSM-IV diagnosed psychiatric disorders such as bipolar disorder, schizophrenia (Zimmerman et al., 1998), and ADHD (Miller et al., 2004), and the high rate of psychiatric disorders in children and adolescents with mental retardation might be a major problem in their functioning and adaptation

(Phelps et al., 2002). The impact of PUFAs for the amelioration of learning, cognition, and behavior-control problems in developmental disorders like ADHD may have implications for the treatment of these same difficulties in people with mental retardation. This is important, particularly because indications show that some forms of mental retardation might be caused by defects in the structure and functioning of neural synapses (Chechlacz & Gleeson, 2003), which are rich in the n-3 PUFA DHA. For a more in-depth discussion of this, see Sinn and Wilson (2006).

## Depression

PUFA deficiency is also implicated in depression. Along with CVD, depression seems to be more prevalent in countries where fish consumption is lower, after controlling for demographic variables and potentially confounding factors such as alcohol intake (Hibbeln et al., 1998a; Hibbeln & Salem, Jr., 1995; Peet, 2004; Tanskanen et al., 2001a; Tanskanen et al., 2001b). It is well established that depression often co-occurs with CVD, which is associated with elevated cholesterol and lower PUFA levels, and studies have confirmed that depression does not result from CVD since it has been found to exist before symptoms of CVD set in (Horrobin & Bennett, 1999). Indicative of a common underlying biological component, higher serum AA:EPA ratios were reported in depressed post-myocardial infarction patients (Schins et al., 2007), and lower total n-3 PUFA and DHA levels were reported in depressed patients recovering from acute coronary syndromes (Frasure-Smith et al., 2004) than similar patients without depression. Shared PUFA abnormalities might further account for the depression that co-occurs with stress, post-natal depression, autoimmune diseases, multiple sclerosis, cancer, diabetes, aging, and osteoporosis (Horrobin & Bennett, 1999). Depression is also very common in alcoholics, which is explained by the lipid oxidation that results from heavy alcohol consumption (Hibbeln & Salem, Jr., 1995).

Research has also found lower levels of serum DHA and total n-3 PUFAs in postpartum depression (De Vriese et al., 2003). However, other research found no difference between the dietary intakes of n-3 PUFAs of depressed and nondepressed Australian women after controlling for age, weight, and smoking status, although average intakes of n-3 PUFAs were below recommendations and rates of depression were higher than expected across the sample (Jacka et al., 2004). A study of 20 moderately to severely depressed patients found a positive relationship between the severity of depression and the AA/EPA (n-6:n-3) phospholipid ratio (Adams et al., 1996). A large, comprehensive epidemiological study also found significantly higher blood ratios of n-6 to n-3 PUFA in elderly people with depressive disorders than in controls (Tiemeier et al., 2003) after controlling for potentially confounding variables. A comparison between 34 volunteers suffering major depression and 14 healthy controls found lower levels of EPA, AA, and the AA/EPA ratio in serum phospholipids as well as a relationship between serum zinc levels (a marker of inflammatory response activation) and n-3 PUFAs EPA and DHA (Maes et al., 1999).

This relationship between n-3 PUFAs, depression, and inflammatory markers is further supported by data from 43 older adults that showed higher n-6:n-3 ratios and tumor necrosis factor-$\alpha$ and interleukin-6 levels as depressive symptoms worsened (Kiecolt-Glaser et al., 2007). In another study, the RBC content and the dietary intake of n-3 PUFAs, notably DHA, were found to be significantly lower in 10 patients diagnosed with a major depressive episode than 14 matched controls, and again there was a significant relationship between the degree of n-3 PUFA deficiency and severity of depression (Edwards et al., 1998). These correlations were not found with any of the n-6 PUFAs. Similarly, Peet et al. (1998) found significantly less n-3 PUFAs, particularly DHA, in depressed patients than in controls, and they further reported evidence of oxidative damage in the depressed patients. Finally, a study into 44 randomly selected patients with a recurrent form of major depressive disorder found lower levels of DPA and DHA in RBCs compared with laboratory reference values even though most of the patients were clinically recovered at the time, suggesting that these fatty acid alterations may represent a biological trait marker for recurrent depression (Assies et al., 2004). A case study reported an improvement in treatment-resistant depression when EPA was added to the conventional treatment, and was associated with reduced neuronal phospholipid turnover and structural brain changes over the nine months of treatment (Puri et al., 2001).

Eight clinical trials have investigated the effects of n-3 PUFA supplementation on unipolar depression, with improvements reported in five of these studies (for reviews, see Sinclair et al., 2007; Stahl et al., 2008). Four of these studies used high EPA supplements. In a small dose-ranging study, treatment with 1 g/day of ethyl-EPA, but not 2 or 4 g/day, was effective in improving depressive symptoms in adults with ongoing depression while continuing their standard medication (Peet & Horrobin, 2002). However, another small study reported positive treatment effects with 2 g of ethyl-EPA as an adjunctive therapy compared with placebo over four weeks (Nemets et al., 2002). Blood samples were not collected in either of the latter studies. After 8 weeks of supplementation with 9.6 g of n-3 PUFAs daily (4.4 g of EPA, 2.2 g of DHA) as an adjunctive therapy (Su et al., 2003), patients in the n-3 PUFA group had significantly lower depression scores than the control group ($P < .001$). Importantly, this team collected blood samples and reported average baseline blood DHA levels of 2.5% of fatty acids in the placebo group and 2.4% in the treatment group (the latter increased to 5.8% in the DHA group after treatment). Finally, some recent evidence shows that 1 g/day of EPA has similar therapeutic effects as 20 mg/day of fluoxetine as a treatment for major depression over eight weeks and that using the two treatments in combination is superior to either of them alone (Jazayeri et al., 2008).

Three larger studies using DHA or DHA-rich oils did not report improvements following n-3 supplementation. One of these studies supplemented patients with 2 g of DHA for only six weeks as a monotherapy (Marangell et al., 2003); one supplied 0.6 g of EPA + 2.4 g of DHA as an adjunctive therapy for 12 weeks (Silvers et al., 2005); and the largest study gave a similar dosage as an adjunctive therapy for 16 weeks (Grenyer et al., 2007). Interestingly though, two of these studies collected blood samples revealing normal baseline n-3 levels; Marangell et al. (2003) reported that the DHA group and the placebo group had 4.15% and 3.78% of DHA as a percentage of total fatty acids at baseline, respectively, and Grenyer et al. (2007) reported baseline DHA as 4.2% of total RBC fatty acids (Meyer et al., 2004). Although reductions in depression scores did not differ between the groups, the latter study reported that increased DHA levels were significantly associated with improvements in depression scores, warranting further research into DHA and depression. Therefore studies using high EPA supplements should also determine to what extent the EPA was converted to DHA and which of these is associated with improvements.

In the largest study to date, Rogers et al. (2008) randomized a community sample of 190 individuals with mild to moderate depression to a combined EPA + DHA supplement (1.5 g/day) or an olive-oil placebo for 12 weeks. They did not report any favorable effects of the supplement on depressed symptoms or a range of outcomes, and concluded that this supports a negligible effect of n-3 on depression. However, they did not use the Hamilton Depression Rating Scales (HDRS) which was generally used as a primary outcome measure by the other studies, thereby reducing comparability. Although they took blood samples, they measured fatty acid levels in plasma rather than RBCs. In any case, note that other studies reporting improvements in depression scores tended to use inpatients with more severe depression, many of whom were treatment-resistant.

## *Bipolar Disorder*

A controlled study comparing RBC PUFA levels in 20 bipolar patients with healthy matched controls found significantly lower AA and DHA levels in the bipolar patients but no difference in EPA, AA/EPA ratios or total n-3 and n-6 fatty acids (Chiu et al., 2003). Clinical variables such as age, age at disease onset, number of episodes, and length of illness were not related to DHA and AA levels, and also no difference was noted between smokers and nonsmokers.

Stoll et al. (1999) conducted one of the pioneering intervention trials on n-3 fatty acids and psychopathology. A placebo-controlled, double-blind clinical trial with bipolar disorder patients produced a significantly greater response to treatment (64%) in the n-3 PUFA group than in those given olive oil placebos (18.8%). In this study, patients received fish-oil capsules containing a total of 6.2 g of EPA and 3.4 g of DHA daily over four months, with no adverse effects overall. Since then, another five studies have been conducted with bipolar patients. Only one of these reported improvements in an open-label study ($n$ = 12) providing 1.5–2 g of ethyl EPA for 24 weeks as an adjunctive therapy in patients diagnosed with bipolar disorder (Osher et al., 2005). Although no control group was used, at one month 7/10 of these previously treatment-resistant patients showed a ≥50% reduction in HDRS scores, and scores in five completers were dramatically reduced at six months. The other placebo-controlled studies all provided ethyl EPA as an adjunctive therapy, supplying

1–2 g for 12 weeks (Frangou et al., 2006), 6 g for 16 weeks (Keck et al., 2006), and 2 g for 12 weeks, with no reported improvements in symptoms. None of these studies took blood samples.

Treatment with n-3 PUFAs in an uncontrolled study with a small group of women with bipolar disorder also found no significant improvement over four weeks, but reported alterations in a marker of membrane fluidity in the n-3 groups compared with bipolar patients not taking n-3s and healthy controls (Hirashima et al., 2004). Therefore, in summary, the only controlled study that improved bipolar symptoms provided a large-dose combination of EPA and DHA over four months.

## Suicidal Ideation

Depression and bipolar disorder are often associated with suicidal ideation. The relationship between PUFAs, increased suicide risk, and related disorders is considered in a review by Brunner and colleagues (2002), who report an association between low cholesterol and a higher risk of suicide. A group of researchers in China investigated this and found significantly lower levels of EPA, DHA, and total n-3 PUFAs in the RBC of suicide-attempt cases compared to matched controls (Huan et al., 2004). These cases also had significantly higher levels of stearic acid, a saturated fat which in excess can reduce membrane fluidity. According to the researchers though, most suicide attempts in China are related to stress rather than to depression.

A recent study investigated an n-3 PUFA supplementation in adults with recurrent nonfatal self-harm, although researchers did not investigate the effect on completed suicide and the recurrence of self-harm due to the large sample size needed, but rather on psychometric measures (Hallahan et al., 2007). Daily supplementation with 2128 mg of EPA and DHA (1.2 g of EPA and 0.9 g of DHA) for 12 weeks improved psychopathology compared with a placebo in 49 participants with recurrent self-harm. Improvements were seen in scores for depression, suicide, and daily stresses. These improvements were not seen in measures of impulsivity, aggression, and hostility, in contrast to studies that indicate an effect of n-3 PUFAs on these measures as discussed in the Aggression, Hostility, Impulsivity, Criminal, and Antisocial Behavior section of this chapter, perhaps because hostility and aggression were not primary problems for this sample. Note that all participants continued to receive standard psychiatric care including changes to their psychotropic medication during the 12 weeks. Therefore, the effects of n-3 PUFA supplementation on self-harm and suicide ideation need further investigation.

## Schizophrenia

Numerous indications suggest that phospholipid abnormalities may help to explain biological underpinnings of schizophrenia (Fenton et al., 2000; Horrobin, 1997, 1998; Peet, 2003; Puri & Richardson, 1998). In particular, low n-3 fatty acid levels in diets or RBCs have consistently been found in people with schizophrenic symptoms compared to controls (Arvindakshan et al., 2003; Assies et al., 2001; Kale et al., 2008;

Peet et al., 1996; Richardson et al., 2003). Interestingly, one of these found similar plasma n-3 PUFA levels between first-episode schizophrenic patients and controls, but lower RBC proportions of DHA in the schizophrenic group, indicating a need for analysis of RBCs rather than plasma. Clinical trials with schizophrenia have reported mostly positive results. In a controlled clinical trial with 20 schizophrenic patients, significant improvements in symptoms were found after daily supplementation with 10 g of fish oil over six weeks. These improvements were correlated with increases in blood levels of n-3 fatty acids (Laugharne et al., 1996). Four other double-blind controlled trials with EPA supplementation also produced significant, positive outcomes (Emsley et al., 2002; Peet et al., 2001; Peet & Horrobin, 2002).

However, another trial found no differences between schizophrenic patients given ethyl EPA and those given placebo over 16 weeks (Fenton et al., 2001). As the researchers noted, participants in this study were older and had experienced symptoms for a longer time than those in previous studies. Horrobin (2003) proposed a number of reasons why an effect was not obtained, including the possibility that ethyl EPA may not have therapeutic benefits. Hibbeln et al. (2003) investigated possible confounding variables using the same data set, and found that PUFA status in schizophrenic patients was predicted by smoking status, gender, and dietary intake of n-3 fatty acids. They concluded that phospholipid abnormalities may be an artifact of these variables. However, Emsley et al. (2002) found significant differences between the active and placebo groups after controlling for age, gender, length of illness, and dietary n-3 intake.

In another recent study (Arvindakshan et al., 2003), schizophrenic patients were matched with healthy controls on a number of factors known to influence PUFA status including age, gender, dietary patterns, smoking, and substance abuse. Schizophrenic patients still had significantly lower levels of EPA and DHA and elevated levels of AA than controls, although few smokers were in these groups. Therefore, other studies with schizophrenic patients found significantly lower PUFA levels that were not accounted for by variables such as age, gender, smoking, or dietary n-3 intake. Arvindakshan et al. (2003) then gave patients in their study a combination of EPA, DHA, and antioxidants (vitamins E and C) over four months; no placebo group was used. The researchers reported significant within-group improvements on various measures of psychopathology between pre- and post-treatment, and these improvements continued for four months after the treatment was discontinued.

## *Aggression, Hostility, Impulsivity, Criminal, and Antisocial Behavior*

A biological basis for criminal-related behavior was indicated by a number of studies. Low concentrations of cerebrospinal fluid 5-hydroxyindoleacetic acid (CSF 5-HIAA), a marker of cerebral serotonin turnover, were consistently associated with impulsive, violent, suicidal, hostile, and aggressive behaviors, as well as an early onset of alcohol dependence and personality disorders (Hallahan & Garland, 2004; Hibbeln et al., 1998b). Low-PUFA status was also associated with deficient serotonergic neurotransmission (Chalon, 2001, 2006), and possibly, low CSF 5-HIAA reflects this deficiency.

A few studies have investigated plasma phospholipids in people with aggressive and related behaviors. An earlier study compared the plasma phospholipid fatty acids between violent, impulsive offenders with intermittent explosive disorder; violent, impulsive offenders with an antisocial personality disorder; and a control group (total $N = 50$) (Virkkunen et al., 1987). Both offender groups had significantly higher levels of n-6 fatty acids DGLA, adrenic acid, and DPA; the latter may be indicative of a DHA deficiency in the brain (Chalon et al., 2001; Hamilton et al., 2000; Lauritzen et al., 2001; Moriguchi et al., 2001; Wainwright et al., 1999; Youdim et al., 2000). Accordingly, the offending groups both had lower plasma DHA levels, although only the antisocial group's levels reached statistical significance.

Hibbeln et al. (1998b) investigated the relationship between CSF 5-HIAA and DHA in blood plasma in a group of alcohol-dependent people with a history of violent/impulsive behavior, compared with a group of nonviolent controls matched for their severity of alcohol dependence. Surprisingly, a negative correlation was found between CSF 5-HIAA and DHA in the violent group only, replicating a previous finding of similar magnitude. They suggested that violent individuals might have a defect in the incorporation of DHA into neural membranes, resulting in a buildup of DHA in plasma, and that supplementation with high doses of DHA may therefore normalize serotonin function among impulsive, violent people. As the authors note, however, these relationships need to be further explored and experimentally tested before any conclusions are drawn.

A similar study compared plasma PUFA levels in cocaine addicts with a history of aggression and nonaggressive cocaine addicts upon admission to an inpatient substance-abuse unit. The aggressive group had significantly lower levels of DPA, DHA and total n-3 EFA, and a higher n-3:n-6 ratio. However, nearly three weeks after admission, the n-3 levels had risen in the aggressive group and the differences became nonsignificant. This may have been due to poor dietary n-3 intake before admission which contributed to their aggression levels (Buydens-Branchey et al., 2003). A large study investigating risk factors for heart disease in 3581 young adults reported an association of fish and PUFA consumption with hostility in a cross-sectional analysis (Iribarren et al., 2004). As with depression, hostility was previously associated with CVD. Consistent with the relationship between violence and low n-3 PUFAs shown in the other studies, a dietary intake of n-3–rich fish was significantly associated with reduced hostility.

A few clinical trials investigated the impact of PUFA supplementation on aggressive behavior. A double-blind, placebo-controlled study measured the effects of daily supplementation with oil containing 49.3% (1.5 g) of DHA, 6.7% of EPA, 7.3% of oleic acid, 3.3% of AA, and other oils for three months on cognitive outcomes and aggression in a group of 41 healthy Japanese students from two different universities (Hamazaki et al., 1996). The placebo capsules contained small amounts of LA and ALA. No differences between groups were observed on cognitive and dementia tests, but a significant difference between the groups was reported in aggression toward others ("extraggression") at the end of the study, which ended in the middle of a highly stressful final-exam period. Extraggression scores significantly increased in the control groups and decreased (though not significantly) in the DHA-supplemented groups. Serum blood analyses confirmed a significant increase in EPA and DHA levels in the treatment groups. Therefore three months' supplementation with n-3 PUFAs seemed to assist students in controlling aggression toward others on a psychological test during a period of high stress.

Another double-blind study tested the effects of supplementation with 1 g of ethyl-EPA daily or a placebo over eight weeks on moderate borderline personality disorder, characterized by emotional reactivity and impulsive aggression, in a group of women (Zanarini & Frankenburg, 2003). The treatment group had a significantly greater decrease in depression and aggression scores at the end of the study.

A randomized, placebo-controlled trial was undertaken with 231 young adult prisoners to investigate the effects of supplementation with micronutrients and EFAs over four to five months on antisocial behavior (Gesch et al., 2002). The participants were given multivitamin/mineral capsules and a fatty acid supplement providing n-3 and n-6 fatty acids (1260 mg of LA, 160 mg of GLA, 80 mg of EPA, and 44 mg of DHA daily) or placebos. Over the period of the trial, the treatment group received significantly fewer disciplinary actions, and the greatest effect was noted for violent behavior. These studies add an important dimension to research with PUFAs in ADHD, which is commonly associated with antisocial behavior, symptomatic of conduct disorder and oppositional defiant disorder in childhood (Colledge & Blair, 2001; Crowley et al., 1998; Root & Resnick, 2003) and criminality and antisocial behavior in late adolescence and adulthood (Biederman et al., 1996; Ingram et al., 1999).

Recently, a small randomized controlled trial involving 24 men with substance abuse found that supplementation with 3 g of n-3 PUFAs for three months improved self-reported scores of anger and anxiety compared to a soybean-oil placebo (Buydens-Branchey et al., 2008; Buydens-Branchey & Branchey, 2008). The active group received five capsules daily, each containing 450 mg of EPA, 100 mg of DHA, and 50 mg of n-3 PUFAs ALA and DPA. Although five participants in both the placebo and active groups were on antidepressant medication during the study, their doses remained stable. Interestingly, the anger ratings remained lower in the active group for three months after the supplementation ceased. Each participant's n-3 PUFA intake was calculated based on a diet questionnaire covering the month preceding the study, and the participants had a daily intake of LC n-3 PUFAs of 148 mg, only 30% of the ISSFAL-recommended intake of 500 mg/day. Furthermore, those participants who reported a history of violent behavior had a significantly lower LC n-3 PUFA intake compared to those who had no history of this behavior. This suggested link between LC n-3 PUFA intake and violence was not seen for short-chain n-3 or any of the n-6 PUFAs. Plasma levels of LC n-3 PUFAs increased only in the treatment group after three months of supplementation (Buydens-Branchey et al., 2008). After the three-month treatment with LC n-3 PUFAs, a low-anxiety score was associated with an increase in EPA but not DHA, whereas a low anger score was associated more strongly with DHA. This indicates a possible variation between the two LC n-3 PUFAs in their effect on psychiatric conditions, and warrants a comparison of them in further research.

## *Dementia and Alzheimer's Disease*

Free radical activity and phospholipid membrane degeneration have been associated with neurodegenerative disorders (Tacconi et al., 1997). With aging, neural membrane fluidity is generally compromised due to an increase in cholesterol, reduced activity level of desaturase enzymes, impaired phospholipid metabolism, and an increased oxidative stress (Yehuda et al., 2002). Such derangements may be associated with dementia and Alzheimer's Disease (AD); for example, autopsied brains of patients who suffered AD showed significantly higher saturated fat and lower PUFA content, particularly DHA, in the hippocampus and frontal lobes compared to aged controls (Söderberg et al., 1991), which is consistent with reports of decreased hippocampus size and function in AD patients (Yehuda et al., 2002).

Prospective cohort/population studies indicate that higher fish consumption is associated with a reduced risk of dementia/AD (Issa et al., 2006). A prospective two-year follow-up of a population-based study with over 5,000 people ages 55+ in Rotterdam found that lower fish consumption at baseline was related to an increased incidence of dementia and AD after controlling for likely confounders (Kalmijn et al., 1997). An increased risk of dementia was also associated with high intakes of total fat, saturated fat, and cholesterol. However, a later follow-up of the same Rotterdam cohort did not find a significant association between high saturated fat/ low-PUFA intake and dementia or AD (Engelhart et al., 2002). Possible methodological issues are discussed such as selective survival (i.e., the possibility that those who did not die of CVD before follow-up were less likely to develop dementia). Also a lower incidence of dementia occurred in survivors, particularly vascular dementia which was previously associated with lower fish consumption. An investigation of data from a Zutphen elderly study found an inverse relationship between fish-oil consumption and cognitive impairment and decline (Kalmijn, 2000). In a prospective study investigating risk factors for AD, participants who ate fish weekly or more had a 60% less chance of developing AD. This outcome became significant after controlling for risk factors such as age, race, education, and total energy intake, and was associated with DHA but not EPA intake (Morris et al., 2003).

Three further studies were published more recently. One study assessed cognitive performance in 404 men and women ages 50–70 over three years and found that those with higher plasma n-3 PUFA levels showed less decline over three years in sensorimotor speed and complex speed but not in memory, information-processing speed, or word fluency. Cross-sectional analyses at baseline showed no associations between n-3 PUFA levels and cognitive performance on these measures (Dullemeijer et al., 2007). A limitation of this study may be that it investigated n-3 PUFAs in plasma and not RBCs. The second study, a cross-sectional investigation of fish intake and cognitive performance in 2031 men and women ages 70–74, found significant associations between higher fish/fish oil intake and a range of cognitive measures including executive function, memory, visuospatial skills, and global cognitive functioning (Mini-Mental State Examination; MMSE) after controlling for multiple confounders (Nurk et al., 2007). The third, a prospective study, found that the consumption of fish was associated with a reduced risk of dementia and AD in 8085 adults of ages over 65, but only in non-apoE ε4 carriers (Barberger-Gateau et al., 2007). This supported the results of another study that found a 28% reduced risk of dementia in 2233 participants, also in those without the apoE ε4 allele (Huang et al., 2005).

A single case report of an elderly dementia patient noted a clinical improvement over several months of increased fish consumption, which led the author to hypothesize that n-3 PUFAs contributed to his improved functioning, although it could have been attributed to numerous other factors associated with admittance to a nursing home (Peers, 1990). An investigation of the n-3 PUFA status in AD patients did find significantly reduced EPA and DHA levels compared to controls, particularly DHA levels which were consistently less than half those in the control group (Tully et al., 2003). These patients also had higher ALA:DHA ratios, suggesting a reduced activity of desaturase enzymes involved in ALA conversion.

Relatively few controlled studies have investigated the effects of n-3 PUFA supplementation on dementia to date. In a short four-week double-blind trial with 100 AD patients, numerous improvements in symptoms were reported in 49 of the 60 patients who received an n-3/n-6 supplement comprised of 0.5 g of ALA and LA in a 1:4 ratio (Yehuda et al., 1996).

Supplementation with 4.32 g of DHA daily for one year improved dementia scores of 10 elderly volunteers with vascular dementia when compared with 10 controls who did not receive capsules (Terano et al., 1999). Another pilot study involving 19 participants with mild to moderate AD treated with 1000 mg/day of EPA for 12 weeks showed no improvement in cognitive functioning, possibly due to the short period of supplementation and/or the nature of the supplement formulation (Boston et al., 2004). Supplementation with a combination of DHA and AA totalling 240 mg/day improved immediate memory and attention in 12 adults with mild cognitive impairment (MCI) but not 8 adults with AD when compared to an olive-oil MCI placebo group (Kotani et al., 2006). In the largest study to date with 174 volunteers with diagnosed AD, only those with very mild AD showed reductions in cognitive decline after adjunctive supplementation with 1700 mg/day of DHA and 600 mg/day of EPA (Freund-Levi et al., 2006). Similarly, a study recently published online also reported improvements relative to placebo in MCI but not AD patients following supplementation with 1.8 g of n-3 PUFAs (1080 mg of EPA, 720 mg of DHA) over

24 weeks (Chiu et al., 2008). These studies indicate that the early stages of cognitive decline may be optimal for an intervention with n-3 PUFAs. MCI is considered a risk factor for AD, with an estimated 16–41% of people with MCI converting to a diagnosis of AD each year and up to 64% after two years. Therefore, MCI is possibly the earliest stage of detectable AD (Gauthier et al., 2006). Furthermore, major and minor depression often occur in MCI (Gabryelewicz et al., 2004) and increase the risk of progressing to AD (Modrego & Ferrández, 2004).

This research highlights the need for further investigation of the role of PUFAs in dementia, focusing on larger sample sizes, the nature of the supplement (e.g., EPA versus DHA), dosage, length of supplementation, baseline RBC n-3 PUFA proportions, response in ApoE ε4 allele carriers, longer-term outcomes, and therapeutic implications. Finally, cardiovascular risk factors for AD led to recent suggestions that lifestyle factors such as inadequate physical activity and/or n-3 PUFA intake may contribute to reduced cerebral blood flow and blood-brain barrier integrity (Hooijmans & Kiliaan, 2008), supporting the notion that one of the primary functions of n-3 PUFAs on mental health may be improved circulatory function (Sinn & Howe, 2008). This should also be explored in future research.

## Conclusion

Growing evidence shows that suboptimal intakes of n-3 PUFAs are associated with psychopathology across the lifespan, and include highly prevalent disorders that present a growing public-health concern. Most clinical trials have been conducted with ADHD in childhood and with major depression in adulthood, but there are growing numbers of interventions with cognitive decline and dementia in older adulthood. Although the causes of these mental-health problems are clearly multifactorial, dietary and lifestyle factors including n-3 PUFAs present modifiable risk factors that individuals can access relatively easily.

The findings of clinical trials have been inconsistent and in some cases inconclusive; methodological differences between studies need to be identified and critically evaluated before drawing conclusions about the efficacy or otherwise of n-3 PUFAs in alleviating symptoms. These include sample size, selection criteria, the dosage of the supplement, the nature of the fatty acids (i.e., EPA- or DHA-rich or combined oil; inclusion of n-6 PUFAs), and length of supplementation. Most importantly, studies need to identify the baseline n-3 PUFA levels in RBCs because they may be a major contributor to different findings between studies. This will assist researchers and clinicians in identifying likely responders. Future research also needs to define long-term outcomes and optimal supplementation strategies including combinations with other nutrients that are consumed suboptimally.

### References

Adams, P.B.; S. Lawson; A. Sanigorski; A.J. Sinclair. Arachidonic acid to eicosapentaenoic acid ratio in blood correlates positively with clinical symptoms of depression. *Lipids* **1996,** *31(Suppl.)*, S157–161.

Aman, M.G.; E.A.Mitchell; S.H. Turbott. The effects of essential fatty acid supplementation by Efamol in hyperactive children. *J. Abnormal Child Psychology* **1987,** *15(1),* 75–90.

Amminger, G.P.; G.E. Berger; M.R. Schäfer; C. Klier; M.H. Friedrich;M. Feucht. Omega-3 fatty acids supplementation in children with autism: A double-blind randomized, placebo-controlled pilot study. *Biol. Psychiatry* **2007,** *61(4)*, 551–553.

Arnold, L.E.; D. Kleykamp; N.A. Votolato; W.A. Taylor; S.B. Kontras; K. Tobin. Gamma-linolenic acid for attention-deficit hyperactivity disorder: placebo-controlled comparison to D-amphetamine. *Biol. Psychiatry* **1989,** *25*, 222–228.

Arvindakshan, M.; M. Ghate; P. Ranjekar; D.R. Evans; S.P. Mahadik. Supplementation with a combination of ω-3 fatty acids and antioxidants (vitamins E and C) improves the outcome of schizophrenia. *Schizophrenia Res.* **2003,** *62*, 195–204.

Assies, J.; R. Lieverse; P. Vreken; R.J.A. Wanders; P.M.J.A. Dingemans; D.H. Linszen. Significantly reduced docosahexaenoic and docosapentaenoic acid concentrations in erythrocyte membranes from schizophrenic patients compared with a carefully matched control group. *Biol. Psychiatry* **2001,** *49(6),* 510–522.

Assies, J.; A. Lok; C.L. Bockting; G.J. Weverling; R. Lieverse; I. Visser; et al. Fatty acids and homocysteine levels in patients with recurrent depression: an explorative pilot study. *Prostaglandins, Leukotrienes Essent. Fatty Acids* **2004,** *70,* 349–356.

Assisi, A.; R. Banzi; C. Buoinocore; F. Capasso; V.D. Muzio; F. Michelacci; et al. Fish oil and mental health: the role of n-3 long-chain polyunsaturated fatty acids in cognitive development and neurological disorders. *Int. Clin. Psychopharmacology* **2006,** *21(6),* 319–336.

Baker, S.M. A biochemical approach to the problem of dyslexia. *J. Learning Disabilities,* **1985,** *18(10),* 581–584.

Barberger-Gateau, P.; C. Raffaitin; L. Letenneur; C. Berr; C. Tzourio;J.F. Dartigues; et al. Dietary patterns and risk of dementia: the three-city cohort study. *Neurology* **2007,** *69,* 1921–1930.

Bell, J.G.; E.E. MacKinlay; J.R. Dick; D.J. MacDonald; R.M. Boyle; A.C.A. Glen. Essential fatty acids and phospholipase A2 in autistic spectrum disorders. *Prostaglandins, Leukotrienes Essent. Fatty Acids* **2004,** *71*, 201–204.

Bell, J.G.; J.R. Sargent; D.R. Tocher; J.R. Dick. Red blood cell fatty acid compositions in a patient with autistic spectrum disorder: a characteristic abnormality in neurodevelopmental disorders? *Prostaglandins, Leukotrienes Essent. Fatty Acids* **2000,** *63(2/1),* 21–25.

Belluzi, A. n-3 fatty acids for the treatment of inflammatory bowel diseases. *Proceedings of the Nutrition Society, 2002*(61).

Biederman, J.; S. Faraone; E. Mick; J. Wozniak; L. Chen; C. Ouellette; et al. Attention-deficit hyperactivity disorder and juvenile mania: an overlooked comorbidity? *J. Am. Academy of Child and Adolescent Psychiatry* **1996,** *35*, 997–1008.

Boston, P.F.; A. Bennett; D.F. Horrobin; C.N. Bennett. Ethyl-EPA in Alzheimer's disease—a pilot study. *Prostaglandins, Leukotrienes Essent. Fatty Acids* **2004,** *71*, 341–346.

Bourre, J.-M.; G. Durand; G. Pascal; A. Youyou. Brain cell and tissue recovery in rats made deficient in n-3 fatty acids by alteration of dietary fat. *J. Nutr.* **1989,** *119*(1), 15–22.

Brunner, J.; K.G. Parhofer; P. Schwandt; T. Bronisch. Cholesterol, essential fatty acids, and suicide. *Pharmacopsychiatry,* **2002,** *35(1),* 1–5.

Burgess, J.R.; L.J. Stevens; W. Zhang; L. Peck. Long-chain polyunsaturated fatty acids in children with attention-deficit hyperactivity disorder. *Am. J. Clin. Nutr.* **2000,** *71(1),* 327–330.

Buydens-Branchey, L.; M. Branchey. Long-chain n-3 polyunsaturated fatty acids decrease feelings of anger in substance abusers. *Psychiatry Res.* **2008,** *157(1–3),* 95–104.

Buydens-Branchey, L.; M. Branchey; J.R. Hibbeln. Associations between increases in plasma n-3 polyunsaturated fatty acids following supplementation and decreases in anger and anxiety in substance abusers. *Prog. Neuropsychopharmacol. Biol. Psychiatry* **2008,** *32(2),* 568–575.

Buydens-Branchey, L.; M. Branchey; D.L. McMakin; J.R. Hibbeln. Polyunsaturated fatty acid status and aggression in cocaine addicts. *Drug and Alcohol Dependence* **2003,** *71,* 319–323.

Chalon, S. Omega-3 fatty acids and monoamine neurotransmission. *Prostaglandins, Leukotrienes Essent. Fatty Acids* **2006,** *75,* 259–269.

Chalon, S.; S. Vancassel; L. Zimmer; D. Guilloteau; G. Durand. Polyunsaturated fatty acids and cerebral function: Focus on monoaminergic neurotransmission. *Lipids* **2001,** *36*(9), 937–944.

Chechlacz, M.; J.G. Gleeson. Is mental retardation a defect of synapse structure and function? *Pediatr. Neurology* **2003,** *29(1),* 11–17.

Chen, J.-R.; S.-F. Hsu; C.-D. Hsu; L.-H. Hwang; S.-C. Yang. Dietary patterns and blood fatty acid composition in children with attention-deficit hyperactivity disorder in Taiwan. *J. Nutr. Biochemistry* **2004,** *15,* 467–472.

Chiu, C.-C.; S.-Y. Huang; K.-P. Su; M.-L. Lu; M.-C. Huang; C.-C. Chen; et al. Polyunsaturated fatty acid deficit in patients with bipolar mania. *European Neuropsychopharmacology* **2003,** *13,* 99–103.

Chiu, C.-C.; K.-P. Su; T.-C. Cheng; H.-C. Liu; C.-J. Chang; M.E. Dewey; et al. The effects of omega-3 fatty acids monotherapy in Alzheimer's disease and mild cognitive impairment: A preliminary randomized double-blind placebo-controlled study. *Progress in Neuro-Psychopharmalogy & Biological Psychiatry* **2008,** *doi: 10.1016/j.pnpbp.2008.05.015.*

Colledge, E.; R.J.R. Blair. The relationship in children between the inattention and impulsivity components of attention deficit and hyperactivity disorder and psychopathic tendencies. *Personality and Individual Differences* **2001,** *30,* 1175–1187.

Colquhoun, I.; S. Bunday. A lack of essential fatty acids as a possible cause of hyperactivity in children. *Med. Hypotheses* **1981,** *7,* 673–679.

Crawford, M.A.; A.J. Sinclair. *Nutritional Influences in the Evolution of Mammalian Brain.* Paper presented at the Lipids, Malnutrition and the Developing Brain; 1971.

Crowley, T.J.; S.K. Mikulich; M. MacDonald; S.E. Young; G.O. Zerbe. Substance-dependent, conduct-disordered adolescent males: severity of diagnosis predicts 2-year outcome. *Drug and Alcohol Dependence* **1998,** *49,* 225–237.

da Silva, A.X.; F. Lavialle; G. Gendrot; P. Guesnet; J.-M. Alessandri;M. Lavialle. Glucos transport and utilization are altered in the brain of rats deficient in n-3 polyunsaturated fatty acids. *J. Neurochem.* **2002,** *81,* 1328–1337.

De Vriese, S.R.; A.B. Christophe; M. Maes. Lowered serum n-3 polyunsaturated fatty acid (PUFA) levels predict the occurrence of postpartum depression: Further evidence that lowered n-PUFAs are related to major depression *Life Sci.* **2003,** *73(25),* 3181–3187.

Dullemeijer, C.; J. Durga; I.A. Brouwer; O. van de Rest; F.J. Kok;R.-J.M. Brummer; et al. n-3

Fatty acid proportions in plasma and cognitive performance in older adults. *Am. J. Clin. Nutr.* **2007,** *86*, 1479–1495.

Edwards, R.; M. Peet; J. Shay; D.F. Horrobin. Omega-3 polyunsaturated fatty acid levels in the diet and in red blood cell membranes of depressed patients. *J. Affective Disorders* **1998,** *48*, 149–155.

Emsley, R.; C. Myburgh; P. Oosthuizen; S.J. van Rensburg. Randomized, placebo-controlled study of ethyl-eicosapentaenoic acid as supplemental treatment in schizophrenia. *Am. J. Psychiatry* **2002,** *159(9),* 1596–1598.

Engelhart, M.J.; M.I. Geerlings; A. Ruitenberg; J.C. van Swieten; A. Hofman; J.C.M. Witteman; et al. Diet and risk of dementia: Does fat matter? *Neurology* **2002,** *59*, 1915–1921.

Fenton, W.S.; F. Dickerson; J. Boronow; J.R. Hibbeln; M. Knable. A placebo-controlled trial of omega-3 fatty acid (ethyl eicosapentaenoic acid) supplementation for residual symptoms and cognitive impairment in schizophrenia. *Am. J. Psychiatry* **2001,** *158*, 2071–2074.

Fenton, W.S.; J.R. Hibbeln; M. Knable. Essential fatty acids, lipid membrane abnormalities, and the diagnosis and treatment of schizophrenia. *Biol. Psychiatry* **2000,** *47*, 8–21.

Frangou, S.; M. Lewis; P. McCrone. Efficacy of ethyl-eicosapentaenoic acid in bipolar depression: randomised double-blind placebo-controlled study. *Br. J. of Psychiatry* **2006,** *188*, 46–50.

Frasure-Smith, N.; F. Lespérance; P. Julien. Major depression is associated with lower omega-3 fatty acid levels in patients with recent acute coronary syndromes. *Biol. Psychiatry* **2004,** *55*, 891–896.

Freund-Levi, Y.; M. Eriksdotter-Jönhagen; T. Cederholm; H. Basun; G. Faxen-Irving; A. Garlind; et al. ω-3 fatty acid treatment in 174 patients with mild to moderate Alzheimer Disease: OmegAD study. *Archives of Neurology* **2006,** *63*, 1402–1408.

Froehlich, J.C. Opioid peptides. *Alcohol Health & Research World* **1997,** *21(2)*, 132–136.

Gabryelewicz, T.; M. Styczynska; A. Pfeffer; B. Wasiak; A. Barczak; E. Luczywek; et al. Prevalence of major and minor depression in elderly persons with mild cognitive impairment—MADRS factor analysis. *International J. Geriatric Psychiatry* **2004,** *19*, 1168–1172.

Gamoh, S.; M. Hashimoto; K. Sugioka; M.S. Hossain; N. Hata; Y. Misawa;, et al. Chronic administration of docosahexaenoic acid improves reference memory-related learning ability in young rats. *Neuroscience* **1999,** *93*(1), 237–241.

Gauthier, S.; B. Reisberg; M. Zaudig; R. Peterson; K. Ritchie; K.Broich; et al. Mild cognitive impairment. *The Lancet* **2006,** *367(9518),* 1262–1270.

Gesch, C.B.; S.M. Hammond; S.E. Hampson; A. Eves; M.J. Crowder. Influence of supplementary vitamins, minerals and essential fatty acids on the behaviour of young adult prisoners. *Br. J. Psychiatry* **2002,** *181*, 22–28.

Grenyer, B.F.S.; T. Crowe; B. Meyer; A.J. Owen; E.M. Grigonis-Deane; P. Caputi; et al. Fish oil supplementation in the treatment of major depression: A randomised double-blind placebo-controlled trial. *Prog. Neuro-Psychopharmacol.Biol. Psychiatry* **2007,** *31*, 1393–1396.

Haag, M. Essential fatty acids and the brain. *Canadian J. Psychiatry* **2003,** *48(3),* 195–203.

Hallahan, B.; M.R. Garland; Essential fatty acids and their role in the treatment of impulsivity disorders. *Prostaglandins, LeukotrienesEssent. Fatty Acids* **2004,** *71*, 211–216.

Hallahan, B.; J.R. Hibbeln; J.M. Davis; M.R. Garland. Omega-3 fatty acid supplementation in patients with recurrent self-harm. Single-centre double-blind randomised controlled trial. *Br. J. Psychiatry* **2007,** *190,* 118–122.

Hamazaki, T.; S. Sawazaki; M. Itomura; E. Asaoka; Y. Nagao; N. Nishimura; et al. The effect of docosahexaenoic acid on aggression in young adults: a placebo controlled double-blind study. *J. Clin. Invest.* **1996,** *97(4),* 1129–1134.

Hamilton, J.; R. Greiner; N. Salem, Jr.; H.-Y. Kim. n-3 fatty acid deficiency decreases phosphatidylserine accumulation selectively in neuronal tissues. *Lipids* **2000,** *35(8),* 863–869.

Hibbeln, J.R.; M. Linnoila; J.C. Umhau; R. Rawlings; D.T. George; N. Salem, Jr. Essential fatty acids predict metabolites of serotonin and dopamine in cerebrospinal fluid among healthy control subjects, and early- and late-onset alcoholics. *Biol. Psychiatry* **1998,** *44,* 235–242.

Hibbeln, J.R.; K.K. Makino; C.E. Martin; F. Dickerson; J. Boronow; W.S. Fenton. Smoking, gender, and dietary influences on erythrocyte essential fatty acid composition among patients with schizophrenia or schizoaffective disorder. *Biol. Psychiatry* **2003,** *53,* 431–441.

Hibbeln, J.R.; N. Salem, Jr. Dietary polyunsaturated fatty acids and depression: When cholesterol does not satisfy. *Am. J. Clin. Nutr.***1995,** *62,* 1–9.

Hibbeln, J.R.; J.C. Umhau; M. Linnoila; D.T. George; P.W. Ragan; S.E. Shoaf; et al. A replication study of violent and nonviolent subjects: cerebrospinal fluid metabolites of serotonin and dopamine are predicted by plasma essential fatty acids. *Biol. Psychiatry* **1998,** *44,* 243–249.

Hirashima, F.; A.M. Parow; A.L. Stoll; C.M. Demopulos; K.E. Damico; M.L. Rohan; et al. Omega-3 fatty acid treatment and T(2) whole brain relaxation times in bipolar disorder. *Am. J. Psychiatry* **2004,** *161(10),* 1922–1924.

Hirayama, S.; T. Hamazaki; K. Terasawa. Effect of docosahexaenoic acid-containing food administration on symptoms of attention-deficit/hyperactivity disorder - a placebo-controlled double-blind study. *Eur. J. Clin. Nutr.* **2004,** *58,* 467–473.

Hooijmans, C.R.; A.J. Kiliaan. Fatty acids, lipid metabolism and Alzheimer pathology. *Eur. J. Pharmacol.* **2008,** *585,* 176–196.

Horrobin, D.F. Schizophrenia and membrane lipids. *Lipids, Health, and Behavior;* M. Hillbrand, R.T. Spitz, Eds.; American Psychological Association: Washington, DC, 1997; pp. 179–194.

Horrobin, D.F. The membrane phospholipid hypothesis as a biochemical basis for the neurodevelopmental concept of schizophrenia. *Schizophrenia Res.* **1998,** *30,* 193–208.

Horrobin, D.F. The phospholipid concept of psychiatric disorders and its relationship to the neurodevelopmental concept of schizophrenia. *Phospholipid Spectrum Disorder in Psychiatry;* M. Peet, I. Glen, D.F. Horrobin, Eds.; Marius Press: Carnforth, 1999; pp. 3–20.

Horrobin, D.F. Omega-3 fatty acid for schizophrenia. *Am. J. Psychiatry* **2003,** *160(1),* 188–189.

Horrobin, D.F.; C.N. Bennett. Depression and bipolar disorder: relationships to impaired fatty acid and phospholipid metabolism and to diabetes, , immunological abnormalities, cancer, ageing and osteoporosis. *Prostaglandins, Leukotrienes Essent. Fatty Acids* **1999,** *60(4),* 217–234.

Horrocks, L.A.; Y.K. Yeo. Health benefits of docosahexaenoic acid (DHA). *Pharmacol. Res.* **1999,** *40(3),* 211–225.

Horvath, K.; J.A. Perman. Autism and gastrointestinal symptoms. *Current Gastroenterology Reports* **2002,** *4(3),* 251–258.

Huan, M.; K. Hamazaki; Y. Sun; M. Itomura; H. Liu; W. Kang; et al. Suicide attempt and n-3 fatty acid levels in red blood cells: A case control study in China. *Biol. Psychiatry* **2004,** *56,* 490–496.

Huang, T.L.; P.P. Zandi; K.L. Tucker; A.L. Fitzpatrick; L.H. Kuller; L.P. Fried; et al. Benefits of fatty fish on dementia risk are stronger for those without *APOE* ε4. *Neurol.* **2005,** *65,* 1409–1414.

Ingram, S.; L. Hechtman; G. Morgenstern. Outcome issues in ADHD: Adolescent and adult long-term outcome. *Mental Retardation and Developmental Disabilities* **1999,** *5,* 243–250.

Iribarren, C.; J.H. Markovitz; D.R. Jacobs, Jr.; P.J. Schreiner; M. Daviglus; J.R. Hibbeln. Dietary intake of n-3, n-6 fatty acids and fish: relationship with hostility in young adults—the CARDIA study. *Eur. J. Clin. Nutr.* **2004,** *58,* 24–31.

Issa, A.M.; W.A. Mojica; S.C. Morton; S. Traina; S.J. Newberry; L.G. Hilton; et al. The efficacy of omega-3 fatty acids on cognitive function in aging and dementia: A systematic review. *Dementia and Geriatric Cognitive Disorders* **2006,** *21,* 88–96.

Jacka, F.N.; J.A. Pasco; M.J. Henry; M.A. Kotowicz; G.C. Nicholson; M. Berk. Dietary omega-3 fatty acids and depression in a community sample. *Nutr. Neurosci.* **2004,** *7(2),* 101–106.

Jazayeri, S.; M. Tehrani-Doost; S.A. Keshavarz; M. Hosseini; A. Djazayery; H. Amini; et al. Comparison of therapeutic effects of omega-3 fatty acid eicosapentaenoic acid and fluoxetine, separately and in combination, in major depressive disorder. *Aust. N Z J. Psychiatry* **2008,** *42(3),* 192–198.

Johnson, S.M.; E. Hollander. Evidence that eicosapentaenoic acid is effective in treating autism. *J. Clin. Psychiatry* **2003,** *64,* 848–849.

Johnson, M.; S. Östlund; G. Fransson; B. Kadesjö; C. Gillberg. Omega-3/omega-6 fatty acids for attention deficit hyperactivity disorder. *J. Attention Disorders* **2008,** *doi: 10.1177/1087054708316261.*

Kale, A.; S. Joshi; N. Naphade; S. Sapkale; M.S. Raju; A. Pillai; et al. Opposite changes in predominantly docosahexaenoic acid (DHA) in cerebrospinal fluid and red blood cells from never-medicated first-episode psychotic patients. *Schizophr. Res.* **2008,** *98(1–3),* 295–301.

Kalmijn, S. Fatty acid intake and the risk of dementia and cognitive decline: a review of clinical and epidemiological studies. *J. Nutr., Health and Aging* **2000,** *4(4).*

Kalmijn, S.; L.J. Launer; A. Ott; J.C.M. Witteman; A. Hofman; M.M.B. Breteler. Dietary fat intake and the risk of incident dementia in the Rotterdam study. *Ann. Neurol.* **1997,** *42(5),* 776–782.

Kaplan, R.J.; C.E. Greenwood. Dietary saturated fatty acids and brain function. *Neurochem. Res.* **1998,** *23(5),* 615–626.

Keck, P.E.; J. Mintz; S.L. McElroy; M.P. Freeman; T. Suppes; M.A.Frye; et al. Double-blind, randomized, placebo-controlled trials of ethyl-eicosapentanoate in the treatment of bipolar depression and rapid cycling bipolar disorder. *Biol. Psychiatry* **2006,** *60,* 1020–1022.

Kiecolt-Glaser, J.; M.A. Belury; K. Porter; D.Q. Beversdorf; S. Lemeshow; R. Glaser. Depressive symptoms, omega-6:omega-3 fatty acids, and inflammation in older adults. *Psychosomatic Med.* **2007,** *69(3),* 217–224.

Kotani, S.; E. Sakaguchi; S. Warashina; N. Matsukawa; Y. Ishikura; Y. Kiso; et al. Dietary supplementation of arachidonic and docosahexaenoic acids improves cognitive dysfunction. *Neurosci. Res.*2006, *56*, 159–164.

Laugharne, J.D.E.; J.E. Mellor; M. Peet. Fatty acids and schizophrenia. *Lipids* **1996,** *31*, S–63–S165.

Lauritzen, L.; H.S. Hansen; M.H. Jørgensen; K.F. Michaelsen. The essentiality of long chain n-3 fatty acids in relation to development and function of the brain and retina. *Progress in Lipid Res.* **2001,** *40*, 1–94.

Leaf, A.; J.X. Kang. Omega-3 fatty acids and . *Nutrition and Fitness: Diet, Genes, Physical Activity and Health;* A.P. Simopoulos, K.N. Pavlou, Eds.; Karger: Basel, 2001; Vol. 89, pp. 161–172.

Lim, S.-Y.; H. Suzuki. Intakes of dietary docosahexaenoic acid ethyl ester and egg phosphatidylcholine improve maze-learning ability in young and old mice. *J. Nutr.* **2000,** *130*, 1629–1632.

Maes, M.; A.B. Christophe; J. Delanghe; C. Altamura; H. Neels; H.Y. Meltzer. Lowered omega3 polyunsaturated fatty acids in serum phospholipids and cholesteryl esters of depressed patients. *Psychiatry Res.* **1999,** *85*, 275–291.

Marangell, L.B.; J.M. Martinez; H.A. Zboyan; B. Kertz; H.F. Seung Kim; L.J. Puryear. A double-blind, placebo-controlled study of the omega-3 fatty acid docosahexaenoic acic in the treatment of major depression. *Am. J. of Psychiatry* **2003,** *160*, 996–998.

Martin, D.S.D.; P. Spencer; D.F. Horrobin; M.A. Lynch. Long-term potentiation in aged rats is restored when the age-related decrease in polyunsaturated fatty acid concentration is reversed. *Prostaglandins, Leukotrienes Essent. Fatty Acids* **2002,** *67*(2–3), 121–130.

Meyer, B.; B.F.S. Grenyer; T. Crowe; A.J. Owen; P.R.C. Howe. (2004, 27 June–1 July). *Improvement of major depression is associated with increased erythrocyte DHA - subset analysis in a double-blind omega-3 supplementation trial.* Paper presented at the International Society for the Study of Fatty Acids and Lipids (ISSFAL), Brighton, UK.

Miller, M.L.; V.E. Fee; A.K. Netterville. Psychometric properties of ADHD rating scales among children with mental retardation I: Reliability. *Res. in Developmental Disabilities* **2004,** *25*, 459–476.

Mitchell, E.A.; M.G. Aman; S.H. Turbott; M. Manku. Clinical characteristics and serum essential fatty acid levels in hyperactive children. *Clin. Pediatrics* **1987,** *26(8),* 406–411.

Mitchell, E.A.; S. Lewis; D.R. Cutler. Essential fatty acids and maladjusted behaviour in children. *Prostaglandins, Leukotrienes Med.* **1983,** *12*, 281–287.

Modrego, P.; J. Ferrández. Depression in patients with mild cognitive impairment increases the risk of developing dementia of Alzheimer type. *Archives of Neurology* **2004,** *61*, 1290–1293.

Mori, T.A.; G.F. Watts; V. Burke; E. Hilme; I.B. Puddey; L.J. Beilin. Differential effects of eicosapentaenoic acid and docosahexaenoic acid on vascular reactivity of the forearm microcirculation in hyperlipidemic, overweight men. *Circulation* **2000,** *102*, 1264–1269.

Moriguchi, T.; J. Loewke; M. Garrison; J.N. Catalan; N. Salem, Jr. Reversal of docosahexaenoic acid deficiency in the rat brain, retina, liver, and serum. *J. Lipid Res.* **2001,** *42*, 419–427.

Morris, M.C.; D.A. Evans; J.L. Bienias; C.C. Tangney; D.A. Bennett; R.S. Wilson; et al. Consumption of fish and n-3 fatty acids and risk of incident Alzheimer Disease. *Archives of Neurology* **2003,** *60(7),* 940–946.

Nemets, B.; Z. Stahl; R.H. Belmaker. Addition of omega-3 fatty acid to maintenance medication treatment for recurrent unipolar depressive disorder. *Am.J. Psychiatry* **2002,** *159*, 477–479.

Nurk, E.; C.A. Drevon; H. Refsum; K. Solvoll; S.E. Vollset; O. Nygård; et al. Cognitive performance among the elderly and dietary fish intake: the Hordaland Health Study. *Am. J. Clin. Nutr.* **2007,** *86*, 1470–1478.

Osher, Y.; Y. Bersudsky; R.H. Belmaker. Omega-3 eicosapentaenoic acid in bipolar depression: Report of a small open-label study. *J. Clin. Psychiatry* **2005,** *66*, 726–729.

Patrick, L.; R. Salik. (2006). Benefits of essential fatty acid supplementation on language and learning skills in children with autism and Asperger's syndrome. *www.nordicnaturals.com/images/pdfs/PatrickStudy05.pdf.*

Peers, R.J. Alzheimer's disease and omega-3 fatty acids: hypothesis. *The Medical J. Australia* **1990,** *153*, 563–564.

Peet, M. Eicosapentaenoic acid in the treatment of schizophrenia and depression: rationale and preliminary double-blind clinical results. *Prostaglandins, Leukotrienes Essent. Fatty Acids* **2003,** *69*, 477–485.

Peet, M. International variations in the outcome of schizophrenia and the prevalence of depression in relation to national dietary practices: an ecological analysis. *Br. J. Psychiatry* **2004,** *184*, 404–408.

Peet, M.; J. Brind; C.N. Ramchand; S. Shah; G.K. Vankar. Two double-blind placebo-controlled pilot studies of eicosapentaenoic acid in the treatment of schizophrenia. *Schizophrenia Res.* **2001,***49*, 243–251.

Peet, M.; D.F. Horrobin. A dose-ranging exploratory study of the effects of ethyl-eicosapentaenoate in patients with persistent schizophrenic symptoms. *J. Psychiatric Res.* **2002,** *36*, 7–18.

Peet, M.; J.D.E. Laugharne; J. Mellor; C.N. Ramchand. Essential fatty acid deficiency in erythrocyte membranes from chronic schizophrenic patients, and the clinical effects of dietary supplementation. *Prostaglandins, Leukotrienes Essent. Fatty Acids* **1996,** *55*(1/2), 71–75.

Peet, M.; B. Murphy; J. Shay; D.F. Horrobin. Depletion of omega-3 fatty acid levels in red blood cell membranes of depressed patients. *Biol. Psychiatry* **1998,** *43*, 315–319.

Phelps, L.; R.T. Brown; T.J. Power. Mental retardation and autistic spectrum disorders. *Pediatric Psychopharmacology: Combining Medical and Psychosocial Interventions;* L.R.T. Phelps, T.J. Brown, Power, et al., Eds.; American Psychological Association: Washington, DC, 2002; pp. 133–161

Pifferi, F.; F. Roux; B. Langelier; J.-M. Alessandri; S. Vancassel; M. Jouin; et al. (n-3) Polyunsaturated fatty acid deficiency reduces the expression of both isoforms of the brain glucose transporter GLUT1 in rats. *J. Nutr.* **2005,** *135*, 2241–2246.

Puri, B.K.; S.J. Counsell; G. Hamilton; A.J. Richardson; D.F. Horrobin. Eicosapentaenoic acid in treatment-resistant depression associated with symptom remission, structural brain changes and reduced neuronal phospholipid turnover. *Int. J. Clin. Pract.* **2001,** *55(8),* 560–563.

Puri, B.K.; A.J. Richardson. Sustained remission of positive and negative symptoms of schizphrenia following treatment with eicosapentaenoic acid. *Arch. General Psychiatry* **1998,** *55(2),* 188–189.

Richardson, A.J. Clinical trials of fatty acid supplementation in ADHD. *Phospholipid Spectrum Disorders in Psychiatry and Neurology;* A.I.M. Glen, M. Peet, D.F. Horrobin, Eds.; Marius Press:

Carnforth, 2003a; pp. 529–541.

Richardson, A.J. Clinical trials of fatty acid treatment in ADHD, dyslexia, dyspraxia and the autistic spectrum. *Prostaglandins, Leukotrienes Essent. Fatty Acids* **2003b,** *70,* 383–390.

Richardson, A.J. Omega-3 fatty acids in ADHD and related neurodevelopmental disorders. *Int. Rev. Psychiatry* **2006,** *18*(6), 155–172.

Richardson, A.J.; C,M. Calvin; C. Clisby; D.R. Schoenheimer; P. Montgomery; J.A. Hall; et al. Fatty acid deficiency signs predict the severity of reading and related difficulties in dyslexic children. *Prostaglandins, Leukotrienes Essent. Fatty Acids* **2000,** *63*(1/2), 69–74.

Richardson, A.J.; I.J. Cox; J. Sargentoni; B.K. Puri. Abnormal cerebral phospholipid metabolism in dyslexia indicated by phosphorus-31 magnetic resonance spectroscopy. *NMR in Biomed.* **1997,** *10,* 309–314.

Richardson, A.J.; E. Cyhlarova; M.A. Ross. Omega-3 and omega-6 fatty acid concentrations in red blood cell membranes relate to schizotypal traits in healthy adults. *Prostaglandins, Leukotrienes Essent. Fatty Acids* **2003,** *69,* 461–466.

Richardson, A.J.; P. Montgomery. The Oxford-Durham study: a randomised, controlled trial of dietary supplementation with fatty acids in children with developmental coordination disorder. *Pediatrics* **2005,** *115,* 1360–1366.

Richardson, A.J.; B.K. Puri. The potential role of fatty acids in attention-deficit/hyperactivity disorder. *Prostaglandins, Leukotrienes Essent. Fatty Acids* **2000,** *63*(1/2), 79–87.

Richardson, A.J.; B.K. Puri. A randomised double-blind, placebo-controlled study of the effects of supplementation with highly unsaturated fatty acids on ADHD-related symptoms in children with specific learning difficulties. *Prog. Neuro-Psychopharmacol. Biol. Psychiatry* **2002,** *26,* 233–239.

Rogers, P.J.; K.M. Appleton; D. Kessler; T.J. Peters; D. Gunnell; R.C. Hayward; et al. No effect of n-3 long-chain polyunsaturated fatty acid (EPA and DHA) supplementation on depressed mood and cognitive function: a randomised controlled trial. *Br. J. Nutr.* **2008,** *99,* 421–431.

Root, R.W.I.; R.J. Resnick. An update on the diagnosis and treatment of attention-deficit/hyperactivity disorder in children. *Professional Psychol.: Res. Practice* **2003,** *34(1),* 34–41.

Salem, N., Jr.; B. Litman; H.-Y. Kim; K. Gawrisch. Mechanisms of action of docosahexaenoic acid. *Lipids* **2001,** *36(9),* 945–959.

Schins, A.; H.J. Crijns; R.J. Brummer; M. Wichers; R. Lousberg; S. Celis; et al. Altered omega-3 polyunsaturated fatty acid status in depressed post-myocardial infarction patients. *Acta Psychiatr. Scand.* **2007,** *115(1),* 35–40.

Silvers, K.M.; C.C. Woolley; F.C. Hamilton; P.M. Watts; R. Watson. Randomised double-blind placebo-controlled trial of fish oil in the treatment of depression. *Prostaglandins, Leukotrienes Essent. Fatty Acids* **2005,** *72,* 211–218.

Simopoulos, A.P. Omega-3 fatty acids in health and disease and in growth and development. *Am. J. Clin. Nutr. 54* **1991,** 438–463.

Sinclair, A.J.; D. Begg; M. Mathai; R.S. Weisinger. Omega 3 fatty acids and the brain: review of studies in depression. *Asia Pacific J. Clin. Nutr.* **2007,** *16(Suppl. 1),* 391–397.

Sinn, N. Physical fatty acid deficiency signs in children with ADHD symptoms. *Prostaglandins, Leukotrienes Essent. Fatty Acids* **2007,** *77(2),* 109–115.

Sinn, N.; J. Bryan. Effect of supplementation with polyunsaturated fatty acids and micronutrients on ADHD-related problems with attention and behavior. *J.Developmental & Behavioral Pediatrics* **2007,** *28(2),* 82–91.

Sinn, N.; J. Bryan; C. Wilson. Cognitive effects of polyunsaturated fatty acids in children with attention deficit hyperactivity disorder symptoms: A randomised controlled trial. *Prostaglandins, Leukotrienes Essent. Fatty Acids* **2008,** *78(4–5),* 311–326.

Sinn, N.; P.R.C. Howe. Mental health benefits of omega-3 fatty acids may be mediated by improvements in cerebral vascular function. *Biosci. Hypotheses* **2008,** *1(2),* 103–108.

Sinn, N.; C. Wilson. Dietary supplementation with highly unsaturated fatty acids: Implications for interventions with persons with mental retardation from research on infant cognitive development, ADHD, and other developmental disabilities. *Int. Rev. Res. Mental Retardation* **2006,** *32,* 159–196.

Söderberg, M.; C. Edlund; K. Kristensson; G. Dallner. Fatty acid composition of brain phospholipids in aging and in Alzheimer's Disease. *Lipids* **1991,** *26(1),* 421–425.

Stahl, L.A.; D.P. Begg; R.S. Weisinger; A.J. Sinclair. The role of omega-3 fatty acids in mood disorders. *Curr. Opinion in Investigational Drugs* **2008,** *9(1),* 57–64.

Stevens, L.J.; S.S. Zentall; M.L. Abate; T. Kuczek; J.R. Burgess. Omega-3 fatty acids in boys with behavior, learning, and health problems. *Physiol. Behavior* **1996,** *59(4/5),* 915–920.

Stevens, L.J.; S.S. Zentall; J.L. Deck; M.L. Abate; B.A. Watkins; S.R. Lipp; et al. Essential fatty acid metabolism in boys with attention-deficit hyperactivity disorder. *Am. J. Clin. Nutr.* **1995,** *62,* 761–768.

Stevens, L.J.; W. Zhang; L. Peck; T. Kuczek; N. Grevstad; A.K. Mahon; et al. EFA supplementation in children with inattention, hyperactivity, and other disruptive behaviors. *Lipids* **2003,** *38(10),* 1007–1021.

Stoll, A. L., Severus, W. E., Freeman, M. P., Rueter, S., Zboyan, H. A., Diamond, E., et al. (1999). Omega 3 fatty acids in bipolar disorder. *Arch. General Psychiatry, 56,* 407–412.

Stordy, B. J. (2000). Dark adaptation, motor skills, docosahexaenoic acid, and dyslexia. *Am. J. Clin. Nutr. 71*(1), 323–326.

Su, K.-P.; S.-Y. Huang; C.-C. Chiu; W.W. Shen. Omega-3 fatty acids in major depressive disorder: A preliminary double-blind, placebo-controlled trial. *Eur. Neuropsychopharmacol.* **2003,** *13,* 267–271.

Tacconi, M.T.; C. Federico; S. Mario. Brain lipids and diet. *Lipids, Health and Behavior;* M. Hillbrand, T. Spitz, Eds.; American Psychological Association: Washington, DC, 1997; pp. 197–226.

Tanskanen, A.; J.R. Hibbeln; J. Hintikka; K. Haatainen. Fish consumption, depression, and suicidality in a general population/in reply. *Arch. General Psychiatry* **2001,** *58(5),* 512.

Tanskanen, A.; J.R. Hibbeln; J. Tuomilehto; A. Uutela; A. Haukkala; H. Viinamaki; et al. Fish consumption and depressive symptoms in the general population in Finland. *Psychiatric Serv. 52*(4), 529–531.

Taylor, K.E.; C.J. Higgins; C.M. Calvin; J.A. Hall; T. Easton; A.M. McDaid; et al. Dyslexia in adults is associated with clinical signs of fatty acid deficiency. *Prostaglandins, Leukotrienes Essent. Fatty Acids* **2000,** *63(1/2),* 75–78.

Taylor, K.E.; A.J. Richardson. Visual function, fatty acids and dyslexia. *Prostaglandins, Leukotrienes Essent. Fatty Acids* **2000,** *63(1/2),* 89–93.

Terano, T.; S. Fujishiro; T. Ban; K. Yamamoto; T. Tanaka; Y. Noguchi; et al. Docosahexaenoic acid supplementation improves the moderately severe dementia from thrombotic cerebrovascular diseases. *Lipids* **1999,** *34(Suppl.),* S345–S346.

Thatcher, R.W. Maturation of the human frontal lobes. Physiological evidence for staging. *Dev. Neuropsychol.* **1991,** *7,* 397–419.

Tiemeier, H.; H.R. van Tuijl; A. Hofman; A.J. Kiliaan; M.M. Breteler. Plasma fatty acid composition and depression are associated in the elderly: the Rotterdam Study. *Am. J. Clin. Nutr.***2003,** *78(1),* 40–46.

Toga, A.W.; P.M. Thompson; E.R. Sowell. Mapping brain maturation. *Trends Neurosci.***2006,** *29(3),* 148–159.

Tully, A.M.; H.M. Roche; R. Doyle; C. Fallon; I. Bruce; B. Lawlor; et al. Low serum cholesteryl ester-docosahexaenoic acid levels in Alzheimer's disease: a case-control study. *Br. J. Nutr.* **2003,** *89,* 483–489.

Vancassel, S.; G. Durand; C. Barthelemy. Plasma fatty acid levels in autistic children. *Prostaglandins, LeukotrienesEssent. Fatty Acids* **2001,** *65,* 1–7.

Virkkunen, M.E.; D.F. Horrobin; D.K. Jenkins; M. Manku. Plasma phospholipid essential fatty acids and prostaglandins in alcoholic, habitually violent, and impulsive offenders. *Biol. Psychiatry* **1987,** *22(11),* 1087–1096.

Voigt, R.G.; A.M. Llorente; C.L. Jensen; J.K. Fraley; M.C. Berretta; W.C. Heird. A randomised, double-blind, placebo-controlled trial of docosahexaenoic acid supplementation in children with attention-deficit/hyperactivity disorder. *J. Pediatrics* **2001,** *139,* 189–196.

Wainwright, P.E.; E. Jalali; L.M. Mutsaers; R. Bell; S. Cvitkovic. An imbalance of dietary essential fatty acids retards behavioural development in mice. *Physiol. Behavior* **1999,** *66*(5), 833–839.

Ward, P.E. Potential diagnostic aids for abnormal fatty acid metabolism in a range of neurodevelopmental disorders. *Prostaglandins, Leukotrienes Essent. Fatty Acids* **2000,** *63(1/2),* 65–68.

WHO. Prevention of mental disorders: effective interventions and policy options. Geneva: World Health Organisation, 2004.

World Health Organization. (2008) Mental health: WHO urges more investments, services for mental health, *http://www.who.int/mental_health/en/.*

Yehuda, S.; S. Rabinovitz; R.L. Carasso; D.I. Mostofsky. Essential fatty acids preparation (SR-3) improves Alzheimer's patients quality of life. *Int. J. Neurosci.* **1996,** *87(3–4),* 141–149.

Yehuda, S.; S. Rabinovitz; R.L. Carasso; D.I. Mostofsky. Fatty acids and brain peptides. *Peptides* **1998.** *19(2),* 407–419.

Yehuda, S.; S. Rabinovitz; R.L. Carasso; D.I. Mostofsky. The role of polyunsaturated fatty acids in restoring the aging neuronal membrane. *Neurobiol. Aging* **2002,** *23,* 843–853.

Youdim, K.A.; A. Martin; J.A. Joseph. Essential fatty acids and the brain: possible health implications. *Int. J. Develop. Neurosci.* **2000,** *18(4–5),* 383–399.

Young, G.; J. Conquer. Omega-3 fatty acids and neuropsychiatric disorders. *Repro. Nutr. Develop.* **2005,** *45,* 1–28.

Zanarini, M.C.; F.R. Frankenburg. Omega-3 fatty acid treatment of women with borderline personality disorder: a double-blind, placebo-controlled pilot study. *Am.J. Psychiatry* **2003,** *160(1),* 167–169.

Zimmer, L.; S. Vancassel; S. Cantagrel; P. Breton; S. Delamanche; D. Guilloteau; et al. The dopamine mesocorticolimbic pathway is affected by deficiency in n-3 polyunsaturated fatty acids. *Am. J. Clin. Nutr.* **2002,** *75,* 662–667.

Zimmerman, A.W.; H.A. Jinnah; P.J. Lockhart. Behavioral Neuropharmacology. *Mental Retardation Develop. Disabilities Res. Rev.* **1998,** *4,* 26–35.

# 25

# The Importance of the Omega-3 and Omega-6 Ratio: Brain Biochemistry, Cognition, and Behavior

**Shlomo Yehuda**
*Psychopharmacology Laboratory, Department of Psychology, Bar Ilan University, Ramat Gan, Israel*

Polyunsaturated essential fatty acids play a pivotal role in mediating cognitive learning and memory functions. We propose that the mode of action is a direct effect of polyunsaturated fatty acids (PUFAs) on the neuronal membrane. PUFAs serve in stabilizing and protecting the structure and functions of the neuronal membrane. PUFAs exert many effects on the brain: on physiology (pain threshold, thermoregulation, and sleep); on brain biochemistry (brain neurotransmitters, cholesterol, myelin, cortisone); and on CNS-related disorders (Alzheimer's Disease, epilepsy, and multiple sclerosis). Many of those functions have effects on the cognitive level. This chapter examines the role and the proposed mode of action of a ratio of an n-3/n-6 mixture on brain related effects. In addition, studies showed that the level of PUFAs is not the only critical factor in maintaining the neuronal membrane—the ratio of the two types of PUFA is, in fact, even more important. We recommend studying the ratio 1:4.

## Introduction

Among the major scientific research efforts recently in the area of neuroscience, the importance of essential fatty acids (EFAs) is recognized. The profound effects of various fatty acids and the equally profound effects of their deficits are appreciated by various disciplines, including (but not necessarily limited to) lipid biochemistry, physiology, nutrition, psychology, psychiatry, and neurosciences at large. Simopoulos (1999) showed the historical shift from a balanced omega-6 and omega-3 ratio diet to a marked and significant reduction in the omega-3 intake, and explained that the general Western diet of today can, in actual fact, be considered an omega-3–deficient diet. Her concern is that this deficiency may lead to coronary heart disease and high cancer mortality.

Linoleic acid (LA; also known as omega-6, ω6, or 18:2ω6) is the parent fatty acid of the omega-6 group. The diet must supply LA to the body because the body is unable to synthesize it. All other members of the omega-6 group are derivatives of LA. Similarly, the parent compound of the omega-3 group is alpha-linolenic acid (ALA; also known as omega-3, ω3, or 18:3ω3). All other members of the omega-3 group are merely derivatives of ALA, and together they form PUFAs. In each group, the derivatives can convert to longer chain fatty acids by using two mechanisms: desaturation and elongation. The enzymes that are involved in these mechanisms have the same functions in the two fatty acid groups, and therefore the omega-6 and omega-3 fatty acids compete for the same enzymes.

While, from a chemical point of view, the differences between omega-6 and omega-3 fatty acids are very small, and may appear insignificant, they exert different and sometimes even opposite effects. These opposing effects are not easily explained. Some recently suggested (Feller et al., 2002) that the distinction between omega-6 and omega-3 PUFAs is based on the differential capacity of protein, in general, and membrane-bound protein, in particular, to "recognize" various PUFAs. The dietary deficiency of omega-3 fatty acids, as well as the particular roles of omega-6 and omega-3, will become obvious as we take a deeper look into the ratio issue.

## The Importance of the Ratio

Several aspects exist as to the issue of the optimal recommended ratio between omega-6 and omega-3 fatty acids. One aspect is the recommendation for total daily dietary intake in various phases of life (e.g., infancy, pregnancy, adulthood, and old age). Another aspect is the optimal ratio of PUFA as a food supplement or treatment. PUFAs are used in the body in a variety of conditions, such as in dermatological diseases and in cardiovascular disorders. One particular area is the role of PUFAs in the brain and the utility of PUFAs to protect and stabilize the neuronal membrane in health and in disease.

One can divide PUFA's effects on brain function into at least five categories: (i) modification of neuronal membrane fluidity, (ii) modification of membrane activity-bound enzymes, (iii) modification of the number and affinity of receptors, (iv) modification of the function of neuronal membrane ionic channels, and (v) modification of the production of neurotransmitters and brain peptides (Yehuda et al., 2001).

Many studies demonstrated that various PUFAs mediate, or are associated with, several aspects of brain activity, ranging from the role of EFAs in neuronal structure and functions, long-term potentiation (LTP), specific brain activation, and prostaglandin activity, to neurological and mental disorders and to mood control. Unfortunately, the vast majority of these studies merely test one or two specific fatty acids, and very few solid studies exist that experimentally examine a wide range of ratios between omega-6 and omega-3. The following review summarizes the areas in which studies on ratios were performed, and subsequently has to leave out some of the most fascinating areas such as depression, psychosis, and pain.

### *EFAs, the Blood-brain Barrier, and the Brain*

Since EFAs must be supplied via the diet, two major issues arise:

- The first issue is: Is it possible for EFAs and PUFAs to cross the blood-brain barrier (BBB)? Recently, Rapoport (2001) and Edmond (2001) provided a detailed discussion on the complex mechanism of the delivery of essential PUFA, as it progresses from the blood into the brain. In two development periods—infancy and aging, the involvement of the BBB is crucial. The human infant is born with an immature BBB, and during these periods the structure and functions of the BBB are not at their optimal levels. Reports exist of structural changes in the BBB complex in aging and in Alzheimer's patients (de la Torre & Mussivand, 1993; Ginsberg et al., 1998), but despite the knowledge about structural changes, the knowledge of functional changes is quite limited. Most of the studies did not find changes in the rate of the transport of PUFAs into the brain during aging (Strosznajder et al., 1994; Terracina et al., 1992). The important, but so far unanswered, question is whether omega-6 and omega-3 fatty acids have different rates of transport into the brain.
- The second issue regarding the BBB is the brain's ability to convert LA and ALA into longer chain fatty acids, arachidonic acid (AA), and docosahexaenoic acid (DHA). Some researchers suspect that the immature brain of the infant is unable to convert those fatty acids to longer chain fatty acids. However, the majority of studies agree that even the infant brain indeed does have such capacity (Rapoport, 2001).

### *Brain Neurotransmitters and PUFA*

The relationships between PUFA ratios and the various neurotransmitters, as described before (Yehuda et al., 1998), are of special interest. Especially note that an omega-3 deficiency induced reduction in dopamine (DA) vesicle density in the cortex (Zimmer et al., 2000), and malfunction of the dopaminergic mesocorticolimbic pathway (Zimmer et al., 2002). The ability to recover from the dopaminergic effects of an omega-3 deficiency is age-dependent (Acar et al., 2003; Chalon et al., 1998; Kodas et al., 2002). Also, the effects of ALAs for recovering from omega-3 deficiency are dependent on spatial configuration. The *trans*-isomer of LAs is inactive, and if not enough *cis*-isomer is supplied, a state of omega-3 deficiency will occur (Acar et al., 2003). Some studies indicate similar effects on the serotonergic system (Farkas et al., 2002).

### *Membrane Fluidity and Myelin*

Before considering the effects of PUFAs on brain-mediated functions, the effects of PUFAs on brain structural components must be elucidated. Fatty acids and lipids are major components in brain structure. Very high levels of fatty acids and lipids are found in two structural components: the neuronal membrane and the myelin sheaths. The neuronal membrane is composed of two lipid layers. The ratio between the proteins and the lipids is about 50%–50%, while lipids (about 70%) constitute the majority in the myelin sheaths. The protein component is especially stable, while the lipid component has a relatively high turnover rate.

To understand the diverse functions, which seem to be mediated by the various PUFAs and by the ratio of omega-6 to omega-3, we (Yehuda et al., 2002) proposed that the membrane-fluidity index is the common denominator for the various effects of PUFAs. Some molecules are able to change the physical state (e.g., the fluidity index) of the membrane. For example, alcohol fluidizes the membrane, while cholesterol hardens it. Two basic questions regarding the hypothesis that PUFAs are able to modify the neuronal membrane- fluidity index are: (i) Would changes in the lipid component of the neuronal membrane (e.g., a different ratio of various fatty acids) lead to changes in the neuronal functions? and (ii) Would the supplementation of various fatty acids affect the composition and the function of the neuronal membrane? Numerous studies show that EFA supplementation, under certain conditions of composition and time, indeed modifies both the structure and membrane function [see summary in Yehuda et al. (1998a)].

The integrity of the myelin is of utmost importance for the proper functions of axons in the nervous system. Breakage or lesions in the myelin can lead to the disintegration of many nervous-system functions. Recent studies emphasize the major role of dietary EFAs in the normal functions of myelin. Moreover, the EFAs are very important in the active phase of myelin synthesis. If EFAs are not available in this phase, or are metabolically blocked, amyelination, or demyelization may occur (Auestad, 2000; Salvati et al., 2000). If EFA deficiency occurs during the postnatal period, a major delay in the myelination process will occur, accompanied by impaired learning, motor, vision, and auditory abnormalities (Stockard et al., 2000). With great interest note that similar impairments in the myelination process and in the cognitive function are also found in postnatally iron-deficient (ID) rodents and humans (Youdim & Yehuda, 2000). Disorders, which are associated with myelin malfunction or with demyelination, can also occur during the adult period. One such disorder is multiple sclerosis. The rate of myelin lipids turnover is age-dependent. The turnover rate is very slow during aging, and therefore the rate of repairing damaged sections of myelin is slower during aging (Ando et al., 2003).

## Cholesterol and Fatty Acids

The membrane-fluidity index is dependent on two major factors: (i) the level, composition, and percentage of the PUFAs in the membrane and (ii) the level of membrane cholesterol. An increase in the PUFA level will result in fluidizing the neuronal membrane, while an increase in cholesterol will harden the membrane. The membrane should be at an optimal physiological gel state. Therefore, cholesterol, which is a complex lipid, is involved in many functions in the membrane. As is well-established, cholesterol decreases the membrane-fluidity index, which affects the activity of ion channels and receptor functions, as well as the DA release. Moreover, cholesterol is a key molecule in the end product of the CRF–ACTH (corticotropin-releasing factor–adrenocorticotropic-hormone) axis. Considering that steroids are derivatives of cholesterol, it is very interesting to find that various fatty acids have differential effects on cholesterol metabolism. Many reliable studies confirm that the administration of omega-6 fatty acids reduces the level of cholesterol in the blood. However, omega-6 fatty acids and omega-3 fatty acids differ in their mode of action in cholesterol reduction: omega-6 fatty acids redistribute cholesterol while omega-3 fatty acids actually reduce the level of cholesterol in the neuronal membrane. This may explain why an increase in the cholesterol level in the blood is found in humans who consume omega-3 fatty acid supplements. Omega-3 EFAs are more effective in reducing cholesterol levels in macrophages than omega-6 EFAs. This is most likely due to the differential effect on the enzyme acyl-coenzyme A (acyl-CoA) activity. However, some studies indicate that cholesterol-esterifying enzymes that incorporate free fatty acids into cholesterol esters, without the participation of CoA, are also present in the rat brain (Horrocks & Harder, 1983).

The mechanism by which omega-6 or omega-3 fatty acids are able to reduce the cholesterol level in the blood or in the neuronal membrane is still unclear, although several hypotheses were proposed. For example, Bourre et al. (1991) claimed that ALA controls the composition of nerve membranes, which implies an inverse relationship between ALA and the cholesterol level. Salem et al. (2001) proposed that DHA controls the level of cholesterol as well as the composition and function of the neuronal membrane. Another approach (unpublished data) suggests that the differential effects of omega-6 or omega-3 on the cholesterol level depend on the activity of PUFAs on reduced low-density lipoprotein (LDL)–receptor activity. A negative correlation was found between membrane cholesterol level and an improvement in learning capacity. Numerous studies provide support for reducing neuronal-membrane cholesterol by dietary supplementation of an omega-6/omega-3 compound in a ratio of 4:1 (Yehuda et al., 1997). Such correlation was not found with other ratios. Possibly, this specific ratio (4:1) optimizes an uptake of PUFAs into the brain and promotes fatty acid incorporation into the neuronal membranes, while displacing cholesterol out of the membrane. The issue of the cholesterol neuronal-membrane level is very important because the level of cholesterol (and cholesterol metabolites) in the aging and in the Alzheimer's patient's brain is very high.

## *Early Development*

Most studies on omega-3 deficiency singled out the early-development periods as an important and almost critical period for brain development. Studies stress the importance of the influence of the fatty acids profile in mothers' milk on brain maturation. Jumpsen et al. (1997a, 1997b) showed that even small changes in the ratio of omega-6 to omega-3 in the diet, during neuronal and glial cell development, have significant effects on the development. He showed that a ratio of 4:1 was the optimal ratio for the development of the frontal cortex, hippocampus, cerebellum, and glial cell number in developing rats. Small changes in the ratio, such as 6:1, impaired the rate of development.

Though the discussion of whether the addition of long-chain (LC) PUFAs to baby formula is recommended is outside the scope of this chapter, the importance of the level of PUFAs and the omega-6/omega-3 ratio in the diet of the infant, in this sensitive development period, is emphasized by a great number of studies (Stockard et al., 2000; Wainwright et al., 1997; Xiang et al., 2000).

### *Attention Deficit/Hyperactivity Disorder (ADHD)*

ADHD is a severe behavioral disorder most commonly diagnosed in children and often continuing into adulthood. The symptoms of inattention, hyperactivity, and impulsivity constitute the core diagnosis of ADHD. The majority of ADHD sufferers are boys. The estimated prevalence of ADHD in England is about 2% and 3–5% in the United States. The etiology of ADHD (which is not a unitary condition) is unknown, although both biological and environmental factors are known to play key roles in the presentation of this disorder.

No single treatment modality for ADHD (e.g., behavior therapy, neurofeedback, medications) is shown to be conclusively effective for all ADHD patients. One of the problems associated with ADHD children is their food-intake habit. They eat at irregular times, and the food is mostly carbohydrates and processed. Not surprisingly, therefore, these children often suffer from malnutrition and nutritional deficits. While the research in this field is not well-developed and while no claim is made that nutritional deficits are the cause of ADHD, most agree that the nutritional deficits may worsen the symptoms of ADHD. Two major nutritional deficits may be of considerable interest, and may suggest the options for undertaking novel interventional alternatives: (i) EFAs deficiency and (ii) ID.

Several studies summarized by Burgess et al. (2000) demonstrate that some of the physical symptoms of ADHD children are similar to those observed in EFA deficiency in animals and humans. Many ADHD children suffer from EFA deficiency (Ross et al., 2003), especially the n-3 subgroup of fatty acids. Moreover, a high correlation exists between the severity of the EFA deficiency and the severity of ADHD symptoms ($r = .80$). Burgess suggested two possible explanations: One is a decrease in EFA intake from food, and the second is the impaired capacity of the ADHD's neurological system to convert EFAs to longer chain fatty acids. Supportive studies showed the relationship between EFA deficiency and ADHD (Farooqui & Horrocks, 2001; Stevens et al., 1995). Richardson (Richardson & Puri, 2000) summarized two studies in which fatty- acid supplements were given to ADHD children: the EFA supplement was effective in one study and had no effect in the other.

Not as much is known about the relationship between ID and ADHD. Burgess et al. (2000) and Kidd (2000) demonstrated the similarities between the effects of ID on the behavior of animals and humans and ADHD symptoms. The fact that many ADHD children were shown to suffer from ID did not lead to a call for treatment, except for in a study by Oner et al. (2008) in which ID was found among ADHD subjects who were then administered an iron-preparation treatment (Ferrocal) for one month that improved the ADHD symptoms.

Recently, a subgroup of ADHD children suffered from an EFA deficiency (Richardson & Puri, 2000). Following the authors' recommendation, we examined the effects of a supplementation of a specific mixture of EFAs on a group of ADHD children. The mixture was created in our laboratory after we experimentally established that the ratio of omega-3 and omega-6 is critical for modulating behavioral and neuropharmacological functions. We used highly purified ALA and LA to avoid the variations that occur in the composition of commercially prepared fatty acid oils that may introduce possible confounding effects of other fatty acids or lipid mixtures. Our animal studies (conducted with rats that were given a normal diet, as recommended by AIN) confirmed that a mixture of ALA and LA with a ratio of 1:4 was the most effective in improving numerous cognitive and physiological indices. Note that preliminary studies with radio-labelled PUFAs showed that the fatty acid ratio is capable of crossing the BBB and maintaining this 1:4 ratio in the neuronal membranes.

To address the ADHD issue, we recruited 44 boys (ages 9–12) who were diagnosed as suffering from ADHD by two independent psychologists. The diagnosis was based on The American Academy of Pediatrics, namely, a child of the age of 6 to 12 years who displayed inattention, hyperactivity, impulsivity, academic underachievement, and/or behavior problems. An independent group of 48 nonaffected boys, of corresponding age and socioeconomic status, served as a control group.

All participants and their parents agreed to participate in the study. Each subject completed a short questionnaire on day 1 of the study. The questions were answered on a "5-point scale" for each of six variables: (i) the level of cooperation with other people, such as parents, teachers, and friends; (ii) the level of good mood in general; (iii) the level of ability to concentrate during the day, mainly at school; (iv) the degree of fatigue, in general, experienced during the day; (v) the percentage of homework completed, in general; and (vi) the quality of sleep.

For each scale, a score of 0 signified a negative and poor status, while a score of 5 signified a positive and excellent status. In addition, a blood assay was taken to measure hemoglobin levels. All participants took two capsules of the 1:4 fatty acid compound while awake, twice daily, for 10 weeks. At the end of the 10 weeks, the subjects were again asked to complete the questionnaire, and their hemoglobin level was tested again.

The results (Table 25.1) show that the administration of the fatty acid ratio mixture for 10 weeks to ADHD children significantly improved their quality of life. The most impressive improvement was in the quality of sleep. The children reported a marked improvement in their ability to concentrate, and they felt less fatigued. In

**Table 25.1. Effects of a Ten-week SR-3 Treatment on ADHD Children**[a]

| Variables | Placebo Before | Placebo After | ADHD Before | ADHD After |
|---|---|---|---|---|
| Cooperation | 4.5 ± 0.6 | 4.9 ± 0.7 | 1.5 ± 0.8 | 2.9 ± 0.6* |
| Good mood | 4.0 ± 0.8 | 4.8 ± 0.8 | 2.2 ± 1.1 | 3.7 ± 0.9* |
| Ability to concentrate | 3.5 ± 0.6 | 4.4 ± 0.5 | 2.0 ± 1.3 | 3.8 ± 0.8** |
| Fatigue during the day | 4.0 ± 0.5 | 4.5 ± 0.8 | 2.3 ± 1.0 | 4.0 ± 0.3** |
| Preparing homework | 4.6 ± 0.6 | 4.8 ± 0.7 | 2.0 ± 1.3 | 3.1 ± 1.2* |
| Quality of sleep | 3.8 ± 1.3 | 4.4 ± 1.0 | 1.2 ± 1.1 | 3.3 ± 0.7** |
| Hemoglobin g/dL | 12.8 ± 1.1 | 13.2 ± 1.2 | 9.9 ± 0.9 | 12.1 ± 1.2** |

[a]There were 48-matched control boys (ages 9–12) and 44 ADHD boys in the study.
Data are presented as means and standard deviations.
* = Statistical significant difference ($P \leq 0.05$) from the "before" value.
** = Statistical significant difference ($P \leq 0.01$) from the "before" value.

addition, their mood and ability to cooperate with other people had improved. Our study shows that ADHD children suffer from ID and that our fatty acid treatment corrected the iron level in their blood. Except for three cases of transient stomach upset and diarrhea and two cases of dizziness, no major side effects were reported. All subjects continued their participation in the study.

The results of this study show that a mixture of EFAs can improve many aspects of the quality of life of ADHD children. While EFAs exert many physiological and behavioral effects, we suggest that the effects of the EFAs on the sleep quality mediate the improvement in ADHD symptomatology and that the improved sleep quality can explain the improvement in the other aspects of their behavior. While the improvement in the iron status of the ADHD children is interesting, we do not attribute direct biochemical effects of the EFAs to iron status, but rather credit the increase in iron level to better food intake. The children look less anorectic and they consumed less "junk food." We do believe that the public- health implications of supplementation using the fatty acid mixture for ADHD, as well as non-ADHD, persons are profound and deserve further study.

## *Learning and Memory*

The above discussion demonstrates that various fatty acids serve different roles in the nervous system and in the body, and as suggested,the nervous system has an absolute molecular-species requirement for proper function. Studies in our laboratory confirm this finding, and even suggest an added qualifying requirement: the need for a proper ratio between the EFAs. Many studies examine the effects of various fatty acids on learning and memory, but very few examine the ratio between various PUFAs. We experimentally tested our hypothesis that the ratio of omega-6 and omega-3 may be a key factor in modulating the behavioral and neuropharmacological effects of PUFAs. Therefore, we attempted to identify the optimal ratio. To avoid the variations that occur in the composition of fatty acids in commercially prepared oils, and to exclude the possible confounding effects of other fatty acids or lipid mixtures, we used highly purified LA and ALA. We tested a wide range of ratios of LA/ALA [3:1, 3.5:1, 4:1, 4.5:1, 5:1, 5.5:1, 6:1 (vol/vol)], which were administered as dietary supplements. All animal studies were conducted on rats fed normal diets, as recommended by the American Institute of Nutrition (AIN). We found that a mixture of LA (omega-6) and ALA (omega-3) with a ratio of 4:1 was the most effective in improving learning performance [as assessed by the Morris Water Maze (MWM) and passive avoidance], elevating pain threshold, improving sleep, and improving thermoregulation (Yehuda & Carasso, 1993). This ratio was also able to correct learning deficits induced by the neurotoxins AF64A and 5,7-dihydroxytryptamine (Yehuda et al., 1995), treatments that decrease the acetylcholine and serotonin brain levels. Similarly, this ratio overcame the learning deficit induced by 6-OH-DA (e.g., a reduction in brain DA level) (Yehuda et al., 1999). Treatment with a single fatty acid was less successful (Ikemoto et al., 2001; Umezawa et al., 1999). On the other hand, a recent review demonstrates that a high-fat diet induces learning deficits (Yehuda et al., 2005).

## EFAs, Aging, and Alzheimer's

Studies show that aging causes a reduction in the levels of PUFAs in the brain due to a reduction in the capacity of those fatty acids to cross the hemato-encephalic barrier and the reduction of delta-6-desaturase, less food intake, absorption difficulties, or a reduced capacity to convert shorter chained fatty acids to longer chained fatty acids. This modifies the brain membrane (Cornford & Oldendorf, 1986). Moreover, the metabolism changes with age, and the increase in the oxidative stress results in a lower concentration of omega-3 in the nervous system. In this case, a diet with plenty of that kind of PUFAs might have an antioxidant function and help reduce age-related impairments.

Aging is a special period during development. The aging brain is different in many aspects from the adult brain. Among the many brain changes (e.g., decrease in the level of most neurotransmitters and hormones and an increase in cholesterol in the neuronal membrane) is that the level and the ratio of EFA is modified. PUFAs are major molecules responsible for regulating cellular differentiation and apoptosis (Sawazaki et al., 1999). Most of the studies on aging report a significant decrease in the level and turnover of PUFAs (Favreliere et al., 2000; Regev et al., 1999; Vreugdenhil et al., 1996; Zaidi & Michaelis, 1999). This major change is a significant decrease in omega-3 fatty acids, such as ALA and DHA (Favreliere et al., 2003). The magnitude of the decrease in the ratio is not uniform in all brain areas. While the decrease is significant in the cortex, striatum, and hypothalamus, the most profound decrease was found in the hippocampus (Ulmann et al., 2001). During aging, a significant change occurs in the transition temperature of the lipids, a change which is more profound in Alzheimer's patients (Giorgi et al., 1998). This change causes the membrane to be more rigid. The most studied fatty acids, in this respect, are DHA (omega-3) and AA (omega-6). While the level of both fatty acids is very low in the neuronal membrane of the aged hippocampus in rats, the treatment with omega-3 fatty acids improves the membrane status (McGahon et al., 1999; Meehan et al., 1995). Basically, two ways can explain the low level of PUFAs in the aging brain, namely, the low rate of transport of PUFAs from the blood into the brain, and the impaired biochemical machinery that normally is expected to incorporate and elongate the fatty acids. These two alternatives are directly related to their respective parent issues: the problem of the BBB and the dynamics of fatty acid brain metabolism.

The brain of an Alzheimer's patient undergoes more severe changes than the brain of a healthy elderly person. Among the major changes that are relevant to our issue are: (i) the decrease in the neurotransmitter acetylcholine in the brain (and in particular in the hippocampus) and (ii) the major double change in the brain lipids, of which one is the significant increase in the cholesterol level in the neuronal membrane, accompanied by a decrease in the total PUFA level; the other is the change in the omega-6 and omega-3 ratio. The level of omega-3 fatty acids (mainly DHA) is severely reduced (Conquer et al., 2000). Those changes have a direct effect on the membrane-fluidity index, causing the membrane to become more rigid and eventually to malfunction.

Alzheimer's Disease is a progressive and degenerative age-related dementia. Among the major symptoms are: short- and long-term memory loss, impairment of speech and language, decline of abstract reasoning, and mood change. The hallmark sign of the Alzheimer's disorder is the loss of spatial orientation. Most researchers agree that the hippocampus is responsible for this function, and indeed postmortem studies showed shrinkage of the hippocampus in Alzheimer's patients. The etiology of this disorder is not known, but many of the theories were summarized by Yehuda et al. (1996). Our preliminary studies show that the administration of a mixture of LA and ALA in a ratio of 4:1 improves the Mini Mental State Examination (MMSE) and quality of life test scores of Alzheimer's patients (Yehuda et al., 1996). Treatments with other ratios did not improve the Alzheimer's patients' condition. Administrations of a single fatty acid (i.e., DHA) did not improve the Alzheimer's condition by much (Das, 2000; Hashimoto et al., 2002). These results reflect similar results that were obtained in animal experimental models of Alzheimer's disease.

## *Seizure*

The relationship between lipids and fatty acid metabolism, on the one hand, and seizures on the other, was previously described (Lauritzen et al., 2001; Yehuda et al., 1994). The general finding shows a gross disturbance in the fatty acid metabolisms (Bazan, 1986; Birkle, 1993; Flynn & Wecker, 1987; Pediconi et al., 1986; Van Rooijen et al., 1986; Visioli et al., 1994 ). One of the effects of a seizure is the transient disruption of the BBB structure and functions (Cervos-Navarro et al., 1998); Cornford & Oldendorf, 1986). A well-known application of fatty acids in the diet for the treatment of epilepsy is represented by the ketogenic diet for children with refractory seizures (Freeman et al., 1998; Stafstrom & Bough, 2003). The promise of therapeutic effects that may be realized from ketogenic diets continues to be reaffirmed by many clinical investigators (Helmstaedter & Kurthen, 2001).

The possible mode of action to account for the involvement of brain lipids in seizures was recently summarized (Yehuda et al., 1994): Lipids are important constituents of the neuronal membrane, and changes in the fatty acid profiles may alter membrane functions:

- EFAs and phospholipids may offset the deleterious effects of substances that induce seizures, such as iron, that increased lipid peroxidation.
- EFAs and phospholipids may offer stability in membrane fluidity that may otherwise be associated with seizures.
- EFAs and phospholipids may control the alteration in neuronal membrane phospholipid metabolism that may result from the high prevalence of excitatory amino-acid receptors in the epileptic focus.
- A genetic link may exist between epilepsy and a PUFA deficit (Søvik et al., 1998), and a mixture of DHA and EPA may provide some measure of correction.
- EFAs may serve as neuroprotectors in the brain, similar to effects observed in the heart, as shown in recent studies where ALA (but not palmitic acid) was found to protect against ischemic-induced neuronal death and to prevent kainic-induced seizures and its associated neuronal death (Lauritzen et al., 2000; Xiao & Li, 1999).

Apart from the interest in a PUFA as a stabilizing agent for the neuronal membrane in seizures, is a growing interest in the use of the ketogenic diet in epileptic children. This diet is high-fat and low-carbohydrate, and is used to control intractable seizures in children. The ketogenic diet was very popular in the past, abandoned, and is currently being re-examined (Cunnane et al., 2002; Klepper et al., 2002; Musa-Veloso et al., 2002; Thavendiranathan et al., 2003 ). Note, however, that conflicting results were obtained in human studies.

## *EFAs and Sleep*

Sleep quality is a major problem in the modern society. Vast numbers of "healthy people" complain about the quality of their sleep. One of the major complaints is that sleep does not refresh them enough. In addition, many disease-states are associated with objective or subjective sleep disturbances. The presumed neurochemical basis for the relationship between EFAs and the different sleep stages was recently reviewed (Yehuda et al., 1998).

We already showed that the particular EFA ratio of 4:1, when given to Alzheimer's patients, significantly reduced their complaints about sleep problems, and indeed, the quality of their sleep improved (Yehuda et al., 1996).

The biological and mental roles and functions of sleep remain vague despite our rapidly increasing understanding of the processes in generating and maintaining the different sleep stages. Special attention was devoted to the Rapid Eye Movement (REM) stage. REM deprivation induces complex effects, which include brain morphological changes such as reduced neurogenesis processes (Mirmiram et al., 1983), and brain neurochemical and hormonal modifications (Andersen et al., 2005).

The finding that REM deprivation induces higher levels of cortisol (or corticosterone in rats) was reported in many studies (e.g., Andersen et al., 2004, 2005; Suchecki et al., 2002). This finding led to the conclusion that REM deprivation might lead to stress and anxiety (e.g., Silva et al., 2004). In addition, those studies examined the effects of REM deprivation on animal behavior in anxiety tests.

The relationship between sleep and lipids in general (Chen & Bazan, 2005), and with EFAs in particular (Yehuda, 2003; Yehuda et al., 1996, 1998, 2002, 2005), were discussed before. Similarly, the relationship between EFAs and stress was reviewed recently (Yehuda et al., 2001, 2006).

The ability of a specific mixture of EFAs [ALA (n-3) and LA (n-6) in a 1:4 ratio (Yehuda, 2003)] to restore sleep disturbances among the elderly and Alzheimer's patients was previously reported (Yehuda et al., 1996). On the other hand, this mixture (SR-3) is also able to reduce elevated cortisol and corticosterone levels (Rabinovitz et al., 2004; Yehuda et al., 2006).

Several techniques are used to measure the animal's anxiety level. One of the techniques is Elevated Plus Maze, which is used to determine the rodent's unconditioned response to a potentially dangerous environment; anxiety-related behavior is measured by the degree to which the rodent avoids the unenclosed arms of the maze. The test is particularly useful in testing the effects of anxiolytic and anxiogenic drugs.

Some types of stress induce hyperthermia. Papakonstantinou et al. (2003) showed that REM deprivation induces hyperthermia. The increase in noradrenaline and DA in REM-deprived rats could explain this hyperthermia (LeBlanc & Ducharme, 2007).

A mixture of EFAs protects rats from the anxiety induced by REM deprivation (Yehuda et al., 2007), and improves sleep complaints about sleep disturbances among test-anxiety students (Yehuda et al., 2005).

Test anxiety is an incapacitating academic syndrome. This study shows that the administration of a PUFA mixture of omega-3 and omega-6 can improve the behavioral variables associated with this type of anxiety (i.e., appetite, mood, mental concentration, fatigue, academic organization, and poor sleep), as well as lower the elevated cortisol level, with a corresponding reduction of anxiety.

Tests and examinations are primary methods of assessing academic performance. Test anxiety can seriously impair academic performance, and the mere anticipation of a critical examination can even hinder the ability to adequately prepare for it. The markers by which anxiety impairs academic performance are seen in the susceptibility to distraction from the task to irrelevant material, elevated cortisol level, sleep disturbances, and decreased appetite. Conventional treatment by anti-anxiety medications is neither effective nor desirable. However, the involvement of n-3 fatty acids in anxiety was suggested in the past, and while the body cannot produce EFAs, dietary intake can [and must] provide them. The many involvements of these fatty acids include retinal functions, learning and memory mechanisms, thermoregulation, pain, stress, and sleep. The influence of EFAs is manifested in the nervous system and in endocrine and immune functions; therefore, they are important in understanding and treating various brain-related disorders including Alzheimer's Disease and epilepsy. We also demonstrated that a specific mixture of ALA (n-3) and LA (n-6) in a ratio of 1:4 (SR-3) improves the quality of life of Alzheimer's patients and exerts beneficial effects in intact aged rats and in rats that were experimentally rendered learning-deficient. The mixture improved the memory, thermoregulation, and sleep in humans and in rats, and was able to rehabilitate the symptoms of induced multiple sclerosis in rats and decreased elevated cortisol level. We previously hypothesized that common to the diverse brain effects is the ability of EFAs to influence and modify the structure and function of the neuronal membrane, namely, the membrane-fluidity index, the functional role of the ionic channels, the activity of membrane-bound enzymes, and the affinity of various receptors.

The aim of the study was to examine the effect of the PUFA mixture on test-taking anxiety among undergraduate college students. Two trained psychologists identified 88 male students as test-anxiety sufferers by using the SMART test (Kleijn et al., 1994). The study was approved by the Bar Ilan University Ethics Committee, Ramat Gan, Israel. Seventy other students (matched for age and education level) from the same classes who did not suffer test anxiety served as the control group. The study started one month before the examination. Morning salivary cortisol samples were collected at 8:00 a.m. while the subjects were still at home. No food intake was allowed 30 minutes before taking the sample. The method of collecting the cortisol was fully described previously (Putignano et al., 2001). Briefly, samples were collected using cotton swabs chewed for 2 minutes, inserted into a plastic test tube, and then transported to a commercially available double-chamber device (Salivette® Sarstedt, Nümbrecht, Germany). After centrifuging and cooling to 4°C and storing at –20°C, the cortisol level was measured by the radio-immunoassay method. All subjects were asked to complete a five-point rating scale for each of the following six dimensions:

1. appetite,
2. overall mood state,
3. concentration during the school day,
4. fatigue experienced during the day,
5. ability to organize materials for the examination, and
6. quality of sleep.

Each subject was instructed to take one capsule of Awake (TransCulture, Tokyo Japan), which contains 225 mg of ALA (omega-3) and LA (omega-6) in a ratio of 1:4, twice daily in the morning and evening, for three weeks. One week before the examination, the cortisol-level samples and the questioners were repeated. Student *t*-tests were used to determine the differences between the groups.

The results (Table 25.2) showed improvement for all the test-anxiety variables following the administration of the EFA preparation. The subjects reported better appetite, improved mood, better ability to concentrate, less fatigue during the day, and better sleep; their ability to organize themselves for the test was much improved.

While test-anxiety students showed an elevated morning cortisol level, the PUFA treatment reduced the elevated level to a normal level. Interestingly, the control group also showed a reduction in the cortisol level. Seventy-eight out of the 88 test-anxiety students reported that even at the conclusion of the study they no longer experienced a state of anxiety. Side effects were minimal: five students reported transient stomach upset, and two reported nausea.

The results of this study demonstrate the multiple properties of the PUFA mixture. One prominent effect is a reduction in elevated cortisol level, beyond the placebo effect, and the other is a remediation of sleep disturbances. Sleep disturbances create a vicious cycle, namely, with a disturbed sleep pattern, the person is fatigued during the day, but the day sleep is not sufficiently refreshing, thereby leading to an exacerbation of the sleep disorder.

We believe this to be the first report on the beneficial effects of PUFAs on test anxiety. The suggested proposed mode of action is the ability of the EFA mixture to improve the neuronal-membrane structure on the serotonergic and gabaminergic

**Table 25.2. Effects of the Fatty Acid Mixture Administration on Behavioral Variables and Cortisol Level of Test-Anxiety Sufferers[a]**

| Variables | Control | | Test anxiety | |
|---|---|---|---|---|
| | Before | After | Before | After |
| Appetite | 4.5 ± 0.6 | 4.9 ± 0.7 | 2.2 ± 0.8 | 3.9 ± 0.6* |
| Good mood | 4.0 ± 0.8 | 4.8 ± 0.8 | 2.2 ± 1.1 | 3.9 ± 0.9* |
| Ability to concentrate | 3.5 ± 0.6 | 4.4 ± 0.5 | 2.0 ± 1.3 | 4.0 ± 0.8** |
| Fatigue during the day | 4.0 ± 0.5 | 4.5 ± 0.8 | 2.3 ± 1.0 | 4.0 ± 0.3** |
| Organizing academic material | 4.6 ± 0.6 | 4.8 ± 0.7 | 2.0 ± 1.3 | 3.9 ± 1.2* |
| Quality of sleep | 3.4 ± 1.3 | 4.6 ± 1.0 | 1.2 ± 1.1 | 3.6 ± 1.0** |
| Morning cortisol level (nmol/L) | 422.8 ± 33 | 414.5 ± 28* | 566.6 ± 48 | 431.6 ± 36** |

[a]There were 70 matched control subjects (ages 20–27) and 88 test-anxiety sufferers in the study. Data are presented as means and standard deviations.

* = Statistical significant difference (*P* ≤ *0.05*) from the "before" value.

** = Statistical significant difference (*P* ≤ *0.01*) from the "before" value.

systems in the brain. Further studies are needed to confirm this finding and to further elucidate the neurochemical basis of this effect.

### Late-onset Depression

"Late-onset depression" is a puzzling medical entity. While the number of late- onset depressive patients is increasing, mainly among the aged female population, it is poorly diagnosed and often confused with dementia, especially Alzheimer's Disease. The distinction between early- and late-onset depression is not clear; however, anti-depressive drugs are less effective in the elderly population.

The etiology of late-onset depression is not yet clear. The discussion whether early- and late-onset depression have a different etiology is still unanswered. Another enigma is whether they share the same phenomenology or whether their phenomenology is also distinct [e.g., a psychotic (delusional) type of depression is more common among late-onset patients]. The connection between depression and fatty acid lipid metabolism was discussed in the past. Changes in the immune system as well as changes in the circadian cycles were also demonstrated in depressed patients.

The repeated demonstrations that PUFAs can modify the production and activity of various components of the immune system left unexplained the mode of action by which they exert their effects. The PUFA mediation of immunological functions and cytokine levels is evident in several disorders such as Alzheimer's Disease and schizophrenia (Yao & van Kammen, 2004). Several mechanisms were proposed, including: (i) membrane fluidity (changes that might affect the capability of cytokines to bind to their respective receptors on the cell membrane); (ii) lipid peroxidation (a decrease in free radical-induced tissue damage); (iii) prostaglandin production (an indirect mechanism whereby prostaglandins, which are derivatives of PUFA, modify cytokine activity); and (iv) the regulation of gene expression (PUFA influences on the signal transudation pathways and modified mRNA activity). The role of PUFA in immune function is complicated by the fact that n-3 and n-6 have differential effects on various immune components. In a recent review, Kuatku (2000) indicated that n-3 fatty acids induce a decrease in lymphocyte proliferation in humans and rats, a decrease in interleukin-1 (IL-1) production, and a decrease in IL-2 production in both humans and animals. In addition, n-3 fatty acid decreases the tumor necrosis factor-α ($TNF_{\alpha}$) production in humans but increases it in mice macrophages, and also decreases natural killer (NK) cell activity. On the other hand, n-6 increases the production of IL-2 in mice and decreases the production of $TNF_{\alpha}$ production and NK cell activity. Still, other studies show that LA (n-6) decreases the activity of IL-2 (Yehuda et al., 1997) and increases IL-1 production and tissue response to cytokines, while n-3 generally decreases IL-1 production and activity (Grimble, 1998). Despite some disagreement among studies, it seems that n-3 fatty acids (ALA, DHA, EPA) decrease the production and activity of the pro-inflammatory cytokines (IL-1, IL-6, $TNF_{\alpha}$) (Blok et al., 1997; Yano et al., 2000) and that the n-6 family has the opposite effect (Caughey et al., 1996; Grimble, 1998; James et al., 2000). The findings about the ability of n-3 PUFA to reduce pro-inflammatory cytokines and prostaglandin (Chavali & Forse, 1999) led to the proposal for the use of fish oil to relieve pain. Fish oil, rich in n-3 PUFA, decreased IL-6, IL-10, IL-12, $TNF_{\alpha}$, and $PGE_2$ (Denisova et al., 2001).

## *Stress, Cortisol, and Learning*

One may appreciate the importance of the differentiation among the various types of fatty acids by noting their effects on immunological and endocrinological factors. For example, omega-3 fatty acids suppress the synthesis of IL-1 and IL-6, and enhance the synthesis of IL-2, while omega-6 fatty acids have the opposite effect. Remember, both IL-6 and IL-1 (and to a lesser degree IL-2) promote the CRF release via AA. However, CRF inhibits the stimulating effect of IL-1 on the prostaglandin synthesis.

Cortisol exerts powerful effects on all body tissues. It increases the level of glucose in the blood, stimulates the breakdown of proteins into amino acids, inhibits the uptake of glucose by muscle tissues (except in the brain), and regulates the response of the cardiovascular system to persistent high blood pressure. All of these actions constitute the "fight or flight" response, which helps the organism to cope with stress situations. Recent studies, however, indicate that cortisol may have some damaging effects, including deterioration of learning and memory. Human studies on normal, aged, depressed Cushing's Syndrome patients, as well as mentally ill patients, demonstrated a strong negative correlation between cortisol levels and learning and memory in a wide range of cognitive tasks. In rats, cortisol induces deterioration in spatial task performance as measured by the MWM test. These negative effects may be explained by the fact that cortisol interferes with physiological mechanisms crucial to the structure and function of the hippocampus. For example, stress is known to cause atrophy of the hippocampal dendrites and damage to the pyramidal neurons, and interferes with synaptic activity. Most likely, this morphological and functional hippocampal damage results from high levels of cortisol.

Recently we demonstrated that a specific mixture of free EFAs [LA (18:2ω6) and ALA (18:3ω3)] is able to reduce the levels of cholesterol in brain neuronal membranes (Yehuda et al., 1996, 1998).

Hippocampal functions, which include spatial-learning abilities, can be assessed through the MWM. This popular test is used to evaluate potential drugs for the Alzheimer's disorder, since Alzheimer's patients exhibit great difficulties in spatial orientation. Independent of hippocampal effects, hypothermia was also shown to impair learning, as evaluated by using various tests, including the MWM performance test, which is especially meant for spatial learning.

Further interest in the relationship between cortisol and learning arose when recent findings showed an increase in the level of cortisol in Alzheimer's patients, who also had elevated levels of IL-6. Note that IL-6 receptors were found in the adrenal cortex, and that the level of cortisol is raised by IL-6, which in turn is increased by general stress and cold.

Our study showed that a mixture of LA and ALA, administered for three weeks prior to an injection of cortisol (10 mg/kg) or prior to the immersion of rats in a 10°C saline bath, blocked the elevation of cortisol and cholesterol blood levels. In addition, this treatment protected the rats from the spatial-learning deficits that usually accompany the stressful conditions in the MWM. Moreover, a recent study showed that certain anti- epileptic drugs induce an increase in the cortisol level. The PUFA mixture at a 4:1 ratio can reduce the elevated cortisol level, and has anti-convalsant effects (Rabinovitz et al., 2004). Only this ratio has the effect of decreasing elevated cortisol levels.

## *ID and Fatty Acids*

Despite some successful interventions and the many research efforts on this topic, ID and anemia remain the most common nutritional disorders in the world. Numerous behavioral manifestations are observed among ID children and adults, such as lethargy, irritability, apathy, restlessness, fatigue, lack of concentration, pathological craving for ice, pica (pervert craving for substance unfit to eat), inattention, hyperactivity, and sleep disturbances. However, the most disturbing functional hallmark of ID is the decrease in mental performance (Youdim & Yehuda, 2000).

While the frequency of ID is greater among children in the Third World, many cases of ID are found at all ages, even among people in wealthy countries (Scrimshaw, 1998). A large number of ID elderly people is found among the Old-Age Homes population (Bourre, 1991). The three high-risk groups for ID are small children, pregnant women, and elderly people. Infants and the elderly are included in the high-risk groups, since in those two periods of life the brain structures and functions undergo rapid changes.

Many ID effects are mediated via brain biochemistry, with a prominent modification in the level and the activity of brain neurotransmitters (mainly DA and DA D2 receptors). In addition, iron plays a major role in fatty acids and lipid metabolism via the family of cytochrome P-450. An important link exists between iron and lipids that affects myelin and all its processes, especially myelin formation and myelin disintegration. An adequate supply of iron and EFAs during the developing periods is required for the normal rate of myelination (Youdim & Yehuda, 2000).

In general, the infancy period is a critical period for the proper development of the central nervous system. Human and animal studies showed that cognitive deficits induced by ID during this period are very difficult to rehabilitate (Lozoff et al., 2000; Youdim et al., 1989).

The long-lasting effects of early ID were recognized by the studies of Lozoff's group (Lozoff et al., 2000). Recently (Yehuda & Yehuda, 2006) the long-term effects of rehabilitated infancy (a 1-year-old) ID were examined at age 10. Despite their normal hematological blood values, those children showed some deficits in their auditory system, reduced I.Q. spatial scores, reduced cortisol level, and an increase in sleep disturbances.

The aim of the study was to explore the possibility of creating an animal model to illustrate the cognitive long-lasting effects of rehabilitated early ID. The cognitive capacities were measured by MWM, and by passive avoidance apparatus. The physiological variable was body temperature, and the levels of iron and hemoglobin were measured. The results showed that ID induced long-lasting effects and a mixture of EFAs can rehabilitate those deficits.

The main finding of this study is the demonstration of the long-lasting cognitive effect of the early period of ID. The former iron-deficient rats, despite the normal values of iron and hemoglobin, normal thermoregulation and normal motor activity level, exhibited severe learning capacities which are not as prominent as iron-deficient rats of their age, but statistically differ from control rats. The second major finding is the ability of a specific mixture of EFAs to rehabilitate the effects of ID.

The same pattern of learning (cognitive) disability was found among children who were diagnosed as iron-deficient at age 1 year, rehabilitated their haematological values, and tested 10 years later (Yehuda & Yehuda, 2006).

It seems that the period between days 21 and 49 included a critical period for an adequate supply of iron to reach the brain in addition to the prenatal and very early development period.

Interestingly, the long-lasting effects of early ID included both MWM and passive avoidance. The first learning is a spatial learning, and the other is inhibitory learning. The common mechanism between those two types of learning and with ID is not yet known.

Treatment with SR-3 improved learning capacity. How fatty acids improve haematological values is unclear. Conceivably, the EFAs facilitate the absorption of iron from the gut and its storage in the blood.

Several hypotheses explain the long-lasting effect of early ID despite the rehabilitation of the hematological values: (i) One hypothesis is that an early ID period during a critical period can cause damage to the dopaminergic system (i.e., DA production and functions which may last for a long period; (ii) Another hypothesis might be based on Youdin (2008), who found that both MWM and passive avoidance learning are mediated via the hippocampus, and ID induced morphological and functional damage to the hippocampus; or (iii) Assume that the damage to the hippocampus is induced by corticosterone, which releases at the time of ID because ID is considered a stress. Importunely, we do not have enough data to support one of these hypotheses or any other.

In conclusion, we were able to show that the cognitive effects of early ID lasted a long time, and that those deficits can be rehabilitated by a mixture of EFAs. This animal model might serve as a tool to investigate this important phenomena.

## Conclusion

This review related mainly to LA and ALA. Using longer chain fatty acids, such as AA and DHA, can maintain the ratio between omega-6 and omega-3. However, very few studies were carried out on the balance between the LC-PUFAs balance or ratio and brain functions. The few studies that, in fact, did examine this area were recently summarized (Simopoulos, 2000; Youdim et al., 2000); they demonstrated the importance of the ratio between omega-6 and omega-3.

Likely, the required ratio of omega-6 and omega-3 may differ when used for different tissues or functions. One can understand that a ratio of 1:1 is the optimal ratio for preventing cardiovascular diseases, and another ratio would be optimal for cancer prevention. We are merely suggesting that a ratio of 4:1 is the optimal ratio for brain-mediated functions. The question is: How can it be that PUFA is helpful to organisms that are only capable of obtaining it from the diet? Our hypothesis is that omega-6 and omega-3, in a ratio of 4:1, act within the neuronal membrane, and improve the membrane-fluidity index, which is the key to all neuronal activity. Other researchers also recommended the ratio of 4:1. The results of those studies were earlier summarized by Yehuda and Carasso (1993) and again more recently by Horrocks and Yeo (1999). We have difficulty explaining why this particular ratio is best. One possibility is that the preferred ratio for omega-6 and omega-3 PUFAs depends on the competition of the same enzymes for desaturation and elongation. Another possibility is that the PUFAs in this ratio are able to create micellae, which protect them. Whatever the biochemical basis could be, the results showed that the 4:1 ratio has protective and stabilizing effects on the neuronal membrane.

## References

Acar, N.; J.M. Chardigny; M. Darbois; B. Pasquis; J.L. Sebedio. Modification of the dopaminergic neurotransmitters in striatum, frontal cortex and hippocampus of rats fed for 21 months with trans isomers of alpha-linolenic acid. *Neurosci. Res.* **2003**, *45*, 375–382.

Andersen, M.L.; M. Bignitto; R.B. Machado; S. Tufik. Different stress modalities result in distinct steroid hormone responses by male rats. *Braz. J. Med. Biol. Res.* **2004**, *37*, 791–797.

Andersen, M.L.; P.J.F. Martins; V. D'Almeida; M. Bignitto; S. Tufik. Endocrinological and catecholaminergic alterations during sleep deprivation and recovery in male rats. *J. Sleep Res.* **2005**, *14*, 83–90.

Ando, S.; Y. Tanaka; Y. Toyoda; K. Kon. Turnover of myelin lipids in aging brain. *Neurochem. Res.* **2003**, *28*, 5–13.

Auestad, N. Infant nutrition—brain development—disease in later life. *Dev. Neurosci.* **2000,** *22*, 472–473.

Bazan, N.G. The neuromessenger platelet-activating factor in plasticity neurodegeneration. *Prog. Brain Res.* **1986**, *118*, 281–291.

Birkle, D.L. Regional and temporal variations in the accumulation of unesterified fatty acids and diacylglycerols in the rat brain during kainic acid induced limbic seizures. *Brain Res.* **1993**, *613*, 115–122.

Blok, W.L.; J.P. Deslypere; P.N.M. Demacker; J. van der VenJongekrijg; M.P. Hectors; J.W. van der Meer; M.B. Katan. Pro- and anti-inflammatory cytokines in healthy volunteers fed various doses of fish oil for 1 year. *Eur J. Clin. Invest.* **1997**, *25*, 629–638.

Bourre, J.M.; O. Dumont; M. Piciotti; M. Clement; J. Chaudiere; M. Bonneil. Essentiality of Ω–3 fatty acids for brain structure and function. *World Rev. Nutr.* **1991**, *66*, 103–117.

Burgess, J.R.; L. Stevens; W. Zhang; L. Peck. Long-chain polyunsaturated fatty acids in children with attention-deficit hyperactivity disorder. *Am. J. Clin. Nutr.* **2000**, *71*, 327S–330S.

Caughey, G.E.; E. Mantzioris; R.A. Gibson; L.G. Cleland; M.J. James. The effect on human tumour necrosis factor α and interleukin 1β production of diets enriched in n-3 fatty acids from vegetable oil or fish oil. *Am. J. Clin. Nutr.* **1996**, *63*, 116–122.

Cervos-Navarro, J.; S. Kannuki; Y. Nakagawa. Blood-brain barrier (BBB). Review from morphological aspect. *Histol. Histopathol.* **1988**, *3*, 203–213.

Chalon, S.; S. Delion-Vancassel; C. Belzung; D. Guilloteau; A.M. Lequisquet; J.C. Besnard; G. Durand. Dietary fish oil effects monoaminergic neurotransmission and behavior in rats. *J. Nutr.* **1998**, *128*, 2512–2519.

Chavali, S.R.; R.A. Forse. Decreased production of interleukin-6 and prostaglandin E2 associated with inhibition of delta-5 desaturation of omega-6 fatty acids in mice fed safflower oil diets supplemented with sesamol. *Prostaglandins Leukotrienes Essent. Fatty Acids* **1999**, *61*, 347–52.

Chen, C.; N.G. Bazan. Lipid signaling: sleep, synaptic plasticity, and neuroprotection. *Prostaglandins Other Lipid Mediat.* **2005,** *77*, 65–76.

Conquer, J.A.; M.C. Tierney; J. Zecevic; W.J. Bettger; R.H. Fisher. Fatty acid analysis of blood plasma of patients with Alzheimer's disease, other types of dementia, and cognitive impairment. *Lipids* **2000**, 35, 1305–1312.

Cornford, E.M., W.H. Oldendorf. Epilepsy and the blood-brain barrier. *Adv. Neurol.* **1986**, *44*, 787–812.

Cunnane, S.C.; K. Musa; M.A. Ryan; S. Whiting; D.D. Fraser: Potential role of polyunsaturates in seizure protection achieved with the ketogenic diet. *Prostaglandins Leukotrienes Essent. Fatty Acids* **2002**, *67*, 131–135.

Das, UN. Beneficial effect(s) of n-3 fatty acids in cardiovascular diseases: but, why and how? *Prostaglandins Leukotrienes Essent. Fatty Acids* **2000**, *63*, 351–362.

de la Torre, J.C.; T. Mussivand. Can disturbed brain microcirculation cause Alzheimer's disease? *Neurol. Res.* **1993**, *15*, 146–153.

Denisova, N.A; I. Cantuti-Castelvetri; W.N. Hassan; K.E. Paulson; J.A. Joseph. Role of membrane lipids in regulation of vulnerability to oxidative stress in PC12 cells: implication for aging. *Free Radical Biol. Med.* **2001,** *30*, 671–678.

Edmond, J. Essential polyunsaturated fatty acids and the barrier to the brain. *J. Mol. Neurosci.* **2001**, *16*, 181–193.

Farkas, E.; M.C. de Wilde; A. Kiliaan; J. Meijer; J.N. Keijser; P.G.M. Luiten. Dietary long chain PUFAs differentially effect hippocampal muscarinic 1 and serotonergic 1A receptors in experimental cerebral hypoperfusion. *Brain Res.* **2002**, *954*, 32–41.

Farooqu, A.A.; L.A Horrocks. Plasmalogens, phospholipase A2, and docosahexaenoic acid turnover in brain tissue. *J. Mol. Neurosci.* **2001,** *16*, 263–272.

Favreliere, S.; M.C. Perault; F. Huguet; D. De Javel; N. Bertrand; A. Piriou; G. Durand. DHA-enriched phospholipid diets modulate age-related alterations in rat hippocampus. *Neurobiol. Aging* **2003**, *24*, 233–243.

Favreliere, S; S. Stadelman-Ingrand; F. Huguet; D. De Javel, A. Piriou; C. Tallineau. Age-related changes in ethanolamine glycerophospholipid fatty acid levels in rat frontal cortex and hippocampus. *Neurobiol Aging* **2000**, *21*, 653–660.

Feller, S.E.; K. Gawrisch; A.D. MacKerell, Jr. Polyunsaturated fatty acids in lipid bilayers: intrinsic and environmental contributions to their unique physical properties. *J. Am. Chem. Soc.* **2002,** *124*, 318–326.

Flynn, C.J.; L. Wecker. Concomitant increases in the levels of choline and free fatty acids in rat brain: evidence supporting the seizure-induced hydrolysis of phosphatidylcholine. *J. Neurochem.* **1987**, *48*, 1178–1184.

Freeman, J.M.; E.P. Vining; D.J. Pillas; P.L. Pyzik; J.C. Casey; L.M. Kelly. The efficacy of the ketogenic diet-1998: a prospective evaluation of intervention in 150 children. *Pediatrics* **1998,** *102,* 1358–1363.

Ginsberg, L.; J.H. Xeureb; N.L. Gershfeld. Membrane instability plasmalogen content and Alzheimer's disease. *J. Neurochem.* **1998**, *70*, 2533–2538.

Giorgi, P.L.; M. Biraghi; A. Kantar. Effect of desmopressin on rat brain synaptosomal membrane: a pilot study. *Curr. Therap. Res.* **1998,** *59*, 172–178.

Grimble, R.F. Dietary lipids and the inflammatory response. *Proc. Nutr. Soc.* **1998**, *57*, 535–542.

Hashimoto, M; S. Hossain; T. Shimada; K. Sugioka; H. Yamasaki; Y. Fujii, Y. Ishibashi; J.I. Oka; O. Shido. Docosahexaenoic acid provides protection from impairment of learning ability in Alzheimer's disease model rats. *J. Neurochem.* **2002**, *81,* 1084–1091.

Helmstaedter, C; M. Kurthen. Memory and epilepsy: characteristics, course and influence of drugs and surgery. *Curr. Opin. Neurol.* **2001,** *14*, 211–216.

Horrocks, L.A.; H.W. Harder. Fatty acids and cholesterol. *Handbook of Neurochemistry;* A. Lajtha, Ed.; Plenum: New York, 1983; pp. 1–16.

Horrocks, L.A.; Y.K. Yeo. Health benefits of docosahexaenoic acid (DHA). *Pharmacol. Res.* **1999**, *40,* 211–225.

Ikemoto, A; M. Ohishi; Y. Sato; N. Hata; Y. Misawa; Y. Fujii; H. Okuyama. Reversibilityof n-3 fatty acid deficiency-induced alterations of learning behavior in the rat: level of n-6 fatty acids as another critical factor. *J. Lipid Res.* **2001**, *42*, 1655–1663.

James, M.J.; R.A. Gibson; L.G. Cleland. Dietary polyunsaturated fatty acids and inflammatory mediator production. *Am. J. Clin. Nutr.* **2000,** *71(Suppl.)*, 343S–348S.

Jumpsen, J.; E.L. Lien; Y.K. Goh; M.T. Clandinin. Small changes of dietary (n-6) and (n-3)/ fatty acid content ratio alter phosphatidylethanolamine and phosphatidylcholine fatty acid composition during development of neuronal and glial cells in rats. *J. Nutr.* **1997a,** *127,* 724–731.

Jumpsen, J.A.; E.L. Lien; Y.K. Goh; M.T. Clandinin. During neuronal and glial cell development diet n-6 to n-3 fatty acid ratio alters the fatty acid composition of phosphatidylinositol and phosphatidylserine. *Biochim. Biophys. Acta* **1997b**, *1347*, 40–50.

Kidd, P.M. Attention deficit/ hyperactivity disorder (ADHD) in children: rationale for its integrative management. *Alt. Med. Rev.* **2000,** *5*, 402–428.

Kleijn, W.C.; H.M. van der Ploeg; R.M. Topman. Cognition, study habits, test anxiety, and academic performance. *Psychol. Rep.* **1994,** *75,* 1219–1226.

Klepper, J; B. Leiendecker; R. Bredahl; S. Athanassopoulos; F. Heinen; E.E. Gertsen; A. Flörcken; A. Metz; T. Voit. Introduction of a ketogenic diet in young infants. *J. Inherit. Metab. Dis.* **2002**, *25*, 449–460.

Kodas, E.; S. Vancassel; B. Lejeune; D. Guilloteau; S. Chalon. Reversibility of n-3 fatty acid deficiency-induced changes in dopaminergic neurotransmission in rats: critical role of developmental stage. *J. Lipid Res.* **2002**, *43*, 1209–1219.

Kuratku, C.N. Proliferation of colonic lymphocytes in response to inflammatory cytokines is lower in mice fed fish oil than in mice fed corn oil. *Cancer Lett.* **2000,** *148(1),* 27–32.

Lauritzen, I.; N. Blondeau; C. Heurteaux; G.R. Widmann; M. Lazdunski. Polyunsaturated fatty acids are potent neuroprotectors. *EMBO J.* **2000**, *19,* 1784–1793.

Lauritzen, L.; H.S. Hansen; M.H. Jorgensen; K.F. Michaelsen. The essentiality of long chain n-3 fatty acids in relation to development and function of the brain and retina. *Prog. Lipid Res.* **2001**, *40,* 1–94.

LeBlanc, J.; M.B. Ducharme. Plasma dopamine and noradrenaline variations in response to stress. *Phys. Behav.* **2007**. (In Press)

McGahon, B.M.; C.A. Murray; D.F. Horrobin; M.A. Lynch. Age-related changes in oxidative mechanisms and LTP are reversed by dietary manipulation. *Neurobiol. Aging* **1999**, *20,* 643–653.

Meehan, E; F. Beauge; D. Choquart; B.E. Leonard. Influence of an n-6 polyunsaturated fatty acid-enriched diet on the development of tolerance during chronic ethanol administration in rats. *Alcohol Clin. Exp. Res.* **1995,** *1*, 1441–1446.

Mirmmiran, N.;H. B. Uylings; M. H. Corner. Effects of experimental suppression of active (REM) sleep during early development upon adult brain and behavior in the rat. *Brain Res.* **1983,** *283*, 277–286.

Musa-Veloso, K; E.E. Rarama; F. Comeau; R. Curtis; S. Cunnane. Epilepsy and the ketogenic diet: assessment of ketosis in children using breath acetone. *Pediatr. Res.* **2002**, *52,* 443–448.

Oner, O.; O.Y. Alkar; P. Oner. Relation of ferritin levels with symptom ratings and cognitive performance in children with attention deficit-hyperactivity disorder. *Pediatr Int.* **2008,** *50*, 40–44.

Papakonstantinou, E; D.H. Ryan; R.B.S. Harris. Dietary fish oil does not protect rats exposed to restraint or sleep deprivation stress. *Phys. Behav.* **2003**, 78, 759–765.

Pediconi, M.F.; E.B. Rodriguez de Turco; N.G. Bazan. Reduced labeling of brain phosphatidylinositol, triacylglycerols, and diacylglycerols by [C]arachidonic acid after electroconvulsive shock: potentiation of the effect by edrenergic drugs and comparison with palmitic acid labeling. *Neurochem. Res.* **1986**, *11,* 1–14.

Putignano, P; A. Dubini; P. Toja; C. Invitti; S. Bonfanti; G. Redaelli; D. Zappulli; F. Cavagnini. Salivary cortisol measurement in normal-weight, obese and anorexic women: comparison with plasma cortisol. *Eur. J. Endocrinol.* **2001**, *145*, 165–171.

Rabinovitz, S.; D.I. Mostofsky; S. Yehuda. Anticonvulsant efficiency, behavioral performance and cortisol level: A comparison of carbamazepine (CBZ) and a fatty acid compound (SR-3). *Psychoneuroendocrinology* **2004**, *2,* 113–124.

Rapoport, S.I. In vivo fatty acid incorporation into brain phospholipids in relation to plasma availability, signal transduction and membrane remodeling. *J. Mol. Neurosci.* **2001**, *16,*

243–261.

Regev, R.; Y.G. Assaraf; G.D. Eytan. Membrane fluidization by ether other anesthetics, and certain agents abolishes P-glycoprotein ATPase activity and modulates efflux from multidrug-resistant cells. *Eur. J. Biochem.* **1999**, *258*, 18–24.

Richardson, A.J.; B.K. Puri. The potential role of fatty acids in attention-deficit/ hyperactivity disorder. *Prostaglandin, Leukotrienes Essent. Fatty Acids* **2000**, *63*, 79–87.

Ross, B.M.; I. McKenzie; C.P. Bennett. Increased levels of ethane, a non-invasive marker of n-3 fatty acid oxidation, in breath of children with attention deficit hyperactivity disorder. *Nutr. Neurosci.* **2003**, *6*, 277–381.

Salem, N.; T. Moriguchi; R.S. Greiner; K. McBride; A. Ahmad; J.N. Catalan; B. Slotnick. Alterations in brain function after loss of docosahexaenoate due to dietary restriction of n-3 fatty acids. *J. Mol. Neurosci.* **2001**, *16l*, 299–307.

Salvati, S.; L. Attorri; C. Avellino; A. Di Biase; M. Sanchez. Diet, lipids and brain development. *Dev. Neurosci.* **2000,** *22*, 481–487.

Sawazaki, S.; T. Hamazaki; K. Yazawa; M. Kobayashi. The effect of docosahexaenoic acid on plasma catecholamine concentrations and glucose tolerance during long-lasting psychological stress: a double blind placebo-controlled study. *J. Nutr. Neurosci. Vitaminol.* **1999**, *45*, 655–665.

Silva, R.H.; S.R. Kameda; A.L.Takatsu-Coleman; S.T. Niigaki; V.C. Abilio; S. Tufik; R. Frussa-Filho. Anxiogenic effect of sleep deprivation in the elevated plus-maze test in mice. *Psychopharmacology (Berlin, Ger.)* **2004**, *176*, 115–122.

Simopoulos, A.P. Evolutionary aspects of omega-3 fatty acids in the food supply. *Prostaglandins, Leukotrienes Essent. Fatty Acids* **1999**, *60*, 421–429.

Simopoulos, A.P. Human requirement for n-3 polyunsaturated fatty acids. *Poult. Sci.* **2000**, *79*, 961–970.

Stafstrom, C.E.; K.J. Bough. The ketogenic diet for the treatment of epilepsy: a challenge for nutritional neuroscientists. *Nutr. Neurosci.* **2003**, *6*, 67–79.

Stevens, L.J.; S.S. Zebtall; J.L. Deck; M.L. Abate; B.A. Watkins; S.R. Lipp; J.R. Burgess. Essential fatty acid metabolism in boys with attention-deficit hyperactivity disorder. *Am. J. Clin. Nutr.* **1995**, *62*, 761–768.

Stockard, J.E.; M.D. Saste; V.J. Benford; L. Barness; N. Auestad; J.D. Carver. Effect of docosahexaenoic acid content of maternal diet on auditory brainstem conduction times in rat pups. *Dev. Neurosci.* **2000,** *22*, 494–499.

Strosznajder, J.; M. Samochocki; M. Duran. Aging diminishes serotonin-stimulated arachidonic acid uptake and cholinergic receptor-activated acid release in rat brain cortex membrane. *J. Neurochem.* **1994**, *62*, 1048–1054.

Søvik, O.; J.E. Mansson; A.L. Bjorke Monsen; E. Jellum; R.K. Berge. Generalized peroxisomal disorder in male twins: fatty acid composition of serum lipids and response to n-3 fatty acids. *J. Inherit. Metab. Dis.* **1998**, *21*, 662–670.

Suchecki, D; P.A. Tiba, S. Tufik. Paradoxical sleep deprivation facilitates subsequent corticosterone response to a mild stressor in rats. *Neurosci. Lett.* **2002,** *320*, 45–48.

Terracina, L.; M. Brunetti; L. Avellini; G.E. de Medio; G. Trovarelli; A. Gaiti. Linoleic acid metabolism in brain cortex of aged rats. *Ital. J. Biochem.* **1992**, *41*, 225–235.

Thavendiranathan, P.; C. Chow; S. Cunnane, W.M. Burnham. The effect of the 'classic' ketogenic diet on animal seizure models. *Brain Res.* **2003**, *959*, 206–213.

Ulmann, L.; V. Mimouni; S. Roux; R. Porsolt; J.P. Poisson. Brain and hippocampus fatty acid composition in phospholipid classes of aged-relative cognitive deficit rats. *Prostaglandins, Leukotrienes Essent. Fatty Acids* **2001**, *64*, 189–195

Umezawa, M.; K. Kogishi; H. Tojo; S. Yoshimura; N. Seriu; A. Ohta; T. Takeda; M. Hosokawa. High-linoleate and high-alpha-linolenate diets affect learning ability and natural behavior in SAMR1 mice. *J. Nutr.* **1999**, *129*, 431–437.

Van Rooijen, L.A.; R. Vadnal; P. Dobard; N.G. Bazan. Enhanced inositide turnover in brain during bicuculline-induced status epilepticus. *Biochem. Biophys. Res. Commun.* **1986**, *136*, 827–834.

Visioli, F.; E.B. Rodriguez de Turco; N.R. Kreisman; N.G. Bazan. Membrane lipid degradation is related to interictal cortical activity in a series of seizures. *Metab. Brain Dis.* **1994**, *9*, 161–170.

Vreugdenhil, M.; C. Bruehl; R.A. Voskuyl; J.X. Kang; A. Leaf; W.J. Wadman. Polyunsaturated fatty acids modulate sodium and calcium currents in CA1 neurons. *Proc. Natl. Acad. Sci. USA* **1996**, *93*, 12559–12563.

Wainwright, P.E.; H.C. Xing; L. Mutsaers; D. McCutcheon; D. Kyle. Arachidonic acid offsets the effects on mouse brain and behavior of a diet with a low (n-6):(n-3) ratio and very high levels of docosahexaenoic acid. *J. Nutr.* **1997,** *127*, 184–193.

Xiang, M.; G. Alfven; M. Blennow; M. Trygg; R. Zetterstrom. Long-chain polyunsaturated fatty acids in human milk and brain growth during early infancy. *Acta Paediatr.* **2000**, *89*, 142–147.

Xiao, Y.; X. Li. Polyunsaturated fatty acids modify mouse hippocampal neuronal excitability during excitotoxic or convulsant stimulation. *Brain Res.* **1999**, *846*, 112–121.

Yano, M.; E. Kishida; M. Iwasaki; S. Kojo; Y. Masuzawa. Docosahexaenoic acid and vitamin E can reduce human monocytic U937 cell apoptosis induced by tumor necrosis factor. *J. Nutr*. **2000**, *130*, 1095–1101.

Yao, J.K.; D.P. van Kammen. Membrane phospholipids and cytokine interaction in schizophrenia. *Int. Rev. Neurobiol.* **2004**, *59*, 297–326.

Yehuda, S. Omega-6/omega-3 ratio and brain-related functions. *World Rev. Nutr. Diet* **2003**, *92*, 37–56.

Yehuda, S; R.L. Carasso. Modulation of learning, pain thresholds, and thermoregulation in the rat by preparations of free purified α- linolenic and linoleic acids: determination of optimal n-3 to omega-6 ratio. *Proc. Natl. Acad. Sci. USA* **1993**, *90*, 10345–10349.

Yehuda S.; R.L. Carasso; D.I. Mostofsky. Essential fatty acid preparation (1:4 ratio) raises the seizure threshold in rats. *Eur. J. Pharmacol.* **1994,** *254*, 193–198.

Yehuda, S.; R.L. Carasso; D.I. Mostofsky. Essential fatty acid preparation (1:4 ratio) rehabilitates learning deficits induced by AF64A and 5,7-DHT. *NeuroReport* **1995**, *6*, 511–515.

Yehuda, S.; S. Rabinovitz; R.L. Carasso; D.I. Mostofsky. Essential fatty acids preparation (SR-3) improves Alzheimer' patients quality of life. *Int. J. Neurosci.* **1996,** *87*, 141–149.

Yehuda, S.; S. Rabinovitz; R.L. Carasso; D.I. Mostofsky. Fatty acids and brain peptides. *Peptides* **1998**, *19*, 407–419.

Yehuda, S.; S. Rabinovitz; R.L. Carasso; D.I. Mostofsky. The Role of PUFA in restoring the aging neuronal membrane. *Neurobiol. Aging* **2002**, *23*, 843–853.

Yehuda, S.; S. Rabinovitz; D.I. Mostofsky. Effects of essential fatty acids preparation (SR-3) on brain biochemistry and on behavioral and cognitive functions. *Handbook of Essential Fatty Acids Biology: Biochemistry Physiology and Behavioral Neurobiology;* S. Yehuda, D.I. Mostofsky, Eds.; Humana Press: New York, 1997; pp. 427–452.

Yehuda, S.; S. Rabinovitz; D.I. Mostofsky. Essential fatty acids and sleep: mini-review and hypothesis. *Med. Hypothesis* **1998a,** *50*,139–145.

Yehuda, S.; S. Rabinovitz; D.I. Mostofsky. Modulation of learning and neuronal membrane composition in the rat by essential fatty acids preparation: Time course analysis. *Neurochem. Res.* **1998b**, *23*, 631–638.

Yehuda, S.; S. Rabinovitz; D.I. Mostofsky. Essential fatty acids are mediators of brain biochemistry and cognitive functions. *J. Neurosci. Res.* **1999a**, 565–570.

Yehuda, S.; S. Rabinovitz; D.I. Mostofsky. PUFA: Mediators for the nervous, endocrine, and immune system. *Fatty Acids: Physiological and Behavioral Functions;* D.I. Mostofsky, S. Yehuda, N. Salem, Eds.; Humana Press: New York, 2001; pp. 403–420.

Yehuda, S.; S. Rabinovitz; D.I. Mostofsky. Mixture of essential fatty acids lowers test anxiety. *Nutr. Neurosci.* **2005**, *8*, 265–267.

Yehuda, S.; S. Rabinovitz; D.I. Mostofsky. Essential fatty acids and stress. *Nutrients, Stress, and Medical Disorders;* S. Yehuda, D.I. Mostofsky, Eds.; Humana Press: Towota, NJ, 2006; pp. 99–111.

Yehuda, S.; S. Rabinovitz; D.I. Mostofsky. Pretreatment with a mixture of essential fatty acids protects rats from anxiogenic effects of REM deprivation. *Nutr Neurosci.* **2007,** *10*, 269–71.

Yehuda, S.; S. Rabinovitz; D.I. Mostofsky; M. Huberman; B. Sredni. Essential fatty acid preparation improves biochemical and cognitive functions in experimental allergic encephalomyelitis rats. *Eur. J. Pharmacol.* **1997,** *328*, 23–29.

Yehuda, S.; M. Yehuda. Long lasting effects of infancy iron deficiency--preliminary results. *J Neural Transm Suppl.* **2006,** *7,* 1197–2000.

Youdim, K.A.; A. Martin; J.A. Joseph. Essential fatty acids and the brain: possible health implications. *Int. J. Dev. Neurosci.* **2000**, *18*, 383–399.

Youdim, M.B.H.; S. Yehuda. The neurochemical basis of cognitive deficits induced by brain iron deficiency: involvement of dopamine-opiate system. *Cell Mol. Biol.* **2000,** *46*, 491–500.

Youdim, M.B.H. Brain iron deficiency and excess; cognitive impairment and neurodegenration with involvement of striatum and hippocampus. *Neurotox Res.* **2008,** *14*, 45–56.

Zaidi, A.; M.L. Michaelis. Effects of reactive oxygen species on brain synapticplasma membrane Ca(2+)-ATPase. *Free Radical Biol. Med.* **1999,** *27,* 810–821.

Zimmer, L.; S. Delpal; D. Guilloteau; J. Aioun; G. Durand. Chronic n-3 polyunsaturated fatty acid deficiency alters dopamine vesicle density in the rat frontal cortex. *Neurosci. Lett.* **2000**, *284*, 25–28.

Zimmer, L.; S. Vancassel; S. Cantagrel; P. Breton; S. Delamanche; D. Guilloteau; G. Durand; S. Chalon. The dopamine mesocorticolimbic pathway is affected by deficiency in n-3 polyunsaturated fatty acids. *Am. J. Clin. Nutr.* **2002**, *75*, 662–667.

# 26

# The Opposing Effects of Dietary Omega-3 and *trans* Fatty Acids on Health: A Yin-Yang Effect at the Molecular Level?

**Jørn Dyerberg and Steen Stender**
*Department of Clinical Biochemistry, Gentofte University Hospital; Copenhagen, Denmark*

## Introduction

During the recent decade, interest focused on positive health effects, especially on ischemic heart disease (IHD) risk, of an increased intake of long-chain omega-3 fatty acids, eicosapentaenoic acid (EPA; C20:5n-3), and docosahexaenoic acid (DHA; C22:6n-3) from seafood (e.g., Wang et al., 2006). Certain diseases and physiological processes, such as inflammatory disorders, dementia, and cognitive development were also beneficially associated with seafood and omega-3 fatty acid intake (Ruxton et al., 2007). This led to a recommendation to increase the intake of long-chain omega-3 fatty acids (American Heart Association Nutrition Committee, 2006).

During the same time period, attention also focused on the association between a high intake of *trans* fatty acids (TFAs) of industrial origin (IP-TFAs), such as elaidic acid (C18:1n-9*t*), and negative health outcomes, especially IHD (Mozaffarian et al, 2006; Stender & Dyerberg, 2004). This led to a recommendation to reduce the intake of TFAs (Dietary Guidelines for Americans, 2005). Because humans do not synthesize neither omega-3 fatty acids nor TFAs, the presence of these fatty acids in the body depends exclusively on their availability in the diet.

The risk of IHD, associated with the intake of IP-TFAs, is as estimated from prospective epidemiological studies, substantially greater than that accounted for by the effect of these fatty acids on blood lipids and lipoproteins (Ascherio et al., 1999; Mozaffarian et al., 2006; Oomen et al., 2001). Similarily, the findings of a decreased mortality of cardiovascular disease (CVD) after supplementation with omega-3 fatty acids could not be explained by a beneficial effect on blood lipids (GISSI-Preventione Investigators, 1999; Harris et al., 2008).

The intake of IP-TFAs and omega-3 fatty acids does, however, affect many biological functions other than those related to the cardiovascular system. They are generally associated with disease prevalence in opposite ways, similar to their relationship in IHD (Fig. 26.1).

Here we focus on this "yin-yang" aspect of the two types of fatty acids by reviewing observational epidemiological data and results from intervention studies. We also offer a hypothesis on the mechanisms of action at the molecular level for this phenomenon.

Be aware that the positive and negative health effects dealt with in this review are mainly based on associations between intakes and health effects obtained from observational studies, not from intervention trials. This opens the possibility for observational bias. Effects on risk factors such as plasma lipids were, however, generally based on intervention trials.

# Omega-3 and *trans* Fatty Acids in Our Food

## *Omega-3 Fatty Acids*

Two families exist of essential fatty acids: omega-3 (or n-3) and omega-6 (or n-6). The polyunsaturated fatty acids from each of these two families are essential since the body cannot synthesize a polyunsaturated fatty acid, nor can it convert a member of one polyunsaturated family to one of the other family. Human metabolism does, however, convert one member of each family to another of the same family. The two fatty acid families are termed "essential" because each was more or less able to meet the growth requirements of rats given fat-free diets. They were originally designated as vitamin F when they were discovered as essential nutrients in 1923. In 1930, Burr and Burr showed that they were more qualified to be with the fats than with the vitamins (Burr & Burr, 1930). The omega-3 family of fatty acids is found in vegetable sources, such as flax oil, in the form of alpha-linolenic acid (ALA) (C18:3n-3), and

| | omega-3 | *trans* |
|---|---|---|
| Ischemic heart disease | ↓ | ↑ |
| Gestation length | ↑ | ↓ |
| Birth outcome | ↑ | ↓ |
| Inflammation | ↓ | ↑ |
| Dementia (Alzheimer's) | ↓ | ↑ |
| Cancer | ↓ | ↑ |
| Type 2 diabetes | ↓ | ↑ |
| Allergy | ↓ | ↑ |

**Fig. 26.1.** Opposing risks of health associated with a daily intake of a few grams of long-chain omega-3 fatty acids or *trans* fatty acids.

in oils from fish and marine mammals, such as seals and whales, in the form of the 20- and 22-carbon fatty acids, EPA and DHA (Ackman, 1989). ALA can be chain-elongated and desaturated in humans to EPA and DHA. In the present-day fatty acid diet, however, the amount of ingested ALA that is converted to EPA and DHA is low to negligible (Burdge & Calder, 2005; Plourde & Cunnane, 2007). The biological effects of omega-3 fatty acids are nearly all associated with the effects of EPA and DHA and their metabolites, which are the focus of this review.

## Trans *Fatty Acids*

The double bonds in most naturally occurring unsaturated fatty acids are stereoisomerically in a so-called *cis*-configuration. TFAs are unsaturated fatty acids with at least one double bond in the *trans* configuration. The *trans* double bonds cannot be made in humans. TFAs have no function as vitamins or essential fatty acids. Humans can, however, metabolize and use TFA as a source of calories.

TFAs in human food stem from two different sources: (i) industrial hardening or hydrogenation of unsaturated fatty acids (industrially produced *trans* fatty acids or IP-TFAs) and (ii) ruminant fat (ruminant produced *trans* fatty acids or RP-TFAs). IP-TFAs are made by the partial hydrogenation of vegetable fat and, to a minor extent, of marine oils by heating under high pressure and with the addition of different catalysts. IP-TFAs are used in a variety of food products, especially margarines, spreads, baked goods, and fast-food. RP-TFAs are made by the bacterial metabolism of polyunsaturated fatty acids in the rumen of ruminants such as cows, sheep, and goats. They are absorbed into the intestine of the ruminants and are consequently present in all fats from these animals.

Whereas the concentration of IP-TFAs in partially hydrogenated fat may be as high as 60%, the maximal content of RP-TFAs in ruminant fat is about 6% of the fatty acid component. In milk, RP-TFAs constitute 4–6% of the fat. One liter of whole milk thus contains about 1 gram of RP-TFA.

During industrial hydrogenation, *trans* double bonds are formed all along the molecules of the fatty acid from position 6 and higher. For fatty acids with 18 carbon atoms, a peak concentration of *trans* double bonds is found at position 9, as elaidic acid, with a Gaussian distribution of fatty acids with the *trans* bond in the other positions. The bacterial desaturation of polyunsaturated fatty acids from grass and vegetables in the rumen also produces *trans* double bonds all over the fatty acid molecules, with a distinct preference for position 11 of the 18-carbon fatty acids, forming vaccenic acid (C18:1n-7*t*).

*Trans* 18:1 fatty acids (elaidic and vaccenic acids) contribute 80–90% of the total TFA in human food. Low amounts of TFA from linoleic and linolenic acids with both *cis* and *trans* double bonds together with TFA with 16, 20, and 22 carbon atoms, and so forth are also formed both industrially and in the rumen. Thus, up to 20% of the TFA found in ruminant fat may be 16:1, which does not occur in IP-TFA from vegetable oils. This fatty acid, together with butyric acid and pentadecanoic acid, may be used as markers for RP-TFA in a mixture of RP-TFA and IP-TFA derived from vegetable oil. Hydrogenated marine oils can, however, contain *trans* 16:1.

## Intake of Omega-3 and *trans* Fatty Acids in the Past

### *Omega-3 Fatty Acids*

Throughout the existence of the human genus, omega-3 fatty acids were a consistent part of the diet. The Paleolithic diet, during the hunter–gatherer period at the beginning of the human genus 2 million years ago, was considered to be far richer in these fatty acids than the present diet. Omega-3 fatty acid intake decreased during the agricultural period due to an increased intake in saturated and omega-6 polyunsaturated fatty acids, and during the industrial revolution due to the introduction of processed food, grain-fattened livestock, and the hydrogenation of vegetable fats (Leaf & Weber, 1987) (Fig. 26.2). Perhaps access to shore-based diets containing high amounts of DHA was necessary for hominine encephalization beyond the level seen in the great apes (Crawford, 2002).

### Trans *Fatty Acids*

TFAs were introduced into the human diet approximately ten thousand years ago, during the agricultural period, by the increased intake of ruminant meat and the introduction of dairy products. This trend dramatically increased during the last century as a result of the industrial hydrogenation of vegetable and marine oils. IP-TFAs are used in a variety of manufactured food products due to their high

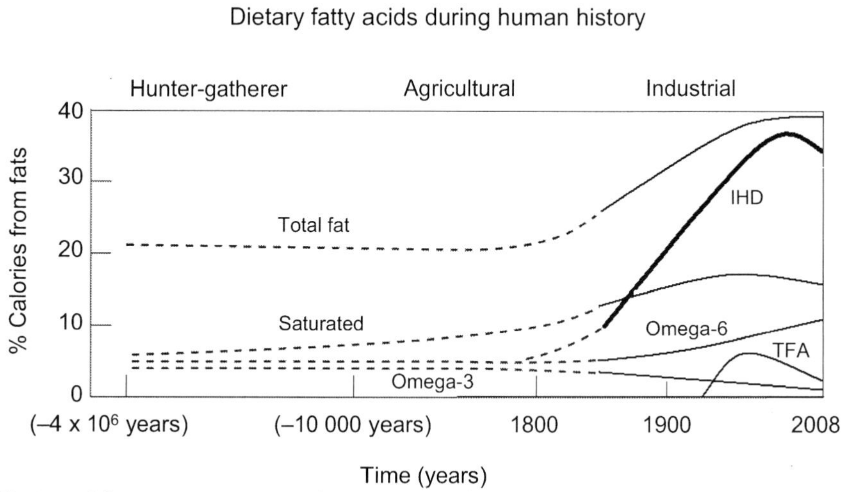


**Fig. 26.2.** Schematic representation, from the origin of the genus to present day, of the dietary content of different types of fatty acids, and the increased prevalence of ischemic heart disease (IHD). TFA = *trans* fatty acids. (Adapted from Leaf & Weber, 1987).

availability, low price, and favorable technical properties such as high melting point, oxidative stability with prolonged shelf-life of food, and the ability to create a specific organoleptic quality.

## Intake of Omega-3 and *trans* Fatty Acids Today

### *Omega-3 Fatty Acids*

The present-day intake of omega-3 fatty acids differs considerably from country to country, and this difference is particularly interesting when related to the intake of EPA and DHA. Dietary data from the MRFIT study from 1982 revealed that the average EPA and DHA intake in the United States was about 175 mg/day, with about 20% of the group reporting zero daily intakes (Dolecek & Grandtis, 1991). In most Western countries, the mean intake of EPA + DHA is currently about 100–300 mg/day, including individuals with zero intakes. These values are considerably lower than the recommended individual intake of at least 500 mg/day (Harris, 2007; Lee et al., 2008).

In populations with a normally high intake of fish (e.g., in Japan and Iceland), the daily intake of EPA and DHA is approximately 1–2 g. An intake of up to several grams daily of long-chain omega-3 fatty acids is not known to have any harmful effects on health (Harris, 2007; Schmidt et al., 1994).

The target DHA and EPA consumption levels are at least 500 mg/day for those without heart disease and 1 g/day for those with known coronary artery disease (Lee et al., 2008).

### Trans *Fatty Acids*

Estimates of the intake of TFA usually rely on the estimates of food consumption and the use of appropriate food composition tables. In that respect, the estimate of food consumption needs to be rather detailed since the content of IP-TFA and of RP-TFA in apparently similar foods may vary considerably from place to place and from time to time. We found that a serving of food at one fast-food chain in Boston in 2006 contained 20 g of IP-TFA, whereas a similar serving contained less than 6 g when bought at the same fast-food chain in New York City (Stender et al., 2006). The amount of IP-TFA in the same brand of food may also vary from time to time depending on market prices for edible fats.

Concentrations of RP-TFA in ruminant fat vary with the feed of the animals and, therefore, vary seasonally (Jakobsen et al., 2006). This variation in grams per serving is, however, much lower than the variation observed for IP-TFA.

The estimates of TFA intake by means of dietary questionnaires are, consequently, likely to be hampered by substantial measurement errors. This is not only because of the limitations inherent in dietary assessment methods that also affect estimates of omega-3 fatty acid intake, but also because food composition tables are much more inaccurate for TFAs than for omega-3 fatty acids. The estimates of TFA intake should consequently be interpreted with great skepticism and should preferably be supported by an analysis of duplicate portions or composite diets, together with measurements of biomarkers for intake, such as TFA in human tissue, including plasma, erythrocytes, subcutaneous fat, and human milk. These inaccuracies may mask associations between the intake of *trans* fat and various diseases, and may underestimate those associations that appear (Clarke et al., 1999).

In the United States, the mean intake of TFA in 1999 was estimated to be 5.3 g/day, with the 90th percentile at 9.4 g/day (Craig-Schmidt, 2006). Previously estimated values were considerably higher (i.e., between 7 and 13 g/day). After mandatory TFA labeling of prepackaged food was instituted in 2006, the current mean intake has, without a doubt, declined further. However, no data are available concerning the present intake (2008) and its distribution.

The total intake of TFA in various European countries was investigated in the "Transfair Study," conducted in 1996 (Hulshof et al., 1999). The average daily intakes varied from 5.4 g in Iceland to about 1.5 g in Greece and Italy. In general, the 90th percentiles were 50–70% above the mean values. These results, together with more recent intake values from Costa Rica (Monge-Rojas et al., 2005), are shown in Fig. 26.3. In Iran, mean IP-TFA intakes of 12–13 g/day were recently reported (Mozaffarian et al., 2007).

Since 1996, the intake of IP-TFA has decreased considerably in Western Europe, including Scandinavia, due to societal pressure on food producers to reduce the content of IP-TFA (Fig. 26.4).

The adult population's average daily intake of RP-TFA in the United States was estimated by the Food and Drug Administration (2008) to be 1.2 g/day for both sexes. This value is similar to the value reported for the intake of RP-TFA in Denmark (Fig. 26.4).

In a series of countries from 2005 to 2007, we investigated whether it was possible to achieve a meal with a high amount of IP-TFA (Stender & Dyerberg, 2007). The results are shown in Fig. 26.5.

The presence of popular foods with high concentrations of IP-TFA in the United States and in other countries means that although the average intake of IP-TFA at the population level may be lower than the recommended maximal level of 2 g per person per day, by 2008 subgroups of the populations will still exist in the United States, Canada, and in most other countries that have an average daily intake of 5 g or more. An average intake of this magnitude —corresponding to 2 E%— is associated with a 25–30% increased risk of cardiovascular disease (Mozaffarian et al., 2006).

## Conclusion Concerning the Intake of Omega-3 and *trans* Fatty Acids

In the United States and most other countries, the average intake in 2008 of omega-3 fatty acids is too low and that of TFA is too high according to the recommended values. This is especially pronounced for certain subgroups of the population.

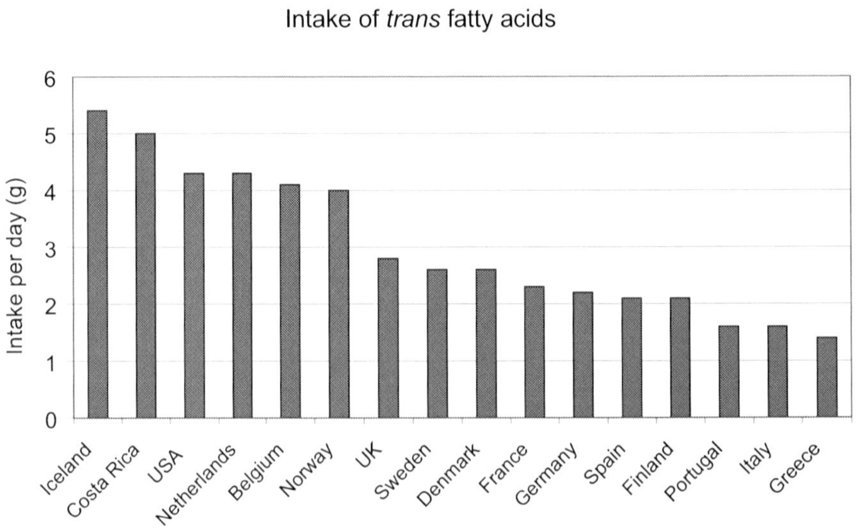


**Fig. 26.3.** Intake of *trans* fatty acids in various countries.

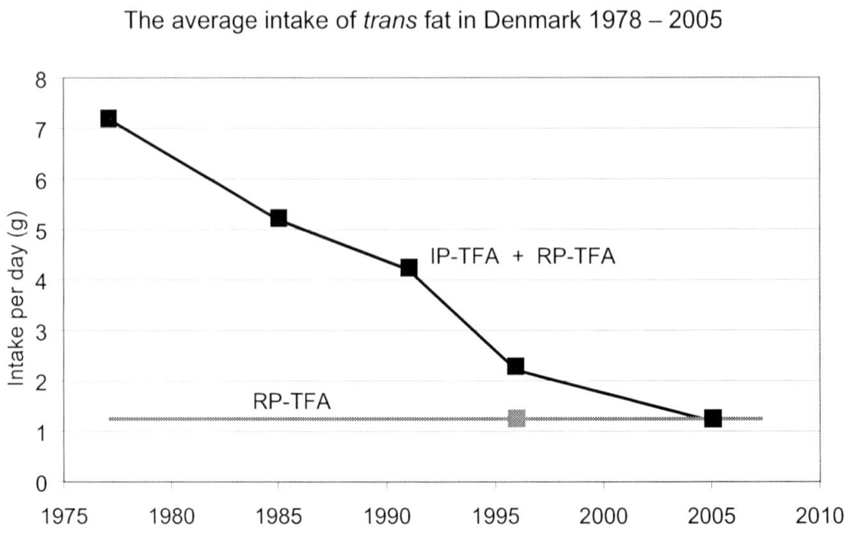


**Fig. 26.4.** Decrease of industrially produced *trans* fatty acids (IP-TFA) in the Danish diet. RP-TFA = ruminant *trans* fatty acids.

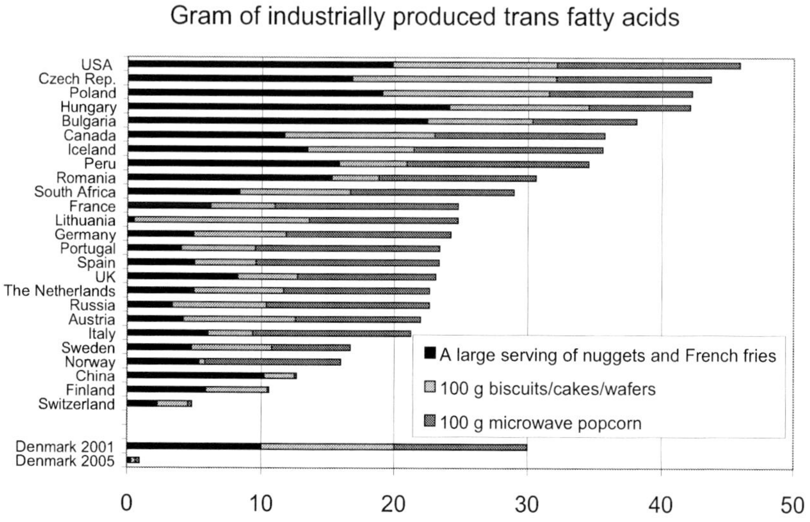


**Fig. 26.5.** Grams of industrially produced *trans* fatty acids in a "high *trans* fat menu."

# Ischemic Heart Disease

Interest in omega-3 fatty acids and IHD is a result of the original observations in Greenland Inuit populations that focused on the antithrombotic effects of a high intake of EPA and DHA (Dyerberg & Bang, 1979). Studies have since indicated that the positive effects on IHD morbidity and mortality may be related more to the hypotriglyceridemic effect of these fatty acids (Bang et al., 1971; Weber & Raederstorff, 2000), in combination with anti-inflammatory and anti-arrhythmic effects (Harris et al., 2008).

After it was discovered that the intake of IP-TFA adversely affected the plasma levels of low- density lipoproteins (LDL) and high-density lipoproteins (HDL) (Mensink et al., 2003; Mensink & Katan, 1990), its relationship to IHD was explored intensively. In several large prospective epidemiological studies, a 25–30% increase in the risk of IHD was associated with a daily TFA intake of approximately 2 E%, which corresponds to approximately 5 g (Mozaffarian et al., 2006).

# Plasma Triglycerides

Triglycerides from plasma do not accumulate in the arterial wall. High concentrations of triglycerides in plasma are considered a marker of cholesterol-containing lipoproteins, such as very low-density lipoprotein (VLDL) remnants. Cholesterol from remnants may accumulate in the arterial wall and promote the formation of atherosclerotic plaque. Some studies suggested that remnants are even more atherogenic than LDL cholesterol (Zilversmit, 1979). Elevated plasma triglycerides are associated with high cardiovascular mortality in patients with familial hypertriglyceridemia (Austin et al., 2000). In recent observational epidemiological studies, an increased risk of IHD events and mortality were associated with elevated nonfasting triglyceride (Bansal et al., 2007; Nordestgaard et al., 2007; Stensvold et al., 1993) and fasting plasma triglyceride (Miller et al., 2008) levels. A raised nonfasting concentration of triglycerides was an independent risk factor for mortality from IHD, cardiovascular disease, and other causes among 24,535 middle-aged Norwegian women who were followed for 14.6 years (Stensvold et al., 1993). The study by Nordestgaard et al. (2007) followed 13,981 Danes for 26 years. Persons with elevated nonfasting triglycerides had hazard ratios for myocardial infarction 2–5 times higher than those with triglycerides <1 mmol/L. In the study by Bansal et al. (2007), nonfasting triglyceride levels in 6,391 women from the Women's Health Study had, during a median follow-up of 11.4 years, a strong independent relationship with cardiovascular events. The incidence of death, myocardial infarction, and recurrent acute coronary syndrome was 1.6% lower for each 0.11 mmol/L of decrement in triglyceride level (Miller et al., 2008).

### *Omega-3 Fatty Acids and Decreased Plasma Triglycerides*

Several studies demonstrated that omega-3 fatty acid supplements from fish oil reduce the plasma triglyceride level substantially (e.g., Goldberg & Sabharwal., 2008). The majority of papers focused on fasting triglyceride levels. A series of studies, however, also investigated the effect on nonfasting triglycerides. In these studies, a diet containing 2–4 g of fish oil per day significantly reduced postprandial triglyceridemia after either a saturated fat or fish oil test meal (Davidson, 2006; Lovegrove et al., 1997; Park & Harris, 2003; Smith et al., 2004). The reduction included both a lowering of the overall triglyceride level as well as an attenuated triglyceridemic response to dietary fats of more than 50%. In general, both EPA and DHA have similar triglyceride-lowering effects (Harris et al., 2008).

### Trans *Fatty Acids and Increased Plasma Triglycerides*

The elevating effect of TFA intake on the concentration of triglycerides in plasma was studied in intervention studies (Ascherio et al., 1999). The effect of IP-TFA is moderate in healthy men (Dyerberg et al., 2004; Motard-Belanger et al., 2008). In women, RP-TFA, compared to IP-TFA, increased plasma triglycerides by about 10% (Chardigny et al., 2008).

### *Mechanism of Action*

The mechanisms behind the triglyceride-lowering effect of EPA and DHA are not completely understood, but they involve reduced hepatic VLDL synthesis and an enhanced triglyceride clearance (Harris et al., 2008). Several mechanisms may play a role in the reduction of hepatic VLDL synthesis. Studies in rats concluded that the effect of EPA and DHA is most likely due to decreased hepatic lipogenesis (Harris

& Bulchandani, 2006). In a study by Park & Harris (2003), healthy subjects were supplemented with 4 g/day of ethyl esters of either EPA or DHA for 4 weeks. Omega-3 fatty acid reduced the postprandial triglyceride and apolipoprotein B concentrations. Chylomicron triglyceride half-lives were reduced, chylomicron particle sizes decreased, and preheparin lipoprotein lipase activity increased during the nonfasting state. Results for EPA and DHA were similar. The results suggest that omega-3 fatty acid accelerates chylomicron triglyceride clearance by increasing lipoprotein lipase activity, and that EPA and DHA are equally effective. Chambrier et al. (2002) found that EPA significantly increased PPARγ mRNA levels in isolated adipocytes. Other tested fatty acids (ALA, DHA, and n-6 PUFA) had no effect. PPARγ mRNA levels in adipocytes were positively associated with lipoprotein lipase activity (Leibowitz et al., 2000).

Peroxisome proliferator-activated receptors (PPARs) are a group of three nuclear receptor isoforms, α, γ, and -σ-PPARs, which are encoded by different genes. PPARs are ligand-regulated transcription factors that control gene expression. The PPARs play a critical physiological role as sensors for glucose and lipid homeostasis, and as regulators of lipid metabolism. Fatty acids and eicosanoids were identified as natural ligands for PPARs. The activation of PPARα lowers lipid levels, PPARγ increases insulin sensitivity, and PPARσ regulates cholesterol and glucose levels. More potent synthetic PPAR ligands, including the fibrates and thiazoledinediones, proved effective in the treatment of hypertriglyceridemia, low HDL concentration, and low plasma glucose.

TFA have the opposite effect on plasma triglycerides compared to drugs such as fibrates and thizoledienediones, which lower plasma triglycerides by enhancing PPAR activity. This indicates that TFA inhibits the PPARs, resulting in an increase in plasma triglycerides and a decrease in HDL, whereas omega-3 fatty acids activate the PPARs.

## Plasma Cholesterol

LDL is considered as the atherogenic cholesterol fraction in plasma. This is based first and foremost on many interventional trials during which a reduction in LDL resulted in a reduction in cardiovascular diseases and death. LDL may be reduced by various drugs, but also with surgical procedures in the intestine such as partial ileal bypass (Buchwald et al., 2002). This suggests that the lowering of LDL, and not the method by which it is lowered, is the important component. The atherosclerotic process depends, however, on many factors other than the plasma LDL level. These include the state of the luminal endothelial cells that form the barrier between the blood and the arterial wall and that cover the predilection sites for the development of atherosclerotic plaques, in the subendothelial space. Also the recruitment of inflammatory cells from the blood and the subsequent formation of foam cells in the subendothelial space are important. This complexity also means that the risk of cardiovascular disease may be positively or negatively affected without corresponding changes in plasma lipoprotein concentrations.

Elevated plasma levels of HDL are associated with the retarded development of atherosclerosis in observational studies. Numerous mechanistic studies in cell cultures and animals suggest that HDL is a core element in the so-called reverse cholesterol transport system, which transfers cholesterol from various tissues to the liver for excretion. Increased levels of lipoprotein (a) [Lp(a)] were, in several studies, associated with an increased risk of IHD. Whether diet or other factors that lead to changes in the concentrations of Lp(a) interfere with the development of atherosclerosis is presently unknown.

## *Omega-3 Fatty Acids and Increased Plasma HDL*

The effect of long-chain omega-3 fatty acids on HDL was estimated by combining the results from 21 trials evaluating lipid outcomes, and fish oil consumption, resulting in a net increase in HDL cholesterol of 0.04 mmol/L (Balk et al., 2006). This increase agrees with our findings of an increase in HDL cholesterol of 0.07 mmol/L in an 8-week intervention trial with a daily intake of approximately 4 g of fish oil (Dyerberg et al., 2004).

The effect of omega-3 fatty acids on LDL is rather modest. The reduction of VLDL caused by the increased intake of long-chain omega-3 fatty acids may result in an elevation in LDL. In a meta-analysis of 23 randomized controlled trials (1,075 participants), the mean dose of omega-3 fatty acids was 3.5 g/day. Among those taking omega-3 fatty acids, LDL cholesterol levels were elevated by 0.11 mmol/L (Hartweg et al., 2008).

In a study of fishermen in Tanzania, an omega-3 fatty acid-rich diet was responsible for low plasma levels of Lp(a) in this population (Marcovina et al., 1999).

## Trans *Fatty Acids and Decreased Plasma HDL*

In a meta-analysis of interventional studies, TFA was found to increase LDL cholesterol and to decrease HDL in plasma (Ascherio et al., 1999; Menzink et al., 2003). HDL cholesterol decreased by 0.06 mmol/L in the TFA group in response to a daily dietary intake of 20 g of *trans* fat in males (Dyerberg et al., 2004) (Fig. 26.6). An increased intake of RP-TFA in males ranging from 4.2 g to 10.2 g per day decreased HDL by 0.06 mmol/L (Motard-Belanger et al., 2008). This decrease was considerably smaller than the decrease of 0.39 mmol/L in HDL in response to an intake of approximately 25 g per day of *trans* fat for 4 weeks in a study by de Roos et al. (2003).

Significant increases in Lp(a) levels were reported after the consumption of diets relatively high in TFA, as compared to either unsaturated or saturated fatty acids. However, the magnitude of change is, for the most part, small (Lichtenstein, 2000).

## *Mechanism of Action*

The effect of omega-3 fatty acids on LDL is considered a result of an increased VLDL metabolism, of which LDL is the metabolic end point. The mechanism behind the

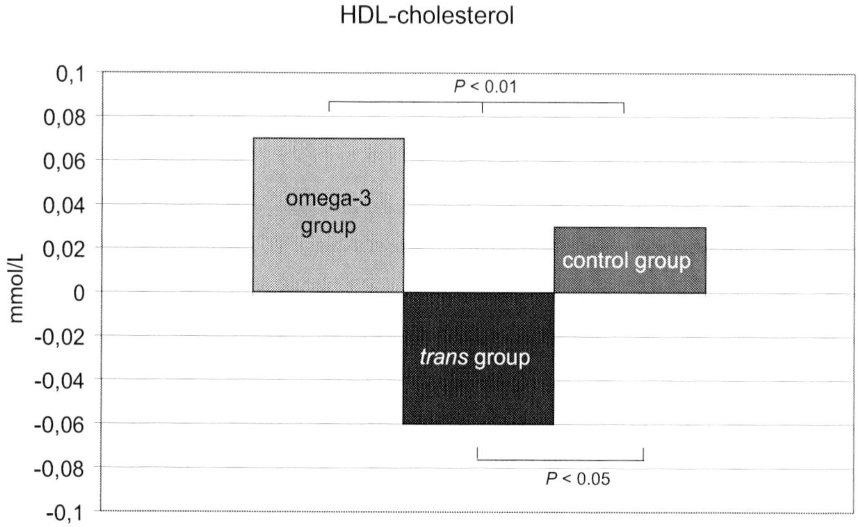


**Fig. 26.6.** Changes in HDL cholesterol 8 weeks after dietary intervention with omega-3 fatty acids, *trans* fatty acids, or control fat (Dyerberg et al., 2004).

increase in HDL is unclear. TFA appears to affect plasma lipids through several mechanisms: by decreasing the rate of LDL apoprotein (apo B-100) catabolism, reducing the size of LDL particles, and increasing the rate of HDL apoprotein (apo-A1) catabolism (Matthan et al., 2004). In humans the consumption of TFA increases the plasma activity of the cholesteryl ester transfer protein (Lagrost, 1992), which transfers cholesterol esters from HDL to LDL and VLDL. This effect was not found in a recent study for either RP-TFA or IP-TFA (Chardigny et al., 2008).

## Inflammation

Inflammatory reactions are considered as important mechanisms in the pathogenesis of atherosclerosis. The accumulation of inflammatory cells in the early plaque, the retardation of clinical symptoms of atherosclerosis by aspirin, and the increased risk of IHD associated with elevated C-reactive protein (CRP) levels in plasma all testify to the importance of chronic inflammation for the development of vulnerable arterial lesions with subsequent plaque rupture. CRP is a marker for both acute and chronic inflammatory activity. Chronic inflammation probably plays a major role during all phases of atherosclerosis. Stable plaques are characterized by chronic inflammatory infiltrate, whereas vulnerable and ruptured plaques are characterized by "active" inflammation involved in the thinning of the fibrous cap, predisposing the plaque to rupture (Spagnoli et al., 2007). The complicated cascades of pro- and anti-inflammatory components (e.g., cytokines, eicosanoids, adhesion molecules, resolvins, and acute phase proteins) involved in the various stages of inflammation are under intense investigation. The inhibition or promotion of key steps in these cascades may significantly interfere with the development of atherosclerosis.

### *Omega-3 Fatty Acids and Decreased Chronic Inflammation*

Several studies demonstrate that omega-3 fatty acid supplementation attenuates the inflammatory process in chronic inflammatory disorders (e.g., rheumatoid arthritis) (Goldberg & Katz, 2007). This effect was used in the treatment of various autoimmune disorders, and it supports the notion of an anti-inflammatory effect of omega-3 fatty acids in IHD prevention and supports the explanation for the unexplained benefit of low doses of omega-3 fatty acids in coronary heart disease.

### Trans *Fatty Acids and Increased Chronic Inflammation*

Evidence from both observational and experimental studies indicates that TFAs are pro-inflammatory (Mozaffarian et al., 2006). In a study of overweight women, a greater intake of TFA was associated with an increased activity of the tumor necrosis factor (TNF) system and increased levels of interleukin-6 (IL-6) and CRP (Lopez-Garcia et al., 2005). In patients with established heart disease, cell membrane levels of TFA were independently associated with the activation of systemic inflammatory responses, including substantially increased levels of interleukin-6, TNF-α, TNF receptors, and monocyte chemoattractant protein (Mozaffarin et al., 2005). These effects on inflammation were seen in either overweight patients or patients with established heart disease. The risk of IHD increases with the increasing levels of CRP found in plasma (Ridker, 2007). In a cross-sectional study of 730 women from the Nurses' Health Study, CRP levels were 73% higher among those in the highest quintile of TFA intake, compared with the lowest quintile, with an average daily intake of 5 g of *trans* fat as compared to about 2 g (Lopez-Garcia et al., 2005). This difference in CRP would, in accordance with the findings of Ridker (2007), correspond to an increase in IHD risk of approximately 30%. The effect on CRP may account much more for the increased risk of IHD associated with the intake of TFA than its effects on plasma lipids. A daily intake of 20 g of TFA for 8 weeks in healthy young men of normal body weight did not change CRP levels (Dyerberg et al., 2004).

### *Mechanism of Action*

The anti-inflammatory effect of long-chain omega-3 fatty acids was first noticed when examining the chemo-tactic potency of leukotrienes generated from EPA compared to the leukotrienes formed from arachidonic acid (Schmidt et al., 1991). Leukotrienes are proinflammatory agents synthesized in the white blood cells (leukocytes) from 20 carbon polyunsaturated fatty acids. Leukotrienes promote, among other things, the migration of leukocytes (chemotaxis). In equal amounts, leukotrienes derived from arachidonic acid exhibit 10- to 30-fold greater chemo tactic potency for human neutrophils than the EPA-derived leukotrienes (Goldman et al., 1983).

The chemotaxis of white blood cells, monocytes, and neutrophils was reduced after an omega-3 fatty acid intake in humans in a dose-dependent fashion, with the majority of the effect observed after the low dose of 1.3 g/day (Schmidt et al., 1991).

The consumption of DHA reduces the endothelial expression of vascular cell adhesion molecules VCAM-1, E-selectin, intercellular adhesion molecule 1 (ICAM-1), IL-6, and IL-8 in response to IL-1, IL-4, TNF, or bacterial endotoxin, in the range of nutritionally achievable plasma concentrations (De Caterina et al., 2000).

New families of locally acting anti-inflammatory mediators generated from omega-3 fatty acids, termed resolvins, protectins, and isoprostanes, were recently identified (Arita et al., 2006; Brooks et al., 2008; Chiang & Serhan, 2006; Serhan, 2006). These components are potent agonists that control the duration and magnitude of inflammation, joining the lipoxins as signals in inflammatory resolution. Given the potent actions of leukotrienes, lipoxins, adhesion molecules, resolvins, and protectins in human disease, the intake of EPA and DHA may attenuate the development of atherosclerotic diseases.

The mechanisms underlying the pro-inflammatory effects of TFA are not well-established, but may involve TFA incorporation into endothelial cells, monocyte/macrophage, or adipocyte cell membranes affecting membrane-signaling pathways relating to inflammation. The activation of inflammatory responses may represent important mediating pathways between TFA consumption and the risk of IHD and sudden cardiac death. The effects of adiposity on the relationship between the intake of *trans* fatty acids and circulating interleukin and CRP levels suggest that the inflammatory effects are partially mediated by adipose tissue. Recently, the effect of membrane-incorporated C18:2 TFA on human aortic endothelial cell (HAEC) function was demonstrated. TFA treatment of HAEC significantly increased the expression of endothelial adhesion molecules and increased HAEC adhesion to fibronectin- or vitronectin-coated plates. TFA treatment also induced the release of monocyte chemo-attractant protein-1 by nearly 3-fold in nonstimulated HAEC (Harvey et al., 2008).

In the studies of animals, the consumption of TFA alters the expression in adipocytes of genes for PPARγ, resistin, and lipoprotein lipase compounds, which have central roles in the metabolism of fatty acids and glucose (Saravanan et al., 2005).

## Endothelial Function

During the last two decades, it was understood that the endothelium is not only the passive inner lining of the vascular system of the organism, but also has a number of fundamental functional properties. It regulates the transfer of macromolecules and blood cells, such as lipoproteins and monocytes, from plasma into the subendothelial space. It regulates the tonus of adjacent smooth muscle cells in the vessels, and it provides a nontrombogenic surface. The functions of the endothelial cells are maintained by the secretion of various molecules that regulate the functions of the secreting cells themselves and of neighboring cells. An important messenger molecule in that connection is nitric oxide (NO) produced from arginine by the endothelial cells. The endothelial cells are considered the gatekeeper for the development of atherosclerosis. In accordance with this concept, dysfunction of the endothelium is the very first step in the process that eventually leads to an atherosclerotic lesion. Dysfunction appears as an impaired ability to produce NO and to increase the production of adhesion molecules.

The hydrolysis of triglyceride-rich lipoproteins by lipoprotein lipases takes place at the luminal endothelial surface and exposes the endothelial cells to particular high concentrations of fatty acids. Fatty acids in the diet may, therefore, interfere with several endothelial functions crucial to the development of atherosclerosis, such as the ability of the endothelial cells to form NO as measured by the so-called flow-mediated vasodilatation (FMD). A low FMD is associated with an increased risk of IHD (Celermajer et al., 1992).

### *Omega-3 Fatty Acids and Increased Flow-mediated Dilatation*

In a four-month treatment period, omega-3 fatty acids at a dose of 4 g/day resulted in a significant improvement in FMD (Goodfellow et al., 2000). In 326 adults, FMD and omega-3 fatty acid levels in plasma and erythrocyte membranes were positively associated (Leeson et al., 2002). In a randomized, placebo-controlled trial, 26 subjects, supplemented with 1 g of fish oil per day for 14 days, showed a significant increase in FMD (Shah et al., 2007). We found however, that a daily supplement of 4 g of omega-3 fatty acids for 8 weeks given to 79 healthy males had no effect on FMD (Dyerberg et al., 2004).

### trans *Fatty Acids and Decreased Flow-mediated Dilatation*

Several studies suggest that *trans* fats cause endothelial dysfunction. After an adjustment for other risk factors, an increased intake of TFA was associated with increased levels of several markers of endothelial dysfunction, including soluble intercellular adhesion molecule 1, soluble vascular-cell adhesion molecule 1, and E-selectin. A Dutch study observed a 30% reduction in brachial artery FMD when an intake of saturated fat was replaced by an intake of *trans* fat (deRoos et al., 2003). This observation was not reproduced in an analogous Danish study (Dyerberg et al., 2004).

### *Mechanism of Action*

Two mechanisms are likely to be mediators for the effects of omega-3 fatty acids and TFA on endothelial cell function. One is a physical–chemical alteration of membrane characteristics caused by the inclusion of omega-3 fatty acids or TFA in membrane bilayers, influencing, for example, the ion-channels in the membranes. The other is a modulation of signaling processes via agonist action on nuclear receptors, such as the PPAR system. Neither of these possibilities was examined in detail relating to endothelial cell function.

## Arrythmia

Sudden cardiac death is the most serious manifestation of IHD. It may appear in conjunction with acute myocardial infarction, which may elicit ventricular fibrillation. The blood supply to the brain becomes insufficient and may, if ventricular fibrillation continues, lead to irreversible brain damage or death within minutes.

### *Omega-3 Fatty Acids and the Reduced Risk of Sudden Cardiac Death*

An anti-arrhythmic effect of omega-3 fatty acids has been the focus of much research. In spite of positive associations in several observational epidemiological studies (Leaf et al., 2005), not all intervention studies found an anti-arrhythmic effect of fish-oil supplementation (Raitt et al., 2005). In an Italian population study, marine omega-3 fatty acid intake was associated with both reduced overall mortality and the incidence of atrial fibrillation in patients hospitalized with myocardial infarction (Macchia et al., 2008). The basis for any stabilizing effect of omega-3 fatty acids on arrhythmic tendencies seems to be related to heart rate variability (Christensen et al., 1996, 1999) and a decrease in heart rate. In randomized controlled trials in humans, fish oil reduces heart rate, particularly in those with higher baseline heart rates (Mozaffarian et al., 2005). Habitual fish and marine omega-3 consumption were associated with beneficial effects on specific heart rate components in older adults (Mozaffarian et al., 2008). In a double-blind, parallel interventional trial, 79 subjects were randomly assigned to 8 weeks of 33 g of a daily intake of experimental fats that contained either partially hydrogenated soy oil with 20 g of TFA, 12 g of fish oil with approximately 4 g of omega-3 fatty acids and 21 g of control fat, or 33 g of control fat. Post-hoc, we did a subgroup analysis of the results from subjects with normal heart-rate variability. In these, 24-hour heart rates were significantly increased by approximately 3 beats/min in the TFA group and decreased by the same magnitude in the omega-3 fatty acid group (Dyerberg et al., 2006) (Fig. 26.7). High heart rate is associated with an increased risk of sudden death (Dallongeville et al., 2003).

### Trans *Fatty Acids and the Increased Risk of Sudden Cardiac Death*

Higher levels of plasma phospholipid *trans*-18:2 fatty acids were associated with a higher risk of fatal IHD and sudden cardiac death in a case-control study nested in the Cardiovascular Health Study (Lemaitre et al., 2006). This is in contrast to the findings of a decreased risk of sudden cardiac death caused by the intake of long-chain omega-3 fatty acids (GISSI-Preventione Investigators, 1999; Lemaitre et al., 2003; Siscovick et al., 1995).

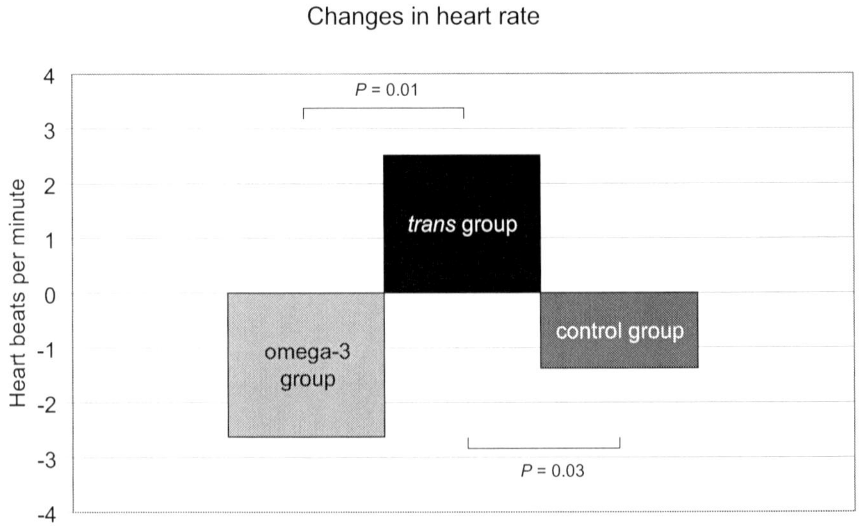


**Fig. 26.7.** Changes in heart rate in subjects with normal heart-rate variability 8 weeks after dietary intake of *trans* fatty acids, omega-3 fatty acids, or control fat (Dyerberg et al., 2004).

### *Mechanism of Action*

Dietary fatty acids incorporated in the phospholipids of cell membranes may change the tertiary structure of proteins in cellular membranes, such as ion-channels. This may also change the function of these channels. Studies of cultured heart cells suggest that the incorporation of omega-3 fatty acids stabilizes rhythm (Leaf, 2007). A possible mechanism for this effect is their ability to affect the activities of cardiac ion channels. The modulation of channel activities, especially $Na^{+}$ and $Ca^{++}$ channels, and hyperpolarization-activated cyclic-nucleotide-modulated channels by the omega-3 fatty acids may explain, at least partially, their antiarrhythmic action (Xiao et al., 2005).

TFA may also modify cellular function by interacting with the hydrophobic regions of membrane proteins (Katz, 2006), thereby affecting ion channels in the membrane and forming the basis for the observed arrythmogenic effect and an increase in sudden cardiac death associated with the intake of TFA (Lemaitre et al., 2006).

## Insulin Sensitivity

### *Omega-3 Fatty Acids and Increased Insulin Sensitivity*

In a study of patients with chronic renal failure regarding maintenance hemodialysis and insulin resistance (IR), the effects of an 8-week supplementation with 2.4 g/day of

EPA and DHA on IR were examined. The values of serum insulin and the calculated IR-index HOMA were significantly reduced after omega-3 fatty acid supplementation (Rasic-Milutinovic et al., 2007). In an 8-week dietary intervention study on insulin resistance in young overweight individuals, omega-3 fatty acid consumption during energy restriction had positive effects on insulin resistance, independent of the changes in body weight (Parra et al., 2008).

### Trans *Fatty Acids and Reduced Insulin Sensitivity*

Among 84,204 women ages 34–59 years with no diabetes, the replacing of 2% of energy from *trans* fatty acids isoenergetically with polyunsaturated fat led to a 40% lower risk of type 2 diabetes during 14 years of follow-up (Salmeron et al. 2001). This association was, however, not observed in all epidemiological observational studies.

In a study on African green monkeys (n = 42), the animals were assigned to diets containing either *cis*-monounsaturated fatty acids or an equivalent diet containing the *trans*-isomers (approximately 8% of energy) for 6 years. The TFA-fed monkeys gained significant weight with increased intra-abdominal fat deposits. Impaired glucose disposal was implied by significant postprandial hyperinsulinemia, elevated fructosamine, and a tendency toward higher glucose concentrations (Kavanagh et al., 2007). Some evidence exists that TFA may impair insulin sensitivity compared to unsaturated fat in insulin-resistant or diabetic individuals. This is especially true for high doses of conjugated TFA (i.e., conjugated linoleic acid) that clearly impairs insulin sensitivity in insulin-resistant and diabetic subjets (Risérus, 2006).

### *Mechanism of Action*

Recent studies suggest that omega-3 fatty acids protect against high-fat, diet-induced insulin resistance through PPARα activation and the subsequent decrease in intracellular lipid abundance (Neschen et al., 2007). Since TFA may interfere with cell membrane function, reasons exist to believe that high TFA intake may affect insulin sensitivity (Risérus, 2006).

## Allergy

### *Omega-3 Fatty Acids and Reduced Allergic Reactions*

The increasing prevalence of atopic eczema is linked to the change in the Western diet, including the reduced consumption of omega-3 fatty acids.

In a prospective birth cohort of 4,089 new-born infants who were followed for 4 years using parental questionnaires at ages 2 months, 1 year, 2 years, and 4 years to collect information on exposure and health effects, regular fish consumption during the first year of life was associated with a reduced risk for allergic disease by age 4 (Kull et al., 2006). In a randomized, double-blind, controlled trial, 53 patients suffering from atopic eczema (ages 18–40 years) received either 5.4 g of DHA daily or an isoenergetic control of saturated fatty acids for 8 weeks. DHA, but not the control treatment, resulted in a significant clinical improvement of atopic eczema (Koch et al., 2008).

### Trans *Fatty Acids and Increased Allergic Reactions*

In an international study of asthma and allergies in childhood (ISSAC) from 1998, the incidence of asthma, allergic cold, and asthmatic eczema in children ages 13–14 years was investigated in 155 places around the world. A positive association was found between the intake of TFA and these diseases (Weiland et al., 1999). The content of *trans* lipid isomers in the erythrocyte and T-lymphocyte membranes of 26 children affected by atopic eczema/dermatitis syndrome was compared with an age-matched control group, and was found to be significantly higher in the children with eczema (Ferreri et al., 2005).

### *Mechanism of Action*

Neither the effect of omega-3 nor TFA on allergy was examined in detail. Likely candidates for disease-modifying effects are changes in membrane lipids by the incorporation of the two fatty acid types into cellular membranes involved in allergic processes. Alternatively, the modification of the cellular cytokine response via an effect on the nuclear PPAR system may mediate the effect.

## Dementia

One of the most interesting nutritional findings in recent decades is the effect of dietary factors on modifying age-related cognitive decline. Membrane fatty acid composition may play a central role in the development of neuronal dysfunction. Arachidonic acid and DHA are highly concentrated in the phospholipid bilayer of the brain and retinal neural membranes; they are important in neuronal function. Interventional trials in human subjects showed that omega-3 fatty acids have possible positive effects in the treatment of various psychiatric disorders, but more data are needed to draw conclusions regarding this correlation. Dietary intake may modulate the ratio of membrane omega-3 to omega-6 fatty acids in the brain. This ratio influences neurotransmission and prostaglandin formation, processes that are vital to the maintenance of normal brain function (Haag, 2003).

### *Omega-3 Fatty Acids and Reduced Cognitive Decline*

The findings of an inverse association between cognitive decline and the ratio of omega-3 to n-6 fatty acids in erythrocyte membranes (Heude et al., 2003) further support the role of omega-3 fatty acids in dementia and Alzheimer's disease. Several observational studies have since found a negative association between the intake of long-chain omega-3 fatty acids and the risk of dementia. Fish intake was associated with a slower rate of cognitive decline in residents 65 years and older who participated in the Chicago Health and Aging Project (Morris et al., 2005). In the Framingham

Heart Study, the top quartile of plasma DHA levels was associated with a significant 47% reduction in the risk of developing dementia (Schaefer et al., 2006). The Atherosclerosis Risk in Communities study indicated that an increase of one standard deviation in dietary long-chain omega-3 fatty acids (percentage of energy intake) decreased the risk of a 6-year decline in verbal fluency with an odds ratio of 0.79 among hypertensives (Beydoun, 2008). In the Zutphen Elderly Study, fish consumers had a significantly less 5-year cognitive decline than did nonconsumers. A linear trend was observed for the relationship between the intake of EPA and DHA and cognitive decline (van Gelder et al., 2007). In the Norwegian Hordaland Health Study, subjects whose mean daily intake of fish and fish products was above 10 g/day had significantly better mean test scores and a lower prevalence of poor cognitive performance than did those whose intake was less than 10 g/day. The association between the total intake of seafood and cognition was strongly dose-dependent; the maximal effect was observed at an intake of approximately 75 g/day (Nurk et al., 2007). In the FACIT trial with men and women ages 50–70 years, the plasma omega-3 fatty acid proportions were associated with a lower decline in speed-related cognitive domains over 3 years (Dullemeijer et al., 2007).

## Trans *Fatty Acids and Increased Cognitive Decline*

Diets high in fat, especially *trans* and saturated fats, are adversely associated with cognition, while those high in fruits, vegetables, cereals, and fish are associated with better cognitive function and a lower risk of dementia (Parrott & Greenwood, 2007). Observational epidemiological studies may sometimes show conflicting results; certain associations were, however, frequently found. A high intake of saturated and *trans*- (hydrogenated) fats was positively associated with an increased risk of Alzheimer's disease, whereas fish consumption is associated with a lower risk of disease in longitudinal cohort studies (Gillette-Guyonnet et al., 2007; Morris et al., 2003).

## *Mechanism of Action*

Environmental and genetic factors contribute to the etiology of Alzheimer's disease. DHA is an essential component of neural tissue and has an unknown turnover rate in the cerebrum. A low dietary intake of omega-3 fatty acids is thus likely to affect cerebral tissue composition, thereby promoting the cognitive decline in dementia. In this respect, likely, as demonstrated in newborns, a competitive influence on DHA availability for the brain is caused by a high intake of IP-TFA. The production from DHA of neuroprotectins, which have essential functional roles and pathophysiological functions in the brain, may also be competitive (Bazan, 2005). Reportedly, DHA significantly increases a neuronal sorting protein, LR11, in a human neuronal line. As reduced LR11 may be a significant genetic cause of Alzheimer's disease, DHA may play an important role in reducing the occurrence of Alzheimer's disease (Ma et al., 2007).

# Reproduction

## Pregnancy

### *Omega-3 Fatty Acids and an Increased Pregnancy Length*

High birth weights, a long duration of pregnancy, and high fish consumption in the Faroe Islands suggest that a high intake of marine-fat-derived omega-3 fatty acids might prolong pregnancy by shifting the balance of production of prostaglandins involved in parturition from the more active type, derived from arachidonic acid, to the less active, EPA derivatives. A Danish study examined the effects of a daily 4-g fish-oil supplementation corresponding to 2.7 g of omega-3 fatty acids on pregnancy duration, birth weight, and birth length in 533 healthy women. Compared to placebo oil consisting of olive oil, the mean length of gestation was 4.0 days longer, and birth weight was 107 g greater in the fish-oil group than in the placebo-oil group (Olsen et al., 1992). In a study in pregnant women with previous pregnancy complications, the same authors found that fish-oil supplementation at the same dose delayed the onset of delivery in low- and middle-, but not in high-level fish consumers (Olsen et al., 2007).

Reports are available on the positive effect of long-chain omega-3 PUFA intake on the risk of developing preeclampsia (Bang & Dyerberg, 1990).

### **Trans** *Fatty Acids and a Reduced Pregnancy Length*

The percentage of TFA elaidic acid in total fatty acids in erythrocytes was 28% higher among 22 preeclamptic women as compared with 40 normotensive pregnant females. After adjusting for confounding factors, women with the highest levels of elaidic acid were 7.4 times more likely to have had their pregnancy complicated by preeclampsia as compared with women with the lowest levels (Williams et al., 1998). In a case-control study from Zimbabwe of 170 women with proteinuric, pregnancy-induced hypertension and 185 normotensive pregnant women, the percentages of omega-3, omega-6, and TFA in fatty acids were measured in erythrocytes. Women in the highest quartile group for total omega-3 fatty acids compared with women in the lowest quartile experienced a 14% reduction in the risk of preeclampsia. A strong statistically significant correlation between di-unsaturated fatty acids with a *trans* double bond and the risk of preeclampsia was observed. The women in the upper quartile of 9-*cis* 12-*trans* octadecanoic acid compared with those in the lowest quartile experienced a three-fold higher risk of preeclampsia (Mahomed et al., 2007).

## Mechanism of Action

The incorporation of fatty acids in the uterus may change its excitability by changing the configuration of the ion channels in the cells, analogous to the hypothesis for the anti-arrythmogenic and arrythmogenic effects in the heart of omega-3 and TFA, respectively. Omega-3 fatty acids incorporated in the muscle cells of the uterus may cause the muscle cells to respond more slowly to a given labor-excitatory stimulus. When TFAs are incorporated in the muscle cells, the response proceeds in the opposite direction (i.e., faster). The final response time is thus influenced by the presence of both types of fatty acids in the membranes.

## Offspring

### *Omega-3 Fatty Acids and an Improved Pregnancy Outcome*

In 11,875 pregnant women, seafood intake during pregnancy of less than 340 g per week was associated with an increased risk of children being in the lowest quartile for verbal intelligence quotient, compared with mothers who consumed more than 340 g per week. Low maternal seafood intake was also associated with an increased risk of suboptimal outcomes for fine motor, communication, and social development scores. For each outcome measured, the lower the intake of seafood during pregnancy, the higher was the risk of a suboptimal developmental outcome (Hibbeln et al., 2007). To investigate the effects on the offspring of mothers who consumed omega-3 fatty acids during pregnancy, pregnant women were given either a DHA-containing functional food providing approximately 200 mg of DHA per day or a placebo food starting from gestation week 24 until delivery, in a double-blind, placebo-controlled, randomized trial. DHA supplementation had significant positive effects on the children's performance of problem-solving tasks at the age of 9 months (Judge et al., 2007). An investigation of the relationship between motor function at 7 years of age and the levels of arachidonic acid and DHA in umbilical venous plasma phospholipids found a significant positive correlation between umbilical plasma DHA concentration and motor-function quality score, but no correlation with arachidonic acid content was found (Bakker et al., 2007).

### **Trans** *Fatty Acids and an Attenuated Pregnancy Outcome*

A study of premature babies found a negative correlation between birth weight and TFA levels in plasma after birth (Koletzko, 1992). In healthy pregnant women, maternal blood at 35 weeks of gestation and umbilical cord blood at birth had TFA concentrations that were inversely proportional to the length of gestation and birth weight, respectively (Elias & Innis, 2001). The results suggest significant negative effects of TFA on the fetal growth and the length of gestation.

## Mechanism of Action

Fatty acids play central roles in growth and development through their roles in membrane lipids, as precursors for eicosanoids and other molecules, and as ligands for nuclear receptors and transcription factors that regulate gene expression. Adverse maternal fatty acid supplies during fetal and child development alter the fatty acid composition of membrane phospholipids with the potential to adversely influence cellular function. These and other findings indicate the need for a sufficient supply of long-chain polyunsaturated fatty acids in the central nervous system during the perinatal central nervous system growth spurt. This also makes it possible that TFAs have negative effects on these processes.

## Fertility

### *Omega-3 Fatty Acids and Improved Fertility*

The effect of omega-3 fatty acids on ovulatory infertility is still unexplored. We predict a beneficial association in observational studies and a positive effect in a randomized trial when compared with other fatty acids.

### **Trans** *Fatty Acids and Reduced Fertility*

Among 18,555 married premenopausal women in the United States without a history of infertility who attempted a pregnancy or became pregnant between 1991 and 1999, some 438 incidents of ovulatory infertility were identified. Whether the intake of total fat, cholesterol, and major types of fatty acids affected the risk of ovulatory infertility was assessed (Chavarro et al., 2007). Diet was assessed twice during the follow-up. Each 2% increase in the intake of energy from TFA as opposed to that from carbohydrates, n-6 polyunsaturated fats, or monounsaturated fats was associated with a 70–230% increased risk of ovulatory infertility after proper adjustment for other risk factors.

### *Mechanism of Action*

Pharmacological activators of PPARγ such as troglitazone (Azziz et al., 2001) and other thiazoledinediones improve dose-dependently signs of ovulatory dysfunction. The opposite effect on ovulatory dysfunction by the intake of *trans* fats can be ascribed to an inhibition of the activity of PPARγ. This hypothesis is supported by the finding that at levels of usual human consumption, TFAs were found to down-regulate the PPARγ expression in vivo by 40% (Saravanan et al., 2005).

## Cancer

### *Omega-3 Fatty Acids and the Reduced Risk of Cancer*

In the New York University Women's Health Study, 14,727 women ages 34–65 years showed a progressive decline in the risk of colorectal cancer with an increased intake of fish and shellfish (Kato et al., 1997). The Nurses' Health Study found no evidence that the intake of specific major types of fat was associated with a decreased risk of breast cancer (Holmes et al., 1999), and a systematic and Cochrane review provided no evidence to suggest a significant association between omega-3 fatty acids and cancer incidence (Hooper et al., 2006; MacLean et al., 2006).

Since then, a national prospective case-control study in Scotland (1999–2006), including 1,455 incident cases and 1,455 matched controls, found a significant dose-dependent reduction in colorectal cancer risk associated with an increased consumption of omega-3 fatty acids and of EPA and DHA (Theodoratou et al., 2007). In a nested case-control study among 14,916 healthy men, whole blood levels of all long-chain omega-3 fatty acids were shown to be inversely related to overall prostate cancer risk (Chavarro et al., 2007). A meta-analysis of prospective cohort studies found that fish consumption was associated with slightly reduced colorectal cancer risk (Geelen et al., 2007). In the Physicians' Health Study, the association between the intake of fish and n-3 fatty acids from fish and colorectal cancer risk in men was recently examined. During 22 years of follow-up, 500 men had a confirmed diagnosis of colorectal cancer. Fish and omega-3 fatty acid intakes were inversely associated with colorectal cancer risk. The relative multivariate risk when comparing the highest and lowest categories of intake was 0.60 and 0.74 for fish and omega-3 fatty acids, respectively. The inverse association was observed for both colon and rectal cancers. The results from this long-term prospective study suggest that the intake of fish and long-chain n-3 fatty acids from fish decreased the risk for colorectal cancer (Hall et al., 2008).

In a study on fatty acid intake and breast cancer risk, no association between omega-3 fatty acid intake and cancer risk was found (Chajes et al., 2008). This is in agreement with most such studies conducted in Western countries (Engeset et al., 2006; Terry et al., 2004). In contrast, results from observational studies conducted in Asian populations showed evidence of a protective effect of fish (Gago-Dominguez et al., 2003) and omega-3 fatty acids against breast cancer risk (Kuriki et al., 2007; Wakai et al., 2005). This discrepancy might be the consequence of higher dietary intakes of omega-3 fatty acids in Asian populations as compared with Western populations. Specifically, in a prospective study conducted in Japan, the mean dietary intake of omega-3 fatty acids in the highest quartile, associated with a 50% reduction in risk for breast cancer, was estimated to be 0.6% of energy consumption, corresponding to about 1 g of omega-3 fatty acids daily (Wakai et al., 2005). Similarly, high intakes were reported in a case-control study carried out in Japan, where the highest mean intake of omega-3 fatty acids, associated with a 50% reduction in the risk of breast cancer, was estimated to be more than 0.55% of energy consumption (Kuriki et al., 2007). A substantially lower dietary intake of long-chain omega-3 fatty acids was found in the French population, where the highest intake reached only 0.23% of energy consumption, corresponding to a daily intake of approximately 0.4 g of EPA and DHA. In this context, a clear inverse relationship may not have been observed in the French population because omega-3 fatty acid intake was below the threshold for a protective effect against breast cancer risk.

## Trans *Fatty Acids and the Increased Risk of Cancer*

A high intake of TFA is associated with an increased risk of postmenopausal breast cancer in a few studies (Kim et al., 2006; Voorrips et al., 2002). The estimates of dietary intake of TFA are hampered by more inaccuracies than estimates of intake of most other dietary fatty acids. This means that only very strong associations are revealed by observational intake studies.

Concentrations of TFA in tissue offer an objective, qualitative measure of bioavailable amounts of these fatty acids regardless of their source in food. In a case-control study nested in a French study of 19,934 females, TFAs in plasma phospholipids were determined in 363 cases of breast cancer documented during an average of 7 years of follow-up after the women provided serum samples, and in samples from appropriate controls from the study (Chajes et al., 2008).

An increased risk of breast cancer was associated with increasing the levels of the *trans*-monounsaturated fatty acids, palmitoleic acid, and elaidic acid (highest quintile versus. lowest).

The TFA that had the strongest association to breast cancer was *trans* palmitoleic acid (C16:1*t*). This acid is usually not present in hydrogenated vegetable oils but only in ruminant fat. It is, however, also present in partially hydrogenated marine oils. Since the authors found no association between the marker for ruminant fat intake of pentadecaneic acid and breast cancer, possibly the presence of C16:1*t* in plasma phospholipids is due to the intake of partially hydrogenated fish oils.

Several studies explored the association between the intake of TFA and prostate cancer. In a case-control study nested within the American Physician Health Study (Chavarro et al., 2008), 476 men diagnosed with prostate cancer during a 13-year follow-up, after the determination of blood fat levels, were compared with matched controls according to age and smoking levels at the baseline. The blood levels of all TFAs examined were unrelated to total prostate cancer risk. When results were divided according to tumor aggressiveness, the blood levels of total TFA, elaidic acid, and three 18:2n-6*t* isomers were positively associated with nonaggressive tumors. Not one TFA examined was associated with aggressive prostate tumors. The authors concluded that their results suggest that some specific TFAs are involved in the early stages of prostate carcinogenesis but do not contribute significantly to disease progression or that they increase risk only for specific tumor types.

## *Mechanism of Action*

Some studies of cancer cells in culture or experimental animals show that the cyclooxygenase and the 5-lipoxygenase pathways of arachidonic acid are required for the invasive and metastatic activities of certain tumor cells (Reich & Martin, 1996). Experimentally, malignant murine melanoma and human fibrosarcoma cells cultured in media supplemented with EPA had a dose- and time-dependent decrease in invasiveness and a reduced ability to metastasize to the lung after intravenous injection (Reich et al., 1989). The mechanisms behind a putative protective effect of diets rich in omega-3 fatty acids against cancer are, however, still unclear. An altered expression of PPAR$\alpha$ and -$\gamma$ by DHA was suggested (Narayanan et al., 2001). Omega-3 fatty acid-enriched LDL modified the production of syndecan-1(SDC-1) in human breast cancer cells. SDC-1 is expressed on the surface of mammary epithelial cells and regulates many biological processes, including growth-factor signaling (Sun et al., 2005). Recent studies show that DHA up-regulates SDC-1 in human breast cancer cells through the activation of PPAR$\gamma$, and that omega-3 fatty acid-induced apoptosis is mediated by SDC-1. This provides a tentative mechanism for the chemo-preventive effects of omega-3 fatty acids in breast cancer (Sun et al., 2008).

Increasing evidence suggests that inflammation is important in prostate carcinogenesis, and chronic inflammatory response is enhanced by TFA intake.

In addition, specific TFAs down-regulate PPARγ in vivo (Saravanna et al., 2005). This is a particularly important finding, considering that PPARγ can modulate inflammation and is expressed in prostate tumors where its agonists have general anti-proliferative effects (Lehrke & Lazar, 2005; Subbarayan et al., 2004).

# Summary

## Health Findings

Many of the studies concerning health effects and fatty acid intake are observational with an inherently limited ability to reveal weak associations due to regression dilutions (Clarke et al., 1999) and the possibility of confounding factors. The general pattern in the results is, however, that the intake of omega-3 fatty acids, when compared with the intake of other fatty acids, is associated with beneficial and neutral health effects with, to the best of our knowledge, no harmful effects, either in the relatively few interventional studies or in the many observational studies.

For TFA, the situation is the opposite. The intake of TFA is associated with either harmful or neutral health effects when compared to the intake of other fatty acids with no beneficial effects.

A direct comparison of the health effects of omega-3 fatty acids and TFA has so far been done only in very few studies, but the findings presented in this review suggest that we are dealing with opposing health effects resulting from the daily intakes of relatively few grams of these nutrients.

## Mechanisms of Action

It seems appropriate to divide the mechanisms of the action of omega-3 fatty acids and TFAs into three categories based on the position of these effects in the cell: in the cell membrane, cytoplasm, and nucleus.

The presence of omega-3 fatty acids in the bilayer of the cell membrane is probably of major significance for the effect of these fatty acids on many organs (e.g., the brain and neural tissue). The TFAs may compete with the omega-3 fatty acids EPA and DHA in the cell membrane, and the resulting change in the fatty acid composition may result in functional changes (i.e., in ion channels and in other membrane functions in the brain), but it may also have an effect on heart rhythm, on pregnancy, and on the initiation of labor.

The presence of these fatty acids in the cytoplasm of the cell may interfere with the formation of various biologically active eicosanoids, cytokines, and other signal components by an enzymatic precursor/product relationship. The shift in balance between various biologically active components may influence the extent of chronic inflammatory reactions in tissues.

Small structural changes in the molecular composition of fatty acids have a great influence on the activation of PPARs. The presence of omega-3 fatty acids and TFAs and their degradation products in the cell nucleus and their interaction with the

PPAR-system may consequently be of importance for the attenuation of chronic inflammation by omega-3 fatty acids and for the promotion of chronic inflammation by TFA. Also the PPAR-mediated effects on a wide spectrum of other metabolic processes may be modulated in an antagonistic way by omega-3 fatty acids and TFAs. These opposing effects may again be important for the effects of omega-3 fatty acids and TFAs on various degenerative diseases, such as atherosclerosis, certain forms of cancer, allergy, type 2 diabetes, and certain forms of infertility.

This topographic separation of the mechanisms of actions for these fatty acids, while only considering omega-3 fatty acids and TFAs in cells, is simplified. The entire plethora of all fatty acids, *cis* and *trans*, of different chain lengths probably should be taken into account to fully describe how changes in the intake of omega-3 fatty acids and TFAs interfere with health and disease.

## Conclusion

Data from hundreds of large and well-conducted studies published during the last decades strongly suggest that an increased intake of omega-3 fatty acids and a decreased intake of TFAs attenuate the development of several serious and prevalent diseases and promote or maintain the function of the human brain—without side effects.

The daily intake of long-chain omega-3 fatty acids should therefore be on the order of grams, not only as a mean average intake for the population but for all individuals in the population. In contrast, the intake of TFA should be as low as possible, not only for the majority of the population, but for all individuals. How this opposing change in the intake of fatty acids may be accomplished is a political issue, but it appears to be possible. Fortification with omega-3 fatty acids and a legislative ban on industriallyproduced TFAs are prudent options.

### References

Ackman, R.G. Nutritional composition of fats in seafoods. *Prog. Food Nutr. Sci.* **1989,** *13,* 161–289.

American Heart Association Nutrition Committee. Diet and lifestyle recommendations revision 2006: a scientific statement from the American Heart Association Nutrition Committee. *Circulation* **2006,** *114,* 82–96.

Arita, M.; S.F. Oh; T. Chonan; S. Hong; S. Elangovan; Y.O. Sun; J. Uddin; N.A. Petasis; C.N. Serhan. Metabolic inactivation of resolvin E1 and stabilization of its anti-inflammatory actions. *J. Biol Chem* **2006,** *281,* 22847–22854.

Ascherio, A.; M.B. Katahn; M.J. Stampfer; W.C. Willett. Trans Fatty Acids and Coronary Heart Disease. Sounding Board. *N. Engl. J. Med.* **1999,** *340,* 1994–1997.

Austin, M.A.; B. McKnight; K.E. Edwards; C.M. Bradley; M.J. McNeely; B.M. Psaty; J.D. Brunzell; A.G. Motulsky. Cardiovascular disease mortality in familial forms of hypertiglyceridemia: A 20-year prospective study. *Circulation* **2000,** *10,* 2777–2782.

Azziz, R; D. Ehrmann; R.S. Legro; R.W. Whitcomb; R. Hanley; SA. G. Fereshetian; M. O'Keefe;

M.N. Ghazzi; PCOS/Troglitazone Study Group. Troglitazone improves ovulation and hirsutism in the polycystic ovary syndrome: a multicenter, double blind, placebo-controlled trial. *J. Clin. Endocrinol. Metab.* **2001**, *86*, 1626–1632

Bakker, E.C.; G. Hornstra; C.E. Blanco; J.S. Vles. Relationship between long-chain polyunsaturated fatty acids at birth and motor function at 7 years of age. *Eur. J. Clin. Nutr.* **2007,** Dec. 19 [Epub ahead of print].

Balk, E.M.; A.H. Lichtenstein; M. Chung; B. Kupelnick; P. Chew; J. Lau. Effects of omega-3 fatty acids on serum markers of cardiovascular disease risk: a systematic review. *Atherosclerosis* **2006,** *189,* 19–30.

Bang, H.O.; J. Dyerberg. Urinary thromboxane metabolites in pre-eclampsia. *Lancet* **1990**, *335,* 1169.

Bang, H.O.; J. Dyerberg; Aa.B. Nielsen. Plasma lipid and lipoprotein pattern in Greenlandic west-coast Eskimos. *Lancet* **1971**, *1,* 1143–1146.

Bansal, S.; J.E. Buring; N. Rifai; S. Mora; F.M. Sacks; P.M. Ridker. Fasting compared with non-fasting triglycerides and risk of cardiovascular events in women. *JAMA* **2007**, *298,* 309–316.

Bazan, N.G. Neuroprotectin D1 (NPD1): a DHA-derived mediator that protects brain and retina against cell injury-induced oxidative stress. *Brain Pathol.* **2005**, *15*, 159–166.

Beydoun, M.A.; J.S. Kaufman; P.D. Sloane; G. Heiss; J. Ibrahim. n-3 Fatty acids, hypertension and risk of cognitive decline among older adults in the Atherosclerosis Risk in Communities (ARIC) study. *Public Health Nutr* **2008**, *11,* 17–29.

Brooks, J.D.; G.L. Milne; H. Yin; S.C. Sanchez; N.A. Porter; J.D. Morrow. Formation of highly reactive cyclopentenone isoprostane compounds (A3/J3-isoprostanes) in vivo from eicosapentaenoic acid. *J. Biol. Chem.* **2008,** *283,* 12043–12055.

Buchwald, H.; S.E. Williams; J.P. Matts; J.R. Boen. Lipid modulation and liver function tests. A report of the Program on the Surgical Control of the Hyperlipidemias (POSCH). *J. Cardiovasc. Risk* **2002**, *9*, 83–87.

Burdge, C.G.; P.C. Calder. Conversion of alpha-linolenic acid to longer-chain polyunsaturated fatty acids in human adults. *Reprod. Nutr. Dev.* **2005**, *45*, 581–597.

Burr, G.O.; M.M. Burr. On the nature and role of the fatty acids essential in nutrition. *J. Biol. Chem.* **1930,** *86*, 587– 621.

Celermajer, D.S.; K.E. Sørensen; V.M. Gooch; D.J. Spiegelhalter; O.I. Miller; I.D. Sullivan; J.K. Lloyd; J.E. Deanfield. Non-invasive detection of endothelial dysfunction in children and adults at risk of atherosclerosis. *Lancet* **1992,** *340,* 1111–1115.

Chajès, V.; A.C. Thiébaut; M. Rotival; E. Gauthier; V. Maillard; M.C. Boutron-Ruault; V. Joulin; G.M. Lenoir; F. Clavel-Chapelon. Association between Serum trans-Monounsaturated Fatty Acids and Breast Cancer Risk in the E3N-EPIC Study. *Am. J. Epidemiol.* **2008,** *167,* 1312–1320.

Chambrier, C.; J.P. Bastard; J. Rieusset; E. Chevillotte; D. Bonnefont-Rousselot; P. Therond; B. Hainque; J.P. Riou; M. Laville; H. Vidal. Eicosapentaenoic acid induces mRNA expression of peroxisome proliferator-activated receptor gamma. *Obes. Res.* **2002**, *10,* 518–525.

Chardigny, J.M.; F. Destaillats; C. Malpuech-Brugère; J. Moulin; D.E. Bauman; A.L. Lock; D.M. Barbano; R.P. Mensink; J.B. Bezelgues; P. Chaumont; et al. Do trans fatty acids from industrially produced sources and from natural sources have the same effect on cardiovascular disease risk factors in healthy subjects? Results of the trans Fatty Acids Collaboration (TRANSFACT) study. *Am. J. Clin. Nutr.* **2008**, *87*, 558–566.

Chavarro, J.E.; M.J. Stampfer; H. Li; H. Campos; T. Kurth; J. Ma. A prospective study of polyunsaturated Fatty Acid levels in blood and prostate cancer risk. *Cancer Epidemiol. Biomarkers Prev* **2007**, *16*, 1364–1370.

Chavarro, J.E.; M.J. Stampfer; H. Campos; T. Kurth; W.C. Willett; J. Ma. A prospective study of trans-fatty acid levels in blood and risk of prostate cancer. *Cancer Epidemiol. Biomarkers Prev.* **2008,** *17*, 95–101.

Chiang, N.; C.N. Serhan. Cell-cell interaction in the transcellular biosynthesis of novel omega-3-derived lipid mediators. *Methods Mol. Biol.* **2006**, *341*, 227–250.

Christensen, J.H.; M.S. Christensen; J. Dyerberg; E.B. Schmidt. Heart rate variability and fatty acid content of blood cell membranes: a dose-response study with n-3 fatty acids. *Am. J. Clin. Nutr.* **1999**, *70*, 331–337.

Christensen, J.H.; P. Gustenhof; E. Korup; J. Aaroee; E. Toft; J. Moeller; C. Rasmussen; J. Dyerberg; E.B. Schmidt. Effect of fish oil on heart rate variability in survivors of myocardial infarction: a double blind randomised controlled trial. *BMJ* **1996**, *312*, 677–678.

Clarke, R.; M. Shipley; S. Lewington; L. Youngman; R. Collins; M. Marmot; R. Peto. Underestimation of risk associations due to regression dilution in long-term follow-up of prospective studies. *Am. J. Epidemiol.* **1999,** *150*, 341–353.

Craig-Schmidt, M.C. World-wide consumption of trans fatty acids. *Atheroscler. Supp.* **2006**, *7*, 1–4.

Crawford, M.A. Cerebral evolution. *Nutr. Health* **2002**, *16*, 29–34.

Dallongeville, J.; J. Yarnell; P. Ducimetière; D. Arveiler; J. Ferrières; M. Montaye; G. Luc; A. Evans; A. Bingham; B. Hass; et al. Fish consumption is associated with lower heart rates. *Circulation* **2003**, *108*, 820–825.

Davidson, M.H. Mechanisms for the hypotriglyceridemic effect of marine omega-3 fatty acids. *Am. J. Cardiol.* **2006**, *98*, 27i–33i.

De Caterina, R; J.K. Liao; P. Libby. Fatty acid modulation of endothelial activation. *Am. J. Clin. Nutr.* **2000** (*1 Suppl*), 213S–223S.

deRoos, N.M.; E.G. Schouten; M.B. Katan. Trans fatty acids, HDL-cholesterol, and cardiovascular disease. Effects of dietary changes on vascular reactivity. *Eur. J. Med. Res.* **2003**, *8*, 355–357.

Dietary Guidelines for Americans 2005, www.health-gov/dietary guidelines. Accessed May 2008.

Dolecek, T.A.; G. Grandtis. Dietary polyunsaturated fatty acids and mortality in the Multiple Risk Factor intervention Trial (MRFIT). In Simopoulos AP et al. (eds): Health Effects of ω3 Polyunsaturated Fatty Acids in Seafoods. *World Rev. Nutr. Diet.* Karger, Basel **1991**; *Vol. 66*, pp. 205–216.

Dullemeijer, C.; J. Durga; I.A. Brouwer; O. van de Rest; F.J. Kok; R.J. Brummer; M.P. van Boxtel; P. Verhoef. n-3 Fatty acid proportions in plasma and cognitive performance in older adults. *Am. J. Clin. Nutr.* **2007**, *86*, 1479–1485.

Dyerberg, J.; H.O. Bang. Haemostatic function and platelet polyunsaturated fatty acids in Eskimos. *Lancet* **1979**, *2*, 433–435.

Dyerberg, J.; J.H. Christensen, D. Eskesen; A. Astrup; S. Stender. *Trans*, and n-3 polyunsaturated fatty acids and vascular function-A yin yang situation? *Atheroscler. Suppl.* **2006**, 33–35.

Dyerberg, J.; D.C. Eskesen; P.W. Andersen; A. Astrup; B. Buemann; J.H. Christensen; P. Clausen; B.F. Rasmussen; E.B. Schmidt; T. Tholstrup; E. Toft; S. Toubro; S. Stender. Effects of trans- and n-3 unsaturated fatty acids on cardiovascular risk markers in healthy males. An 8-week dietary intervention study. *Eur. J. Clin. Nutr.* **2004**, *58,* 1062–1070.

Elias, S.L.; S.M. Innis. Infant plasma trans, n-6, and n-3 fatty acids and conjugated linoleic acids are related to maternal plasma fatty acids, length of gestation, and birth weight and length. *Am. J. Clin. Nutr.* **2001**, *73,* 807–814.

Engeset, D.; E. Alsaker; E. Lund; A. Welch; K.T. Khaw; F. Clavel-Chapelon; A. Thiébaut; V. Chajès; T.J. Key; N.E. Allen; et al. Fish consumption and breast cancer risk. The European Prospective Investigation into Cancer and Nutrition (EPIC). *Int. J. Cancer.* **2006**, *119,*175–182

Ferreri, C; F. Angelini; C. Chatgilialoglu; S. Dellonte; V. Moschese; P. Rossi; L. Chini. Trans fatty acids and atopic eczema/dermatitis syndrome: the relationship with a free radical cis-trans isomerization of membrane lipids. *Lipids* **2005**, *40,* 661–667.

Gago-Dominguez, M; J.M. Yuan; C.L. Sun; H.P. Lee; M.C. Yu. Opposing effects of dietary n-3 and n-6 fatty acids on mammary carcinogenesis: The Singapore Chinese Health Study. *Br. J. Cancer.* **2003**, *89,* 1686–1692.

Geelen, A.; J.M. Schouten; C. Kamphuis; B.E. Stam; J. Burema; J.M. Renkema; E.J. Bakker; P. Van't Veer; E. Kampman. Fish Consumption, n-3 Fatty Acids, and Colorectal Cancer: A Meta-Analysis of Prospective Cohort Studies. *Am. J. Epidemiol.* **2007**, *166,* 1116–1125.

Gillette-Guyonnet, S.; G. Abellan Van Kan; S. Andrieu; P. Barberger Gateau; C. Berr; M. Bonnefoy; J.F. Dartigues; L. de Groot; M. Ferry; P. Galan; et al. IANA task force on nutrition and cognitive decline with aging. *J. Nutr. Health Aging* **2007**, *11,* 132–152.

GISSI-Preventione Investigators. Dietary supplementation with n-3 polyunsaturated fatty acids and Vitamin E after myocardial infarction: results of the GISSI-Prevenzione trial. *Lancet* **1999**, *354,* 447–455.

Goldberg, R.J; J. Katz. A meta-analysis of the analgesic effects of omega-3 polyunsaturated fatty acid supplementation for inflammatory joint pain. *Pain* **2007**, *129,* 210–223.

Goldberg, R.B.; A.K. Sabharwal. Fish oil in the treatment of dyslipidemia. *Curr. Opin. Endocrinol. Diabetes Obes* **2008**, *15,* 167–174.

Goldman, D.W.; W.C. Pickett; E.J. Goetzl. Human neutrophil chemotactic and degranulating activities of leukotriene B5 (LTB5) derived from eicosapentaenoic acid. *Biochem. Biophys. Res. Commun* **1983**, *117,* 282–288.

Goodfellow, J.; M.F. Bellamy; M.W. Ramsey; C.J. Jones; M.J. Lewis. Dietary supplementation with marine omega-3 fatty acids improves systemic large artery endothelial function in subjects with hypercholesterolemia. *J. Am. Coll. Cardiol.* **2000**, *35,* 265–270.

Haag, M. Essential fatty acids and the brain. *Can. J. Psychiatry.* **2003**, *48,* 195–203.

Hall, M.N; J.E. Chavarro; I.M. Lee; W.C. Willett; J. Ma. *Cancer Epidemiol. Biomarkers Prev.* **2008,** *17,* 1136–1143.

Harris, W.S. International recommendations for consumption of long-chain omega-3 fatty acids. *J. Cardiovasc. Med. (Hagerstown).* **2007**,*8* Suppl 1, S50–52.

Harris, W.S.; D. Bulchandani. Why do omega-3 fatty acids lower serum triglycerides? *Curr. Opin. Lipidol.* **2006**, *17,* 387–393.

Harris, W.S.; M. Miller; A.P. Tighe; M.H. Davidson; E.J. Schaefer. Omega-3 fatty acids and coronary heart disease risk: clinical and mechanistic perspectives. *Atherosclerosis* **2008**, *197*, 12–24.

Hartweg, J.; R. Perera; V. Montori; S. Dinneen; H.A. Neil;. A. Farmer. Update of: Cochrane Database Syst Rev. 2001;(3):CD003205. Omega-3 polyunsaturated fatty acids (PUFA) for type 2 diabetes mellitus. *Cochrane Database Syst. Rev.* **2008**, (1):CD003205.

Harvey, K.A.; T. Arnold; T. Rasool; C. Antalis; S.J. Miller; R.A. Siddiqui. Trans-fatty acids induce pro-inflammatory responses and endothelial cell dysfunction. *Br. J. Nutr.* **2008**, *99*, 723–731.

Heude, B.; P. Ducimetière; C. Berr; EVA Study. Cognitive decline and fatty acid composition of erythrocyte membranes—The EVA Study. *Am. J. Clin. Nutr.* **2003**, *77,* 803–808.

Hibbeln, J.R.; J.M. Davis; C. Steer; P. Emmett; I. Rogers; C. Williams; J. Golding. Maternal seafood consumption in pregnancy and neurodevelopmental outcomes in childhood (ALSPAC study): an observational cohort study. *Lancet* **2007**, *369,* 578–585.

Holmes, M.D.; D.J. Hunter; G.A. Colditz; M.J. Stampfer; S.E. Hankinson; F.E. Speizer; B. Rosner; W.C. Willett. Association of dietary intake of fat and fatty acids with risk of breast cancer. *JAMA* **1999**, *281,* 914–920.

Hooper, L.; R.L. Thompson; R.A. Harrison; C.D. Summerbell; A.R. Ness; H.J. Moore; H.V. Worthington; P.N. Durrington; J.P. Higgins; N.E. Capps; R.A. Riemersma; S.B. Ebrahim; G. Davey Smith. Risks and benefits of omega 3 fats for mortality, cardiovascular disease, and cancer: systematic review. *BMJ* **2006**, *332,* 752–760.

Hulshof, K.F.; M.A. van Erp-Baart; M. Anttolainen; W. Becker; S.M. Church; C. Couet; E. Hermann-Kunz; H. Kesteloot; T. Leth; I. Martins; et al. Intake of fatty acids in western Europe with emphasis on trans fatty acids: the TRANSFAIR Study. *Eur. J. Clin. Nutr.* **1999**, *53,* 143–157.

Jakobsen. M.U; A. Bysted; N.L. Andersen; B.L. Heitmann; H.B. Hartkopp; T. Leth; K. Overvad; J. Dyerberg. Intake of ruminant trans fatty acids in the Danish population aged 1–80 years. *Eur. J. Clin. Nutr.* **2006**, *60,* 312–318.

Judge, M.P.; O. Harel; C.J. Lammi-Keefe. Maternal consumption of a docosahexaenoic acid-containing functional food during pregnancy: benefit for infant performance on problem-solving but not on recognition memory tasks at age 9 mo. *Am. J. Clin. Nutr.* **2007**, *85,* 1572–1577.

Kato, I.; A. Akhmedkhanov; K. Koenig; P.G. Toniolo; R.E. Shore; E. Riboli. Prospective study of diet and female colorectal cancer: the New York University Women's Health Study. *Nutr. Cancer* **1997**, *28,* 276–281.

Katz, A.M. Should trans fatty acids be viewed as membrane-active drugs? *Atheroscler. Suppl.* **2006**, *7,* 41–42.

Kavanagh, K.; K.L. Jones; J. Sawyer; K. Kelley; J.J. Carr; J.D. Wagner; L.L. Rudel. Trans fat diet induces abdominal obesity and changes in insulin sensitivity in monkeys. *Obesity (Silver Spring)* **2007**, *15,* 1675–1684.

Kim, E.H.; W.C. Willett; G.A. Colditz; S.E. Hankinson; M.J. Stampfer; D.J. Hunter; B. Rosner; M.D. Holmes. Dietary fat and risk of postmenopausal breast cancer in a 20-year follow-up. *Am. J. Epidemiol.* **2006**, *164,* 990–997.

Koch, C; S. Dölle; M. Metzger; C. Rasche; H. Jungclas; R. Rühl; H. Renz; M. Worm. Docosahexaenoic acid (DHA) supplementation in atopic eczema: a randomized, double-blind, controlled trial. *Br. J. Dermatol.* **2008**, *158*, 786–792.

Koletzko, B. Trans fatty acids may impair biosynthesis of long-chain polyunsaturates and growth in man. *Acta Paediatr.* **1992**, *81,* 302–306.

Kull, I; A. Bergstrom; G. Lilja; G. Pershagen; M. Wickman. Fish consumption during the first year of life and development of allergic diseases during childhood. *Allergy* **2006**, *61*, 1009–1015.

Kuriki, K.; K. Hirose; K. Wakai; K. Matsuo; H. Ito; T. Suzuki; A. Hiraki; T. Saito; H. Iwata; M. Tatematsu; K. Tajima. Breast cancer risk and erythrocyte compositions of n-3 highly unsaturated fatty acids in Japanese. *Int. J. Cancer* **2007**, *121*, 377–385.

Lagrost, L. Differential effects of cis and trans fatty acid isomers, oleic and elaidic acids, on the cholesteryl ester transfer protein activity. *Biochim. Biophys. Acta.* **1992**, *1124*, 159–162.

Leaf, A. Omega-3 fatty acids and prevention of arrhythmias. *Curr. Opin. Lipidol.* **2007**, *18*, 31–34.

Leaf, A.; C.M. Albert; M. Josephson; D. Steinhaus; J. Kluger; J.X. Kang; B. Cox; H. Zhang; D. Schoenfeld. Fatty Acid Antiarrhythmia Trial Investigators. Prevention of fatal arrhythmias in high-risk subjects by fish oil n-3 fatty acid intake. *Circulation* **2005**, *112,* 2762–2768.

Leaf, A.; P.C. Weber. A new era for science in nutrition. *Am. J. Clin. Nutr.* **1987,** *45* (5 Suppl), 1048–1053.

Lee, J.H.; J.H. O'Keefe; C.J. Lavie; R. Marchioli; W.S. Harris. Omega3 Fatty acids for cardioprotection. *Mayo Clin. Proc.* **2008**, *83*, 324–332.

Leeson, C.P.; A. Mann; M. Kattenhorn; J.E. Deanfield; A. Lucas; D.P. Muller. Relationship between circulating n-3 fatty acid concentrations and endothelial function in early adulthood. *Eur. Heart J.* **2002**, *23*, 216–222.

Leibowitz, M.D.; C. Fiévet; N. Hennuyer; et al. Activation of PPARdelta alters lipid metabolism in db/db mice. *FEBS Lett.* **2000**, *473,* 333–336.

Lehrke, M.; M.A. Lazar. The many faces of PPARgamma. *Cell* **2005**, *123*, 993–999.

Lemaitre, R.N.; I.B. King; D. Mozaffarian; L.H. Kuller; R.P. Tracy; D.S. Siscovick. n-3 Polyunsaturated fatty acids, fatal ischemic heart disease, and nonfatal myocardial infarction in older adults: the Cardiovascular Health Study. *Am. J. Clin. Nutr.* **2003**, *77,* 319–325.

Lemaitre, R.N.; I.B. King; D. Mozaffarian; N. Sotoodehnia; T.D. Rea; L.H. Kuller; R.P. Tracy; D.S. Siscovick. Plasma phospholipid trans fatty acids, fatal ischemic heart disease, and sudden cardiac death in older adults: the cardiovascular health study. *Circulation* **2006,** *114,* 209–215.

Lichtenstein, A.H. Dietary trans fatty acid. *J. Cardiopulm. Rehabil.* **2000,** *20,* 143–146.

Lopez-Garcia, E; M.B. Schulze; J.B. Meigs; J.E. Manson; N. Rifai; M.J. Stampfer; W.C. Willett; F.B. Hu. Consumption of trans fatty acids is related to plasma biomarkers of inflammation and endothelial dysfunction. *J. Nutr.* **2005,** *135*, 562–566.

Lovegrove, J.A.; C.N. Brooks; M.C. Murphy; B.J. Gould; C.M. Williams. Use of manufactured foods enriched with fish oils as a means of increasing long-chain n-3 polyunsaturated fatty acid intake. *Br. J. Nutr.* **1997**, *78*, 223–236.

Ma, Q.L.; B. Teter; O.J. Ubeda; T. Morihara; D. Dhoot; M.D. Nyby; M.L. Tuck; S.A. Frautschy. Omega-3 fatty acid docosahexaenoic acid increases SorLA/LR11, a sorting protein with reduced expression in sporadic Alzheimer's disease (AD): relevance to AD prevention. *J. Neurosci.* **2007,** *27,* 14299–14307.

Macchia, A.; S. Monte; F. Pellegrini; M. Romero; D. Ferrante; H. Doval; A. D'Ettorre; A. P. Maggioni; G. Tognoni. Omega-3 fatty acid supplementation reduces one-year risk of atrial fibrillation in patients hospitalized with myocardial infarction. *Eur. J. Clin. Pharmacol.* **2008,** *Feb. 29.* [Epub ahead of print]

MacLean, C.H.; S.J. Newberry; W.A. Mojica; P. Khanna; A.M. Issa; M.J. Suttorp; Y.W. Lim; S.B. Traina; L. Hilton; R. Garland; S.C. Morton. Effects of omega-3 fatty acids on cancer risk: a systematic review. *JAMA* **2006**, *295,* 403–415.

Mahomed, K.; M.A. Williams; I.B. King; S. Mudzamiri; G.B. Woelk. Erythrocyte omega-3, omega-6 and trans fatty acids in relation to risk of preeclampsia among women delivering at Harare Maternity Hospital, Zimbabwe. *Physiol. Res.* **2007**, *56,* 37–50.

Marcovina, S.M.; H. Kennedy; B.G. Bittolo; G. Cazzolato; C. Galli; E. Casiglia; M. Puato; P. Pauletto. Fish intake, independent of apo(a) size, accounts for lower plasma lipoprotein(a) levels in Bantu fishermen of Tanzania: The Lugalawa Study. *Arterioscler. Thromb. Vasc. Biol.* **1999**, *19,* 1250–1256.

Matthan, N.R.; F.K. Welty; P.H. Barrett; C. Harausz; G.G. Dolnikowski; J.S. Parks; R.H. Eckel; E.J. Schaefer; A.H. Lichtenstein. Dietary hydrogenated fat increases high-density lipoprotein apoA-I catabolism and decreases low-density lipoprotein apoB-100 catabolism in hypercholesterolemic women. *Aterioscler. Thromb. Vasc. Biol.* **2004**, *24,* 1092–1097.

Mensink, R.P.; M.B. Katan. Effect of dietary trans fatty acids on high-density and low-density lipoprotein cholesterol levels in healthy subjects. *N. Engl. J. Med.* **1990**, *323,* 439–445.

Mensink, R.P.; P.L. Zock; A.D. Kester; M.B. Katan. Effects of dietary fatty acids and carbohydrates on the ratio of serum total to HDL cholesterol and on serum lipids and apolipoproteins: a meta-analysis of 60 controlled trials. *Am. J. Clin. Nutr.* **2003**, *77,* 1146–1155.

Miller, M.; P. Cannon; S A. Murphy; J. Qin; K.K. Ray; E. Braunwald. Impact of triglyceride levels beyond low-density lipoprotein cholesterol after acute coronary syndrome in the PROVE IT-TIMI 22 trial. *J. Am. Coll. Cardiol.* **2008**, *51,* 724–730.

Monge-Rojas, R; H. Campos; X. Fernández Rojas. Saturated and cis- and trans-unsaturated fatty acids intake in rural and urban Costa Rican adolescents. *J. Am. Coll. Nutr.* **2005**, *24,* 286–293.

Morris, M.C.; D.A. Evans; J.L. Bienias; C.C. Tangney; D.A. Bennett; N. Aggarwal; J. Schneider; R.S. Wilson. Dietary fats and the risk of incident Alzheimer's disease. *Arch. Neurol.* **2003**, *60,* 194–200.

Morris, M.C.; D.A. Evans; C.C. Tangney; J.L. Bienias; R.S. Wilson. Fish consumption and cognitive decline with age in a large community study. *Arch. Neurol.* **2005**, *62,* 1849–1853.

Motard-Bélanger, A.; A. Charest; G. Grenier; P. Paquin; Y. Chouinard; S. Lemieux; P. Couture; B. Lamarche. Study of the effect of trans fatty acids from ruminants on blood lipids and other risk factors for cardiovascular disease. *Am. J. Clin. Nutr.* **2008,** *87,* 593–599.

Mozaffarian, D. Trans fatty acids—effects on systemic inflammation and endothelial function. *Atheroscler. Suppl.* **2006**, *7,* 29–32.

Mozaffarian, D.; M. Abdollahi; H. Campos; A. Houshiarrad; W.C. Willet. Consumption of trans fats and estimated effects on coronary heart disease in Iran. *Eur. J. Clin. Nutr.* **2007**, *61,*

1004–1010.

Mozaffarian, D.; A. Geelen; I.A. Brouwer; J.M. Geleijnse; P.L. Zock; M.B. Katan. Effect of fish oil on heart rate in humans: a meta-analysis of randomized controlled trials. *Circulation* **2005**, *112,* 1945–1952.

Mozaffarian, D.; M.B. Katan; A. Ascherio; M.J. Stampfer; W.C. Willett. Trans fatty acids and cardiovascular disease. *N. Engl. J. Med.* **2006**, *354,* 1601–1613.

Mozaffarian, D.; P.K. Stein; R.J. Prineas; D.S. Siscovick. Dietary fish and omega-3 fatty acid consumption and heart rate variability in US adults. *Circulation* **2008**, *117,* 1130–1137.

Narayanan, B.A.; N.K. Narayanan; B.S. Reddy. Docosahexaenoic acid regulated genes and transcription factors inducing apoptosis in human colon cancer cells. *Int. J. Oncol.* **2001**, *19,* 1255–1262.

Neschen S.; K. Morino; J. Dong; Y. Wang-Fischer; G.W. Cline; A.J. Romanelli; J.C. Rossbacher; I.K. Moore; W. Regittnig; D.S. Munoz; et al,. Fatty acids preserve insulin sensitivity in vivo in a peroxisome proliferator-activated receptor-alpha-dependent manner. *Diabetes*. **2007,** *56,* 1034–41.

Nordestgaard, B.G.; M. Benn; P. Schnohr; A. Tybjaerg-Hansen. Nonfasting triglycerides and risk of myocardial infarction, ischemic heart disease, and death in men and women. *JAMA* **2007**, *298,* 299–308.

Nurk, E.; C.A. Drevon; H. Refsum; K. Solvoll; S.E. Vollset; O. Nygård; H.A. Nygaard; K. Engedal; G.S. Tell; A.D. Smith. Cognitive performance among the elderly and dietary fish intake: the Hordaland Health Study. *Am. J. Clin. Nutr.* **2007**, *86,* 1470–1478.

Olsen, S.F.; M.L. Østerdal; J.D. Salvig; T. Weber; A. Tabor; N.J. Secher. Duration of pregnancy in relation to fish oil supplementation and habitual fish intake: a randomised clinical trial with fish oil. *Eur. J. Clin. Nutr.* **2007**, *61,* 976–985.

Olsen, S.F.; J.D. Sørensen; N.J. Secher; M. Hedegaard; T.B. Henriksen; H.S. Hansen; A. Grant. Randomised controlled trial of effect of fish-oil supplementation on pregnancy duration. *Lancet* **1992**, *339,* 1003–1007.

Oomen, C.M.; M.C. Ocké; E.J.M. Feskens; M.J. van Erp-Baart; F.J. Kok; D. Kromhout. Association between trans fatty acid intake and 10-year risk of coronary heart disease in the Zutphen Elderly study: a prospective population-based study. *Lancet* **2001**, *357,* 746–751.

Park, Y.; W.S. Harris. Omega-3 fatty acid supplementation accelerates chylomicron triglyceride clearance. *J. Lipid Res.* **2003**, *44,* 455–463.

Parra D.; A. Ramel; N. Bandarra; M. Kiely; J.A. Martínez; I. Thorsdottir. A diet rich in long chain omega-3 fatty acids modulates satiety in overweight and obese volunteers during weight loss. *Appetite*. 2008 Jun 14. [Epub ahead of print]

Parrott, M.D.; C.E. Greenwood. Dietary influences on cognitive function with aging: from high-fat diets to healthful eating. *Ann. NY Acad. Sci.* **2007**, *1114,* 389–397.

Plourde, M; S.C. Cunnane. Extremely limited synthesis of long chain polyunsaturates in adults: implications for their dietary essentiality and use as supplements. *Appl. Physiol. Nutr. Metab.* **2007**, *32,* 619–634.

Raitt, M.H.; W.E. Connor; C. Morris; J. Kron; B. Halperin; S.S. Chugh; J. McClelland; J. Cook; K. MacMurdy; R. McAnulty; et al.. Fish oil supplementation and risk of ventricular tachycardia and ventricular fibrillation in patients with implantable defibrillators: a randomized controlled trial. *JAMA* **2005**, *293,* 2884–2891.

Rasic-Milutinovic, Z.; G. Perunicic; S. Pljesa; Z. Gluvic; S. Sobajic; I. Djuric; D. Ristic. Effects of n-3 PUFAs supplementation on insulin resistance and inflammatory biomarkers in hemodialysis patients. *Ren. Fail.* **2007**, *29,* 321–329.

Reich, R.; G.R. Martin. Identification of arachidonic acid pathways required for the invasive and metastatic activity of malignant tumor cells. *Prostaglandins* **1996**, *51,* 1–17.

Reich, R.; L. Royce; G.R. Martin. Eicosapentaenoic acid reduces the invasive and metastatic activities of malignant tumor cells. *Biochem. Biophys. Res. Comm.* **1989**, *160,* 559–564.

Ridker, P.M. C-reactive protein and the prediction of cardiovascular events among those at intermediate risk: moving an inflammatory hypothesis toward consensus. *J. Am. Coll. Cardiol.* **2007**, *49,* 2129–2138.

Risérus, U. Trans fatty acids and insulin resistance. *Atheroscler. Suppl.* **2006**, *7,* 37–39.

Ruxton, C.H.; S.C. Reed; M.J. Simpson; K.J. Millington. The health benefits of omega-3 polyunsaturated fatty acids: a review of the evidence. *J. Hum. Nutr. Diet* **2007**, *20,* 275–285.

Salmerón, J.; F.B. Hu; J.E. Manson; M.J. Stampfer; G.A Colditz; E.B. Rimm; W.C. Willett;. Dietary fat intake and risk of type 2 diabetes in women. *Am. J. Clin. Nutr.* **2001,** *73,* 1019–1026.

Saravanan, N.; A. Haseeb; N.Z. Ehtesham; Ghafoorunissa. Differential effects of dietary saturated and trans-fatty acids on expression of genes associated with insulin sensitivity in rat adipose tissue. *Eur. J. Endocrinol.* **2005**, *153,* 159–165.

Schaefer, E.J.; V. Bongard; A.S. Beiser; S. Lamon-Fava; S.J. Robins; R. Au; K.L. Tucker; D.J. Kyle; P.W. Wilson; P.A. Wolf. Plasma phosphatidylcholine docosahexaenoic acid content and risk of dementia and Alzheimer disease: the Framingham Heart Study. *Arch. Neurol.* **2006**, *63,* 1545–1550.

Schmidt, E.B.; J.M. Moeller; N. Svaneborg; J. Dyerberg. Safety aspects of fish oils. Experiences with an n-3 concentrate of re-esterified triglycerides (Pikasol). *Drug Invest.* **1994**, *7,* 215–220.

Schmidt, E.B.; J.O. Pedersen; K. Varming; E. Ernst; C. Jersild; N. Grunnet; J. Dyerberg. n-3 Fatty acids and leukocyte chemotaxis. Effects in hyperlipidemia and dose-response studies in healthy men. *Arterioscler. Thromb.* **1991**, *11,* 429–435.

Serhan, C.N. Novel chemical mediators in the resolution of inflammation: resolvins and protectins. *Anesthesiol. Clin.* **2006**, *24,* 341–364.

Shah, A.P.; A.M. Ichiuji; J.K. Han; M. Traina; A. El-Bialy; S.K. Meymandi; J. Wachsner. Cardiovascular and endothelial effects of fish oil supplementation in healthy volunteers. *Cardiovasc. Pharmacol. Ther.* **2007**, *12,* 213–219.

Siscovick, D.S.; T.E. Raghunathan; I. King; S. Weinmann; K.G. Wicklund; J. Albright; V. Bovbjerg; P. Arbogast; H. Smith; L.H. Kushi; et al.. Dietary intake of long-chain omega-3 polyunsaturated fatty acids and the risk of primary cardiac arrest. *JAMA* **1995**, *247,* 1363–1367.

Smith, B.K; G.Y. Sun; O.M. Donahue; T.R. Thomas. Exercise plus n-3 fatty acids: additive effect on postprandial lipemia. *Metabolism* **2004**, *53,* 1365–1371.

Spagnoli, L.G.; E. Bonanno; G. Sangiorgi; A. Mauriello. Role of inflammation in atherosclerosis. *J. Nucl. Med.* **2007**, *48,* 1800–1815.

Stender, S.; J. Dyerberg. Influence of trans fatty acids on health. *Ann. Nutr. Metab.* **2004**, *48*, 61–66.

Stender, S.; J. Dyerberg; A. Astrup. High levels of industrially produced trans fat in popular fast foods. *N. Engl. J. Med.* **2006**, *354*, 1650–1652.

Stender, S; J. Dyerberg; A. Astrup. Fast food: unfriendly and unhealthy. *Int. J. Obes. (Lond).* **2007**, *31*, 887–890.

Stensvold, I.; Aa. Tverdal; P. Urdal; S. Graff-Iversen. Non-fasting serum triglyceride concentration and mortality from coronary heart disease and any cause in middle aged Norwegian women. *BMJ* **1993**, *307*, 1318–1322.

Subbarayan, V.; A.L. Sabichi; J. Kim; N. Llansa; C.J. Logothetis; S.M. Lippman; D.G. Menter. Differential peroxisome proliferator-activated receptor-gamma isoform expression and agonist effects in normal and malignant prostate cells. *Cancer Epidemiol. Biomarkers Prev.* **2004**, *13*, 1710–1716.

Sun, H.; I.M. Berquin; I.J. Edwards. Omega-3 polyunsaturated fatty acids regulate syndecan-1 expression in human breast cancer cells. *Cancer Res.* **2005**, *65*, 4442–4447.

Sun, H.; I.M. Berquin; R.T. Owens; J.T. O'Flaherty; I. J. Edwards. Peroxisome proliferator-activated receptor gamma-mediated up-regulation of syndecan-1 by n-3 fatty acids promotes apoptosis of human breast cancer cells. *Cancer Res.* **2008**, *68*, 2912–2919.

Terry, P.D.; J.B. Terry; T.E. Rohan;. Long-chain (n-3) fatty acid intake and risk of cancers of the breast and the prostate: recent epidemiological studies, biological mechanisms, and directions for future research. *J. Nutr.* **2004**, *134*(12 Suppl), 3412S–3420S.

Theodoratou, E.; G. McNeill; R. Cetnarskyj; S.M. Farrington; A. Tenesa; R. Barnetson; M. Porteous; M. Dunlop; H. Campbell. Dietary fatty acids and colorectal cancer: a case-control study. *Am. J. Epidemiol.* **2007**, *166*, 181-195.

van Gelder, B.M.; M. Tijhuis; S. Kalmijn; D. Kromhout. Fish consumption, n-3 fatty acids, and subsequent 5-y cognitive decline in elderly men: the Zutphen Elderly Study. *Am. J. Clin. Nutr.* **2007**, *85*, 1142–1147.

Voorrips, L.E.; H.A. Brants; A.F. Kardinaal; G.J. Hiddink; P.A. van den Brandt; R.A. Goldbohm. Intake of conjugated linoleic acid, fat, and other fatty acids in relation to postmenopausal breast cancer: the Netherlands Cohort Study on Diet and Cancer. *Am. J. Clin. Nutr.* **2002**, *76*, 873–882.

Wakai, K.; K. Tamakoshi; C. Date; M. Fukui; S. Suzuki; Y. Lin; Y. Niwa; K. Nishio; H. Yatsuya; et al. JACC Study Group. Dietary intakes of fat and fatty acids and risk of breast cancer: a prospective study in Japan. *Cancer Sci.* **2005**, *96*, 590–599.

Wang, C.; M. Chung; A. Lichtenstein; E. Balk; B. Kupelnick; D. DeVine; A. Lawrence; J. Lau. Effects of omega-3 fatty acids on cardiovascular disease. Summary, Evidence Report/Technology Assessment: Number 94. (Prepared by Tufts-New England Medical Center Evidence-based Practice Center, under Contract No. 290-02-0022). *AHRQ Publication Number 04-E009-1*, **2004**. Agency for Healthcare Research and Quality, Rockville, MD.

Wang, C.; W.S. Harris; M. Chung: A.H. Lichtenstein; E.M. Balk; B. Kupelnick; H.S. Jordan; J. Lau. n-3 Fatty acids from fish or fish-oil supplements, but not alfa-linolenic acid, benefit cardiovascular disease outcomes in primary- and secondary-prevention studies: a systematic review. *Am. J. Clin. Nutr.* **2006**, *84*, 5–17.

Weber, P.; D. Raederstorff. Triglyceride-lowering effect of omega-3 LC-polyunsaturated fatty acids—a review. *Nutr. Metab. Cardiovasc. Dis.* **2000**, *10,* 28–37.

Weiland, S.K.; E. von Mutius; A. Hüsing; M.I. Asher. Intake of trans fatty acids and prevalence of childhood asthma and allergies in Europe. ISAAC Steering Committee. *Lancet* **1999**, *353,* 2040–2041.

Williams, M.A.; I.B. King; T.K. Sorensen; R.W. Zingheim; B.L. Troyer; A.M. Zebelman; D.A. Luthy. Risk of preeclampsia in relation to elaidic acid (trans fatty acid) in maternal erythrocytes. *Gynecol. Obstet. Invest.* **1998**, *46,* 84–87.

Xiao, Y.F.; D.C. Sigg; A. Leaf. The antiarrhythmic effect of n-3 polyunsaturated fatty acids: modulation of cardiac ion channels as a potential mechanism. *J. Membr. Biol.* **2005**, *206,* 141–154.

Zilversmit, D.B. Atherogenesis: a postprandial phenomenon. *Circulation.* **1979**, *60*, 473–485

27

# Polyunsaturated Fatty Acids: Effects on Steroid-hormone Biosynthesis

**D.R.E. Abayasekara, L.M. Barton, and D.C. Wathes**
*Department of Veterinary Basic Sciences, Royal Veterinary College, Hawkshead Lane, North Mymms, Herts AL9 7TA, United Kingdom*

## Introduction

This chapter focuses on how polyunsaturated fatty acids (PUFAs) and their metabolites impact steroid-hormone synthesis. As such, it is not a comprehensive guide to fatty acids and their eicosanoid metabolites and includes only a brief overview of fatty acids and their eicosanoid metabolites. Fatty acids are carboxylic acids with long-chain hydrocarbon side groups, usually containing an even number of carbon atoms, and are described as "saturated," "monounsaturated," or "polyunsaturated" (Fig. 27.1). One can subdivide unsaturated fatty acids into monounsaturated fatty acids and PUFAs. Then one can further classify unsaturated fatty acids on the basis of their chemical structures according to the position of the first double bond in the structure, commencing from the methyl end of the molecule. In effect, three groups of PUFAs exist: omega-3 (n-3), omega-6 (n-6), and omega-9 (n-9), where the first double bond is located 3 carbons, 6 carbons, or 9 carbons, respectively, from the methyl end of the molecule (Fig. 27.1). When more than one double bond is present within the molecule, it is referred to as "polyunsaturated."

## Steroid Hormones and their Biosynthesis

Steroid hormones are lipid molecules whose synthesis is generally considered to be restricted to the classical steroidogenic tissues, namely ovary, testis, adrenal cortex, and placenta. The array of steroids generated by the main steroidogenic tissues exert a multiplicity of functions, ranging from regulating electrolyte balance (aldosterone), to maintaining pregnancy (progesterone), and through to inducing the formation and maintenance of male internal and external genitalia (testosterone). The plethora of actions exerted by the steroids amply illustrates the importance of this group of lipid molecules. Predictably, aspects of steroid-hormone biosynthesis are tissue-specific.

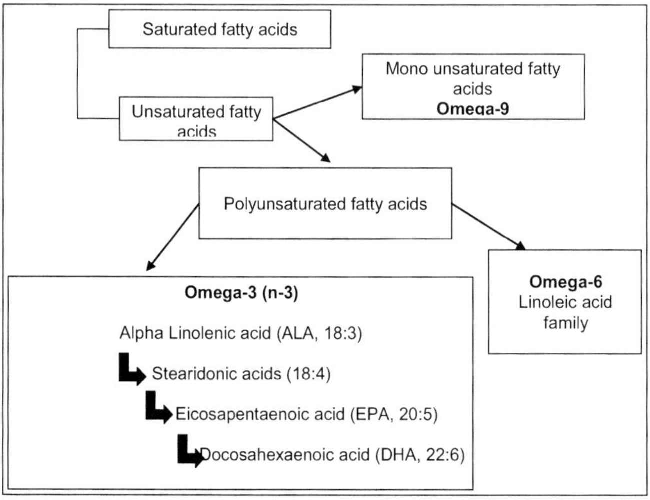


**Fig. 27.1.** Main fatty acid families. The main families of fatty acids are listed, and the omega-3 fatty acids are listed further (adapted from Bourre, 2005).

However, many elements, including the organization of the biosynthetic pathways, and the control mechanisms that regulate the activity of the various enzymes involved in steroid biosynthesis are common to all steroidogenic tissues.

In this chapter, we outline the general principles of steroid-hormone formation, before considering detailed aspects of how PUFAs and their eicosanoid metabolites impact steroid-hormone biosynthesis in the various steroidogenic tissues. The chapter opens with a consideration of the general structures of steroid hormones since relatively minor differences in steroid structures have a profound impact on the biological actions of each steroid hormone.

All steroid hormones are synthesized from a common precursor, cholesterol, which contains 27 carbon atoms (Fig. 27.2). In steroid-producing tissues (gonads, placenta, adrenal cortex), cholesterol is transported into mitochondria, where it is converted to the first steroid, pregnenolone, through the action of the cytochrome P450 cholesterol side-chain cleavage enzyme (P450cscc), which resides on the inner mitochondrial membrane (Miller, 1988; Simpson & Boyd, 1967; Tuckey, 2005). Pregnenolone is then further converted to various steroid hormones in a tissue-specific manner via pathways involving a whole array of enzymes (Fig. 27.3).

Steroid hormones are classified into five families depending on the number of carbon (C) atoms and the identity of chemical groups present at key carbon residues. All steroid hormones with 21 carbon atoms are collectively termed "pregnenes." This category of steroid hormones is subdivided into three steroid families: the progestins (e.g., progesterone), glucocorticoids (e.g., cortisol), and mineralocorticoids (e.g., aldosterone). While the progestins are secreted predominantly from the ovary, the

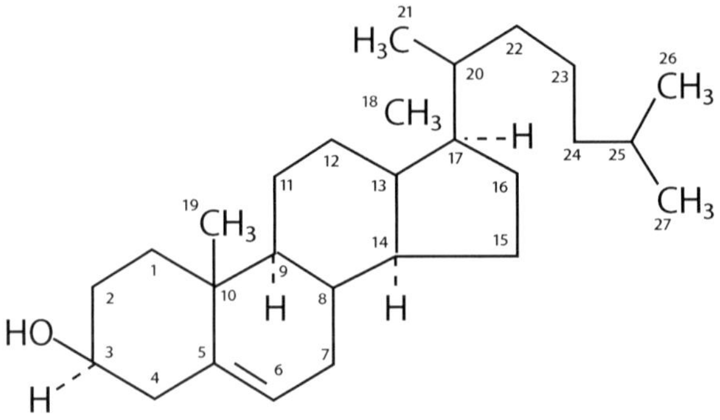


Fig. 27.2. The molecular structure of cholesterol.

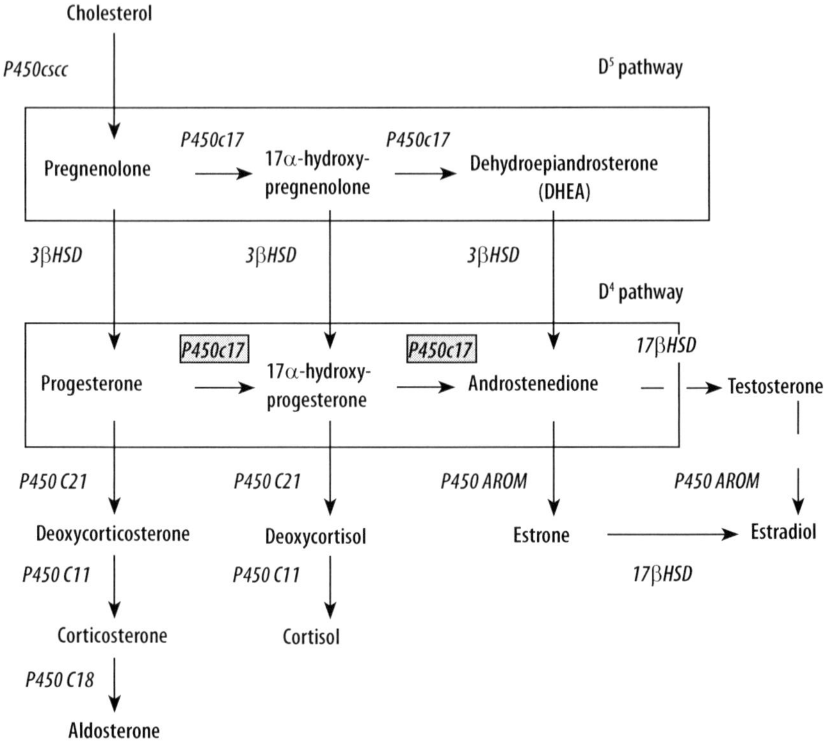


Fig. 27.3. Steroid biosynthetic pathway.

glucocorticoids and mineralocorticoids are collectively termed "corticosteroids," and are secreted mainly by the adrenal cortex. The major structural difference between the three pregnene families is that while progestins possess a methyl group ($CH_3$) at position C21, both glucocorticoids and mineralocorticoids possess a hydroxyl group ($CH_2OH$) at the same position.

The C21 progestins are metabolized to generate C19 steroids: the androgens dehydroepiandrosterone (DHEA), androstenedione ($A_4$), and testosterone. The site(s) of synthesis of androgens vary considerably, with testosterone being synthesized mainly by the Leydig cells of the testes, while DHEA and $A_4$ (also termed "adrenal androgens") are formed principally by the zona reticularis cells of the adrenal cortex (Vinson et al., 1992). The fifth and final family of steroids is the estrogens (e.g., estradiol-17ß, estrone, and estriol), which contain 18 carbon atoms and are generated from androgens primarily within the ovary of the nonpregnant female.

## *Substrate for Steroid-hormone Biosynthesis—Cholesterol Sources and Utilization*

Cholesterol (Fig. 27.2) is a sterol that can exist as a free sterol or is esterified with a long-chain fatty acid. It is an important molecule that regulates the fluidity of mammalian plasma membranes; it can constitute up to 25% of some membrane lipids, and, as already stated, is the precursor for steroid-hormone synthesis (as well as bile-acid synthesis).

The level of "free cholesterol" within a cell is highly regulated within narrow limits through a balance of influx, synthesis, catabolism, and efflux because excess is toxic to most cells (Azhar et al., 2003). The cholesterol utilized for steroidogenesis is obtained from three main sources: (i) de novo synthesis, (ii) cholesterol esters, and (iii) circulating lipoproteins (Fig. 27.4) (Andersen & Dietschy, 1978; Azhar & Reaven, 2002; Brown et al., 1979; Flint et al., 1973; Gwynne & Strauss, 1982). Cholesterol can be synthesized de novo from acetate as outlined in Fig. 27.5. One can divide the biosynthesis of cholesterol into five stages. Stage 1 involves the formation of mevalonate, a compound containing 6 carbon atoms. The initial step in Stage 1 is the conversion of acetyl-coenzyme A (CoA) to 3-hydroxy-3-methylglutaryl-CoA (HMG-CoA) catalyzed by HMG-CoA synthase. The acetyl-CoA utilized for cholesterol biosynthesis is derived from an oxidation reaction (i.e., fatty acid or pyruvate) in the mitochondria, which is transported to the cytoplasm. The HMG-CoA intermediate is then reduced to mevalonate, a process catalyzed by the enzyme HMG-CoA reductase, an integral membrane protein of the endoplasmic reticulum (ER). The synthesis of mevalonate is the committed step in the formation of cholesterol. In Stage 2, isoprenoid units are formed from mevalonate through the loss of $CO_2$. The condensation of six isoprenoid units to form squalene constitutes Stage 3, while the formation of lanosterol through the cyclization of squalene is Stage 4. Stage 5, the final stage, is a multistep process involving the removal of three methyl groups from lanosterol, the reduction of one double bond, and the migration of the other, all of which leads to the

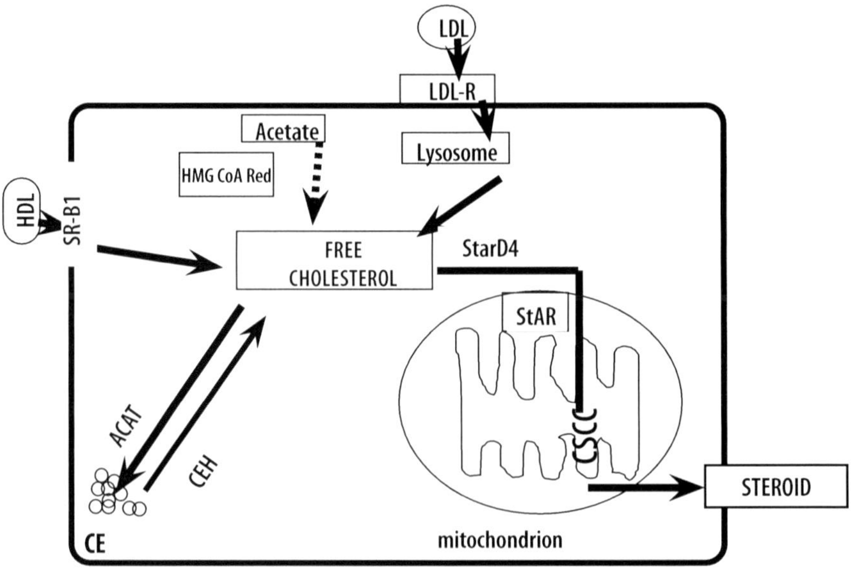


Fig. 27.4. Cholesterol utilization—pathways by which cholesterol can be acquired, for use in steroid biosynthesis. LDL (low-density lipoprotein), LDL-R (low- density lipoprotein receptor), HDL (high-density lipoprotein), SR-B1 (scavenger receptor, class B type I), CSCC (cytochrome P450-dependent cholesterol side-chain cleavage), HMG-CoA red (3-hydroxy-3-methylglutaryl coenzyme A reductase), ACAT (acyl Co-A:cholesterol acyl transferase), CEH (cholesterol-ester hydrolase).

formation of cholesterol. However, this method of generating cholesterol contributes negligibly to the "cholesterol pool" that is utilized in steroid-hormone biosynthesis in most steroidogenic tissues in the normal physiological state (Christenson & Devoto, 2003). However, its contribution becomes more significant when other sources of cholesterol are compromised (Brown et al., 1979). In contrast, esterified cholesterol found in lipid droplets (a characteristic of many steroidogenic cells) acts as a store of cholesterol substrate to enable the cells to mount a rapid steroidogenic response to acute trophic hormone stimulation (Azhar & Reaven, 2002). Free cholesterol that is not utilized to synthesize steroids is rapidly esterified into lipid droplets through a process catalyzed by cholesterol-ester synthetase (acyl CoA:cholesteroacyl transferase: ACAT) (Azhar et al., 2003). When required, cholesterol-ester hydrolase, a hormone-sensitive lipase, can convert these stored cholesterol esters back to free cholesterol (Azhar et al., 2003; Kraemer, 2007). Apart from cholesterol esters stored within lipid droplets, circulating lipoproteins also make an important contribution to the intracellular free-cholesterol pool. The type of lipoprotein that supplies cholesterol from the circulation to the intracellular cholesterol pool appears to depend on both the tissue and the species (Gwynne & Strauss, 1982). Receptor-mediated endocytosis can internalize cholesterol-rich low-density lipoproteins (LDL). The lipoprotein

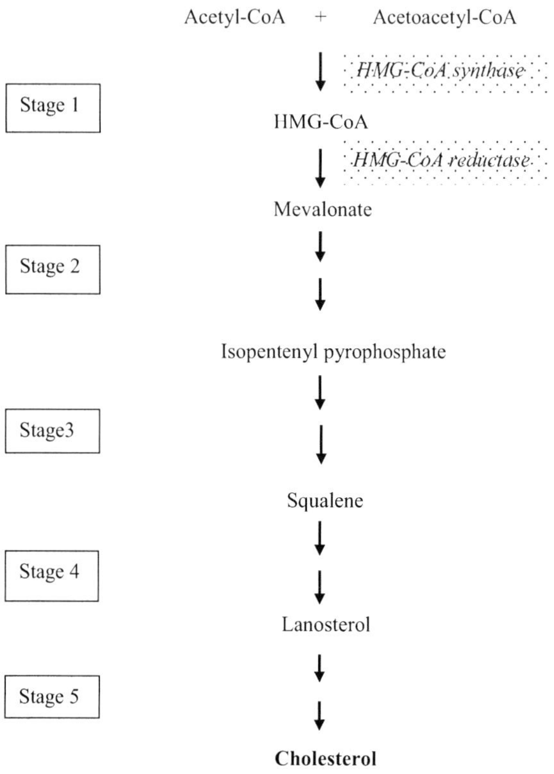


**Fig. 27.5.** Outline of cholesterol biosynthetic pathway.

binds to the LDL receptor (LDL-R), and the LDL-R complex is internalized and fuses with the lysosome. The LDL dissociates from the receptor, and is broken down by lysosomal enzymes, releasing free cholesterol, allowing the receptor to be recycled back to the cell surface or degraded (Kraemer, 2007). This free cholesterol generated from the breakdown of lipoproteins can be used as the substrate for steroid-hormone synthesis, or if not required immediately, can be stored in intracellular lipid droplets, primarily as cholesterol esters (Kraemer, 2007). Cholesterol can also be derived from high-density lipoproteins (HDLs). HDL-sterol uptake is mediated by the scavenger receptor BI (SR-BI): this receptor facilitates the "selective" uptake of cholesterol esters from HDL (Azhar et al., 2003; Kraemer, 2007). Cholesterol-ester hydrolase (CEH) can convert the released cholesterol ester to free cholesterol.

While crucial for steroidogenesis, the availability of the cholesterol precursor is only part of the story in synthesizing steroids. The cholesterol that is to be utilized for hormone production needs to be accessible to enzymes that will, in turn, convert it to steroid hormones. Having a large amount of substrate would be pointless unless relevant enzymes could act upon it. Therefore, to be converted to pregnenolone (the first steroid in the biosynthetic pathway), the cholesterol must move to the mitochondria [a process historically suggested to involve cytoskeletal elements (Hall & Almahbobi, 1997), but more recently thought to require StarD4 (StarD4: steroidogenic acute regulatory protein (StAR) related proteins that play a role in intracellular cholesterol; Miller, 2007c; Soccio & Breslow, 2003)], and then traverse the outer mitochondrial membrane to gain access to the enzyme cytochrome P450cscc, which resides on the inner membrane. The transport of cholesterol across the mitochondrial membrane, which is considered the rate-limiting step in steroid biosynthesis, is mediated by a protein named "StAR" (Clark et al., 1994; Stocco & Clark, 1996). Cholesterol is then converted to pregnenolone by the cholesterol side-chain cleavage reaction, which is the first enzymatic step in the production of steroid hormones (Simpson & Boyd, 1967).

### *Steroidogenic Acute Regulatory Protein (StAR)*

Growing evidence suggests that the rate-limiting step in steroidogenesis is the transport of cholesterol from the relatively cholesterol-rich outer mitochondrial membrane to the cholesterol-poor inner membrane, where the P450cscc enzyme is located (Christenson & Devoto, 2003; Simpson & Boyd, 1967). This step depends on the expression of StAR (Jones et al., 2000; Petrescu et al., 2001; Stocco & Clark, 1997). The importance of StAR for steroidogenesis was conclusively demonstrated through the study of individuals who suffer from a potentially lethal condition called congenital lipoid adrenal hyperplasia (CAH), which is a rare, autosomal recessive disease that results from the almost complete inability to synthesize steroids (Stocco, 2002). The observation of large adrenals containing high levels of cholesterol in individuals with CAH initially led to the mistaken conclusion that this disease was due to a deficiency in P450cscc. However, since both the gene and protein for P450cscc were normal (Lin et al., 1991; Sakai et al., 1994), clearly, the problem was at the level of cholesterol transport (i.e., StAR rather than cholesterol metabolism). This was evident when StAR cDNA of affected patients shown to contain nonsense mutations, and expression studies of these mutant StAR cDNAs in COS-1 cells led to a significantly lower level of steroid synthesis (Stocco & Clark, 1996). Complementary in vitro studies (including a demonstration of the sensitivity of StAR-protein expression and steroidogenesis to the protein-synthesis inhibitor cycloheximide, and the temporal association between the appearance of StAR and steroid output-reviewed in Stocco & Clark, 1996) helped to clinch the case for StAR as the protein that mediates the transfer of cholesterol to the inner mitochondrial membrane.

However, much debate persists regarding the manner by which StAR exerts this action. Four distinct models can explain the mode of action of StAR (Miller, 2007a): (i) Contact sites: A model was proposed suggesting that StAR forms contact sites between the outer and inner mitochondrial membranes. In this model, StAR could be synthesized in the cytoplasm as a short-lived 37 kDa form, which loses its

N-terminal leader sequence upon import into the mitochondria to yield a 30kDa intramitochondrial form to yield a mature 30 kDa intramitochondrial form. The 37 kDa form became the contact sites which served as a channel through which cholesterol could move down a concentration gradient to the inner mitochondrial membrane (Stocco, 2000). A deletion in the N-terminal of the StAR protein by as many as 62 amino acids did not render the protein inactive. The deletion of 62 amino-terminal amino acids resulted in a cytoplasmic form of StAR (N-62 StAR). This form retained activity and appeared to interact with the outer mitochondrial membrane, although without being imported, and this form of StAR was able to support full steroidogenesis (Stocco, 2000). Deletions to the C-terminal of the protein, however, resulted in the complete loss of steroid synthesis with the removal of as little as 28 amino acids in the C-terminal of the protein rendering it inactive, suggesting that this region of the protein harbors domains crucial for biological activity (Bose et al., 1999; Stocco, 2000). (ii) Desorption: A second model of StAR action was proposed, suggesting that StAR can act as a sterol-transfer protein, enhancing sterol desorption from one membrane to another (Stocco, 2000). In this model, StAR is directed to the mitochondria via its N-terminal import sequence, and then via C-terminal sequences it somehow produces alterations in the outer mitochondrial membrane to facilitate the "desorption" of cholesterol in the form of microdroplets of cholesterol, from the outer to the inner mitochondrial membrane (Christenson & Strauss III, 2001). (iii) Intramembranous space (ims) shuttle: Another hypothesis emerged as a result of the characterization of MLN64 (metastatic lymph node clone 64), a protein related to StAR, which has a 35% identity with the StAR lipid-transfer (START) domain (Petrescu et al., 2001). MLN64 played a StAR-like role in the promotion of steroidogenesis in the placenta and the brain (Bose et al., 1999). X-ray crystallography and molecular modelling revealed that the MLN64 START domain contained a hydrophobic tunnel. This was able to accommodate a cholesterol molecule (Petrescu et al., 2001); the geometry and dimensions of the pocket, approximately 26Å deep and 10Å wide at its deepest diameter, was appropriate for the binding of a single molecule of cholesterol (Miller, 2007c). These findings led to the proposal of the intermembrane shuttle hypothesis, whereby StAR protein binds and solubilizes one cholesterol molecule at a time, and then shuttles it across the intermembrane space of the mitochondria. However, this model is not able to account for the rapid increases in steroid seen in response to tropic hormone stimulation. Evidence suggests that the StAR protein becomes inactivated very rapidly; therefore, if StAR is only capable of transferring one cholesterol molecule at a time, then it could not possibly generate large quantities of steroid. Another flaw with this hypothesis is that the sterol-binding pocket may very well comfortably fit one molecule of cholesterol; however, apparent access channels to the pocket are too small to allow a cholesterol molecule to enter or exit (Miller, 2007c). This led to the proposition that StAR may act to bind cholesterol as a result of a conformational change which then led directly to the molten-globule hypothesis (iv) Molten globule: The idea that StAR undergoes a transition to a molten globule, induced by acid pH was proposed (Bose et al., 1999; Miller, 2007a). A molten globule is an intermediate form of a protein, which has a high degree of secondary structure, but lacks defined tertiary structure (Bose et al., 1999). Acidic conditions exist at the outer mitochondrial membrane as a result of the expulsion of protons from the mitochondrial matrix (an intact mitochondrial proton pump was required for StAR activity–King et al., 1999) and the presence of negatively charged phospholipid head groups in the outer mitochondrial membrane (Bose et al., 1999). This acidic environment could therefore result in the conformational change in StAR to a molten globule, and thus allow cholesterol to access the sterol-binding pocket. Suggesting that the mechanism of StAR action could be a combination of the molten-globule hypothesis and the intermembrane-shuttle hypothesis.

The translocator protein (18 kDa: TSPO), previously known as the peripheral benzodiazepine receptor (PBR), has also been suggested to play a role in the mitochondrial import of cholesterol (Hauet et al, 2005, Papadopoulos, 1993). StAR was originally envisaged to provide cholesterol to TSPO, which in turn transported it to P450cscc on the inner mitochondrial membrane. However, the fact that bacterially expressed StAR on its own supported steroid synthesis by isolated mitochondria argues against a simple linear-delivery model. Instead, a complex consisting of StAR, TSPO, PAP7 (PBR-associated protein), and PKAR1α (the regulatory subunit R1α of cyclic AMP-dependent-protein kinase A) was localized to the outer mitochondrial membrane (Liu et al., 2006). In this complex, PAP7 acts to bring together PKAR1α and TSPO, which in turn attracts StAR. The four-component complex then acts to transport cholesterol via a mechanism that remains to be elucidated. Support for this model comes from the finding that the disruption of the interaction between either PKAR1α and PAP7 or PAP7 and TSPO leads to the loss of a gonadotrophin-stimulated steroid output (Liu et al., 2006). From the aforementioned information, clearly, although numerous models have been proposed for the mode of action of StAR, the precise mechanism still remains elusive.

On the other hand, more is known regarding the nature of StAR regulation. StAR expression is governed by a whole array of transcription factors that include steroidogenic factor 1 (SF-1), a nuclear receptor that plays a pivotal role in the regulation of reproductive endocrine function at numerous levels (Manna et al., 2003). The importance of SF-1 became apparent when it was revealed that SF-1 null mice exhibited a complete absence of adrenal glands and gonads (Parker, 1998). The StAR promoter (for a number of different species) contained several SF-1 binding motifs (Manna et al., 2003). Although SF-1 has an important role in the regulation of StAR, it is by no means the only transcription factor involved in StAR regulation. Recent evidence suggests that: (i) sterol regulatory element-binding proteins (SREBPs) (shown in a later section) can regulate StAR expression, (ii) the 5' flanking region of the StAR gene contains recognition motifs for SREBP, and (iii)mutations in the SREBP-binding sites decrease StAR-reporter activity (Manna et al., 2003). Apart from the possible role(s) in StAR synthesis, SREBPs could also influence steroid synthesis through their actions on cholesterol and fatty acid synthesis (Horton et al., 2002). More recently, a family of nuclear receptors Liver X receptors (LXRs) (see later section for details) were shown to be involved in the regulation of StAR (Cummins et al., 2006; Nilsson et al., 2007; Volle & Lobaccaro, 2007). The mouse StAR promoter contains an LXR response element-like sequence, including a hexanucleotide repeat separated by four base pairs (Cummins et al., 2006). Since SREBPS are at the fulcrum of factors that govern the levels of intracellular cholesterol (Horton et al., 2002), and since LXRs affect SREBPs, it is possible that they provide the link between cholesterol metabolism/mobilization and fatty acid synthesis within the steroidogenic cells.

### Steroidogenic Enzymes

The pathway of steroid-hormone biosynthesis (illustrated in Fig. 27.3) at first sight appears to be somewhat complex. However, the fact that the eight major steroidogenic enzymes that are required to convert cholesterol to estradiol-17β can be grouped into just two enzyme families (the cytochrome P450 enzymes and the hydroxysteroid dehydrogenases) makes the whole pathway easier to decipher.

The steroidogenic cytochrome P450 enzymes are members of a far larger family of cytochrome P450 oxidases. Each of which is encoded by a *CYP* gene and catalyzes the introduction of atomic oxygen into a hydrocarbon (C-H) bond to generate a hydroxyl group (C-O-H) using NADPH as a donor of electrons (Miller, 1988; Nebert & Russell, 2002). The nonsteroidogenic cytochrome P450 enzymes include those hepatic enzymes responsible for the inactivation and clearance of a wide range of drugs. Each of the cytochrome P450 enzymes within the steroidogenic pathway catalyzes the hydroxylation of a steroid substrate at a specific carbon position. For example, P450cscc acts in the inner membrane of the mitochondria to catalyze the rate-limiting reaction in steroid synthesis: the conversion of cholesterol to pregnenolone. P450cscc hydroxylates two adjacent carbons (C20 and C22) in the side-chain of cholesterol, facilitating the cleavage of this side-chain between C20 and C22 to leave the C21 steroid, pregnenolone (Miller, 1988).

The second family of steroidogenic enzymes is comprised of hydroxysteroid dehydrogenase (HSD) enzymes encoded by *HSD* genes (reviewed in Miller, 1988; Penning, 1997). Each member of this family catalyzes the interconversion of a hydroxyl group with a ketone to influence the affinity of the steroid for intracellular receptors (Penning, 1997). Each HSD enzyme is specified by a number and a Greek letter: the number denotes the position of the carbon atom at which the enzyme acts, and the Greek letter indicates the orientation of the OH group relative to the steroid molecule (where α and ß indicate bonds below and above the plane of the molecule, respectively).

Two significant HSD enzymes are involved in steroid-hormone production: (i) 3ßHSD converts the 3ß-hydroxyl group to a ketone (Miller, 1988; Penning,

1997). Hence, 3ßHSD converts pregnenolone to progesterone, and DHEA to androstenedione. (ii) In contrast, 17ßHSD acts at position C17 where it catalyzes not oxidation, but reduction, converting a ketone at C17 to a ß-oriented hydroxyl group (Miller, 1988; Penning, 1997).

# Polyunsaturated Fatty Acids and their Actions

## Polyunsaturated Fatty Acids (PUFAs)

Of all fats found in food, the n-3 PUFA, α-linolenic acid (ALA; *cis*-9,12,15-octadecatrienoic acid), and the n-6 PUFA, linoleic acid (LA; *cis*-9,12-octadecadienoic acid), cannot be synthesized within mammals, and therefore need to be provided in the diet because they are absolutely necessary for numerous processes, including the maintenance of growth, reproduction, vision, and brain development (Abayasekara & Wathes, 1999; Burr & Burr, 1930; Schimtz & Ecker, 2008; Smith, 2008; Wathes et al., 2007). As such, ALA and LA are designated as essential fatty acids (EFAs) that are converted in the liver to long-chain PUFAs (LC-PUFAs), which have a higher number of carbon atoms and double bonds. Animals can synthesize n-9 but not n-6 or n-3 fatty acids since they do not have the appropriate desaturase enzymes to insert the n-6 or n-3 double bonds. The metabolic pathways of all families of PUFAs share common desaturation and elongation enzyme systems. The most important dietary n-3 PUFA and the main precursor for longer chain PUFAs of the n-3 family is ALA, and this is found mainly in the chloroplasts of green vegetables and grass. The n-3 PUFAs, eicosapentaenoic acid (EPA) (*cis*-5,8,11,14,17-EPA) and docosahexaenoic acid (DHA) (*cis*-4,7,10,13,16,19-DHA) may be supplied directly from fish oils, thereby bypassing the need for desaturation and elongation (Gurr et al., 2002). The most important dietary n-6 PUFA and the main precursor for LC-PUFAs of the n-6 family is LA, which is abundant in vegetable oils such as corn, safflower, sunflower, and rapeseed oils (Gurr et al., 2002). The saturated fatty acid content of the diet was implicated as a major factor in cardiovascular disease. As a result, Western populations are tending to reduce saturated- fatty acid intake in favor of unsaturated fatty acids. However, while diets high in PUFAs are supposed to be healthier, most people consume quantities of n-6 PUFAs far in excess of those needed for normal physiological functioning. Supposedly, man evolved on a diet with an n-6:n-3 PUFA ratio of 1:1, but modern dietary trends have resulted in a massive increase in the ratio of n-6:n-3 PUFAs in Western diets where it ranges from 10:1 to 25:1 at present (Simopoulous, 2008).

### *Role of PUFAs in Prostaglandin Synthesis*

At a cellular level, PUFAs can act as precursors for eicosanoid synthesis including prostaglandins (PGs) (Schmitz & Ecker, 2008; Wathes et al., 2007). Eicosanoids derived from 20-carbon PUFAs are the direct precursors of a large group of physiologically active compounds. These compounds are unique: they are only detectable at very low levels in tissues, having a rapid metabolic turnover, while being capable of exerting very potent biological effects. The eicosanoids generally act as local hormones via specific receptors in the cell membranes. Eicosanoids are so named because they are synthesized from C20 eicosanoic acids derived from EFAs LA and ALA or directly from arachidonic acid (AA; all-*cis* 5,8,11,15-eicosatetraenoic acid) and EPA. While these PUFA precursors can give rise to a range of eicosanoids (e.g., PGs, thromboxanes, leukotrienes, and lipoxins) (Needleman et al., 1986; Schmitz & Ecker, 2008), in the context of this review, the products of the cyclooxygenase (COX) enzymes, PGs, are the eicosanoids of principal interest and are shown in Fig. 27.6. The precise biochemical structure of a PG that is synthesized is determined by the structure of its PUFA precursors, which, in turn, determines its relative biological potency (Smith, 2005).

The synthesis of PGs in tissues throughout the body is very tightly regulated. The initial step in PG synthesis is the generation of the PUFA substrate, in the case of 2-series PGs, AA within the cell. In most cells, AA is present in various phospholipids in an esterified form. AA can be liberated from the phospholipids directly by the

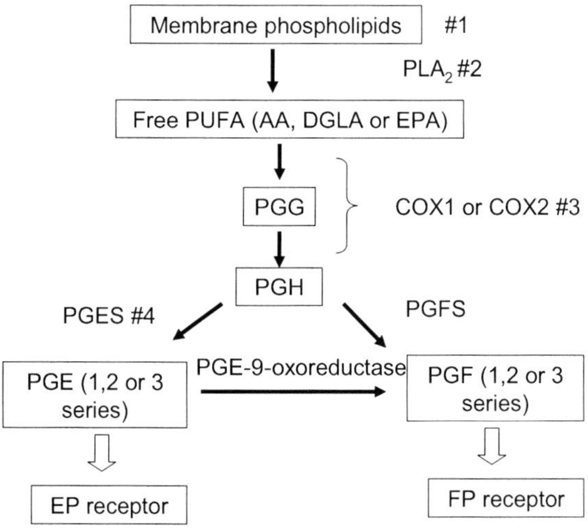


**Fig. 27.6.** Synthesis and action of prostaglandins (PGs). Points at which PG synthesis can be regulated by PUFAs are denoted by #.
**#1 = PUFA composition in membrane phospholipids**
**#2 = release of PUFA from phospholipids by phospholipase A2**
**#3 = metabolism of PUFA by cyclooxygenases 1 and 2 to generate PGH**
**#4 = metabolism of PGH to PGE via membrane prostaglandin E synthase 1 (mPGES-1).**
**(Wathes et al., 2007)**

action of phospholipase $A_2$ (Diaz & Arm, 2003) or indirectly via the coordinate actions of phospholipase C (Tang et al., 2006).

The free AA generated is metabolized to the intermediate prostaglandin $H_2$ ($PGH_2$) by COX, also known as prostaglandin H synthase (PGHS) enzymes, referred to hereafter as COX. Since the early 1990s, two isoforms of COX, COX-1 and COX-2, have been described in the literature. Although COX-1 and COX-2 fulfill the same function, they are encoded by different genes, regulated differentially, expressed in a cell-specific manner, and found in different subcellular compartments (Smith & Lagenbach, 2001). These enzymes provide PGH to PGE and PGF synthases in a spatially segregated manner (Ueno et al., 2005). The preferred substrate for COX catalysis by either COX-1 or COX-2 is AA (Smith, 2005; Wada et al., 2007). Although EPA is also a substrate for COX-1 and COX-2, its metabolism via COX-1 is poor which means that its ability to generate 3-series PGs is also poor (Smith, 2005). In addition, EPA is also an inhibitor of COX-1 activity. Taken together, this means that EPA not only inhibits 2-series PG generation, but does not, as expected induce a concomitant increase in 3-series PG generation via COX-1. These findings clearly illustrate that the type of PG generated by COX enzymes, when presented with a mixture of n-3 and n-6 PUFAs, is very difficult to predict.

## PUFAs and Gene Transcription

Growing evidence shows that PUFAs, in addition to their role as structural components of membrane lipids and precursors of eicosanoids, can also act as second messengers and regulators of signal-transduction molecules (Hwang & Rhee, 1999). In addition, PUFAs also have the ability to regulate gene expression (Jump et al., 1996, 2005). Fatty acids can have pronounced effects on gene expression, leading to changes in metabolism, cell growth, and differentiation (Jump et al., 1996). Therefore, fatty acids are no longer merely regarded as energy-providing molecules, but can, in fact, be thought of as metabolic regulators (Benatti et al., 2004). Such gene regulation is achieved in two general ways. The fatty acid may regulate transcription-factor function through binding directly to the transcription factor. In this instance, the fatty acids act as ligands for nuclear receptors such as peroxisome proliferator-activated receptor alpha (PPARα), LXRα, and retinoid X receptor α (RXRα) (Jump et al., 2005). The other mechanism is through affecting the nuclear expression of transcription factors such as SREBPs (Jump et al., 2005). How fatty acids induce expression remains a mystery, but it is thought not to involve the binding of the fatty acid to the transcription factor.

### *Liver X Receptor (LXR)*

LXRs are cholesterol-sensing transcription factors that play central roles in regulating lipid metabolism (Schultz et al., 2000; Zelcer & Tontonoz, 2006). Two isoforms exist: LXRα and LXRβ; both are ligand-activated receptors. The expression of the two isoforms differs in that LXRα is principally expressed in the liver, kidney, intestine, adipose tissue, and the adrenal gland: that is to say, it is predominantly expressed in tissues that play an important role in lipid metabolism (Ulven et al., 2005), whereas the expression of LXRβ is ubiquitous.

In the liver, fatty acids induce the expression of LXRα, where this appears to be a direct result of the induction of LXRα gene expression, mediated through a fatty acid response element located in the proximal LXRα 5'-flanking region (Tobin et al., 2000). Contrasting results, however, were observed where LXRα activity is suppressed by PUFAs through inhibiting the formation of the LXR/RXR heterodimers (Kersten, 2002). Furthermore, PUFAs compete with oxysterols for binding to LXR, which suggests that the PUFAs could also behave as LXR antagonists (Kersten, 2002).

LXRs are also regulated by oxysterols such as 22 (*S*)-hydroxycholesterol and 25-epoxycholesterol that are produced through the actions of P450 enzymes in various metabolic pathways (Lehmann et al., 1997). They are known to reflect cellular cholesterol content (Jankowski et al., 1999), and are believed to be important in many different processes such as cholesterol regulation, synthesis of steroid hormones and bile acids, and apoptosis (Alberti et al., 2000). LXRs regulate cyp7a1, the rate-limiting enzyme, in bile-acid synthesis (Peet et al., 1998) and cholesterol efflux through affecting adenosine triphosphate (ATP)-binding cassette (ABC) genes such as ABCA1, ABCG1, and ABCG5 (Schultz et al., 2000; Ulven et al., 2005; Zelcer & Tontonoz, 2006). In addition, LXRs also regulate genes involved in fatty acid metabolism including SREBPs (Repa et al., 2000; Ulven et al., 2005). Changes in levels of cholesterol metabolites can be sensed by LXRα which in turn can modulate transcription i.e. LXR could operate as a cholesterol sensor (Tobin et al., 2000). That is, LXRs can respond to elevated sterol concentration by inducing the transactivation of genes governing transport, catabolism, and the elimination of cholesterol (Chawla et al., 2001). Moreover, the activation of LXRs with a synthetic ligand influenced the regulation of a number of steroidogenic genes: LXR activation results in an increased mRNA expression of StAR, P450cscc, and 3βHSD (Cummins et al., 2006). Paradoxically, $LXR\alpha\beta^{-/-}$ mice exhibit increased StAR expression and corticosterone output from adrenals under basal conditions (Cummins et al., 2006). However, steroid output from the testis (testosterone) is decreased in $LXR\alpha\beta^{-/-}$ mice (Volle et al., 2007). The striking difference in steroid output from the two organs highlights the fact that although the basic mechanisms governing steroid regulation are similar in steroidogenic tissues, the presence/absence of different co-activators/co-repressors in each particular milieu could lead to different outcomes.

The majority of LXR proteins are localized in the nucleus, and to be functional, they require heterodimerization with a RXR (Peet et al., 1998). The LXR/RXR heterodimer binds to DNA target sequences upstream of target genes, at specific sites on the DNA known as LXREs (Ulven et al., 2005).

As stated previously, one target gene of LXR is SREBP. Perhaps, many of the effects of PUFAs are mediated through the inhibition of LXR via activated SREBP. Several studies report the PUFA-induced suppression of SREBP through inhibiting LXR/RXR-binding to the LXRE in the promoter region (Yoshikawa et al., 2002).

SREBP is therefore another important protein to consider in terms of PUFAs and their influence on steroid synthesis via the modulation of cholesterol-metabolizing machinery.

***Sterol Regulatory Element-binding Proteins (SREBPs)***

SREBPs are unique transcription factors that have the ability to regulate cholesterol homeostasis in mammals. To date, three isoforms of SREBP have been identified so far: SREBP-1a, SREBP-1c, and SREBP-2, with SREBP-1a and SREBP-1c being important for lipid-synthesis genes, whereas SREBP-2 is mainly important for genes involved in cholesterol homeostasis (Osborne, 2000). They belong to the basic helix-loop-helix-leucine zipper (bHLH-Zip) family of transcription factors (Horton et al., 2002). They are synthesized as inactive precursors, with a molecular weight of 125 kDa. To regulate gene transcription, they must undergo proteolytic cleavage to a mature 68 kDa form, where they are capable of entering the nucleus and controlling the regulation of numerous genes involved in cholesterol biosynthesis, uptake, and metabolism (Christenson et al., 2001; Horton et al., 2002). Such genes include HMG-CoA synthase and reductase, squalene synthase, LDL-receptor, and cholesteryl-ester transfer protein (CETP) (Christenson et al., 2001). In addition, SREBP may also be involved in the regulation of StAR, as the StAR promoter contains potential SREBP binding sites. This could provide a link between cholesterol homeostasis (and metabolism) and steroidogenesis (Stocco, 2000).

The SREBP regulation of gene transcription involves the control of its nuclear abundance (nSREBP). This is regulated via two post-translational mechanisms: proteolytic processing (Horton et al., 2002) and proteasomal degradation (Sundqvist et al., 2005). The well-known PUFA-induced decrease in lipid synthesis may be a result of the suppression of SREBP-1 (Jump & Clarke, 1999), which is possibly due to the ability of PUFAs to suppress nSREBP1 but not nSREBP-2 (Xu et al., 1999). Of those fatty acids studied, DHA, the n-3 PUFA, is the most potent PUFA in suppressing SREBP-1, and is therefore the most likely regulator of the nuclear abundance of SREBP-1 in vivo (Jump et al., 2008). While the PUFA-induced inhibition of genes involved in lipid generation has a requirement for SREBP-1c, PUFA effects on a range of other genes are mediated through PPARs [e.g., stearoyl-CoA desaturase 1 (SCD1) (Miller & Ntambi, 1996) and COX-2 (Sheldrick et al., 2007)].

***Peroxisome Proliferator-activated Receptors (PPARs)***

PPARs are a subfamily of nuclear receptors that belong to the steroid receptor superfamily (Feige et al., 2006; Komar, 2005). In the early 1990s, PPARs were first identified as nuclear receptors that mediate the effects of synthetic compounds known as peroxisome proliferators due to their ability to induce peroxisomal proliferation in the liver of rodents (Feige et al., 2006).

The three known subtypes of PPAR [PPAR$\alpha$, PPAR$\beta$ (also called PPAR$\delta$), PPAR$\gamma$] are expressed in a tissue-specific manner and the pattern of expression of each contributes to its specific function (Wahli, 2002). PPARα is predominantly expressed in the liver and brown adipose tissue, with lower-level expression in the heart and kidneys (Wahli, 2002). PPARβ expression is much more ubiquitous, and is often expressed at a much higher level than the other two subtypes; however, much less is known about this particular PPAR, and its function remains elusive at present. PPARγ is expressed at its highest levels in adipocytes and macrophages, and is essential for the differentiation of both (Khan & Vanden Heuvel, 2003). Both PPARα and -γ play important roles in the storage and catabolism of fatty acids (Berger et al., 2002).

To bind DNA, PPARs must form a dimer with RXR. The PPAR/RXR complex regulates the expression of genes by binding to specific sites on the DNA, PPREs, located upstream of target genes (Khan & Vanden Heuvel, 2003). PPARs bind to a DR1 motif, which is a direct repeat of a hexanucleotide sequence AGGTCA, separated by one nucleotide (Berger et al., 2002).

Among the endogenous ligands for PPARs are long-chain unsaturated-, polyunsaturated-, and branched-chain fatty acids (Khan & Vanden Heuvel, 2003). PPARs are preferentially activated by 18C and 20C fatty acids, since those that are shorter or longer will not fit correctly into the binding pocket (Berger et al., 2002). These long-chain fatty acids preferentially activated PPARα although they are also capable of activating the other two forms. PGs also activated all PPAR family members, with 15-deoxy-$\Delta^{12,14}$-prostaglandin $J_2$ ($PGJ_2$) preferentially activating PPARγ (Komar, 2005).

PPARs are important mediators of steroidogenesis because they can induce the expression of a variety of genes whose encoded proteins are involved in the biosynthesis and metabolism of cholesterol and fatty acids (Lohrke et al., 1998). PPARs have the ability to regulate the expression of 3-HMG-CoA synthase, an enzyme involved in cholesterol synthesis (Fig. 27.5), which is also regulated by SREBP (Lohrke et al., 1998), and could therefore have the potential to modulate the availability of the cholesterol precursor for steroid-hormone synthesis. The activation of PPARγ in cultured ovarian cells leads to either an increase (human granulosa cells) or decrease (porcine theca and bovine luteal cells) in steroid synthesis (Banerjee & Komar, 2006; Komar, 2005). PPARα agonists convincingly inhibited testicular steroidogenesis, an effect ascribed to an inhibition of TSPO protein expression (Gazouli et al., 2003). Although pioglitazone, a PPARγ agonist, inhibited androgen secretion in human adrenal NCI-H295R cells, these effects were PPARγ-independent (Kempna et al., 2007). Hence, although the activation of PPAR can affect steroid synthesis, since these effects are clearly dependent on PPAR subtype, species, and cell-type, to make generalized statements regarding the role of PPARs in regulating steroid synthesis is difficult.

## PUFAs and Steroid-hormone Synthesis

### *Effect of PUFAs and their Metabolites*

As PUFAs have the capacity to affect cholesterol homeostasis and since cholesterol is the precursor for all steroid hormones, PUFAs should be able to affect steroid-hormone synthesis. As such, the n-6 PUFA AA and its COX, lipoxygenase (LOX) and epoxygenase metabolites (Abayasekara et al., 1993; Dix et al., 1984; Van Voorhis et al., 1993) modulated steroid synthesis. In fact, the ability of PUFAs and their metabolites to modulate steroid synthesis in adrenal and gonadal cells has been known for many years (testis: Abayasekara et al., 1990; ovary: Wang & Leung, 1989; adrenal: Wang et al., 2000a). In terms of ovarian steroid synthesis, $PGE_2$ stimulated progesterone secretion by cyclic corpora lutea, whereas in the corpora lutea of pregnancy, $PGE_1$ was more potent than $PGE_2$ in stimulating progesterone secretion (Weems et al., 1997). Cows fed a diet high in either n-3 PUFAs (ALA) or n-6 PUFAs (LA) had altered levels of ovarian steroids; those fed n-3 PUFAs had elevated levels of estradiol and lower progesterone levels (Robinson et al., 2002). This suggests that n-3 or n-6 PUFAs in vivo can affect ovarian steroidogenesis either directly or indirectly (via metabolites, e.g., PGs) (for review, see Mattos et al., 2000). The finding that n-3 PUFAs in vitro inhibit bovine luteal cell progesterone secretion (Hinckley et al., 1996) supports the notion that PUFAs and/or their metabolites affect steroid synthesis. The recent observations that inhibitors of phospholipase $A_2$, COX, and LOX activity inhibit gonadotrophin-stimulated progesterone secretion in rat corpora luteal cells tend to point to the involvement of PUFAs themselves (Kurusu et al., 2007).

More recently, the StAR protein, which plays a critical role in regulating steroid synthesis (see earlier section in this chapter), was affected by AA and its metabolites (Wang & Stocco, 1999). The inhibition of the endogenous release of AA inhibited dibutyryl cyclic AMP (dbcAMP)-induced steroid synthesis as well as StAR- promoter activity, StAR mRNA and StAR protein, whereas the addition of exogenous AA reversed all these effects (Wang et al., 2000b). Cyclic AMP increased the generation of the three cytochrome P450-dependent epoxygenase metabolites of AA, epoxyeicostrienoic acids (EET) (5,6-EET, 8,9- EET, and 11,12-EET) in MA10 cells (Wang et al., 2006). The addition of these EETs in the presence of dibutyryl cyclic AMP to MA10 cells increased StAR expression and steroid output (Wang et al., 2006). The enhancement in StAR expression and steroid output induced by EETs was abolished through the inhibition of protein kinase A (PKA) activity. The presence of active cyclic AMP-dependent PKA appears to be an absolute requirement for AA and its epoxygenase metabolites to exert their stimulatory actions on StAR expression and steroid output. This is supported by the finding that PUFAs (both n-3 and n-6 PUFAs, i.e., EPA and AA) affected ovarian-steroid synthesis at a site post-generation of cyclic AMP (Mercure & Van Der Kraak, 1995). In contrast, n-3 PUFAs were able to stimulate StAR expression and steroid output in Y1 mouse-tumor adrenocortical cells in the presence of basal levels of cyclic AMP (Barton et al., 2008).

The observation that a specific inhibition of COX-2 is associated with an increase in StAR expression and steroid output in MA-10 Leydig cells (Wang et al., 2003a) is consistent with the notion that a product of COX-2 action on AA is responsible for the tonic inhibition of StAR expression and steroid output. The inhibitory effects of COX-2 product(s) on StAR were possibly brought about by $PGF_{2\alpha}$ since this prostanoid inhibits StAR-protein expression (Fiedler et al., 1999) consistent with its well-established role in inhibiting luteal progesterone synthesis (Niswender, 2002). As the inhibition of thromboxane A synthase leads to the enhancement of StAR expression and steroid output (Wang et al., 2008), thromboxane A joins $PGF_{2\alpha}$ as another candidate eicosanoid to mediate the PUFA-induced inhibition of steroid output. As the increase in StAR expression was associated with decreased DAX-1 (a dosage-sensitive sex-reversal-adrenal hypoplasia gene on the X-chromosome gene 1) protein, a powerful repressor of StAR gene transcription, this provides another potential target for mediating the inhibitory effects of PUFAs on transcription within steroidogenic cells.

The action of two enzymes, acyl-CoA synthetase (ACS4) and mitochondrial acyl-CoA thioesterase (ARTISt or MTE1: Maloberti et al., 2007), can also regulate the level of free AA within steroidogenic cells. ACS4 converts AA to arachidonyl CoA (AA-CoA) which binds to acyl-CoA binding protein which in turn binds to TSPO in mitochondria. The adrenocorticotrophic hormone (ACTH) stimulates the expression of ACS4 (Cornejo Maciel et al., 2005), and the siRNA knockdown of ACS4 leads to abrogation of steroid synthesis (Maloberti et al., 2005). So ACS4, by providing AA-CoA which can interact with mitochondrial TSPO (which complexes with StAR, PAP7, and PKAR1α to transport cholesterol across the mitochondrial membrane; see earlier section), can promote steroid synthesis. ARTISt, on the other hand, is a mitochondrial enzyme that converts AA-CoA to free AA (Hunt & Alexson, 2002) which, in turn, stimulates StAR gene expression (Stocco et al., 2005). Therefore, not surprisingly, a decreased expression of ARTISt is also associated with decreased steroidogenesis (Maloberti et al., 2005). These two enzymes (ACS4 and ARTISt) join an ever-increasing band of molecules that have an impact on steroidogenesis through affecting PUFA levels in cells. PUFAs other than AA were also implicated in modulating steroid synthesis. LA stimulated basal-corticosterone synthesis (Sarel & Widmaier, 1995), whereas ACTH-stimulated steroid synthesis, and cyclic AMP generation was inhibited (Matthys & Widmaier, 1998). More recently, an oxidized metabolite of LA, 12,13-epoxy-9-keto-10(*trans*)-octadecenoic acid (EKODE) stimulated both basal and ACTH-stimulated corticosterone production by rat-adrenal cells (Bruder et al., 2003). In the same study, submaximal cyclic AMP-stimulated steroid synthesis was enhanced by EKODE, while maximal cAMP-induced corticosterone synthesis was inhibited by EKODE (Bruder at al., 2003). Levels of EKODE in obese individuals were found to be higher than in their lean counterparts, and these increased levels were correlated with an increase in the circulating levels of aldosterone and systolic blood pressure (Goodfriend et al., 2004). The increase in aldosterone output is mediated via an increase in intracellular calcium because EKODE was able to mobilize intracellular calcium in rat-adrenal glomerulosa cells (Payet et al., 2006). The n-3 PUFA ALA and the n-6 PUFA AA inhibited angiotensin II-induced aldosterone synthesis by bovine zona glomerulosa cells (Goodfriend et al., 1991). In addition to the effects of n-6 PUFAs and metabolites reviewed above, n-3 PUFAs also affected adrenal-steroid synthesis in both mammalian (Chin et al., 2006; Hinckley et al., 1996; Hodges et al., 2006) and nonmammalian species (Ganga et al., 2006). The effects of AA on steroid synthesis are not restricted to StAR—direct inhibitory effects of AA on 17β hydroxysteroid dehydrogenase activity in Leydig cells were also reported (Marinero et al., 1998). From the preceding, clearly, while PUFAs and their metabolites affect steroid synthesis in a variety of steroidogenic tissues, no simple unifying model can explain the mode of action.

## Conclusion

So, seemingly, much evidence supports the idea that PUFAs affect steroid output. But how do they exert their actions on steroid synthesis? The simple answer is: we don't know. However, we can make some informed observations that might help us along the way to unravelling a very complex story. First, do PUFAs affect steroid synthesis directly or do they exert their actions via PUFA metabolites (e.g., PGs)? One can cite evidence to support both ideas. For starters, both PUFAs and PUFA metabolites stimulate/inhibit StAR expression, and these actions on StAR are inevitably associated with either an increase or a decrease in steroid output (see Stocco et al., 2005 for review). The evidence for AA rather than its metabolites being able to stimulate StAR and steroid output is quite powerful (Wang & Stocco, 1999). However, the inhibition of 5-LOX being able to block some of the effects of AA suggests that the conversion to LOX metabolites is required, which means that it does not quite clinch it for the PUFA rather than the metabolites (Wang et al., 2003b). The intriguing idea that AA-CoA forms a complex with StAR, TSPO, PAP 7, and PKAR1α, which together act to transport cholesterol across the mitochondrial membrane, would seem almost the only aspect of PUFA action on steroid synthesis that was not replicated by a PUFA metabolite (Maloberti et al., 2007). So, if AA-CoA is used to transport cholesterol along with StAR, where does that leave the other PUFAs, especially those n-3 PUFAs that have stimulatory effects on steroid output? The n-3 PUFAs can stimulate StAR output (Ganga et al., 2006; Hodges et al., 2006). How do they do this? The n-3 PUFAs are able to directly activate a range of transcription factors (Jump et al., 2008), at least two (LXRs and SREBPs) which stimulate StAR-protein expression (Cummins et al., 2006; Manna et al., 2003). To identify which of these transcription factors mediates the n-3 PUFA-induced stimulatory effect on StAR expression, one must perform experiments with n-3 PUFAs on StAR expression in SREBP and LXR null mice. Some such studies were performed that show that the LXR agonists are able to stimulate StAR expression in adrenals of wild-type but not in LXRαβ$^{-/-}$ mice (Cummins et al., 2006). Although these observations support a role for LXR in mediating StAR expression, they do not provide any direct evidence to support a role for LXR in mediating the actions of n-3 PUFAs on StAR. Since both SREBP and LXR share a heterodimerization partner, RXR (Yoshikawa et al., 2002), possibly, both SREBPs and LXRs contribute to the steroidogenic actions of n-3 PUFAs (Fig. 27.7). PUFAs clearly modulate steroid synthesis. The mechanistic nature of this modulation remains to be elucidated. The possible sites at which PUFAs could interact with the steroidogenic cascade is illustrated in Fig 27.7.

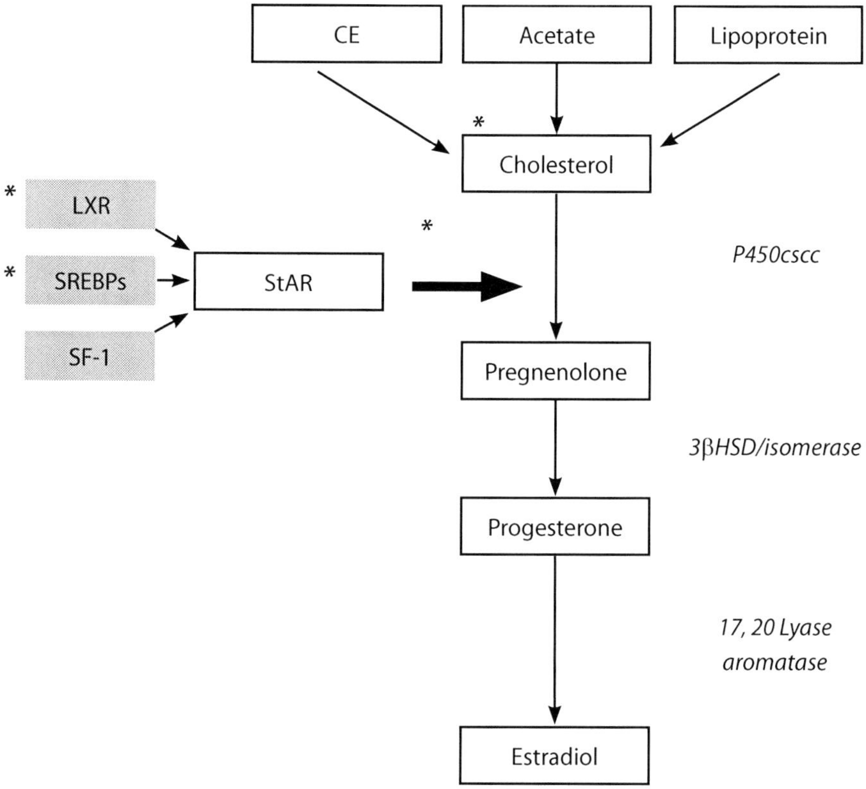


**Fig. 27.7.** Steroid biosynthesis and PUFAs. Points at which steroid synthesis can be regulated by PUFAs are denoted by *. CE-cholesterol esters, P450cscc-cytochrome P450 cholesterol side-chain cleavage enzyme, StAR-steroidogenic acute regulatory protein, 3βHSD/isomerase-3beta hydroxysteroid dehydrogenase/isomerase

## References


Abayasekara, D.R.E.; A.M. Band; B.A. Cooke. Evidence for the involvement of phospholipase A2 in the regulation of luteinizing hormone-stimulated steroidogenesis in rat testis Leydig cells. *Mol. Cell. Endocrinol.* **1990**, *70*, 147–153.

Abayasekara, D.R.E.; A.E. Michael; G.E. Webley; A.P.F. Flint. Mode of action of prostaglandin F2 alpha in human luteinized granulose cells: role of protein kinase C. *Mol. Cell. Endocrinol.* **1993**, *97*, 81–91.

Abayasekara, D.R.E.; D.C. Wathes. Effects of altering dietary fatty acid composition on prostaglandin synthesis and fertility. *Prostaglandins, Leukotrienes Essent. Fatty Acids* **1999** *61,* 275–287.

Alberti, S.; K.R. Steffensen; J.A. Gustafsson. Structural characterisation of the mouse nuclear oxysterol receptor genes LXRalpha and LXRbeta. *Gene* **2000**, *243*, 93–103.

Andersen, J.M.; J.M. Dietschy. Relative importance of high and low density lipoproteins in the regulation of cholesterol synthesis in the adrenal gland, ovary and testis of the rat. *J. Biol. Chem.* **1978**, *253*, 9024–9032.

Azhar, S.; S. Leers-Sucheta; E. Reaven. Cholesterol uptake in adrenal and gonadal tissues: The SR-B1 and "selective" pathway connection. *Front. Biosci.* **2003**, *8*, 998–1029.

Azhar, S.; E. Reaven. Scavenger receptor class B1 and selective cholesteryl ester uptake: partners in the regulation of steroidogenesis. *Mol. Cell. Endocrinol.* **2002**, *195*, 1–26.

Banerjee, J.; C.M. Komar. Effects of luteinizing hormone on peroxisome proliferator-activated receptor gamma in the rat ovary before and after the gonadotropin surge. *Reproduction* **2006**, *131*, 93–101.

Barton, L.; P. Jones, C. Wathes; R. Abayasekara. Do polyunsaturated fatty acids stimulate steroid secretion through affecting the expression of the Liver X receptor? *Endocrinol. Abst.* **2008**, *15,* OC31.

Benatti, P.; G. Peluso; R. Nicolai; M. Calvani. Polyunsaturated Fatty Acids: Biochemical, Nutritional and Epigenetic Properties. *J. Am. Coll. Nutr.* **2004**, *23*, 281–302.

Berger, A.D.; M. Mutch; J.B. German; M.A. Roberts. Dietary effects of arachidonate-rich fungal oil and fish oil on murine hepatic and hippocampal gene expression. *Lipids Health Dis.* **2002**, *1,* 2.

Bose, H.S.; R.M. Whittal; M.A. Baldwin; W.L. Miller. The active form of the steroidogenic acute regulatory protein, StAR, appears to be a molten globule. *Proc. Natl. Acad. Sci. U.S.A.* **1999,** *96*, 7250–7255.

Bourre, J.M. Where to find omega-3 fatty acids and how feeding animals with diet enriched in omega-3 fatty acids to increase nutritional value of derived products for human: what is actually useful? *J. Nutr. Health Aging* **2005**, *9*, 232–242.

Brown, M.S.; P.T. Kovanen; J.L. Goldstein. Receptor-mediated uptake of lipoprotein-cholesterol and its utilization in the adrenal cortex. *Recent Prog. Horm. Res.* **1979,** *35*, 215–257.

Bruder, E.D.; D.L. Ball; T.L. Goodfriend; H. Raff. An oxidized metabolite of linolenic acid stimulates corticosterone production by rat adrenal cells. *Am. J. Physiol.* **2003** *284,* R1631–R1635.

Burr, G.O.; M.M. Burr. On the nature and role of fatty acids in essential nutrition. *J. Biol. Chem.* **1930**, *86*, 587–621.

Chawla, A.; J.J. Repa; R.M. Evans; D.J. Mangelsdorf. Nuclear receptors and lipid physiology:

opening the X-files. *Science* **2001**, *294*, 1866–1870.

Chin, E.C.; J.M. Naddafy; Z. Cheng; J. Brickell; D.C. Wathes; D.R.E. Abayasekara. Dietary polyunsaturated fatty acid supplementation *in vivo* stimulates ovine adrenal steroidogenesis *in vitro*. *Endocrinol. Abst.* **2006**, *11*, P750.

Christenson, L.K.; L. Devoto. Cholesterol transport and steroidogenesis by the corpus luteum. *Reprod. Biol. Endocrinol.* **2003**, *1*, 90.

Christenson, L.K.; T.F. Osborne; J.M. MacAllister; J.F. Strauss III. Conditional response of the human steroidogenic acute regulatory protein gene promoter to sterol regulatory element binding protein-1a. *Endocrinology* **2001**, *142*, 28–36.

Christenson, L.K.; J.F. Strauss III. Steroidogenic acute regulatory protein: an update on its regulation and mechanism of action. *Arch. Med. Res.* **2001**, *32*, 576–586.

Clark, B.J.; J. Wells; S.R. King; D.M. Stocco. The purification, cloning and expression of a novel LH-induced mitochondrial protein in MA-10 mouse Leydig tumour cells: characterization of the steroidogenic acute regulatory protein (StAR). *J. Biol. Chem.* **1994**, *269*, 28314–28322.

Corneja Maciel, F.; P. Maloberti; I. Neuman; F. Cano; R. Castilla; F. Castillo; C. Paz; E.J. Podesta. An arachidonic acid preferring acyl-CoA synthetase is a hormone-dependent and obligatory protein in the signal transduction of steroidogenic hormones. *J. Mol. Endocrinol.* **2005**, *34*, 655–666.

Cummins, C.L.; D.H. Volle; J.G. McDonald; B. Sion; A.M. Lefrancois-Martinez; F. Caira; G. Veyssiere; D.L. Mangelsdorf; J.M. Lobaccaro. Liver X receptors regulate adrenal cholesterol balance. *J. Clin. Invest.* **2006**, *116*, 1902–1912.

Diaz, B.L.; J.P. Arm. Phospholipase $A_2$. *Prostaglandins, Leukotrienes Essent. Fatty Acids* **2003**, *69*, 87–97.

Dix, C.J.; A.D. Haberfield; M.H.F. Sullivan; B.A. Cooke. Inhibition of steroid production in Leydig cells by non-steroidal anti-inflammatory and related compounds: evidence for the involvement of lipoxygenase products in steroidogenesis. *Biochem. J.* **1984**, *219*, 529–537.

Feige, J.N.; L. Gelman; L. Michalik; B. Desvergne; W. Wahli. From molecular action to physiological outputs: Peroxisome proliferator-activated receptors are nuclear receptors at the crossroads of key cellular functions. *Prog. Lipid. Res.* **2006**, *45*, 120–159.

Fiedler, E.P.; F. Plouffe, Jr.; D.B. Hales; K.H. Hales; I. Khan. Prostaglandin F (2alpha) induces a rapid decline in progesterone production and steroidogenic acute regulatory protein expression in isolated rat corpus luteum without altering messenger ribonucleic acid expression. *Biol. Reprod.* **1999**, *61*, 643–650.

Flint, A.P.F.; D.L. Grinwich; D.T. Armstrong. Control of ovarian cholesterol ester synthesis. *Biochem. J.* **1973,** *132*, 313–321.

Ganga, R.; L. Tort; L. Acerete; D. Montero; M.S. Izuquiredo. Modulation of ACTH-induced cortisol release by polyunsaturated fatty acids in interrenal cells from gilthead seabream, *Sparus aurata*. *J. Endocrinol.* **2006**, *190*, 39–45.

Gazouli, M.; Z.X. Yao; N. Boujrad; J.C. Corton; M. Culty; V. Papadopoulos. Effect of peroxisome proliferators on Leydig cell peripheral-type benzodiazepine receptor gene expression, hormone-stimulated cholesterol transport, and steroidogenesis: role of the peroxisome proliferator-activator receptor alpha. *Endocrinology* **2003**, *143*, 2571–2583.

Goodfriend, T.L.; D.L. Ball; B.M. Egan; W.B. Campbell; K. Nithipatikom. Fatty acids are potential regulators of aldosterone secretion. *Hypertension* **2004**, *43*, 358–363.

Goodfriend, T.L.; D.L. Ball; M.E. Elliott; A.R. Morrison; M.A. Evenson. Fatty acids are potential regulators of aldosterone secretion. *Endocrinology* **1991**, *128*, 2511–2519.

Gurr, M.I.; J.L. Harwood; K.N. Frayn. *Lipid Biochemistry: An Introduction,* 5th ed.; Blackwell Science Ltd.: Oxford, UK, 2002.

Gwynne, G.T.; J.F. Strauss III. The role of lipoproteins in steroidogenesis and cholesterol metabolism in steroidogenic glands. *Endocrinol. Rev.* **1982,** *3*, 299–329.

Hall, P.F.; G. Almahbobi. Roles of microfilaments and intermediate filaments in adrenal steroidogenesis. *Microsc. Res. Tech.* **1997**, *36*, 463–479.

Hauet, T.; Z-X. Yao; H.S. Bose; C.T. Wall; Z. Han; W. Li; D.B. Hales; W.L. Miller; M. Cult; V. Papadopoulos. Peripheral-type benzodiazepine receptor-mediated action of steroidogenic acute regulatory protein on cholesterol entry in Leydig cell mitochondria. *Mol. Endocrinol.* **2005**, *19*, 550–554.

Hinckley, T., Sr.; R.M. Clark; S.L. Bushmich; R.A. Milvae. Long chain polyunsaturated fatty acids and bovine luteal cell function. *Biol. Reprod.* **1996**, *55*, 445–449.

Hodges, L.M.; E.C. Chin; J.M. Nadaffy; J. Brickell; Z. Cheng; E.L. Sheldrick; A.P.F. Flint; D.C. Wathes; D.R.E. Aabayasekara. Polyunsaturated fatty acids in vivo and in vitro affect expression of steroidogenic acute regulatory protein in steroidogenic tissues. *Endocrinol. Abst.* **2006**, *11*, P98.

Horton, J.D.; J.L. Goldstein; M.S. Brown. SREBPs:activators for the complete program of cholesterol and fatty acid synthesis in the liver. *J. Clin. Invest.* **2002**, *109,* 1125–1131.

Hunt, M.C.; S.E. Alexson. The role acyl CoA thioesterases play in mediating intracellular lipid metabolism. *Prog. Lipid. Res.* **2002**, *41*, 99–130.

Hwang, D.; S.H. Rhee. Receptor-mediated signaling pathways: potential targets of modulation by dietary fatty acids. *Am. J. Clin. Nutr.* **1999,** *70*, 545–556.

Jankowski, B.A.; M.J. Grogan; S.A. Jones; G.B. Wisely; S.A. Kliewer; E.J. Corey; D.J. Mangelsdorf. Structural requirements of ligands for the oxysterol liver x receptors LXR alpha and LXR beta. *Proc. Natl. Acad. Sci. U.S.A.* **1999**, *96*, 266–271.

Jones, P.M.; S. Sayed; S.J. Persaud; C.J. Burns; S Gyles; B.J. Whitehouse. Cyclic AMP-induced expression of steroidogenic acute regulatory protein is dependent upon phosphoprotein phosphatase activities. *J. Mol. Endocrinol.* **2000,** *24*, 233–239.

Jump, D.B.; D. Botolin; Y. Wang; J. Xu; B. Christian; O. Demeure. Fatty acid regulation of hepatic gene transcription. *J. Nutr.* **2005**, *135*, 2503–2506.

Jump, D.B.; D. Botolin; Y. Wang; J. Xu; O. Demeure; B. Christian. Docosahexaenoic acid (DHA) and hepatic gene transcription. *Chem. Phys. Lipids* **2008**, 153, 3–13.

Jump, D.B.; S.D. Clarke. Regulation of gene expression by dietary fat. *Ann. Rev. Nutr.* **1999**, *19*, 63–90.

Jump, D.B.; S.D. Clarke; A. Thelen; M. Liimatta; B. Ren; M. Badin. Dietary polyunsaturated fatty acid regulation of gene transcription. *Prog. Lipid. Res.* **1996**, *35*, 227–241.

Kempna, P.; G. Hofer; P.E. Mullis; C.E. Fluck. Pioglitazone inhibits androgen production in

NCI-H295R cells by regulating gene expression of cyp17 and HSD3β2. *Mol. Pharmacol.* **2007**, *71*, 787–798.

Kersten, S. Effects of fatty acids on gene expression: role of peroxisome proliferator-activated receptor alpha, liver X receptor alpha and sterol regulatory element-binding protein-1c. *Proc. Nutr. Soc.* **2002**, *61*, 371–374.

Khan, S.A.; J.P. Vanden Heuvel. Role of nuclear receptors in the regulation of gene expression by dietary fatty acids (review). *J. Nutr. Biochem.* **2003**, *14*, 554–567.

King, S.R.; Z. Liu; J. Zoh; S. Eimerl; J. Orly; D.M. Stocco. Effects of disruption of the mitochondrial electrochemical gradient on steroidogenesis and the steroidogenic acute regulatory protein. *J. Steroid Biochem. Mol. Biol.* **1999**, *69*, 143–154.

Komar, C.M. Peroxisome proliferator-activated receptors (PPARs) and ovarian function—implications for regulating steroidogenesis, differentiation, and tissue remodeling. *Reprod. Biol. Endocrinol.* **2005**, *3*, 41.

Kraemer, F.B. Adrenal cholesterol utilization. *Mol. Cell. Endocrinol.* **2007**, 265–266, 42–45.

Kurusu, S.; M. Ohkawa; M. Kawaminami. Effects of arachidonate metabolism inhibitors on basal and human chorionic gonadotrophin-stimulated progesterone secretion by the rat corpus luteum. *Prostglandins, Other Lipid Mediat.* **2007**, *83*, 139–145.

Lehmann, J.M.; S.A. Kliewer; L.B. Moore; T.A. Smith-Oliver; B.B. Oliver; J.L. Su; S.S. Sundseth; D.A. Winegar; D.E. Blanchard; T.A. Spencer; T.M. Willson. Activation of the nuclear receptor LXR by oxysterols defines a new hormone response pathway. *J. Biol. Chem.* **1997**, *272*, 3137–3140.

Lin, D.; S.E. Gitelman; P. Saenger; W.L. Miller. Normal genes for the cholesterol side chain cleavage enzyme, $P450_{scc}$, in congenital lipoid adrenal hyperplasia. *J. Clin. Invest.* **1991**, *88*, 1955–1962.

Liu, J.; M.R. Rone; V. Papdopoulos. Protein-protein interactions mediate mitochondrial cholesterol transport and steroid biosynthesis. *J. Biol. Chem.* **2006**, *281*, 38879–38893.

Lohrke, B.; T. Viergutz; S.K. Shahi; L. Pohland; K. Wollenhaupt; T. Goldhammer; H. Walzel; W. Kanitz. Detection and functional characterisation of the transcription factor peroxisome proliferator-activated receptor gamma in lutein cells. *J. Endocrinol.* **1998**, *159*, 429–439.

Maloberti, P.; R. Castilla; A.F. Castillo; F.C. Maciel; C.F. Mendez; C. Paz; E.J. Podesta. Silencing the expression of mitochondrial acyl-CoA thioesterase I and acyl-Co-A synthetase 4 inhibits hormone-induced steroidogenesis. *FEBS J.* **2005**, *272*, 1804–1814.

Maloberti, P.; F. Cornejo Maciel; A.F. Castillo; R. Castilla; A. Duarte; M.F. Toledo; F. Meuli; P. Mele; C. Paz; E.J. Podesta. Enzymes involved in arachidonic acid release in adrenal and Leydig cells. *Mol. Cell. Endocrinol.* **2007**, *265–266*, 113–120.

Manna, P.R.; X-J. Wang; D.M. Stocco. Involvement of multiple transcription factors in the regulation of steroidogenic acute regulatory protein gene expression. *Steroids* **2003,** *68*, 1125–1134.

Marinero, M.J.; V. Penalva; J.L. Oliva; B. Colas; J.C. Prieto; M.P. Lopez-Ruiz. Specific effect of arachidonic acid on 17β-hydroxysteroid dehydrogenase in rat Leydig cells. *FEBS Lett.* **1998**, *422*, 10–14.

Matthys, L.A.; E.P. Widmaier. Fatty acids inhibit adrenocorticotropin-induced adrenal steroidogenesis. *Horm. Metab. Res.* **1998**, *30*, 80–83.

Mattos, R.; C.R. Staples; W.W. Thatcher. Effects of dietary fatty acids on reproduction in ruminants. *Rev. Reprod.* **2000**, *5*, 38–45.

Mercure, F.; G. Van Der Kraak. Inhibition of gonadotrophin-stimulated ovarian steroid production by polyunsaturated fatty acids in teleost fish. *Lipids* **1995**, *30*, 547–554.

Miller, W.L. Molecular biology of steroid hormone synthesis. *Endocrinol. Rev.* **1988** *3*, 295–318.

Miller, W.L. Mechanism of StAR's regulation of mitochondrial cholesterol import. *Mol. Cell. Endocrinol.* **2007a,** *265–266*, 46–50.

Miller, W.L. Steroidogenic acute regulatory protein (StAR), a novel mitochondrial cholesterol transporter. *Biochim. Biophys. Acta* **2007b**, *1771*, 663–676.

Miller, W.L. StAR search—what we know about how the steroidogenic acute regulatory protein mediates mitochondrial cholesterol import. *Mol. Endocrinol.* **2007c,** *21*, 589–601.

Miller, C.W.; J.M. Ntambi. Peroxisome proliferators induce mouse liver stearoyl-CoA desaturase 1 gene expression. *Proc. Natl. Acad. Sci. U.S.A.* **1996**, *93*, 9443–9448.

Nebert, D.W.; D.W. Russell. Clinical importance of cytochromes P450. *Lancet* **2002**, *9340*, 1155–1162.

Needleman, P.; J. Turk; B.A. Jakschik; A.R. Morrison; J.B. Lefkowith. Arachidonic acid metabolism. *Annu. Rev. Biochem.* **1986**, *55*, 69–102.

Nilsson, M.; T.L. Stulnig; C-Y. Lin; P. Nowotny; E.T. Liu; K.R. Steffensen. Liver X receptors regulate adrenal steroidogenesis and hypothalamic-pituitary adrenal feedback. *Mol. Endocrinol.* **2007**, *21*, 126–137.

Niswender, G.D. Molecular control of luteal progesterone secretion. *Reproduction* **2002**, *123*, 333–339.

Osborne, T.F. Sterol regulatory element binding proteins (SREBPs): key regulators of nutritional homeostasis and action. *J. Biol. Chem.* **2000,** *275*, 32379–32382.

Papadopoulos, V. Peripheral-type benzodiazepine/diazepam binding inhibitor receptor: biological role in steroidogenic function. *Endocrinol. Rev.* **1993**, *14*, 222–240.

Parker, K.L. The roles of steroidogenic factor 1 in endocrine development and function. *Mol. Cell. Endocrinol.* **1998**, *25*, 59–63.

Payet, M.D.; T.L. Goodfriend; L. Bilodeau; C. Mackendale; L. Chouinard; N. Galo-Payet. An oxidized metabolite of linolenic acid increases intracellular calcium in rat adrenal glomerulosa cells. *Am. J. Physiol. Endocrinol. Metab.* **2006**, *291*, E1160–E1167.

Peet, D.J.; S.D. Turley; W. Ma; B.A. Jankowski; J-M. A. Lobaccaro; R.E. Hammer; D.J. Mangelsdorf. Cholesterol and bile acid metabolism are impaired in mice lacking the nuclear oxysterol recep tor LXRα. *Cell* **1998**, *93*, 693–704.

Penning, T.M. Molecular endocrinology of hydroxysteroid dehydrogenases. *Endocrinol. Rev.* **1997**, *18*, 281–305.

Petrescu, A.D.; A.M. Gallegos; Y. Okamura; J.F. Strauss III; F. Schroeder. Steroidogenic acute regulatory protein binds cholesterol and modulates mitochondrial membrane sterol domain dynamics. *J. Biol. Chem.* **2001**, *276*, 36970–36982.

Repa, J.J.; G. Liang; J. Ou; Y. Basmakov; J-M.A. Lobaccaro; I. Shimomura; B. Shan; M.S. Brown; J.L. Goldstein; D.J. Mangelsdorf. Regulation of mouse sterol regulatory element binding protein-1c (SREBP-1c) by oxysterol receptors LXRα and LXRβ. *Genes Dev.* **2000**, *14*, 2819–2830.

Robinson, R.S.; P.G. Pushpakumara; Z. Cheng; A.R. Peters; D.R.E. Aabayasekara; D.C. Wathes. Effects of dietary polyunsaturated fatty acids on ovarian and uterine function in lactating dairy cows. *Reproduction* **2002**, *124*, 119–131.

Sakai, Y.; T. Yanase; Y. Okabe; T. Hara; M.R. Waterman; R. Takayanagi; M. Haji; H. Nawata. No mutations in cytochrome P450 side chain cleavage in a patient with congenital lipoid adrenal hyperplasia. *J. Clin. Endocrinol. Metab.* **1994**, *79*, 1198–1201.

Sarel, I.; E.P. Widmaier. Stimulation of sterodogenesis in cultured rat adrenocortical cells by unsaturated fatty acids. *Am. J. Physiol.* **1995**, *268*, R1484–R1490.

Schmitz, G.; J. Ecker. The opposing effects of n-3 and n-6 fatty acids. *Prog. Lipid. Res.* **2008**, *47*, 147–155.

Schultz, J.R.; H. Tu; A. Luk; J.J. Repa; J.C. Medina; L. Li; S. Schwender; S. Wang; M. Thoolen; D.J. Mangelsdorf; K.D. Lustig; B. Shan. Role of LXRs in control of lipogenesis. *Genes Dev.* **2000**, *14*, 2831–2838.

Sheldrick E.L.; K. Derecka; E. Marshall; E.C. Chin; L. Hodges; D.C. Wathes; D.R.E. Abayasekara; A.P.F. Flint. Peroxisome-proliferator activated receptors and the control of prostaglandin endoperoxide synthase 2 by arachidonic acid. *Biochem. J.* **2007**, *406*, 175–183.

Simopoulos, A.P. The importance of omega-6/omega-3 fatty acid ratio in cardiovascular disease and other chronic diseases. *Exp. Biol. Med.* **2008**, *233*, 674–688.

Simpson, E.R.; G.S. Boyd. The cholesterol side chain cleavage system of the adrenal cortex. *Eur. J. Biochem.* **1967**, *2*, 275–285.

Smith, W.L. Cyclooxygenases, peroxide and the allure of fish oil. *Curr. Opin. Cell. Biol.* **2005**, *17*, 174–182.

Smith, W.L. Nutritionally essential fatty acids and biologically indispensable cyclooxygenases. *Trends Bicochem. Sci.* **2008**, *33*, 27–37.

Smith, W.L.; R. Lagenbach. Why there are two cylcooxygenase enzymes. *J. Clin. Invest.* **2001**, *107*, 1491–1495.Soccio, R.E.; J.L. Breslow. StAR related lipid transfer (START) proteins: mediators of intracellular lipid metabolism. *J. Biol. Chem.* **2003**, *278*, 22183–22186.

Stocco, D.M. The role of the StAR protein in steroidogenesis: challenges for the future. *J. Endocrinol.* **2000,** *164*, 247–253.

Stocco, D.M. Clinical disorders associated with abnormal cholesterol transport:mutations in the steroidogenic acute regulatory protein. *Mol. Cell. Endocrinol.* **2002**, *191*, 19–25.

Stocco, D.M.; B.J. Clark. Regulation of the acute production of steroids in steroidogenic cells. *Endocrinol. Rev.* **1996** *17*, 221–244.

Stocco, D.M; B.J. Clark. The role of the steroidogenic acute regulatory protein in steroidogenesis. *Steroids* **1997**, *62*, 29–36.

Stocco, D.M.; X. Wang; Y. Jo; P.R. Manna. Multiple signaling pathways regulating steroidogenesis and steroidogenic acute regulatory protein expression: more complicated than we thought. *Mol Endocrinol.* **2005,** *19*, 2647–59.

Sundqvist, A.; M.T. Bengoechea-Alonso; X. Ye; J. Lukiyanchuk; J.W. Harper; J. Ericsson. Control of lipid metabolism by phosphorylation-dependent degradation of the SREBP family of transcription factors by SCGFBW7. *Cell. Metab.* **2005**, *1*, 379–391.

Tang, X.; E.M. Edwards; B.B. Holmes; J.R. Falck; W.B. Campbell. *Am. J. Physiol. Heart Circ. Physiol.* **2006**, *290*, H37–H45.

Tobin, K.A.; H.H. Steineger; S. Alberti; O. Spydevold; J. Auwerx; J.A. Gustafsson; H.I. Nebb. Cross-talk between fatty acid and cholesterol metabolism mediated by liver X receptor-alpha. *Mol. Endocrinol.* **2000**, *14*, 741–752.

Tuckey, R.C. Progesterone synthesis by the human placenta. *Placenta* **2005**, *26*, 273–281.

Ueno, N.; Y. Takegoshi; D. Kamei; I. Kudo; M. Murakami. Coupling between cyclooxygneases and terminal prostanoid synthases. *Biochem. Biophys. Res. Commun.* **2005**, *338*, 70–76.

Ulven, S.M.; K.T. Dalen; J.A. Gustafsson; H.I. Nebb. LXR is crucial in lipid metabolism. *Prostaglandins, Leukotrienes Essent. Fatty Acids* **2005**, *73*, 59–63.

Van Voorhis B.J.; M.S. Dunn; J.R. Falck; R.K. Bhatt; M. VanRollins; G.D. Snyder. Metabolism of arachidonic acid to epoxyeicostrienoic acids by human granulose cells may mediate steroidogenesis. *J. Clin. Endocrinol. Metab.* **1993,** *76,* 1555–1559.

Vinson, G.P.; B.J. Whitehouse; J.P. Hinson. *The Adrenal Cortex.* Prentice Hall: U.K., 1992.

Volle, D.H.; J-M.A. Lobaccaro. Role of the nuclear receptors for oxysterols LXR in steroidogenic tissues: Beyond the "foie gras", the steroids and sex? *Mol. Cell. Endocrinol.* **2007**, *265–266*, 183–189.

Volle, D.H.; K. Mouzat; R. Duggavathi; B. Siddeek; P. Dechelotte; B. Sion; G. Veyssiere; M. Benahmed; J-M.A. Lobaccaro. Multiple roles of the nuclear receptors for oxysterols liver X receptor to maintain male fertility. *Mol. Endocrinol.* **2007**, *21*, 1014–1027.

Wada, M.; C.J. DeLong; Y.H. Hong; C.J. Rieke; I. Song; R.S. Sidhu; C. Yuan; M. Warnock; A.H. Schmaier; C. Yokoyama; et al. Enzymes and receptors of prostaglandin pathways with arachidonic acid-derived versus eicosapentaenoic acid-derived substrates and products. *J. Biol. Chem.* **2007**, *282*, 22254–22266.

Wahli, W. Peroxisome proliferator-activated receptors (PPARs): from metabolic control to epidermal wound healing. *Swiss. Med. Wkly.* **2002,** *132*, 83–91.

Wang, X.J.; M.T. Dyson; Y. Jo; D.M. Stocco. Inhibition of cyclooxygenase-2 activity enhances steroidogenesis and steroidogeneic acute regulatory gene expression in MA-10 mouse Leydig cells. *Endocrinology* **2003**a, *144*, 3368–3375.

Wang, X.J.; M.T. Dyson; Y. Jo; D.M. Stocco. Involvement of 5-lipoxygenase metabolites of arachidonic acid in cyclic AMP-stimulated steroidogenesis and steroidogenic acute regulatory protein gene expression. *J. Steroid. Biochem. Mol. Biol.* **2003b** *85*, 159–166.

Wang, J.; P.C.K. Leung. Arachidonic acid as a stimulatory mediator of luteinizing hormone-releasing hormone action in the rat ovary. *Endocrinology* **1989**, *124*, 1973–1979.

Wang, X.J.; C-L. Shen; M.T. Dyson; X. Xianlin; R.B. Schiffer; P. Grammas; D.M. Stocco. The involvement of epoxygenase metabolites of arachidonic acid in cAMP-stimulated steroidogenesis and steroidogenic acute regulatory protein gene expression. *J. Endocrinol.* **2006**, *190*, 871–878.

Wang, X.J.; D.M. Stocco. Cyclic AMP and arachidonic acid: a tale of two pathways. *Mol. Cell. Endocrinol.* **1999**, *158*, 7–12.

Wang, H.; S.W. Walker; J.I. Mason; S.D. Morley; B.C. Williams. Role of arachidonic acid metabolism in ACTH-induced cortisol secretion by bovine adrenocortical cells. *Endocrinol. Res.* **2000a**, *26*, 705–709.

Wang, X.J.; L.P. Walsh; A.J. Reinhart; D.M. Stocco. The role of arachidonic acid in steroidogenesis and steroidogenic acute regulatory (StAR) gene and protein expression. *J. Biol. Chem.* **2000b**, *275*, 20204–20209.

Wang, X.J.; X. Xianlin; R.B. Schiffer; S.R. King; D.M. Stocco; P. Grammas. Inhibition of thromboxane A synthase activity enhances steroidogenesis and steroidogenic acute regulatory gene expression in MA-10 mouse Leydig cells. *Endocrinology* **2008**, *149*, 851–857.

Wathes, D.C.; D.R.E. Abayasekara; R.J. Aitken. Polyunsaturated fatty acids in male and female reproduction. *Biol. Reprod.* **2007**, *77*, 190–201.

Weems, Y.S.; P.J. Bridges; Y. Tanaka; R.G. Sasser; B.R. LeaMaster; D.L. Vincent; C.W. Weems. PGE1 or PGE2 not LH regulates secretion of progesterone in vitro by the 88-90 day ovine corpus luteum of pregnancy. *Prostaglandins* **1997**, *53*, 337–353.

Xu, J.; M.N. Nakamura; H.P. Cho; S. Clarke. Sterol regulatory element binding protein-1 expression is suppressed by dietary polyunsaturated fatty acids. *J. Biol. Chem.* **1999,** *274*, 23577–23583.

Yoshikawa, T.; H. Shimano; N. Yahagi; T. Ide; M. Amemiya-Kudo; T. Matzukaka; M. Nakakuki; S. Tomita; H. Okazaki; Y. Tamura, et al. Polyunsaturated fatty acids suppress sterol regulatory element-binding protein 1c promoter activity by inhibition of liver X receptor (LXR) binding to LXR response elements. *J. Biol. Chem.* **2002**, *277*, 1705–1711.

Zelcer, N.; P. Tontonoz. Liver X receptors as integrators of metabolic and inflammatory signalling. *J. Clin. Invest.* **2006**, *116*, 607–614.

# 28

# Dietary Fat and Fatty Acids in Exercise and Athletic Performance

**Stephen M. Cornish[1], Philip D. Chilibeck[1], Craig Pinkoski[1], and Gordon A. Zello[2]**
*College of Kinesiology[1] and College of Pharmacy and Nutrition[2], University of Saskatchewan, Saskatoon, Canada*

## Introduction

Individuals who engage in physical activity or exercise predominantly rely on fats/lipids and carbohydrates to sustain energy production. During high-intensity exercise, carbohydrate (in the form of glycogen and glucose) is the main form of energy utilized to sustain activity. During low- and moderate-intensity exercise, a combination of carbohydrate and lipids (in the form of fatty acids) is utilized to sustain activity. The purposes of this chapter are to: (i) explain the transport and utilization of fatty acids for energy during exercise; (ii) delineate the differences in fat oxidation and utilization between trained and untrained (sedentary) individuals; (iii) clarify the requirements for fat and fatty acids (i.e., Dietary Reference Intakes) when considering exercise and athletic performance; and (iv) discuss the health and ergogenic benefits of consuming differing amounts of fat or various types of fatty acids in combination with exercise.

## Fatty Acid Metabolism During Exercise

Fatty acids are utilized as substrates for exercise predominantly during low- or moderate-intensity exercise (up to an intensity corresponding to ≈65% of maximal oxygen uptake or $VO_2max$), with the absolute amount of fatty acid utilization maximized with moderate-intensity exercise (Romijn et al., 1993). The utilization of fatty acids during exercise can come from various sources, including adipose-tissue stores, intramuscular triacylglyceride (IMTG), free fatty acids (FFAs) in plasma, chylomicrons, and very low density lipoprotein (Spriet, 2002). Of these sources, the liberation of FFAs from adipose tissue and IMTG provides the greatest amount of fatty acids during exercise (Spriet, 2002; van Loon, 2004). During exercise, energy expenditure is increased due to skeletal muscle contraction. As an individual begins to exercise, more fuel in the form of adenosine triphosphate (ATP) is needed to provide substrate to the working skeletal musculature. Fatty acids provide this fuel via their entry into the tricarboxycylic acid (TCA) cycle in the form of acetyl coenzyme A (CoA). Before fatty acids can enter the TCA cycle, lipolysis of triacylglyceride (TAG) must occur. This occurs by an increase in the phosphorylation of hormone-sensitive lipase to stimulate the breakdown of TAG into three fatty acids and glycerol. As exercise commences, epinephrine, norepinephrine, and growth hormone are released, resulting in the phosphorylation of hormone-sensitive lipase which stimulates the breakdown of TAG. Once TAG is broken down, the FFAs are bound to albumin in the blood and carried to skeletal muscle where they are oxidized. Skeletal muscle also contains hormone-sensitive lipase, which is also activated by growth hormone. This hormone-sensitive lipase can break down TAGs that are in the blood (i.e., as occurs shortly after a meal). Specific carrier proteins, fatty-acid-binding protein (FABP) and fatty-acid-transport protein (FAT/CD36), transport fatty acids across the muscle cell membrane. Once inside the cell, the FFA is bound to a carnitine complex to allow for entry into the mitochondria of the cell. After the FFA is transported by the carnitine complex into the mitochondria of the cell, it undergoes a transformational change in which the large carbon-chain molecule is broken down into smaller 2-carbon skeletons. This occurs via the process of β-oxidation within the mitochondrial matrix, which is a series of cyclic steps designed to break down the large fatty acid molecule. The β-oxidation process results in the formation of acetyl CoA, which is the main entry point for the TCA cycle. Once acetyl CoA is formed, it enters the TCA cycle, which generates NADH and $FADH_2$ coenzymes that act as temporary energy-storage molecules. These coenzymes advance to the electron-transport chain, and drive the formation of ATP from adenosine 5′-diphosphate (ADP) and inorganic phosphate via oxidative phosphorylation. Additional recommended reading includes an indepth review of fat oxidation in exercising humans (Spriet, 2002) and an excellent review on IMTG-substrate use during exercise (van Loon, 2004).

One main difference between carbohydrate oxidation and fat oxidation is that fat oxidation is a completely aerobic process requiring oxygen as the final electron acceptor during oxidative phosphorylation. Carbohydrate oxidation can generate energy in the form of ATP without requiring oxygen via glycolysis. This is one reason that as exercise intensity increases, a corresponding shift in substrate utilization occurs. That is, carbohydrate oxidation is predominantly utilized for energy production with increasing exercise intensity, especially high-intensity exercise, as it is a more efficient substrate (i.e., supplies more energy per liter of oxygen consumed). Although carbohydrate is considered a more efficient substrate for exercise, the amount of energy from fat stores in the human body greatly exceeds the energy stored as carbohydrate in the form of glycogen, and thus, is able to provide energy for low- to moderate-intensity exercise for an indefinite period of time. The amount of fat stores in the human body becomes an essential component of exercise performance for long-duration activities such as ultramarathons (>100 miles) or ultraadventure racing where athletes are required to carry food with them and race for long periods of time (usually >24 hours). So, the utilization of fat during exercise mainly depends on the duration, intensity, and type of exercise in which the individual is participating. The following sections review the scientific literature on the effects of training on the use of fatty acids and the utilization of fatty acids for specific durations, intensities, and types of activity in humans.

### Effect of Training Status on Fatty Acid Oxidation

Fat oxidation is higher in trained versus untrained individuals during moderate- and high-intensity exercises, with no difference at a low-exercise intensity (Stisen et al., 2006). Adaptations to exercise training explain the differences in fat oxidation between trained and untrained individuals. These adaptations include a rise in enzyme activity (i.e., an increase of proteins that stimulate the breakdown of fat in muscle, including citrate synthase, β-hydroxyacyl-CoA dehydrogenase, hormone-sensitive lipase, and carnitine palmitoyl transferase I), improvements in FAT/CD36 that allow fats to be transported into muscle, and a greater reliance on IMTG during exercise (Helge et al., 2006; Schrauwen et al., 1999; Stisen et al., 2006; Tunstall et al., 2002). Training also increases the proximity of mitochondria to IMTG (i.e., a greater number of mitochondria is observed to be in contact with IMTG following training) (Tarnopolsky et al., 2007b). This allows more efficient transport of fats and the use of fats by the mitochondria during exercise. Training also increases muscle capillarization, which allows an increased delivery of blood-borne triglycerides or fatty acids to skeletal muscle (Henriksson, 1992).

### Effect of Duration of Exercise on Fat Metabolism

Endurance athletes may be at increased risk of health and performance detriments due to an inadequate dietary intake of total kilocalories, especially fat (Horvath et al., 2000). The general consensus with energy expenditure is that the longer the duration of the activity, the more fat is utilized to sustain muscle contraction. Although this concept seems intuitively correct, during high-intensity exercise, this may not always hold true. The processes involved in fat oxidation (i.e., stimulation of hormone-sensitive lipase at the adipose tissue and muscle, transport of fatty acids to skeletal muscle, uptake by skeletal muscle, translocation to the mitochondria, and then metabolism through β-oxidation, the TCA cycle, and the electron transport chain) are relatively slow; therefore, long-duration exercise is usually recommended for mobilizing and oxidizing fats. When exercise is performed at a low intensity (i.e., 50% of $VO_2$max), the appearance of fatty acids and glycerol in the blood increases over time, with levels increasing until at least 150 minutes into exercise (Zinker et al., 1990). With longer exercise sessions at moderate intensities (i.e., 70% of anaerobic threshold), the rate of fat oxidation rises up to 4 hours into exercise (Meyer et al., 2003). Therefore, the longer the duration of exercise, the greater the contribution of fat oxidation to energy needs.

### Effect of Exercise Intensity on Fat Metabolism

In a classic study of intensity on fat and carbohydrate metabolism during exercise, Romijn et al. (1993) demonstrated that in men exercising at a moderate intensity of exercise (65% of $VO_2$max, equivalent to fast walking or an easy jog), the oxidation of FFAs derived from the hydrolysis of TAG stores in adipose tissue progressively increased over a 2-hour time period, whereas IMTG and intramuscular glycogen oxidation decreased at this intensity. The results of the aforementioned study were also evaluated in trained women with identical results (Romijn et al., 2000). The researchers concluded that the absolute amount of fat oxidation was maximized at ≈65% of $VO_2$max. Later research corroborated these findings: (i) fat oxidation is maximized at 64 ± 4% of $VO_2$max, while a range between 55 ± 3 and 72 ± 4% of $VO_2$max results in significant fat oxidation, and (ii) any exercise intensity above 89 ± 3% of $VO_2$max results in minimal or no fat oxidation (Achten et al., 2002). Further research from the same group found that feeding carbohydrate before exercise blunts both the intensity at which fat oxidation is maximized by 14% and total-fat oxidation by 28% (Achten & Jeukendrup, 2003).

From the previous section, the indication was that the longer the duration of exercise, the greater the fatty acid oxidation. Then, sensibly, low- to moderate-intensity exercise is optimal for stimulating fatty acid oxidation because one cannot sustain high intensities of exercise for long durations. The effect of exercise intensity on fatty acid oxidation is, however, complex. For example, Romijn et al. (1993) found that TAG lipolysis from adipose tissue was maximal at a very low exercise intensity (25% of $VO_2$ max); however, the hydrolysis of TAG stored in skeletal muscle was only stimulated at higher intensities (i.e., 65–85% of $VO_2$max). Furthermore, during recovery from high-intensity exercise, the rate of release of fatty acids into plasma increased, indicating that fatty acid oxidation might be stimulated during recovery from high-intensity exercise. Several studies indicate that high-intensity training might up-regulate the metabolic machinery (i.e., enzymes) involved in fatty acid oxidation, and this would promote the use of fats and, in turn, reduce body fatness.

Tremblay et al. (1994) compared a low-intensity training program of 20 weeks to a higher intensity intermittent training program of 15 weeks. The low-intensity program involved more than double the energy expenditure; however, the high-intensity program resulted in a greater reduction in subcutaneous fat (measured by skinfolds) and a greater increase in 3-hydroxyacyl CoA dehydrogenase, a marker enzyme of β-oxidation (i.e., a major enzyme involved in the breakdown of fat). Comparing similar exercise programs in rats, Chilibeck et al. (1998) found that direct measures of fatty acid oxidation by mitochondria, the organelles in a muscle cell that are involved in fat oxidation, were increased to a greater extent following a high-intensity intermittent exercise program compared to a low-intensity, long-duration program. This occurred even though the low-intensity, long-duration program involved twice the energy expenditure. Recently, the extremes of exercise duration/intensity were more thoroughly evaluated. Burgomaster et al. (2008) compared 6 weeks of sprint–interval training to traditional low-intensity, long-duration training. The sprint–interval training consisted of 4–6 repetitions of 30-second "all-out" sprints on a cycle ergometer, with a 4.5-minute rest between sprints, performed 3 times per week, whereas the traditional low-intensity, long-duration training involved 40–60 minutes of exercise at 65% of $VO_2$ max carried out 5 times per week. The low-intensity, long-duration program involved approximately 10 times the energy expenditure as compared to the sprint–interval training. Both programs resulted in similar and significant increases in 3-hydroxyacyl CoA dehydrogenase and a protein called the peroxisome proliferator-activated receptor (PPAR)-$\gamma$ coactivator 1$\alpha$, which is involved in "turning on" the synthesis of new mitochondria.

Additional research on exercise intensity suggests that high- intensity interval training is beneficial for promoting fat metabolism at submaximal exercise intensities (Talanian et al., 2007). In one study, untrained women performed 7 high-intensity interval-training sessions over 2 weeks (10 × 4 minutes at 90% of $VO_2$max with 2 minutes of rest between work bouts). The researchers demonstrated a significant improvement in mitochondrial 3-hydroxyacyl CoA dehydrogenase (32% increase), citrate synthase (a TCA-cycle enzyme) (20% increase), and FABP content (25% increase), suggesting a vast improvement in the ability of muscle tissue to oxidize fat. Further, during a submaximal 60-minute exercise task (60% of $VO_2$max at baseline), a 36% improvement in whole-body fat oxidation was demonstrated. These results indicate that in untrained women, significant changes in the ability to oxidize fat can be accomplished within a relatively short period of time with high-intensity training.

The above studies indicate that the traditionally prescribed low-intensity, long-duration endurance exercise for oxidizing fats may not be the only type of exercise that may be of benefit for reducing fat mass. When prescribing a type of exercise, one would have to take into consideration the initial health status and motivation of an exercising individual. For example, to prescribe maximal interval training to someone who is obese and unmotivated may not be prudent; however, evidence shows that exercise not traditionally prescribed for reducing fat mass (i.e., high-intensity resistance training) can be effective for significantly reducing fat mass in such populations (Chilibeck et al., 2002).

## *Effect of Sex on Fat Metabolism during Exercise*

Sex differences in substrate utilization also exist, with females able to oxidize more fat and less carbohydrate and protein when compared to equally trained males during endurance running (Tarnopolsky et al., 1990). This may confer a performance advantage for females during extremely long endurance events (i.e., ultramarathon running) because a greater ability to oxidize fats would preserve muscle glycogen (carbohydrate), which is important for sustaining endurance performance (Speechly et al., 1996). The reason for females' greater ability to oxidize fats may be related to several factors. Estrogen appears to play a role because estrogen supplementation in males enhances their ability to oxidize fats during endurance exercise (Hamadeh et al., 2005). Also, some evidence exists showing that higher estrogen levels during the luteal phase of the menstrual cycle result in a greater ability to oxidize fats compared to the follicular phase (Zderic et al., 2001). However, this may depend on the intensity of the exercise. At lower intensity exercise (70% of anaerobic threshold), no difference was noted in the rate of fat oxidation between menstrual-cycle phases, but at higher intensities (90% of anaerobic threshold), a difference was apparent. This implies a possible small performance advantage for women in the luteal phase of the menstrual cycle because a greater fat oxidation could preserve muscle glycogen (Devries et al., 2006).

Morphological or metabolic differences in skeletal muscle may explain the greater ability of females to oxidize fats during endurance exercise. Women have a greater storage of IMTG, and they use a greater amount of IMTG during endurance exercise compared to males (Roepstorff et al., 2006a). Women also have higher amounts of muscle hormone-sensitive lipase compared to males, indicating they may be better at breaking down TAG in the blood for use in the muscle (Roepstorff et al., 2006a). The higher rate of fat oxidation in females is also partially explained by their greater muscle capillarization and type I fiber percentage compared to males (Roepstorff et al., 2006b). A higher capillarization would enhance fatty acid delivery to skeletal muscle and type I ("slow") muscle fibers are characterized as having higher mitochondrial content, and therefore greater metabolic machinery for oxidizing fats, compared to other muscle-fiber types.

## Effects of Dietary Fat and Fatty Acids on Exercise Performance

The amount of fat intake and the types of fatty acids consumed have important health implications in both inactive and exercising individuals. In the next section, the current dietary recommendations for fat and fatty acids are presented, and investigations in which fat and fatty acid intakes were manipulated to improve exercise performance are discussed.

### *Current Dietary Recommendations for Fat and Fatty Acids and Implications for Exercise*

The Dietary Reference Intakes (DRIs) are the North American reference standards for nutrients in the diets of healthy individuals of both sexes at all stages of the life cycle. The macronutrient DRI report includes the standards for energy, fat and fatty acids, carbohydrate and fiber, and protein and amino acids (IOM, 2005). The DRIs for the macronutrients are presented as recommended daily allowances (RDAs) or adequate intakes (AIs), as well as acceptable macronutrient distribution ranges (AMDRs), and were determined by considering both nutrient inadequacies and excesses. As healthy individuals include those engaged in various levels of physical activity, the DRIs should apply to exercising individuals and address their nutrient needs. In fact, the expert committees assembled to determine the DRIs were instructed to consider physical activity as a factor in determining requirements (IOM, 2005). In general, consensus was that "with minor exception, dietary recommendations for athletes are not distinguished from the general population, or vice versa" (IOM, 2005).

Many athletes and exercising individuals, however, have daily nutritional requirements that differ from the general population, due to the nature of the exercises that are involved (e.g., type, intensity, and duration). Therefore, one should have a good understanding of the DRIs themselves (Barr, 2006) before examining specific dietary intervention studies involving exercise in which the intakes of total fat or fatty acids may be below or above the DRI values. Additionally, a detailed review of the DRIs for the macronutrients and the implications for the athlete was published (Zello, 2006), with the relevant information on fat and fatty acids summarized below.

***Dietary Reference Intakes (DRIs) for Fat and Fatty Acids***

For total dietary fat, an AI or an RDA was not set because of insufficient scientific data to determine a defined level of fat intake at which the risk of inadequacy or the prevention of chronic disease occurs. For the two dietary essential fatty acids: (i) α-linolenic acid (ALA), an 18-carbon ω-3 (omega-3, n-3) polyunsaturated fatty acid (PUFA, 18:3ω3) and the parent to longer carbon chain ω-3 fatty acids, and (ii) linoleic acid LA, an 18-carbon ω-6 (omega-6, n-6) PUFA (18:2ω6) and precursor to arachidonic acid (AA, 20:4ω6), AIs were set for all age groups. ALA functions as a precursor to other ω-3 fatty acids such as eicosapentaenoic acid (EPA, 20:5ω3) and docosahexaenoic acid (DHA, 22:6ω3) via carbon- chain elongation and further desaturation (Burdge, 2004). The 20-carbon-chain fatty acids in the ω-3 and ω-6 families are the precursors to the prostaglandin 3-series and the prostaglandin 1- and 2-series, respectively, as well as the thromboxanes and leukotrienes. These eicosanoids have important roles in immune function, gastric secretions, smooth-muscle contraction, platelet aggregation, and as vasodilators or vasoconstrictors. DHA, a 22-carbon-chain fatty acid, is an important component of membrane phospholipids and the cerebellum. Therefore, in the adult, the AIs for the dietary essential ω-3 and ω-6 PUFA ranges are 1.1–1.6 $g{\cdot}d^{-1}$ and 14–17 $g{\cdot}d^{-1}$, respectively. Most of the ω-3 fatty acids in the diet come from certain plant oils as ALA (e.g., canola, flaxseed, and soybean); however, good sources of EPA and DHA are fatty-fish or fish-liver oils. Dietary sources of the ω-6 fatty acids include seed oils such as LA (e.g., sunflower, corn, and safflower), with meat being a source of AA.

Monounsaturated fat, such as oleic acid (18:1ω9), although important in the diet for health and found in plant oils (e.g., olive, canola, and peanut), is produced by the body, and therefore is not required in specific amounts in the diet (i.e., no AI and RDA). Likewise, cholesterol is a fat synthesized in the liver and is not essential in the diet.

A Tolerable Upper Intake Level (i.e., intake above which a risk for adverse effects exists) was not set for total fat, different types of fatty acids, and cholesterol because no one could establish specific intakes at which adverse events occur. However, the associated negative effects on lipid profiles [e.g., increased low-density lipoprotein (LDL) cholesterol and decreased high-density lipoprotein (HDL) cholesterol] of increasing intakes of dietary saturated and *trans* fatty acids, as well as cholesterol, resulted in the DRI committee recommending that the intakes of these compounds be as low as possible while consuming a nutritionally adequate diet.

***Acceptable Macronutrient Distribution Range (AMDR) for Dietary Fat***

An important distinction between macronutrients and micronutrients is that in addition to supplying nutrients to meet the body's need for specific physiological functions, macronutrients also provide the energy needs of the body. As individual macronutrients can, to some extent, substitute for one another as energy sources and still supply sufficient amounts of required nutrients, a range of intakes exists for carbohydrates, fats, and protein, known as the "acceptable macronutrient distribution range" (AMDR) that is associated with reduced chronic disease (Barr, 2006). The AMDRs in adults are 45–65% of total energy from carbohydrates, 20–35% from fats, and 10%–35% from protein (IOM, 2005). The justification for setting the AMDR for carbohydrate was that below 45% of energy the AI for fiber, which is mainly found in carbohydrate foods, would be difficult to meet. Also, certain other nutrients (i.e., vitamins) would be inadequate at a low-carbohydrate intake. Above 65% of energy as carbohydrate, fat and protein intakes would be too low to meet nutrient needs (e.g., essential fatty acids and indispensable amino acids), and the risk of hypertriglyceridemia is increased (IOM, 2005). In addition to supplying the essential fatty acids, dietary fat is a major source of energy, and assists in the absorption of vitamins and the development of tissues. Along with an AMDR for fat, AMDRs were established for the essential fatty acids at 0.6–1.2% of energy for the ω-3 fatty acids and 5–10% of energy for the ω-6 fatty acids.

The AMDRs differ somewhat from previous guidelines (Health and Welfare Canada, 1990; NRC, 1989) which recommended dietary intakes of 50–55% of energy from carbohydrates and 30% or less from fat. Protein recommendations are essentially unchanged. Therefore, the AMDR ranges are clearly more liberal, thus making them useful for dietary planning and application (Barr, 2006). Any macronutrient needs, including that of fat, of an exercising individual should also fit within these ranges. Since many intervention studies involving macronutrient manipulations result in the consumption of dietary intakes below or above the AMDR, the discussion of such studies in the DRI report is scant. However, when considering exercise performance, the report does suggest that athletes may not be able to train as effectively on short-term intakes (i.e., a few days) of a high-fat diet when compared to a high-carbohydrate diet as endogenous glycogen stores would be depleted. Further, in the report, mention is made that high-fat diets close to 70% of energy did not negatively affect performance in endurance-trained athletes, although this type of dietary pattern would not normally be recommended because it exceeds the AMDR for total fat. Nonetheless, athletes are interested in enhancing performance, and modifying typical dietary intake is frequently used in an attempt to provide an ergogenic effect. In the next part of the chapter, specific intervention studies—in which total fat or the fatty acid composition of the diet is changed to examine the effects on exercise performance—are discussed.

### Dietary Intervention Studies Investigating the Effects of Fat on Exercise Performance

Research recently investigated the effects of fat-loading dietary interventions on endurance performance. "Fat-loading" is defined as increasing the total amount of fat in the diet above 30% of total kilocalories from dietary fat (Erlenbusch et al., 2005). The hypothesis is that fat-loading will increase the utilization of FFAs for energy production during exercise which, in turn, will result in carbohydrate-sparing which may have a performance-enhancing effect. Fat-loading strategies are utilized for research purposes to evaluate whether consuming a high-fat diet will be beneficial for endurance performance. The majority of the research evaluating the effects of fat-loading on endurance performance utilized highly trained individuals (Burke et al., 2000, 2002; Burke & Hawley, 2002; Carey et al., 2001; Coyle et al., 2001; Hawley et al., 2000; Helge et al., 1998; Horvath et al., 2000; Lambert et al., 1994, 2001; Okano et al., 1998; Pitsiladis et al., 1999; Rowlands & Hopkins, 2002a, 2002b; Staudacher et al., 2001; Stepto et al., 2002; Zderic et al., 2004; Zehnder et al., 2006), while limited research evaluated the effects of fat-loading in untrained individuals (Fleming et al, 2003). In the following section, the efficacy of dietary interventions utilizing fat-loading for improving endurance- exercise performance is evaluated.

Early research suggested that the perception of fatigue (exhaustion) was lessened in a 34-km march (6–8 hours of exercise) with a 25-kg backpack when subjects ingested food containing fat (almonds) versus sugar cubes or control (Arieli et al., 1985). A reduction in the respiratory exchange ratio (RER, an indicator of both carbohydrate and fat oxidation) and carbohydrate oxidation with a corresponding increase in fat oxidation and power output was noted in a group of highly trained cyclists consuming a high-fat diet versus a high-carbohydrate diet for 6 days prior to a 4-hour submaximal ergometer test followed by a 1-hour time trial (Carey et al., 2001). Although the study noted some adaptations to metabolism of the fuel source, the results indicated no significant improvement to the performance in the time trial. Untrained men on a high-fat diet (61% of total kilocalories) who performed a battery of exercise tests ($VO_2$max, 2 × 30-second maximal-intensity cycling sprints, and a 45-minute time-trial cycle task) demonstrated increased fat oxidation and rating of perceived exertion with a corresponding decrease in peak-power output and endurance performance when compared to a control diet (Fleming et al., 2003). Helge et al. (1998) demonstrated a lower RER (indicating a higher amount of fat oxidized compared to carbohydrate) in a submaximal-endurance exercise task after 2 and 4 weeks of a high-fat diet, but no difference in time-to-exhaustion when compared to a high-carbohydrate diet in untrained men, suggesting no performance enhancement with high-fat diets in this population. Also, untrained healthy males showed no benefit or detriment from submaximal- and maximal-endurance performances when comparing a low-fat (15% kilocalories from fat), high-fat (55% kilocalories from fat), or "spontaneous" fat (30% kilocalories from fat) diet, suggesting no effect of substrate availability on performance (Pogliaghi & Veicsteinas, 1999). Trained endurance cyclists demonstrated improved time to exhaustion and lowered RER at a moderate submaximal-exercise intensity (60% of $VO_2$max) but no improvement to a high-intensity exercise task (90% of $VO_2$max) after 2 weeks of a high-fat diet (70% of total kilocalories) (Lambert et al., 1994). Zderic et al. (2004) studied the effects of a 2-day high-fat diet (60% of total kilocalories) on submaximal exercise, and found that IMTG stores were higher pre-exercise and that fat oxidation was increased in the high-fat diet. The researchers speculated that the increased IMTG stores were utilized for substrate during the exercise task.

Men randomized to either a high-fat diet (62, 21, and 17% kilocalories from fat, carbohydrate, and protein, respectively) or a high-carbohydrate diet (20, 65, and 15% kilocalories from fat, carbohydrate, and protein, respectively) for 4 weeks were evaluated by a time-to-exhaustion test at a predetermined exercise intensity both before and after the dietary intervention (Helge et al., 1998). Time-to-exhaustion increased similarly in both groups, while RER was decreased in the men on the high-fat diet, suggesting an increased oxidation of fatty acids after adaptation to a high-fat diet. Research supported these data, indicating that moderate-intensity exercise (60% of $VO_2$max) performed after 2 weeks of either a high-fat diet (70 and 7% kilocalories from fat and carbohydrate, respectively) or a high-carbohydrate diet (12 and 74% kilocalories from fat and carbohydrate, respectively) resulted in improved endurance performance and lowered RER values in trained cyclists (Lambert et al., 1994).

Burke et al. (2000) evaluated the effects of either a high-fat diet (2.4 $g \cdot kg^{-1} \cdot d^{-1}$ of carbohydrate, 4.0 $g \cdot kg^{-1} \cdot d^{-1}$ of fat) or a high- carbohydrate diet (9.6 $g \cdot kg^{-1} \cdot d^{-1}$ of carbohydrate, 0.7 $g \cdot kg^{-1} \cdot d^{-1}$ of fat) for 5 days followed by a high-carbohydrate diet on day 6 and a performance test-to-exhaustion on day 7 in well-trained cyclists. During steady-state exercise (70% of $VO_2$max) for 2 hours, the high-fat diet reduced RER, indicating that the amount of fat oxidized increased and carbohydrate oxidation decreased. No significant difference in time-to-exhaustion was noted between dietary groups although the high-carbohydrate diet group performed approximately 3.5 more minutes of exercise when compared to the high-fat diet group.

Improving endurance time-to-exhaustion was also attempted with a single high-fat meal (Okano et al., 1998). In this study, subjects were highly trained, and ingested either a high-fat meal (61, 30, and 9% kilocalories from fat, carbohydrate, and protein, respectively) or a control meal (31, 58, and 11 kilocalories from fat, carbohydrate, and protein, respectively) 4 hours prior to exercise. Subjects exercised at 67% of $VO_2$max for 120 minutes, and then increased intensity to 78% of $VO_2$max until volitional exhaustion. The high-fat meal resulted in a significant increase in plasma FFAs with a corresponding decrease in RER during the first 60 minutes of activity but no improvement in time- to-exhaustion when compared to the control diet. Pitsiladis et al. (1999) performed a similar study, but utilized a 3.5-day carbohydrate-loading regime (70% carbohydrate diet) before an isocaloric single meal of either high fat (90% fat) or high carbohydrate (70% carbohydrate) was ingested by well-trained males. The outcome indicated no difference in RER, volume of oxygen consumed, heart rate, or rating of perceived exertion between the two diets although a significant increase existed in time-to-exhaustion with the high-fat diet, sustaining activity for approximately 10 minutes longer. Interpret this study with caution since the researchers injected heparin into subjects before exercise to stimulate an increased release of FFAs into the plasma.

A recent meta-analysis of the topic concluded that no benefit is given to a performance in untrained individuals who fat load, while a clear benefit is given if they carbohydrate load (Erlenbusch et al., 2005). Further, the meta-analysis concluded that insufficient data are available to determine whether or not fat-loading is ergogenic (i.e., beneficial for performance) for highly trained endurance athletes (Erlenbusch et al., 2005). Since the training state does influence the oxidative abilities of both fat and carbohydrate, the following section briefly reviews this topic in relation to the oxidation of fat during endurance exercise.

***Differences between Trained versus Untrained Individuals in Response to High-fat Diets***

Sedentary individuals do not seem to respond in the same manner to endurance exercise tasks with a dietary manipulation of fat as do highly trained individuals (Pogliaghi & Veicsteinas, 1999). Pogliaghi & Veicsteinas (1999) determined $VO_2max$ and time-to-exhaustion at 75% of $VO_2max$ in a within-subjects design where sedentary males consumed either a low (15%), high (55%), or spontaneous (30%) eucaloric-fat diet for 4 weeks before testing. $VO_2$, RER, or endurance time-to-exhaustion were not different between diets. Further, 6 weeks of a high-fat diet (61% of total kilocalories) increased fat oxidation and the rating of perceived exertion, but decreased peak-power production on a high-intensity exercise task (i.e., Wingate Anaerobic Test) and an endurance-performance task when compared to a control diet in untrained men (Fleming et al., 2003).

Some research does suggest that highly trained individuals possess the ability to maintain or enhance performance with high- fat diets (Horvath et al., 2000; Lambert et al., 1994; Muoio et al., 1994; Venkatraman et al., 2001) although a limitation of this research is that a high-fat diet will lower muscle and liver glycogen stores, which could be detrimental to performance at a higher intensity. Burke and colleagues (Burke et al., 2000, 2002; Burke & Hawley, 2002; Hawley et al., 2000; Lambert et al., 2001) addressed this limitation by performing a series of studies that examined the adaptive effects of a 5–6-day high-fat diet and then a 1-day carbohydrate load, which restored muscle glycogen content, on high-intensity endurance performance in highly trained endurance athletes. The researchers suggest that highly trained athletes are able to adapt to a high-fat diet and maintain performance by increasing the oxidation of fatty acids but that clear evidence is lacking in relationship to enhanced endurance performance in endurance and ultraendurance events (Burke & Hawley, 2002). A recent meta-analysis concluded that untrained subjects lack the metabolic adjustments necessary to enhance FFA oxidation necessary but that future research should continue to investigate the likelihood of a positive effect of a high-fat diet on endurance performance in trained individuals (Erlenbusch et al., 2005). Recent evidence from older men indicates that, with increasing exercise intensity, a corresponding increase occurs in carbohydrate oxidation with no difference in fat oxidation between trained and untrained subjects (Bassami et al., 2007). This suggests that the same metabolic adaptations may not occur in older adults compared to younger adults when evaluating substrate oxidation patterns.

## Dietary Intervention Studies Investigating the Effects of Fatty Acids on Exercise Performance

In addition to the exercise research which studied the effects of varying the amounts of dietary fat on macronutrient utilization and performance, investigations were carried out focusing on the effects that differing types of fatty acids have on exercise performance. Most of these studies concentrated on the dietary essential ω-3 fatty acids (i.e., ALA, EPA, and DHA); however, some examined novel fatty acids, such as conjugated linoleic acid (CLA), as ergogenic aids in aerobic and strength-training exercises.

### *Aerobic Exercise and Fatty Acid Supplementation*

Supplementation with ω-3 fatty acids was hypothesized to enhance aerobic performance by reducing the viscosity of red blood cells and by altering prostaglandin synthesis, resulting in increased vasodilation which will improve oxygen deliverability to working musculature. This hypothesis was tested on highly trained soccer athletes by having the athletes ingest a fish-oil supplement containing 1.6 $g{\cdot}d^{-1}$ of EPA and 1.04 $g{\cdot}d^{-1}$ of DHA or placebo (corn oil) for 10 weeks before and after a maximal aerobic fitness test (Raastad et al., 1997). Although the subjects in the fish-oil group had a significant decrease in TAG at rest, no performance differences were noted between the groups before or after the supplementation period. Also, fish-oil supplementation (50 $mL{\cdot}d^{-1}$) for 12 weeks did not result in an improvement in $VO_2max$ when compared to fish oil combined with aerobic exercise or a control group (Warner et al., 1989). Oostenbrug et al. (1997) found no effects of 3 weeks of fish-oil supplementation (6 $g{\cdot}d^{-1}$) on endurance performance as measured by a cycle ergometer time trial at a prefixed workload before or after supplementation. In accord with the preceding research, Huffman et al. (2004) found no effect on running performance after 4 weeks of supplementation with 300 $mg{\cdot}d^{-1}$ and 200 $mg{\cdot}d^{-1}$ of EPA in recreationally active men and women, respectively. From the available research supplementation with ω-3 fatty acids (EPA and DHA) does not confer any aerobic-exercise ergogenic potential to exercising adults. Future research should consider the effects of ω-3 fatty acid supplementation in other highly trained athletes such as those who compete in sports that predominantly rely on aerobic- energy metabolism such as running, cycling, and triathlons.

***Strength-training Exercise and Fatty Acid Supplementation***

CLA was theorized to act in an ergogenic manner in athletes completing strength-training programs. CLA encompasses a group of 18-carbon PUFA isomers derived from the essential ω-6 fatty acid, LA. CLA is found in the meat and dairy products of ruminant animals. Studies using animal models demonstrated that supplementing with CLA increases lean body mass (Dugan et al., 1997, 1999; Kashiwazaki et al., 1990) and reduces fat mass (Azain et al., 2000; DeLany et al., 1999; Du & Ahn, 2002) possibly through an increase in fatty acid oxidation (Nagao et al., 2003; Ohnuki et al., 2001; West et al., 1998). We recently showed that CLA supplementation (5 $g{\cdot}d^{-1}$) combined with strength training for 7 weeks significantly increased muscle mass and strength, and reduced fat mass over resistance training alone (Pinkoski et al., 2006). Contrary to our results, Kreider et al. (2002) did not demonstrate efficacy with 4 weeks of CLA supplementation (3 $g{\cdot}d^{-1}$) on body composition, strength, or general biochemical markers of catabolism in experienced strength-training athletes. The dose and length of supplementation and the isoform of CLA used were different between the two studies, which may explain the discrepancy in the results. Tarnopolsky et al. (2007a) completed a 6-month intervention of combined CLA (6 $g{\cdot}d^{-1}$) and creatine (5 $g{\cdot}d^{-1}$) supplementation in older adults completing a strength- training program that demonstrated effective increases in muscular endurance and strength as well as a greater improvement in fat-free mass and a greater reduction in fat mass versus placebo. We recently completed a study of supplementation with CLA, creatine, and protein in young strength-trained adults (Cornish et al., 2007). In this study, we randomized subjects to one of three groups that received: protein only, creatine and protein, or CLA, creatine, and protein for 5 weeks while completing a high-volume strength-training program. The results from this research indicate that the addition of CLA to the other two supplements effectively increased strength and hypertrophy while demonstrating some efficacy in reducing markers of myofibrillar protein breakdown (3-methylhistidine) and bone resorption (*N*-telopeptides of cross-linked collagen). The majority of research carried out to date on the combined effects of CLA supplementation and strength training demonstrates some efficacy in promoting strength gains as well as favorable changes in body composition.

Several mechanisms can account for the effects of CLA. When CLA is fed to mice or applied to fat cells, it increases the activity of carnitine palmitoyl transferase, an enzyme involved in transporting fatty acids across the mitochondria so they can be oxidized for energy. CLA also reduces the activity of lipoprotein lipase, an enzyme that breaks down TAG in the blood so they can be stored in fat tissue. This enzyme promotes fat storage. CLA therefore increases enzymes involved in fat breakdown and decreases enzymes involved in fat storage (Park et al., 1997).

In animal models, CLA seems to stimulate energy expenditure and reduce energy intake (West et al., 1998). CLA may increase the activity of "uncoupling proteins" in the mitochondria of animals, proteins that allow the dissipation of energy as heat instead of being directed toward producing ATP (Ryder et al., 2001). CLA influences a protein called PPAR which controls energy metabolism and determines whether cells are stimulated to divide and develop or die. Through its action on PPAR, CLA may influence metabolism and decrease the proliferation and development of fat cells (Brown et al., 2003). Finally, CLA may influence muscle mass by reducing inflammation, which is sometimes involved in the breakdown of muscle tissue. CLA interferes with the metabolism of other fatty acids (i.e., AA) involved in the formation of inflammatory proteins (Iwakiri et al., 2002). This might account for the reduced muscle-protein breakdown and increased muscle mass and strength in individuals consuming CLA during a resistance-training program (Pinkoski et al., 2006).

Inflammation was implicated as one contributor to the etiology of sarcopenia (i.e., the loss of muscle mass during aging) (Dirks & Leeuwenburgh, 2006; Pistilli et al., 2006). Increasing the exogenous consumption of ALA (18:3ω-3), with the associated increase in EPA, will reduce inflammation by competing for the same enzymatic pathways (cyclooxygenase and 5-lipoxygenase) as AA (a major ω-6 fatty acid), and will decrease the more potent pro-inflammatory eicosanoids (such as the 2-series prostaglandins and thromboxanes and 4-series leukotrienes) produced during an inflammatory reaction with a corresponding decrease in inflammatory cytokines such as tumor necrosis factor alpha (TNF-α) and interleukin-6 (IL-6) (Pedersen et al., 2000). We recently completed research (Cornish & Chilibeck, 2008) to examine the effect of 12 weeks of ALA (14 $g{\cdot}d^{-1}$) supplementation (from flaxseed oil) on TNF-α and IL-6 and measures of strength in older adults completing a strength-training program. Results demonstrated efficacy in lowering the IL-6 concentration in older men supplementing with ALA, with no difference in women supplementing with ALA compared to placebo (corn oil), but no greater improvement in strength, muscle size, or lean tissue mass when comparing the ALA to the placebo group.

## Conclusion

This chapter reviewed the effects of altering dietary-fat amounts on exercise performance in a variety of populations. As concluded, increasing dietary-fat consumption above the AMDR for fat consumption (i.e., above 35% of the dietary kilocalories from fat) will result in a detriment to exercise performance in untrained individuals. Also, highly trained individuals likely will not benefit in terms of exercise performance from fat-loading, but no negative effect of fat-loading is noted on exercise performance as long as carbohydrate stores are replenished after a fat-loading protocol. Participating in a structured exercise program of sufficient intensity and duration will stimulate an increase in the ability of the human body to oxidize fats as a fuel source which may lead to a beneficial effect on performance or may benefit health. Supplementing with specific fatty acids, such as CLA, while completing structured strength training seems to impart health benefits above and beyond strength training alone (i.e., an increase in overall strength and improvement in body composition). More research on combining the interventions of supplementation with various fatty acids and exercise training is warranted as additive or synergistic effects on health or exercise performance may result.

## References

Achten, J.; M. Gleeson; A.E. Jeukendrup. Determination of the exercise intensity that elicits maximal fat oxidation. *Med. Sci. Sports Exerc.* **2002**, *34*, 92–97.

Achten, J.; A.E. Jeukendrup. The effect of pre-exercise carbohydrate feedings on the intensity that elicits maximal fat oxidation. *J. Sports Sci.* **2003**, *21*, 1017–1024.

Arieli, A.; Y. Epstein; S. Brill; M. Winer; Y. Shapiro. Effect of food intake on exercise fatigue in trained and untrained subjects. *Eur. J. Appl. Physiol. Occup. Physiol.* **1985**, *54*, 297–300.

Azain, M.J.; D.B. Hausman; M.B. Sisk; W.P. Flatt; D.E. Jewell. Dietary conjugated linoleic acid reduces rat adipose tissue cell size rather than cell number. *J. Nutr.* **2000**, *130*, 1548–1554.

Barr, S.I. Introduction to dietary reference intakes. *Appl. Physiol. Nutr. Metab.* **2006**, *31*, 61–65.

Bassami, M.; S. Ahmadizad; D. Doran; D.P. Maclaren. Effects of exercise intensity and duration on fat metabolism in trained and untrained older males. *Eur. J. Appl. Physiol.* **2007**, *101*, 525–532.

Brown, J.M.; M.S. Boysen; S.S. Jensen; R.F. Morrison; J. Storkson; R. Lea-Currie; M. Pariza; S. Mandrup; M.K. McIntosh. Isomer-specific regulation of metabolism and PPARgamma signaling by CLA in human preadipocytes. *J. Lipid Res.* **2003**, *44*, 1287–1300.

Burdge, G. Alpha-linolenic acid metabolism in men and women: nutritional and biological implications. *Curr. Opin. Clin. Nutr. Metab. Care* **2004**, *7*, 137–144.

Burgomaster, K.A.; K.R. Howarth; S.M. Phillips; M. Rakobowchuk; M.J. Macdonald; S.L. McGee; M.J. Gibala. Similar metabolic adaptations during exercise after low volume sprint interval and traditional endurance training in humans. *J. Physiol.* **2008**, *586*, 151–160.

Burke, L.M.; D.J. Angus; G.R. Cox; N.K. Cummings; M.A. Febbraio; K. Gawthorn; J.A. Hawley; M. Minehan; D.T. Martin; M. Hargreaves. Effect of fat adaptation and carbohydrate restoration on metabolism and performance during prolonged cycling. *J. Appl. Physiol.* **2000**, *89*, 2413–2421.

Burke, L.M.; J.A. Hawley. Effects of short-term fat adaptation on metabolism and performance of prolonged exercise. *Med. Sci. Sports Exerc.* **2002**, *34*, 1492–1498.

Burke, L.M.; J.A. Hawley; D.J. Angus; G.R. Cox; S.A. Clark; N.K. Cummings; B. Desbrow; M. Hargreaves. Adaptations to short-term high-fat diet persist during exercise despite high carbohydrate availability. *Med. Sci. Sports Exerc.* **2002**, *34*, 83–91.

Carey, A.L.; H.M. Staudacher; N.K. Cummings; N.K. Stepto; V. Nikolopoulos; L.M. Burke; J.A. Hawley. Effects of fat adaptation and carbohydrate restoration on prolonged endurance exercise. *J. Appl. Physiol.* **2001**, *91*, 115–122.

Chilibeck, P.D.; G.J. Bell; R.P. Farrar; T.P. Martin. Higher mitochondrial fatty acid oxidation following intermittent versus continuous endurance exercise training. *Can. J. Physiol. Pharmacol.* **1998**, *76*, 891–894.

Chilibeck, P.D.; K.S. Davison; S.J. Whiting; Y. Suzuki; C.L. Janzen; P. Peloso. The effect of strength training combined with bisphosphonate (etidronate) therapy on bone mineral, lean tissue, and fat mass in postmenopausal women. *Can. J. Physiol. Pharmacol.* **2002**, *80*, 941–950.

Cornish, S.M.; D.G. Candow; P.D. Chilibeck; N.T. Jantz; K. Jones; S. Forbes; J.P. Little. Effect of supplementing with conjugated linoleic acid, creatine monohydrate, and whey protein during high intensity resistance training in young adults. *Appl. Physiol. Nutr. Metab.* **2007**, *32(Suppl.*

*S1)*. S21.

Cornish, S.M.; P.D. Chilibeck. Effects of alpha-linolenic acid supplementation on cytokines during resistance training in older adults. *Med. Sci. Sports Exerc.* **2008**, *40*, Supplement: S402.

Coyle, E.F.; A.E. Jeukendrup; M.C. Oseto; B.J. Hodgkinson; T.W. Zderic. Low-fat diet alters intramuscular substrates and reduces lipolysis and fat oxidation during exercise. *Am. J. Physiol. Endocrinol. Metab.* **2001**, *280*, E391–398.

DeLany, J.P.; F. Blohm; A.A. Truett; J.A. Scimeca; D.B. West. Conjugated linoleic acid rapidly reduces body fat content in mice without affecting energy intake. *Am. J. Physiol.* **1999**, *276*, R1172–1179.

Devries, M.C.; M.J. Hamadeh; S.M. Phillips; M.A. Tarnopolsky. Menstrual cycle phase and sex influence muscle glycogen utilization and glucose turnover during moderate-intensity endurance exercise. *Am. J. Physiol.* **2006**, *291*, R1120–1128.

Dirks, A.J.; C. Leeuwenburgh. Tumor necrosis factor alpha signaling in skeletal muscle: effects of age and caloric restriction. *J. Nutr. Biochem.* **2006**, *17*, 501–508.

Du, M.; D.U. Ahn. Effect of dietary conjugated linoleic acid on the growth rate of live birds and on the abdominal fat content and quality of broiler meat. *Poult. Sci.* **2002**, *81*, 428–433.

Dugan, M.; J. Aalhus; L. Jeremiah; J. Kramer; A. Schaefer. The effects of feeding conjugated linoleic acid on subsequent pork quality. *Can. J. Animal Sci.* **1999**, *79*, 45–51.

Dugan, M.; J. Aalhus; A. Schaefer; J. Kramer. The effect of feeding conjugated linoleic acid on fat to lean repartitioning and feed conversion in pigs. *Can. J. Animal Sci.* **1997**, *77*, 723–725.

Erlenbusch, M.; M. Haub; K. Munoz; S. MacConnie; B. Stillwell. Effect of high-fat or high-carbohydrate diets on endurance exercise: a meta-analysis. *Int. J. Sport Nutr. Exerc. Metab.* **2005**, *15*, 1–14.

Fleming, J.; M.J. Sharman; N.G. Avery; D.M. Love; A.L. Gomez; T.P. Scheett; W.J. Kraemer; J.S. Volek. Endurance capacity and high-intensity exercise performance responses to a high fat diet. *Int. J. Sport Nutr. Exerc. Metab.* **2003**, *13*, 466–478.

Hamadeh, M.J.; M.C. Devries; M.A. Tarnopolsky. Estrogen supplementation reduces whole body leucine and carbohydrate oxidation and increases lipid oxidation in men during endurance exercise. *J. Clin. Endocrinol. Metab.* **2005**, *90*, 3592–3599.

Hawley, J.A.; L.M. Burke; D.J. Angus; K.E. Fallon; D.T. Martin; M.A. Febbraio. Effect of altering substrate availability on metabolism and performance during intense exercise. *Br. J. Nutr.* **2000**, *84*, 829–838.

Health and Welfare Canada. *Nutrition recommendations: The report of the scientific review committee;* Health and Welfare Canada: Ottawa, Ontario, 1990.

Helge, J.W.; T.O. Biba; H. Galbo; M. Gaster; M. Donsmark. Muscle triacylglycerol and hormone-sensitive lipase activity in untrained and trained human muscles. *Eur. J. Appl. Physiol.* **2006**, *97*, 566–572.

Helge, J.W.; B. Wulff; B. Kiens. Impact of a fat-rich diet on endurance in man: role of the dietary period. *Med. Sci. Sports Exerc.***1998**, *30*, 456–461.

Henriksson, J. Effects of physical training on the metabolism of skeletal muscle. *Diabetes Care* **1992**, *15*, 1701–1711.

Horvath, P.J.; C.K. Eagen; S.D. Ryer-Calvin; D.R. Pendergast. The effects of varying dietary fat on the nutrient intake in male and female runners. *J. Am. Coll. Nutr.* **2000**, *19*, 42–51.

Huffman, D.M.; T.S. Altena; T.P. Mawhinney; T.R. Thomas. Effect of n-3 fatty acids on free tryptophan and exercise fatigue. *Eur. J. Appl. Physiol.* **2004**, *92*, 584–591.

Institute of Medicine. *Dietary Reference Intakes for Energy, Carbohydrate, Fiber, Fat, Fatty Acids, Cholesterol, Protein, and Amino Acids;* National Academies Press: Washington, D.C., 2005.

Iwakiri, Y.; D.A. Sampson; K.G. Allen. Suppression of cyclooxygenase-2 and inducible nitric oxide synthase expression by conjugated linoleic acid in murine macrophages. *Prostaglandins, Leukotrienes Essent. Fatty Acids* **2002**, *67*, 435–443.

Kashiwazaki, H.; Y. Dejima; T. Suzuki. Influence of upper and lower thermoneutral room temperatures (20 degrees C and 25 degrees C) on fasting and post-prandial resting metabolism under different outdoor temperatures. *Eur. J. Clin. Nutr.* **1990**, *44*, 405–413.

Kreider, R.B.; M.P. Ferreira; M. Greenwood; M. Wilson; A.L. Almada. Effects of conjugated linoleic acid supplementation during resistance training on body composition, bone density, strength, and selected hematological markers. *J. Strength Cond. Res.* **2002**, *16*, 325–334.

Lambert, E.V.; J.H. Goedecke; C. Zyle; K. Murphy; J.A. Hawley; S.C. Dennis; T.D. Noakes. High-fat diet versus habitual diet prior to carbohydrate loading: effects of exercise metabolism and cycling performance. *Int. J. Sport Nutr. Exerc. Metab.* **2001**, *11*, 209–225.

Lambert, E.V.; D.P. Speechly; S.C. Dennis; T.D. Noakes. Enhanced endurance in trained cyclists during moderate intensity exercise following 2 weeks adaptation to a high fat diet. *Eur. J. Appl. Physiol. Occup. Physiol.* **1994**, *69*, 287–293.

Meyer, T.; H.H. Gabriel; M. Auracher; J. Scharhag; W. Kindermann. Metabolic profile of 4 h cycling in the field with varying amounts of carbohydrate supply. *Eur. J. Appl. Physiol.* **2003**, *88*, 431–437.

Muoio, D.M.; J.J. Leddy; P.J. Horvath; A.B. Awad; D.R. Pendergast. Effect of dietary fat on metabolic adjustments to maximal VO2 and endurance in runners. *Med. Sci. Sports Exerc.* **1994**, *26*, 81–88.

Nagao, K.; Y.M. Wang; N. Inoue; S.Y. Han; Y. Buang; T. Noda; N. Kouda; H. Okamatsu; T. Yanagita. The 10trans, 12cis isomer of conjugated linoleic acid promotes energy metabolism in OLETF rats. *Nutrition* **2003**, *19*, 652–656.

National Research Council. *Recommended Dietary Allowances,* 10th ed; National Academies Press: Washington, D.C., 1989.

Ohnuki, K.; S. Haramizu; K. Ishihara; T. Fushiki. Increased energy metabolism and suppressed body fat accumulation in mice by a low concentration of conjugated linoleic acid. *Biosci. Biotechnol. Biochem.* **2001**, *65*, 2200–2204.

Okano, G.; Y. Sato; Y. Murata. Effect of elevated blood FFA levels on endurance performance after a single fat meal ingestion. *Med. Sci. Sports Exerc.* **1998**, *30*, 763–768.

Oostenbrug, G.S.; R.P. Mensink; M.R. Hardeman; T. De Vries; F. Brouns; G. Hornstra. Exercise performance, red blood cell deformability, and lipid peroxidation: effects of fish oil and vitamin E. *J. Appl. Physiol.* **1997**, *83*, 746–752.

Park, Y.; K.J. Albright; W. Liu; J.M. Storkson; M.E. Cook; M.W. Pariza. Effect of conjugated linoleic acid on body composition in mice. *Lipids* **1997**, *32*, 853–858.

Pedersen, B.K.; H. Bruunsgaard; K. Ostrowski; K. Krabbe; H. Hansen; K. Krzywkowski; A. Toft; S.R. Sondergaard; E.W. Petersen; T. Ibfelt; P. Schjerling. Cytokines in aging and exercise. *Int. J. Sports Med.* **2000**, *21( Suppl. 1)*, S4–9.

Pinkoski, C.; P.D. Chilibeck; D.G. Candow; D. Esliger; J.B. Ewaschuk; M. Facci; J.P. Farthing; G.A. Zello. The effects of conjugated linoleic acid supplementation during resistance training. *Med. Sci. Sports Exerc.* **2006**, *38*, 339–348.

Pistilli, E.E.; J.R. Jackson; S.E. Alway. Death receptor-associated pro-apoptotic signaling in aged skeletal muscle. *Apoptosis* **2006**, *11*, 2115–2126.

Pitsiladis, Y.P.; I. Smith; R.J. Maughan. Increased fat availability enhances the capacity of trained individuals to perform prolonged exercise. *Med. Sci. Sports Exerc.***1999**, *31*, 1570–1579.

Pogliaghi, S.; A. Veicsteinas. Influence of low and high dietary fat on physical performance in untrained males. *Med. Sci. Sports Exerc.* **1999**, *31*, 149–155.

Raastad, T.; A.T. Hostmark; S.B. Stromme. Omega-3 fatty acid supplementation does not improve maximal aerobic power, anaerobic threshold and running performance in well-trained soccer players. *Scand. J. Med. Sci. Sports* **1997**, *7*, 25–31.

Roepstorff, C.; M. Donsmark; M. Thiele; B. Vistisen; G. Stewart; K. Vissing; P. Schjerling; D.G. Hardie; H. Galbo; B. Kiens. Sex differences in hormone-sensitive lipase expression, activity, and phosphorylation in skeletal muscle at rest and during exercise. *Am. J. Physiol. Endocrinol. Metab.* **2006a**, *291*, E1106–1114.

Roepstorff, C.; M. Thiele; T. Hillig; H. Pilegaard; E.A. Richter; J.F. Wojtaszewski; B. Kiens. Higher skeletal muscle alpha2AMPK activation and lower energy charge and fat oxidation in men than in women during submaximal exercise. *J. Physiol.* **2006b**, *574*, 125–138.

Romijn, J.A.; E.F. Coyle; L.S. Sidossis; A. Gastaldelli; J.F. Horowitz; E. Endert; R.R. Wolfe. Regulation of endogenous fat and carbohydrate metabolism in relation to exercise intensity and duration. *Am. J. Physiol.* **1993**, *265*, E380–391.

Romijn, J.A.; E.F. Coyle; L.S. Sidossis; J. Rosenblatt; R.R. Wolfe. Substrate metabolism during different exercise intensities in endurance-trained women. *J. Appl. Physiol.* **2000**, *88*, 1707–1714.

Rowlands, D.S.; W.G. Hopkins. Effect of high-fat, high-carbohydrate, and high-protein meals on metabolism and performance during endurance cycling. *Int. J. Sport Nutr. Exerc. Metab.* **2002a**, *12*, 318–335.

Rowlands, D.S.; W.G. Hopkins. Effects of high-fat and high-carbohydrate diets on metabolism and performance in cycling. *Metabolism* **2002b**, *51*, 678–690.

Ryder, J.W.; C.P. Portocarrero; X.M. Song; L. Cui; M. Yu; T. Combatsiaris; D. Galuska; D.E. Bauman; D.M. Barbano; M.J. Charron; J.R. Zierath; K.L. Houseknecht. Isomer-specific antidiabetic properties of conjugated linoleic acid. Improved glucose tolerance, skeletal muscle insulin action, and UCP-2 gene expression. *Diabetes* **2001**, *50*, 1149–1157.

Schrauwen, P.; F.J. Troost; J. Xia; E. Ravussin; W.H. Saris. Skeletal muscle UCP2 and UCP3 expression in trained and untrained male subjects. *Int. J. Obes. Relat. Metab. Disord.* **1999**, *23*, 966–972.

Speechly, D.P.; S.R. Taylor; G.G. Rogers. Differences in ultra-endurance exercise in performance-matched male and female runners. *Med. Sci. Sports Exerc.* **1996**, *28*, 359–365.

Spriet, L.L. Regulation of skeletal muscle fat oxidation during exercise in humans. *Med. Sci. Sports Exerc.* **2002**, *34*, 1477–1484.

Staudacher, H.M.; A.L. Carey; N.K. Cummings; J.A. Hawley; L.M. Burke. Short-term high-fat diet alters substrate utilization during exercise but not glucose tolerance in highly trained athletes. *Int. J. Sport Nutr. Exerc. Metab.* **2001**, *11*, 273–286.

Stepto, N.K.; A.L. Carey; H.M. Staudacher; N.K. Cummings; L.M. Burke; J.A. Hawley. Effect of short-term fat adaptation on high-intensity training. *Med. Sci. Sports Exerc.* **2002**, *34*, 449–455.

Stisen, A.B.; O. Stougaard; J. Langfort; J.W. Helge; K. Sahlin; K. Madsen. Maximal fat oxidation rates in endurance trained and untrained women. *Eur. J. Appl. Physiol.* **2006**, *98*, 497–506.

Talanian, J.L.; S.D. Galloway; G.J. Heigenhauser; A. Bonen; L.L. Spriet. Two weeks of high-intensity aerobic interval training increases the capacity for fat oxidation during exercise in women. *J. Appl. Physiol.* **2007**, *102*, 1439–1447.

Tarnopolsky, L.J.; J.D. MacDougall; S.A. Atkinson; M.A. Tarnopolsky; J.R. Sutton. Gender differences in substrate for endurance exercise. *J. Appl. Physiol.* **1990**, *68*, 302–308.

Tarnopolsky, M.A.; C.D. Rennie; H.A. Robertshaw; S.N. Fedak-Tarnopolsky; M.C. Devries; M.J. Hamadeh. Influence of endurance exercise training and sex on intramyocellular lipid and mitochondrial ultrastructure, substrate use, and mitochondrial enzyme activity. *Am. J. Physiol.* **2007b**, *292*, R1271–1278.

Tarnopolsky, M.; A. Zimmer; J. Paikin; A. Safdar; A. Aboud; E. Pearce; B. Roy; T. Doherty. Creatine monohydrate and conjugated linoleic acid improve strength and body composition following resistance exercise in older adults. *PLoS ONE* **2007a**, *2*, e991.

Tremblay, A.; J.A. Simoneau; C. Bouchard. Impact of exercise intensity on body fatness and skeletal muscle metabolism. *Metabolism* **1994**, *43*, 814–818.

Tunstall, R.J.; K.A. Mehan; G.D. Wadley; G.R. Collier; A. Bonen; M. Hargreaves; D. Cameron-Smith. Exercise training increases lipid metabolism gene expression in human skeletal muscle. *Am. J. Physiol. Endocrinol. Metab.* **2002**, *283*, E66–72.

van Loon, L.J. Use of intramuscular triacylglycerol as a substrate source during exercise in humans. *J. Appl. Physiol.* **2004**, *97*, 1170–1187.

Venkatraman, J.T.; X. Feng; D. Pendergast. Effects of dietary fat and endurance exercise on plasma cortisol, prostaglandin E2, interferon-gamma and lipid peroxides in runners. *J. Am. Coll. Nutr.* **2001**, *20*, 529–536.

Warner, J.G., Jr.; I.H. Ullrich; M.J. Albrink; R.A. Yeater. Combined effects of aerobic exercise and omega-3 fatty acids in hyperlipidemic persons. *Med. Sci. Sports Exerc.* **1989**, *21*, 498–505.

West, D.B.; J.P. Delany; P.M. Camet; F. Blohm; A.A. Truett; J. Scimeca. Effects of conjugated linoleic acid on body fat and energy metabolism in the mouse. *Am. J. Physiol.* **1998**, *275*, R667–672.

Zderic, T.W.; A.R. Coggan; B.C. Ruby. Glucose kinetics and substrate oxidation during exercise in the follicular and luteal phases. *J. Appl. Physiol.* **2001**, *90*, 447–453.

Zderic, T.W.; C.J. Davidson; S. Schenk; L.O. Byerley; E.F. Coyle. High-fat diet elevates resting intramuscular triglyceride concentration and whole body lipolysis during exercise. *Am. J. Physiol. Endocrinol. Metab.* **2004**, *286*, E217–225.

Zehnder, M.; E.R. Christ; M. Ith; K.J. Acheson; E. Pouteau; R. Kreis; R. Trepp; P. Diem; C.

Boesch; J. Decombaz. Intramyocellular lipid stores increase markedly in athletes after 1.5 days lipid supplementation and are utilized during exercise in proportion to their content. *Eur. J. Appl. Physiol.* **2006**, *98*, 341–354.

Zello, G.A. Dietary Reference Intakes for the macronutrients and energy: considerations for physical activity. *Appl. Physiol. Nutr. Metab.* **2006**, *31*, 74–79.

Zinker, B.A.; K. Britz; G.A. Brooks. Effects of a 36-hour fast on human endurance and substrate utilization. *J. Appl. Physiol.* **1990**, *69*, 1849–1855.

# 29

# Omega-3 versus Omega-6 Fatty Acid Intake and Immunity

**Gabriel Keith Harris**
*Assistant Professor, North Carolina State University, Department of Food, Bioprocessing, and Nutrition Science, Campus Box 7624, Raleigh, NC 27695-7624*

## Introduction

### *Omega-3 and Omega-6 Fatty Acids*

Omega-3 and omega-6 fatty acids are important components of a human's diet, both as essential nutrients and as potential mediators of immunity. In recent years, omega-3 fatty acids have become popular in three areas: (i) as natural components of oily fish (e.g., salmon) or of oilseeds (e.g., flax and soy); (ii) as additives to foods, ranging from baby formula to orange juice and ice cream; and (iii) as supplements for the prevention of chronic diseases. Various beneficial properties have been reported for omega-3 fatty acids, including anti-inflammatory, anti-hypertensive, and anti-allergenic effects (Calder, 2001; Dunstan et al., 2003). The omega-3 fatty acids eicosapentaenoic acid (EPA) and docosahexaenoic acid (DHA) have gained particular notoriety. In 2004, a Qualified Health Claim was approved for EPA and DHA for the reduction of the risk for coronary heart disease (FDA, 2008). In addition, DHA and the omega-6 fatty acid arachidonate are now commonly used as ingredients in infant formula to mimic the fatty acid composition and the developmental benefits of human breast milk.

Omega-6 fatty acids are now viewed somewhat negatively since they contribute to inflammation and to the etiology of chronic diseases in Western societies, where their consumption levels are high. What appears to be missing from public perception, however, is the importance of establishing an appropriate balance between both omega-3 and omega-6 fatty acid consumption for the maintenance of appropriate immune responses. Arachidonic acid (AA), an omega-6 fatty acid stored in cell membranes, is a source of many pro-inflammatory mediators, but it is also involved in normal, "healthy" immune function. Over time, the omega-3:omega-6 ratio has decreased in Western diets, leading to speculation that this might result in dysfunctional immune responses and an increased chronic-disease risk.

This chapter examines the roles of omega-3 and omega-6 fatty acids in immunity by first considering dietary and supplemental sources, then fatty acid metabolism, and finally, the roles of these fatty acids in immune function in health and disease. With regard to immunity, we will consider these key questions:

- How are omega-3 and omega-6 fatty acids metabolized differently to form unique mediators of immunity?
- What is the current scientific understanding of the effects of omega-3 and omega-6 fatty acids on immunity?
- Can the consumption of the appropriate types and levels of fatty acids affect immune function in healthy adults?
- Can omega-3 fatty acids affect immunity in either an inflammatory or an immune-suppressed disease state?

***Description and Dietary Sources***

Before we begin to discuss the dietary sources of omega-3 and omega-6 fatty acids, we must define these terms. Parts A, B, and C of Fig. 29.1 show the basic structure of a saturated fatty acid, an omega-3 unsaturated fatty acid, and an omega-6 unsaturated fatty acid, respectively. Horizontal arrows indicate that the fatty acids vary in the number of carbons they contain. All fatty acids have two ends, designated alpha and omega. The alpha end terminates with a carboxylic-acid group. The omega end terminates in a methyl group. Omega-3 and omega-6 fatty acids, also referred to as n-3 and n-6 fatty acids, are unsaturated, that is, their carbon chain is interrupted by double bonds, as indicated by the vertical arrows in parts B and C of Fig. 29.1.

The difference between the omega-3 (Fig. 29.1B) and omega-6 (Fig. 29.1C) fatty acids is the placement of the double bond closer to the methyl (omega) end of the fatty acid. Omega-3 fatty acids have double bonds situated three carbons from the methyl end. In omega-6 fatty acids, the first double bond is located six carbons from the methyl end. The differences in biological effects between omega-3 and omega-6 fatty acids are driven by this difference in structure.

Two fatty acids, alpha-linolenic acid (ALA) and linoleic acid (LA) (Fig. 29.2, A and B, respectively), are considered essential for humans for two reasons: (i) they serve as precursors to important signaling molecules and (ii) the body cannot synthesize them from other nutrients. Both of these fatty acids contain 18 carbons. ALA is an omega-3 fatty acid with 3 double bonds, while LA is an omega-6 fatty acid with 2 double bonds. ALA is a precursor of both DHA and EPA, while LA is a precursor of AA.

Although diet and food-consumption patterns vary considerably worldwide, omega-3 fatty acids represent a smaller proportion of the total dietary fat than omega-6 fatty acids. Table 29.1 shows major dietary sources of omega-3 and omega-6

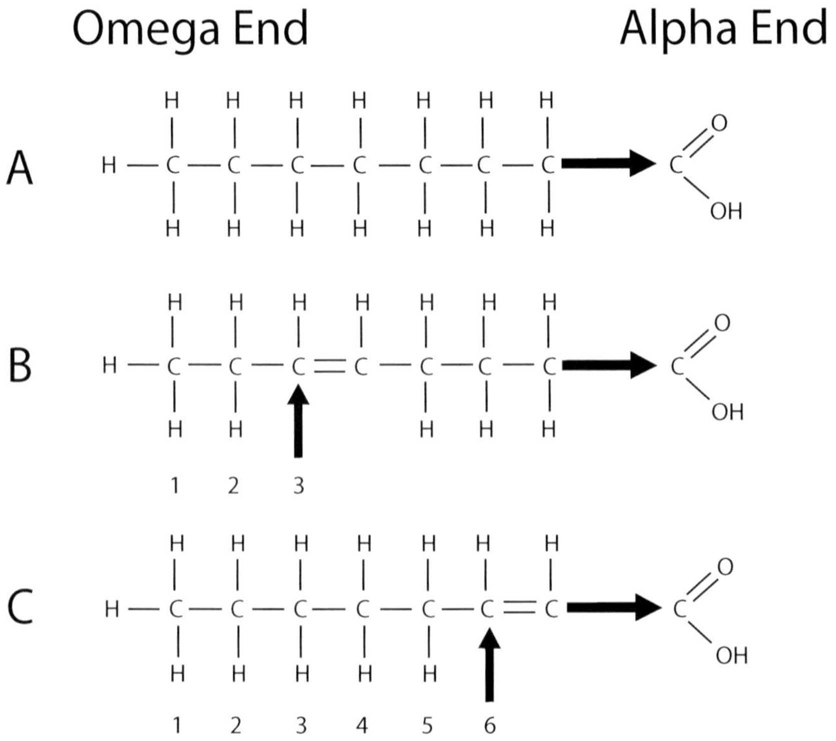


**Fig. 29.1.** Structural comparison of saturated (A), omega-3 (B), and omega-6 (C) fatty acids.

fatty acids. Notice that numerous foods common in Western diets, including meat, dairy, and soybean oil, are sources of omega-6 fatty acids.

In Western societies where fish consumption is low, estimates of the ratio of omega-3 to omega-6 fatty acids vary between 1:7 and 1:50 (Calder, 2001). In Japan, Iceland, and other countries where fish consumption is high, omega-3's represent a larger part of the total fat intake, so that the omega-3:omega-6 ratio may be as high as 1:2 (Caramia, 2008; Olafsdottir et al., 2006). Differences in the consumption levels of omega-3 fatty acids change the fatty acid composition of cell membranes. Since cell membranes serve as reservoirs for the formation of products with profound immune effects, these changes may have important health implications, as reflected in a study by Yamagashi et al. (2008), This was a prospective Japanese study that surveyed 57,972 men and women about their fish-consumption habits over 12.7 years, and reported an 18–19% reduction in cardiovascular-disease mortality in those that consumed the most fish as opposed to those that consumed the least fish. On the basis of eight epidemiological studies and two clinical trials, the Food and Drug Administration (FDA) concluded in 2004 that "supportive, but not conclusive" research indicates that the consumption of the omega-3 fatty acids EPA and DHA may reduce heart-disease risk, and allowed for a Qualified Health Claim on this basis (FDA, 2008).

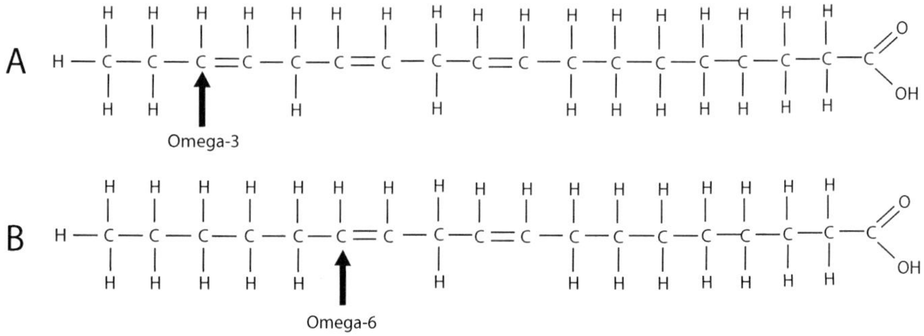


**Fig. 29.2**. Alpha-linolenic (ALA; A) and linoleic acid (LA; B) structures.

**Table 29.1. Dietary and Supplementary Sources of Omega-3 and Omega-6 Fatty Acids**

| Fatty acid types | Major sources |
|---|---|
| Omega-3 fatty acids | |
| Alpha-linolenic acid (C18:2) | Flaxseed, walnut, canola, and soybean oils; flaxseed; English walnuts |
| Eicosapentaenoic acid (C20:5) Docosahexaenoic acid (C22:6) | Salmon, sardines, herring, trout, oysters, fish-oil and algae-derived supplements |
| Docosapentaenoic acid (C22:5) | Fish oils and red meat |
| Omega-6 fatty acids | |
| Linoleic acid (C18:3) | Sunflower, safflower, corn, and soybean oils |
| Gamma-linolenic acid (C18:3) | Evening primrose, black currant, and borage oils |
| Arachidonic acid (C20:4) | Meat, poultry, eggs, milk products |

Sources: Howe et al. (2006); Institute of Medicine (2006); Kris-Etherton et al., (2002).

### *Metabolism*

When consumed in the diet, the essential omega-3 fatty acid ALA and the essential omega-6 fatty acid LA are converted to a variety of lipid products via shared desaturase and elongase enzymes. These enzymes serve to insert double bonds and to extend fatty acid chain length by two carbons, respectively. Fig. 29.3 shows a summary of these metabolic pathways.

Since omega-3 and omega-6 fatty acids compete for the same enzymes, changing the omega-3:omega-6 ratio can also result in changes in the relative quantities of metabolites that are formed. As shown in Fig. 29.3, ALA can be converted to EPA and DHA, but this conversion is inefficient, partly due to the body's use of ALA and pathway intermediates as energy sources, and partly due to the inefficiency of the enzymes themselves. Estimates vary, but the conversion of ALA to EPA and DHA in men ranges from 0.2% to 6.0% (Burdge, 2006). For this reason, the

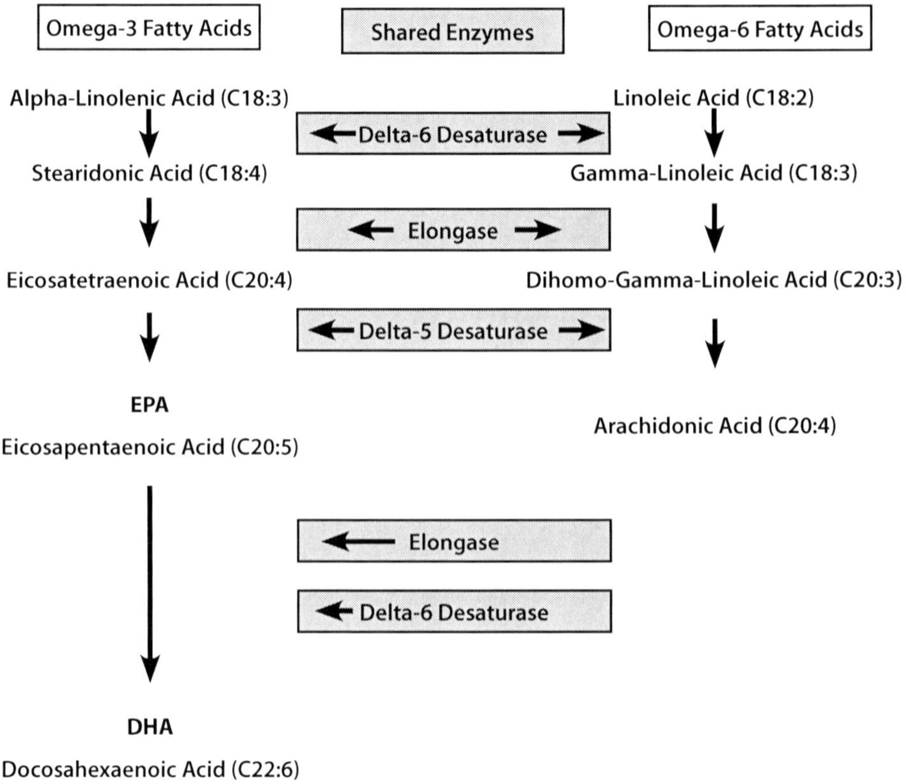


**Fig. 29.3.** Omega-3 and omega-6 fatty acids: common metabolic pathways.

direct consumption of EPA and DHA in fatty fish or of fish-oil- or algae-derived supplements is more effective for increasing their concentration in the body than is the consumption of ALA. A recent study by Welch et al. (2008) reported that this conversion is more efficient in nonfish consumers than in fish consumers.

Both intermediates and end products of omega-3 and omega-6 metabolism can serve as substrates for the formation of biologically active compounds via the action of cyclooxygenase, monooxygenase, lipooxygenase, and other enzymes (Table 29.2).

What are the mechanisms by which omega-3 fatty acids exert their immune effects? Based on current literature, we can divide these mechanisms into two broad categories: direct and indirect. Direct effects refer to the biological activity of the fatty acids themselves. These effects include modulating cell-membrane fluidity, signal transduction, glucose metabolism, and serving as receptor ligands (Pompeia et al., 2000; Shaikh & Edidin, 2006; Wendel et al., 2007). Indirect effects are those produced by omega-3 and omega-6 metabolites. Table 29.3 provides a general summary of these indirect effects.

**Table 29.2. Products of Omega-3 and Omega-6 Fatty Acids**

| Fatty acid precursors | Metabolites |
|---|---|
| Omega-3 fatty acids | |
| EPA | 3-Series prostaglandins and thromboxanes 5-series leukotrienes, resolvins |
| DHA | Resolvins neuroprotectins |
| Omega-6 fatty acids Dihomo-gamma-linolenic acid | 1-Series prostaglandins and thromboxanes |
| Arachidonic acid | 2-Series prostaglandins and thromboxanes, 4-series leukotrienes |

Sources: Aterburn et al. (2006); Kidd (2007).

Two products of the omega-3 metabolic pathway, EPA and DHA, serve as substrates for the formation of a variety of products, including prostaglandins, thromboxanes, leukotrienes, and resolvins. The overall effect of these omega-3 metabolites is to dampen inflammation and immune responses. Likewise, two products of the omega-6 pathway, dihomo-gamma-linolenic acid (DGLA) and AA, serve as substrates for the formation of similar types of metabolites. Like omega-3 metabolites, the prostaglandins and thromboxanes formed from DGLA generally have anti-inflammatory properties. In contrast, the metabolites of AA tend to promote enhanced immune responses and inflammation. One should note that some components of these pathways, such as Prostaglandin $E_2$, have both pro- and anti-inflammatory activities (Calder, 2006). Overall, the impression is one of a complex system of checks and balances.

***Immune Effects***

Since omega-3 fatty acid intake is generally low compared to omega-6 intake, most human studies examining the effects of these fatty acids on immunity have focused on increasing omega-3 intake via dietary supplements. Increased omega-3 fatty acid consumption affects human immunity in both healthy and diseased individuals. Omega-3 fatty acids also affect biomarkers of immunity during fetal development in infants, as well as in breast-feeding mothers. Here, we examine the reported effects of omega-3 fatty acids in healthy and diseased adults and during early development.

Altering omega-3:omega-6 ratios may affect immune function in healthy adult subjects. The questions arise as to whether these effects may be beneficial (by preventing long-term, low-grade inflammation, thus potentially reducing chronic-disease risk) or whether they might lower immune defenses to the point where healthy individuals are more susceptible to infection and disease. Three studies, primarily involving the effects of omega-3 supplementation on natural-killer (NK) cell activity (a type of innate immune response associated with resistance to infection and the rejection of tumors), have examined these questions (Kim, 2000). A 12-week supplement study involving the consumption of EPA-, stearidonic acid-, and gamma-linolenic acid

**Table 29.3. Bioactivities of the Metabolites of Omega-3 and Omega-6 Fatty Acids**

| Metabolites | Pro-inflammatory versus anti-inflammatory effects |
|---|---|
| Docosanoids | |
| Resolvins | Resolution of acute inflammation |
| Prostaglandins | |
| 1-Series prostaglandins | Anti-inflammatory |
| 2-Series prostaglandins | Pro-inflammatory |
| 3-Series prostaglandins | Anti-inflammatory (or less inflammatory than 2-series prostaglandins) |
| Leukotrienes | |
| 4-Series leukotrienes | Pro-inflammatory |
| 5-Series leukotrienes | Anti-inflammatory (or less inflammatory than 4-series leukotrienes) |
| Thromboxanes | |
| 1-Series thromboxanes | Anti-inflammatory |
| 2-Series thromboxanes | Pro-inflammatory |
| 3-Series thromboxanes | Anti-inflammatory |

Sources: Calder (2006); Serhan (2005).

(GLA)-containing oils reported a reduction in the number of NK cells with EPA and GLA (omega-6) supplementation. These treatments corresponded to an increase in the levels of these two fatty acids in monocytes (Miles et al., 2004). A second, double-blinded, randomized, parallel study by the same group, involving men of 18 to 42 years of age, found little effect of EPA supplementation on any measure of immune response, including NK cell activity (Miles et al., 2006). In an earlier study, EPA specifically suppressed NK cell activity by 48% in a randomized, double-blinded, parallel study of a group of subjects of 55–75 years of age. Study subjects were given a variety of omega-3 (ALA, EPA, and DHA) and omega-6 (GLA and AA) supplements in capsule form. Only EPA had an immunosuppressive effect in this study (Thies et al., 2001). A single clinical trial examined the effects of increasing omega-3 fatty acid intake by dietary, rather than supplementary, intervention in healthy adults. A group of 10 men (31–65 years of age) ate salmon, a mixed source of EPA and DHA, as part of a crossover study. The study involved a 20-day washout period, after which half of the men were placed on a salmon-containing diet, increasing their omega-3 intake by more than fivefold and changing their omega-3:omega-6 ratio to 1:4. The other half of the men consumed a low omega-3 reference diet with an omega-3:omega-6 ratio of 1:20. Salmon consumption was reported to lower PGE-M, a urinary marker of inflammation, by 24% (Ferreti et al., 1991). Based on the limited data available from these supplement and dietary studies, ascertaining the effects of increased omega-3 consumption on immunity in healthy adults is difficult.

Just as inflammation (which one can view as an overreaction of the immune system) can have negative health consequences, so can immune suppression. Major surgery or trauma can simultaneously increase some markers of inflammation, and suppress markers of immune function. Seven studies examined the effects of "immunonutrition" formulas containing omega-3 fatty acids (often with other ingredients, such as arginine and RNA) on post-surgical infections, inflammation, and immune suppression. A study involving 122 men and 59 women reported lower mortality and fewer infections in sepsis patients receiving omega-3-containing formulas, especially for patients with less severe sepsis (Galban et al., 2000). In a second study, an omega-3-containing formula completely prevented post-surgical infections in a group of 33 well-nourished colon-cancer patients, compared to 34 well-nourished control patients without other health problems (Horie et al., 2006).

Five studies reported that omega-3 supplementation may suppress post-operative inflammation. A study of 19 patients who underwent surgery for esophageal cancer reported that the administration of EPA as part of a total parenteral nutrition feeding reduced interleukin-6 (a marker of inflammation) 1, 2, and 6 hours after surgery and improved immune function after 3 weeks, compared to patients who did not receive supplemental EPA (Tashiro et al., 1998). A randomized, double-blinded study of stomach- and colorectal-cancer patients given enteral formula containing omega-3 fatty acids, arginine, and RNA reported that subjects receiving the omega-3-supplemented formula experienced less post-operative inflammation, as indicated by lower interleukin-6 and interleukin-1 levels, than patients not supplemented with the omega-3 formula (Gianotti et al., 1999). An enteral nutrition formula with an omega-3:omega-6 ratio of 1:3 increased the anti-inflammatory marker leukotriene-B5 in 14 treated patients compared to 16 controls after major abdominal surgery (Koller et al., 2003). A formula containing omega-3 fatty acids, along with glutamine and arginine, increased markers of immunity, including CD4 cell counts; increased CD4:CD8 ratios; and reduced markers of inflammation, including interleukin-6 and tumor necrosis factor-alpha in a study of 20 post-operative stomach-cancer patients, compared to 20 control patients (Chen et al., 2005). In contrast to the effects of omega-3-containing formulas, enteral formulas containing high levels of omega-6 fatty acids increased post-operative inflammatory markers in gastric-, colon-, and esophageal-cancer surgical patients (Furukawa, 2002). Based on this limited data, omega-3 fatty acids may play some role in normalizing immune responses and inhibiting inflammation during sepsis or after surgery. The difficulty, however, may occur in separating the effects of omega-3 fatty acids from those of the other ingredients in "immunonutrition" formulas.

Numerous studies have examined the effects of omega-3 fatty acids on inflammatory and autoimmune diseases, including inflammatory bowel disease, rheumatoid arthritis, and type I diabetes. A meta-analysis by MacLean et al.

(2004) examined the effects of omega-3 fatty acids on inflammatory bowel disease and rheumatoid arthritis. Based on 13 studies, omega-3 fatty acids did not affect inflammatory bowel disease. Based on 9 studies, omega-3 fatty acids may, however, have some beneficial effect on joint tenderness in rheumatoid arthritis patients. Type I diabetes is considered to be an autoimmune disease. Omega-3 fatty acid intake was inversely correlated with the onset of type I diabetes in a group of 1770 children as part of the DAISY (Diabetes Autoimmunity Study in the Young) cohort. Children at a high risk of type I diabetes as a result of having one diabetic parent or sibling or a high-risk HLA (human leukocyte antigen) genotype were followed for 12 years. Fatty acid consumption was then determined either by dietary survey or by blood sample in a smaller cohort of 244 children (Norris et al., 2007). Overall, the effects of omega-3 fatty acids are mild. This may be due to the fact that omega-3 metabolites, such as 3-series prostaglandins, 5-series leukotrienes, and 3-series thromboxanes, still allow inflammation to occur, although at a lower level.

Supplementing pregnant or breast-feeding women with omega-3 fatty acids affects the fatty acid profiles in breast milk, as well as in maternal and fetal blood cells. The effects of omega-3 fatty acids on fetal and neonatal immune responses are not clear, however. Icelandic women who consume diets high in fish and cod-liver oil express higher levels of the omega-3 fatty acids DHA and EPA, as well as docosapentaenoic acid, in their breast milk (Olafsdottir et al., 2006). A study of 83 women indicated that omega-3 fatty acid supplementation during pregnancy increased the omega-3 fatty acid content of neonatal red blood cell membranes. The authors postulated that this may affect neonatal immunity and allergenicity (Dunstan et al., 2003). In a randomized, double-blinded, placebo-controlled, 2 x 2 factorial, supplements combining folate and omega-3 fatty acid (fish oil) from week 22 of pregnancy through birth not only enhanced omega-3 levels in fetal plasma, but also reduced the depletion of the mother's stores to a greater degree than fish oil alone (Krauss-Etschmann et al., 2007). Both omega-3 and omega-6 fatty acids can cause immune-cell death in monocytes drawn from umbilical-cord blood when given at high doses ex vivo (blood cells are drawn, isolated, and treated). DHA was the most potent of these, causing cell death at 100 μM (Sweeney et al., 2001). Although logically, the altering of neonatal fatty acid profiles would influence immunity, more studies are needed to examine this question.

## Conclusion

While some evidence from human studies shows that increasing the omega-3:omega-6 ratio via an increased consumption of, or supplementation with, omega-3 fatty acids may affect immune response, relatively few studies are available for individual diseases or health conditions. Potential effects must be confirmed through further clinical studies. Relative to the questions proposed at the beginning of this chapter, we asked: Can the consumption of the appropriate types and levels of fatty acids improve immune function in healthy adults? Based on the limited data available, omega-3 fatty acid supplementation does not appear to affect immunity in healthy adults. Since evidence shows that increased omega-3 intake may reduce heart-disease risk, its consumption may still be warranted. We also asked: Do omega-3 fatty acids affect immunity in either inflammatory or immune-suppressed states? The answer to this question is a qualified "yes." Omega-3 fatty acid supplementation does appear to reduce the rate of post-surgical infections and inflammation, and may be of some benefit to rheumatoid arthritis patients. Overall, bringing the omega-3:omega-6 ratio closer to parity may play a role in "normalizing" immunity, rather than enhancing it per se. Also note that dramatically increasing omega-3 fatty acid consumption may not be beneficial and may actually be harmful for some individuals suffering from immune-suppression and blood-clotting disorders.

## References

Arterburn, L.; B. Hall; H. Oken. Distribution, interconversion, and dose response of n-3 fatty acids in humans. *Am. J. Clin. Nutr.* **2006**, *83,* 467S–476S.

Burdge, G.C. Metabolism of alpha-linolenic acid in humans. *Prostaglandins, Leukotrienes Essent. Fatty Acids* **2006**, *75,* 161–168.

Calder, P.C. Polyunsaturated fatty acids, inflammation, and immunity. *Lipids*, **2001**, *36,* 1007–1024.

Calder, P.C. n-3 Polyunsaturated fatty acids, inflammation, and inflammatory diseases. *Am. J. Clin. Nutr.* **2006**, *83,* 1505S–1509S.

Caramia, G. The essential fatty acids omega-6 and omega-3: from their discovery to their use in therapy. *Minerva Pediatr.* **2008**, *60,* 219–233.

Chen, D.W.; Z. Wei Fei; Y.C. Zhang; J.M. Ou; J. Xu. Role of enteral immunonutrition in patients with gastric carcinoma undergoing major surgery. *Asian J. Surg.* **2005**, *28,* 121–124.

Dunstan, J.A., T.A. Mori; A. Barden; L.J. Beilin; A.L. Taylor; P.G. Holt; S.L. Prescott. Fish oil supplementation in pregnancy modifies neonatal allergen-specific immune responses and clinical outcomes in infants at high risk of atopy: a randomized, controlled trial. *J. Allergy Clin. Immunol.* **2003**, *112,* 1178–1184.

Ferretti, A.; G.J. Nelson; P.C. Schmidt. Salmon-rich diet inhibits arachidonate cyclooxygenation in healthy men. *J. Nutr. Biochem.* **1991**, *2,* 547.

Food and Drug Administration. FDA Announces Qualified Health Claims for Omega-3 Fatty Acids Accessed September 23, 2008. http://www.fda.gov/bbs/topics/news/2004/NEW01115.html

Galban, C.; J.C. Montejo; A. Mesejo; P. Marco; S. Celaya; J.M. Sanchez-Segura; M. Farre; D.J. Bryg. An immune-enhancing enteral diet reduces mortality rate and episodes of bacteremia in septic intensive care unit patients. *Crit. Care Med.* **2000**, *28,* 643–648.

Gianotti, L.; M. Braga; C. Fortis; L. Soldini; A. Vignali; S. Colombo; G. Radaelli; V. Di Carlo. A prospective, randomized clinical trial on perioperative feeding with an arginine-, omega-3 fatty acid-, and RNA-enriched enteral diet: effect on host response and nutritional status. *J. Parenter. Enteral Nutr.* **1999**, *23,* 314–320.

Horie, H.; M. Okada; M. Kojima; H. Nagai. Favorable effects of preoperative enteral immunonutrition on a surgical site infection in patients with colorectal cancer without malnutrition. *Surg.*

*Today* **2006**, *36,* 1063–1068.

Howe, P.; B. Meyer; S. Record; K. Baghurst. Dietary intake of long-chain omega-3 polyunsaturated fatty acids: contribution of meat sources. *Nutrition* **2006**, *22,* 47–53.

Institute of Medicine of the National Academies. Dietary fat: total fat and fatty acids. *Dietary Reference Intakes;* J.J. Otten, J.P. Hellwig, L.D. Meyers, Eds.; The National Academies Press: Washington, D.C., 2006; pp. 122–139.

Kidd, P. Omega-3 DHA and EPA for cognition, behavior, and mood: clinical findings and structural–functional synergies with cell membrane phospholipids. *Altern. Med. Rev.* **2007**, *12,* 207–227.

Koller, M.; M. Senkal; M. Kemen; W. Konig; V. Zumtobel; G. Muhr. Impact of omega-3 fatty acid enriched TPN on leukotriene synthesis by leukocytes after major surgery. *Clin. Nutr.* **2003**, *22,* 59.

Krauss-Etschmann, S.; R. Shadid; C. Campoy; E. Hoster; H. Demmelmair; M. Jimenez; A. Gil; M. Rivero; B. Veszpremi; T. Decsi; B.V. Koletzko. Effects of fish-oil and folate supplementation of pregnant women on maternal and fetal plasma concentrations of docosahexaenoic acid and eicosapentaenoic acid: a European randomized multicenter trial. *Am. J. Clin. Nutr.* **2007**, *85,* 1392–1400.

Kris-Etherton, P.M.; W.S. Harris; L.J. Appel.; C. Fish. Consumption, fish oil, omega-3 fatty acids, and cardiovascular disease. *Circulation* **2002**, *106,* 2747–2757.

MacLean, C.H.; W.A. Mojica; S.C. Morton; J. Pencharz; R. Hasenfeld Garland; W. Tu; S.J. Newberry; L.K. Jungvig; J. Grossman; P. Khanna; S. Rhodes; P. Shekelle. Effects of omega-3 fatty acids on lipids and glycemic control in type II diabetes and the metabolic syndrome and on inflammatory bowel disease, rheumatoid arthritis, renal disease, systemic lupus erythematosus, and osteoporosis. *Evid. Rep. Technol. Assess* **2004**, *89,* 1–4.

Miles, E.A.; T. Banerjee; M.M. Dooper; L. M'Rabet; Y.M. Graus; P.C. Calder.The influence of different combinations of gamma-linolenic acid, stearidonic acid and EPA on immune function in healthy young male subjects. *Br. J. Nutr.* **2004**, *91,* 893–903.

Miles, E.A.; T. Banerjee; S.J. Wells; P.C. Calder. Limited effect of eicosapentaenoic acid on T-lymphocyte and natural killer cell numbers and functions in healthy young males. *Nutrition* **2006**, *22,* 512–519.

Norris, J.M.; X. Yin; M.M. Lamb; K. Barriga; J. Seifert; M. Hoffman; H.D. Orton; A.E. Baron; M. Clare-Salzler; H.P. Chase; et al. Omega-3 polyunsaturated fatty acid intake and islet autoimmunity in children at increased risk for type 1 diabetes. *JAMA* **2007**, *298,* 1420–1428.

Olafsdottir, A.S.; I. Thorsdottir; K.H. Wagner; I. Elmadfa. Polyunsaturated fatty acids in the diet and breast milk of lactating Icelandic women with traditional fish and cod liver oil consumption. *Ann. Nutr. Metab.* **2006**, *50,* 270–276.

Pompeia, C.; L.R. Lopes; C.K. Miyasaka; J. Procapio; P. Sannomiya; R. Curi. Effect of fatty acids on leukocyte function. *Braz. J. Med. Biol. Res.* **2000**, *33,* 1255–1268.

Serhan, C.N. Novel eicosanoid and docosanoid mediators: resolvins, docosatrienes, and neuroprotectins. *Curr. Opin. Clin. Nutr.* **2005**, *8,* 115–121.

Shaikh, S.R.; M. Edidin. Polyunsaturated fatty acids, membrane organization, T cells, and antigen presentation. *Am. J. Clin. Nutr.* **2006**, *84,* 1277–1289.

Sweeney, B.; P. Puri; D.J. Reen. Polyunsaturated fatty acids influence neonatal monocyte survival. *Pediatr. Surg. Int.* **2001**, *17,* 254–258.

Tashiro, T.; H. Yamamori; K. Takagi; N. Hayashi; K. Furukawa; N. Nakajima. n-3 versus n-6 polyunsaturated fatty acids in critical illness. *Nutrition* **1998**, *14,* 551–553.

Thies, F.; G. Nebe-von-Caron; J.R. Powell; P. Yaqoob; E.A. Newsholme; P.C. Calder. Dietary supplementation with eicosapentaenoic acid, but not with other long-chain n-3 or n-6 polyunsaturated fatty acids, decreases natural killer cell activity in healthy subjects aged >55 y. *Am. J. Clin. Nutr.* **2001**, *73,* 539–548.

Welch, A.A.; S.A. Binghma; K.T. Khaw. Estimated conversion of alpha-linolenic acid to long chain n-3 polyunsaturated fatty acids is greater than expected in non fish-eating vegetarians and non fish-eating meat-eaters than in fish-eaters. *J. Human Nutr. Diet* **2008**, *21,* 404.

Wendel, M.; R. Paul; A.R. Heller. Lipoproteins in inflammation and sepsis. II. Clinical aspects. *Intensive Care Med.* **2007**, *33,* 25–35

Yamagishi, K.; H. Iso; C. Date; M. Fukui; K. Wakai; S. Kikuchi; Y. Inaba; N. Tanabe; A. Tamakoshi; J.S.G. Fish. Omega-3 polyunsaturated fatty acids, and mortality from cardiovascular diseases in a nationwide community-based cohort of Japanese men and women: The JACC (Japan Collaborative Cohort Study for Evaluation of Cancer Risk) Study. *J. Am. Coll. Cardiol.* **2008**, *52,* 988–996.

# 30

# Omega-3 Long-chain Polyunsaturated Fatty Acids and Obesity

**Jonathan David Buckley and Peter R.C. Howe**
*Nutritional Physiology Research Centre and Australian Technology Network Centre for Metabolic Fitness, University of South Australia, Adelaide, Australia*

## Introduction

Obesity is increasing in epidemic proportions throughout the developed and developing world (Dunstan et al., 2002; Flegel et al., 1998) bringing with it increased morbidity and mortality (Must et al., 1999; Visscher & Seidell, 2001). If we are to avoid prohibitive increases in health costs and catastrophic health consequences for an increasing proportion of society, feasible and affordable strategies to combat the rising prevalence of obesity must be found.

Current recommendations from most public-health bodies for reducing body fat are based on increasing physical activity (Department of Health and Ageing, 1999) and eating a healthy balanced diet (National Health and Medical Research Council, 2003). However, many people have difficulty complying with these lifestyle changes, particularly over the longer term. Indeed, a recent meta-analysis showed that almost half of any initial weight loss achieved through diet or exercise is regained after one year (Curioni & Lourenco, 2005). Hence, despite widespread recommendations from public-health bodies to improve diet and physical-activity habits, the prevalence of obesity continues to rise. Accordingly, more acceptable and sustainable strategies for reducing body fat must be found.

Considerable efforts were directed toward investigating the benefits of the omega-3 long-chain polyunsaturated fatty acids (n-3 LC-PUFAs), notably eicosapentaenoic acid (EPA) and docosahexaenoic acid (DHA), for improving cardiovascular health and reducing cardiovascular disease (CVD) risk. However, despite the current obesity epidemic and a growing body of evidence indicating that the regular consumption of these fatty acids may be effective in reducing adiposity, less attention was paid to the potential for EPA and DHA to reduce obesity.

## n-3 LC-PUFA and Body Fat Reduction in Animals

### *Protection against Body Fat Gain*

A growing number of studies show that incorporating n-3 LC-PUFA into high-fat obesogenic diets fed to rodents reduces body fat accumulation (Baillie et al., 1999; Belzung et al., 1993; Cunnane et al., 1986; Hainault et al., 1993; Ruzickova et al., 2004), although one study in diabetic rats reported that supplementing a high-fat diet with n-3 LC-PUFA exacerbated, rather than reduced, weight gain (Todoric et al., 2006).

Cunnane et al. (1986) fed 6-week-old male *ln/ln* and *ob/ob* C57BL/6J mice synthetic diets that were supplemented with 10% (w/w) of evening-primrose oil [predominantly n-6 fatty acids (n-6)] or 10% of cod-liver oil (predominantly n-3 LC-PUFA) for 16 weeks. Overall, the *ob/ob* mice gained significantly more weight than the *ln/ln* mice, irrespective of the diet consumed. The increase was attenuated in the *ob/ob* mice consuming the cod-liver oil, but due to a slight difference in starting weights, the attenuation of weight gain did not reach statistical significance, even though the *ob/ob* mice that consumed the cod-liver oil finished the study with a significantly lower body weight than the *ob/ob* mice that consumed the evening-primrose oil. The difference in body weight between treatment groups was not related to differences in energy intake; instead, the authors ascribed the effect to a difference in incorporation of n-3 LC-PUFAs and n-6 fatty acids into liver, brown-adipose tissue, and white-adipose tissue, with the ob/ob mice fed the cod-liver oil demonstrating a greater incorporation of n-3 LC-PUFAs and a reduced incorporation of n-6 into these tissues. The greater incorporation of LC-PUFAs, particularly n-3 LC-PUFA, has the potential to influence gene expression in these tissues, and thus alter their metabolic activity, leading to reductions in body fat accumulation (Clarke, 2000).

Hainault et al. (1993) subsequently fed six-week-old male Wistar rats one of three high-fat diets (50% of energy) or a low- fat control diet (10% of corn oil, 20% of casein, 70% of starch) ad libitum for 16–20 days. The high–fat diets consisted of a high-lard diet (48% of lard, 2% of corn oil), a lard–corn-oil diet (35% of lard, 15% of corn oil), and a lard–corn-oil–fish-oil diet (33% of lard, 2% of corn oil, and 15% of fish oil), with the balance consisting of 20% of casein and 30% of starch. Food intake and body weight were similar for all diets, but rats consuming the fish-oil diet had 20 and 30% lower weights of subcutaneous (inguinal) and visceral (retroperitoneal and epididymal) adipose tissue, respectively, by the end of the study period, suggesting that the fish oil had provided a protective benefit against the accumulation of body fat.

While Hainault et al. (1993) demonstrated that a fish-oil diet rich in n-3 LC-PUFA protected against the accumulation of body fat in male Wistar rats fed a high-fat diet, Belzung et al. (1993) demonstrated that this protective effect exhibited a dose-response relationship. Belzung and co-workers (1993) fed 1-week-old male Wistar rats for 4 weeks on either a control diet (standard chow) or three high-fat diets (20% of fat, w/w) containing high, medium, and low n-3 LC-PUFA content (40.6, 18.6, and 0.7% of fatty acids, respectively). The three high-fat diets resulted in greater body fat accumulation compared with the control diet, with no differences in increases in body weight, subcutaneous fat, or mesenteric fat. However, the accumulation of epididymal fat was less in the high n-3 LC-PUFA group, and a dose- dependent reduction occurred in the magnitude of increase in the retroperitoneal fat mass. These differences in epididymal and retroperitoneal fat were due primarily to reduced hypertrophy of existing fat cells rather than to any effects on cell hyperplasia, and the authors proposed that the reduced-fat deposition was possibly mediated by a lowering of circulating triglycerides. This reduction in adipose-cell hypertrophy rather than hyperplasia is consistent with the findings of an earlier study by Parrish et al. (1990), who fed male Wistar Rats high-fat diets containing 20% of triglycerides from fish oil or 20% of triglycerides from lard for 3 weeks and found no difference in body weight, but significantly less perirenal and epididymal fat in the fish-oil-fed group as a result of a reduced adipocyte size with no difference in adipocyte number. Thus, one may achieve the protective benefits of n-3 LC-PUFA against the accumulation of body fat through a lesser accumulation of fat in existing adipocytes, with these effects being primarily evident in visceral fat depots and exhibiting a dose-response relationship.

This preferential reduction in the accumulation of visceral fat was confirmed in two subsequent studies (Baillie et al., 1999; Ruzickova et al., 2004), with the latter of these studies also determining that the effect was mediated primarily by DHA. Baillie et al. (1999) fed two groups of 3–4-week-old male Fisher 344 rats a high- fat diet containing 40% of energy as either fish oil or corn oil for 6 weeks. Epididymal-fat pads from rats fed the fish-oil diet weighed 25% less than those of the rats fed corn oil by the end of the 6-week study period. Ruzickova et al. (2004) subsequently fed 3–4-month-old male C57BL/6 mice a low-fat control diet, one of two high-fat control diets (20 and 35% of fat, w/w), or one of seven experimental diets which consisted of the high-fat control diets admixed with varying levels of EPA and DHA for 5 weeks. By the end of the study period, EPA and DHA attenuated the accumulation of epididymal fat, but had a limited effect on the accumulation of subcutaneous fat. Importantly, further determination showed that this effect was promoted by a low ratio of EPA/DHA (i.e., more DHA relative to EPA), suggesting that DHA, rather than EPA, was primarily responsible for promoting the anti-obesity effect of an increased n-3 LC-PUFA intake.

Therefore, numerous studies in rodents indicate that the dietary intake of n-3 LC-PUFA can attenuate increases in dietary-induced obesity, particularly increases in visceral (epidiymal fat). However, in a recent study (Todoric et al., 2006)—a comparison of the effect of feeding different high-fat diets for 6 weeks on the development of obesity in male C57BL/KsJ-lepr$^{db}$/lepr$^{db}$ diabetic mice and their nondiabetic littermates—findings showed that compared with feeding a high-fat diet (30% of energy) containing safflower oil (rich in n-6 fatty acids), a similar high-fat diet containing a concentrate of n-3 LC-PUFA exacerbated weight gain. This exacerbation of weight gain only occurred in diabetic mice, since in nondiabetic mice while the safflower diet resulted in increased weight gain compared with a low-fat control diet, the n-3 LC-PUFA diet did not result in any greater weight gain. This study did not assess the changes in body fat content, making it difficult to determine whether the differences in weight gain between diets were due to differences in body fat deposition. Nevertheless, the increased weight gain experienced by the diabetic mice fed the n-3 LC-PUFA diet suggests that these fatty acids may exert quite different metabolic effects in diabetes, at least in diabetic mice.

### *n-3 LC-PUFA for Reducing Existing Obesity*

While numerous studies in rodents show that the incorporation of n-3 LC-PUFA into an obesogenic diet can ameliorate the accumulation of body fat, at least in nondiabetic animals, limited studies have examined the effect of incorporating n-3 LC-PUFA into a diet to reduce obesity that has already developed. In the only study to specifically examine this question, Huang et al. (2004) demonstrated that the intake of n-3 LC-PUFA could reduce body fat in mice that were made obese by prior feeding of a high-fat diet. In this study, male C57B1/l mice were fed a high-fat diet (59% of energy) for 13 weeks or a low-fat control diet (10% of energy). The mice were then classified as diet-induced obese or diet-resistant according to whether they fell within the upper or lower tertiles of body-weight gain. The diet-induced obese mice were then subjected to a 6-week dietary intervention which consisted of feeding one of these diets: the original high-fat diet, a high-fat diet with a high n-3 LC-PUFA content (59% of energy from fish oil), or the low-fat control diet. After switching the diet-induced obese mice to the n-3 LC-PUFA or the low-fat diet, their body weights were reduced to the level of the diet-resistant mice and the controls that were maintained on the low-fat control diet, indicating that both the n-3 LC-PUFA and the low-fat diet were effective for weight loss. The loss of body weight after the mice were switched to the n-3 LC-PUFA diet could not be attributed to a reduction in food intake because, despite an initial reduction in energy intake during the first week after the dietary change, for the remaining 5 weeks of the dietary-intervention period, the energy intake of these mice did not differ from that of the other treatment groups. However, the mice that were switched to the n-3 LC-PUFA diet exhibited the lowest food efficiencies (i.e., lowest weight gain per unit of energy intake), indicating that the n-3 LC-PUFA reduced metabolic efficiency.

Therefore, apparently, in rodent models, the dietary intake of n-3 LC-PUFA may be effective for reducing body-weight and body fat gain during the consumption of an obesogenic diet, and for reducing body weight in animals that are already obese. However, evidence, although somewhat limited, shows that the dietary intake of n-3 LC-PUFA may exert different metabolic effects in diabetic animals, resulting in an exacerbation of weight gain when a high-fat obesogenic diet is consumed.

## n-3 LC-PUFA and Body Fat Reduction in Humans

While evidence from a considerable number of animal studies shows that n-3 LC-PUFA can reduce body fat, the impact of n-3 LC-PUFA intake on body composition in humans is less certain due to a lack of studies of adequate size and duration. Furthermore, despite dietary energy restriction and/or exercise being the cornerstones of treatment for obesity, few studies have investigated the efficacy of n-3 LC-PUFA for reducing body fat when combined with these treatments.

### *Observational Studies—Relationships between n-3 LC-PUFA Intake and Body Weight*

Numerous large, long-term, prospective cohort studies have examined the effects of n-3 LC-PUFA supplementation on cardiovascular health, but none have specifically examined the effects on body weight or body fat. Nevertheless, the Health Professional Follow-Up Study, a prospective cohort study with 12 years of follow-up which examined the effects of n-3 LC-PUFA intake on the risk of stroke in 43,671 men (He et al., 2002), reported that, at baseline, men with high fish consumption were less likely to be overweight than those with low fish consumption, and the percentage of overweight volunteers was inversely related to the n-3 LC-PUFA intake. Conversely, in the Nurses' Health Study (Iso et al., 2001), which was a prospective cohort study in 79,839 women with a 14-year follow-up which examined the relationship between the intake of fish and omega-3 fatty acids on the risk of stroke, higher intakes of fish and n-3 LC-PUFA were associated with a higher prevalence of obesity. While the higher prevalence of obesity associated with fish intake could be accounted for by a higher energy intake, this was not the case for n-3 LC-PUFA intake.

Thus, the limited evidence available from large, prospective cohort studies regarding the potential relationships between n-3 LC-PUFA intake and body weight is conflicting. Unclear is whether the different findings of the two studies that have investigated this issue are due to confounding or to gender differences in the effect of n-3 LC-PUFA on body fat. The Health Professional Follow-Up Study (which showed an inverse relationship between n-3 LC-PUFA intake and body weight) was conducted in men, while the Nurses' Health Study (which showed that a higher intake of n-3 LC-PUFA was associated with a higher prevalence of obesity) was conducted in women, raising the possibility that the effect of n-3 LC-PUFA on reducing body weight and/or body fat may be limited to males. The possibility of any gender effects cannot be determined from the data available from rodent studies because these studies were conducted exclusively in male rodents (Baillie et al., 1999; Belzung et al., 1993; Cunnane et al., 1986; Hainault et al., 1993; Huang et al., 2004; Ruzickova et al., 2004).

### *Randomized Controlled Trials*

While the two cohort studies that provided information relating to the relationship between n-3 LC-PUFA intake and body weight have provided conflicting evidence, randomized controlled trials also produced conflicting results. The randomized controlled trials that were carried out to examine the effects of increasing n-3 LC-PUFA intake on body composition are few in number and, as such, little information is available regarding the efficacy of n-3 LC-PUFA for improving body composition when consumed either alone or in conjunction with dietary energy restriction and/or regular exercise.

### *Effect of n-3 LC-PUFA Intake Alone on Body Composition*

Couet et al. (1997) used a single-blind intervention in which six healthy adults (five male, one female) consumed a control diet for 3 weeks, and then, after a 10–12-week washout, consumed the same diet but with 6 g/day of visible fat replaced with fish oil (predominantly DHA). At the beginning and end of each dietary period, the resting metabolic rate and fat oxidation were measured by indirect calorimetry, and body composition was assessed by dual-energy x-ray absorptiometry (DXA). Dietary intakes (7-day recall) and physical activity (by activity recall) were completed 2 weeks prior to each experimental period to monitor any changes in diet or physical activity. Resting fat oxidation was increased (22%), and body fat was reduced (–0.88 kg) on the fish-oil diet; these differences were not accounted for by any differences in dietary intake or physical activity. However, one major limitation of this study was that, rather than balancing the order in which the dietary treatments were undertaken, all volunteers consumed the control diet followed by the fish-oil diet, and this may have introduced an order effect which may have potentially confounded the outcome.

In a well-designed and controlled study, Groh-Wargo et al. (2005) showed that feeding formula supplemented with arachidonic acid and n-3 LC-PUFA (DHA) to pre-term infants until 12 months of gestation-corrected age resulted in a greater increase in lean body mass and less body fat accumulation compared with controls who were fed formula that was not supplemented with arachidonic acid or DHA. Indeed, in this study, a 15% difference in body fat occurred between treatment and control by the end of the study period, with the greatest differences in body composition occurring during the final 6 months of supplementation. The findings of this study are consistent with those of numerous rodent studies which also reported less body fat accumulation during growth in animals fed diets supplemented with n-3 LC-PUFA (Baillie et al., 1999; Belzung et al., 1993; Cunnane et al., 1986; Hainault et al., 1993; Ruzickova et al., 2004). However, the design of the study did not allow for the determination of whether the effect on body composition was mediated by DHA or arachidonic acid because the treatment groups received both. Nevertheless, this is the only human study that lasted more than 3 months, and the finding of an increasing difference in body fat levels between intervention and control groups during the final 6 months of the study suggests that, if the effect was mediated by DHA, the improvements in body composition may become greater with an increasing duration of supplementation. However, to extrapolate the results of this developmental study to potential effects on body composition in adults is difficult.

Subsequently, Kabir et al. (2007) studied the effects of supplementation with n-3 LC-PUFA on body composition in overweight and obese female postmenopausal volunteers with type 2 diabetes. Twenty-seven participants were randomized in a double-blind, parallel study design to consume 3 g/day of EPA-rich fish oil (1.08 g of EPA, 0.72 g of DHA) or 3 g/day of paraffin oil for 2 months. Body composition was assessed by DXA, and subcutaneous- and visceral-fat areas were determined by a single-slice computerized tomography scan at the L4-L5 disc space level. A biopsy of subcutaneous, periumbilical adipose tissue was also collected. By the end of the study period, neither treatment group had reduced its body weight, and no changes were noted in subcutaneous- or visceral-fat areas. However, the n-3 LC-PUFA group reduced their body fat mass significantly (~1.6 kg); this reduction was primarily due to a loss of trunk fat. Participants randomized to the fish-oil treatment also experienced a reduction in adipocyte diameter, whereas this did not change in the control group. The finding of a reduction in adiposity in these postmenopausal women with type 2 diabetes is in contrast to the earlier study by Todoric et al. (2006) in mice which showed that the dietary intake of n-3 LC-PUFA exacerbated increases in body fat during high-fat feeding. The reason for the discrepancy in findings between these two studies is not clear, but possibly the effects of n-3 LC-PUFA on body composition are regulated differently in mice that are genetically predisposed to diabetes and humans who develop type 2 diabetes as a result of lifestyle habits. Additionally, this study demonstrated that n-3 LC-PUFAs are effective in reducing body fat in females, indicating that the conflicting findings of the earlier cohort studies—where the study in males reported an inverse association between n-3 LC-PUFA intake and body weight (He et al., 2002), and the study in females reported a positive association (Iso et al., 2001)—were unlikely due to differential gender effects.

### *Effect of n-3 LC-PUFA Intake Combined with Dietary Energy Restriction on Body Composition*

Dietary energy restriction is widely accepted as a cornerstone in the management of obesity, and numerous studies have examined whether supplementing the diet with n-3 LC-PUFA can enhance the weight loss that one can achieve through dietary restriction.

Fontani et al. (2005) investigated the effects of n-3 LC-PUFA supplementation against a background of body fat reduction by using two different controlled diets. Thirty-three noncompetitive athletes were randomized to consume either a low-carbohydrate Zone diet (40% of carbohydrate, 30% of protein, 30% of fat) or a diet recommended by the Italian National Research Institute for Nutrition and Foods (55% of carbohydrate, 15% of protein, 30% of fat) for 70 days. Half of the volunteers on each dietary pattern were further randomized to consume 4 g/day of fish oil (1.6 g of EPA, 0.8 g of DHA) or 4 g/day of olive oil in a crossover design (i.e., consumed fish oil for 35 days and then crossed over to olive oil, or vice versa). Body fat was assessed by skinfolds at baseline, and at the end of each 35-day period. The two diets both reduced body fat (–7%), but no additional effect of n-3 LC-PUFA supplementation was observed. However, the important limitations of this study were: the oil-supplementation periods were short (35 days), and some volunteers were supplemented with n-3 LC-PUFA during the first 35-day period before crossing over to the olive oil for the second 35-day period. Possibly, a carryover effect of n-3 LC-PUFA accumulation in various tissues occurred which might have confounded the outcome in these volunteers. The incorporation of n-3 LC-PUFA into tissues (e.g., erythrocyte membranes) increased as much as 150% when provided at a similar dose to that employed by Fontani et al. (2005) for the same 35-day period (Buckley et al., 2008), and retention of n-3 LC-PUFA into these tissues is very prolonged, with levels staying elevated for up to 18 weeks (Brown et al., 1991). Thus, any metabolic effects of the incorporation of n-3 LC-PUFA into tissue membranes in volunteers who were provided with fish oil during the first 35-day dosing period in the study by Fontani et al. (2005) were likely to have persisted during the second 35-day dosing period when these volunteers were consuming olive oil, possibly confounding the ability to identify a difference between the n-3 LC-PUFA and olive-oil treatments.

More recently, Krebs et al. (2006) examined the effect of adding n-3 LC-PUFA to a low-fat high-carbohydrate weight-loss diet on body weight and body composition in overweight women. Ninety-three overweight women completed the study in which they were randomized to: (i) the weight-loss diet (3.3–3.8 MJ/day) combined with n-3 LC-PUFA (5 g of fish oil containing 1.3 g of EPA, 2.9 g of DHA per day), (ii) the weight-loss diet combined with placebo (5 g of oil containing 2.8 g of linoleic acid, 1.4 g of oleic acid per day), or (iii) a control condition (no weight-loss diet) for 24 weeks. Body composition was assessed at baseline, and after 12 and 24 weeks by DXA. Body weight did not change in the control group, but was reduced ~12% in both dietary treatment groups, with no difference in the magnitude of weight loss between the weight-loss diet combined with n-3 LC-PUFA and that combined with the placebo. Similarly, body fat did not change in the control group, but was reduced by a similar amount in both diet groups. Therefore, the findings of this study did not provide any support for greater weight loss or differential changes in body composition when n-3 LC-PUFA supplementation is combined with an energy-restricted diet in overweight women.

In the most recent study to examine the effects of n-3 LC-PUFA intake on body composition when consumed in conjunction with an energy-restricted diet, Thorsdottir et al. (2007) investigated the effects of fish and fish-oil consumption on weight loss during caloric restriction. Two hundred and seventy-eight overweight men and women completed an 8-week dietary intervention study in which they were randomly assigned to one of four isocaloric energy-restricted diets (2500 kJ/day of caloric restriction, 50% of carbohydrate, 20% of protein, 30% of fat). The diets consisted of: (i) a control diet containing no seafood, (ii) a diet containing lean fish (150 g of cod three times per week, 0.3 g of n-3 LC-PUFA per day), (iii) a diet containing fatty fish (150 g of salmon three times per week, 3.0 g of n-3 LC-PUFA per day), or (iv) required volunteers consuming six fish-oil capsules per day (1.5 g of n-3 LC-PUFA per day). The average weight loss was 6.5 kg for men (~7% of body weight) and 4.2 kg for women (~5% of body weight). Weight loss and reductions in waist circumference were significantly greater in the groups receiving fish or fish oil compared with controls (~1 kg greater weight loss over the first 4 weeks for both of these diets), but these differences were limited to male volunteers. The finding of additional weight loss—not only with the fish-oil diet but also with the lean and fatty-fish diets—was interpreted by the authors as suggesting that weight loss might have been facilitated in the fish diets by fish protein rich in the amino acid taurine, since taurine decreased body weight in mice (Fujihira et al., 1970). However, the fatty-fish and fish-oil diets (which provided a higher n-3 LC-PUFA intake) tended to provide greater weight loss than the lean-fish diet even though no significant difference was seen in the weight loss achieved between the fish and fish-oil diets. This suggests that n-3 LC-PUFA may provide some small additional benefit for weight loss.

The finding of a significantly greater weight loss in male volunteers only in the study by Thorsdottir et al. (2007) suggests that the lack of any additional weight loss in the study by Krebs et al. (2006) when n-3 LC-PUFAs were added to an energy-restricted diet may have been because only females were evaluated. However, too few studies were conducted to date to confirm any gender-related difference in the efficacy of n-3 LC-PUFA to promote additional improvements in body composition when combined with an energy-restricted diet.

### *Effect of n-3 LC-PUFA Intake Combined with Regular Exercise on Body Composition*

While dietary energy restriction is a cornerstone in the treatment of obesity, increasing physical activity is also widely advocated to assist with improving body composition in obesity. As a result, numerous studies have examined whether combining n-3 LC-PUFA supplementation with a program of regular exercise provides any additional improvements in body composition beyond what might be achieved through exercise alone.

Warner et al. (1989) randomized thirty-four dyslipidemic adults with ~30% of body fat to either a control group or to one of three treatment groups. For 12 weeks, the treatment groups consumed 50 mL of corn oil per day, 50 mL of fish oil per day (17% of EPA, 12% of DHA), or 50 mL of fish oil plus undertook a progressive aerobic-exercise program which consisted of walking or jogging 3 days per week for 45–50 minutes at 70–85% of maximal heart rate. Body composition was determined by hydrostatic weighing at baseline and after the 12-week intervention, and dietary intake was assessed by a 48-hour dietary recall. The volunteers who undertook the exercise program in conjunction with consuming the fish oil exhibited a 3% reduction in body fat, while body fat was unchanged in the other groups. However, because the study lacked an exercise control (i.e., no group undertook an exercise-only intervention), to determine whether the reduction in body fat was due to the exercise alone or to some interaction between the fish oil and exercise was impossible, although no change occurred in body fat in the fish-oil treatment group which suggests that the former was more likely.

Brilla and Landerholm (1990) subsequently investigated the effects of 10 weeks of fish-oil supplementation and exercise on body composition in healthy, previously sedentary, young males, but included an exercise control group in the study design. Thirty-two healthy young male volunteers were randomized to four groups: control, fish oil, exercise, or fish oil and exercise. The fish-oil groups consumed 4 g/day of n-3 LC-PUFA. The exercise groups performed aerobic exercise for 1 hour three times per week. The percentage of body fat (hydrostatic weighing) and dietary intake (3-day diet records) were assessed at baseline and after 10 weeks. Body fat did not decrease significantly in any treatment group. Unlike previous studies in which n-3 LC-PUFA reduced body fat in overweight and obese volunteers, the young male volunteers studied by Brilla and Landerholm (1990) were lean (15–20% of body fat), and the use of a lean population may have limited the capacity for the n-3 LC-PUFA to provide any reduction of body fat. Indeed, the use of a lean population also appeared to limit the ability to demonstrate an effect of exercise, given that body fat did not reduce significantly in the exercise group either.

In the most recent study that examined the potential for supplementation with n-3 LC-PUFA to enhance the benefits of exercise for improving body composition, Hill et al. (2007) used a study design similar to that employed by Brilla and Landerholm (1990), but studied the effects in overweight and obese adults. In the study by Hill et al. (2007), sixty-five overweight or obese adults completed a 12-week intervention in which they were randomized (double-blind) to consume 6 g/day of fish oil containing ~1.9 g of n-3 LC-PUFA (26% of DHA, 6% of EPA) or 6 g/day of sunflower oil. Half of the volunteers in each oil-treatment group were further randomized to maintain their usual physical activity or to undertake a program of regular exercise which involved walking three times per week for 45 minutes at 75% of their age-predicted maximal heart rate. Energy intake was assessed using 3-day weighed food records, and indicated that no differences were noted in energy intake between treatment groups. Body weight was reduced by the exercise, but no effect was noted of n-3 LC-PUFA. However, both exercise and n-3 LC-PUFA supplementation exerted independent (but additive) effects on body fat reduction, with the volunteers who undertook exercise and n-3 LC-PUFA supplementation losing ~1.6 kg of body fat over the 12-week intervention period. The subjects who were randomized to sunflower-oil supplementation alone experienced a small increase in body fat (~600 g), possibly as a result of continuing to consume the same diet that made them overweight/obese in the first place, but the magnitude of this increase was attenuated in the volunteers who consumed the n-3 LC-PUFA (~180-g increase) (see Fig. 30.1). These data indicate that regular supplementation with ~1.9 g/day of n-3 LC-PUFA can reduce body fat accumulation in overweight/obese adults, but the magnitude of this effect was modest, at least with this relatively low dose of n-3 LC-PUFA over a 12-week time frame. Further studies should evaluate the effects of higher doses of n-3 LC-PUFA over longer time frames on body fat reduction in overweight and obese populations.

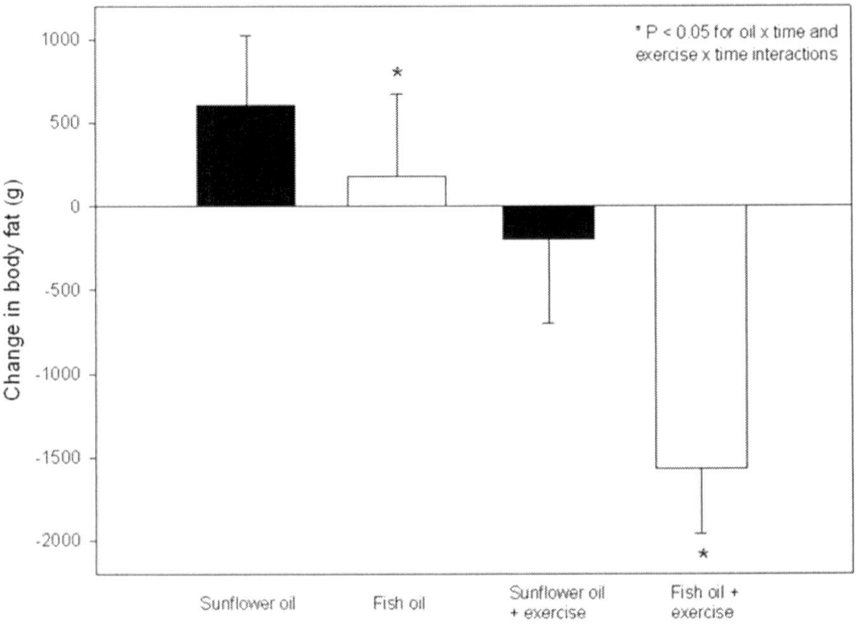


**Fig. 30.1.** Dual-energy x-ray absorptiometry assessed changes in body fat mass after supplementation with 6 g/day of docosahexaenoic acid-rich fish oil, 6 g/day of sunflower oil, and fish oil and exercise or sunflower oil and exercise for 12 weeks in overweight and obese adults. Significant oil x time and exercise x time interactions were detected ($P < 0.05$). (Adapted from Hill et al. (2007) with permission of the American Society for Nutrition).

### *Effect of n-3 LC-PUFA Intake Combined with Dietary Energy Restriction and Regular Exercise on Body Composition*

While some studies examined whether combining n-3 LC-PUFA with diet or exercise provides any additional benefit for improving body composition, only one study examined whether n-3 LC-PUFA provides any additional benefit for improving body composition when combined with both dietary energy restriction and a program of regular exercise. Kunešová et al. (2006) reported a 1.5-kg greater weight loss over a 3-week period in severely obese women who undertook a regular exercise program combined with consuming a very low-calorie diet that was supplemented with 2.8 g/day of n-3 LC-PUFA (predominantly EPA) compared with those undertaking the exercise program while consuming the very low-calorie diet but receiving a placebo rather than the n-3 LC-PUFA. Twenty-seven severely obese women underwent a 1-week outpatient weight-stabilization period, followed by a 3-week inpatient weight-reduction period. During the weight-reduction period, volunteers undertook 60 minutes/day of light to moderate physical activity, and were randomly assigned to consume either a very low calorie diet (2200 kJ/day) supplemented with 2.8 g/day of n-3 LC-PUFA (2:1 ratio of EPA to DHA) or a very low calorie diet supplemented with saline solution. Weight loss was greater in the n-3 LC-PUFA-supplemented group but did not quite reach statistical significance (7.6 ± 1.8 versus 6.1 ± 2.2 kg, $P < 0.10$), whereas significantly greater reductions occurred in the body-mass index (2.8 ± 0.6 versus 2.2 ± 0.7 kg/m$^2$, $P < 0.05$) and hip circumference (4.8 ± 1.8 versus 2.5 ± 2.5 cm, $P < 0.05$) in this treatment group compared with controls. The reduction in the body-mass index was inversely related to the incorporation of DHA into plasma phospholipids ($r = -0.60$, $P < 0.008$). While body fat changes were not reported, the authors did find a greater increase in serum β-hydroxybutyrate in the n-3 LC-PUFA-supplemented group compared with control, and interpreted this as providing evidence of greater fat oxidation in this treatment group. These findings indicate that the addition of n-3 LC-PUFA to a relatively short (3 weeks) weight-loss program comprised of severe caloric restriction and exercise may increase fat oxidation, leading to a greater improvement in body composition.

The finding of this study contrasts with the study by Krebs et al. (2006), which reported no additional reduction in body weight when n-3 LC-PUFAs were combined with caloric restriction. The reason for the discrepant findings between these two studies is not immediately obvious because both studies combined caloric restriction with 3–4 g/day of n-3 LC-PUFA to achieve weight loss in overweight and/or obese women. A possible explanation for the discrepant findings of these two studies may lie in the magnitude of weight loss achieved, with the study by Krebs et al. (2006) achieving approximately double the weight loss reported in the study by Kunešová et al. (2006) (12% of body weight versus 6% of body weight). Therefore, possibly, the much larger weight loss achieved in the study by Krebs et al. (2006) may have masked any additional weight loss that might have been achieved as a result of n-3 LC-PUFA supplementation.

## *Summary of Effects of n-3 LC-PUFA Intake on Body Composition in Humans*

In summary, most evidence indicating that n-3 LC-PUFA intake is effective for reducing body weight and improving body composition in humans comes from short-term studies (3–12 weeks). These studies have, for the most part, showed that n-3 LC-PUFAs promote modest reductions in body weight and improvements in body composition when taken either alone or in conjunction with an energy-restricted diet. The longest study to date which has examined the effects of n-3 LC-PUFA supplementation on body composition was conducted by Groh-Wargo et al. (2005) in preterm infants, and showed that the greatest improvements in body composition were achieved during the final 6 months of a 12-month supplementation period. This study also demonstrated the greatest differential in body fat between treatment and control (15% difference in body fat). However, because this study was conducted in pre-term infants, it reflects the attenuation of adiposity during early growth and development. The findings may not be generalizable to the regression of adiposity in overweight or obese adults. With regular n-3 LC-PUFA consumption, tissue levels will continue to increase beyond 12 weeks (Harris et al., 2007), suggesting that improvements in body composition associated with an increased bioavailability of n-3 LC-PUFA may continue to accrue over the longer term. Accordingly, an important need exists to examine the longer-term effects of n-3 LC-PUFA supplementation on body fat in overweight and obese adults and thereby determine if n-3 LC-PUFA supplementation may be an effective long-term strategy for body fat reduction in these populations.

## Mechanisms of Body fat Reduction with n-3 LC-PUFA

The dietary intake of n-3 LC-PUFA may assist with body-weight and body fat reduction by multiple mechanisms. One mechanism is through an enhancement of postprandial satiety which might lead to reduced food intake. Another mechanism, the one with the most evidence, is through alterations in the expression of genes involved in: (i) the regulation of fat oxidation in adipose, liver, cardiac, intestinal, and skeletal muscle tissue and (ii) the regulation of adipogenesis in adipose tissue, with these effects on gene expression favoring enhanced fat oxidation and reduced-fat deposition.

### *Appetite Effects*

Most studies in animals and humans show the effects of n-3 LC-PUFA on body weight and/or body composition are independent of energy intake (Cunnane et al., 1986; Hainault et al., 1993; Hill et al., 2007; Huang et al., 2004). However, a recent subanalysis (Parra et al., 2008) of a larger weight-loss study (Thorsdottir et al., 2007)—which showed that weight loss achieved through caloric restriction was enhanced when fish or fish oil was included in the diet—indicated that the intake of n-3 LC-PUFA was associated with a greater satiety immediately after, and 120 minutes after a test meal. Of the 278 volunteers, 233 completed the original study and participated in the subanalysis of the effects of n-3 LC-PUFA intake on postprandial satiety. Appetite was assessed during the final 2 weeks of the 8-week dietary intervention in which volunteers were randomly assigned to one of four isocaloric energy-restricted diets consisting of: (i) a control diet that contained no seafood, (ii) a diet containing lean fish (0.3 g of n-3 LC-PUFA per day), (iii) a diet containing fatty fish (3.0 g of n-3 LC-PUFA per day), or (iv) a diet including 6 fish-oil capsules per day (1.5 g of n-3 LC-PUFA per day). Weight loss and a decrease in waist circumference were significantly greater in the groups receiving fish or fish oil compared with controls (~1 kg greater weight loss over the first 4 weeks) but in male volunteers only. For the substudy, a validated visual analog scale was used to assess hunger sensations (fullness, hunger) directly after and 2 hours after a test meal consisting of 22% of protein, 30% of fat, and 48% of carbohydrate. The test meal supplied 35% of the prescribed daily energy intake (1.8–2.9 MJ), and food included in the test meals was representative of the different group-specific diets with regard to the inclusion of lean or fatty fish and n-3 LC-PUFA intake. The visual analog-scale assessment revealed higher sensations of fullness in the volunteers who consumed the higher n-3 LC-PUFA-content meals (fatty fish and fish oil) compared with those who consumed the lower n-3 LC-PUFA-content meals (control and lean-fish groups) immediately after and 2 hours after consuming the meal. Feelings of hunger were also lower in the higher n-3 LC-PUFA groups 2 hours after the test meal. The authors concluded that n-3 LC-PUFA intake modulates postprandial satiety in overweight and obese volunteers during weight loss, and postulated that this might improve compliance with the nutritional treatment of overweight and obesity. Thus, possibly increased feelings of satiety following a meal containing a high n-3 LC-PUFA content might reduce subsequent food intake, leading to improvements in weight loss and body composition, but additional research is required.

## *Effects on Expression of Genes Regulating Metabolic Pathways*

Animal studies show that feeding n-3 LC-PUFA up-regulates the expression of genes and proteins involved in fatty acid oxidation in liver, intestine, cardiac muscle, and skeletal muscle, and down-regulates the expression of genes involved in lipogenesis in adipose tissue. These changes may contribute to reductions in body fat by shifting the metabolic profile toward one which favors fat oxidation and reduces fat storage.

Mitochondrial carnitine palmitoyl transferase I (CPT-I) exchanges coenzyme A (CoA) for carnitine to facilitate the transfer of acyl groups into the mitochondria for ß-oxidation in liver, cardiac muscle, and skeletal muscle cells, and is the main control point for ß-oxidation. The mitochondrial expression of CPT-I is regulated by peroxisome proliferator-activated receptors (PPARs) (Mascaro et al., 1998), and increases when the dietary intake of n-3 LC-PUFA increases (Power & Newsholme, 1997). Power and Newsholme (1997) fed male weanling Lewis rats ad libitum for up to 10 weeks on either a nonpurified low-fat diet (25 g of fat/kg) or one of five high-fat diets (200 g of fat/kg). The low-fat diet provided the fat content as corn oil, while the high-fat diets contained hydrogenated coconut oil, olive oil, safflower oil, evening-primrose oil, or EPA-rich menhaden (fish) oil. Groups of 12–18 rats were provided with each diet, and groups of 4–6 animals were removed after 2, 4, and 10 weeks for the analysis of heart CPT-I, and after 4 and 10 weeks for the analysis of skeletal muscle CPT-I. Rats fed the EPA-rich menhaden oil had a significantly greater heart- and skeletal muscle CPT-I specific activity (nmol of product formed/min·mg mitochondrial protein) and a significantly greater skeletal muscle tissue capacity (nmol of product formed/min·mg tissue) compared with rats fed the low-fat diet. While some of the safflower-oil and evening-primrose-oil diets also increased CPT-I specific activity in the heart, only menhaden oil increased mithochondrial CPT-I activity in skeletal muscle. In rats fed menhaden oil, heart, and skeletal muscle CPT-I had lower sensitivity to inhibition by malonyl CoA, compared with rats fed the low-fat diet. This lower sensitivity of CPT-I would also be likely to contribute to increased fat oxidation by maintaining a higher CPT-I activity in the face of other dietary effects on CPT-I regulation by malonyl CoA (Elayan & Winder, 1991). The increased expression of CPT-I in heart and skeletal muscles as a result of increased n-3 LC-PUFA intake is likely to contribute to the regulation of the balance between fat and carbohydrate oxidation by promoting an increased transport of fatty acids into the mitochondria and their subsequent oxidation.

Apart from increases in heart- and skeletal muscle CPT-I, supplementing the diet of rats with n-3 LC-PUFA increased the expression of uncoupling protein 3 (UCP-3) mRNA in skeletal muscle and the expression of peroxisomal acyl-CoA oxidase in skeletal muscle, liver, and heart (Baillie et al., 1999). Baillie et al. (1999) fed two groups of 3–4-week-old male Fisher 344 rats ($n$ = 5 per group) a diet containing 40% of energy from corn oil or fish oil for 6 weeks. By the end of the 6 weeks, the epididymal (i.e., visceral) fat pads from the rats fed the fish-oil diet weighed 25% less than those of the rats fed the corn oil. This decrease in fat deposition was associated with a significant increase in the abundance of skeletal muscle UCP-3 mRNA and an increase in peroxisomal acyl-CoA oxidase gene expression in liver, skeletal muscle, and heart. An increase in peroxisomal fatty acid oxidation is important in terms of regulating energy balance because it is a much less efficient method for oxidizing fats than mitochondrial ß-oxidation, yielding 30–40% more heat and 30% less adenosine triphosphate (ATP) than mitochondrial oxidation (Reddy & Mannaerts, 1994). An increase in peroxisomal acyl-CoA oxidase gene expression suggests that n-3 LC-PUFAs increase the oxidative capacity of this less efficient method of fatty acid oxidation. Additionally, UCPs reduce the efficiency of mitochondrial oxidative phosphorylation by inducing mitochondrial proton leakage, resulting in a reduced ATP yield from oxidative phosphorylation and an increase in heat production. Thus, the combination of an increase in the expression of UCPs and peroxisomal acyl-CoA oxidase would be expected to result in a reduction in overall metabolic efficiency, thereby potentially contributing to an increased loss of energy in the form of heat and less storage of energy in the form of fat.

In addition to these studies which have demonstrated alterations in gene expression in skeletal muscle, liver, and cardiac muscle, Mori et al. (2007) examined the effects of supplementing the diet with n-3 LC-PUFA on body fat accumulation, and the potential role of changes in intestinal gene expression in mediating a reduction in body fat accumulation. Mori and coworkers (2007) divided obesity-prone C57BL/6J mice into five treatment groups and fed them a low-fat diet (5% of triglyceride by weight) or one of four high-fat diets (30% by weight) for 5 months. The high-fat diets consisted of 30% of triglyceride, or 2, 4, or 8% of fish oil with the balance made up of triglyceride. The animals supplemented with 8% of fish oil + 22% of triglyceride exhibited an attenuation ($P < 0.05$) of body-weight increase [13.7 ± 5.3 g increase (mean ± SD)] compared with the 30% of triglyceride diet (20.8 ± 3.7 g increase). The increase in body weight in this treatment group did not differ from that of the mice fed the low-fat (5%) diet (14.6 ± 2.9 g). The differences in body -weight gain between the 8% of fish-oil group and the 30% of triglyceride group could not be accounted for by differences in energy intake. However, the attenuation of weight gain in the 8% of fish-oil group was associated with an increased intestinal expression of genes coding for CPT-Ia, cytochrome P450 4A10, and malic enzyme and 1.2-, 1.6-, and 1.7-fold increases in enzymes of ß-oxidation, ω-oxidation, and malic enzyme, respectively, compared to those receiving the 30% of triglyceride diet. The authors concluded that the anti-obesity effect of fish oil was associated with an up-regulation of intestinal lipid oxidation.

Therefore, part of the mechanism by which n-3 LC-PUFAs reduce body fat may be through the promotion of fat oxidation and, in particular, the less efficient peroxisomal oxidation of fat combined with less efficient mitochondrial substrate oxidation due to the up-regulation of UCPs in liver, cardiac muscle, and particularly skeletal muscle which is a major site for whole-body lipid metabolism (Dagenais et al., 1976), as well as through an increase in intestinal lipid oxidation. Taken together, these effects would be expected to lead to increased, but less efficient, fat oxidation (and potentially less efficient mitochondrial oxidation of other substrates), contributing to a reduced availability of substrate for uptake and storage of fat by adipose cells.

While these effects on intestinal tissue, skeletal muscle, liver, and heart may promote fat oxidation and reduce metabolic efficiency in these tissues, contributing to a reduction in substrate availability for storage by adipose cells, also evidence shows that feeding fish oil influences fat metabolism in adipose tissue itself. Indeed, evidence shows that n-3 LC-PUFA results in changes in gene expression in adipose tissue which favor the oxidation of fat and reduce the capacity to synthesize fat in visceral-fat depots.

Flachs et al. (2005) fed 4-month-old male C57BL/6J mice for 4 weeks on two diets containing 20% of fat (w/w), with the fat in these diets consisting of either flaxseed oil [rich in α-linolenic acid (ALA, a short-chain n-3 PUFA)] or flaxseed oil admixed with an n-3 LC-PUFA concentrate (6% of EPA, 51% of DHA). Two more groups of mice were fed for 5 weeks on two diets containing 35% of fat (w/w), one very low in n-3 LC-PUFA and the other admixed with an n-3 LC-PUFA concentrate which replaced 15% of the dietary lipids. Mice on the n-3 LC-PUFA-supplemented diets had significantly lower body weights and epididymal-fat (i.e., visceral fat) weights by the end of the study periods compared with mice on the non-n-3 LC-PUFA-supplemented diets, but no differences were noted in dorsolumbar-fat (i.e., subcutaneous fat) weights. The greater reduction in epididymal fat with the n-3 LC-PUFA-supplemented diets was associated with increased ß-oxidation and decreased fatty- acid synthesis in epididymal fat and the up-regulation of a number of genes coding for mitochondrial proteins. In particular, an up-regulation of PPAR gamma coactivator 1 α (PGC-1α), CPT-I, and nuclear respiratory factor-1 (NRF-1) occurred in epididymal fat but not in subcutaneous fat. Given that PGC-1α is an upstream regulator of mitochondrial biogenesis and oxidative metabolism, while CPT-I regulates fatty acid entry to the mitochondria and NRF-1 regulates mitochondrial biogenesis (Kelly & Cscarpulla, 2004), these changes in gene expression would be expected to increase the capacity of epididymal fat to oxidize fatty acids, and this was observed as an increase in ß-oxidation in this tissue, as assessed by the release of radioactivity into tissue-culture medium from fragments of adipose tissue prelabeled with [9,10(n)-$^3$H]oleic acid. The diets admixed with n-3 LC-PUFA also resulted in a reduction in expression of stearoyl-CoA desaturase mRNA (a key enzyme in the lipogenic pathway) in epididymal fat, and this was associated with a reduction in fatty acid synthesis in this tissue as assessed by $^3H_20$ incorporation into saponifiable fatty acids. Thus, taken together, the findings of this study by Flachs et al. (2005) indicate that n-3 LC-PUFAs increase the expression of genes in epididymal (i.e., visceral) fat which favor fatty acid oxidation and reduce fatty acid synthesis.

Overall, an increased oxidation of fat in heart, liver, skeletal muscle, and visceral fat would lead to a reduction in the availability of substrate for deposition in adipose tissue, while a reduced capacity to store fat as a result of reduced expression of lipogenic genes in this tissue would contribute to an overall reduction in body fat. While the aforementioned alterations in gene expression would favor a reduction in body fat, many of these changes are not necessarily specific for individual n-3 LC-PUFAs. A recent preliminary study using microarray analysis of genes regulated by dietary fatty acids showed considerable overlap in the influence of different PUFAs on PPARs and other nuclear receptors (Vanden Heuvel, 2008). Therefore, the net influence on fat metabolism will be determined by a complex integration of the effects of individual PUFAs on gene expression.

## Conclusion

A considerable body of evidence was acquired from rodent studies, indicating that supplementing the diet with n-3 LC-PUFA can attenuate weight gain and reduce body fat, particularly epididymal (visceral) fat. Similarly, in human studies, a growing body of evidence indicates that an increased intake of n-3 LC-PUFA can reduce body weight and body fat in overweight and obese individuals.

The mechanism by which an increased intake of n-3 LC-PUFA may improve body composition is most likely an altered gene expression favoring increased fat oxidation in adipose, liver, cardiac, intestinal- and skeletal muscle tissues and reduced fat deposition in adipose tissue. Some preliminary evidence was noted from a recent human study that n-3 LC-PUFA intake might also attenuate postprandial sensations of hunger, although the majority of studies in both rodents and humans which reported that an increased n-3 LC-PUFA intake improved body composition have not reported any reduction in food (i.e., energy) intake.

While growing evidence demonstrates that n-3 LC-PUFA can improve body composition in humans, the majority of studies were of relatively short duration, and the magnitude of the improvements was modest. Accordingly, an urgent need exists for longer term studies to determine the feasibility of using n-3 LC-PUFA supplementation as a strategy to improve body composition in overweight and obese populations.

## References


Baillie, R.; R. Takada; M. Nakamura; S. Clarke. Coordinate induction of peroxisomal acyl-CoA oxidase and UCP-3 by dietary fishoil: a mechanism for decreased body fat deposition. *Prostaglandins, Leukotrienes Essent. Fatty Acids* **1999**, *60,* 351–356.

Belzung, F.; T. Raclot; R. Groscolas. Fish oil n-3 fatty acids selectively limit the hypertrophy of abdominal fat depots in growing rats fed high-fat diets. *Am. J. Physiol.* **1993**, *264,* R1111–R1118.

Brilla, L.; T. Landerholm. Effect of fish oil supplementation and exercise on serum lipids and aerobic fitness. *J. Sports Med. Phys. Fitness* **1990**, *30,* 173–180.

Brown, A.; E. Pang; D. Roberts. Persistent changes in the fatty acid composition of erythrocyte membranes after moderate intake of n-3 polyunsaturated fatty acids: study design implications. *Am. J. Clin. Nutr.* **1991**, *54,* 668–673.

Buckley, J.; S. Burgess; K. Murphy; P. Howe. DHA-rich fish oil lowers heart rate during submaximal exercise in elite Australian Rules footballers. *J. Sci. Med. Sport* **2008** (in press).

Clarke, S. Polyunsaturated fatty acid regulation of gene transcription: a mechanism to improve energy balance and insulin resistance. *Br. J. Nutr.* **2000**, *83,* S59–S66.

Couet, C.; J. Delarue; P. Ritz; J.-M. Antoine; F. Lamisse. Effect of dietary fish oil on body fat mass and basal fat oxidation in healthy adults. *Int. J. Obesity* **1997**, *21,* 637–643.

Cunnane, S.; K. Mcadoo; D. Horrobin. n-3 essential fatty acids decrease weight gain in genetically obese mice. *Br. J. Nutr.* **1986**, *56,* 87–95.

Curioni, C.C.; P.M. Lourenco. Long-term weight loss after diet and exercise: a systematic review. *Int. J. Obes. Relat. Metab. Disord.* **2005**, *29,* 1168–1174.

Dagenais, G.; R. Tancredi; K. Zierler. Free fatty acid oxidation by forearm muscle at rest, and evidence for an intramuscular lipid pool in the human forearm. *J. Clin. Invest.* **1976**, *58,* 421–431.

Dunstan, D.W.; P.Z. Zimmet; T.A. Welborn; M.P. DeCourten; A.J. Cameron; R.A. Sicree; T. Dwyer; S. Colagiuri; D. Jolley; M. Knuiman; et al. The rising prevalence of diabetes and impaired glucose tolerance: the Australian diabetes, obesity and lifestyle study. *Diab. Care* **2002,** *25,* 829–834.

Department of Health and Ageing (1999). National Physical Activity Guidelines for Australians. Canberra, Australia.

Elayan, I.; W. Winder. Effect of glucose infusion on muscle malonyl-CoA during exercise. *J. Appl. Physiol.* **1991**, *70,* 1495–1499.

Flegel, K.; M. Carroll; R. Kuczmarski; C. Johnson. Overweight and obesity in the United States: prevalence and trends, 1960–1994. *Int. J. Obes.* **1998,** *22,* 39–47.

Flachs, P.; O. Horakova; P. Brauner; M. Rossmeisl; P. Pecina; N. Franssen-Van Hal; J. Ruzickova; J. Sponarova; Z. Drahota; C. Vlcek; et al. Polyunsaturated fatty acids of marine origin upregulate mitochondrial biogenesis and induce β-oxidation in white fat. *Diabetologica* **2005**, *48,* 2365–75.

Fontani, G.; F. Corradeschi; A. Felici; F. Alfatti; R. Bugarini; A.I. Fiaschi; D. Cerretani; G. Montorfano; A.M. Rizzo; B. Berra. Blood profiles, body fat and mood state in healthy subjects on different diets supplemented with Omega-3 polyunsaturated fatty acids. *Eur. J. Clin. Invest.* **2005**, *35,* 499–507.

Fujihira, E.; H. Takahashi; M. Nakazawa. Effect of long-term feeding of taurine in hereditary hyperglycemic obese mice. *Chem. Pharm. Bull. (Tokyo)* **1970**, *18,* 1636–1642.

Groh-Wargo, S.; J. Jacobs; N. Auestad; D.L. O'connor; J.J. Moore; E. Lerner. Body composition in preterm infants who are fed long chain polyunsaturated fatty acids: a prospective, randomized, controlled trial. *Pediatr. Res.* **2005**, *57,* 712–718.

Hainault, I.; M. Carlotti; E. Hajduch; C. Guichard; M. Lavau. Fish oil in a high lard diet prevents obesity, hyperlipidemia, and adipocyte insulin resistance in rats. *Ann. N. Y. Acad. Sci.* **1993**, *683,* 98–101.

Harris, W.S.; J.V. Pottala; S.A. Sands; P.G. Jones. Comparison of the effects of fish and fish-oil capsules on the n 3 fatty acid content of blood cells and plasma phospholipids. *Am. J. Clin. Nutr.* **2007**, *86,* 1621–1625.

He, K.; E. Rimm; A. Merchant; B. Rosner; M. Stampfer; W. Willett; A. Ascherio. Fish consumption and risk of stroke in men. *JAMA* **2002**, *288,* 3130–3136.

Hill, A.; J. Buckley; K. Murphy; P. Howe. Combining fish oil supplementation with regular aerobic exercise improves body composition and cardiovascular risk factors. *Am. J. Clin. Nutr.* **2007**, *85,* 1267–1274.

Huang, X.F.; X. Xin; P. Mclennan; L. Storlien. Role of fat amount and type in ameliorating diet-induced obesity: insights at the level of hypothalamic arcuate nucleus leptin receptor, neuropeptide Y and pro-opiomelanocortin mRNA expression. *Diab. Obes. Metab.* **2004**, *6,* 35–44.

Iso, H.; K.M. Rexrode; M.J. Stampfer; J.E. Manson; G.A. Colditz; F.E. Speizer; C.H. Hennekens; W.C. Willett. Intake of fish and omega-3 fatty acids and risk of stroke in women. *JAMA* **2001**, *285,* 304–312.

Kabir, M.; G. Skurnik; N. Naour; V. Pechtner; E. Meugnier; S. Rome; A. Quignard-Boulange; H. Vidal; G. Slama; K. Clement; et al. Treatment for 2 mo with n-3 polyunsaturated fatty acids reduces adiposity and some atherogenic factors but does not improve insulin sensitivity in women with type 2 diabetes: a randomized controlled study. *Am. J. Clin. Nutr.* **2007**, *86,* 1670–1679.

Kelly, D.; R. Cscarpulla. Transcriptional regulatory circuits controlling mitochondrial biogenesis and function. *Genes Dev.* **2004**, *18,* 357–368.

Krebs, J.; L. Browning; N. Mclean; J. Rothwell; G. Mishra; C. Moore; S. Jebb. Additive benefits of long chain n-3 polyunsaturated fatty acids and weight-loss in the management of cardiovascular disease risk in overweight hyperinsulinaemic women. *Int. J. Obes.* **2006**, *30,* 1535–1544.

Kunešová, M.; R. Braunerová; P. Hlavatý; E. Tvrzická; B. Staňková; J. Škrha; J. Hilgertová; M. Hill; J. Kopecký; M. Wagenchnecht; et al. The influence of n-3 polyunsaturated fatty acids and very low calorie diet during a short-term weight reducing regimen on weight loss and serum fatty acid composition in severely obese women. *Physiol. Res.* **2006**, *55,* 63–72.

Mascaro, C.; E. Acosta; J. Ortiz; P. Marrero; F. Hegardt; D. Haro. Control of human muscle-type carnitine palmitoyltransferase I gene transcription by peroxisome proliferator-activated receptor. *J. Biol. Chem.* **1998**, *273,* 8560–8563.

Mori, T.; H. Kondo; T. Hase; I. Tokimitsu; T. Murase. Dietary fish oil upregulates intestinal lipid metabolism and reduces body Weight gain in C57BL/6J mice. *J. Nutr.* **2007**, *137,* 2629–2634.

Must, A.; J. Spadano; E.H. Coakley; A.E. Field; G. Colditz; W.H. Dietz. The disease burden associated with overweight and obesity. *JAMA* **1999**, *282,* 1523–1529.

National Health and Medical Research Council. *Dietary Guidelines for Australian Adults*; Commonwealth of Australia, 2003.

Parra, D.; A. Ramel; N. Bandarra; M. Kiely; J. Martinez; I. Thorsdottir. A diet rich in long chain omega 3 fatty acids modulates satiety in overweight and obese volunteers during weight loss. *Appetite* **2008**, doi:10.1016/j.appet.2008.06.003.

Parrish, C.; D. Pathy; J. Parkes; A. Angel. Dietary fish oils limit adipose tissue hypertrophy in rats. *Metabolism* **1990**, *39,* 217–219.

Power, G.; E. Newsholme. Dietary fatty acids influence the activity and metabolic control of mitochondrial carnitine palmitoyltransferase I in rat heart and skeletal muscle. *J. Nutr.* **1997**, *127,* 2142–2150.

Reddy, J.; G. Mannaerts. Peroxisomal lipid metabolism. *Ann. Rev. Nutr.* **1994**, *14,* 343–370.

Ruzickova, J.; M. Rossmeisl; T. Prazak; P. Flachs; J. Sponarova; M. Veck; E. Tvrzicka; M. Bryhn; J. Kopecky. Omega-3 PUFA of marine origin limit diet-induced obesity in mice by reducing cellularity of adipose tissue. *Lipids* **2004**, *39,* 1177–1185.

Thorsdottir, I.; H. Tomasson; I. Gunnarsdottir; E. Gisladottir; M. Kiely; M. Parra; N. Bandarra; G. Schaafsma; J. Martine. Randomized trial of weight-loss-diets for young adults varying in fish and fish oil content. *Int. J. Obes.* **2007**, doi:10.1038/sj.ijo.0803643.

Todoric, J.; M. Löffler; J. Huber; M. Bilban; M. Reimers; A. Kadl; M. Zeyda; W. Waldhäusl; T. Stulnig. Adipose tissue inflammation induced by high-fat diet in obese diabetic mice is prevented by n-3 polyunsaturated fatty acids. *Diabetologia* **2006**, *49,* 2109–2119.

Vanden Heuvel, J. Fatty acid transcriptomics. *Proceedings of the International Society for the Study of Fatty Acids and Lipids,* Kansas City; 2008.

Visscher, T.L.; J.C. Seidell. The public health impact of obesity. *Annu. Rev. Public Health* **2001**, *22,* 355–375.

Warner, J.; I. Ullrich; M. Albrink; R. Yeater. Combined effects of aerobic exercise and omega-3 fatty acids in hyperlipidemic persons. *Med. Sci. Sports Exerc.* **1989**, *21*, 498–505.

# 31

# Food Sources and Intakes of Omega-3 Fatty Acids

**Karen J. Murphy and Peter R.C. Howe**
*Nutritional Physiology Research Centre, Division of Health Sciences, University of South Australia, Adelaide, SA 5000*

## Health Benefits of n-3 LC-PUFA

Early population studies by (Bang & Dyerberg, 1972; Sinclair et al., 1994) and others first indicated that consumption of seafood rich in omega-3 long chain polyunsaturated fatty acids (n-3 LC-PUFA) is beneficial for cardiovascular (CV) health. Extensive literature has since shown that a high intake of n-3 LC-PUFA is cardioprotective through reduction of risk factors such as hypertension, dyslipidemia and thrombosis (Hu & Willett, 2002; Wijendran & Hayes, 2004), improvement of arterial compliance, endothelial vasodilator function and heart rate variability (Nestel, 2001; Nestel et al., 2002; Christensen, 2003), and prevention of arrhythmia and sudden cardiac death (McLennan et al., 1996; Marchioli, 1999).

The most investigated n-3 LC-PUFA are eicosapentaenoic acid (EPA, 20:5n-3) and docosahexaenoic acid (DHA, 22:6n-3), which are obtained primarily through regular consumption of fatty fish and become incorporated in tissues throughout the body. Harris and Von Schacky (2004) have shown that the level of EPA + DHA in erythrocytes (Omega-3 Index), a readily measurable biomarker of n-3 LC-PUFA status, is inversely related to the risk of CV morbidity and mortality. Fish also contains lower proportions of docosapentaenoic acid (DPA, 22:5n-3), an intermediate n-3 LC-PUFA. Although less is known about its health benefits, DPA is also found in meat and there is emerging evidence to support cardioprotective and possibly mental health benefits (Conquer et al., 1999; Akiba et al., 2000).

Other studies have shown the beneficial effect of raised blood levels of n-3 LC-PUFA for neural development in infants (Bourre, 2005a; Smithers et al., 2008), for mental fitness, including cognition and psychological well-being, in adults (Sinn, 2008; Sinn, 2008; Sinn et al., 2008) and for inflammatory conditions such as arthritis and psoriasis (James et al., 2000; Cleland et al., 2006; Proudman et al., 2008).

The rapid growth of the brain in the last trimester of pregnancy and the first two years of infancy is largely dependent upon maternal intake of n-3 LC-PUFA, particularly DHA (Innis, 2008). Effects of maternal DHA consumption on neurodevelopment have been investigated in a number of observational and randomized controlled trials.

The latter have shown that increasing maternal intake of n-3 LC-PUFA through supplementation with fish oil results in higher blood levels of n-3 LC-PUFA in the infant and may aid growth and development (Simmer et al., 2008). In a meta-analysis of 14 trials, DHA supplementation was associated with improvements in visual acuity in a dose response manner (Uauy et al., 2003). Similarly, other studies have shown improvements in child IQ scores, mental processing scores, language, and behavioral attention scores (Helland et al., 2003; Colombo et al., 2004; Daniels et al., 2004; Cohen et al., 2005; Oken et al., 2005).

Neural and mental development continues to occur rapidly for the first year necessitating an adequate supply of n-3 LC-PUFA, which is why a number of infant formulas have been fortified with n-3 LC-PUFA. n-3 LC-PUFA are essential nutrients that are incorporated into the grey matter of the brain where they influence several functions including cognition (Bourre, 2005a). Emerging evidence is slowly identifying inverse associations between fish consumption and the prevention of psychiatric disorders such as depression, manic depression, and dementia (Bourre, 2005a; Sinn, 2008). Recent studies have shown improvements in cognitive function including attention and behaviour in children with attention deficit hyperactivity disorder (Sinn, 2008; Sinn et al., 2008). However more research is required in this area to fully understand the relationship between n-3 LC-PUFA and mental and psychological health.

## n-3 LC-PUFA Intake Recommendations

Various recommendations have been proposed by governments and international professional organisations for n-3 LC-PUFA intake requirements at different stages of life. While these recommendations reflect a general consensus on the importance of n-3 LC-PUFA consumption, the requirements vary considerably and there is uncertainty as to their scientific justification. For this reason, the United States and Canada declined to make official recommendations for n-3 LC-PUFA intake. The joint US/Canada dietary reference values (DRV) released in 2002 confirmed the need for α-linolenic acid (ALA, 18:3n-3) but not EPA and DHA (FNB, 2002). Nevertheless they allowed for the latter to be consumed at up to 10% of the requirement for ALA. Additionally the American Heart Association (AHA) have not specified an intake requirement of n-3 LC-PUFA for a normal healthy population, although they recommend eating at least two fatty-fish meals per week, equating to 400-500mg/day n-3 LC-PUFA to maintain CV health (Kris-Etherton et al., 2003).

A number of other public health organisations have also recommended regular consumption of fatty fish and suggested n-3 LC-PUFA equivalents without specifying actual recommendations for the latter (see Table 31.1).

An International Society for the Study of Fatty Acids and Lipids ISSFAL sponsored consensus workshop held at NIH in 1999 recommended a daily intake of 650mg n-3 LC-PUFA. This recommendation was based on the Multiple Risk Factor Intervention Trial (MRFIT) of 12,866 males (Dolecek, 1992) and represents the median intake of

**Table 31.1. Various international recommendations for n-3 LC-PUFA intake (mg/d)**

| | n-3 LC-PUFA mg/d | Serves of fish (n-3 LC-PUFA equivalent ) |
|---|---|---|
| North Atlantic Treaty Organisation (NATO), 1989 (Simopoulos et al. 1999) | 800 | |
| British Nutrition Foundation, 1992 (BNF 1992) | 400–1000[a] | |
| UK Committee on Medical Aspects of Food Policy, 1994 (COMA 1994) | 200 | |
| Japanese, 1996 (Ministry of Health Labor and Welfare 1999) | 1600 | |
| ISSFAL Expert workshop, 1999 (Simopoulos et al. 1999) | 650 | |
| Crete Eurodiet-nutrition, 2000 (Bourre 2005b) | 200 | |
| France, CNERNA-CNRS; AFSSA, 2001(Martin 2001) | 400 (F) 500 (M) | |
| Health Council of the Netherlands, 2001 (1991) | 200 | |
| European Academy of Nutritional Sciences, Expert Workshop, 1997 (de Deckere et al. 1998) | | 1 serve/wk (200mg/d) |
| American Heart Association, 2002 (Kris-Etherton et al. 2003) | | 2 serves/wk (400-500mg/d) |
| World Health Organisation, Food & Agriculture Organisation, 2003 (WHO 2003) | | 1-2 fish meals/wk |
| UK Scientific Advisory Committee on Nutrition, 2004 | | 2 serves/wk (450mg/d) |
| ISSFAL, 2004 (ISSFAL. 2004) | 500 | |
| National Health Medical Research Council, Australia, 2005 (NHMRC 2006) | 430 (F) 610 (M)[b] | |
| National Heart Foundation of Australia, 2008 (Colquhoun et al. 2008) | 500 | |

F, females, M, males
[a] EPA 0.2% - 0.5% dietary energy, DHA 0.5% dietary energy
[b] suggested daily target

the highest quintile which showed a significantly lower risk of CV mortality. In 2004, the leading professional body in lipid and fatty acid research, ISSFAL recommended the consumption of 500mg per day of EPA+DHA for CV health. This recommendation was based on evidence from major epidemiological studies conducted in the United States in which the intakes of n-3 LC-PUFA among healthy adults were estimated and the subsequent risk for death from coronary heart disease (CHD) was determined. A meta-analysis of these studies identified a significant relationship between risk for CHD mortality and EPA+DHA intake (ISSFAL). The relative risk reduction in the highest vs. the lowest intake groups was 37%, and the intake in that quintile averaged 566 mg EPA+DHA per day. Based on large prospective population studies and case-control studies, an intake of about 500 mg of EPA+DHA per day has been estimated to significantly reduce risk for death from CHD in healthy adults. This intake is achievable by diet alone, particularly for fish eating populations, and has shown to be safe even for pregnant and lactating women for whom mercury intake can be an issue.

In fact doses lower than 500mg of n-3 LC-PUFA may be sufficient to improve CV health. The Nurses' Health Study (Hu et al., 2002) shows that in 84,688 healthy women aged 34–59 yrs, median intakes in each quintile of 30mg, 50mg, 80mg, 140mg, and 240mg n-3 LC-PUFA were associated with relative risk of CHD of 1.0, 0.93, 0.78, 0.68, and 0.67, respectively ($P < 0.001$ for trend). Moreover Mozaffarian and Rimm (2006) have shown in a number of prospective cohort studies and randomized clinical trials that the threshold intake for relative risk of CHD death is approximately 250mg of EPA + DHA per day. These data taken together show that a dose of less than 500mg of n-3 LC-PUFA might in fact be beneficial to health as well as being an easier dietary target intake level, particularly for non-fish eating populations like Australia and the United States.

## Official Recommendations for Australia and New Zealand

Australia and New Zealand are among the first countries to have official Government recommendations for n-3 LC-PUFA intakes. The growing evidence relating n-3 LC-PUFA consumption to health prompted the Australian National Health and Medical Research Council (NHMRC) to include nutrient reference values (NRVs) for n-3 LC-PUFA for the first time when revising its nutrient intake recommendations in 2005 (NHMRC, 2006). These NRVs, which were based on population intakes estimated from the 1995 Australian National Nutrition Survey (Howe et al., 2007), have been officially adopted by the Australian and New Zealand governments. The recommendations for adults are summarised in Table 31.2. Although the essentiality of n-3 LC-PUFA, for health was recognised, there was insufficient evidence to establish a recommended dietary intake (RDI) for n-3 LC-PUFA. Hence the NHMRC set an adequate intake (AI) based on the median population intake of n-3 LC-PUFA including EPA+DPA+DHA, of the Australian population.

Recognising that a higher intake of n-3 LC-PUFA (higher than the AI) was likely to be beneficial for the prevention of chronic disease, the NHMRC established suggested dietary targets (SDT) for EPA+DPA+DHA (610mg and 430mg in males and females, respectively). Those intake levels represent the 90$^{th}$ percentile of intakes. The SDTs were not based on a precise estimation of requirement but were set at a level that was being consumed readily and with apparent safety by the top decile of the population.

**Table 31.2. National Health and Medical Research Council Nutrient Reference Values for Australia and New Zealand.**

| Group (Adults) | n-3 LC-PUFA (EPA+DPA+DHA) mg/day | | |
|---|---|---|---|
| | Adequate Intake (AI) | Suggested Dietary Target (SDT) | Upper Level of Intake (UL) |
| Males | 160 | 610 | 3000 |
| Females | 90 | 430 | 3000 |

## Current Dietary Intakes

While there is considerable evidence supporting the health benefits of increased consumption of n-3 LC-PUFA, there is little information regarding current intakes and the contribution of various food groups to intake levels. There appears to have been a large evolutionary change in intake of dietary fat and PUFA consumption. Our paleolithic ancestors had a lower intake of total fat, saturated fat, and omega-6 (n-6) PUFA; it is estimated that these ancestors consumed around 8.8g/d of linoleic acid and 12.6g/d of ALA ie. a n-6:n-3 intake of ≈0.7. This is vastly different to the 10:1 ratio estimated for Western diets today (Eaton et al., 1998). Hunter-gatherer diets were reported to contain around 1100mg/d for n-3 LC-PUFA, which is thought to be much higher than intakes of Western populations such as the United States and Australia. However, reliable information on population intakes of n-3 LC-PUFA has been sadly lacking.

The lack of information on population intakes is due primarily to a lack of dietary databases containing detailed and reliable information on the fatty acid compositions of foods and beverages. To address this, Mann and colleagues (2003) updated the NUTTAB95 dietary database with fatty acid composition profiles for a range of commonly eaten foods in Australia. The information used in extending this database was derived from an extensive search of the literature post 1990 to locate published fatty acid profiles of foods. This was combined with data collected from government bodies, industry sources, and research groups and food analysed in the author's laboratory to produce a comprehensive fatty acid database for 1044 foods. Utilising this comprehensive database, Meyer and colleagues (2003) analysed the dietary intake data of 10,851 Australian adults from the 1995 National Nutrition Survey (McLennan & Podger, 1997) and reported that the average intake of n-3 LC-PUFA was 189mg/d (56mg EPA, 26mg DPA, 106mg DHA). As expected, fish and seafood were the main contributors to n-3 LC-PUFA intake (71%). Interestingly however, meat was identified as a major contributor (≈20%) to total n-3 LC-PUFA consumption.

This potentially important role for meat in meeting n-3 LC-PUFA intake requirements prompted the same authors to re-evaluate dietary intakes and food sources with a sharper focus on the relative contribution of meat. The authors extended the database with additional analyses of the EPA, DPA, and DHA contents of different cuts of meat, thus expanding the database to 4550 foods (Howe et al., 2006). Using this expanded database, the mean intake of n-3 LC-PUFA (EPA+DPA+DHA) estimated from the NNS95 was revised upwards to 246mg/d; EPA was 75mg/d, DPA 71mg/d, and DHA 100mg/d. Fish and seafood products and dishes were then found to contribute 48% of n-3 LC-PUFA intake, with 50%, 15%, and 70% of this intake comprising EPA, DPA, and DHA intake, respectively, while meat, poultry, and game products and dishes contributed 43% of the n-3 LC-PUFA intake. The intakes of EPA and DHA, predominantly from fish and seafood, were similar in both studies (Meyer et al., 2003; Howe et al., 2006). However, the re-evaluation of the contribution of meat to n-3 LC-PUFA intake in the second study (Howe et al., 2006) was notably different, indicating that meat was the main source of DPA, providing 71mg/d, compared with the estimate of 26mg/d in the earlier study by Meyer et al. (2003), thus increasing the estimated intake of n-3 LC-PUFA from 189mg/d to 246mg/d. Given the emerging evidence for health benefits associated with DPA, these data highlight the importance of including the contribution of DPA to n-3 LC-PUFA intake, especially for meat eating populations.

Based on the data from Howe et al. (2006), there is a clear indication that Australians are eating less n-3 LC-PUFA than other Western populations except for the United States where they are consuming ≤200mg/d (EPA+DHA) (Kris-Etherton et al. 2000). Fish eating populations have considerably higher intakes. For example, Greenland Eskimos reportedly consumed around 7000mg of n-3 LC-PUFA per day (Dyerberg and Jorgensen 1982; Dyerberg 1986). Similarly, the Japanese are reported to be consuming an average of 1600mg n-3 LC-PUFA per day with a median intake of 900mg (Sugano, 1996) and Norwegians are consuming approximately 369mg/d (Bonaa et al., 1992). Like Australia and the United States, the French are eating less than a half of their recommended dietary allowance (Meyer et al., 2004).

## Sources of n-3 LC-PUFA

### *Seafood*

Seafood is arguably the best and safest source of n-3 LC-PUFA and is also an excellent source of protein and vitamins and minerals including iodine, zinc, iron, magnesium, selenium, and fluoride. Shellfish, particularly crustaceans, contain around twice as much cholesterol as typical finfish, however they also contain a lot of non-cholesterol sterols such as brassicasterol and dinosterol (Murphy et al., 2003) which may have anti-inflammatory activity (Bouic & Lamprecht, 1999; Gomez et al., 1999). The Heart Foundation of Australia, like the AHA, has traditionally recommended that we eat two fatty fish meals per week, but Australians eat six times as much meat as fish contributing to low n-3 LC-PUFA intakes. Additionally, popular fish in Australia have relatively low fat content which further impacts on low n-3 LC-PUFA intake. Seafood consumption rates vary substantially from country to country. Iceland is notably the highest fish eating population around the world at approximately 91kg per capita per annum, followed by Japan (66kg), Guyana (64kg), Malaysia (56kg),

Korea and Norway (51kg), Gabon (45kg), Spain (41kg), Senegal (36kg), Finland (33kg), (30kg), United States (21kg), Canada (22kg), and New Zealand (24kg) (York & Gossard, 2004). These are based on figures of food sold whereas the actual fish consumed might be considerably less. For example according to the NNS95 Australians consume 26g of fish and seafood products and dishes per day which equates to 9.4kg/year (McLennan & Podger, 1997). This rate of consumption is lower than the recommended fish consumption of two serves per week (equivalent to 30–40g per day).

Why don't we eat more fish? Is it just because we are unsure of how to prepare and cook it or is it more to do with consumer attitudes? The Fisheries Research and Development Corporation in Australia reported on consumer's attitudes towards purchasing fish. It was noted that when fish and seafood was purchased for in-home consumption, consumers expected the physical condition of the retailer to be clean and hygienic and the presentation and speed and efficiency of the staff was also expected to be of high standard. They also preferred to purchase fresh, not frozen, local product of high quality when either dining at home or out of home, and outlets offering completely boneless fillets and products ready to eat were also attractive to consumers (FRDC, 2002). One of the most interesting trends in Australia in the 1990s was the move to eateries such as cafes, fast food outlets, and eat-in fish and chip shops which tend to be cheaper and more casual than restaurant dining (FRDC, 2002). Sushi consumption was on the increase in 1999, probably due to the expansion of franchised sushi stores.

The choice of fish to consume is important in determining n-3 LC-PUFA intake as not all fish and seafood are the same in terms of their n-3 LC-PUFA composition. As a rule plant eating finfish (aquatic vertebrates with gills, fins, and elongated body with scales) have less n-3 LC-PUFA than carnivorous finfish, whereas tuna, salmon, sardine, swordfish, and trout are rich in n-3 LC-PUFA (Nichols, 2004).

### *Over-fishing*

Serious concerns have been raised about the widespread global decline of major fish stocks and the effects of overfishing on these communities. It is becoming apparent that global fish stocks will be insufficient to meet human nutritional requirements in the not too distant future. Abeywardena et al. (2005) reported that Pacific Ocean stocks of up to 60 species are already under pressure from environmental degradation and over fishing. These concerns have sparked a United Nations resolution to restore fisheries and marine ecosystems to healthy levels. An analysis conducted by Myers and Worm (2003) has shown pronounced declines of entire communities across widely varying ecosystems and the global ocean has lost over 90% of large predatory fishes.

Freshwater or farmed fish have the ability to convert the shorter chain precursor ALA to EPA and DHA, unlike deep sea fish which have poor endogenous conversion of precursor n-3 PUFA and must obtain their n-3 LC-PUFA from algae, phytoplankton, and other small fish (Sargent, 1997). Interestingly, different parts of fish have different n-3 LC-PUFA composition. Table 31.3 shows that the edible portions of fish, e.g. fillets, have about half the amount of n-3 LC-PUFA as the skin and about a fifth of the n-3 LC-PUFA content present in the viscera. The inedible parts of the fish, including skin, head, frame, and viscera, are byproducts of processing which are very rich sources of n-3 LC-PUFA. This byproduct is utilised to produce fish oil and fishmeal which can then be used for human consumption to enrich livestock feeds (Howe et al., 2002) and for aquaculture feed.

### *Safety Concerns*

There is a growing concern regarding environmental factors such as contaminants including heavy metals notably mercury and methyl mercury, dioxins, and polychlorinated biphenyls in fish and seafood and potential detrimental health benefits. This environmental concern is perhaps a major deterrent for consumers to increase their fish intake. However a study by Weil and colleagues (2005) found that blood mercury level and neurobehavioral function were not significantly related in a population of 50–70 year olds. The median blood mercury level was lower than the 'acceptable' level for women of childbearing age and children as established by the U.S. Environmental Protection Agency and National Research Council.

The mercury issue has been overstated at times and consumers confuse the warnings surrounding the increased consumption of large fish and regard the warnings for all fish. Large predatory fish like swordfish, tuna, marlin, bass, and shark tend to accumulate higher levels of mercury than smaller fish like herring, catfish, shrimp, or tilapia, crustaceans, and molluscs which, in turn, eat smaller plant eating fish. Moreover, fish and seafood contain selenium which counteracts the effects of mercury (FRDC, 2004). The FDA in the United States and FSANZ in Australia have now established specific guidelines for consumers to follow in relation to fish consumption to mercury concerns.

## Alternative Dietary Sources of n-3 LC-PUFA

The increasing worldwide demand for n-3 LC-PUFA, combined with the reduction in the world's fish stocks (Myers & Worm, 2003; Abeywardena et al., 2005) necessitates

**Table 31.3. n-3 LC-PUFA Composition of Australian Seafood (mg/100g, wet weight).**

| Food (Tasmanian Atlantic salmon (farmed)) | n-3 LC-PUFA (mainly EPA+DHA) mg/100g (wet weight) |
|---|---|
| Whole fillet | 1930 |
| Skin | 4050 |
| Head | 5370 |
| Frame | 5240 |
| Belly flap/viscera | 10270 |

* based on figures for Australian fish.
Adapted from Nichols et al. (1998).

the identification of new sources of n-3 LC-PUFA. A rapidly increasing market for alternative n-3 LC-PUFA sources is being developed which includes processed foods enriched with microencapsulated fish oil or microalgal oils, farmed fish and meat and eggs enriched through manipulation of aquaculture feeds, and livestock feeds with fish oil, fishmeal, plant sources of ALA, and plants genetically modified to produce LC n3 PUFA . These sources of n-3 LC-PUFA are illustrated in Fig. 31.1. Consumer acceptance of the enriched sources will depend on a range of factors including taste, quality, stability, price, and the potential for producers to make health claims.

Suitable sensory qualities of n-3 LC-PUFA enriched foods are the primary determinant of consumer acceptability. Consumers can readily detect subtle changes in appearance, odour, taste, texture, mouthfeel, and aftertaste of foods that have been modified in some way. Similarly the cost of the product and value for money will also be considered by the consumer. These considerations are the most important characteristics when choosing the type of food to enrich and the level of enrichment to maintain shelf life and sensory qualities. Most importantly consumers will consider what type of food has been enriched with n-3 LC-PUFA. Would consumers choose to buy n-3 LC-PUFA enriched beer or water?

## *Meat*

Meat tends to be overlooked as a source of n-3 LC-PUFA. Most of the evidence substantiating the health benefits of n-3 LC-PUFA is based on dietary supplementation trials with fish or fish oils rich in EPA and/or DHA. However meat contains relatively greater amounts of DPA. Table 31.4 shows the relative proportions of EPA, DPA, and DHA in meat and fish, weighted according to the relative rates of consumption of different meat and fish products in Australia. DPA accounts for 29% of the total dietary intake of n-3 LC-PUFA of Australian adults.

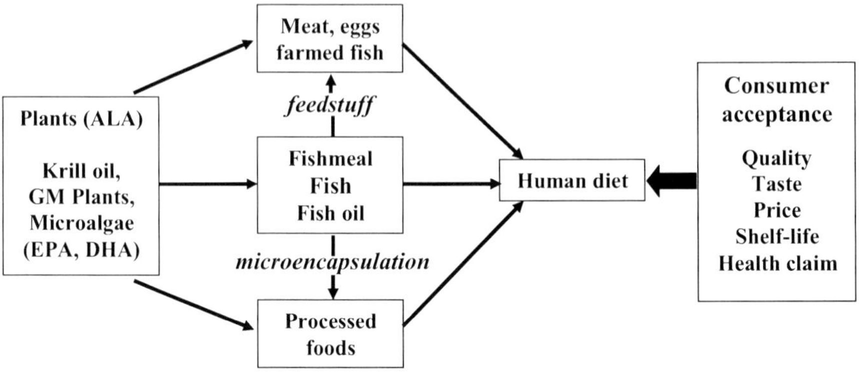


**Fig. 31.1.** Sources of n-3 LC-PUFA.

## *Fish Oil Supplements*

Over the past decade there have been significant improvements in both the production and encapsulation of fish oils leading to improvements in the color and odor and the reduction of the 'fishy' taste and 'fishy burps.' As consumers are becoming more aware of the health benefits of n-3 LC-PUFA, they appear to be increasing their use of fish oil supplements and including n-3 LC-PUFA enriched foods in their diet. Marine sources are the main source for n-3 LC-PUFA, while only a small percentage of n-3 LC-PUFA is derived from microalgae. The most common sources are tuna oil, salmon oil, menhaden oil, and cod liver oil. However, additional sources are being introduced to the market, which include krill oil, seal oil (DPA rich), and shark liver oil (Nichols, 2007). Interestingly only 3% of the fish oil produced is used for human consumption, of which nearly three quarters is used in nutritional supplements, while 13% being used in functional foods and 9% used in other applications (Daniells, 2008).

A study by Harris et al. (2007) investigated the bioequivalence of fish vs. fish oil. Harris and colleagues found the consumption of equivalent quantity of n-3 LC-PUFA in salmon and tuna (485mg) compared with fish oil supplements provided the same level of incorporation of EPA and DHA into erythrocytes, raising the Omega-3 Index by ≈2% after 16 weeks of consumption.

Given that the bioavailability of n-3 LC-PUFA is the same for fish and fish oil, fish oil may be a good option for individuals who are unable to eat fish and seafood for various reasons such as taste, vegetarian diet, fish protein allergy, or for individuals unable to eat the suggested number of fish serves per week required to provide health benefits. Fish oil can be purchased either as oil or capsules with differing doses of n-3 LC-PUFA ranging from 300mg EPA+DHA/g, typically menhaden oil with EPA (180mg) and DHA (120mg) in triglyceride form, to more concentrated preparations of methyl and ethyl ester derivatives eg. Omacor (850mg EPA+DHA/g). Larger doses of n-3 LC-PUFA (up to 30mL/d) may be more conveniently consumed as bottled fish oil.

## *Single Cell Oils*

Environmental concerns and declining global fish stocks have encouraged the recent market entry of products derived from single cell organisms like algae and fungi.

**Table 31.4. Relative n-3 LC-PUFA Composition of Meat and Fish (mg/100g).**

| Food (mg/100g), raw | EPA | DPA | DHA | n-3 LC-PUFA |
|---|---|---|---|---|
| Fish* | 247 | 66 | 415 | 728 |
| Beef | 45 | 71 | 13 | 129 |
| Lamb | 40 | 83 | 20 | 143 |
| Pork | 14 | 28 | 16 | 58 |
| Poultry | 14 | 18 | 15 | 47 |

*contributions of different types of meat and fish were weighted according to their relative rates of consumption in the Australian National Nutrition Survey (NNS,1995) (McLennan & Podger, 1997).

Adapted from Howe et al. (2007).

Ratledge and Cohen (2008). The productivity of microorganisms and algae (biomass and oil) is much higher than that of plants, however their production costs using fermentation technology is far more expensive at present (Ratledge and Cohen 2008).

Common microalgae utilized for their n-3 LC-PUFA content include dinoflagellates and thraustochytrids which are grown in fermenters to produce n-3 LC-PUFA. These algal sources of n-3 LC-PUFA have been used in supplementation studies and dietary intervention studies with algal n-3 LC-PUFA derived enriched foods. An early study by Conquer et al. (1999) demonstrated the efficacy of an algae source of DHA (DHASCO®) on serum and platelet fatty acid status and CV risk factors in healthy vegetarians. Similarly, Arterburn et al. (2007) demonstrated the bioequivalence of two different strains of microalgal oils (DHASCO®) and a microalgal oil enriched snack bar.

Microalgal sources provide useful bioavailable alternatives for fish and seafood consumption for vegetarians (Conquer et al., 1999; Arterburn et al., 2007; Arterburn et al., 2008) and can be added to food products including bread (Serna-Saldivar et al., 2006). A natural golden marine algae has also been used as a poultry ration supplement for the production of shell eggs rich in n-3 LC-PUFA (Herber & Van Elswyk, 1996) while some single cell n-3 LC-PUFA rich oils have been used in infant formula (Fleith & Clandinin, 2005). n-3 LC-PUFA are considered essential nutrients for not only neurodevelopment in the term infant, but for the infant born prematurely. Attempts are being made to match fatty acid profiles of formula and breast milk. Infants born prematurely miss part of the accretion of n-3 LC-PUFA, particularly arachidonic acid (AA, 20:4n-6) and DHA during the last trimester of pregnancy (Clandinin et al., 1980). A study by (Makrides et al., 1994) showed a lower content of DHA in brain and retina in infants fed formula devoid of n-3 LC-PUFA than infants fed human milk containing n-3 LC-PUFA. The demand for n-3 LC-PUFA during gestation and the first few years of life for brain development as well as the extra demand for pre-term infants highlights the need for formulas enriched with n-3 LC-PUFA.

It has recently been shown that crude glycerol is a suitable carbon source for algal fermentation. The crude glycerol-derived algal biomass had a high level of DHA and a nutritional profile similar to that of commercial algal biomass, suggesting a great potential for using crude glycerol-derived algae in n-3 LC-PUFA fortified food or feed (Pyle et al., 2008).

## *Krill Oil*

Neptune krill oil is increasing in terms of its ability to provide a viable source of n-3 LC-PUFA in phospholipid form and it is becoming increasingly available on the world market (Nichols, 2007). Krill oil is extracted from Antarctic krill which is considered to be the most abundant biomass on the planet (Kock et al., 2007). The annual production of Antarctic krill is thought to be several hundred million tonnes of which 85 million tonnes is consumed by Antarctic baleen whales. Krill oil is composed of at least 30% EPA+DHA (by weight) and is approximately 40% phospholipid (mainly phosphatidylcholine) which is in contrast to regular fish body oils which are in triglyceride form. A recent review by Massrieh (2008) shows that krill oil (at approximately the same EPA+DHA dose) can increase high density lipoprotein cholesterol, can lower triglyceride and low density lipoprotein cholesterol levels, and is more effective in lowering total cholesterol than fish oil in subjects with hypertriglyceridemia and hypercholesterolemia (Massrieh, 2008).

## *Genetically Modified Land Plant Sources*

More recently several research groups have begun the development of enriching land plants with n-3 LC-PUFA using genetic engineering technology. The prospects for new land plant sources of n-3 LC-PUFA appear promising and offer hope for alternative and sustainable sources of these fatty acids. Several authors have published reviews in this area (Domergue et al., 2005; Singh et al., 2005; Robert, 2006).

All higher plants have the ability to synthesise the medium chain n-6 and n-3 precursor fatty acids linoleic acid (LA, 18:2n-6) and ALA, respectively (Robert et al., 2005). While most major oilseed crops produce n-6 PUFA in their seeds, linseed plants can produce high levels of ALA, but some other plants can only produce low levels of ALA in their green tissue. However, land plants generally lack the enzymes required to further elongate and desaturate the medium chain precursors to produce n-3 LC-PUFA. Genes coding for the required elongation and desaturation enzymes for LC-PUFA synthesis are present in a range of organisms including microalgae, thraustochytrids, fungi, mosses, and bacteria (Robert et al., 2005; Zhou et al., 2007) and can synthesise LC-PUFA via a number of pathways including through a series of chain elongation and desaturation. To produce n-3 LC-PUFA, ALA is metabolised to produce 18:4n-3, stearidonic acid, 20:4n-3, 20:5n-3 EPA, 22:5n-3 DPA, and 22:6n-3 DHA (Fig. 31.2). Compared to higher plants like canola, lower plants like microalgae can synthesise EPA and DHA from ALA through a number of desaturation (adding a double bond) and elongation (adding two carbons) steps. Genes encoding the desaturase and elongase enzymes have now been cloned from a number of microalgae and introduced into higher plants to give these plants the ability to synthesise n-3 LC-PUFA from medium chain n-3 PUFA precursors. This work has been summarised in an excellent mini-review (Robert et al., 2005; Robert, 2006).

Qi et al. (2004) have led the way in transferring fatty acid synthetic pathway genes into terrestrial plants. The authors were able to constitutively express an elongase gene and two desaturase genes (isolated from microalga and fungi) and express them in the Arabidopsis thaliana plant. This transfer of genes resulted in the production of low levels of EPA and arachidonic acid (AA, 20:4n-6) in the leaf tissue. Similarly, in a study by Abbadi et al. (2004), the authors were able to transfer a delta 6 desaturase (D6D) and a delta 5 desaturase (D5D) from a diatom and a D6 elongase from a fungus to a flax plant to produce EPA. Low but significant levels of AA and EPA were produced in the flax seed, however the low levels were thought to be due to the use of phosphatidylcholine linked fatty acids as substrates by algal desaturases and elongases use fatty acids esterified to coenzyme A (CoA). Robert et al. (2005) transferred four genes: D5D/D6D, an elongase with D6D activity, and a D5E/D4D into Arabidopsis thaliana.

The authors demonstrated the production of low levels of AA (≈1%), EPA (≈3%), and DHA (0.5%). Low levels were perhaps thought to be due to a low level of ALA as a substrate for D6D. Similarly, Kinney et al. (2004) were successful in producing high levels of n-3 LC-PUFA in soy seed and embryos, ≈20% EPA, ≈3% DHA. The authors used a D17D which was able to shunt the majority of biosynthesis in the n-6 pathway to the n-3 pathway. Similarly, Wu et al. (2005) transferred genes into Brassica juncea and produced high levels of AA (25%) as well as EPA (15%), but low levels of DHA (1.5%). More recently Robert et al. (2005) have for the first time demonstrated the production of DHA in the model plant Arabidopsis thaliana. The levels of n-3 LC-PUFA produced were less than those found in fish and seafood however there is potential to further increase the concentration in plant seeds by further modulating the genetic capability of the plant.

There is now increased understanding of the complexities involved in transferring biosynthetic enzymes to plants to express genes that encode the fatty acid synthetic pathways (Singh et al., 2005). The development of n-3 LC-PUFA containing plant seeds is an exciting opportunity for the future food supply. This technology will provide the opportunity to enhance the nutritional value of foods which can be passed on to consumers as well as reducing the stress on already depleted global fish stocks.

## Enriching Foods with n-3 LC-PUFA

### *What are the Drivers for Enrichment?*

The United States Food and Drug Administration (FDA) introduced a health claim for foods containing n-3 LC-PUFA in 2004 which indicated that "Supportive but not conclusive research shows that consumption of EPA and DHA n-3 fatty acids may reduce the risk of CHD. One serving of (food name) provides (X) grams of EPA or DHA n-3 fatty acids" (Starling, 2008). The introduction of this health claim boosted the US market for sales of n-3 LC-PUFA enriched foods. The introduction of a similar health claim in Australia and New Zealand by The Food Standards Australia New Zealand (FSANZ) is currently under consideration and will allow a general level claim indicating that foods which are a good source of n-3 LC-PUFA may promote heart health. A similar claim is also under consideration by European Union Member States (Starling, 2008).

The approval of a general level health claim for n-3 LC-PUFA will extend their previous introduction of a nutrition claim where only food sources containing EPA and DHA could qualify as a 'good source' of n-3 LC-PUFA (FSANZ, 2008). A claim for a good source of n-3 PUFA can only be made if the food contains at least 60mg EPA and/or DHA per serving (FSANZ, 2008). The introduction of this nutrition claim has encouraged the food industry to produce food products that contain EPA

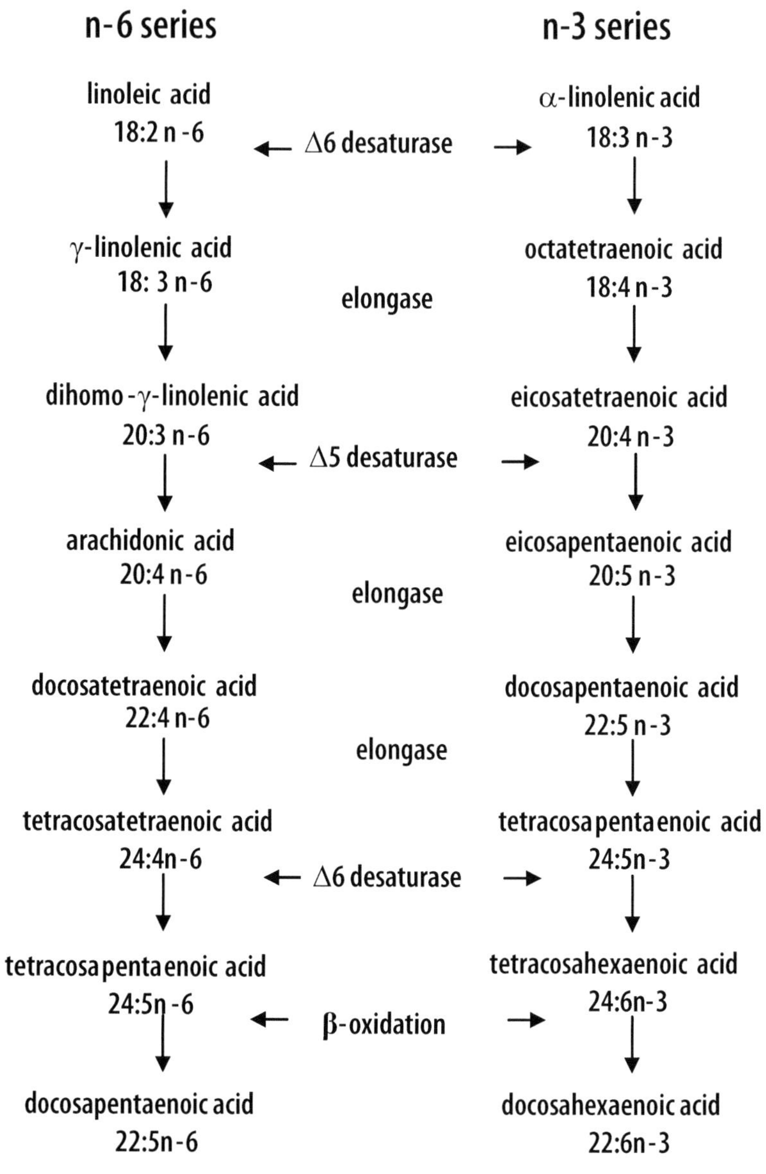


**Fig. 31.2.** Metabolism of essential fatty acids from precursor fatty acids 18:3 n-3 (alpha-linolenic acid) to produce n-3 LC-PUFA 20:5n-3 (eicosapentaenoic acid), 22:5n-3 (docosapentaenoic acid) and 22:6n-3 (docosahexaenoic acid) and from and 18:2 n-6 (linoleic acid) to produce 20:4n-6 (arachidonic acid) and 22:5n-6 (docosapentaenoic acid n-6).

and DHA rather than ALA. This has resulted in increased availability of n-3 LC-PUFA which will potentially translate into increased consumption of n-3 LC-PUFA and subsequent health benefits.

A 1998 survey by AC Neilsen asked 1400 Australian consumers 'which foods would be of interest' for enrichment of processed foods with n-3 LC-PUFA. Bread was the most desired food with 53% of responses indicating this was the most preferred food for n-3 LC-PUFA enrichment, followed by milk, pasta, margarine, and yoghurt with 45%, 43%, 41%, and 40%, respectively, and juice, crackers, and fitness bars with 37%, 28%, and 20%, respectively. These responses suggest that consumers would prefer the enrichment of staple foods with n-3 LC-PUFA which would facilitate a greater increase in n-3 LC-PUFA intake by increasing n-3 LC-PUFA availability in foods which could be consumed on a daily basis. To this end food companies have increased their efforts to develop n-3 LC-PUFA enriched staple foods including chicken meat (Lopez-Ferrer et al., 2001; Lopez-Ferrer et al., 2001), pork (Howe, 1998; Howe et al., 2002; Coates et al., 2008; Sioutis et al., 2008), and eggs (Jiang & Sim, 1993; Farrell, 1994; Farrell, 1998; Lewis et al., 2000; Makrides et al., 2002; Shapira et al., 2008).

***Aquaculture***

Aquaculture refers to the farming of freshwater and saltwater fish and seafood including molluscs, crustaceans, and aquatic plants under controlled conditions. Cultured seafood is an excellent source of n-3 LC-PUFA as feed oils can be manipulated to increase lipid levels which may result in increases in n-3 LC-PUFA content by up to 10 fold compared with wild caught fish and seafood (Nichols, 2004). Many reports are indicating that plant-based oils are being increasingly utilised as replacements for fish oil in feed stocks. This is leading to a decline in the n-3 LC-PUFA content of farmed species.

## Enrichment of Primary Produce

### *Pork, Poultry, and Eggs*

Meat and eggs can be enriched with n-3 LC-PUFA by supplementing the feeds of single-stomached animals such as pigs and chickens with appropriate sources which can be incorporated into triglyceride stores in adipose and skeletal muscle phospholipids giving rise to even greater acquisition of n-3 LC-PUFA intake through regular consumption of a range of animal products (Coates et al., 2008). Sources such as fish oil and tuna fishmeal have been manipulated to produce a high quality DHA-rich product which has been demonstrated to enrich chicken and pork meat without tainting of the product (Howe, 1998; Howe et al., 2002). Previous studies have enriched animal products with plant sources of fatty acids including ALA, fish oil, fishmeal, or a combination of these sources with varying degrees of success (Howe, 1998). Enriching livestock feeds comes with its problems including increased cost of livestock feeds, tainting of meat through fat oxidation, minimal enrichment of n-3

LC-PUFA due to poor endogenous conversion of ALA to EPA and DHA, and poor sensory properties of the meat. However several studies have been able to successfully enrich meat products using stabilised forms of n-3 LC-PUFA such as fishmeal (Howe et al., 2002; Coates et al., 2008; Sioutis et al., 2008) and when eaten together with other n-3 LC-PUFA fortified foods, we are likely to consume close to our target intake level.

## Studies on Pork Enrichment

A study by Sioutis et al. (2008) fed an enriched feed containing 15% tuna fishmeal for six weeks. Animals were slaughtered and meat processed to produce a range of cuts. The authors found based on an average serving size of 100g, the total EPA+DHA in steak was 48 mg, stir-fry 53 mg, diced 66 mg, mince 180 mg, and sausage 177 mg (Table 31.5). Enriching these cuts had no effect on sensory attributes or storage time and quality of meat. In fact the pigs fed the tuna fishmeal diet had a 12% lower feed conversion ratio than pigs fed the control feed. Furthermore, a study by Coates and colleagues (Coates et al., 2008) investigated the effects of regular consumption of lean n-3 LC-PUFA enriched pork versus regular pork for 12 weeks on erythrocyte EPA and DHA incorporation and cardiometabolic risk factors including blood triglycerides and serum thromboxane $B_2$. Volunteers received a range of cuts of n-3 LC-PUFA enriched pork which delivered 1300mg of n-3 LC-PUFA weekly (equivalent to 58–226mg/100g serve). After 12 weeks of consumption of enriched pork, there were significant elevations in the n-3 LC-PUFA content of erythrocytes as well as reductions in serum triglycerides and thromboxane $B_2$.

## Studies on Poultry Enrichment

The n-3 LC-PUFA composition of broiler meat can be modified by adding ALA using vegetable oils, fish meal, and fish oil. However enriched meat with the medium chain n-3 PUFA such as ALA exhibits poorer sensory properties compared with products enriched with n-3 LC-PUFA from fishmeal or fish oils. A study by Lopez-Ferrer et al. (2001) enriched the diets of chickens with fish oil at a dose level of 0, 2, or 4% plus tallow up to 8% added fat throughout a 38 day growth period. 4% was then replaced by a mixture of fish oil, linseed oil, and tallow at a dose of 1%, 3%, and 4%, respectively, for 1 wk or 2 wks prior to slaughter. The authors demonstrated when high fish oil concentrations were incorporated into feeds, the level of saturated and monounsaturated fatty acids decreased in the thigh samples. The amount of n-3 LC-PUFA (EPA+DPA+DHA) increased when added to the diet. In addition there were no sensory differences detected between meats with different fish oil enrichment levels and the control diet. In a similar study the authors enriched feeds with ALA rich linseed oil and found no peripheral tissue accumulation of n-3 LC-PUFA in chickens using a longer feeding time. This was despite the chickens' ability to convert ALA to n-3 LC-PUFA in the liver at 24 d of age (Lopez-Ferrer et al., 2001). Chickens appear to have a higher D6D activity than mammals and are therefore better able to convert ALA to EPA and DHA.

Howe and colleagues (Howe et al., 2002) evaluated the use of PorcOmega™ (POM), a stabilized tuna fishmeal formulation, as a source of DHA for enrichment of pork and poultry products. Pigs, broilers, and laying hens were fed rations containing varying levels of POM for varying time periods and subsequently pork and chicken products, including chops, sausages, and eggs were produced. The authors found increases of up to sevenfold of n-3 LC-PUFA, predominantly DHA when using up to 10% POM in rations. Using modest feeding levels of 5–10% of POM provided palatable products with reasonable levels of enrichment whereas feeding greater than 15% of POM in meat and 10% in eggs gave poor sensory outcomes. The increases in n-3 LC-PUFA in meat and eggs were retained following cooking. A similar study by Hulan et al. (1989) investigated the effect of feeding redfish meal (RFM) on performance and n-3 LC-PUFA content of edible meat and skin lipids of broiler chickens. The four diets included (control) 0%, 4.0%, 8.0%, and 12.0% RFM. The authors found additions of RFM to the diets resulted in a substantial dietary enrichment of n-3 LC-PUFA especially EPA and DHA. Moreover the authors calculated that consumption of 100g of chicken that has been fed 12% RFM would contribute nearly 200mg of n-3 LC-PUFA (EPA+DPA+DHA) compared with approximately 140mg of n-3 LC-PUFA obtained from the consumption of 100g of cod fish.

## *Studies on Egg Enrichment*

Eggs were possibly one of the first foods to be enriched with n-3 LC-PUFA. n-3 LC-PUFA enriched eggs are available all over the world but with varying n-3 LC-PUFA content (Whelan & Rust, 2006). Eggs have been enriched with n-3 LC-PUFA using marine microalgal products (Herber-McNeill & Van Elswyk, 1998), fish and fish oils (Farrell, 1998) without compromising taste or storage life of the eggs and no degradation of n-3 LC-PUFA in eggs is observed during cooking (Van Elswyk et al., 1992; Farrell, 1998). Herber-McNeill and Van Elswyk (1998) have shown that feeding a minimum of 2.4% of marine microalgal oil to laying hens results in the production of an egg with as much n-3 PUFA as a serving of lean fish.

Shapira and colleagues (2008) enriched eggs using 5% linseed (ALA rich seed) for 5 weeks and showed a 3.8 fold increase in n-3 PUFA which included a 6.4 fold increase in ALA and 2.4 fold increase in DHA. Regular consumption of these eggs

**Table 31.5. EPA+DHA composition of n-3 LC-PUFA enriched pork and control pork (mg/100g).**

| | EPA+DHA (mg) | |
|---|---|---|
| Pork cut (per 100g serve) | n-3 enriched | Control |
| Steak | 58 | 19 |
| Stir Fry | 64 | 22 |
| Diced | 77 | 20 |
| Mince | 226 | 37 |
| Sausage | 223 | 46 |

may help increase n-3 LC-PUFA intakes and provide health benefits; however, when feeding hens an ALA rich source you will also increase the level of ALA present. Conversion of ALA from DHA is limited due to the sharing of the D6D enzyme by both ALA and DHA. However this study suggested there was some conversion of ALA to DHA.

Eggs have received an unhealthy image in the past due their cholesterol content and the link between dietary cholesterol, blood lipid levels, and CV risk resulting in recommendations to limit egg intake. However several studies have demonstrated that regular consumption of eggs does not raise blood cholesterol. Farrell (1994) showed that when subjects ate 14 eggs per week for 9 weeks, plasma cholesterol and triacylglycerol did not rise significantly. Similarly, in a later study (Farrell, 1998), there were no significant increases in blood cholesterol or triacylglycerol in subjects who consumed seven n-3 enriched eggs per week for 24 weeks. In fact Ferrier et al. (1994) showed reductions in triacylglycerol and increases in HDL when subjects ate four n-3 LC-PUFA enriched eggs per day for 2 weeks compared with non-enriched eggs. Similarly, Makrides et al. (2002) have demonstrated that feeding n-3 LC-PUFA enriched eggs to infants can significantly increase erythrocyte levels of DHA (by 30-40%) to a greater extent than feeding with regular eggs. Hoffman et al. (2004) also demonstrated increases in erythrocyte DHA following feeding with baby food containing egg yolk enriched DHA and improvements in visual-evoked potential acuity.

## Enrichment of Foods During Processing

### *Microencapsulation*

Oils containing n-3 LC-PUFA can theoretically be delivered in a wide range of processed foods; however, the physical and sensory qualities of the foods may be adversely affected. Issues that may affect the quality of enriched foods include the quality of oil used for enrichment, resistance to oxidative degradation of n-3 LC-PUFA during manufacturing due to heat and or shear stress, during storage (poor shelf life), or during cooking such as baking or toasting. There are several ways to help to protect the n-3 LC-PUFA against oxidation, including addition of appropriate antioxidants or emulsification, microencapsulation, or chemical complexing with cyclodextrin.

Microencapsulation is the process where microdroplets of oil (≈300μm diameter) are emulsified in a gelatine/sucrose complex and protected from oxidation by encapsulation in a food starch layer and addition of tocopherols and ascorbic acid. Clover Corporation Australia has developed a microencapsulation system achieving 60% fish oil in dry powder. In their patented emulsification process the aqueous phase comprises stable protein-sugar complex. Wacker Chemie GmbH have produced a γ-cyclodextrin which can stabilise n-3 LC-PUFA against heat and oxidation and increase resistance to shear force. The type of system used to stabilise and protect n-3 LC-PUFA varies depending on the product and specific requirements including degree of enrichment, sensory qualities, and price.

Fortified foods can contain varying amounts of EPA and DHA, depending on the source of these fatty acids. A variety of foods including yoghurt (Let et al., 2007), ice-cream (Rudolph et al.), bread (Yep et al., 2002; Serna-Saldivar et al., 2006), caviar paste (Engstrom et al., 2003), spreads (Roche & Gibney, 1994; Kolanowski et al., 2001; Borneo et al., 2007; Porsgaard et al., 2007), dips (Garg et al., 2007), cookies (Borneo et al., 2007), beverages, dairy (Borneo et al., 2007; Let et al., 2007), and other processed products (Lovegrove et al., 1997; Metcalf et al., 2003; Ramaprasad et al., 2006; Murphy et al., 2007) have now been enriched with n-3 LC-PUFA. Some foods have been enriched for evaluation in research trials while others have been successfully introduced to the market place.

***Dairy***

Dairy is a suitable food for enriching with n-3 LC-PUFA. Milk is generally around 4% fat of which is mainly saturated fat and enriching with n-3 LC-PUFA may produce a healthier fat profile. Only a handful of studies have enriched dairy with n-3 LC-PUFA. A study by Let et al. (2007) enriched milk (1% fish oil by weight) and yoghurt (1% fish oil by weight) with neat fish oil or a fish oil-emulsion. Milk had poor oxidative stability and poor sensory properties with a pronounced fishy flavour initially and after 30 days of storage. Similarly, yoghurt tended to increase in fishy flavour following prolonged periods of storage. The poor sensory properties may be due to the amount of fish oil that was added to produce the n-3 LC-PUFA enriched products. A study by Metcalf et al. (2003) enriched a range of foods with fish oil including long life milk to provide 175mg of EPA+DHA per 250mL serving of milk. This product was the second most popular enriched product behind canola oil, flaxseed products, and margarine with subjects consuming about 285mL per day. Together with a range of other n-3 LC-PUFA enriched products and fish and seafood the authors were able to increase plasma and platelet phospholipid levels of EPA and DHA.

Lovegrove et al. (1997) fortified a number of food products including milkshake powder, milkshake, and ice cream. Each food portion was assigned an exchange value where one exchange was equivalent to 200mg EPA+DHA. Subjects were asked to consume nine exchange values daily plus 113g of mackerel pate per week. The authors found no difference in palatability between enriched foods and non-enriched foods and there was a significant increase in EPA+DHA in plasma phospholipids and free fatty acids following consumption of the enriched foods. Similarly, Hlavaty et al. (2008) showed that daily consumption of n-3 LC-PUFA enriched yogurt (620mg EPA+DHA/day) significantly increased serum levels of EPA and DHA after 3 weeks of supplementation compared with non-enriched yoghurt. Rudolph et al. (personal communication) fortified reduced fat ice-cream with n-3 LC-PUFA from a range of sources including refined menhaden oil or microencapsulated oils including marine oil, sardine and anchovy oil, DHA from microalgae, and $\gamma$-cyclodextrin/refined menhaden oil complex, at a concentration of 250mg/100g serve. The authors reported that the two ice-creams fortified with microencapsulated sardine and anchovy oil and unencapsulated menhaden oil tasted more similar to the control than the other sources of n-3 LC-PUFA tested. In fact the microencapsulated DHA from microalgae appeared to perform the best with better sensory properties including flavor, fullness, and least fishy aroma.

***Dips, Pastes, and Salad Dressing***

Foods like dips, pastes, and salad dressings have a relatively high fat content thus substitution of some of the less healthy saturated and *trans* fats in these products by increasing the n-3 LC-PUFA content could produce a range of more nutritionally acceptable food products. Caviar paste (cod roe paste) is a good choice for enrichment with n-3 fish oil as the food already tastes fishy. However, foods such as caviar paste are more commonly eaten in their country of origin (Engstrom et al., 2003). Dips are another suitable vehicle for added n-3 LC-PUFA. Recently Garg and colleagues (2007) demonstrated that daily consumption of a humus based dip enriched with approximately 1.4g of n-3 LC-PUFA per 100g for 6 weeks significantly increased plasma n-3 LC-PUFA. A standard serve size (approximately 30g) delivered 420mg of n-3 LC-PUFA. However, a study by Let et al. (2007) enriched salad dressing with 15% rapeseed oil and 10% fish oil by weight and found an increase in a fishy flavour following prolonged periods of storage.

***Cookies and Biscuits***

A variety of biscuits have been enriched with n-3 LC-PUFA by various researchers (Borneo et al., 2007; Murphy et al., 2007). Borneo and colleagues (2007) were able to enrich cream-filled sandwich cookies with 400mg of n-3 LC-PUFA without impacting negatively on taste or shelf life. In fact the results demonstrate that cookies fortified with n-3 LC-PUFA were liked as much as cookies without the n-3 LC-PUFA.

***Spreads***

There are currently a variety of spreads available on markets world-wide which have been enriched with the plant derived n-3 PUFA, ALA, or marine derived n-3 LC-PUFA. Kew et al. (2003) has demonstrated that regular consumption of n-3 LC-PUFA enriched spread together with fish oil capsules increased the level of EPA and DHA in peripheral blood mononuclear cells over a 6 month period without altering the functional responses of inflammatory and immune cells. In an animal study (Porsgaard et al., 2007) hamsters were fed with an interesterified butter blend enriched with fish oil (equivalent to 220 mg n-3 LC-PUFA per 20 g serve) for 6 weeks which led to elevated levels of plasma and erythrocyte n-3 LC-PUFA.

***Bread***

Bread is a popular vehicle for introducing n-3 LC-PUFA as it is a common food for most countries and the current fat source can be substituted with an n-3 LC-PUFA source. However, it is difficult to introduce high levels of n-3 LC-PUFA from fish oil into bread without affecting sensory properties. Serna-Saldivar et al. (2006) was able to enrich white bread with up to 70 mg DHA per 32 g slice of bread using either fish oil, algae oil or microencapsulated powders, but found that the most suitable bread in terms of nutritional properties and functional properties was the bread enriched with 50 mg DHA from algae oil. Similarly, Patch et al. (2005) enriched bread enriched with cod fish oil such that it contained 125 mg of n-3 LC-PUFA per two slices of bread but subjects reported adverse sensory properties. Yep and colleagues (2002) demonstrated that when white bread enriched with n-3 LC-PUFA rich microencapsulated tuna oil was either consumed acutely (80 mg dose) or chronically (60 mg dose daily for three weeks) it could increase plasma levels of n-3 LC-PUFA without adverse sensory responses.

**Can Enriched Foods Meet the n-3 LC-PUFA Intake Requirements?**

One of the first studies to demonstrate that a range of processed foods can be enriched with n-3 LC-PUFA without affecting the sensory properties was a study by Murphy et al. (2007). The aim of this study was to determine whether regular consumption of a range of foods enriched with n-3 LC-PUFA were palatable and had suitable sensory properties and if regular consumption could improve n-3 LC-PUFA levels in erythrocytes and CV health outcomes. Volunteers were randomized to consume control foods (n=44) or n-3 LC-PUFA (cod fish oil) enriched foods (n=42). Foods enriched with n-3 LC-PUFA and matching control foods and EPA+DHA composition are listed in Table 31.6. Study participants were asked to consume 8 servings of foods per day for 6 months by replacing customary foods with study food equivalents. Each serving of the n-3 LC-PUFA enriched foods was intended to provide approximately 125 mg EPA + DHA, i.e. a total of 1000mg of EPA+DHA/day.

Daily logs and food compliance questionnaires revealed that the control group consumed approximately 6.8 servings/d and the n-3 enriched group consumed 6.2 servings/d (equivalent to 775mg EPA+DHA) which was slightly below the target of 8 servings/d, but sustained throughout the 6-month study period (Patch et al., 2005). However, as seen in Table 31.6, the actual EPA+DHA content of randomly sampled n-3 LC-PUFA enriched foods varied markedly from the intended 125 mg/serving and was taken into account in estimating individual intakes of fatty acids from weighed food records, as described by Patch et al (2005). While the n-3 LC-PUFA varied vastly from foods, the n-3 LC-PUFA enriched group was still obtaining approximately 810mg/d of n-3 LC-PUFA on average which based on 6.2 serves per day equates to approximately 130mg/serving of n-3 enriched food.

Upon completion of the study, participants rated the acceptability of the study foods on a 7-point Likert scale ranging from extremely dislike (-3) to extremely like (+3) as described by Patch et al. (2005). The n-3 LC-PUFA enriched group rated the oats and milk slightly favorably (1·4 and 0·5, respectively) whereas they rated the bread as quite unfavorable (-0·3), which was significantly different ($P$ <0·05) from the control group (1·1). The salad dressing was also rated unfavorably (-0·3 for both groups). All other food items were rated favorably with no reported significant differences between the groups.

This study not only showed that the majority of foods enriched were acceptable to the study volunteers, but regular consumption of a variety of n-3 LC-PUFA enriched products over a 6 month period raised the blood level of n-3 LC-PUFA in erythrocytes to a level where heart health benefits may be expected. Total n-3 LC-PUFA content of erythrocytes in the n-3 group increased by 43% and 60% at 3 and 6 months of the intervention, respectively ($P < 0.05$) (Fig. 31.3). EPA and DHA content of erythrocytes increased by 82% and 53%, respectively, at 3 months and 111% and 76% at 6 months ($P < 0.05$). There were no changes in n-3 LC-PUFA content of erythrocytes in the control group. Erythrocyte EPA and DHA levels were not related to intakes at baseline in the whole group (n=80) perhaps due to the difficulties in dietary assessment methodology (Patch et al., 2005). However there was a significant correlation between the calculated intake of EPA+DHA from foods and erythrocyte levels of EPA+DHA in individuals at 3 months (r=0.35; $P < 0.01$), which became stronger after 6 months (r=0.69; $P < 0.001$), reflecting the progressive incorporation of n-3 LC-PUFA from food into erythrocytes.

This study indicated that it was possible to increase n-3 LC-PUFA intake to approximately 800mg/d by replacing habitual foods with a variety of n-3 LC-PUFA enriched study foods other than fish. Moreover, the 5-fold increase in n-3 LC-PUFA

**Table 31.6. Content (mg/serve) of EPA and DHA in n-3 enriched foods and control foods**

| | | EPA+DHA (mg) | |
|---|---|---|---|
| Food | Serving size | Control | n-3 enriched |
| Anzac Biscuit | 2 biscuits (40g) | 2 | 111 |
| Ginger Biscuit | 2 biscuits (40g | 1 | 119 |
| Bread | 2 slices (90g) | ND | 103 |
| Cheese spread | 15g | 4 | 114 |
| Chocolate | 25g | ND | 42 |
| Tomato Salsa Dip | 25g | ND | 97 |
| Cracked Pepper Dip | 30g | 6 | 124 |
| Tzatziki Dip | 30g | 2 | 96 |
| Egg | 2 ≈ 90g | 62 | 158 |
| Margarine | 20g | ND | 146 |
| Skim Milk | 250mL | ND | 89 |
| Muesli | 30g | 1 | 13 |
| Muffin | 1 ≈ 75g) | ND | 151 |
| Porridge | 30g | 1 | 3 |
| Pancake | 3 pikelet ≈ 30g | ND | 55 |
| Salad dressing | 40mL | 7 | 93 |
| Laksa Soup mix | 1 sachet ≈ 85g | 11 | 371 |
| Vegetable Soup mix | 1 sachet ≈ 85g | 1 | 442 |

ND, not detected

intake could be maintained for a long duration (i.e. 6 month intervention period). The level of EPA and DHA in erythrocytes increased from 4% of total fatty acids at baseline to 7% of total fatty acids at 6 months which is nearly double. According to the Omega-3 Index, an erythrocyte level of 8% EPA+DHA and above is considered cardioprotective (Harris & Von Schacky, 2004). As the 7% seen in the study by Murphy et al. (2007) was not a peak value it is assumed the erythrocyte level of EPA+DHA would have continued to rise to a threshold point in the region of the Omega-3 Index for greatest protection from SCD. This study is important for the food industry as it shows that a range of foods can be produced to help increase the intake level to meet recommendations.

## Conclusion

This chapter has discussed n-3 LC-PUFA consumption recommendations for good health throughout life, dietary intakes, and sources including seafood, fish, enriched meats and eggs, terrestrial plant sources, microalgal sources, fish oil, and a range of processed foods that can be enriched with n-3 LC-PUFA. It appears that supplementation with fish oil or consumption of enriched foods can increase the omega-3 index and reduce CV risk, as indicated by increases in the omega-3 index. Meaningful increases can be achieved with the generally recommended intake of 500mg EPA+DHA per day.

Even though few countries have official government recommendations for n-3 LC-PUFA consumption at present, food manufacturers recognize the need to develop a range of n-3 LC-PUFA enriched foods to enable the regular consumption of a variety of these foods to meet the recommendations for good health. Improvements in technology associated with microencapsulation and oil production, including genetically modified plant sources, will further expand the n-3 LC-PUFA functional

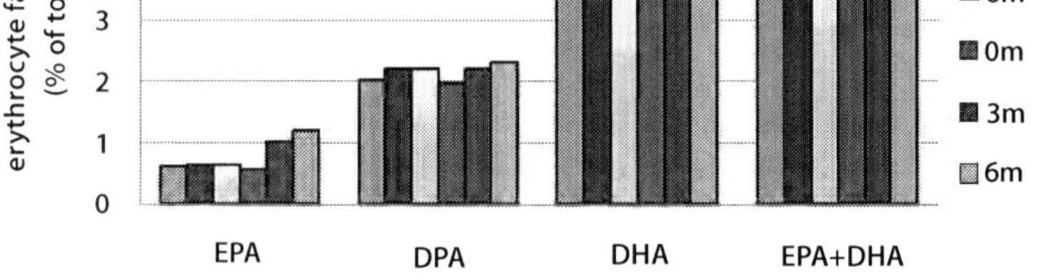


Fig. 31.3. n-3 LC-PUFA composition of erythrocytes (% of total fatty acids) at baseline and after 3 and 6 months after consuming n-3 enriched foods.

food range. There are a number of n-3 LC-PUFA enriched products now available on the market including breads, spreads, milk, eggs, and meat which are otherwise comparable to conventional products. Such products have already been shown to have the capacity to enable consumers to achieve intake recommendations for n3 LC PUFA.

## Acknowledgement

We would like to thank Associate Professor Jon Buckley for his assistance with the preparation of the chapter.

### References

Abbadi, A.; F. Domergue; J. Bauer; J. A. Napier; R. Welti; U. Zahringer; P. Cirpus; E. Heinz. "Biosynthesis of very-long-chain polyunsaturated fatty acids in transgenic oilseeds: constraints on their accumulation." *Plant Cell* **2004**, *16(10)*: 2734–48.

Abeywardena, M.; P. D. Nichols; S. P. Singh. Future Omega-3s. World of Food Ingredients: 2005, 50–54.

Akiba, S.; T. Murata; K. Kitatani; T. Sato. "Involvement of lipoxygenase pathway in docosapentaenoic acid-induced inhibition of platelet aggregation." *Biol. Pharm. Bull.* **2000**, *23(11)*: 1293–7.

Albert, C. M.; H. Campos; M. J. Stampfer; P. M. Ridker; J. E. Manson; W. C. Willett; J. Ma. "Blood levels of long-chain n-3 fatty acids and the risk of sudden death." *N. Engl. J. Med.* **2002**, *346(15)*: 1113–8.

Arterburn, L. M.; H. A. Oken; E. Bailey Hall; J. Hamersley; C. N. Kuratko; J. P. Hoffman. "Algal-oil capsules and cooked salmon: nutritionally equivalent sources of docosahexaenoic acid." *J. Am. Diet Assoc.* **2008**, *108(7)*: 1204–9.

Arterburn, L. M.; H. A. Oken; J. P. Hoffman; E. Bailey-Hall; G. Chung; D. Rom; J. Hamersley; D. McCarthy. "Bioequivalence of Docosahexaenoic acid from different algal oils in capsules and in a DHA-fortified food." *Lipids* **2007**, *42(11)*: 1011–24.

Bang, H. O.; J. Dyerberg. "Plasma lipids and lipoproteins in Greenlandic West-coast Eskimos." *Acta Medica Scandinavica* **1972**, *4*: 210–217.

BNF (1992). British Nutrition Foundation. Unsaturated fatty acids nutritional and physiological significance: the report of the British Nutrition Foundation's task force.

Bonaa, K. H.; K. S. Bjerve; A. Nordoy. "Habitual fish consumption, plasma phospholipid fatty acids, and serum lipids: the Tromso study." *Am. J. Clin. Nutr.* **1992**, *55(6)*: 1126–34.

Borneo, R.; D. Kocer; G. Ghai; B. J. Tepper; M. V. Karwe. "Stability and consumer acceptance of long-chain omega-3 fatty acids (eicosapentaenoic acid, 20:5, n-3 and docosahexaenoic acid, 22:6, n-3) in cream-filled sandwich cookies." *J. Food Sci.* **2007**, *72(1)*: S049–54.

Bouic, P. J.; J. H. Lamprecht. "Plant sterols and sterolins: a review of their immune-modulating properties." *Altern. Med. Rev.* **1999**, *4(3)*: 170–7.

Bourre, J. M. "Dietary omega-3 Fatty acids and psychiatry: mood, behaviour, stress, depression, dementia and aging." *J. Nutr. Health Aging* **2005a**, *9(1)*: 31–8.

Bourre, J. M. "Where to find omega-3 fatty acids and how feeding animals with diet enriched in omega-3 fatty acids to increase nutritional value of derived products for human: what is actually useful ?" *J. Nutr .Health Aging* **2005b**, *9(4)*: 232–42.

Christensen, J. H. "n-3 fatty acids and the risk of sudden cardiac death. Emphasis on heart rate variability." *Dan. Med. Bull.* **2003**, *50(4)*: 347–67.

Clandinin, M. T.; J. E. Chappell; S. Leong; T. Heim; P. R. Swyer; G. W. Chance. "Intrauterine fatty acid accretion rates in human brain: implications for fatty acid requirements." *Early Hum. Dev.* **1980**, *4(2)*: 121–9.

Cleland, L. G.; G. E. Caughey; M. J. James; S. M. Proudman. "Reduction of cardiovascular risk factors with longterm fish oil treatment in early rheumatoid arthritis." *J. Rheumatol.* **2006**, *33(10)*: 1973–9.

Coates, A. M.; S. Sioutis; J. D. Buckley; P. R. Howe. "Regular consumption of n-3 fatty acid-enriched pork modifies cardiovascular risk factors." *Br. J. Nutr.* **2008**, 1–6.

Cohen, J. T.; D. C. Bellinger; W. E. Connor; B. A. Shaywitz. "A quantitative analysis of prenatal intake of n-3 polyunsaturated fatty acids and cognitive development." *Am. J. Prev. Med.* **2005**, *29(4)*: 366–74.

Colombo, J.; K. N. Kannass; D. J. Shaddy; S. Kundurthi; J. M. Maikranz; C. J. Anderson; O. M. Blaga; S. E. Carlson. "Maternal DHA and the development of attention in infancy and toddlerhood." *Child Dev.* **2004**, *75(4)*: 1254–67.

Colquhoun, D.; A. Ferreira-Jardim; T. Udell; B. Eden; a. t. N. a. M. C. o. t. H. Foundation (2008). Review of evidence: Fish, fish oils, n-3 polyunsaturated fatty acids and cardiovascular health N. H. F. o. Australia. Canberra.

COMA (1994). COMA Cardiovascular Review Group. Report on health and social subjects. nutritional aspects of cardiovascular disease.

Conquer, J. A.; L. A. Cheryk; E. Chan; P. A. Gentry; B. J. Holub. "Effect of supplementation with dietary seal oil on selected cardiovascular risk factors and hemostatic variables in healthy male subjects." *Thromb. Res.* **1999**, *96(3)*: 239–50.

Daniells, S. (2008). European omega-3 market to grow by 24 percent: analyst. Nutraingredients. com Europe

Daniels, J. L.; M. P. Longnecker; A. S. Rowland; J. Golding. "Fish intake during pregnancy and early cognitive development of offspring." *Epidemiology* **2004**, *15(4)*: 394–402.

de Deckere, E. A.; O. Korver; P. M. Verschuren; M. B. Katan. "Health aspects of fish and n-3 polyunsaturated fatty acids from plant and marine origin." *Eur. J. Clin. Nutr.* **1998**, *52(10)*: 749–53.

Dolecek, T. A. "Epidemiological evidence of relationships between dietary polyunsaturated fatty acids and mortality in the multiple risk factor intervention trial." *Proc. Soc. Exp. Biol. Med.* **1992**, *200(2)*: 177–82.

Domergue, F.; A. Abbadi; E. Heinz. "Relief for fish stocks: oceanic fatty acids in transgenic oilseeds." *Trends Plant Sci.* **2005**, *10(3)*: 112–6.

Dyerberg, J. "Linolenate-derived polyunsaturated fatty acids and prevention of atherosclerosis." *Nutr. Rev.* **1986**, *44(4)*: 125–34.

Dyerberg, J. and K. A. Jorgensen. "Marine oils and thrombogenesis." *Prog. Lipid Res.* **1982**, *21(4)*: 255–69.

Eaton, S. B.; S. B. Eaton 3rd; A. J. Sinclair; L. Cordain; N. J. Mann. "Dietary intake of long-chain polyunsaturated fatty acids during the paleolithic." *World Rev. Nutr. Diet* **1998**, *83*: 12–23.

Engstrom, K.; R. Wallin; T. Saldeen. "Effects of Scandinavian caviar paste enriched with a stable fish oil on plasma phospholipid fatty acids and lipid peroxidation." *Eur. J. Clin. Nutr.* **2003**, *57(9)*: 1052–9.

Farrell, D., Ed. (1994). The fortification of hens' eggs with omega-3 fatty acids and their effects in humans. In: Egg uses and processing technologies: new developments. , Oxon, United Kingdom: CAB International.

Farrell, D. J. "Enrichment of hen eggs with n-3 long-chain fatty acids and evaluation of enriched eggs in humans." *Am. J. Clin. Nutr.* **1998**, *68(3)*: 538–44.

Ferrier, L.; S. Leeson; B. Holub; L. Catson; D. Squires, Eds. (1994). High linolenic acid eggs and their influence on blood lipids in man. In: Egg uses and processing technologies new developments., Oxon, United Kingdom: CAB International

Fleith, M.; M. T. Clandinin. "Dietary PUFA for preterm and term infants: review of clinical studies." *Crit. Rev. Food Sci. Nutr.* **2005**, *45(3)*: 205–29.

Food and Nutrition Board, Institute of Medicine. Dietary Reference Intakes for Energy, Carbohydrate, Fiber, Fat, Fatty Acids, Cholesterol, Protein and Amino Acids (Macronutrients). National Academies Press, Washington DC, 2002. http://www.iom.edu/board.asp?id=3788

FRDC (2002). Retail sale and consumption of seafood.

FRDC, F. R. a. D. C. (2004). What's so healthy about seafood? A guide for seafood marketers. ACT, Fisheries Research and Development Corporation.

FSANZ (2008). Claims in relation to omega fatty acid content of foods.

Garg, M. L.; R. J. Blake; E. Clayton; I. A. Munro; L. Macdonald-Wicks; H. Singh; P. J. Moughan. "Consumption of an n-3 polyunsaturated fatty acid-enriched dip modulates plasma lipid profile in subjects with diabetes type II." *Eur. J. Clin. Nutr.* **2007**, *61(11)*: 1312–7.

Gomez, M. A.; M. T. Saenz; M. D. Garcia; M. A. Fernandez. "Study of the topical anti-inflammatory activity of Achillea ageratum on chronic and acute inflammation models." *Z Naturforsch [C]* **1999**, *54(11)*: 937–41.

Harris, W. S.; J. V. Pottala; S. A. Sands; P. G. Jones. "Comparison of the effects of fish and fish-oil capsules on the n 3 fatty acid content of blood cells and plasma phospholipids." *Am. J. Clin. Nutr.* **2007**, *86(6)*: 1621–5.

Harris, W. S.; C. Von Schacky. "The Omega-3 Index: a new risk factor for death from coronary heart disease?" *Prev. Med.* **2004**, *39(1)*: 212–20.

Health Council of The Netherlands. Dietary reference intakes: energy, proteins, fats and digestible carbohydrates. Report 19. The Hague, Netherlands: Health Council of the Netherlands. Publication no. 2001/1999. (WHO, 2003).

Helland, I. B.; L. Smith; K. Saarem; O. D. Saugstad; C. A. Drevon. "Maternal supplementation with very-long-chain n-3 fatty acids during pregnancy and lactation augments children's IQ at 4 years of age." *Pediatrics* **2003**, *111(1)*: e39–44.

Herber-McNeill, S. M.; M. E. Van Elswyk. "Dietary marine algae maintains egg consumer acceptability while enhancing yolk color." *Poult. Sci.* **1998**, *77(3)*: 493–6.

Herber, S. M.; M. E. Van Elswyk. "Dietary marine algae promotes efficient deposition of n-3 fatty acids for the production of enriched shell eggs." *Poult. Sci.* **1996**, *75(12)*: 1501–7.

Hlavaty, P.; M. Kunesova; M. Gojova; E. Tvrzicka; M. Vecka; P. Roubal; M. Hill; K. Hlavata; P. Kalouskova; V. Hainer; A. Zak; J. Drbohlav. "Change in fatty acid composition of serum lipids in obese females after short-term weight-reducing regimen with the addition of n-3 long chain polyunsaturated fatty acids in comparison to controls." *Physiol. Res.* **2008**, *57* Suppl 1: S57–65.

Hoffman, D. R.; R. C. Theuer; Y. S. Castaneda; D. H. Wheaton; R. G. Bosworth; A. R. O'Connor; S. E. Morale; L. E. Wiedemann; E. E. Birch. "Maturation of visual acuity is accelerated in breast-fed term infants fed baby food containing DHA-enriched egg yolk." *J. Nutr.* **2004**, *134(9)*: 2307–13.

Howe, P.; J. D. Buckley; B. Meyer. "Long chain omega-3 fatty acids in red meat." *Nutrition and Dietetics* **2007**, *64(4)*: S135–S139.

Howe, P.; B. Meyer; S. Record; K. Baghurst. "Dietary intake of long-chain omega-3 polyunsaturated fatty acids: contribution of meat sources." *Nutrition* **2006**, *22(1)*: 47–53.

Howe, P. R. "Omega 3-enriched pork." *World Rev. Nutr. Diet* **1998**, *83*: 132–43.

Howe, P. R.; J. A. Downing; B. F. Grenyer; E. M. Grigonis-Deane; W. L. Bryden. "Tuna fishmeal as a source of DHA for n-3 PUFA enrichment of pork, chicken, and eggs." *Lipids* **2002**, *37(11)*: 1067–76.

Hu, F. B.; L. Bronner; W. C. Willett; M. J. Stampfer; K. M. Rexrode; C. M. Albert; D. Hunter; J. E. Manson. "Fish and omega-3 fatty acid intake and risk of coronary heart disease in women." *JAMA* **2002**, *287(14)*: 1815–21.

Hu, F. B.; W. C. Willett. "Optimal diets for prevention of coronary heart disease." *JAMA* **2002**, *288(20)*: 2569–78.

Innis, S. M. "Dietary omega 3 fatty acids and the developing brain." *Brain Res.* **2008**.

ISSFAL. "International Society for the Study of Fatty Acids and Lipids. Statement 3 PUFA in Adults. For cardiovascular health, a minimum intake of eicosapentaenoic acid and docosahexaenoic acid combined of: 500 mg/day." http://www.issfal.org.uk/lipid-matters/issfal-policy-statements/statement-3-pufa-in-adults-2.html.

ISSFAL. "Recommendations for intake of polyunsatured fatty acids in healthy adults. Internet: http://www.issfal.org.uk/Welcome/PolicyStatement3.asp." (2004).

James, M. J.; R. A. Gibson; L. G. Cleland. "Dietary polyunsaturated fatty acids and inflammatory mediator production." *Am. J. Clin. Nutr.* **2000**, *71*(1 Suppl): 343S–8S.

Jiang, Z.; J. S. Sim. "Consumption of n-3 polyunsaturated fatty acid-enriched eggs and changes in plasma lipids of human subjects." *Nutrition* **1993**, *9(6)*: 513–8.

Kew, S.; T. Banerjee; A. M. Minihane; Y. E. Finnegan; R. Muggli; R. Albers; C. M. Williams; P. C. Calder. "Lack of effect of foods enriched with plant- or marine-derived n-3 fatty acids on human immune function." *Am. J. Clin. Nutr.* **2003**, *77(5)*: 1287–95.

Kinney, A. J.; E. B. Cahoon; H. G. Damude; W. D. Hitz; Z. B. Liu; C. Kolar. "Production of very long chain polyunsaturated fatty acids in oilseed plants." *Patent WO 2004/071467 A2 E.I DuPont de Nemours, Company* **2004**.

Kock, K. H.; K. Reid; J. Croxall; S. Nicol. "Fisheries in the Southern Ocean: an ecosystem approach." *Philos. Trans. R. Soc. Lond. B. Biol. Sci.* **2007**, *362(1488)*: 2333–49.

Kolanowski, W.; F. Swiderski; E. Lis; S. Berger. "Enrichment of spreadable fats with polyunsaturated fatty acids omega-3 using fish oil." *Int. J. Food. Sci. Nutr.* **2001**, *52(6)*: 469–76.

Kris-Etherton, P. M.; W. S. Harris; L. J. Appel. "Omega-3 fatty acids and cardiovascular disease: new recommendations from the American Heart Association." *Arterioscler Thromb. Vasc. Biol.* **2003**, *23(2)*: 151–2.

Kris-Etherton, P. M.; D. S. Taylor; S. Yu-Poth; P. Huth; K. Moriarty; V. Fishell; R. L. Hargrove; G. Zhao; T. D. Etherton. "Polyunsaturated fatty acids in the food chain in the United States." *Am. J. Clin. Nutr.* **2000**, *71*(1 Suppl): 179S–88S.

Let, M. B.; C. Jacobsen; A. S. Meyer. "Lipid oxidation in milk, yoghurt, and salad dressing enriched with neat fish oil or pre-emulsified fish oil." *J. Agric. Food Chem.* **2007**, *55(19)*: 7802–9.

Lewis, N. M.; S. Seburg; N. L. Flanagan. "Enriched eggs as a source of N-3 polyunsaturated fatty acids for humans." *Poult. Sci.* **2000**, *79(7)*: 971–4.

Lopez-Ferrer, S.; M. D. Baucells; A. C. Barroeta; J. Galobart; M. A. Grashorn. "n-3 enrichment of chicken meat. 2. Use of precursors of long-chain polyunsaturated fatty acids: linseed oil." *Poult. Sci.* **2001** *80(6)*: 753–61.

Lopez-Ferrer, S.; M. D. Baucells; A. C. Barroeta; M. A. Grashorn. "n-3 enrichment of chicken meat. 1. Use of very long-chain fatty acids in chicken diets and their influence on meat quality: fish oil." *Poult. Sci.* **2001**, *80(6)*: 741–52.

Lovegrove, J. A.; C. N. Brooks; M. C. Murphy; B. J. Gould; C. M. Williams. "Use of manufactured foods enriched with fish oils as a means of increasing long-chain n-3 polyunsaturated fatty acid intake." *Br. J. Nutr.* **1997**, *78(2)*: 223–36.

Makrides, M.; J. S. Hawkes; M. A. Neumann; R. A. Gibson. "Nutritional effect of including egg yolk in the weaning diet of breast-fed and formula-fed infants: a randomized controlled trial." *Am. J. Clin. Nutr.* **2002**, *75(6)*: 1084–92.

Makrides, M.; M. A. Neumann; R. W. Byard; K. Simmer; R. A. Gibson. "Fatty acid composition of brain, retina, and erythrocytes in breast- and formula-fed infants." *Am. J. Clin. Nutr.* **1994**, *60(2)*: 189–94.

Mann, N. J.; A. J. Sinclair; P. Percival; J. L. Lewis; B. J. Meyer; P. R. C. Howe. "Development of a database of fatty acids in Australian foods." *Nutrition and Dietetics* **2003**, *60(1)*: 42–45.

Marchioli, R. "[Results of GISSI Prevenzione: diet, drugs, and cardiovascular risk. Researchers of GISSI Prevenzione]." *Cardiologia* **1999**, *44* Suppl 1(Pt 2): 745–6.

Martin, A. (2001). Apports nutritionnels conseilles pour la population Francaise.

Massrieh, W. "Health benefits of omega-3 fatty acids from Neptune krill oil. ." *Lipid Technology* **2008**, *20(5)*: 108–111.

McLennan, P.; P. Howe; M. Abeywardena; R. Muggli; D. Raederstorff; M. Mano; T. Rayner; R. Head. "The cardiovascular protective role of docosahexaenoic acid." *Eur. J. Pharmacol.* **1996**, *300(1-2)*: 83–9.

McLennan, W.; A. Podger (1997). National nutrition survey, selected highlights.

Metcalf, R. G.; M. J. James; E. Mantzioris; L. G. Cleland. "A practical approach to increasing intakes of n-3 polyunsaturated fatty acids: use of novel foods enriched with n-3 fats." *Eur. J. Clin. Nutr.* **2003**, *57(12)*: 1605–12.

Meyer, B. J.; T. A. Larkin; A. J. Owen; L. B. Astheimer; L. C. Tapsell; P. R. Howe. "Limited lipid-lowering effects of regular consumption of whole soybean foods." *Ann. Nutr. Metab.* **2004**, *48(2)*: 67–78.

Meyer, B. J.; N. J. Mann; J. L. Lewis; G. C. Milligan; A. J. Sinclair; P. R. Howe. "Dietary intakes and food sources of omega-6 and omega-3 polyunsaturated fatty acids." *Lipids* **2003**, *38(4)*: 391–8.

Ministry of Health Labor and Welfare, J. (1999). Nutrition requirements for Japanese. 6th edition.

Mozaffarian, D.; E. B. Rimm. "Fish intake, contaminants, and human health: evaluating the risks and the benefits." *JAMA* **2006**, *296(15)*: 1885–99.

Murphy, K. J.; N. J. Mann; A. J. Sinclair. "Fatty acid and sterol composition of frozen and freeze-dried New Zealand Green Lipped Mussel (Perna canaliculus) from three sites in New Zealand." *Asia Pac. J. Clin. Nutr.* **2003**, *12(1)*: 50–60.

Murphy, K. J.; B. J. Meyer; T. A. Mori; V. Burke; J. Mansour; C. S. Patch; L. C. Tapsell; M. Noakes; P. A. Clifton; A. Barden; I. B. Puddey; L. J. Beilin; P. R. Howe. "Impact of foods enriched with n-3 long-chain polyunsaturated fatty acids on erythrocyte n-3 levels and cardiovascular risk factors." *Br. J. Nutr.* **2007**, *97(4)*: 749–57.

Myers, R. A.; B. Worm. "Rapid worldwide depletion of predatory fish communities." *Nature* **2003**, *423(6937)*: 280–3.

Nestel, P. "Fish oil fatty acids beneficially modulate vascular function." *World Rev. Nutr. Diet* **2001**, *88*: 86–9.

Nestel, P.; H. Shige; S. Pomeroy; M. Cehun; M. Abbey; D. Raederstorff. "The n-3 fatty acids eicosapentaenoic acid and docosahexaenoic acid increase systemic arterial compliance in humans." *Am. J. Clin. Nutr.* **2002**, *76(2)*: 326–30.

NHMRC, N. H. a. M. R. C. (2006). Nutrient Reference Values for Australia and New Zealand_ Canberra.

Nichols, P. "Sources of long-chain omega-3 oils." *Lipid Technology* **2004**, *16(11)*: 247–251.

Nichols, P. D. (2007). Fish oil sources. Long-Chain Omega-3 Specialty Oils. H. Breivik. Bridgwater, England, The Oily Press: 23–42.

Nichols, P. D.; P. Virtue; B.D. Mooney; E. NG; Y. GK (1998). Seafood the Good Food. The Oil Content and Composition of Australian Commercial Fishes, Shellfishes and Crustaceans. FRDC Project 95/122. Guide prepared for the Fisheries Research and Development Corporation. Hobart, Tasmania, Australia: CSIRO Publication.

Oken, E.; R. O. Wright; K. P. Kleinman; D. Bellinger; C. J. Amarasiriwardena; H. Hu; J. W. Rich-Edwards; M. W. Gillman. "Maternal fish consumption, hair mercury, and infant cognition in a U.S. Cohort." *Environ. Health Perspect.* **2005**, *113(10)*: 1376–80.

Patch, C. S.; L. C. Tapsell; T. A. Mori; B. J. Meyer; K. J. Murphy; J. Mansour; M. Noakes; P. M. Clifton; I. B. Puddey; L. J. Beilin; G. Annison; P. R. Howe. "The use of novel foods enriched with long-chain n-3 fatty acids to increase dietary intake: a comparison of methodologies assessing nutrient intake." *J. Am. Diet Assoc.* **2005**, *105(12)*: 1918–26.

Porsgaard, T.; J. Overgaard; A. L. Krogh; M. B. Jensen; Z. Guo; H. Mu. "Butter blend containing fish oil improves the level of n-3 fatty acids in biological tissues of hamster." *J. Agric. Food Chem.*

**2007**, *55(18)*: 7615–9.

Proudman, S. M.; L. G. Cleland; M. J. James. "Dietary omega-3 fats for treatment of inflammatory joint disease: efficacy and utility." *Rheum. Dis. Clin. North Am.* **2008**, *34(2)*: 469–79.

Pyle, D. J.; R. A. Garcia; Z. Wen. "Producing docosahexaenoic acid (DHA)-rich algae from biodiesel-derived crude glycerol: effects of impurities on DHA production and algal biomass composition." *J. Agric. Food Chem.* **2008**, *56(11)*: 3933–9.

Qi, B.; T. Fraser; S. Mugford; G. Dobson; O. Sayanova; J. Butler; J. A. Napier; A. K. Stobart; C. M. Lazarus. "Production of very long chain polyunsaturated omega-3 and omega-6 fatty acids in plants." *Nat. Biotechnol.* **2004**, *22(6)*: 739–45.

Ramaprasad, T. R.; K. Srinivasan; V. Baskaran; K. Sambaiah; B. R. Lokesh. "Spray-dried milk supplemented with alpha-linolenic acid or eicosapentaenoic acid and docosahexaenoic acid decreases HMG Co A reductase activity and increases biliary secretion of lipids in rats." *Steroids* **2006**, *71(5)*: 409–15.

Ratledge, C.; Z. Cohen. "Microbial and algal oils: Do they have a future for biodiesel or as commodity oils?" *Lipid Technology* **2008**, *20(7)*: 155–160.

Robert, S. S. "Production of eicosapentaenoic and docosahexaenoic acid-containing oils in transgenic land plants for human and aquaculture nutrition." *Mar. Biotechnol. (NY)* **2006**, *8(2)*: 103–9.

Robert, S. S.; S. P. Singh; X. R. Zhou; J. R. Petrie; S. I. Blackburn; P. M. Mansour; P. D. Nichols; Q. Liu; A. G. Green. "Metabolic engineering of Arabidopsis to produce nutritionally important DHA in seed oil. ." *Functional Plant Biology* **2005**, *32* 473–479.

Roche, H.; M. J. Gibney. "The effect of consumption of fish oil-enriched spreadable fats on platelet phospholipid fatty acid composition in human volunteers." *Int. J. Vitam. Nutr. Res.* **1994**, *64(3)*: 237–42.

Rudolph, M.; Y. Huang; G. Lobo; S. Lowry; C. Kuesten; R. Little. "Fortification of reduced fat ice cream with omega-3 long chain polyunsaturated fatty acids." *DSM, Personal communication with RD Little.*

Sargent, J. R. "Fish oils and human diet." *Br. J. Nutr.* **1997**, *78*(Suppl 1): S5–S13.

Serna-Saldivar, S. O.; R. Zorrilla; C. De La Parra; G. Stagnitti; R. Abril. "Effect of DHA containing oils and powders on baking performance and quality of white pan bread." *Plant Foods Hum Nutr* **2006**, *61(3)*: 121–9.

Shapira, N.; P. Weill; R. Loewenbach. "Egg fortification with n-3 polyunsaturated fatty acids (PUFA): nutritional benefits versus high n-6 PUFA western diets, and consumer acceptance." *Isr. Med. Assoc. J.* **2008**, *10(4)*: 262–5.

Simmer, K.; S. M. Schulzke; S. Patole. "Longchain polyunsaturated fatty acid supplementation in preterm infants." *Cochrane Database Syst. Rev.* **2008**, *(1)*: CD000375.

Simopoulos, A. P.; A. Leaf; N. Salem Jr. "Workshop on the essentiality of and recommended dietary intakes for omega-6 and omega-3 fatty acids." *Food Australia* **1999**, *51(8)*: 332–333.

Sinclair, A. J.; L. Johnson; K. O'Dea; R. T. Holman. "Diets rich in lean beef increase arachidonic acid and long-chain omega 3 polyunsaturated fatty acid levels in plasma phospholipids." *Lipids* **1994**, *29(5)*: 337–43.

Singh, S. P.; X. R. Zhou; Q. Liu; S. Stymne; A. G. Green. "Metabolic engineering of new fatty acids in plants." *Curr. Opin. Plant Biol.* **2005**, *8(2)*: 197–203.

Sinn, N. "Nutritional and dietary influences on attention deficit hyperactivity disorder." *Nutr. Rev.* **2008**, *66(10)*: 558–68.

Sinn, N.; J. Bryan; C. Wilson. "Cognitive effects of polyunsaturated fatty acids in children with attention deficit hyperactivity disorder symptoms: a randomised controlled trial." *Prostaglandins Leukot. Essent. Fatty Acids* **2008**, *78(4-5)*: 311–26.

Sinn, N.; P.R.C. Howe; "Mental health benefits of omega-3 fatty acids may be mediated by improvements in cerebral vascular function." *Bioscience Hypotheses* **2008**, *1*: 103–108.

Sioutis, S.; A. M. Coates; J. D. Buckley; T. W. Murphy; H. A. Channon; P. R. C. Howe. "N-3 enrichment of pork with fishmeal: Effects on production and consumer acceptability." *European Journal of Lipid Science and Technology* **2008**, *110*: 701–706.

Smithers, L. G.; R. A. Gibson; A. McPhee; M. Makrides. "Effect of long-chain polyunsaturated fatty acid supplementation of preterm infants on disease risk and neurodevelopment: a systematic review of randomized controlled trials." *Am. J. Clin. Nutr.* **2008**, *87(4)*: 912–20.

Starling, S. "Regulation: Omega-3 ready for RDIs and further health claims." *Nutraingredients.com* (2008).

Sugano, M. "Characteristics of fats in Japanese diets and current recommendations." *Lipids* **1996**, *31* Suppl: S283–6.

Uauy, R.; D. R. Hoffman; P. Mena; A. Llanos; E. E. Birch. "Term infant studies of DHA and ARA supplementation on neurodevelopment: results of randomized controlled trials." *J. Pediatr.* **2003**, *143(4 Suppl)*: S17–25.

"UK Scientific Advisory Committee on Nutrition. Internet: http://www.sacn.gov.uk/reports/." (1991).

Van Elswyk, M. E.; A. R. Sams; P. S. Hargis. "Composition, functionality, and sensory evaluation of eggs from hens fed dietary menhaden oil." *J. Food Sci.* **1992**, *57*: 342–344.

Weil, M.; J. Bressler; P. Parsons; K. Bolla; T. Glass; B. Schwartz. "Blood mercury levels and neurobehavioral function." *JAMA* **2005**, *293(15)*: 1875–82.

Whelan, J.; C. Rust. "Innovative dietary sources of n-3 fatty acids." *Annu. Rev. Nutr.* **2006**, *26*: 75–103.

Wijendran, V.; K. C. Hayes. "Dietary n-6 and n-3 fatty acid balance and cardiovascular health." *Annu. Rev. Nutr.* **2004**, *24*: 597–615.

Wu, G.; M. Truksa; N. Datla; P. Vrinten; J. Bauer; T. Zank; P. Cirpus; E. Heinz; X. Qui. "Stepwise engineering to produce high yields of very long-chain polyunsaturated fatty acids in plants. " *Nat. Biotechnol.* **2005**, *23*: 1013–1017.

Yep, Y. L.; D. Li; N. J. Mann; O. Bode; A. J. Sinclair. "Bread enriched with microencapsulated tuna oil increases plasma docosahexaenoic acid and total omega-3 fatty acids in humans." *Asia. Pac. J. Clin. Nutr.* **2002**, *11(4)*: 285–91.

York, R.; M. Gossard. "Cross-national meat and fish consumption: exploring the effects of modernization and ecological context." *Ecological Economics* **2004**, *48*: 293–302.

Zhou, X. R.; S. S. Robert; J. R. Petrie; D. M. Frampton; M. P. Mansour; S. I. Blackburn; P. D. Nichols; A. G. Green; S. P. Singh. "Isolation and characterization of genes from the marine microalga Pavlova salina encoding three front-end desaturases involved in docosahexaenoic acid biosynthesis." *Phytochemistry* **2007**, *68(6)*: 785–96.

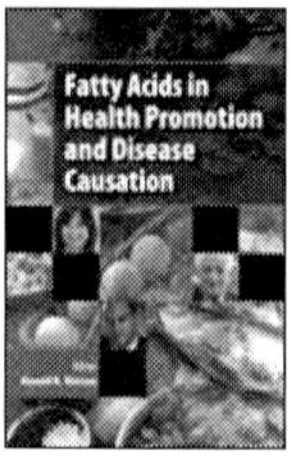


# Index

## B

## E

# F

## G

## H

## M

## O

## S

## Z